Targeted Delivery of Small and Macromolecular Drugs

Targeted Delivery of Small and Macromolecular Drugs

Edited by
Ajit S. Narang | Ram I. Mahato

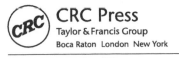

CRC Press
Taylor & Francis Group
Boca Raton London New York

CRC Press is an imprint of the
Taylor & Francis Group, an **informa** business

CRC Press
Taylor & Francis Group
6000 Broken Sound Parkway NW, Suite 300
Boca Raton, FL 33487-2742

First issued in paperback 2017

© 2010 by Taylor and Francis Group, LLC
CRC Press is an imprint of Taylor & Francis Group, an Informa business

No claim to original U.S. Government works

ISBN-13: 978-1-4200-8772-7 (hbk)
ISBN-13: 978-1-138-11451-7 (pbk)

Library of Congress Cataloging-in-Publication Data

Targeted delivery of small and macromolecular drugs / [edited by] Ram I. Mahato and Ajit S. Narang.
     p. ; cm.
   Includes bibliographical references and index.
   ISBN 978-1-4200-8772-7 (alk. paper)
   1. Drug targeting. I. Mahato, Ram I. II. Narang, Ajit S.
   [DNLM: 1. Drug Delivery Systems. 2. Drug Administration Routes. 3. Drug Carriers. 4. Macromolecular Substances--administration & dosage. 5. Molecular Weight. QV 785 T1845 2010]

   RM301.63.T365 2010
   615'.7--dc22
                                                                      2010002143

Visit the Taylor & Francis Web site at
http://www.taylorandfrancis.com

and the CRC Press Web site at
http://www.crcpress.com

I dedicate this work to the sacrifices of my parents, Mr. Tirath Singh and Mrs. Gurdip Kaur, and my wife, Swayamjot; to the love of my brother, Supreet, and son, Manvir; and to the encouragement and confidence bestowed on me by my teachers and mentors.

Ajit S. Narang

To my wife Subhashini, my children Kalika and Vivek for their love and support, my mother for believing in me, and my students and mentors who have always helped me in my quest for learning.

Ram I. Mahato

*****

The many benefits and potentials of

targeted drug delivery

is just one of the outcomes of

the entrepreneurial spirit of the innovators

and

our quest for

finding novel solutions to known challenges.

*****

Contents

PART III   Intracellular/Organelle-Specific Strategies

PART IV   Prodrug Strategies

PART V   Organ- or Tissue-Specific Drug Delivery

PART VI   Polymer–Drug Conjugates and Micelles

PART VII   Stimuli-Responsive Systems

Editors

Ajit S. Narang works for the Bristol-Myers Squibb, Co. in New Brunswick, New Jersey, in the biopharmaceutical aspects of drug delivery. He has over eight years of experience in the pharmaceutical industry in the development of oral dosage forms and drug delivery platforms. In addition to the Bristol-Myers Squibb, Co., he has worked for Ranbaxy Research Labs (currently a subsidiary of Daiichi Sankyo, Japan) in Gurgaon, India, and Morton Grove Pharmaceuticals (currently a subsidiary of Wockhardt USA LLC, Parsippany, New Jersey) in Vernon Hills, Illinois. He graduated from the University of Delhi in India and completed his postgraduate studies at the Banaras Hindu University in India and at the University of Tennessee Health Science Center, Memphis. His current research interests include innovations in drug product development and drug delivery technologies that enable the pharmaceutical development of challenging molecules to resolve stability, pharmacokinetic, and pharmacodynamic issues. He has more than 35 publications and 3 pending patent applications, and has contributed to the development of several marketed drug products.

Ram I. Mahato is a full-time professor in the Department of Pharmaceutical Sciences at the University of Health Science Center, Memphis, Tennessee. He was a research assistant professor at the University of Utah, Salt Lake City; a senior scientist at GeneMedicine, Inc., The Woodland, Texas; and a postdoctoral fellow at the University of Southern California in Los Angeles, Washington University in St. Louis, and Kyoto University, Japan. He received his BS in pharmaceutics from China Pharmaceutical University, Nanjin in 1989 and his PhD in pharmaceutics and drug delivery from the University of Strathclyde, Glasgow in 1992. He is an author or coauthor of 79 peer-reviewed articles and book chapters, and has edited/written three books. He is also a special features editor of *Pharmaceutical Research* and serves on the editorial boards of the *Journal of Drug Targeting*, *Expert Opinion on Drug Delivery*, and *Transplantation and Risk Management*. His research includes delivery and targeting of small molecules, oligonucleotides, siRNA, and genes.

Contributors

Fakhrul Ahsan
Department of Pharmaceutical Sciences
School of Pharmacy
Texas Tech University Health Sciences Center
Amarillo, Texas

Nurmamet Amet
Department of Pharmacology and
    Pharmaceutical Sciences
School of Pharmacy
University of Southern California
Los Angeles, California

Mansoor Amiji
Department of Pharmaceutical Sciences
School of Pharmacy
Northeastern University
Boston, Massachusetts

Narsinha M. Andurkar
Organic Chemistry Synthesis Laboratory
Dnyanopasak College
Parbhani, India

Feride Cengelli
Centre Hospitalier Universitaire Vaudois
University Institute of Pathology
University of Lausanne
Lausanne, Switzerland

Rae Sung Chang
School of Life Sciences and Biotechnology
Korea University
Seoul, Korea

Xiaoying Chen
Department of Pharmacology and
    Pharmaceutical Sciences
School of Pharmacy
University of Southern California
Los Angeles, California

Satish A. Dake
Organic Chemistry Synthesis Laboratory
Dnyanopasak College
Parbhani, India

Roberto Diaz
Department of Radiation Oncology
Emory University School of Medicine
Atlanta, Georgia

Abraham J. Domb
Institute of Drug Research
School of Pharmacy
The Hebrew University of Jerusalem
Jerusalem, Israel

Gerard G. M. D'Souza
Department of Pharmaceutical Sciences
Massachusetts College of Pharmacy and Health
    Sciences
Boston, Massachusetts

Mark D. Erion
Merck & Co., Inc.
Rahway, New Jersey

and

Metabasis Therapeutics, Inc.
La Jolla, California

Lanyan Fang
Division of Pharmaceutics
College of Pharmacy
The Ohio State University
Columbus, Ohio

Srinivas Ganta
Department of Pharmaceutical Sciences
School of Pharmacy
Northeastern University
Boston, Massachusetts

Ripal Gaudana
Division of Pharmaceutical Sciences
School of Pharmacy
University of Missouri-Kansas City
Kansas City, Missouri

Vivek Gupta
Department of Pharmaceutical Sciences
School of Pharmacy
Texas Tech University Health Sciences Center
Amarillo, Texas

Dennis E. Hallahan
Department of Radiation Oncology
Washington University School of Medicine
St. Louis, Missouri

Bing Han
Division of Pharmacology
College of Pharmacy
The Ohio State University
Columbus, Ohio

Kristiina Huttunen
School of Pharmacy
University of Eastern Finland
Kuopio, Finland

Arun Iyer
Department of Radiology and Biomedical
    Imaging
School of Medicine
University of California at San Francisco
San Francisco, California

Lucienne Juillerat-Jeanneret
Centre Hospitalier Universitaire Vaudois
University Institute of Pathology
University of Lausanne
Lausanne, Switzerland

Hyun Ah Kim
Department of Bioengineering
College of Engineering
Hanyang University
Seoul, Republic of Korea

Eun-Joong Kim
School of Pharmacy
Seoul National University
Seoul, Korea

Sungwon Kim
Department of Biomedical Engineering
Purdue University
West Lafayette, Indiana

and

Department of Pharmaceutics
Purdue University
West Lafayette, Indiana

Krista Laine
School of Pharmacy
University of Eastern Finland
Kuopio, Finland

Han Young Lee
School of Life Sciences and Biotechnology
Korea University
Seoul, Korea

Hsin-Fang Lee
Department of Pharmacology and
    Pharmaceutical Sciences
School of Pharmacy
University of Southern California
Los Angeles, California

Minhyung Lee
Department of Bioengineering
College of Engineering
Hanyang University
Seoul, Republic of Korea

John M. Luk
Department of Pharmacology
National University Health System
National University of Singapore
Singapore, Singapore

and

Department of Surgery
National University Health System
National University of Singapore
Singapore, Singapore

and

Department of Surgery
Queen Mary Hospital
Hong Kong, China

Ram I. Mahato
Department of Pharmaceutical Sciences
University of Tennessee Health Science Center
Memphis, Tennessee

Gyan P. Mishra
Division of Pharmaceutical Sciences
School of Pharmacy
University of Missouri-Kansas City
Kansas City, Missouri

Ashim K. Mitra
Division of Pharmaceutical Sciences
School of Pharmacy
University of Missouri-Kansas City
Kansas City, Missouri

Ajit S. Narang
Pharmaceutical Development
Bristol-Myers Squibb, Co.
New Brunswick, New Jersey

Yu-Kyoung Oh
College of Pharmacy
Seoul National University
Seoul, Korea

Ravikiran Panakanti
Department of Pharmaceutical Sciences
University of Tennessee Health Science Center
Memphis, Tennessee

Hui Pang
Department of Pharmaceutics
China Pharmaceutical University
Nanjing, People's Republic of China

Kinam Park
Department of Biomedical Engineering
Purdue University
West Lafayette, Indiana

and

Department of Pharmaceutics
Purdue University
West Lafayette, Indiana

Rajendra P. Pawar
Department of Chemistry
Deogiri College
Aurangabad, India

Jarkko Rautio
School of Pharmacy
University of Eastern Finland
Kuopio, Finland

Wei-Chiang Shen
Department of Pharmacology and
    Pharmaceutical Sciences
School of Pharmacy
University of Southern California
Los Angeles, California

Yan Shen
Department of Pharmaceutics
China Pharmaceutical University
Nanjing, People's Republic of China

Ga Yong Shim
School of Life Sciences and Biotechnology
Korea University
Seoul, Korea

Niteen R. Shinde
Organic Chemistry Synthesis Laboratory
Dnyanopasak College
Parbhani, India

Brian Storrie
Department of Physiology and Biophysics
University of Arkansas for Medical Sciences
Little Rock, Arkansas

Duxin Sun
Department of Pharmaceutical Science
College of Pharmacy
The University of Michigan
Ann Arbor, Michigan

Viral M. Tamboli
Division of Pharmaceutical Sciences
School of Pharmacy
University of Missouri-Kansas City
Kansas City, Missouri

Maria Teresa Tarragó-Trani
Department of Biochemistry
Virginia Polytechnic Institute and State
    University
Blacksburg, Virginia

Chandan Thomas
Department of Pharmaceutical Sciences
School of Pharmacy
Texas Tech University Health Sciences Center
Amarillo, Texas

Jiasheng Tu
Department of Pharmaceutics
China Pharmaceutical University
Nanjing, People's Republic of China

Arto Urtti
Centre for Drug Research
University of Helsinki
Helsinki, Finland

Volkmar Weissig
Department of Pharmaceutical Sciences
College of Pharmacy Glendale
Midwestern University
Glendale, Arizona

Kwong-Fai Wong
Department of Pharmacology
National University Health System
National University of Singapore
Singapore, Singapore

and

Department of Surgery
National University Health System
National University of Singapore
Singapore, Singapore

and

Department of Surgery
Queen Mary Hospital
Hong Kong, China

Ningning Yang
Department of Pharmaceutical Sciences
University of Tennessee Health Science Center
Memphis, Tennessee

Yubing Yu
Department of Pharmaceutics
China Pharmaceutical University
Nanjing, People's Republic of China

Jennica Zaro
Department of Pharmacology and
    Pharmaceutical Sciences
School of Pharmacy
University of Southern California
Los Angeles, California

Li Zhou
Department of Radiation Oncology
Vanderbilt University Medical Center
Nashville, Tennessee

1 Therapeutic Potential of Targeted Drug Delivery

Ajit S. Narang and Ram I. Mahato

CONTENTS

1.1 INTRODUCTION

Maximizing the safety and efficacy of drug treatment is the key goal of pharmaceutical scientists and physicians. To this end, drug targeting is being actively pursued in several areas. Some of these approaches involve drug design toward molecular pathways relevant to the pathophysiology of the disease. In other cases, drug delivery systems are designed to transport the therapeutic moiety preferentially to the target organ, tissue, cell, and/or the intracellular disease target(s) after systemic administration. The delivery systems can also be designed for local delivery to the site of the disease to minimize systemic exposure and toxicity. In this book, we focus on the targeted drug delivery technologies that utilize both systemic and local routes of administration.

Targeted delivery is one of the most exciting contributions pharmaceutical sciences can make to drug therapy. The preferred clinical use of advanced drug delivery systems over conventional formulations testifies to their potential. This is well exemplified by the clinical success of liposomal doxorubicin, an anthracycline anticancer agent. Irreversible and cumulative cardiac damage is its major dose-limiting toxicity, which limits the total lifetime dose to a patient. Its liposomal encapsulation is intended to increase safety while maintaining efficacy. Liposomal and PEGylated liposomal formulations of anthracycline anticancer agents have significantly reduced cardiotoxicity. These formulations include liposomal daunorubicin (DaunoXome®, Gilead Sciences, Inc., San Dimas, California), liposomal doxorubicin (D-99, Myocet®, Elan Pharmaceuticals, Princeton, New Jersey), and PEGylated liposomal doxorubicin (Doxil®, Ortho Biotech Products, LP, Bridgewater, New Jersey and Caelyx®, Schering Plough Corp., Kenilworth, New Jersey, utilizing STEALTH® liposomes).[1] The STEALTH® liposomes are composed of *N*-(carbonyl-methoxypolyethylene glycol 2000)-1,2-distearoyl-*sn*-glycero-3-phosphoethanolamine (MPEG-DSPE), fully hydrogenated soy phosphatidylcholine (PC), and cholesterol.[2]

1

In contrast to the nonencapsulated drug, doxorubicin encapsulated in PEGylated liposomes has a slow rate of distribution to the extra vascular space, leading to high drug concentrations in the intravascular tissue. The cardiotoxicity advantage of PEGylated liposomal doxorubicin vis-à-vis the nonencapsulated drug was shown in a phase III clinical trial.[3] The PEGylated liposomal doxorubicin showed a lower incidence of reduction in the left ventricular ejection fraction (LVEF) in association with the signs and symptoms of congestive heart failure (CHF) as well as without the CHF symptoms. The median percentage reduction in the LVEF was significantly lower in patients who received PEGylated liposomal doxorubicin. The reduction in cardiotoxicity with liposomal doxorubicin is attributed to its greater size and inability to escape the vascular space in tissues with tight capillary junctions, such as the cardiac muscle. In addition, the avoidance of phagocytosis and the extension of plasma half-life (to >55 h) ensures drug availability for permeation through the relatively porous endothelial barriers of growing tumors leading to the enhanced permeation and retention (EPR) effect at the target site. In another study, the tumor drug exposure of PEGylated liposomal doxorubicin was six-fold higher than the unencapsulated drug.[4]

> Targeted delivery is one of the most exciting contributions pharmaceutical sciences can make to drug therapy. The preferred clinical use of advanced drug delivery systems over conventional formulations testifies to their potential. This is well exemplified by the clinical success of liposomal doxorubicin, an anthracycline anticancer agent.

In addition to some of the well-established targeted drug delivery products, such as the liposomal doxorubicin discussed above, several approaches are in the earlier stages of investigation. In this book, we exemplify some promising strategies for drug targeting. Leading experts in each area of investigation discuss targeted drug delivery platforms and technologies at various stages of clinical and preclinical development.

1.2   STRATEGIES AND PLATFORMS FOR TARGETED DRUG DELIVERY

In the following sections, we describe the specific topics of discussion in this book, divided into the mentioned subsections.

1.2.1   ACTIVE TARGETING

Amet et al. describe the application of **transferrin receptor–mediated** transcytosis in the intestinal epithelial cells and its application to the gastrointestinal absorption of protein drugs. The authors exemplify its application to the delivery of recombinant human growth hormone and granulocyte colony stimulating factor.

Luk and Wong discuss **antibody therapies** for liver malignancy and transplantation. The authors describe antibody engineering, phage display technologies, and the application of monoclonal antibodies for the treatment of liver diseases.

Diaz et al. describe the use of **ionizing radiation** for tumor-targeted drug delivery. The authors provide a perspective on the induction of neoantigens in target tissues by radiation and the use of ligands in drug delivery vehicles that target these antigens. They further discuss biomarker development using phage display technology and exemplify case studies of ionizing the radiation-facilitated tumor targeting of drugs.

1.2.2   NUCLEIC ACID DELIVERY AND TARGETING

Nucleic acids present special challenges to targeted delivery since they are large, anionic, hydrophilic molecules that poorly extravasate and attract greater regulatory attention because of their potential to influence the cellular genetic processes in addition to safety and immunogenicity concerns. Thus, concerted cross-disciplinary efforts and new therapeutic paradigms are needed to turn nucleic acids into therapeutics.

Urtti provides a commentary on the **cellular barriers** for nucleic acid delivery and targeting. The author discusses the factors affecting, and unanswered questions surrounding, the cellular uptake; intracellular dissociation kinetics and fate of the delivery system; and transgene expression.

Panakanti and Mahato introduce the basics of **gene delivery and expression systems**. The authors describe the basic components of both nonviral plasmid vectors and various types of recombinant viruses commonly used for gene delivery—these include the adenoviral, adeno-associated viral, retroviral, and lentiviral systems. They also discuss various gene delivery platforms such as the liposomes and the peptide and protein-based gene delivery.

Yang and Mahato describe the basic concepts of the delivery and targeting of **oligonucleotides and siRNA**. They describe how bioconjugation and electrostatic complexation have been used to overcome the barriers to oligonucleotide delivery. They further discuss the clinical examples of these delivery systems along with their targeting aspects such as pharmacokinetics and biodistribution.

Tu et al. describe the use of **liposomes** for nonviral gene delivery. They describe the use of cationic, wrapped, and fusogenic liposomes. The authors further describe the merits of anionic lipoplexes and fluidosomes, approaches to increase liposome circulation times, and their targeting strategies. The strategies discussed include active targeting via antibodies or ligands that target receptors or integrin. In addition, they describe stimuli-responsive liposomes that release their payload in response to triggers such as acid, light, heat, enzymes, oxidation potential, or ultrasound.

Shim et al. provide an overview of targeted delivery systems for nonviral nucleic acid–based therapeutics. The authors describe active targeting strategies that include the **use of ligands** targeting receptors such as transferrin and folate receptors. They also describe the use of monoclonal antibodies, and cell-mediated and stimulus-triggered targeted delivery systems.

1.2.3 Intracellular/Organelle-Specific Strategies

Weissig and D'Souza describe drug targeting to the **mitochondria** for cancer chemotherapy. The characteristics of mitochondriotropic molecules are discussed followed by a case study on the use of the dequalinium-derived liposome-like vesicles (DQAsomes) for mitochondrial targeting. The authors also describe the surface modification of liposomes with mitochondriotropic molecules such as methyltriphenylphosphonium (MTPP)[5] and the mitochondria-targeted delivery of liposomal ceramide for antiapoptotic activity.[6]

Tarragó-Trani and Storrie provide a perspective on intracellular drug delivery that highlights the importance of understanding the physiology to design novel targeting approaches. The authors provide an in-depth review of molecular pathways as the basis of emerging intracellular targeting and drug delivery strategies. Using a case study on Alzheimer's disease, the authors describe the drug **delivery to the lipid rafts** within the endosomal cell membranes. In addition, using the knowledge of trafficking pathways identified in the research on Shiga toxins and Shiga-like toxins, they describe declawed toxin subunits as potential tumor cell–targeting ligands.

1.2.4 Prodrug Strategies

Drugs are to be converted to bioreversible derivatives, or prodrugs, to overcome specific formulation and therapeutic barriers, or to enhance drug safety or efficacy by targeting.[7]

Rautio et al. discuss the **enzyme-activated prodrug strategies** for targeted drug action. In addition to the utilization of endogenous enzymes, prodrugs can be designed for bioactivation by exogenous enzymes selectively delivered via monoclonal antibodies (the antibody-directed enzyme prodrug therapy, **ADEPT**). The authors discuss design elements and component selection criteria for ADEPT and exemplify these with some specific preclinical and clinical examples of their application.

> Drugs can be converted to bioreversible deriva- tives, called prodrugs, to overcome specific formulation and therapeutic barriers, or to enhance drug safety or efficacy. One such class of prodrugs, called HepDirect prodrugs, are aryl- substituted cyclic prodrugs of phosphates and phosphonates that undergo an oxidative-cleavage reaction in the liver.

Erion discusses the case of **site-specific prodrug activation strategy for liver targeting using HepDirect prodrugs**. HepDirect prodrugs are aryl-substituted cyclic prodrugs of phosphates and phosphonates that undergo an oxidative-cleavage reaction in the liver.[8] In addition, the author describes other prodrug strategies for tumor and organ selective targeting.

1.2.5 ORGAN OR TISSUE-SPECIFIC DRUG DELIVERY

Ahsan and associates discuss the principles and practice of **pulmonary** drug delivery. The authors provide a detailed background of the physiology of the airways and the factors affecting particle deposition in and drug absorption from the lungs. Drug delivery to the lungs requires a close match and parallel development of both the drug product and the delivery device. The authors discuss the drug delivery devices and absorption enhancement strategies with examples from both small and large molecule drugs.

Mitra and associates describe the role of transporters, receptors, and nanocarriers in **ocular** drug delivery. The authors describe the anatomy and physiology of the eye, and the barriers and routes of ocular drug administration. They further describe the presence and physiological role of influx and efflux transporters within the eye, and how they can be exploited to target drugs to ocular segments using strategies such as prodrugs, implants, hydrogels, nanocarriers, and iontophoresis.

Narang and Mahato describe the importance of pathophysiological considerations in the design of organ- and tissue-targeted drug delivery systems, as exemplified by **colon** and **kidney** targeting.

1.2.6 DRUG–POLYMER CONJUGATES AND MICELLES

Domb and associates describe **injectable polymers** for regional and systemic drug therapy. The authors discuss disease conditions that can benefit from regional drug therapy. *In situ* drug depot systems, such as thermoplastic pastes, polymer precipitation or linking, and thermally induced gell- ing systems, are described. Examples of natural and synthetic biodegradable polymeric carriers are discussed in detail along with their biocompatibility considerations.

Juillerat-Jeanneret and Cengelli discuss the challenges and opportunities in the use of **polymeric drug conjugates**. In addition to conjugation strategies and the biopharmaceutical evaluation of these delivery systems, the authors discuss several examples of targeted drug delivery advantages achieved through the use of these systems.

Kim and Park describe the basic concepts in the use of **polymeric micelles** for drug solubiliza- tion and delivery. They describe the thermodynamic and kinetic stability of polymeric micelles in water, buffers, and the biological environment. They discuss the micelle stabilization strategies, micelle-cell interaction, and the *in vivo* stability of polymeric micelles.

1.2.7 STIMULI-RESPONSIVE SYSTEMS

Ganta et al. describe the use of **stimuli-responsive nanoparticles** for targeted drug release. They describe nanoparticles that respond to stimuli such as pH, temperature, oxidation potential, and electromagnetic waves and conclude with an overview of the development considerations of such carriers.

Kim and Lee describe **physiological stress responsive gene regulation systems** for tissue targeting. The use of hypoxia, heat shock, and glucose levels as responses for the design of gene regulation systems are described along with their therapeutic applications.

1.3 TARGETED DRUG DELIVERY PARADIGM: ENABLING PHARMACEUTICAL DEVELOPMENT

In the current drug discovery and development paradigm, targeted drug delivery is usually applied to well-established drugs to improve or extend their clinical outcome. It is seen as an innovation-driven strategy whose clinical benefit helps extend the life cycle of existing drug molecules. The requirements for the demonstration of clinical benefit and the proof-of-concept (that the clinical benefit is a direct result of the targeting intervention) impose significant financial, resource, and time commitment needs on the developer. Not surprisingly, most companies focusing on targeted drug delivery are different from the companies involved in new drug discovery and development. Table 1.1 lists some targeted drug delivery companies and exemplifies their technologies. In the current paradigm, most of the innovator companies have developed intense focus, specialization, and in-depth expertise in specific disease areas and the identification of lead structural elements and prototypes for synthetic drugs.

> In the current drug discovery and development paradigm, targeted drug delivery is usually applied to well-established drugs to improve or extend their clinical profile. It is seen as an innovation-driven strategy whose clinical benefit helps extend the life cycle of existing drug molecules.

> A paradigm shift with greater focus on innovation-driven pharmaceutics approaches will enable the development of the most challenging and clinically valuable drug molecules. The drug candidates that have been dropped from development can be reinvestigated as research candidates to build a repertoire of targeted delivery and dosage forms to improve their safety and efficacy.

A drug candidate must meet the minimum requirements of safety, efficacy, potency, chemical stability, and pharmaceutical developability to transition through the various stages of drug development through regulatory registration and commercialization. The multiparametric requirements for optimal performance often results in drug candidates being dropped from the development pipeline for various reasons, including, in many cases, a lack of efficacy and the presence of undesired side effect(s) or toxicity at nontarget site(s). The exploration of nonconventional and sophisticated drug delivery approaches is not preferred, often because of the cost, complexity, and development risks. Nevertheless, certain disease states and therapeutic areas with significant unmet clinical needs and commercial potential, such as anticancer drug development,[9] can make the development costs, risks, and efforts worthwhile—especially when they can make a difference to a drug candidate being dropped versus being considered developable. Table 1.2 lists some examples of the nonconventional delivery strategies used for anticancer drugs.

Several of the concerns that compromise drug developability can be addressed with biopharmaceutical approaches such as targeted delivery and the use of nonconventional dosage form platforms.

We hypothesize that a paradigm shift with greater focus on innovation-driven pharmaceutics approaches for increasing the safety and efficacy of drug candidates will enable the pharmaceutical development of some of the most challenging and clinically valuable drug molecules. The drug candidates that have been dropped from development can be reinvestigated as research candidates to build a repertoire of targeted delivery and dosage to form a platform for improving safety and efficacy aspects. For example, colonic delivery approaches can help reduce the gastrointestinal side effects of drugs, nanoparticulate systems can help improve oral absorption, targeting of mesangial cells can mitigate the extra-renal side effects of drugs, and coadministration of low molecular weight proteins (LMWPs) can help reduce renal toxicity and allow high-dose administration of anticancer drugs.[10]

TABLE 1.1

Examples of Targeted Drug Delivery Companies and Technologies

Company	Example(s) of Drug-Targeting Technology	Web Site Reference
Abraxis Bioscience	Albumin nanocapsules encapsulating the drug	www.abraxisbio.com
Access Pharmaceuticals	Nanopolymer-based targeted delivery for cancer and dermatology. Targeted delivery to cancer subtypes via folate, vitamin B12, and biotin conjugation to polymeric vehicles	www.accesspharma.com
Alza Corporation (J&J)	Alza has oral, implantable, transdermal, and liposomal technology platforms and has more than 30 marketed products	www.biospace.com/company_profile.aspx?CompanyId=1588
Avidimer Therapeutics	Focused on cancer detection and treatment, the company utilizes nanometer sized dendrimeric polymers with simultaneously attached targeting vectors, drugs, and /or imaging agents	www.biospace.com/company_profile.aspx?CompanyId=949320
Calando Pharmaceuticals	Cyclodextrin-based polymeric nanoparticles for targeted small molecules and small interfering RNA (siRNA) for oncology applications	www.calandopharma.com
Cell Therapeutics	Polyglutamate polymers for the delivery of anticancer drugs such as paclitaxel (polyglutamate–paclitaxel conjugate)	www.celltherapeutics.com
Copernicus Therapeutics	Nonviral nucleic acid delivery through the formation of condensed nanoparticles	www.cgsys.com
Enzon Pharmaceuticals	Protein PEGylation technology using specific linkers	www.enzon.com
Endocyte	Drug–folate conjugates through a linker for tumor targeting	www.endocyte.com
Eurand	Hyaluronic acid for tumor drug targeting by drug conjugation directly or through a polymer	www.eurand.com
ImmunoGen	Tumor-targeting monoclonal antibody conjugated with a cytotoxic agent	www.immunogen.com
ImaRx Therapeutics	Microbubble (lipid shell incorporating inert gas) technology for vascular occlusions that utilizes ultrasound-mediated cavitation of microbubbles to break up blood clots	www.imarx.com
Calando Pharmaceuticals	Cyclodextrin-based cationic polymers for making siRNA nanoparticles for tumor targeting by electrostatic interaction, with the incorporation of a stabilizer and a targeting ligand	www.insertt.com
NanoBioMagnetics	Magnetically responsive nanoparticles for site-specific drug delivery	www.nanobmi.com
Nanobiotix	Tumor-targeted nanoparticles that get activated with external x-ray application and generate free radicals that help destroy tumors	www.nanobiotix.com
NanoCarrier	Micellar nanoparticles using block copolymers of hydrophilic polyethylene glycol and hydrophobic polyamino acid for drug encapsulation and delivery	www.nanocarrier.co.jp
NeoPharm	Recombinant protein, cintredekin besudotox, which consists of a single molecule composed of two parts: a tumor-targeting molecule (IL13) and a cytotoxic agent (PE38) for tumor targeting	www.neopharm.com
Novosom AG	Negatively charged liposomes that get protonated and fuse with the endosomal membrane to release cargo upon cell internalization	www.novosom.com
PCI Biotech AS	Light induced rupture of endocytic vesicles by the use of photosensitizing compounds	www.pcibiotech.no
Quest PharmaTech	Photodynamic and sonodynamic therapy for oncology and dermatology applications	www.questpharmatech.com
Seattle Genetics	Genetically engineered monoclonal antibodies and antibody–drug conjugates for cancer therapy	www.seagen.com
Starpharma	Lysine-based polymeric dendrimers for drug delivery	www.starpharma.com
Supratek Pharma	Copolymer encapsulation of drugs for targeting	www.supratek.com
Tekmira Pharmaceuticals	siRNA delivery using PEGylated polycationic lipid nanoparticles	www.tekmirapharm.com

TABLE 1.2
Examples of Parenteral Formulations of Cytotoxic Anticancer Agents

S. No.	Example of Drug	Formulation Details	Remarks
		Simple aqueous solutions for drugs with high solubility and stability in water	
1	Tetraplatin	Solution in normal saline	Platinum analog
2	CHIP, *cis*-dichloro, *trans*-dihydroxybis-iso-propylamine platinum IV	Solution in normal saline	Platinum analog
3	Topotecan	5 mg/mL base solution in 0.1 M gluconate buffer at pH 3.0	Topoisomerase I inhibitor. Acidic pH of the solution prevents hydrolysis of the lactone ring
		Solubility improvement using cosolvent and surfactant	
1	Etoposide (Vepesid®)	Drug formulated with polysorbate 80, PEG 300, and ethanol along with benzyl alcohol as preservative and citric acid for pH adjustment	Large doses of IV ethanol can cause phlebitis. The amount of ethanol that can be administered per hour depends on its rate of metabolism, which is up to 10 g/h
2	Teniposide (Vumon®)	Drug formulation contains *N,N*-dimethyl acetamide, Cremophor EL, and ethanol for solubilization in addition to maleic acid for pH adjustment	High dose teniposide could lead to ethanol intoxication and toxicity due to Cremophor EL
3	Paclitaxel (Taxol®)	Solution in 1:1 mixture of Cremophor EL and ethanol	IV Cremophor EL can cause hypersensitivity reactions
4	Carzelesin Adozelesin Bizelesin	Uses PEG 400, ethanol, and Tween 80 for solubilization	Must be diluted in the IV infusion fluid before administration
		Solubility improvement using cosolvents	
1	Busulfan	Aqueous solutions of 40% PEG 400 in normal saline	
2	2-Amino-5-bromo-6-phenyl-4(3)-pyrimidone (ABPP)	Aqueous solution in sodium carbonate buffer containing *N,N*-dimethylacetamide (DMA)	
3	2-Chloro-2′,3′-dideoxyadenosine (2-CIDDA)	Phosphate-buffered solution containing 60% propylene glycol and 10% ethanol	Propylene glycol is hemolytic *in vitro* and should be administered at less than 40% concentration
4	Melphalan	Aqueous solution containing 60% propylene glycol and 5% ethanol	It is diluted with normal saline before administration

(continued)

TABLE 1.2 (continued)
Examples of Parenteral Formulations of Cytotoxic Anticancer Agents

S. No.	Example of Drug	Formulation Details	Remarks
		Complexation to improve aqueous solubility and stability	
1	N-nitrosourea-based anticancer agents	Form complex with Tris buffer (Tris(hydroxyethyl)amino ethane)	Rate of degradation of drug in the complex is slower than free drug
2	5-Fluorouracil	Formulated in Tris buffer	Cardiotoxicity observed upon IV administration. Attributed to the presence of adducts of two degradation products of the drug with Tris
3	Erbuzole Benzaldehyde	Complexation with cyclodextrins	
		Hydrotropic solubilizing agents	
1	Etoposide	Formulated in sodium salicylate solution. Planar orientation of both the drug and the salicylate salt tend to improve solubility in aqueous solution	
2	Doxorubicin Epirubicin	Use parabens in the lyophilized formulation	Drug has a tendency to form dimeric and polymeric self-aggregates, increasing the time required to dissolve the lyophilized vial. Incorporating parabens facilitates drug-paraben complexation, reduces drug self-aggregation, and facilitates rapid dissolution of the drug
		Liposomes for improving PK profile, drug activity, and drug targeting	
1	Doxorubicin	Commercially available as a stable, lyophilized liposomal formulation	IV administered liposomes concentrate in fenestrated capillaries such as liver, spleen, and the bone marrow. IV doxorubicin liposomes has been shown to reduce its cardiotoxicity
2	Camptothecin (CPT) 9-amino CPT (9-ACPT)	Formulated as liposomes of cholesterol, phosphatidyl serine (PS), and phosphatidyl choline (PC)	Freebase of CPT has ~10-fold higher activity than the sodium salt. Therefore, formulation in liposomes provided higher activity
3	Tin protoporphyrin (SnPP)	Formulated as liposomes	IV administration increased drug accumulation in spleen due to its high concentration of reticuloendothelial cells
		Microencapsulation for improving toxicity profile, controlled release	
1	Merbarone	Microdispersion of nanoparticles at neutral pH	IV administration of the N-methyl glucamine salt solution at pH 10 caused injection site vasculitis, which was overcome with the nanoparticle formulation

2	Methotrexate	Methotrexate was conjugated with gelatin and incorporated in gelatin microspheres	Reduced renal toxicity compared with the free drug
Parenteral emulsion formulations for improvement in solubility, stability, local irritation or toxicity, and/or compatibility issues			
1	Hexamethyl melamine (HMM)	Ethanol or DMA solubilized drug to be diluted in intralipid parenteral emulsion before administration	Overcomes drug solubility problems
2	Perrila ketone	Drug formulated in propylene glycol, ethanol, and water; to be diluted in a parenteral emulsion before IV administration	IV administration in 5% dextrose led to loss of 20%–60% drug by adsorption to the polyvinylchloride (PVC) of the infusion tubing. This problem was overcome in IV emulsion formulation
Lipoproteins for tumor targeting			
1	Prednimustine	Drug microemulsion complexed with the apo B receptor of the low-density lipoprotein (LDL) particle	Its cytotoxic activity against breast cancer cells was higher than the free drug. This was attributed to the up-regulation of LDL receptors on tumor cells
2	Vincristine	LDL-associated vincristine compared with free drug	Reduced neurotoxicity with the LDL formulation
Prodrug approaches to increase drug activity and aqueous solubility			
1	1-β-D-Arabinofuranosylcytosine (ara-C)	Lipophilic prodrug prepared by conjugation with phosphatidic acid	Significant increase in the lifespan of mice with L1210 and P388 leukemia
2	Chlorambucil	Drug conjugation to α, β-poly(N-hydroxyethyl-DL-aspartamide) by ester linkage	Increased water solubility
Lyophilization to improve drug stability			
1	Bryostatin I	Bryostatin lyophilized from butanolic solution with povidone; to be dissolved in PEG 400, ethanol, and Tween 80 mixture (PET diluent) followed by dilution in normal saline immediately before administration	Improved drug solubility with reduced requirement of cosolvents for administration and improved shelf-life of the lyophilized formulation
2	Tumor necrosis factor-α (TNF-α)	Lyophilized solution with mannitol and the sugar-based amorphous protectant dextran, sucrose, or cyclodextrin in citrate buffer	Stabilization of solution from tendency for dimeric and polymeric self-aggregation, leading to the formation of particulates in solution

Source: Reproduced from Narang, A.S. and Desai, D.D., Anticancer drug development: Unique aspects of pharmaceutical development, in Mahato, R.I. and Lu, Y. (eds.), *Pharmaceutical Perspectives of Cancer Therapeutics*, AAPS-Springer Publishing Program, New York, 2009, 78–81. With permission.

Note: These cases exemplify that certain disease states and therapeutic areas with significant unmet clinical need and commercial potential, such as anticancer drug development, can make the development costs, risks, and efforts required for nonconventional drug delivery technologies worthwhile.

The enthusiasm for targeted drug delivery is often subdued by the time, cost, and resource requirements for the clinical requirement of proving efficacy and proof-of-concept. In addition, the regulatory agencies treat prodrugs and drug conjugates as new chemical entities, which helps with the patent life extension of existing drug molecules but also encumbers the new drug application (NDA) sponsor with the data generation and characterization requirements equivalent to new drug molecules. Therefore, the value proposition of pharmaceutics approaches to increasing the safety and/or efficacy of drugs would vary on a case-by-case basis and depend on the level of unmet medical need and the projected commercial prospects of the drug candidate.

REFERENCES

1. Safra, T. Cardiac safety of liposomal anthracyclines. *The Oncologist* 2003; **8**(Suppl 2): 17–24.
2. Ortho Biotech Products, Prescribing information, Doxil® (doxorubicin HCl liposome injection), available at http://www.doxil.com/common/prescribing_information/DOXIL/PDF/DOXIL_PI_Booklet.pdf (2001).
3. Wigler, N, O'Brien, M, and Rosso, R. Reduced cardiac toxicity and comparable efficacy in a phase III trial of pegylated liposomal doxorubicin (Caelyx®/Doxil®) vs. doxorubicin for first-line treatment of metastatic breast cancer. In *Conference Proceeding: American Society of Clinical Oncology*, 2002, Orlando, FL.
4. Colbern, G, Vaage, J, Donovan, D et al. Tumor uptake and therapeutic effects of drugs encapsulated in long-circulating pegylated stealth liposomes. *J Liposome Res* 2000; **10**(1): 81–92.
5. Liberman, EA, Topaly, VP, Tsofina, LM et al. Mechanism of coupling of oxidative phosphorylation and the membrane potential of mitochondria. *Nature* 1969; **222**(5198): 1076–1078.
6. Boddapati, SV, D'Souza, GG, Erdogan, S et al. Organelle-targeted nanocarriers: Specific delivery of liposomal ceramide to mitochondria enhances its cytotoxicity in vitro and in vivo. *Nano Lett* 2008; **8**(8): 2559–2563.
7. Stella, VJ. Prodrugs as therapeutics. *Exp Opin Ther Pat* 2004; **14**(3): 277–280.
8. Erion, MD, Reddy, KR, Boyer, SH et al. Design, synthesis, and characterization of a series of cytochrome P(450) 3A-activated prodrugs (HepDirect prodrugs) useful for targeting phosph(on)ate-based drugs to the liver. *J Am Chem Soc* 2004; **126**(16): 5154–5163.
9. Narang, AS and Desai, DD. Anticancer drug development: Unique aspects of pharmaceutical development. In RI Mahato and Y Lu (Eds.), *Pharmaceutical Perspectives of Cancer Therapeutics* (AAPS-Springer Publishing Program, New York, 2009).
10. Nishikawa, M, Nagatomi, H, Chang, BJ et al. Targeting superoxide dismutase to renal proximal tubule cells inhibits mitochondrial injury and renal dysfunction induced by cisplatin. *Arch Biochem Biophys* 2001; **387**(1): 78–84.

Part I

Active Targeting

2 Antibody Therapies for Liver Malignancy and Transplantation

John M. Luk and Kwong-Fai Wong

CONTENTS

2.1 INTRODUCTION

The first treatment of human disease with an antibody can be dated back to 1890, when an antiserum against a bacterial toxin was used to treat diphtheria.[1] The success of this "immunotherapy" prompted medical communities to explore further the usefulness of antiserum or antibody therapies in the treatment of various human diseases. Disappointingly, little therapeutic success has been achieved with the administration of polyclonal antiserum because of its heterogeneous quality and potential immunogenicity in human patients. Research on antibody therapy continued, and gained momentum in 1975 with the advent of hybridoma fusion technology that enabled the production of antibodies with defined specificity. In this technology, antibody-producing cells (lymphocytes) from an animal (e.g., mouse), which had been immunized with a particular antigen, were fused with immortalized myeloma cells to form a hybridoma. Each hybridoma secretes a single immunoglobulin population whose specificity is restricted to a single, specific epitope on antigen. The antibodies that are produced by these hybridomas are named monoclonal antibodies because of the monoclonal nature of the hybridoma.

With the advent of hybridoma fusion technology, a panel of monoclonal antibodies with proven therapeutic efficacy has been produced. However, two major drawbacks of these monoclonal antibodies need to be overcome before they are approved for clinical use in human patients: (1) poor delivery of the antibody to the targeted antigen and (2) potential immunogenicity in human patients.

One of the purposes of this chapter is to introduce methods that are aimed at overcoming these two major drawbacks. In order to improve the delivery of a therapeutic antibody to its target site, a single-chain variable fragment (scFv) has been developed as a replacement for the monoclonal antibody. In order to minimize immunogenicity, different antibody engineering strategies have been developed to "humanize" monoclonal antibodies that are raised usually in nonhuman animals. In this chapter, we limit our discussion to the following humanization strategies: mouse–human chimeric antibody, complementarity-determining region (CDR) grafting, and specificity-determining residues (SDR) grafting.

In addition to these antibody "humanization" technologies, expression systems that facilitate *in vitro* affinity maturation of recombinantly made antibodies are also discussed. Both cell-based (phages, bacteria, and yeast) and cell-free (*in vitro* transcription/translation [IVTT]) expression systems are used currently by the antibody manufacturing industry. Capitalizing on these molecular display schemes, therapeutic antibodies, whose avidity has been enhanced a 1000-fold, have been developed.

Section 2.4 describes how the advancement of antibody engineering has benefited the clinical management of various diseases. For this purpose, antibodies that target hepatocellular carcinoma (HCC) and graft rejection will be used as examples. HCC is a liver malignancy that affects different regions of the world, and hepatectomy is the only curative intervention. However, the high rate of tumor recurrence after surgery results in an unacceptable 5 year survival rate among the HCC cohorts. Due to the improved understanding of the molecular biology of HCC, antibodies that target specific signaling molecules and/or pathways in cancerous hepatocytes and are essential for cancer progression and survival are now being evaluated in HCC patients. The clinical results on the combined use of chemotherapeutic drugs and antibody-directed immunotherapy in HCC are promising and encouraging. Monoclonal antibodies that are capable of blocking or antagonizing the graft rejection response following organ transplantation are now also available in the market. Prophylactic treatment with these antibodies can minimize the dosages of the conventional immunosuppressive drugs, whose long-term and high-dose administration to transplant recipients can result in many unwanted clinical manifestations.

> Antibodies that target specific signaling molecules and/or pathways in cancerous hepatocytes are now being evaluated in HCC patients. A combination therapy of chemotherapeutic drugs and antibody-directed immunotherapy is promising for the treatment of HCC.

Collectively, this chapter provides a review of the antibody engineering strategies that have been developed for improving the efficacy of therapeutic antibodies in the treatment of diseases. Therapeutic monoclonal antibodies that are used to treat patients with HCC as well as prevent graft rejection are also discussed.

2.2 ANTIBODY ENGINEERING

The pharmacodynamics and pharmacokinetics of a therapeutic antibody are the key determinants for the successful immunotherapy of a disease. Both these attributes are, in turn, influenced by the intrinsic properties of the antibody. These intrinsic properties include molecular structure and conformation, amino acid composition, and physicochemical properties, such as isoelectric point.

Recent advances in recombinant DNA technology have enabled the genetic manipulation of these properties, and even the introduction of new properties, such as multivalency. In addition, increasing knowledge about the molecular structure of the antibody/antigen complex has resulted in more accurate *in silico* modeling. This enables protein engineering to improve antibody humanization. Furthermore, different molecular display systems have been developed for affinity maturation of an antibody *in vitro*. Having outlined the goals of antibody engineering as above, Sections 2.2.1 and 2.2.2 focus on the various approaches that are used currently for antibody engineering with their key attributes, applications, and limitations.

However, before discussing the methods for improving antibody efficacy, the molecular architecture of an antibody will be described first. Specifically, the discussion will focus on immunoglobulin G (IgG) because most therapeutic monoclonal antibodies that are in current clinical use or under development belong to the IgG family.

IgG is a glycoprotein with a molecular weight of approximately 150 kDa. Although there are different subclasses of IgG, most IgG antibodies conform to the basic molecular structure of an immunoglobulin. Figure 2.1 depicts a model showing the molecular structure of an IgG. The basic structural units of immunoglobulin are the light and heavy chains, for each chain has two copies in an immunoglobulin. These chains are held together by interchain disulfide bridges and weak noncovalent interactions. In addition to the interchain disulfide bridges, intrachain disulfide bridges are present to facilitate domain formation within both chains. The light chains have variable (V_L) and constant (C_L) domains, while the heavy chains have four domains: V_H, C_H1, C_H2, and C_H3.

The two key functions of an antibody are antigen binding and effector function (e.g., fixation of complement). These functions are mediated by the antigen-binding fragment (Fab) and constant crystallizable fragment (Fc), which are distinct structural subunits of immunoglobulins. Fab harbors the antigen-binding domains, and these are the sites where the antibody epitope interacts with the antigen. The Fc harbors those domains that contribute to the binding of the antibody to complement receptor and cellular Fc receptor.

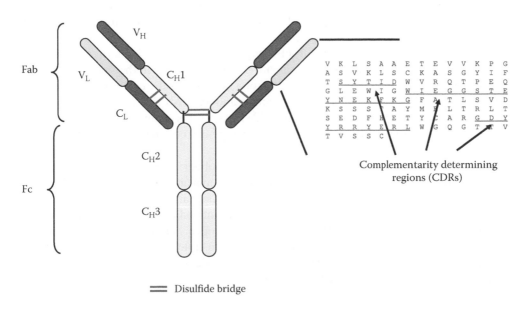

FIGURE 2.1 Schematic diagram showing molecular structure of IgG. Each immunoglobulin consists of two heavy and two light chains. Light chain consists of variable domain (V_L) and constant domain (C_L); while heavy chain consists of V_H, C_H1, C_H2, and C_H3. The variable regions of both chains bind epitope on antigen at the CDRs.

2.2.1 Single-Chain Variable Fragment

A therapeutic monoclonal antibody represents a good candidate for high affinity and protein-based binding agents for the treatment of various cancers. However, the success of antibody therapy in cancer patients is limited usually by the undesirable biodistribution of antibody in noncancerous tissues. This results in the poor delivery of the therapeutic antibody to the tumor. As already noted, the constant Fc of an antibody can bind to the cell surface Fc receptors in cancerous and noncancerous tissues and is another reason for monoclonal antibody accumulation in noncancerous tissues.

The delivery of therapeutic monoclonal antibodies to solid tumors faces another problem due to the high molecular weight of the immunoglobulin. The tumor is surrounded by an extracellular matrix whose major constituent is collagen. Collagen deposition is up-regulated in cancer patients.[2] The excessively formed network of collagen significantly hampers the passage of macromolecules, such as therapeutic monoclonal antibodies with a typical molecular weight of approximately 150 kDa, through the extracellular matrix.

To overcome the poor tissue penetration and undesirable distribution and accumulation of existing therapeutic Fc antibodies, scFvs, which are monoclonal antibodies without the entire constant Fc region and are sometimes called the single-chain antibody, have been developed. In this process, the antibody-binding domains of the light and heavy chains of immunoglobulin are genetically engineered together by a flexible peptide linker, such as the widely used (GlyGlyGlySer)$_3$.[3,4] In order to increase the avidity of a single scFv toward its targeted antigen, a multivalent scFv is sometimes constructed under certain circumstances. Bivalent scFvs (diabodies) and trivalent scFvs (triabodies) can be constructed by linking several single scFvs (Figure 2.2). Chemical linking can be used to construct a multivalent scFv. For example, scFv fragments were joined to give diabody and triabody by cross-linking maleimide that is located in the linker.[5]

The production of multivalent scFvs is of clinical significance. A multivalent scFv usually has a higher avidity toward its targeted antigen when compared with that of its single scFv counterpart. This results in a longer duration of action and retention in tumor masses.[6] The relationship between the valency of the antibody and its retention in the tumor is simply depicted in Figure 2.2. Nevertheless, any significant increase in the molecular weight of a multivalent scFv is likely to reduce its tissue penetrability. Therefore, the balance between tissue penetrability and affinity needs to be weighed carefully when developing efficacious therapeutic scFvs.

In addition to multivalent scFvs, several scFv fragments can be joined to form a bi-specific scFv that can target two different antigens or two nonoverlapping epitopes in the same antigen. Gruber and colleagues have reported that the construction of a bi-specific scFv can be done genetically.[7] In his early study, two different scFv fragments, namely, anti-TCR Ab 1B2 and anti-fluorescein, were linked to form a bi-specific scFv by a flexible peptide linker that is comprised of 25 amino acid residues. In addition to bi-specificity, this engineering strategy can obtain scFv with enhanced affinity and avidity toward its antigen.[8]

Given these advantages over traditional therapeutic antibodies, scFvs that aim to treat various liver diseases like viral hepatitis are currently under development. The risk of developing liver cirrhosis and HCC is high in individuals with hepatitis C. There are currently no effective interventions to completely resolve the viral infection. Therefore, antibodies that can potentially inhibit the proliferation of the hepatitis C virus (HCV) are being developed. An example of this development is scFv42C—a monoclonal antibody that targets the HCV core protein—which has been implicated in the pathogenesis of HCV hepatitis and HCC. The scFv42C significantly decreased the intracellular levels of the HCV core protein in a hepatoma cell line.[9]

2.2.2 Humanized Therapeutic Antibodies

A vast repertoire of monoclonal antibodies of murine origin can now be produced, and are being used clinically, as a result of the pioneering work of Köhler and Milstein, the inventors of hybridoma

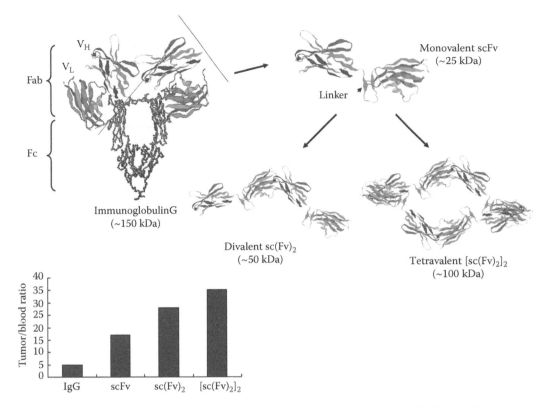

FIGURE 2.2 Schematic diagram showing construction of scFv, di-scFv, and tri-scFv. Each scFv consists of the variable regions of the antigen-binding domains of heavy and light chains. Both chains are linked by a flexible peptide linker. Single scFv can be joined to give di-scFv and tri-scFv to increase the valency of scFv for enhancement of affinity toward targeted antigen. Depicted also is the effect of antibody valency on tumor retention of scFv. Multivalency generally increases the tumor retention of scFv. (From Goel, A. et al., *Cancer Res.*, 60, 6964, 2000. With permission.)

fusion technology.[10] However, these monoclonal antibodies are potentially immunogenic because they can elicit a host immune response, which is referred to as the human anti-mouse antibody (HAMA) response.[11,12] The HAMA response prevents the repetitive administration of a therapeutic antibody because it may lead to a fatal anaphylactic shock.

Many factors such as the amino acid composition of the antibody, the nature of vehicle, and the genetic background and disease status of the patient can contribute to the immunogenicity of a therapeutic antibody. Generally, it is assumed that the immunogenicity of a therapeutic monoclonal antibody is proportional to its mouse content.[13] Therefore, minimizing the mouse content in the therapeutic monoclonal antibodies of murine origin and still retaining affinity have become one of the important goals in the engineering of therapeutic monoclonal antibodies. The approaches to chimerize or humanize monoclonal antibodies are summarized in Figure 2.3 and described in Sections 2.2.2.1 through 2.2.2.3. Using these technologies, more than 15 monoclonal antibodies of low immunogenicity have been approved for clinical use (Table 2.1).

2.2.2.1 Mouse–Human Chimeric Antibodies

In the early 1980s, mouse–human chimeric antibodies were developed. To construct a mouse–human chimera, the antigen-binding variable domains of the heavy (V_H) and light chains (V_L) of mouse immunoglobulin are linked to the constant Fc region of human immunoglobulin. Usually, the V_L is linked to human C_L, and the V_H is linked to human C_H1–C_H2–C_H3 of the light and heavy chains in

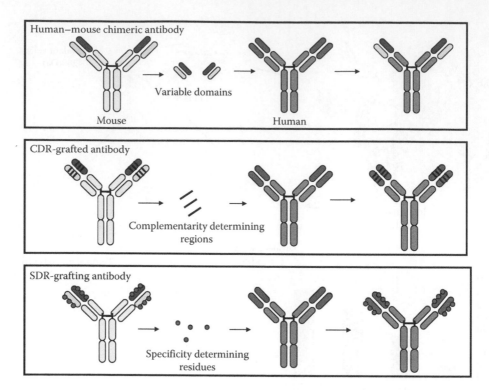

FIGURE 2.3 Schematic diagram showing the different approaches for minimizing the immunogenicity of therapeutic antibodies of murine origin. For the mouse–human chimeric antibody, the antigen-binding domains of murine monoclonal antibody of both heavy and light immunoglobulin chains are grafted into a human immunoglobulin framework. In order to further eradicate the sequence content of mouse antibody in the therapeutic antibody, techniques for the grafting of CDR and SDR of mouse antibody to human immunoglobulin have been developed.

human immunoglobulin.[14] Using this technology, many therapeutic monoclonal antibodies of murine origin have been humanized and are now used to treat different diseases. Examples of these antibodies include rituximab (Rituxan®; Genentech, South San Francisco, California) for the treatment of B cell non-Hodgkin's lymphoma and basiliximab (Simulect®; Novartis, East Hanover, New Jersey) for the prevention of acute rejection in renal transplantation.

2.2.2.2 Complementarity-Determining Region-Grafted Antibodies

Since mouse–human chimeric antibodies contain considerable amounts of mouse antibody polypeptide, which is potentially immunogenic in humans, further minimization of the content of mouse antibody in therapeutic monoclonal antibodies is desired. The CDRs within the variable antigen-binding domains of the light and heavy chains of immunoglobulin are the molecular determinants of antigen specificity. Based on this finding, a therapeutic antibody that retains the specificity of mouse monoclonal antibodies but shows little immunogenicity can be generated by grafting the CDRs of mouse antibody into a human immunoglobulin framework. The resulting CDR-grafted antibody has been found to be less immunogenic when compared with the mouse–human chimeric antibody.[15]

CDR-grafted antibodies have been approved for the clinical treatment of different diseases. In 1997, the United States Food and Drug Administration (FDA) approved the clinical use of daclizumab (Zenapax®; Hoffman-La Roche, Inc., Nutley, New Jersey) to prevent graft rejection after organ transplantation, especially for renal transplantation.

TABLE 2.1
Chimeric and CDR-Grafted Monoclonal Antibodies on the Market

Nature	Monoclonal Antibody	Indication	Date of Approval
Chimeric	Abciximab (ReoPro®; Lilly, Indianapolis, Indiana)	Percutaneous coronary intervention (PCI) adjunct	December 1994
	Rituximab (Rituxan®; Genentech, Vacaville, California)	Non-Hodgkin's lymphoma	November 1997
	Basiliximab (Simulect®; Novartis, East Hanover, New Jersey)	Graft rejection prophylaxis	May 1998
	Infliximab (Remicade®; Centocor, Horsham, Pennsylvania)	Crohn's disease, Rheumatoid arthritis	August 1998
	Cetuximab (Erbitux®; Bristol-Myers Squibb/ImClone, Princeton, New Jersey)	Colorectal cancer	February 2004
CDR-grafted	Daclizumab (Zenapax®; Hoffman-La Roche, Inc., Nutley, New Jersey)	Graft rejection prophylaxis	December 1997
	Palivizumab (Synagis®; MedImmune, Gaithersburg, Maryland)	Respiratory syncytial virus (RSV) infection	June 1998
	Trastuzumab (Herceptin®; Genentech, Vacaville, California)	Metastatic breast cancer	September 1998
	Gemtuzumab (Mylotarg®; Wyeth, Madison, New Jersey)	Acute myeloid leukemia	May 2000
	Alemtuzumab (Campath®; Bayer Pharmaceuticals, Wayne, New Jersey)	Chronic lymphocytic leukemia	July 2001
	Omalizumab (Xolair®; Genentech-Novartis, East Hanover, New Jersey)	Asthma	June 2003
	Efalizumab (Raptiva®; Genentech, Vacaville, California)	Psoriasis	October 2003
	Bevacizumab (Avastin®; Genentech, Vacaville, California)	Colorectal cancer	February 2004
	Natalizumab (Tysabri®; Biogen-Idec, Research Triangle Park, North Carolina)	Multiple sclerosis	November 2004
	Ranibizumab (Lucentis®; Genentech, Vacaville, California)	Wet age-related macular degeneration	June 2006
	Eculizumab (Soliris®; Alexion, Cheshire, Connecticut)	Paroxysmal nocturnal hemoglobinuria	March 2007

However, the CDR-grafted antibodies can still be immunogenic in humans because the number of amino acid residues of mouse origin was still substantial[16] and capable of causing harmful immune responses, as was reported by Sharkey et al.[17] They reported that the administration of a CDR-grafted monoclonal antibody against the carcinoembryonic antigen (CEA) provoked an adverse humoral response in patients with advanced CEA-producing tumors.

2.2.2.3 Specificity-Determining Residue-Grafted Antibodies

Due to the fact that CDR-grafted antibodies can sometimes be immunogenic, new approaches to minimize the content of murine residues in therapeutic antibodies are being evaluated. One such approach is to graft only the amino acid residues that are involved in the antibody–antigen interaction (SDRs), but not the entire CDR, to the human immunoglobulin scaffold. The key challenge to this grafting approach is to select SDRs for grafting. Detailed information about the binding between the antibody and the antigen is inferred usually from the molecular structure of the antibody–antigen complex after x-ray crystallography or *in silico* modeling of the complex.[18]

2.3 *IN VITRO* AFFINITY MATURATION

The genetic engineering of monoclonal antibodies has yielded therapeutic monoclonal antibodies with enhanced tissue penetrability and specificity, and reduced immunogenicity. However, these advantages are always accompanied with decreased binding affinity. The affinity of a monoclonal antibody toward its targeted antigen can be maximized by selecting a high-affinity antibody from a pool of recombinant antibodies by a process called panning or biopanning. Since this process mimics the physiological affinity maturation of an antibody, it is also called *in vitro* affinity maturation.

> Recent advances in antibody engineering have made it possible to overcome the shortcomings of monoclonal antibodies of murine origin, such as potential immunogenicity, ineffective tissue penetration, and undesirable biodistribution. The humanization of therapeutic monoclonal antibodies of murine origin has allowed their use in the treatment of many human diseases.

The same basic principle is shared by all methods of biopanning. To select a high-affinity antibody by biopanning, the target antigen is first immobilized on a solid support. Recombinant antibodies of differential affinity are then incubated with the immobilized antigen. After removing any unbound antibodies, the bound antibodies are eluted and allowed to bind again to the antigen. This process is repeated several times in order to identify the antibody with the highest affinity.

For successful biopanning, antibodies need to be expressed and made accessible to the immobilized antigen. For this purpose, different molecular display systems have been developed. These systems can be categorized into two types: a cell-surface display system and a cell-free display system. A cell-surface display system utilizes a phage (e.g., M13 bacteriophage), a bacterium (e.g., *E. coli*), or yeast to synthesize recombinant antibodies that are then expressed on the cell surface. In a cell-free display system, recombinant antibodies are synthesized by an IVTT system. The advantages and disadvantages of these different methods are summarized in Table 2.2.

TABLE 2.2
Advantages and Disadvantages of the Different Molecular Display Systems

Display System	Advantages	Disadvantages
Cell surface display		
Phage display	Rapid and easy screening	Limited size of displayed protein
Bacterial display	Large library size	Lack of posttranslational quality control over protein folding
	Use of FACS to monitor antibody binding to antigen in solution	Codon usage is different from mammalian
Yeast display	Possesses posttranslational quality control over protein folding, which is very similar to that in mammalian cells	Different glycosylation from mammalian cells
	Possesses a codon usage that is very similar to that in mammalian cells	Relative low transformation efficiency when compared with bacteria
	Easy handling and manipulation	
	Use of FASC to monitor antibody binding to antigen in solution	
Cell-free display		
Ribosome display	Largest library size of all display systems	Requires immobilized antigen on solid support
	Allows recursive mutagenesis, in which selected antibodies are repeatedly mutated to result higher specificity and avidity toward the targeted antigen	Bacterial codon bias

2.3.1 PHAGE DISPLAY

Phage display is the oldest and probably the most commonly used approach. In short, antibodies of interest are packaged and displayed by phages, and then subjected to selection that is based on the differential binding affinities toward the targeted antigen. Although many bacteriophages such as the filamentous phage, T4, T7, and lambda phage can be used for phage display, the M13 bacteriophage is the mostly commonly used. The M13 bacteriophage is a filamentous bacteriophage with a viral genome of approximately 6407 nucleotides, from which one major (P8) and three minor (P9, P6, and P3) coat proteins are encoded. Of these proteins, the P3 minor coat protein is used to facilitate phage docking on *E. coli*, thereby allowing the phagemid, to which genes of the antibodies have been ligated, to be rescued, expressed, and displayed.[19]

Most phage display protocols follow the same principle as described in Figure 2.4. To produce phage-displayed antibodies, antibody genes are ligated first to the P3 gene in a phagemid that is subsequently transformed into a competent *E. coli* such as TG1. Transformed bacterial cells are then infected with M13 bacteriophages, and recombinant M13 phages are produced. Due to the fact that the antibody genes are ligated to the P3 minor coat protein, the antibodies are expressed or displayed on the tips of phages, and are accessible to the immobilized antigen. Using phage display, Schier et al. reported that they were able to achieve a 1230-fold increase in the affinity of a scFv against the tumor antigen c-*erb*-2.[20]

2.3.2 BACTERIAL DISPLAY

Bacterial display is another commonly used cell-based display system and has two advantages over phage display. First, a larger-sized library can be generated quickly because of the rapid transformation and growth rate of bacteria. Second, fluorescence activated cell sorting (FACS) can be used to

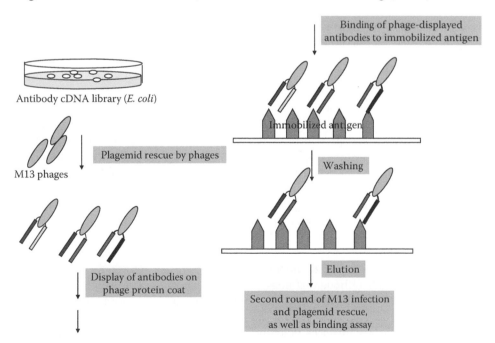

FIGURE 2.4 Schematic diagram showing the procedure for biopanning. In order to display antibodies, genes of antibodies are ligated into phagemid, which is then transformed into *E. coli*. Bacteriophages (e.g., M13) are then allowed to infect bacteria. The resulting recombinant M13 phages with antibodies displayed on their protein coats are incubated with immobilized antigen, and after washing, bound recombinant M13 phages are used to reinfect *E. coli* for another round of screening.

monitor the binding of antibodies to a fluorescently labeled antigen in solution. This eliminates the need to immobilize the antigen on a solid support. Owing to the fact that the antibody–antigen interaction takes place in solution, nonspecific binding of the antibody to the solid support does not occur.

In spite of these advantages, the display of many mammalian proteins in bacterial display can sometimes be problematic. The reason for this drawback is due to the lack of posttranslational control over protein folding and modification, as well as the difference in codon usages between bacteria and mammalian.[21] In view of this, eukaryotic display systems like yeast are usually employed to display mammalian protein for affinity enhancement.

2.3.3   YEAST DISPLAY

Yeast possesses a protein-folding machinery and a codon usage that are very similar to those in mammalian cell.[22] Therefore, yeast is an ideal system for displaying mammalian proteins for biopanning. The production of improperly folded variants due to bacterial codon bias can be circumvented by using yeast display.[20] Another advantage of yeast display is the ease of manipulating yeast reproduction, which allows the generation of a large repertoire library. A typical yeast library harbors 10^6–10^7 repertoires. The library size can be expanded. For example, by mating two different yeast strains, each of which was capable of expressing the V_H and V_L library, Blaise et al. and Weaver-Feldhaus et al. were able to build a Fab library with 3×10^9 different repertoires.[23,24]

2.3.4   RIBOSOME DISPLAY

Ribosome display is a cell-free display system in which an IVTT system is used to display proteins for biopanning. For this purpose, RNA polymerase is used to transcribe the antibody-coding gene into an mRNA transcript. Based on the coding sequence of the resulting mRNA, a polypeptide chain is synthesized by bacterial ribosomes *in vitro*. Since a stop codon is lacking in the mRNA transcript, the nascent polypeptide is trapped in the mRNA-ribosome complex, thus forming a polypeptide-ribosome complex that is accessible to the immobilized antigen. After removing the unbound complex, the mRNA transcripts of the bound complexes are then reverse-transcribed to cDNAs. The cDNAs can be transcribed again. Polypeptides are again synthesized, and then subjected to another round of selection.

There are two features that distinguish the ribosome display from the cell-based display systems. The transformation and growth of cells are not required for expressing proteins in ribosome display. Therefore, ribosome display can usually generate a large library (approximately 10^{12} proteins per library), a size that is considerably larger than those generated by cell-based display systems. In addition, ribosome displays have the potential for affinity maturation through recursive mutagenesis to produce high affinity antibodies. Hanes and colleagues were the first group to report a 65-fold enhancement of the binding affinity of an scFv to its target antigen by recursive mutagenesis-coupled panning.[25]

Although ribosome display allows recursive mutagenesis to produce antibodies of enhanced affinity, the requirement for a solid support to immobilize the antigen for antibody selection potentially increases the likelihood that nonspecific binding will occur. Another drawback of the ribosomal system is that bacterial codon bias may lead to the improper folding of mammalian proteins.

To summarize, the recent advances in antibody engineering have made it possible to overcome the existing shortcomings of therapeutic monoclonal antibodies of murine origin that restricted their widespread clinical use, namely, potential immunogenicity, ineffective tissue penetration, and undesirable biodistribution. With the introduction of methods to humanize therapeutic monoclonal antibodies of murine origin, humanized monoclonal antibodies are now available and have become part of a wide choice of pharmacological therapies to treat many human diseases. In Section 2.4, the uses of engineered antibodies in the management of patients with liver malignancy and liver transplant recipients will be discussed.

2.4 MONOCLONAL ANTIBODIES FOR TREATING LIVER DISEASES

2.4.1 HEPATOCELLULAR CARCINOMA

HCC is endemic in Asia and Africa because of the high prevalence of infection with hepatitis B and C viruses. It is the third most common cause of cancer-related deaths. Although the number of cases is relatively low in the United States and Europe, its rate of incidence has been increasing. Thus, HCC is becoming a major health problem worldwide.[26]

Partial hepatectomy and liver transplantation are the only two curative interventions for HCC. However, the effectiveness of these two interventions is greatly hampered by the low resectability rate, the high postoperative recurrence rate, and the shortage of liver tissue for grafting. Several palliative interventions, such as transarterial radioembolization, transarterial chemoembolization, and local ablative therapy, have been developed. However, the clinical benefits of these interventions remain to be established.[27]

Recent advancements in our understanding of the biology of liver cancer have paved the way for the treatment of cancers with monoclonal antibodies. The progression of a malignant tumor requires that the cancer cells be constitutively stimulated with an aberrant growth signal and also supplied with oxygen and nutrients. The aberrant growth signal to cancer cells in liver results from the uncontrolled activation of the epithermal growth factor receptor (EGFR), which is a result of mutations that cause tyrosine kinase of EGFR to be constitutively active.[28] The EGFR-mediated signaling pathways are, therefore, activated, and many of these pathways favor the progression of cancer cells by promoting unchecked cellular proliferation, cellular motility, and angiogenesis. On the other hand, the supply of oxygen and other nutrients is maintained by angiogenesis, which is driven mainly by vascular endothelial growth factor (VEGF), among other proteins. The underlying mechanism of VEGF action is to increase the permeability of the microvasculature and the extravasation of plasma fibrinogen. This leads to the formation of fibrin deposits in the extracellular matrix. These deposits serve as a building scaffold for the formation of a new capillary network.[29] Cellular signaling resulting from the activation of EGF and VEGF receptors are described in Figure 2.5.

In this context, monoclonal antibodies against the EGFR, such as cetuximab, and against VEGF, such as bevacizumab, have been developed. Their uses are approved by the FDA to treat various cancers. Although their FDA approval for treating HCC is still pending, evaluation of the efficacy of cetuximab and bevacizumab in patients with HCC is underway in several experimental studies and clinical trials. Table 2.3 summarizes the therapeutic monoclonal antibodies studied for treating HCC and liver transplantation.

> Monoclonal antibodies against the EGFR, such as cetuximab, and against VEGF, such as bevacizumab, have been approved by the FDA to treat various cancers. Although their FDA approval for treating HCC is still pending, evaluation of the efficacy of cetuximab and bevacizumab in patients with HCC is underway in several experimental studies and clinical trials.

2.4.1.1 Cetuximab

Over-expression of EGFR has been reported in HCC, which is related with tumor recurrence and extrahepatic metastasis.[30] Cetuximab (Erbitux®; Bristol-Myers Squibb/ImClone, Princeton, New Jersey) is a mouse–human chimeric monoclonal antibody against EGFR. It is approved for use in the treatment of colorectal cancer and head and neck cancers. In addition, studies on its efficacy in HCC are underway.

Huether and colleagues reported that cetuximab could prevent HCC cells from proliferating by inducing cell cycle arrest *in vitro*.[31] Despite the substantial therapeutic effect of cetuximab *in vitro*, the clinical benefits of cetuximab in HCC patients remain to be fully established. Recently, Zhu and

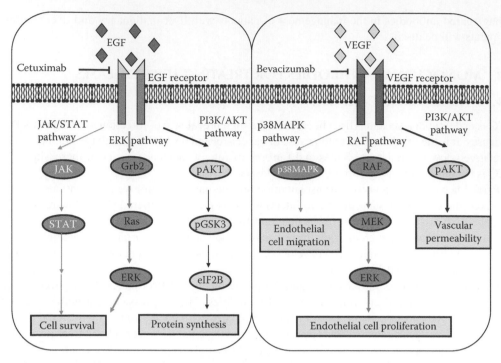

FIGURE 2.5 Schematic diagram showing the downstream cellular effects resulted from activation of EGF and VEGF receptors. Binding of EGF and VEGF triggers dimerization of their respective receptors, and leads to activation on many downstream signaling pathways. Binding of EGF activates PI3K/AKT pathway, ERK pathway and JAK/STAT pathway, promoting survival and protein survival of cancer cells. Binding of VEGF activates PI3K/AKT pathway, RAF pathway, and p38MAPK pathway, promoting proliferation and migration of endothelial cells, as well as increasing endothelial permeability.

colleagues reported that no antitumor effects were found in patients with advanced HCC following treatment with cetuximab alone. They also found that there was no correlation between EGFR expression and the response to therapy.[32] Although the reasons for this disappointing result are unknown, the promise of cetuximab in HCC may not be fulfilled when it is used as the sole therapeutic agent, but rather when it is part of a combination therapy. In 2007, Paule et al. reported that treating nine

TABLE 2.3
Examples of Antibodies Used for the Treatment of HCC and Liver Graft Rejection

	Monoclonal Antibody	Nature	Target Antigen	References
HCC	Bevacizumab (Avastin)	Humanized	VEGF	[38,39]
	Cetuximab (Erbitux)	Human–mouse chimeric	Epidermal growth factor receptor	[31,32,34]
Liver graft rejection	Alemtuzumab	Humanized	CD52 of B and T cells, monocyte, natural killer cells	[54,55]
	Basiliximab (Simulect)	Human–mouse chimeric	IL-2 receptor α-chain (CD25)	[48,49]
	Rituximab (Rituxan)	Human–mouse chimeric	CD20 of B-lymphocyte	[51,52]

patients with intrahepatic cholangiocarcinomas with cetuximab in combination with a gemcitabine plus oxaliplatin (GEMOX) regimen could circumvent chemo-resistance with benefits of patient survival.[33] In 2008, Asnacios et al. reported the results of a phase II clinical trial in which 45 patients with advanced-stage progressive HCC were treated with cetuximab in combination with a GEMOX regimen.[34] The combined therapy resulted in a progression-free survival of 4.7 months without any undesirable drug toxicity. This result is encouraging because the progression-free survival rate following cetuximab monotherapy in HCC patients is 1.4 months.[32] Based on the results of these studies, it seems that cetuximab can be administered to patients with advanced liver malignancy as a palliative treatment.

2.4.1.2 Bevacizumab

Bevacizumab (Avastin®; Genentech, Vacaville, California) is a humanized monoclonal antibody against VEGF and is used to treat patients with metastatic cancers. It was the first monoclonal antibody designed to inhibit angiogenesis in tumors. Blocking the action of VEGF results in the destruction of the blood vessel network that provides the nutrients and oxygen supply to tumor cells, and eventually causes cancer cell death and tumor regression.[35]

The FDA approved the use of bevacizumab for the treatment of colorectal cancer in 2004, lung cancer in 2006, and breast cancer in 2008. Although it has not been approved for the treatment of HCC, it is generally believed that bevacizumab will be effective in treating HCC because HCC tumors are highly vascularized. This is supported by the correlation between VEGF levels with the prognosis of HCC. Intrahepatic VEGF levels in patients with HCC are significantly elevated when compared with those with hepatitis and cirrhosis.[36] El-Assal and colleagues reported that the elevated transcript level of hepatic VEGF is correlated with HCC tumor invasion and metastasis.[37]

Based on these findings, experimental studies and clinical trials on the efficacy of bevacizumab were initiated, and the results are now being reported. For example, Finn and colleagues examined the anti-angiogenic effect of bevacizumab in human HCC cells that were grown and developed into tumors in a mouse orthotopic model of human HCC. They showed that an intraperitoneal injection of bevacizumab (5 mg/kg) significantly decreased microvessel density in the tumor and the rate of tumor progression.[38] Siegel and colleagues reported the results of a phase II clinical trial on the use of bevacizumab in patients with unresectable HCC.[39] The patients were given bevacizumab (5 or 10 mg/kg) every 2 weeks until they showed symptoms of drug toxicity. Treatment with bevacizumab was associated with a significant reduction in tumor enhancement, assessed by dynamic contrast-enhanced magnetic resonance imaging (MRI). It also reduced the circulating VEGF-A and stromal-derived factor-1 levels. Despite these beneficial effects, the patients had undesirable clinical symptoms that included hemorrhage, hypertension, and thrombosis.

In another study, the combined use of bevacizumab with cytotoxic drugs was tested in HCC patients. In this phase II study, Zhu and colleagues demonstrated that patients with advanced HCC treated with bevacizumab in combination with GEMOX had significant reductions in surrogate markers of angiogenesis, as assessed by computed tomography perfusion scans of the liver.[40]

2.4.2 Potential Targets for Antibody Therapy of HCC

The success of bevacizumab and cetuximab has been a stimulus for new investigations to identify specific tumor biomarkers for HCC. The identification of such specific markers can be further exploited to develop a HCC-specific drug delivery system. Different technology platforms are currently available, and Figure 2.6 summarizes the general approach for identifying protein biomarkers from various types of samples like the tissue and blood of a patient, as well as cancer

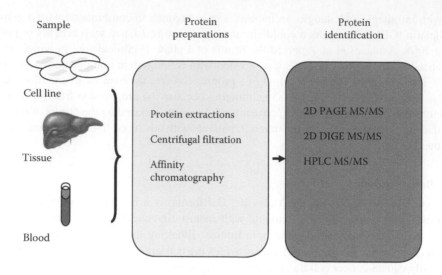

FIGURE 2.6 Schematic workflow for protein biomarker identification from cell line and samples from patients. 2D-DIGE, two-dimensional fluorescence difference gel analysis; 2D-PAGE, two-dimensional polyacrylamide gel electrophoresis; HPLC, high-performance liquid chromatography; MS, mass spectrometry.

cell lines. Over the years, many proteins have been identified whose expressions are specific to patients with HCC and different stages of the disease.[41] Antibodies against these proteins have been generated.

For example, Mohr and colleagues identified a 180 kDa glycoprotein whose expression was found exclusively in HCC tissue, but not in adjacent nontumor tissues. They raised an antibody, AF-20, against this glycoprotein and found that it was a good carrier molecule for the selective delivery of cytotoxic drugs to tumor tissues. When AF-20 was conjugated with a chemotherapeutic drug or a tumoricidal gene and bound to glycoprotein, the antibody–drug complex was internalized and cancer cell death ensued *in vitro* and in animal models.[42]

To search for a HCC-specific biomarker/antigen, we recently conducted a large-scale proteomic study on HCC patients (>100). In this study, we generated a monoclonal antibody against HCC tumor tissue lysate, named CLD3. We found that the epitope of CLD3 is also present in the heterodimeric Ku70/Ku80 autoantigen.[43] This epitope could be a very promising target for the treatment of HCC because Ku antigens contribute to cell proliferation and resistance to irradiation.[44]

2.4.3 LIVER GRAFT REJECTION

Liver transplantation is the only curative treatment for HCC and cirrhosis. The prevention of a rejection of the transplanted liver is critical for successful treatment. Thus, immunosuppressants, such as cyclosporine A, are usually administered to prevent graft rejection. However, immunosuppression can result in many undesirable clinical outcomes such as opportunistic infection[45] and post-transplant lymphoproliferative disorders.[46] Therefore, the following section will describe the development of many mouse–human chimeric and humanized monoclonal antibodies that target the specific effectors of the host immunity in order to prolong graft survival with minimal side effects. In general, these monoclonal antibodies prevent graft rejection by the elimination of alloreactive T lymphocytes, suppression of the humoral response, or induction of donor-specific tolerance.

2.4.3.1 Basiliximab

The infiltration of alloreactive T lymphocytes into a graft can cause tissue damage and graft failure. Therefore, the elimination of this population of T lymphocytes should prevent graft rejection. The binding of interleukin (IL)-2 to its receptor on T lymphocytes results in immune cell proliferation.[47] A monoclonal antibody against the α-chain of the IL-2 receptor (CD25 antigen) has been developed to antagonize the binding of IL-2 to its receptor. Basiliximab (Simulect) is an FDA-approved human–mouse chimeric monoclonal antibody for use in renal transplantation. The combined use of basiliximab and tacrolimus resulted in a significant reduction in the number of acute rejection episodes and infectious complications[48] and the occurrence of postoperative lymphoproliferative disorders.[49]

2.4.3.2 Rituximab

The thymus (T) cell-mediated immune response is one of the key effector mechanisms of graft rejection. However, the B lymphocyte-mediated humoral immune response can be the cause of graft failure in certain circumstances, such as ABO-incompatible (ABO-I) transplantations.[50] Thus, a therapeutic agent that can specifically suppress the activity of B cells is required for this type of transplantation. Rituximab (Rituxan) is a mouse–human chimeric monoclonal antibody against the CD20 antigen of B lymphocytes. It was approved by the US FDA in 1997 for treating B cell non-Hodgkin's lymphoma because of its ability to eradicate B lymphocytes. The successful prevention of graft rejection in ABO-I transplantation by rituximab has been reported in patients with high preoperative circulating levels of antibody against ABO.[51] Recently, the prophylactic administration of rituximab seven days before transplantation effectively eliminated both effector and memory B lymphocytes. This resulted in a low rejection rate and a low peak IgG titers in ABO-I patients who received liver grafts.[52]

2.4.3.3 Alemtuzumab

The induction of donor-specific tolerance in a graft recipient is another strategy in preventing graft rejection.[53] In this approach, tolerance toward the transplanted graft is induced during the first few postoperative weeks by the migration of leucocytes from the graft to the recipient's lymphoid organs. To develop tolerance, the host immune response against the alloantigen needs to be depleted before exposure to the donor's leucocytes. For this purpose, Campath-H1®, a monoclonal antibody against CD52, which is a protein expressed on T cells, B cells, natural killer cells, and monocytes, was developed by the Cambridge University.[54] Subsequently, Campath-H1 was humanized and named alemtuzumab. When used as an anti-lymphoid agent in liver transplantation, a single preoperative administration of alemtuzumab significantly improved graft survival compared with conventional postoperative immunosuppressants.[55] Despite its beneficial effects, opportunistic infections following alemtuzumab administration have been reported in patients following organ transplantation.[56–58] Thus, the prophylactic administration of antimicrobial agents before treatment with alemtuzumab is usually recommended to patients who are scheduled to undergo organ transplantation.

2.5 CONCLUDING REMARKS

Treating malignancies and immune disorders with therapeutic monoclonal antibodies is becoming more widespread clinically because of the significant improvements in their specificity, reduced immunogenicity, and improved biodistribution. These improvements are the result of recombinant DNA technologies that allow the humanization of therapeutic monoclonal antibodies of murine origin by CDR- and SDR-grafting and molecular display systems that express recombinant antibodies for *in vitro* affinity maturation by biopanning. Associated with the development of these technologies are the discoveries of many proteins and/or biomarkers whose expressions are correlated specifically with the stages of diseases and their prognosis.

Immune modulation of the graft rejection response after organ transplantation by monoclonal antibodies has resulted in significant clinical benefits such as those that have been discussed in this chapter. However, the treatment of solid tumors and/or cancers such as HCC with therapeutic antibodies thus far has not yielded encouraging results. As discussed, scFv has emerged as a new technology to enhance antibody delivery to the tumor site and its retention in the tumor. Nevertheless, in our opinion, the discovery of new tumor-specific biomarkers will be beneficial for antibody therapy for HCC. Biomarkers that are capable of differentiating the different stages or/and the different etiologies of HCC would be particularly useful. Therefore, large scale genome- and proteome-wide analyses on the differential expression of mRNA and protein in both circulation and the liver are important. Indeed, these studies are being performed by different centers including our group. Also, Dougan and Dranoff in their review on immune therapy for cancer suggested that in addition to the most commonly used parameters on the efficacy of antibody therapy such as patient survival and tumor size, other criteria such as tumor composition should be incorporated into the assessment in order to provide a more meaningful evaluation on their efficacy.[35] In summary, Table 2.3 highlights the current successful and marketed mAbs in liver transplantation and HCCs.

> Immune modulation of the graft rejection response after organ transplantation by monoclonal antibodies has resulted in significant clinical benefits with fewer undesirable outcomes as compared to the conventional immunosuppressive agents. However, the treatment of solid tumors and/or cancers such as HCC with therapeutic antibodies thus far has not yielded encouraging results.

REFERENCES

1. von Behring EAS, Kitasoto K. Ueber das zustandekommen der diphtherie-immunaitat und der tetanus-immunitar bei thieren. *Ttsch Med Wochenschr* 1890; 16:113–114.
2. Netti PA, Berk DA, Swartz MA et al. Role of extracellular matrix assembly in interstitial transport in solid tumors. *Cancer Res* 2000; 60(9):2497–2503.
3. Hoogenboom HR, Marks JD, Griffiths AD et al. Building antibodies from their genes. *Immunol Rev* 1992; 130:41–68.
4. Marks JD, Hoogenboom HR, Bonnert TP et al. By-passing immunization. Human antibodies from V-gene libraries displayed on phage. *J Mol Biol* 1991; 222(3):581–597.
5. King DJ, Turner A, Farnsworth AP et al. Improved tumor targeting with chemically cross-linked recombinant antibody fragments. *Cancer Res* 1994; 54(23):6176–6185.
6. Goel A, Colcher D, Baranowska-Kortylewicz J et al. Genetically engineered tetravalent single-chain Fv of the pancarcinoma monoclonal antibody CC49: Improved biodistribution and potential for therapeutic application. *Cancer Res* 2000; 60(24):6964–6971.
7. Gruber M, Schodin BA, Wilson ER et al. Efficient tumor cell lysis mediated by a bispecific single chain antibody expressed in *Escherichia coli*. *J Immunol* 1994; 152(11):5368–5374.
8. Zhou HX. Quantitative account of the enhanced affinity of two linked scFvs specific for different epitopes on the same antigen. *J Mol Biol* 2003; 329(1):1–8.
9. Karthe J, Tessmann K, Li J et al. Specific targeting of hepatitis C virus core protein by an intracellular single-chain antibody of human origin. *Hepatology* 2008; 48(3):702–712.
10. Kohler G, Milstein C. Continuous cultures of fused cells secreting antibody of predefined specificity. *Nature* 1975; 256(5517):495–497.
11. Schroff RW, Foon KA, Beatty SM et al. Human anti-murine immunoglobulin responses in patients receiving monoclonal antibody therapy. *Cancer Res* 1985; 45(2):879–885.
12. Shawler DL, Bartholomew RM, Smith LM et al. Human immune response to multiple injections of murine monoclonal IgG. *J Immunol* 1985; 135(2):1530–1535.
13. Abhinandan KR, Martin AC. Analyzing the "degree of humanness" of antibody sequences. *J Mol Biol* 2007; 369(3):852–862.
14. Boulianne GL, Hozumi N, Shulman MJ. Production of functional chimaeric mouse/human antibody. *Nature* 1984; 312(5995):643–646.

15. Jones PT, Dear PH, Foote J et al. Replacing the complementarity-determining regions in a human antibody with those from a mouse. *Nature* 1986; 321(6069):522–525.
16. Vaughan TJ, Osbourn JK, Tempest PR. Human antibodies by design. *Nat Biotechnol* 1998; 16(6):535–539.
17. Sharkey RM, Juweid M, Shevitz J et al. Evaluation of a complementarity-determining region-grafted (humanized) anti-carcinoembryonic antigen monoclonal antibody in preclinical and clinical studies. *Cancer Res* 1995; 55(23 Suppl):5935s–5945s.
18. Kashmiri SV, De Pascalis R, Gonzales NR et al. SDR grafting—A new approach to antibody humanization. *Methods* 2005; 36(1):25–34.
19. Vieira J, Messing J. Production of single-stranded plasmid DNA. *Methods Enzymol* 1987; 153:3–11.
20. Schier R, McCall A, Adams GP et al. Isolation of picomolar affinity anti-c-erbB-2 single-chain Fv by molecular evolution of the complementarity determining regions in the center of the antibody binding site. *J Mol Biol* 1996; 263(4):551–567.
21. Schirrmann T, Al-Halabi L, Dubel S et al. Production systems for recombinant antibodies. *Front Biosci* 2008; 13:4576–4594.
22. Cho BK, Kieke MC, Boder ET et al. A yeast surface display system for the discovery of ligands that trigger cell activation. *J Immunol Methods* 1998; 220(1–2):179–188.
23. Blaise L, Wehnert A, Steukers MP et al. Construction and diversification of yeast cell surface displayed libraries by yeast mating: Application to the affinity maturation of Fab antibody fragments. *Gene* 2004; 342(2):211–218.
24. Weaver-Feldhaus JM, Lou J, Coleman JR et al. Yeast mating for combinatorial Fab library generation and surface display. *FEBS Lett* 2004; 564(1–2):24–34.
25. Hanes J, Jermutus L, Weber-Bornhauser S et al. Ribosome display efficiently selects and evolves high-affinity antibodies in vitro from immune libraries. *Proc Natl Acad Sci USA* 1998; 95(24):14130–14135.
26. Llovet JM, Burroughs A, Bruix J. Hepatocellular carcinoma. *Lancet* 2003; 362(9399):1907–1917.
27. El-Serag HB, Marrero JA, Rudolph L et al. Diagnosis and treatment of hepatocellular carcinoma. *Gastroenterology* 2008; 134(6):1752–1763.
28. Adjei AA, Hidalgo M. Intracellular signal transduction pathway proteins as targets for cancer therapy. *J Clin Oncol* 2005; 23(23):5386–5403.
29. Thomas MB, Abbruzzese JL. Opportunities for targeted therapies in hepatocellular carcinoma. *J Clin Oncol* 2005; 23(31):8093–8108.
30. Kira S, Nakanishi T, Suemori S et al. Expression of transforming growth factor alpha and epidermal growth factor receptor in human hepatocellular carcinoma. *Liver* 1997; 17(4):177–182.
31. Huether A, Hopfner M, Baradari V et al. EGFR blockade by cetuximab alone or as combination therapy for growth control of hepatocellular cancer. *Biochem Pharmacol* 2005; 70(11):1568–1578.
32. Zhu AX, Stuart K, Blaszkowsky LS et al. Phase 2 study of cetuximab in patients with advanced hepatocellular carcinoma. *Cancer* 2007; 110(3):581–589.
33. Paule B, Herelle MO, Rage E et al. Cetuximab plus gemcitabine-oxaliplatin (GEMOX) in patients with refractory advanced intrahepatic cholangiocarcinomas. *Oncology* 2007; 72(1–2):105–110.
34. Asnacios A, Fartoux L, Romano O et al. Gemcitabine plus oxaliplatin (GEMOX) combined with cetuximab in patients with progressive advanced stage hepatocellular carcinoma: Results of a multicenter phase 2 study. *Cancer* 2008; 112(12):2733–2739.
35. Dougan M, Dranoff G. Immune therapy for cancer. *Annu Rev Immunol* 2008; 27:83–117.
36. Park YN, Kim YB, Yang KM et al. Increased expression of vascular endothelial growth factor and angiogenesis in the early stage of multistep hepatocarcinogenesis. *Arch Pathol Lab Med* 2000; 124(7):1061–1065.
37. El-Assal ON, Yamanoi A, Soda Y et al. Clinical significance of microvessel density and vascular endothelial growth factor expression in hepatocellular carcinoma and surrounding liver: Possible involvement of vascular endothelial growth factor in the angiogenesis of cirrhotic liver. *Hepatology* 1998; 27(6):1554–1562.
38. Finn RS, Bentley G, Britten CD et al. Targeting vascular endothelial growth factor with the monoclonal antibody bevacizumab inhibits human hepatocellular carcinoma cells growing in an orthotopic mouse model. *Liver Int* 2008; 29(2):284–290.
39. Siegel AB, Cohen EI, Ocean A et al. Phase II trial evaluating the clinical and biologic effects of bevacizumab in unresectable hepatocellular carcinoma. *J Clin Oncol* 2008; 26(18):2992–2998.
40. Zhu AX, Holalkere NS, Muzikansky A et al. Early antiangiogenic activity of bevacizumab evaluated by computed tomography perfusion scan in patients with advanced hepatocellular carcinoma. *Oncologist* 2008; 13(2):120–125.

41. Sun S, Lee NP, Poon RT et al. Oncoproteomics of hepatocellular carcinoma: From cancer markers' discovery to functional pathways. *Liver Int* 2007; 27(8):1021–1038.
42. Mohr L, Yeung A, Aloman C et al. Antibody-directed therapy for human hepatocellular carcinoma. *Gastroenterology* 2004; 127(5 Suppl 1):S225–S231.
43. Luk JM, Su YC, Lam SC et al. Proteomic identification of Ku70/Ku80 autoantigen recognized by monoclonal antibody against hepatocellular carcinoma. *Proteomics* 2005; 5(7):1980–1986.
44. Fewell JW, Kuff EL. Intracellular redistribution of Ku immunoreactivity in response to cell-cell contact and growth modulating components in the medium. *J Cell Sci* 1996; 109(Pt 7):1937–1946.
45. Jamil B, Nicholls K, Becker GJ et al. Impact of acute rejection therapy on infections and malignancies in renal transplant recipients. *Transplantation* 1999; 68(10):1597–1603.
46. Shroff R, Rees L. The post-transplant lymphoproliferative disorder—A literature review. *Pediatr Nephrol* 2004; 19(4):369–377.
47. Morgan DA, Ruscetti FW, Gallo R. Selective in vitro growth of T lymphocytes from normal human bone marrows. *Science* 1976; 193(4257):1007–1008.
48. Spada M, Petz W, Bertani A et al. Randomized trial of basiliximab induction versus steroid therapy in pediatric liver allograft recipients under tacrolimus immunosuppression. *Am J Transplant* 2006; 6(8):1913–1921.
49. Marino IR, Doria C, Scott VL et al. Efficacy and safety of basiliximab with a tacrolimus-based regimen in liver transplant recipients. *Transplantation* 2004; 78(6):886–891.
50. Demetris AJ, Jaffe R, Tzakis A et al. Antibody-mediated rejection of human orthotopic liver allografts. A study of liver transplantation across ABO blood group barriers. *Am J Pathol* 1988; 132(3):489–502.
51. Usuda M, Fujimori K, Koyamada N et al. Successful use of anti-CD20 monoclonal antibody (rituximab) for ABO-incompatible living-related liver transplantation. *Transplantation* 2005; 79(1):12–16.
52. Egawa H, Ohmori K, Haga H et al. B-cell surface marker analysis for improvement of rituximab prophylaxis in ABO-incompatible adult living donor liver transplantation. *Liver Transplant* 2007; 13(4):579–588.
53. Starzl TE, Zinkernagel RM. Transplantation tolerance from a historical perspective. *Nat Rev Immunol* 2001; 1(3):233–239.
54. Hale G, Bright S, Chumbley G et al. Removal of T cells from bone marrow for transplantation: A monoclonal antilymphocyte antibody that fixes human complement. *Blood* 1983; 62(4):873–882.
55. Marcos A, Eghtesad B, Fung JJ et al. Use of alemtuzumab and tacrolimus monotherapy for cadaveric liver transplantation: With particular reference to hepatitis C virus. *Transplantation* 2004; 78(7):966–971.
56. Peleg AY, Husain S, Kwak EJ et al. Opportunistic infections in 547 organ transplant recipients receiving alemtuzumab, a humanized monoclonal CD-52 antibody. *Clin Infect Dis* 2007; 44(2):204–212.
57. Silveira FP, Husain S. Fungal infections in solid organ transplantation. *Med Mycol* 2007; 45(4):305–320.
58. Silveira FP, Husain S, Kwak EJ et al. Cryptococcosis in liver and kidney transplant recipients receiving anti-thymocyte globulin or alemtuzumab. *Transpl Infect Dis* 2007; 9(1):22–27.

3 Transferrin Receptor–Mediated Transcytosis in Intestinal Epithelial Cells for Gastrointestinal Absorption of Protein Drugs

Nurmamet Amet, Xiaoying Chen, Hsin-Fang Lee,
Jennica Zaro, and Wei-Chiang Shen

CONTENTS

3.1   INTRODUCTION

The advances in molecular biology and recombinant DNA technology over the past 30 years has made it possible for the biopharmaceutical industry to develop protein and peptide drugs, such as human insulin (In), human growth hormone (hGH), human granulocyte colony-stimulating factor (G-CSF), and human erythropoietin (EPO).[1,2] The peptide and protein drugs have been available for clinical use in the market for many years.[3] However, one drawback of these drugs is that patients have to take them either subcutaneously (s.c.), intramuscularly (i.m.), or intravenously (i.v.) by injection. These invasive techniques are associated with pain, unwanted site effects, and low patient compliance. Therefore, noninvasive routes, such as oral, nasal, rectal, ocular, and pulmonary routes, have long been sought after by the pharmaceutical industry, but with little success.[4]

The development of an oral delivery system, among other noninvasive routes, for peptide and protein drugs remains an attractive option for the biopharmaceutical industry. Unfortunately, many difficulties exist in the development of an oral delivery system: (1) these drugs are not stable in the gastrointestinal (GI) tract; (2) they are susceptible to enzymatic breakdown by proteolytic enzymes such as trypsin, chymotrypsin, and pepsin; and (3) large molecular weight and high hydrophilicity prevents them from being absorbed by the GI epithelium. Approaches to overcome these obstacles include the use of penetration enhancers to improve absorption across the GI epithelium, enzyme inhibitors to prevent proteolysis by GI enzymes, enteric coating, and entrapment of protein drugs in microspheres to protect them from harsh environment. However, these approaches are associated with unwanted side effects including irritancy, nonspecific absorption of additional molecules, and absorption of the enhancers in the bloodstream. The negative side effects can be intensified when the protein drugs are given over a long period of time, for example, in the case of In.[5,6]

Using receptors as targets and receptor-binding ligands as vectors for transcellular transport is a promising way of achieving a selective delivery of peptide and protein drugs across the intestinal epithelium.[7] This process, termed receptor-mediated transcytosis, is highly specific because it enhances only the transport of molecules that are conjugated to receptor-binding ligands.[8] Receptor-mediated transcytosis is an inherent cellular process in epithelial and endothelial cells.[9] Unlike most other approaches as mentioned above, a receptor-mediated transcytotic process does not change the structure of the plasma membranes or the intercellular junctions, and conceivably has fewer unwanted side effects and safety concerns. The receptor of vitamin B-12-intrinsic factor complex expressed on the surface of intestinal epithelial cells has been explored for peptide and protein delivery via receptor-mediated transcytosis.[10] In this chapter, we focus on the transepithelial transport of transferrin (Tf)-fusion proteins as a pathway for oral delivery of protein drugs.

3.2   TRANSFERRIN

Human serum Tf is a single-chain glycoprotein consisting of 679 amino acids with an 80 kDa molecular weight.[11] The glycoprotein has two lobes, connected by a short peptide linker (Figure 3.1).[12,13] Each lobe further divides into two domains, designated as N1 and N2 for the N-lobe domains, and C1 and C2 for the C-lobe domains. The cavities between the domains in each lobe form the binding sites for ferric iron (Fe^{3+}). Therefore, one molecule of Tf has two iron-binding sites. Four amino acids, including two tyrosines, one aspartate, and one histidine, and two anionic carbonates are involved in Fe^{3+} binding.[14] The iron bound Tf (diferric-Tf) and ironless Tf (apo-Tf) have different affinities to the transferrin receptor (TfR), with the latter having a much lower affinity to TfR at neutral pH due to its unfavorable conformation.[15]

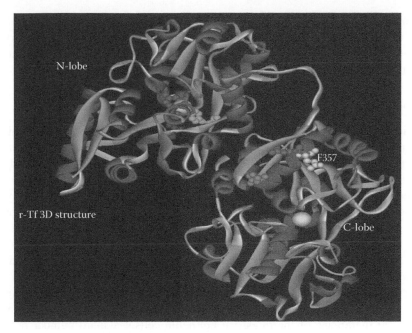

FIGURE 3.1 Three-dimensional structure of rabbit serum Tf (r-Tf) binding to TfR. r-Tf binds to human TfR, and shares 79% amino acid sequence identity with human diferric Tf.[12,13] The x-ray crystal structure for the human diferric-Tf has not been resolved. This figure illustrates the structural attributes of Tf including the N and C lobes, 4 domains (N1, N2, C1, and C2), two bound iron atoms and crucial amino acids that may be important in both Tf–TfR interaction and TfR-dependent transcytosis. The Protein Data Bank (PDB) reference ID and URL are 1JNF and www.pdb.org, respectively.

3.2.1 TRANSFERRIN RECEPTOR

TfRs are expressed in almost all types of cells except mature erythrocytes and terminally differentiated cells. Transferrin receptor 1 (TfR1) is a classical functional receptor with expression particularly in blood–brain barrier endothelial cells, and GI and alveolar epithelial cells, all of which require iron for their physiological functions. Transferrin receptor 2 (TfR2), a homologue of TfR1, is predominantly expressed in the liver.[16] Both TfR1 and TfR2 bind Tf in a pH-dependent manner, with TfR2 binding with a lower affinity.[17–19]

TfR is a homodimer consisting of two identical units, each of 90 kDa molecular weight. It is composed of a protease-like domain, an apical domain, and a helical domain. The TfR homodimer binds two Tf molecules, and thus transports up to four Fe^{3+} molecules into cells per receptor. The crystal structure derived from the Tf–TfR complex reveals that the apical domain of TfR interacts with the C1-Tf domain as the primary contact, while the helical and protease-like domains interact, to a weaker extent, with the N1 and N2-Tf domains, respectively. The involvement of the C2 domain of Tf in the TfR binding is minor.[14,15]

There are many studies published on immunohistochemical detection for the tissue distribution of TfR, both TfR1 and TfR2, each indicating the presence of the receptors in the small intestine. Generally, TfR staining is strongest in the crypt region and decreases moving along the entire villous axis.[20] However, perhaps due to differences in tissue isolation and fixation methods, localization differs slightly.[21] Due to the area of localization in intestinal epithelial cells, it is generally believed that TfR is not directly involved in the major iron absorption from the diet.[22] However, recent findings indicate that TfR can serve as a regulator of iron absorption in GI epithelia via the TfR-mediated endocytosis/transcytosis pathway, although the exact molecular mechanisms have not been established.[23] Furthermore, the possibility of a transient appearance of TfR on the luminal side as a result of membrane missorting due to the recycling protein transport pathway in intestinal epithelial cells[24] can also induce an apical-to-basolateral TfR-mediated transcytosis for the GI absorption of protein drugs.

3.2.2 Transferrin Receptor–Mediated Transcytosis

At physiological pH (~7.4), Tf binds two Fe^{3+} and subsequently becomes diferric-Tf, which leads to a conformational change favorable for receptor binding. After binding to its receptor expressed on the cell surface, the iron and receptor-bound Tf is then internalized by receptor-mediated endocytosis (RME). The low pH (~5.5) environment of the endosome induces another conformational change in the Tf–TfR complex, leading to the release of iron, which may be transported to the cytosol by the divalent metal transporter 1 (DMT1). The apo-Tf-TfR complex recycles back to the plasma membrane where the higher pH (~7.4) causes the dissociation of apo-Tf from its receptor. This whole cycle repeats to provide sufficient iron needed in cellular physiology.

In polarized cells, RME can occur from both the apical and the basolateral plasma membranes through vesicles termed apical endosomes (AE) and basolateral endosomes (BE), respectively.[9] Additionally, a vesicle that is accessible by both apically and basolaterally endocytosed ligands, termed the common endosome (CE), has been described.[25] While a majority of TfRs are localized at the basolateral membrane of the intestinal epithelial cells,[18] a small number of TfRs appear at the apical membrane, likely due to missorting of TfRs internalized in the BE.[18,26] When a Tf-ligand conjugate is administered orally, it can bind TfRs at the apical membrane and internalize into the AE, where the diferric-Tf discharges the bound iron and subsequently becomes an apo-Tf. Apo-Tf may accumulate in the CE of intestinal epithelial cells for a prolonged time.[27] As the divalent metal transporter DMT1 transports iron across the apical membrane via endocytosis, some iron atoms may reach the CE[28] and bind to apo-Tf. This conversion from apo-Tf to diferric-Tf in the CE could induce the transcytosis of Tf–TfR complex across the basolateral membrane,[29] ultimately resulting in the delivery of the ligand conjugated to Tf into the systemic circulation. However, the exact mechanism that causes the transcytosis of Tf–TfR complexes in the GI epithelial cells is still not well established. The overall Tf transcytosis scheme is illustrated in Figure 3.2.

3.2.3 Approaches to Improve Efficiency of TfR-Mediated Transcytosis

Since TfR-mediated transcytosis is a slow process, the enhanced understanding of the pathways and molecular regulators of this transepithelial transport can help achieve higher efficiency in the oral delivery of Tf-conjugated macromolecule drugs. To improve the efficiency of Tf-ligand absorption across intestinal epithelial cells, the investigation of the mechanism of Tf–TfR recycling and trafficking following internalization in endosomes is of paramount importance.

3.2.3.1 Transferrin Oligomerization

The effect of TfR cross-linking induced by Tf-oligomers has been previously investigated in Chinese-hamster ovary (CHO) cells.[30] More recently, Tf-oligomers have been further studied both in Caco-2 cells and *in vivo* experiments in order to demonstrate whether the oligomerization of Tf can improve Tf–TfR-mediated transcytosis, and subsequently enhance the bioavailability of the Tf-conjugated ligand. To form Tf oligomers, an average of 3.5 Tf molecules per aggregate were crosslinked either by using a homobifunctional linker [1,11-bismaleimidotetra-ethyleneglycol, BM(PEO)4], or a heterobifunction linker [succinimidyl 4-(-p-maleimidophenyl)-butyrate, SMPB]. The resulting Tf oligomer-In conjugates showed a twofold enhancement in the absorption and bioactivity in Caco-2 cells and in diabetic mice.[31] This indicated that the oligomerization of

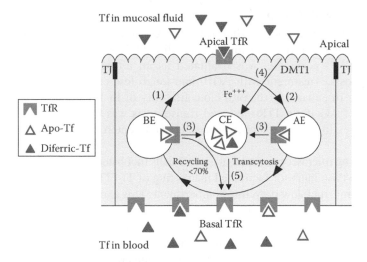

FIGURE 3.2 A hypothetical scheme of the regulatory mechanism for the transport of Tf from the mucosal side of the intestinal epithelial cells to the blood. (1) Missorting of basolateral membrane in basolateral endosomes (BE) would allow a small number of TfR to appear on the apical surface. (2) Orally administered Tf would bind to apical TfR and internalized to AE, where diferric Tf would be converted to apo-Tf due to the acidification. (3) Apo-Tf in AE would be transported to a CE by a similar process that has been described for apo-Tf in BE. Apo-Tf would be accumulated in CE for a prolonged time. (4) Iron uptake from the mucosal surface via divalent metal transporter 1 (DMT1) could reach CE due to the endocytosis of DMT1. (5) The conversion of Apo-Tf to diferric Tf in CE would accelerate the transport of diferric Tf from CE to the basolateral membrane *via* exocytosis, and eventually to be released to the blood.

Tf could enhance the delivery efficiency of conjugated macromolecules, including peptide and protein drugs.

3.2.3.2 Treatment with Brefeldin A

The effect of the fungal metabolite brefeldin A (BFA) on Tf transcellular transport and TfR distribution has been evaluated in filter-grown Madin–Darby canine kidney (MDCK) and in Caco-2 cells using radioactively labeled iron (^{59}Fe) and Tf (^{125}I-Tf). Treatment with BFA enhanced Tf transcytosis in both the apical-to-basal and the basal-to-apical directions. The enhancement was not accompanied by a concurrent increase in the transcytosis of a fluid phase marker, horseradish peroxidase, indicating that BFA treatment did not induce leakage or other damage to the cell monolayers. The results also demonstrated a decrease in the recycling of TfRs back to the basolateral membrane, a decrease in the number of TfRs expressed at the basolateral surface accompanied by an increase in the number of TfRs expressed at the apical surface, and an increase in the extent of the endocytosis of Tf at the apical surface. Taken together, the results indicated that BFA alters the traffic of Tf–TfR complexes by decreasing receptor recycling and diverting the non-recycled fraction to the transcytotic pathway.[26,32] Therefore, treatment with BFA could potentially improve the oral efficacy of Tf-bioactive drug conjugates by increasing the amount of drug conjugate delivered to the systemic circulation.

One of the concerns of using BFA as a transcytosis enhancer is that it can cause alterations at many intracellular sites, including endosomes, *trans*-Golgi cisterni, and lysosomes.[33] Therefore, other unwanted side effects may result if BFA is used *in vivo*. Agents with a specific and selective effect on TfR-mediated transcytosis would be more desirable for the development of a practical formulation that will enhance the absorption of Tf-conjugates across intestinal epithelial cells.

3.2.3.3 Treatment with AG-10

The effect of a GTPase inhibitor AG-10 (tyrphostin A8, or 4-hydroxybenzylidene-malononitrile) on the internalization, the trafficking, and the recycling of fluorescently labeled Tf, Tf-fluorescein isothiocyanate (FITC) conjugate, was evaluated as an alternative enhancing agent for TfR-mediated transcytosis. Treatment with AG10 had much less effect on cellular physiology, and was more effective in enhancing the oral bioavailability of In-Tf conjugates.[34] Furthermore, the enhancing effect of AG-10 on TfR-mediated transcytosis was found only in Caco-2, but not in MDCK cells, suggesting that it may be more selective to enterocytes than other types of epithelial cells.[34]

Confocal scanning microscopy results in Caco-2 cells incubated with Tf in the presence of AG-10 showed that the GTPase inhibitor facilitated the sorting of Tf-FITC to the Rab11 positive compartment, a late endosomal and slow recycling compartment. This alteration in Tf sorting could possibly contribute to the slow recycling of Tf-FITC back to the apical membrane, or to the exocytosis of Tf-FITC through the basolateral membrane,[35] both of which could increase the efficiency of the oral absorption of a Tf-conjugated ligand into the systemic circulation. Taken together, these findings indicate that the coadministration of AG10 with Tf-conjugates could improve oral bioavailability and conceivably enhance the bioactivity of the conjugated drug.

3.3 TRANSFERRIN RECEPTOR–MEDIATED DRUG DELIVERY

> Tf has been widely used as a targeting ligand for the delivery of small molecule drugs, peptides, proteins, and genes to target tissues and cancer cells. Tf-mediated drug delivery offers several advantages including the capability of Tf to pass through the GI epithelium or across the blood–brain barrier by transcytosis, the resistance of Tf to enzymatic digestion by trypsin and chymotrypsin, and the abundant expression of TfRs in human GI epithelium.

Tf has been widely applied as a vehicle to deliver small molecule drugs, peptides, proteins, and genes to target tissues.[36,37] Tf-mediated drug delivery offers several advantages including the capability of Tf to pass through the GI epithelium or across the blood–brain barrier by transcytosis, the resistance of Tf to enzymatic digestion by trypsin and chymotrypsin,[38] and the abundant expression of TfRs in human GI epithelium. These advantages make Tf a rational choice as a carrier for the oral delivery of protein drugs.

3.4 CHEMICAL CONJUGATION OF TRANSFERRIN AND PROTEIN DRUGS

Tf has been chemically conjugated to various biological macromolecules. One such study described the design of an oral delivery system consisting of In conjugated to Tf (In-Tf). In is a 51-amino acid peptide hormone with a molecular weight of 5808 Da. This peptide has long been used medically to treat diabetes mellitus primarily via subcutaneous injection.[39] In was chemically conjugated to Tf by first blocking the α-amino groups of In with dimethylmaleic anhydride (DMMA). The ε-amino groups were then modified with N-succimidyl-3-(2-pyridyldithio) propionate (SPDP), and subsequently conjugated to SPDP-modified Tf via a disulfide linkage. When the In-Tf conjugate was administered orally to streptozotocin (STZ)-induced diabetic mice, a prolonged hypoglycemic effect was observed. Further, In-Tf was detected in the serum 4 h after oral administration, indicating that the conjugate was absorbed from the GI epithelium.[34]

Another study described the generation of Tf conjugated to G-CSF. G-CSF is a member of the growth factor family that regulates hematopoetic cell proliferation and differentiation. This glycoprotein consists of 174 amino acids with a molecular weight of approximately 20 kDa.[40] Human G-CSF is protective in a broad variety of animal infection models in terms of improved survival, reduced bacterial loads, enhanced neutrophil action, and immigration into infected sites.[41]

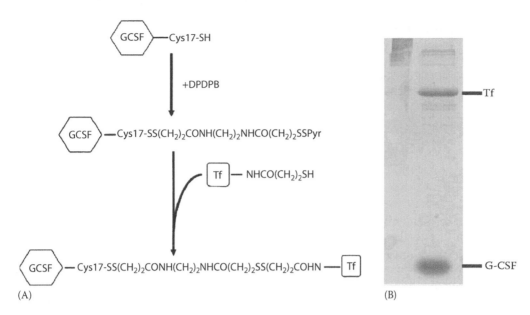

(A)   (B)

FIGURE 3.3 Preparation and characterization of G-CSF-Tf conjugates. (A) The Cys-17 residue of G-CSF was first modified with the cleavable, sulfhydryl-reactive crosslinker, 1,4-di-[3′-(2′-pyridyldithio)-propionamido] butane (DPDPB), and subsequently coupled with SPDP-modified and reduced Tf. The product was purified by gel filtration chromatography.[26] (B) PAGE, a technique used to separate proteins by their molecular weight differences, was used to evaluate the final conjugation product. As shown in lane 1, the predominant bands were located at the top of the gel, indicating that the conjugates were predominately large molecular weight aggregates. The conjugate was then treated with DTT, a strong disulfide-reducing agent, which can cleave the disulfide bond between GCSF and Tf. As shown in lane 2, two bands were observed at the corresponding molecular weights for Tf and G-CSF, indicating that they were linked by disulfide bonds.

G-CSF was conjugated to a SPDP-modified Tf via the Cys-17 residue of G-CSF to form a disulfide linkage between the two proteins (Figure 3.3A). The oral biological activity of the resulting GCSF-Tf conjugate was examined in a BDF1 mice, an animal known for their stimulatory response to human G-CSF.[42] Following oral administration, the number of neutrophils were significantly increased as compared to control without treatment.[43] These results demonstrated that Tf could be effectively used as a carrier for oral delivery.

The In and G-CSF Tf-conjugates described in this section were made by chemically cross-linking the protein drugs to Tf via a disulfide bridge. Unfortunately, this approach is associated with some problems ranging from low yield and low quality to heterogeneous products, thus rendering it unsuitable for therapeutic application (Figure 3.3B). Although some studies applied recombinant DNA approach to engineer a protein consisting of Tf and a therapeutic domain for drug targeting,[44,45] the delivery of therapeutic protein is still limited to injection. To overcome limitations arising from the chemical conjugation approach and to demonstrate TfR-mediated oral absorption of protein drugs, subsequent sections will describe the use of recombinant fusion protein technology for the preparation of Tf-protein drug conjugates.

3.5 RECOMBINANT TRANSFERRIN-FUSION PROTEINS

With the advancement of recombinant DNA technology, the Tf platform for protein delivery moved forward from chemical conjugates to recombinant fusion proteins. Recombinant fusion proteins are proteins that are synthesized by joining two genes coded for separate proteins using recombinant DNA technology. As previously described, the In-Tf and G-CSF-Tf chemical conjugates were orally effective and elicited a pharmacological response. However, a major obstacle for the chemical conjugation approach is that their compositions and sizes are heterogeneous, which is unaccept-able for therapeutic use. In comparison, recombinant fusion proteins can be precisely constructed and produced as homogenous products by molecular biology technologies. Recombinant G-CSF-Tf fusion protein was the first example that the recombinant Tf fusion proteins were orally available and had therapeutic effects.[46]

3.6 RECOMBINANT GRANULOCYTE COLONY-STIMULATING FACTOR

Recombinant G-CSF (rh-GCSF) was first cloned from the bladder carcinoma cell line 5637 and expressed in *E. coli*.[47] This drug, with the commercial name Filgrastim® (Amgen, Inc., Thousand Oaks, California) was approved by the FDA in 1991 for the treatment of chemotherapy-induced neutropenia in cancer patients. Another recombinant G-CSF cloned from human squamous carcinoma CHU-II and expressed in COS (monkey kidney *C*V-1 *O*rigin *S*imian virus-40) cells has also been developed (Lenograstim®; Chugai Pharmaceuticals, Tokyo, Japan). Both forms have similar bioavailability and bioactivities following subcutaneous or intravenous administration.[48,49] G-CSF is an important drug for the treatment of several immune disorders and com-plications associated with cancer chemotherapy. The administration of G-CSF is typically at doses of 1–20 mg/kg per day. Higher doses may be required in patients with severe congenital neutropenia (SCN).

To improve the bioactivity of G-CSF, one approach uses recombinant G-CSF fused to human albumin (Albugranin). This drug was reported to have prolonged myelopoietic effects in mice and monkeys.[42] Albugranin has a long terminal half-life and mean residence time, and a slower clear-ance in mice. In addition, a polyethylene glycol (PEG)-conjugated (PEGylated) form of G-CSF (Neulasta®, Amgen, Inc., Thousand Oaks, California) has been approved by the FDA as a long-lasting G-CSF.[50] Even though the modified versions of G-CSF exhibited better pharmacokinetic profiles, they still need to be injected.

3.6.1 Recombinant G-CSF-Transferrin-Fusion Protein

Recombinant G-CSF-Tf fusion protein was produced by engineering an expression plasmid con-taining G-CSF fused in-frame with Tf with either a short dipeptide linker, a helical linker, or a disulfide–cyclopeptide linker between the two domains. The expression plasmids were then used to transiently transfect human embryonic kidney (HEK) 293 cells. The identity of the isolated fusion proteins was confirmed by Western blot, as both anti-G-CSF and anti-Tf antibodies rec-ognized the protein. Figures 3.4 and 3.5 illustrate the expression plasmid, representative Western blot, and a computer–generated molecular model for the G-CSF-Tf fusion protein containing a short dipeptide linker, Leu-Glu (LE). Next, the *in vitro* biological activities of the fusion proteins were assayed for both the G-CSF and the Tf domains. For its G-CSF activity, the fusion pro-teins were able to induce the proliferation of NFS-60 cells, a murine myeloblastic cell line that responds to G-CSF stimulation. For the demonstration of Tf activity, the fusion proteins were able to compete with the binding of Tf to TfR in cultured Caco-2 cells, a human epithelial colorectal adenocarcinoma cell line with close morphological and functional similarities to the intestinal epithelium. The *in vitro* assays confirmed that the G-CSF-Tf fusion proteins were correctly pro-duced and biologically active.

3.6.2 Fusion Protein Linkers

The insertion of various linkers between protein domains in recombinant fusion proteins provides multiple functions, such as linkage, separation, and flexibility.[51] Additionally, the linkers affect the folding, the stability, the proteolytic resistance, and the solubility of the fusion proteins.[52] The most commonly used linker between fusion domains, especially for single-chain Fv domains of

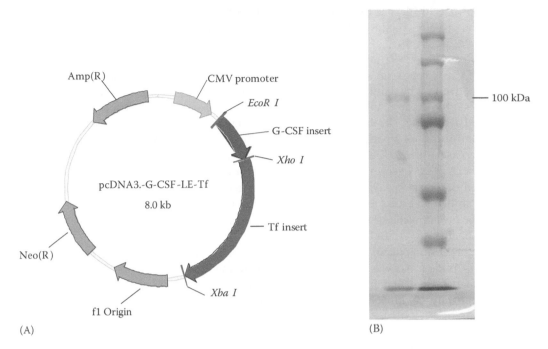

(A)

(B)

FIGURE 3.4 The construction and characterization of G-CSF-LE-Tf fusion protein. (A) The genes encoding G-CSF-LE-Tf fusion protein were inserted into mammalian expression vector pcDNA3.0. (B) The G-CSF-LE-Tf fusion protein was produced from HEK293 cells and analyzed by SDS-PAGE. Lane 1, G-CSF-LE-Tf fusion protein; lane 2, molecular weight marker.

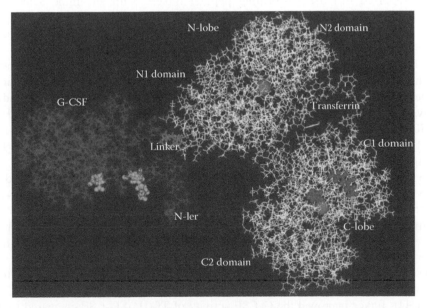

FIGURE 3.5 Computer generated molecular model for G-CSF-Tf fusion protein connected by a short linker. Highlighted are amino acids known to play an important role in receptor binding, and two iron atoms positioned in the iron-binding pocket. The structure was generated using WebLab Viewer and Insight II molecular modeling programs. The coordinates used in this model are 1GNC for G-CSF and 1JNF for rat-Tf, both obtained from the PDB.

immunoglobulin, is the flexible linker, (GGGGS)$_3$.[53] However, optimal linker sequences are selected for each fusion protein to optimize the production and biological activity.

3.6.2.1 Dipeptide Linker

The G-CSF-Tf fusion protein with a short dipeptide linker, G-CSF-LE-Tf, demonstrated *in vivo* activity as determined by daily absolute neutrophil counts (ANC) following administration. At a dose of 5 mg/kg, the s.c. injected fusion protein elicited a comparable myelopoietic response as free G-CSF in the BDF1 mice. The dramatic effect of the fusion protein as a myelopoietic agent was seen in the oral administration experiments. At a dose of 50 mg/kg, the fusion protein induced more than a fourfold increase of the ANC in the blood. In contrast, the orally administered free G-CSF failed to increase the ANC. Moreover, the myelopoietic effect of the orally administered fusion protein was prolonged, lasting 4–5 days. To confirm that the transport of the fusion protein was due to its TfR-binding ability, an excess amount of Tf was coadministered orally with the fusion protein. The decrease of the myelopoietic effect with an excess of Tf demonstrated that the transport of the fusion protein was specifically via the TfR.[46]

Although this fusion protein successfully elicited myelopoiesis in BDF1 mice via oral administration, the dipeptide linker was not optimal for maintaining the biological activity. With this short linker, the fusion protein only retained about 1/10th of the G-CSF activity and about 1/16th of the TfR-binding affinity *in vitro*.[46] There are two possible reasons that account for the low activity of the fusion protein. First, the protein domains may have had steric hindrance between each other due to the short linkage. Second, the extended peptide sequences on the N- or C-terminus of the functional domains may have partially blocked their receptor-binding sites. In any case, the orally administered recombinant G-CSF-Tf fusion protein was bioavailable, and exhibited sustained effect on myelopoiesis in BDF1 mice, which opens up possibilities for the optimization and application of Tf fusion proteins for the oral delivery of other protein drugs.

3.6.2.2 Helical Linkers

It has been reported that α-helix-forming peptide linkers, with an amino acid sequence of A(EAAAK)$_n$A ($n = 2$–5), increased the distance between functional domains in fusion protein and reduced their interference.[54] These helical linkers can effectively separate the domains at a distance that can be controlled by changing the repetitions of the EAAAK motif.

α-Helix-forming peptide linkers were inserted in G-CSF-Tf fusion proteins to better separate the functional domains. The G-CSF and Tf activities of fusion proteins with various sizes of linker peptides were assayed by the NFS-60 cell proliferation assay and TfR binding assay, respectively. Among the α-helix-forming linkers tested, fusion protein with the (H4)$_2$ linker (A(EAAAK)$_4$ALEA(EAAAK)$_4$A) had the highest G-CSF activity, approximately 10-fold higher than that of G-CSF-Tf. On the other hand, the TfR binding affinity of G-CSF-(H4)$_2$-Tf was not improved significantly.

With the improvement of the intrinsic G-CSF activity, G-CSF-(H4)$_2$-Tf also displayed a superior *in vivo* activity compared to G-CSF-Tf. The subcutaneously administered G-CSF-(H4)$_2$-Tf induced a higher ANC than G-CSF-Tf and free G-CSF. More strikingly, at a relatively low dose of 20 mg/kg, orally administered G-CSF-(H4)$_2$-Tf exhibited a good efficacy, while the G-CSF-Tf did not have a significant effect. In comparison, G-CSF-Tf only induced an increase of ANC at a higher dose of 50 mg/kg in previous studies.

A fusion protein with Tf located at the N-terminus (Tf-(H4)$_n$-G-CSF) was also constructed and compared with the C-terminally located Tf fusion protein. Similar to G-CSF-(H4)$_2$-Tf, the insertion of the (H4)$_2$ linker improved the G-CSF activity of Tf-(H4)$_2$-G-CSF compared to Tf-G-CSF (Table 3.1). Although the potency, as measured by the half-maximal effective concentration (EC$_{50}$), of the fusion protein without the linker, Tf–LE-G-CSF, was lower than Tf-(H4)$_2$-G-CSF, the maximum biological effect (E_{max}) of Tf-(H4)$_2$-G-CSF was similar to G-CSF. Tf-LE-GCSF retained less than 50% biological activity.

TABLE 3.1
Summary of *In Vitro* and *In Vivo* Activities in Different G-CSF-Tf Fusion Proteins

Fusion Protein	E_{max}[a]	Dose Ratio[b]
Tf-LE-GCSF	0.69	15.7
Tf-(H4)$_2$-GCSF	1.53	30
GCSF-LE-Tf	1.36	54
GCSF-(H4)$_2$-Tf	1.44	29
GCSF	1.6	1

[a] E_{max}, maximal effect, as determined by the MTT (3-(4,5-dimethylthiazol-2-yl)-2,5-diphenyltetrazolium bromide) assay for NSF-60 cell proliferation. The MTT assay is a colorimetric assay based on the reduction of MTT to purple formazan in the mitochondria of living cells.

[b] Dose ratio = The half-maximal effective concentration (EC_{50}) obtained for the fusion protein divided by the G-CSF control {(EC_{50} of fusion protein)/(EC_{50} of GCSF)}.

The improvement of G-CSF activity following the insertion of the (H4)$_2$ linker indicates that the steric hindrance between domains limited the G-CSF receptor–binding ability. However, the TfR-binding affinity did not increase following the insertion of the (H4)$_2$ linker. Since the orientation of G-CSF and Tf did not significantly affect the *in vitro* activity for the fusion proteins, the blockage of either the N- or the C-terminus of the Tf domain may have a similar impact to the TfR-binding affinity. Further data on the *in vivo* activity of G-CSF-(H4)$_2$-Tf and Tf-(H4)$_2$-G-CSF will aid in the elucidation of the best orientation for an optimal effect.

3.6.2.3 Effect of Helical Linkers on Fusion Protein Production Levels

Another interesting finding for the use of α-helix linkers is that they may increase fusion protein production levels.[55] For the production of Tf-(H4)$_n$-G-CSF from HEK-293 cells, the insertion of H4 linkers induced a dose-dependent increase in the expression of the recombinant protein (Figure 3.6). With H4 linkers, the better separation of protein domains may facilitate the correct

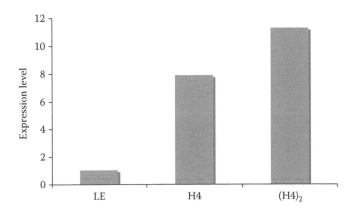

FIGURE 3.6 Expression level of Tf-(H4)$_n$-G-CSF ($n = 0$–2) fusion proteins. The expression level of fusion proteins containing a short peptide linker, LE, and one or two copies of a helical linker, H4 and (H4)$_2$, respectively, was determined by Western blot using anti-G-CSF and anti-Tf antibodies. The data are presented as the fold-increase of fusion protein concentration compared to the fusion protein without the peptide linker (LE).

folding of the functional domains and thus increase the efficiency of protein production. Similar results were also observed in the expression of hGH-Tf fusion proteins as described in the next section.[55]

In conclusion, the helical linkers improved the G-CSF activity of the fusion proteins, possibly by separating the functional domains, and also increased the fusion protein production. These linkers may also be applied in other recombinant fusion proteins to improve their intrinsic biological activities.

3.6.2.4 Disulfide Linker

Another class of linkers, which utilize the reversible nature of the disulfide bond, has been applied in the G-CSF-Tf fusion proteins. As previously discussed, the addition of an $(H4)_2$ linker greatly enhanced the *in vitro* and *in vivo* activity of the G-CSF-Tf fusion protein by spatially separating the functional domains. However, several limitations are still present for stable peptide linkers. First, the steric hindrance is almost inevitable as long as the domains are linked together. Second, the extended peptide linker blocks either the N- or the C-terminus of Tf. These reasons may account for the decreased biological activity of fusion proteins. Third, for a therapeutic purpose, the attachment of Tf affects the biodistribution and *in vivo* metabolism of the protein drug. Therefore, the addition of an *in vivo*-cleavable linker between the functional domains will allow the protein drug to be released from the Tf carrier and regain its full biological activity, biodistribution, and pharmacokinetic properties.

The reversible disulfide linkage has been widely used for drug delivery and drug targeting.[56] A well-known example is immunotoxin, in which a cytotoxic toxin is conjugated to an antibody via a disulfide bond. It was reported that the disulfide bond in this immunotoxin was not stable and was reduced *in vivo*.[57–59] Therefore, the reversible disulfide bond approach was applied to the Tf fusion proteins.

To produce the fusion protein, a disulfide–cyclopeptide linker was inserted between the G-CSF and Tf-protein domains (Figure 3.7). The cyclopeptide linker was designed to contain (1) two cysteine residues on the cyclopeptide linker that naturally form a disulfide bond and (2) a specific protease sequence for the *in vitro* cleavage of the peptide linker before the *in vivo* administration. Therefore, after the *in vitro* protease treatment, G-CSF and Tf were linked by the reversible disulfide bond, which is cleavable *in vivo*.

The *in vitro* reversibility of the disulfide–cyclopeptide linker between G-CSF and Tf was demonstrated by first cleaving the linker by a specific protease and followed by reduction using the strong reducing agent, dithiothreitol (DTT), to break the disulfide bond. After these treatments, G-CSF was released from the fusion protein as determined by Western blot (Figure 3.8). This cleaved and reduced fusion protein exhibited about a 10-fold increase of *in vitro* biological activity, with an EC_{50} of 0.6 ng/mL, compared to the non-cleaved, non-reduced fusion protein (EC_{50} = 6 ng/mL), as determined by the NFS-60 cell proliferation assay. The reversibility of the disulfide bond in G-CSF-cyclo-Tf fusion protein was also demonstrated *in vivo* in CF1 mice, where the results demonstrated that free G-CSF was released from the fusion protein in the plasma, possibly due to the reduction of the disulfide bond between G-CSF and Tf.

In summary, two different classes of linkers, helix linkers and disulfide linkers have been applied in the recombinant G-CSF-Tf fusion proteins. The helix linkers reduced the steric

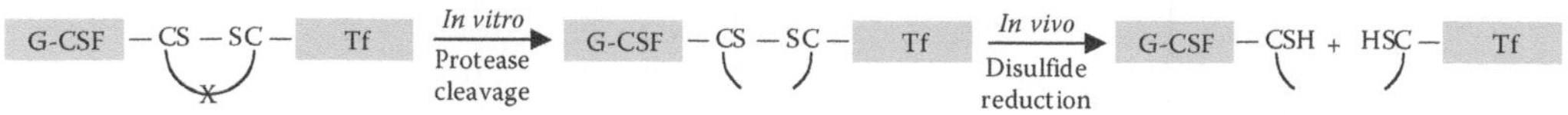

FIGURE 3.7 Illustration of the activation of disulfide–cyclopeptide linker inserted between G-CSF and Tf. The G-CSF-Tf fusion protein containing the disulfide–cyclopeptide linker is first cleaved *in vitro* at the specific protease cleavage sequence (X). Following *in vivo* administration, the disulfide bond is cleaved, resulting in the release of free G-CSF from the fusion protein.

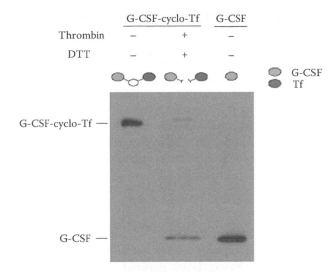

FIGURE 3.8 Release of free G-CSF from the G-CSF-cyclo-Tf increased its biological activity. G-CSF-cyclo-Tf fusion protein was analyzed by Western blot using anti-G-CSF antibody. The fusion protein was treated with thrombin and DTT to determine the release of free G-CSF following protease cleavage and DTT reduction, respectively. Lane 1, G-CSF-cyclo-Tf; lane 2, G-CSF-cyclo-Tf following treatment with thrombin and DTT; lane 3, G-CSF (control).

hindrance in the fusion proteins by spatially separating the functional domains. The use of the linkers increased the protein production, as well as the *in vitro* and *in vivo* biological activities for G-CSF-Tf fusion proteins. The reversible disulfide linkers were shown to release free G-CSF from the fusion protein *in vivo*. Therefore, G-CSF may regain its full activity,

> The production of G-CSF-Tf fusion proteins using helix linkers and disulfide linkers increased the protein production as well as biological activity. The reversible disulfide linkers allow the release of G-CSF from the fusion protein. Thus, G-CSF may regain its full activity.

biodistribution, and pharmacokinetics *in vivo* after release from the Tf carrier. Depending on the application of the protein drug, or the required pharmacokinetic properties, different linkers can be applied in the recombinant Tf fusion proteins for the optimal therapeutic effect. In addition, these linkers can also be applied to other recombinant fusion proteins, such as hGH-Tf fusion proteins.

3.7 RECOMBINANT HUMAN GROWTH HORMONE

hGH is a 191-amino acid, single polypeptide with 22 kDa molecular weight.[60] The successful cloning and expression of hGH gene[61] paved the way for its subsequent application as a therapeutic protein to treat patients with hGH deficiency. In 1991, Cunningham et al. resolved the crystal structure of hGH bound to its receptor (hGH-R), a member of class I cytokine receptors.[62] In 1996, Sundstrom et al. further investigated the crystal structure of hGH bound to the soluble portion of its receptor, called hGH-binding protein (hGHbp), and shed light on the details of hGH–hGHbp interactions.[63]

hGH is an important regulator of metabolism. It stimulates growth and differentiation in the target tissues including muscle, bone, cartilage, and liver. It exerts its effect of growth promotion both directly, and indirectly via the In-like growth factor-I (IGF-I) by binding hGH-R and subsequent activation of down stream signaling molecules such as JAK2 (Janus kinase 2)[64] and STAT5 (signal transducer and activator of transcription 5).[65,66] The signal transduction pathway for hGH was nicely illustrated elsewhere.[65,67] The deficiency in hGH production is associated with short stature, turner syndrome, chronic kidney disease, abnormal metabolism, and abnormal body composition. If left untreated, these clinical conditions may pose significant health risk to patients, including both children and adults.[48,68,69]

Patients with growth hormone deficiency were treated using hGH extracted from pituitary gland of human cadavers until Genentech, Inc. (South San Francisco, California) obtained U.S. Food and Drug Administration (FDA) approval for recombinant hGH in 1985.[70] Since then, many patients with hGH deficiency have benefited from this recombinant protein drug. Like other peptide and protein drugs, the administration of hGH is limited to injection, which could lead to insufficient compliance, especially among children with hGH deficiency. Therefore, developing an hGH analogue with an oral dosage form may help enhance its efficacy and, importantly, improve the quality of life.

3.7.1 Recombinant Growth Hormone-Tf Fusion Protein

Similar to the recombinant GCSF-Tf fusion proteins, recombinant growth hormone-Tf fusion proteins were produced by engineering an expression plasmid containing hGH fused in-frame with Tf with a short dipeptide linker, LE, between the two domains (Figure 3.9).

Recombinant proteins including hGH, hGH-Tf, and Tf-hGH were produced in a serum-free media by HEK293/293T cells that were transfected with the respective plasmid constructs. Based on a sodium dodecyl sulfate (SDS)-polyacrylamide gel electrophoresis (PAGE) analysis of conditioned media collected from transfected cells, both fusion proteins and hGH were expressed well and relatively pure with major bands corresponding to a 100 and 22 kDa molecular weight, respectively (Figure 3.10). The identity of the fusion proteins was confirmed by Western blot analysis of conditioned media using either anti-hGH (Figure 3.11A) or anti-Tf (Figure 3.11B) antibody. Fusion protein bands with about 100 kDa were detected, indicating that fusion protein is composed of both hGH- and Tf-domains.

Both the hGH-Tf and the Tf-hGH fusion proteins were produced to contain a helical linker $(H4)_2$ between hGH- and Tf- domains. Similar to the results obtained for the G-CSF helical linker fusion proteins, these new fusion proteins with the inserted helical linker also expressed at a higher level compared to the fusion proteins without the helical linker.

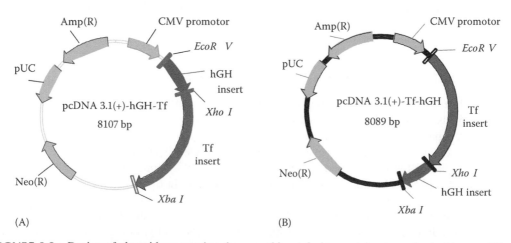

FIGURE 3.9 Design of plasmids expressing the recombinant fusion proteins comprised of human Tf and growth hormone in mammalian vector pcDNA3.1. (A) Plasmid construct that produces hGH-Tf fusion protein. (B) Plasmid construct that produces Tf-hGH fusion protein.

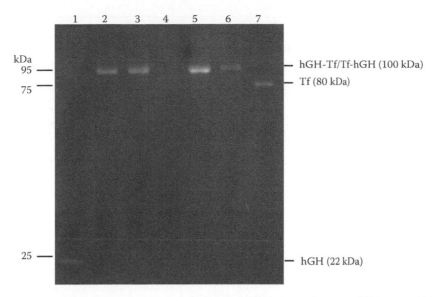

FIGURE 3.10 SDS-PAGE (7.5%) showing the expression of fusion proteins and hGH in HEK293 cells after silver stain. 50 μL conditioned media without concentration and 50 ng of pure Tf as a control were fractionated on the gel, followed by silver staining. The gel image was captured by Discovery Series System from Bio-Rad, Hercules, California. Lanes 1 and 4, hGH; lanes 2 and 5, hGH-Tf; lanes 3 and 6, Tf-hGH; lane 7, Tf (Sigma).

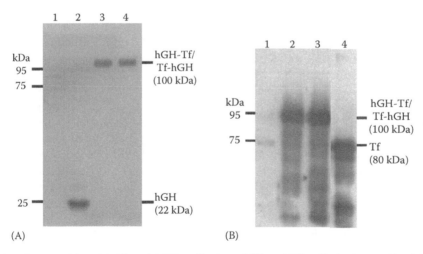

FIGURE 3.11 Western blot with (A) anti-hGH antibody and (B) anti-Tf antibody detected both hGH-Tf and Tf-hGH fusion proteins. (A) SDS-PAGE (10%) was used to fractionate conditioned media. Lane 1, Tf (Sigma, negative control); lane 2, hGH; lane 3, hGH-Tf; lane 4, Tf-hGH. (B) SDS-PAGE (7.5%) was used to fractionate conditioned media. Lane 1, hGH (negative control); lane 2, hGH-Tf; lane 3, Tf-hGH; lane 4, Tf.

3.7.2 GROWTH HORMONE-TF FUSION PROTEIN BIOLOGICAL ACTIVITY

Following characterization for expression and identity, both hGH-Tf and Tf-hGH fusion proteins were assessed for dual *in vitro* biological activity by utilizing TfR-binding and hGH-dependent Nb2 cell proliferation assays.[71] TfR competition binding in the presence of radioactively labeled Tf (^{125}I-Tf) by both fusion proteins indicated that they retained the biological function of Tf (Table 3.2). Correspondingly, treatment with either fusion protein led to the proliferation of Nb2

TABLE 3.2

Human Growth Hormone-Tf Recombinant Fusion Protein Produced in Mammalian Cells Show Both *In Vitro* and *In Vivo* Bioactivity in Hypophysectomized Rats

| | *In Vitro* Biological Activity | | *In Vivo* Biological Activity | |
| | TfR[a] Binding | Nb2 Cell Proliferation | Weight Gain in Hypophysectomized Rats after 7-Daily Administration | |
Fusion Protein	$(IC_{50}/IC_{50}\,Tf)^{b}$	$(EC_{50})^{c}$	Subcutaneous Administration	Oral Administration
hGH-Tf	25	2 ng/mL	12 g	NS[d]
Tf-hGH	18	N/A[e]	N/A	N/A
hGH-(H4)$_2$-Tf	25	1 ng/mL	16 g	2.5 g
Tf-(H4)$_2$-hGH	18	1 ng/mL	16 g	NS

[a] TfR, transferrin receptor.

[b] IC_{50}, half-maximal inhibitor concentration for TfR binding, expressed as IC_{50} obtained for the fusion protein divided by the IC_{50} obtained for the Tf control.

[c] EC_{50}, half-maximal effective concentration for cell proliferation.

[d] NS, not significant.

[e] N/A, data not available.

cells in a dose-dependent fashion, suggesting both fusion proteins maintained the biological activity of hGH (Table 3.2).

The *in vitro* biological activity of the hGH fusion proteins containing a helical linker was also evaluated. Remarkably, the hGH-(H4)$_2$-Tf and Tf-(H4)$_2$-hGH fusion proteins demonstrated an enhanced Nb2 cell proliferation with lower ED_{50} value when compared to the fusion proteins without the helical linker (Table 3.2).

The fusion proteins were also evaluated for their *in vivo* biological activity using hypophysectomized rats. These animals have had their pituitary gland, which secretes rat growth hormone, surgically removed. Thus hypophysectomized rats are common choice for testing the *in vivo* bioactivity of the recombinant hGH as an animal model since they are GH-deficient. To determine the *in vivo* biological activity, fusion proteins were administered both s.c. at a dose of 1.25 mg/kg and orally (p.o.) at a dose of 12.5 mg/kg for seven consecutive days. The s.c. administration produced a significant weight gain of 16 g by both hGH-(H4)$_2$-Tf and Tf-(H4)$_2$-hGH fusion proteins, and 12 g by hGH-Tf fusion protein, as compared to control rats receiving mannitol–phosphate buffer only (Table 3.2). This result showed that the insertion of helical linker increased not only the yield of expression but also the *in vivo* biological activity of hGH-domain in the fusion protein. The oral efficacy evaluation demonstrated that only the hGH-(H4)$_2$-Tf fusion protein, but neither Tf-(H4)$_2$-hGH nor hGH-Tf, induced a modest body weight gain of 2.5 g (Table 3.2) compared to the control rats administered with either hGH or mannitol-phosphate buffer orally, which did not gain weight. This modest weight gain by the oral administration of select fusion proteins indicates that oral efficacy could be achieved in an hGH animal model, and thus provides further evidence for the feasibility of using the Tf-based fusion protein approach to develop a potential oral dosage form for therapeutic proteins, including G-CSF and hGH.

3.8   CONCLUDING REMARKS

During recent years, TfR has been developed as a potential binding site to enable drug targeting and delivery of therapeutic agents that would normally suffer from poor pharmacokinetic characteristics.[72] TfR-directed targeting has enabled the efficient delivery of therapeutic agents to sites of interest, including the central nervous system[73] and malignant tissues.[74,75] In addition, by utilizing the knowledge of the intracellular sorting and recycling pathways of TfR, one can maximize the transepithelial delivery of peptide-based therapeutics.

Depending upon the desired result, apparently paradoxical effects can be achieved. For example, TfR-based strategies can selectively achieve either an accumulation of the carried drug within targeted tissues, or the delivery of the therapeutic entity across tissues of interest.[76] TfR can be utilized for the development of orally administered, receptor-mediated delivery systems for peptide and protein drugs for several reasons. First, TfR density is very high in human[18] and rat GI epithelium.[77] The utilization of even a fraction of this receptor pool can potentially result in a significant delivery of Tf-conjugated peptides across the GI mucosal barrier. The high density of TfR in intestinal epithelial cells makes TfR a better vehicle than other receptors with low density, such as cobalamin-intrinsic factor receptors,[78] for the GI absorption of a therapeutically effective dose of peptide drugs. Second, Tf is a natural carrier protein for iron.[79] Hence, unlike the binding of hormones or growth factors to their receptors, the binding of Tf to TfR will not alter any major metabolic or physiologic functions within the cell. Third, diferric Tf has been found to be a relatively stable glycoprotein in the GI tract. Enzymes such as chymotrypsin, which are responsible for the degradation of a majority of the proteins and peptides in the GI tract, have a low degradative action on the Tf molecule.[38] Finally, the mechanism in which Tf deposits iron in the cells has been well characterized.[21]

TfR has been used as a biological marker for drug delivery. In cancer chemotherapy, TfR has been investigated extensively as a marker of tumor cells for the targeted delivery of anticancer drugs.[75,80,81] In addition, TfR has been exploited as a vehicle for the transendothelial transport of macromolecules to cross the blood–brain barrier.[17] One of the limitations for targeting to TfR in systemic drug delivery is the high level of endogenous Tf in the blood and physiological fluids.[82] Therefore, many of the approaches that targeted to TfR for systemic drug delivery used the anti-TfR antibodies rather than the receptor-binding ligand, Tf.[73,83–86]

On the other hand, for the intestinal absorption route, Tf is a suitable carrier for other protein drugs, either as a conjugate form or as a fusion protein. The concentration of Tf in the lumen in the GI tract is very low, therefore the competition for the binding to TfR on the surface of intestinal epithelium is minimal. TfR is expressed in high level in intestinal epithelium. It is generally believed that TfR is localized predominately on the basolateral surface of the intestinal epithelial cells.[18] However, we have detected a low level of TfR-mediated transcytosis in highly differentiated and polarized Caco-2 cell monolayers.[87] The occurrence of the apical-to-basolateral transcytosis of TfR could be due to several reasons. First, the membrane sorting in intestinal epithelial cells is carried out by pathways of both the direct-sorting, as in kidney epithelial cells, and the indirect-sorting, as in hepatocytes.[88–90] Some of the TfR may be missorted to the apical surface where, subsequently, it will be endocytosed and delivered to the basolateral surface.[91] Second, the intestinal epithelial cells are differentiated from nonpolarized stem cells in the cryptic area to the fully polarized absorptive epithelial and goblet cells on the villi. This process is constantly going on because fully differentiated epithelial cells will shed from the tip of the villi in about 2–3 days.[92,93] It is very likely that some of the epithelial cells that are not fully differentiated will express TfR on the apical surface. This possibility is supported by the immunohistological studies using anti-TfR antibodies in rat intestine, which showed the existence of TfR on the apical surface of epithelium at lower part of the villi (Figure 3.12). Therefore, while one of the problems associated with TfR-mediated drug delivery is the basolateral localization of the TfRs, this drawback can be overcome by taking advantage of the sorting mechanisms.

This innovative transport process of Tf-fusion proteins provides a unique opportunity to develop a new generation of protein drugs that can be administered via the oral route for treating human diseases. The impact of such a drug delivery system on cost-effectiveness and patient compliance in

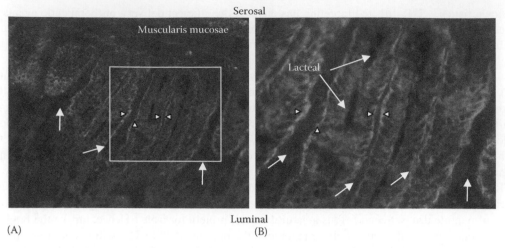

FIGURE 3.12 Immunofluorescent staining of TfR in a representative frozen section of rat small intestine using anti-rat TfR antibody. The top of the panel is the serosal side and crypt region; the bottom, the luminal side and villi. Arrows indicate the intervillous space and triangles indicate positive TfR staining of enterocytes on the luminal side, predominantly in the lower villous and crypt areas. (A) 20× magnification. (B) 40× magnification of boxed area in A.

long-term pharmaceutical care, to say the least, would be enormous. Even though the feasibility of using Tf-fusion proteins as oral drugs has been demonstrated, there are several issues including the preservation of the *in vitro* biological activities of both Tf and the attached protein drug, the *in vivo* stability of the drug delivery systems, and the potential immunogenicity of the proteins, that need to be addressed before this delivery system can be applied toward future clinical utilization.

> TfR-based strategies can selectively achieve either an accumulation of the carried drug within targeted tissues, or the delivery of the therapeutic entity across tissues of interest.

ACKNOWLEDGMENTS

Work described in this chapter from the authors' laboratories was partially supported by grants from the National Institutes of Health (GM 063647) and the American Diabetes Association (ADA 98–01), and from a contract from Pfizer, Inc., New York.

REFERENCES

1. Aggarwal, S. 2007. What's fueling the biotech engine? *Nature Biotechnology* 25:1097–1104.
2. Walsh, G. 2006. Biopharmaceutical benchmarks 2006. *Nature Biotechnology* 24:769–776.
3. Pavlou, A. K. and J. M. Reichert. 2004. Recombinant protein therapeutics—Success rates, market trends and values to 2010. *Nature Biotechnology* 22:1513–1519.
4. Shen, W. C. 2003. Oral peptide and protein delivery: Unfulfilled promises? *Drug Discovery Today* 8(14):607–608.
5. Lee, V. H., A. Yamamoto, and U. B. Kompella. 1991. Mucosal penetration enhancers for facilitation of peptide and protein drug absorption. *Critical Reviews in Therapeutic Drug Carrier System* 8(2):91–192.
6. Carino, G. P. and E. Mathiowitz. 1999. Oral insulin delivery. *Advanced Drug Delivery Reviews* 35(2–3):249–257.
7. Swaan, P. W. 1998. Recent advances in intestinal macromolecular drug delivery via receptor-mediated transport pathways. *Pharmaceutical Research* 15(6):826–834.

8. Shen, W. C., J. S. Wan, and H. Ekrami. 1992. Enhancement of polypeptide and protein-absorption by macromolecular carriers via endocytosis and transcytosis. 3. *Advanced Drug Delivery Reviews* 8(1):93–113.

9. Mostov, K. E. 1995. Regulation of protein traffic in polarized epithelial-cells. *Histology and Histopathology* 10(2):423–431.

10. Sennett, C., L. E. Rosenberg, and I. S. Mellman. 1981. Transmembrane transport of cobalamin in prokaryotic and eukaryotic cells. *Annual Review of Biochemistry* 50:1053–1086.

11. Yang, F., J. B. Lum, J. R. McGill, C. M. Moore, S. L. Naylor, P. H. van Bragt, W. D. Baldwin, and B. H. Bowman. 1984. Human transferrin: cDNA characterization and chromosomal localization. *Proceedings of the National Academy of Sciences of the United States of America* 81(9):2752.

12. Hall, D. R., J. M. Hadden, G. A. Leonard, S. Bailey, M. Neu, M. Winn, and P. F. Lindley. 2002. The crystal and molecular structures of diferric porcine and rabbit serum transferrins at resolutions of 2.15 and 2.60 A, respectively. *Acta Crystallographica Section D* 58(1):70–80.

13. Wally, J., P. J. Halbrooks, C. Vonrhein, M. A. Rould, S. J. Everse, A. B. Mason, and S. K. Buchanan. 2006. The crystal structure of iron-free human serum transferrin provides insight into inter-lobe communication and receptor binding. *Journal of Biological Chemistry* 281(34):24934.

14. Lawrence, C. M., S. Ray, M. Babyonyshev, R. Galluser, D. W. Borhani, and S. C. Harrison. 1999. Crystal structure of the ectodomain of human transferrin receptor. *Science* 286(5440):779.

15. Cheng, Y., O. Zak, P. Aisen, S. C. Harrison, and T. Walz. 2004. Structure of the human transferrin receptor-transferrin complex. *Cell* 116(4):565–576.

16. Kawabata, H., R. Yang, T. Hirama, P. T. Vuong, S. Kawano, A. F. Gombart, and H. P. Koeffler. 1999. Molecular cloning of transferrin receptor 2 A new member of the transferrin receptor-like family. *Journal of Biological Chemistry* 274(30):20826–20832.

17. Jefferies, W. A., M. R. Brandon, S. V. Hunt, A. F. Williams, K. C. Gatter, and D. Y. Mason. 1984. Transferrin receptor on endothelium of brain capillaries. *Nature* 312(5990):162–163.

18. Banerjee, D., P. R. Flanagan, J. Cluett, and L. S. Valberg. 1986. Transferrin receptors in the human gastrointestinal tract. Relationship to body iron stores. *Gastroenterology* 91(4):861–869.

19. West, A. P., M. J. Bennett, V. M. Sellers, N. C. Andrews, C. A. Enns, and P. J. Bjorkman. 2000. Comparison of the interactions of transferrin receptor and transferrin receptor 2 with transferrin and the hereditary hemochromatosis protein HFE. *Journal of Biological Chemistry* 275(49):38135–38138.

20. Griffiths, W. J. H. and T. M. Cox. 2003. Co-localization of the mammalian hemochromatosis gene product (HFE) and a newly identified transferrin receptor (TfR2) in intestinal tissue and cells. *Journal of Histochemistry and Cytochemistry* 51(5):613–623.

21. Morgan, E. H. and P. S. Oates. 2002. Mechanisms and regulation of intestinal iron absorption. *Blood Cells Molecules and Diseases* 29(3):384–399.

22. Fleming, R. E. 2005. Advances in understanding the molecular basis for the regulation of dietary iron absorption. *Current Opinion in Gastroenterology* 21(2):201–206.

23. Parkkila, S., O. Niemela, R. S. Britton, R. E. Fleming, A. Waheed, B. R. Bacon, and W. S. Sly. 2001. Molecular aspects of iron absorption and HFE expression. *Gastroenterology* 121(6):1489–1496.

24. Rodriguez-Boulan, E. and W. J. Nelson. 1989. Morphogenesis of the polarized epithelial-cell phenotype. *Science* 245(4919):718–725.

25. Hughson, E. J. 1990. Endocytic pathways in polarized Caco-2 cells: Identification of an endosomal compartment accessible from both apical and basolateral surfaces. *The Journal of Cell Biology* 110(2):337–348.

26. Widera, A., K. J. J. Kim, E. D. Crandall, and W. C. Shen. 2003. Transcytosis of GCSF-transferrin across rat alveolar epithelial cell monolayers. *Pharmaceutical Research* 20(8):1231–1238.

27. Lim, C. J., F. Norouziyan, and W. C. Shen. 2007. Accumulation of transferrin in Caco-2 cells: A possible mechanism of intestinal transferrin absorption. *Journal of Controlled Release* 122(3):393–398.

28. Ma, Y., R. D. Specian, K. Y. Yeh, M. Yeh, J. Rodriguez-Paris, and J. Glass. 2002. The transcytosis of divalent metal transporter 1 and apo-transferrin during iron uptake in intestinal epithelium. *American Journal of Physiology—Gastrointestinal and Liver Physiology* 283(4):965–974.

29. Odorizzi, G., A. Pearse, D. Domingo, I. S. Trowbridge, and C. R. Hopkins. 1996. Apical and basolateral endosomes of MDCK cells are interconnected and contain a polarized sorting mechanism. *Journal of Cell Biology* 135(1):139–152.

30. Marsh, E. W., P. L. Leopold, N. L. Jones, and F. R. Maxfield. 1995. Oligomerized transferrin receptors are selectively retained by a lumenal sorting signal in a long-lived endocytic recycling compartment. *Journal of Cell Biology* 129(6):1509–1522.

31. Lim, C. J. and W. C. Shen. 2004. Transferrin-oligomers as potential carriers in anticancer drug delivery. *Pharmaceutical Research* 21(11):1985–1992.

32. Wan, J. S., M. E. Taub, D. Shah, and W. C. Shen. 1992. Brefeldin-A enhances receptor-mediated transcytosis of transferrin in filter-grown Madin-Darby canine kidney-cells. *Journal of Biological Chemistry* 267(19):13446–13450.

33. Klausner, R. D., J. G. Donaldson, and J. Lippincott-Schwartz. 1992. Brefeldin-A—Insights into the control of membrane traffic and organelle structure. *Journal of Cell Biology* 116(5):1071–1080.

34. Xia, C. Q., J. Wang, and W. C. Shen. 2000. Hypoglycemic effect of insulin-transferrin conjugate in streptozotocin-induced diabetic rats. *Journal of Pharmacology and Experimental Therapeutics* 295(2):594.

35. Norouziyan, F., W. C. Shen, and S. F. Hamm-Alvarez. 2008. Tyrphostin A8 stimulates a novel trafficking pathway of apically endocytosed transferrin through Rab11-enriched compartments in Caco-2 cells. *American Journal of Physiology—Cell Physiology* 294(1):C7.

36. Gomme, P. T., K. B. McCann, and J. Bertolini. 2005. Transferrin: Structure, function and potential therapeutic actions. *Drug Discovery Today* 10(4):267–273.

37. Qian, Z. M., H. Li, H. Sun, and K. Ho. 2002. Targeted drug delivery via the transferrin receptor-mediated endocytosis pathway. *Pharmacological Reviews* 54(4):561.

38. Azari, P. R. and R. E. Feeney. 1958. Resistance of metal complexes of Conalbumin and transferrin to proteolysis and to thermal denaturation. *Journal of Biological Chemistry* 232(1):293–302.

39. Rosenfeld, L. 2002. Insulin: Discovery and controversy. *Clinical Chemistry* 48(12):2270–2288.

40. Nicola, N. A., D. Metcalf, M. Matsumoto, and G. R. Johnson. 1983. Purification of a factor inducing differentiation in murine myelomonocytic leukemia-cells—Identification as granulocyte colony-stimulating factor. *Journal of Biological Chemistry* 258(14):9017–9023.

41. Nicola, N. A. 1990. Granulocyte colony-stimulating factor. In *Immunology Series, Vol. 49. Colony-Stimulating Factors: Molecular and Cellular Biology*, Xvi+475p. Dexter, T. M., J. M. Garland, and N. G. Testa (Eds.), Marcel Dekker, Inc., New York, *Illus*:77–110.

42. Halpern, W., T. A. Riccobene, H. Agostini, K. Baker, D. Stolow, M. L. Gu, J. Hirsch, A. Mahoney, J. Carrell, and E. Boyd. 2002. Albugranin TM, a recombinant human granulocyte colony stimulating factor (G-CSF) genetically fused to recombinant human albumin induces prolonged myelopoietic effects in mice and monkeys. *Pharmaceutical Research* 19(11):1720–1729.

43. Widera, A., Y. Bai, and W. C. Shen. 2004. The transepithelial transport of a G-CSF-transferrin conjugate in Caco-2 cells and its myelopoietic effect in BDF1 mice. *Pharmaceutical Research* 21(2):278–284.

44. Ali, S. A., H. C. Joao, F. Hammerschmid, J. Eder, and A. Steinkasserer. 1999. Transferrin Trojan horses as a rational approach for the biological delivery of therapeutic peptide domains. *Journal of Biological Chemistry* 274(34):24066–24073.

45. Park, E., R. M. Starzyk, J. P. McGrath, T. Lee, J. George, A. J. Schutz, P. Lynch, and S. D. Putney. 1998. Production and characterization of fusion proteins containing transferrin and nerve growth factor. *Journal of Drug Targeting* 6(1):53–64.

46. Bai, Y., D. K. Ann, and W.-C. Shen. 2005. Recombinant granulocyte colony-stimulating factor-transferrin fusion protein as an oral myelopoietic agent. *Proceedings of the National Academy of Sciences* 102(20):7292–7296.

47. Souza, L. M., T. C. Boone, J. Gabrilove, P. H. Lai, K. M. Zsebo, D. C. Murdock, V. R. Chazin, J. Bruszewski, H. Lu, K. K. Chen, J. Barendt, E. Platzer, M. A. S. Moore, R. Mertelsmann, and K. Welte. 1986. Recombinant human granulocyte colony-stimulating factor—Effects on normal and leukemic myeloid cells. *Science* 232(4746):61–65.

48. Takahashi, Y., H. Shirono, O. Arisaka, K. Takahashi, T. Yagi, J. Koga, H. Kaji, Y. Okimura, H. Abe, and T. Tanaka. 1997. Biologically inactive growth hormone caused by an amino acid substitution. *Journal of Clinical Investigation* 100(5):1159–1165.

49. Bonig, H., S. Silbermann, S. Weller, R. Kirschke, D. Korholz, G. Janssen, U. Gobel, and W. Nurnberger. 2001. Glycosylated vs non-glycosylated granulocyte colony-stimulating factor (G-CSF)—Results of a prospective randomised monocentre study. *Bone Marrow Transplantation* 28(3):259–264.

50. Lord, B. I., L. B. Woolford, and G. Molineux. 2001. Kinetics of neutrophil production in normal and neutropenic animals during the response to filgrastim (r-metHu G-CSF) or filgrastim SD/01 (PEG-r-metHu G-CSF). *Clinical Cancer Research* 7(7):2085–2090.

51. Argos, P. 1990. An investigation of oligopeptides linking domains in protein tertiary structures and possible candidates for general gene fusion. *Journal of Molecular Biology* 211(4):943–958.

52. Robinson, C. R. and R. T. Sauer. 1998. Optimizing the stability of single-chain proteins by linker length and composition mutagenesis. *Proceedings of the National Academy of Sciences* 95(11):5929–5934.

53. Lo, A. S. Y., Q. Zhu, and W. A. Marasco. 2008. Intracellular antibodies (intrabodies) and their therapeutic potential. In *Handbook of Experimental Pharmacology*. Y. Chernajovsky and A. Nissim (Eds.), Springer-Verlag, Berlin, Germany.

54. Arai, R., H. Ueda, A. Kitayama, N. Kamiya, and T. Nagamune. 2001. Design of the linkers which effectively separate domains of a bifunctional fusion protein. *Protein Engineering* 14(8):529–532.

55. Amet, N., H. F. Lee, and W. C. Shen. 2009. Insertion of the designed helical linker led to increased expression of Tf-based fusion proteins. *Pharmaceutical Research* 26(3):523–528.

56. Shen, W. C. 1999. Emerging targeting concepts membrane-associated protein thiol-disulfide interchange activity: A potential target for anti-viral and anti-tumor drug design. *Journal of Drug Targeting* 6(6):387–389.

57. Gilliland, D. G., R. J. Collier, J. M. Moehring, and T. J. Moehring. 1978. Chimeric toxins—Toxic, disulfide-linked conjugate of Concanavalin-A with fragment A from diphtheria-toxin. *Proceedings of the National Academy of Sciences of the United States of America* 75(11):5319–5323.

58. King, T. P., Y. Li, and L. Kochoumian. 1978. Preparation of protein conjugates via intermolecular disulfide bond formation. *Biochemistry* 17(8):1499–1506.

59. Chang, T. M. and D. M. Neville. 1977. Artificial hybrid protein containing a toxic protein fragment and a cell-membrane receptor-binding moiety in a disulfide conjugate. 1. Synthesis of diphtheria-toxin fragment A-S-S-human placental lactogen with methyl-5-bromovalerimidate. *Journal of Biological Chemistry* 252(4):1505–1514.

60. Roskam, W. G. and F. Rougeon. 1979. Molecular cloning and nucleotide sequence of the human growth hormone structural gene. *Nucleic Acids Research* 7(2):305.

61. Martial, J. A., R. A. Hallewell, J. D. Baxter, and H. M. Goodman. 1979. Human growth hormone: Complementary DNA cloning and expression in bacteria. *Science* 205(4406):602.

62. Cunningham, B. C., M. Ultsch, A. M. De Vos, M. G. Mulkerrin, K. R. Clauser, and J. A. Wells. 1991. Dimerization of the extracellular domain of the human growth hormone receptor by a single hormone molecule. *Science* 254(5033):821–825.

63. Sundstrom, M., T. Lundqvist, J. Rodin, L. B. Giebel, D. Milligan, and G. Norstedt. 1996. Crystal structure of an antagonist mutant of human growth hormone, G120R, in complex with its receptor at 2.9 A resolution. *Journal of Biological Chemistry* 271(50):32197.

64. Argetsinger, L. S., G. S. Campbell, X. Yang, B. A. Witthuhn, O. Silvennoinen, J. N. Ihle, and C. Carter-Su. 1993. Identification of JAK2 as a growth hormone receptor-associated tyrosine kinase. *Cell* 74(2):237–244.

65. Herrington, J., L. S. Smit, J. Schwartz, and C. Carter-Su. 2000. The role of STAT proteins in growth hormone signaling. *Space* 19(21):2585–2597.

66. Huang, Y., S. O. Kim, N. Yang, J. Jiang, and S. J. Frank. 2004. Physical and functional interaction of growth hormone and insulin-like growth factor-I signaling elements. *Molecular Endocrinology* 18(6):1471–1485.

67. Carter-Su, C., J. Schwartz, and L. J. Smit. 1996. Molecular mechanism of growth hormone action. *Annual Reviews in Physiology* 58(1):187–207.

68. Staub, J. M., B. Garcia, J. Graves, P. T. J. Hajdukiewicz, P. Hunter, N. Nehra, V. Paradkar, M. Schlittler, J. A. Carroll, L. Spatola, D. Ward, G. N. Ye, and D. A. Russell. 2000. High-yield production of a human therapeutic protein in tobacco chloroplasts. *Nature Biotechnology* 18(3):333–338.

69. Takahashi, Y., H. Kaji, Y. Okimura, K. Goji, H. Abe, and K. Chihara. 1996. Short stature caused by a mutant growth hormone. *New England Journal of Medicine* 334(7):432.

70. Glaser, V. 1995. Pharmacia challenges Genentech in rhGH market. *Biotechnology (NY)* 13:1038–1040.

71. Amet, N., W. Wang, and W. C. Shen. 2010. Human growth hormone-transferrin fusion protein for oral delivery in hypophysectomized rats. *Journal of Controlled Release* 141(2):177–182.

72. Widera, A., F. Norouziyan, and W. C. Shen. 2003. Mechanisms of TfR-mediated transcytosis and sorting in epithelial cells and applications toward drug delivery. *Advanced Drug Delivery Reviews* 55(11):1439–1466.

73. Friden, P. M. 1994. Receptor-mediated transport of therapeutics across the blood–brain-barrier. *Neurosurgery* 35(2):294–298.

74. Weaver, M. and D. W. Laske. 2003. Transferrin receptor ligand-targeted toxin conjugate (Tf-CRM107) for therapy of malignant gliomas. *Journal of Neuro-Oncology* 65(1):3–13.

75. Singh, M. 1999. Transferrin as a targeting ligand for liposomes and anticancer drugs. *Current Pharmaceutical Design* 5(6):443–451.

76. Shah, D. and W. C. Shen. 1995. The paradox of transferrin receptor-mediated drug delivery—Intracellular targeting or transcellular transport? *Journal of Drug Targeting* 3(4):243–245.

77. Anderson, G. J., L. W. Powell, and J. W. Halliday. 1990. Transferrin receptor distribution and regulation in the rat small-intestine—Effect of iron stores and erythropoiesis. *Gastroenterology* 98(3):576–585.

78. Russell-Jones, G. J. 1998. Use of vitamin B-12 conjugates to deliver protein drugs by the oral route. *Critical Reviews in Therapeutic Drug Carrier Systems* 15(6):557–586.

79. Crichton, R. R. 1990. Proteins of iron storage and transport. In *Advances in Protein Chemistry*, Vol. 40, Vi+403p. Anfinsen, C. B. et al. (Ed.), Academic Press, Inc., San Diego, CA; London, U.K. *Illus*:281–364.

80. Prost, A. C., F. Menegaux, P. Langlois, J. M. Vidal, M. Koulibaly, J. L. Jost, J. J. Duron, J. P. Chigot, P. Vayre, A. Aurengo, J. C. Legrand, G. Rosselin, and C. Gespach. 1998. Differential transferrin receptor density in human colorectal cancer: A potential probe for diagnosis and therapy. *International Journal of Oncology* 13(4):871–875.

81. Shindelman, J. E., A. E. Ortmeyer, and H. H. Sussman. 1981. Demonstration of the transferrin receptor in human-breast cancer-tissue—Potential marker for identifying dividing cells. *International Journal of Cancer* 27(3):329–334.

82. Huebers, H. A. and C. A. Finch. 1987. The physiology of transferrin and transferrin receptors. *Physiological Reviews* 67(2):520–582.

83. Moos, T. and E. H. Morgan. 2001. Restricted transport of anti-transferrin receptor antibody (OX26) through the blood–brain barrier in the rat. *Journal of Neurochemistry* 79(1):119–129.

84. Kordower, J. H., V. Charles, R. Bayer, R. T. Bartus, S. Putney, L. R. Walus, and P. M. Friden. 1994. Intravenous administration of a transferrin receptor antibody nerve growth-factor conjugate prevents the degeneration of cholinergic striatal neurons in a model of Huntington disease. *Proceedings of the National Academy of Sciences of the United States of America* 91(19):9077–9080.

85. Pardridge, W. M., J. L. Buciak, and P. M. Friden. 1991. Selective transport of an antitransferrin receptor antibody through the blood–brain-barrier in vivo. *Journal of Pharmacology and Experimental Therapeutics* 259(1):66–70.

86. Bickel, U., T. Yoshikawa, and W. M. Pardridge. 2001. Delivery of peptides and proteins through the blood–brain barrier. *Advanced Drug Delivery Reviews* 46(1–3):247–279.

87. Shah, D and W. C. Shen. 1996. Transcellular delivery of an insulin-transferrin conjugate in enterocyte-like Caco-2 cells. *Journal of Pharmaceutical Sciences* 85(12):1306–1311.

88. Bartles, J. R., H. M. Feracci, B. Stieger, and A. L. Hubbard. 1987. Biogenesis of the rat hepatocyte plasma-membrane in vivo—Comparison of the pathways taken by apical and basolateral proteins using subcellular fractionation. *Journal of Cell Biology* 105(3):1241–1251.

89. Wandingerness, A., M. K. Bennett, C. Antony, and K. Simons. 1990. Distinct transport vesicles mediate the delivery of plasma-membrane proteins to the apical and basolateral domains of Mdck cells. *Journal of Cell Biology* 111(3):987–1000.

90. Simons, K. and A. Wandingerness. 1990. Polarized sorting in epithelia. *Cell* 62(2):207–210.

91. Widera, A. S., K.-J. Kim, Z. Borok, E. D. Crandall, and W.-C. Shen. 2003. Enhancement of transferrin-protein drug transcytosis across rat alveolar epithelial cell monolayers. *FASEB Journal* 17(4–5):104.2.

92. Cheng, H. and C. P. Leblond. 1974. Origin, differentiation and renewal of 4 main epithelial-cell types in mouse small intestine. 5. Unitarian theory of origin of 4 epithelial-cell types. *American Journal of Anatomy* 141(4):537–561.

93. Okamoto, R. and M. Watanabe. 2004. Molecular and clinical basis for the regeneration of human gastro-intestinal epithelia. *Journal of Gastroenterology* 39(1):1–6.

4 Ionizing Radiation for Tumor-Targeted Drug Delivery

Roberto Diaz, Li Zhou, and Dennis E. Hallahan

CONTENTS

4.1 INTRODUCTION

Current treatments of solid tumors often involve using both chemotherapy and radiotherapy in parallel. Concomitant chemotherapy and radiation therapy is the standard of care for patients with advanced (stages III and IV) head and neck cancer[1,2] and non-small-cell lung cancer.[3,4]

Chemotherapeutic agents generally utilized include radiosensitizing agents like taxanes (e.g., paclitaxel) and platinum compounds (e.g., carboplatin). This approach has improved local control and median survival in these patients.

Paclitaxel is a member of a family of drugs called taxanes, which stabilize microtubules causing mitotic arrest.[5] Taxanes show broad-spectrum activity in solid tumors, including non-small-cell lung cancer.[6,7] However, their use has been limited by their solvent-based formulations, which may lead to serious toxicities. The development of paclitaxel[8] was, in fact, delayed because of problems in drug formulation.[9] The most viable option for improving paclitaxel's solubility was found to be a vehicle composed of polyethoxylated castor oil (Cremophor®) and ethanol. Unfortunately, Cremophor can also cause neutropenia[10–13] and prolonged, sometimes irreversible, peripheral neuropathy, which may be associated with axonal degeneration.[14–18]

Targeting chemotherapeutic compounds specifically to the tumor can avoid systemic organ toxicity without compromising the drug's therapeutic effects. New research done in the last decade has shown that the use of ionizing radiation (IR) can induce neoantigens, to which delivery vehicles and ligands carrying chemotherapeutic agents can bind and improve the targeting of various drug therapies. By using radiation treatment as a means to "mark" the tumor for drug delivery, this new potential form of treatment hopes to dramatically reduce the systemic toxicity that is typically associated with cancer drugs, while simultaneously increasing the biodistribution of these drugs to the tumor region.

4.1.1 CURRENT LIMITATIONS OF DRUG THERAPY ON SOLID TUMORS

Solid tumors contain a unique microenvironment that is often not conducive to drug distribution. In order for drugs to become available to all of the cancer cells, there are many obstacles that need to be overcome, the first of which is tissue penetration.[19,20]

Drugs often reach tumor sites by penetrating across the endothelial linings of the capillaries (extravasation), but different pressure gradients inside the tumor influence the ability of drugs to extravasate. First, in normal tissues, the oncotic pressure (the osmotic pressure exerted by proteins dissolved in blood plasma) of the vasculature and interstitial space are around 20–25 and 5–15 mmHg, respectively.[21,22] However, it has been measured that tumor xenografts such as rhabdomyosarcoma may have oncotic pressures of around 24.2 mmHg.[23] This elevated oncotic pressure is consistent with the observed elevated levels of interstitial fluid pressure in tumors compared with normal tissue (whose interstitial pressure is close to zero). As a result, one of the primary means through which extravasation occurs—convection, which is proportional to the difference in the hydrostatic pressure within a blood vessel and interstitial pressure within the target tissue—would be reduced. The extravasation of macromolecules is particularly difficult under these conditions and even worse in central regions of tumors, which have an interstitial fluid pressure similar to the microvascular pressure.[24–26]

> Oncotic pressure is the osmotic pressure exerted by proteins dissolved in blood plasma. The oncotic pressure of the vasculature and interstitial space are around 20–25 and 5–15 mmHg, respectively. Tumor xenografts may have oncotic pressures of around 24.2 mmHg, resulting in reduced convection. The extravasation of macromolecules is inefficient under these conditions and even worse in central regions of tumors, which have an interstitial fluid pressure similar to the microvascular pressure. In light of these hurdles, targeted therapy becomes a necessity.

4.1.2 ROLE OF TUMOR VASCULATURE

In light of these hurdles, targeted therapy becomes a necessity. However, an important aspect of this goal is the part of the tumor that the drugs ought to be targeting. In 1971, Dr. Judah Folkman proposed the idea that lying at the heart of cancer growth is its dependence on angiogenesis. The theory was that for tumors to grow and progress, a network of microvessels that is produced through neovascularization is necessary.[27] Now, it is widely accepted that solid tumors cannot reach a size larger than approximately 1 mm³ in the absence of a vascular network.[28] Accordingly, experiments blocking the activity of certain pro-growth receptors on vascular endothelial cells, such as the vascular endothelial growth factor receptor (VEGF-R), have shown the inhibition of tumor growth.[29,30] The inalienability of angiogenesis from tumor progression has laid the foundation of a strategy for targeting tumor vasculature as a method for treating cancer.

Another principle guiding the rationale in targeting tumor vasculature is the adaptive resistance often observed with the treatment of cancer. Due to the genetic instability of the tumor, mutations often arise, which produce cancer cells and subsequent clonal populations on which drugs have attenuated efficacy. Often, these resistances are due to the selection of cells that develop multi-drug resistance as a result of the selection for ABC (ATP-binding cassette) transporters that aid in the transport of antineoplastic agents out of the cell. One example of these drug extrusion pumps is the breast cancer resistance protein (BCRP). The expression of BCRP was found in different normal tissues such as the colon, small and large intestine, venous endothelium, hepatocytes and biliary canaliculi, and many others.[31,32] *In vitro* models revealed the presence of BCRP in atypical multidrug-resistant cancer cell lines that were selected against mitoxantrone.[33] In contrast, tumor-related blood vessels are made primarily of "normal" cells, which have less chances of becoming drug resistant because of their genomic stability. Therefore, targeting tumor vasculature would allow the destruction of those blood vessels without the risk of adaptive resistance to drugs. It must be noted, however, that the microvascular expression of markers differs based on the environment to which it is exposed. For example, tumor vasculature expresses different markers than those on normal vasculature, and each type of tumor expresses its own cocktail of extracellular factors to influence its own microvasculature. Endothelium that is proliferating, as is usually the case with most growing solid tumors, may have a unique expression of cell adhesion molecules that have a different response to stimuli as compared with nonproliferating (most of the body's endothelium) vessels.[34,35]

Investigators have tried to take advantage of this molecular diversity within the tumor associated vasculature. One product of this research has been the identification of recombinant peptide markers. Certain peptides that bind to organ-specific active proteins of tumor vasculature have been isolated using phage display technology (described later in this chapter). These peptides are used to control, identify, and image various tumors, including malignant leukemia and melanoma, prostate cancer, glioblastoma, and thyroid tumors.[36–40] While this method is effective against individual tumor vasculature, more recent developments have suggested a method for targeting not just a single type of tumor vasculature, but also various (and potentially all) types of tumor-associated vasculature. Furthermore, in light of the diversity found between various tumor environments, researchers have tried to "normalize" tumor vasculature.[41]

4.2 PARADIGM OF RADIATION-GUIDED TUMOR-TARGETED THERAPY

The process of developing drugs for radiation-induced tumor-targeted delivery involves three major steps:

1. Radiation-induction of neoantigens
2. Identification of these receptors and receptor ligands
3. Conjugation of a drug delivery vehicle to ligands

In our discussion of these steps, we address some of the recent advances in biotechnology that have significantly improved and expedited this process.

4.2.1 RADIATION INDUCTION OF NEOANTIGENS

The primary use of radiation therapy as a form of cancer treatment has remained essentially unchanged since its inception. It induces sufficient DNA damage within the cell to either cause immediate cell death or delayed cell death after several rounds of cell division. However, more recent studies have shown the ability of radiation to induce the formation of neoantigens in tumor vasculature.[42–44] Radiation can induce the expression of cellular adhesion molecules (CAM) such as ICAM-1, E-selectin, and P-selectin on tumor vasculature.[42–49] The expression of molecules such as P-selectin are localized to areas of the vasculature exposed to radiation as part of an inflammatory response.[50,51] Furthermore, the vascular endothelium responds to these radiation-induced oxidative stresses in a very similar, or possibly identical, manner in all tumor models.

4.2.1.1   Mechanisms of Radiation-Induced Damage

Radiation produces biological effects principally from its damage to the cellular DNA but the means of action varies depending on the radiation source. When using radiation that has high linear energy transfer (including neutrons or α-particles), there is a high probability of what is known as the direct action of radiation. Direct action occurs when the DNA is directly affected by these radiation particles.

In contrast, other forms of radiation affect DNA by the ionization of the solvent (predominantly water) in which DNA is dissolved. This is known as the indirect action of radiation. Water is ionized according to the reaction $H_2O \rightarrow H_2O^+ + e^-$, $H_2O^+ + H_2O \rightarrow H_3O^+ + OH^\bullet$. The $OH^\bullet$ is a hydroxyl radical that is thought to cause about two-thirds of the x-ray damage done to mammalian DNA.

> Radiation can cause DNA damage. Single-stranded breaks are usually not lethal and can be repaired if the other strand is used as a template. However, mutations may occur if the strand is incorrectly repaired. More detrimental to the cell is a double-stranded DNA break. This may occur if two single-stranded breaks occur on opposite strands and are only separated by several base pairs.

Radiation can cause two forms of DNA damage, single- or double-stranded damage. Single-stranded breaks are usually not lethal and can usually be repaired if the other strand is used as a template. However, mutations may occur if the strand is incorrectly repaired. More detrimental to the cell is a double-stranded DNA break. This may occur if two single-stranded breaks occur on opposite strands and are only separated by several base pairs.

4.2.1.2   Mechanisms of Adhesion Molecule Induction by Radiation

In response to radiation injury, the tumor vasculature responds to preserve barrier function and maintaining homeostasis. Various adhesion molecules are activated, which leads to the activation of platelet aggregation and inflammation. Both direct and indirect mechanisms have been proposed for the altered expression of adhesion molecules following radiation treatment. Radiation produces reactive oxygen intermediates (ROI), which oxidize various parts of the cell, including DNA and phospholipids. The resulting biological response occurs at various levels, including changes in transcription factors, adhesion molecules, and cytokines.[52,53] An example of this is the ROI activation of the NFκB (nuclear factor kappa-light-chain-enhancer of activated B cells) transcription factor, one of the participants in inducing ICAM-1, VAMC-1, and E-selectin. This proposed mechanism is supported by the antioxidant inhibition of radiation-induced NFκB-dependent transcriptional activation of ICAM-1 and the radiation-mediated activation of NFκB[52–55] (Figure 4.1).

Another proposed mechanism is the increase in cytokine secretion, which, in turn, causes the indirect up-regulation of irradiated tissues' adhesion molecules. Krykamides et al. suggested that tumor necrosis factor α (TNF-α) and interleukin-1 (IL-1) could be required for the induction of ICAM-1 in astrocytes.[56] Hong et al. have found that the expression of ICAM-1 after irradiation is not directly related to the expression of TNF-α and IL-1.[57] Also, Hallahan et al. have shown that in the absence of TNF-α and IL-1, cell adhesion molecules are induced by radiation in human umbilical vein endothelial cells (HUVEC).[43] Together, these data suggest that both cytokine-independent and cytokine-dependent pathways may be responsible for enhancing cell adhesion interactions.

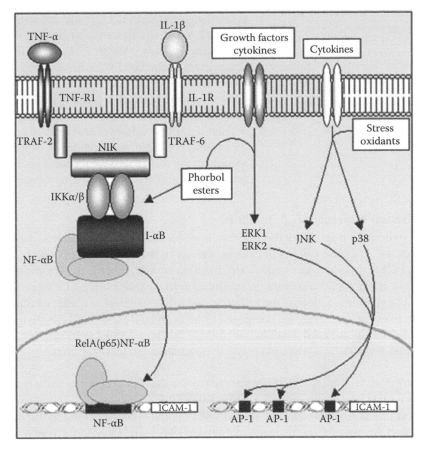

FIGURE 4.1 Schematic of ICAM-1 upregulation. (From Niessen, H.W. et al., *Ann. NY Acad. Sci.*, 973, 573, 2002. With permission.)

4.2.1.3 Adhesion Molecule: P-Selectin

P-selectin is a cell adhesion molecule of particular interest because its expression in response to radiation is both rapid and reversible.[58,59] P-selectin is an integral glycoprotein (embedded in the cell membrane) with a molecular weight of 140 kDa. It is in platelets (where it was originally discovered) as well as endothelial cells.[60,61] Normally, it is sequestered in α-granules (granules containing growth factors and clotting proteins) and Weibel-Palade bodies (organelles made of von Willebrand Factor and P-selectin) in platelets and endothelial cells, respectively.[58,62] When exposed to radiation, these storage vesicles fuse with their cell membranes.[58] Following radiation, the vascular endothelial cells of the vasculature lumen transiently express P-selectin and subsides after inflammation, P-selectin returns back to the interior of the cell.[58]

Antibodies that confer the benefit of high specificity were developed to bind this adhesion molecule. In contrast to the monoclonal antibodies, which have the drawbacks of slow blood clearance and sizes too large to penetrate tumor tissue, the single chain variable fragment (scFv) region of the antibody could be used alone. The scFv are smaller (~30 kDa), which allows for a faster renal clearance and an improved penetration into tumor tissues, and these are properties that make them preferred candidates.[63,64] Faster clearance prevents the undesirable side effects of systemic toxicity in normal organs and can result in a higher tumor:blood ratio of antibody localization. Another benefit is the antibody's lack of the constant fragment (Fc) domain, which makes it less immunogenic.[63–66]

The scFv antibody specificity was demonstrated by the visualization of Cy-7 labeled antibody against P-selectin. This was administered through tail vein injection and showed significant binding to

In contrast to the monoclonal antibodies, which have the drawbacks of slow blood clearance and sizes too large to penetrate tumor tissue, the smaller (~30 kDa) scFv region of the antibody could be used, which has faster renal clearance and an improved penetration into tumor tissues. Faster clearance prevents the undesirable side effects of systemic toxicity in normal organs and can result in a higher tumor:blood ratio of antibody localization. The lack of a Fc domain makes antibodies less immunogenic.

Lewis lung carcinoma (LLC) cells that were xenografted into nude mice and treated with 6 Gy of radiation over unirradiated tumors.[46] P-selectin localizes in the vascular lumen in rat glioma cell lines when exposed to radiation.[44] In the same study done by Hallahan et al., it was found that the localization for P-selectin to the lumen of the vasculature was specific to those of malignant glioma and did not manifest in the vessels of an irradiated normal brain.[44] As a result, P-selectin was identified as an inducible target specific to the malignant vasculature. This makes it a target of consideration for targeted drug therapy.

4.2.1.4 Adhesion Molecule: $\alpha_{2b}\beta_3$ Integrin

Integrins are cell surface receptors that are essential for various intracellular signals. They play a major role in the attachment between cells as well as in the attachment of cells to the extracellular matrix (ECM). Integrins can control the function of various growth factor receptors, cytoplasmic kinases, the organization of the intracellular actin cytoskeleton, and various ion channels. Additionally, integrins also influence the cell cycle and help to determine whether a cell proliferates, differentiates, lives, or dies. They are composed of an α and a β subunit. There are currently 19 α and 8 β known subunits and each combination of these two types produces its own binding specificity and signaling properties. It was discovered that radiation induces $\alpha_{2b}\beta_3$ integrins in melanoma cells.[67]

Peptides targeting $\alpha_{2b}\beta_3$ integrins were identified by the use of phage display technology. Hallahan et al. irradiated mice bearing either GL261 (glioma) or LLC (lung carcinoma) tumors.[68] After irradiation, a library of phages was injected into circulation and allowed to bind to these tumors. The tumors were then recovered from mice and the phages that were bound to them were reintroduced back into the circulation of another irradiated mouse bearing xenografted tumors. These rounds of selection were repeated several times to enrich the phage display peptides that were specific for these tumors. In addition, the use of this *in vivo* selection is advantageous due to the spatial separation of organs in the mouse. This allows for any peptide that binds in regions outside of the tumor to be discarded from the list of candidates.

The amino acid sequence of phage-displayed peptides that was isolated from multiple tumor models and also bound within the vascular lumen of tumors following irradiation was RGDGSSV. Protein sequence matching with the known databases using Blast and Swisspro searches found that the RGD sequence within the recovered peptide had the greatest matches. From this, putative receptors were proposed that would bind the RGD peptide, including the β_1, β_3, and β_5 chains that heterodimerize with α_{2b} chains on platelets or with α_v chain in other tissues[48]. Immunohistochemistry revealed an increase in $\alpha_{2b}\beta_3$ in the microvasculature of tumors 6 h after irradiation. In contrast, α_v did not show an increase in levels after irradiation[68]. This study showed that the physiologic response of the vasculature of different tumor models (B16 melanomas, GL261 gliomas, LLC lung carcinomas) are similar[68] meaning that upregulating with radiation $\alpha_{2b}\beta_3$ could be a potential multitumor drug targeting paradigm.

4.2.2 Identifying Potential Targeting Moieties/Receptor Ligands

Following irradiation, the changes in endothelial cells occur on many levels, including gene transcription, altered conformations of proteins, and various intra/intercellular translocations. Currently, there are multiple strategies that can be used to identify these differences in expression including bioinformatics and microarray. One method that has been showing great promise in recent years is known as phage-display technology, which we will discuss below.

4.2.2.1 Phage-Display Technology

Phage display is a method used to discover peptide ligands while minimizing and optimizing the structure and function of proteins.[69–71] The premise of phage display is the ability to produce a massive number of phages, up to 10^{10} variant phages, simultaneously, each with a different peptide sequence encoded on the surface of the phage capsid. This multitude of peptide sequences is introduced into these phages as a DNA library and the expression of these different sequences constitutes a phage library.

> Phage-displayed peptide libraries are a valuable research tool because the amino acid sequence on the capsid is encoded by the recombinant DNA. This DNA can be amplified within bacteria infected with the recombinant bacteriophage. Phage DNA can then be sequenced to determine the amino acid sequence of peptides on the capsid that have been panned on specific sites, such as tumor blood vessels.

The vehicle for carrying these various sequences is bacteriophages. These viruses are made of an elongated cylindrical protein capsid that is 6.5 nm in diameter and 930 nm in length. The structure encapsulates an approximately 6400 nucleotide genome that consists of 11 genes. For the purposes of phage display, the pVIII and pIII regions of the bacteriophage genome are of greatest interest because the proteins encoded by these regions are expressed on the surface. In most common usages of phage display, the N-terminus of these two proteins is used to display antigenic peptides with binding affinity for the chosen foreign peptide or protein.[72] The pIII protein can display 3–5 copies of an individual peptide (up to 38 amino acids long),[73] while the pVIII region can display up to 2700 copies of peptides of up to six amino acids in length.[74]

The process of using the bacteriophages to isolate peptides of interest is known as "bio-panning." The isolation of phages of interest involves the following steps. A primary library is prepared or an existing library is amplified by

1. The phage particles being exposed to the target surface of interest
2. Nonspecific binders being removed using washing or perfusion
3. Target phage being recovered
4. The above steps are repeated using recovered phages

The phage is used as a scaffold to display the libraries of recombinant peptides. It provides a means for recovering and amplifying the peptides that bind to putative receptor molecules *in vivo*. The *in vivo* selection simultaneously provides positive and subtractive screens because organs and tissues, such as tumors, are spatially separated. Phages that specifically bind within the vasculature of organs and tissues other than the tumor are discarded (subtractive screening), while phages homing to irradiated tumors become enriched through serial rounds of bio-panning (positive screening).

Phage-displayed peptide libraries are a valuable research tool because the amino acid sequence on the capsid is encoded by the recombinant DNA. This DNA can be amplified within bacteria infected with the recombinant bacteriophage. Phage DNA can then be sequenced to determine the amino acid sequence of peptides on the capsid that have been panned on specific sites, such as tumor blood vessels.[48,75,76] Repeating this process multiple times allows for the enrichment of peptides of interest. When a peptide is isolated and sequenced, one can reproduce the sequence by making synthetic or recombinant peptides. This can help identify the ligands that bind to the target receptors of interest.[77] Nowadays, displayed moieties include complementary DNA (cDNA) products made from mRNA pools,[78] DNA encoded short peptides, and non-natural amino acids or other building blocks.[79]

4.2.3 Conjugation of a Drug Delivery Vehicle to Ligands

Among the many drug-delivery vehicles that are currently available, nanoparticles are one of the most popularly used. Nanoparticles can be designed to meet the requirements of stability, size, active targeting, and solubility.[80–82] Nanoparticles smaller than 20 nm can penetrate through blood vessel walls, the blood–brain barrier, and the stomach epithelium,[83] and can simultaneously avoid rapid clearance by the liver and the spleen.[84]

Compared with small molecule drugs, which are easily diffusible through the capillary walls into tissues, the limited pore size of endothelial walls prevents nanoparticles from freely diffusing into untargeted areas within the body. Nanoparticles, therefore, rely on gaps between the endothelium in order to bypass this barrier. Fortunately, one of the properties of tumor endothelium is their increased capillary permeability, thus showing an increased uptake of nanoparticles. This phenomenon has been termed the enhanced permeability and retention (EPR) effect.[85]

The EPR effect is the phenomenon whereby molecules of a certain size, typically liposomes or macromolecular drugs, tend to accumulate in tumor tissues much more than they do in normal tissues.[86–88] The newly formed tumor vessels are usually abnormal in form and architecture. They have poorly-aligned endothelial cells with wide fenestrations, lack a smooth muscle layer, and have a wider lumen. These factors lead to abnormal molecular and fluid transport dynamics, especially for macromolecular drugs. This effect is further enhanced by pathophysiological factors that increase the extravasation of macromolecules in solid tumor tissues. Examples of these factors include bradykinin, nitric oxide, prostaglandins, vascular permeability factor (also known as vascular endothelial growth factor, VEGF), tumor necrosis factor, and others.[89]

In Sections 4.2.3.1 and 4.2.3.2, we will describe a few types of nanoparticles. These nanoparticles can be coated with targeting ligands to improve tumor-targeting. Nanoparticles may be either natural or synthetic depending upon the origin of their key structural and functional components.

4.2.3.1 Natural Nanoparticles

A key benefit of the natural nanoparticle is the higher probability of mimicking the phospholipid bilayer on the cell surface (as in the case of liposomes) and/or biocompatibility. Natural nanoparticles include nanoalbumin and various biologically compatible polymers such as chitosan and alginate.

Liposomes consist of a lipid bilayer that separates the external aqueous environment from the vehicle's internal aqueous compartment. This vehicle has been used extensively in the past 10 years as carriers of many anticancer drugs, such as platinum compounds, cytarabine,[90] anthracyclines,[91] camptothecin,[92] and vincristine.[93] Encapsulation in liposomes can improve the pharmacokinetic profile of a drug and reduce systemic toxicity.[94] For example, a study using PEG-liposomal doxorubicin showed a 5.2–11.4-fold increase in the amount of drug delivered to patients with AIDS-related Kaposi's sarcoma.[95]

Similarly, chitosan, a polysaccharide with structural similarities to cellulose, has also shown improved therapeutic efficacy and reduced toxicity when carrying a cargo of doxorubicin-dextran in comparison with treatment with doxorubicin itself.[96]

In the search for potential ligands that would bind to the $\alpha_{2b}\beta_3$ receptor, fibrinogen became a leading candidate as it had two RGD peptides on its α chain that could bind to the activated $\alpha_{2b}\beta_3$ receptor. It was found that fibrinogen colocalizes with α_{2b} in the tumor vascular lumen. With both the inducible receptor and the ligand that binds to it identified, Hallahan et al. conjugated fibrinogen with albumin nanoparticles. In this study, fibrinogen-conjugated nanoparticles bound to the $\alpha_{2b}\beta_3$ receptor obliterated tumor blood flow and significantly increased regression and growth delay in tumors treated with radiation (Figure 4.2).[68]

Presently, nanoalbumin and liposomes do not achieve tumor-specific drug delivery. For example, Abraxane® (nanoparticle albumin-bound (nab) paclitaxel) and Doxil® (liposomal doxorubicin) do not have tumor-targeting ligands. Peptide ligands that specifically target radiation-inducible receptors in cancer tissue could improve the delivery of chemotherapeutic drugs to tumor sites. The most widely used radiation sensitizing drugs include platinum-based compounds (e.g., cisplatin and carboplatin) and taxanes (paclitaxel). These drugs are administered during radiotherapy for epidermoid carcinomas. Concomitant therapy with radiation and platins or taxanes has improved local control in diseases such as lung cancer, head and neck cancer, and cervical carcinoma.

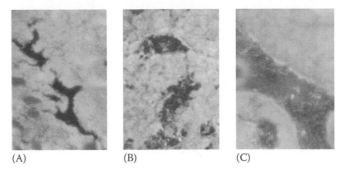

FIGURE 4.2 Fibrinogen-liposome conjugates localize to irradiated tumors. Thiolated fibrinogen was conjugated to maleimide-containing liposome vesicles. Liposomes were labeled with Dil fluorescent marker and administered by tail vein injection to tumor bearing mice. Tumors were treated with 4 Gy radiation either prior to or after the administration of fibrinogen-liposome conjugates. Tumors were fixed and sectioned at 24 h following irradiation. Shown are tumor sections of (A) sham irradiated, (B) irradiation prior to fibrinogen-liposome administration, and (C) irradiation after fibrinogen-liposome administration. Fluorescence was imaged by UV microscopy (100×). (From Hallahan, D. et al., *Cancer Cell*, 3, 63, 2003. With permission.)

Nanoalbumin binds to the albumin receptor, a cell surface, 60 kDa glycoprotein (gp60), in caveolae that delivers nanoalbumin to cancer through a process termed transendothelial transport. Albumin has features that make it an appropriate vehicle for targeted drug delivery in oncology. It is a natural carrier of hydrophobic molecules, to which it binds by noncovalent bonds. Binding of hydrophobic substances to albumin is reversible and allows for transport in the body and release at the cell surface.[97,98] In addition, albumin facilitates endothelial transcytosis of albumin-bound plasma constituents into the extravascular space. This process is initiated by the binding of albumin to gp60, which activates the binding of gp60 with an intracellular protein (caveolin-1) and subsequent invagination of the cell membrane to form transcytotic vesicles, referred to as caveolae.[99–102]

Radiolabeled paclitaxel transport across the endothelial cell monolayer was 4.2-fold higher with nab-paclitaxel compared with Cremophor-paclitaxel.[99] Methyl β-cyclodextrin completely inhibited endothelial transcytosis of nab-paclitaxel, indicating active transport via gp60-mediated caveolar-albumin transport.[99] Albumin also provided the preferential intratumoral accumulation of paclitaxel. The intratumor paclitaxel accumulation was 33% higher for nab-paclitaxel compared with Cremophor-paclitaxel for equal doses of paclitaxel.[99] The higher concentrations of paclitaxel delivered by nanoalbumin slightly improved bioavailability to cancer and thereby improved median survival rate as compared with the standard Cremophor formulation. Overall, the tolerability of intravenous nab-paclitaxel 260 mg/m^2 was generally similar to that of Cremophor-paclitaxel 175 mg/m^2 in a phase III clinical trial.[103] Almost all patients reported at least one adverse event. Nab-paclitaxel recipients experienced significantly more sensory neuropathy and gastrointestinal disturbances and less neutropenia and skin flushing than Cremophor-paclitaxel recipients.[104] No severe hypersensitivity reactions were reported in nab-paclitaxel recipients.[104]

However, a drawback of this strategy is that the albumin receptor is present in all tissues. Clinical studies evaluating Abraxane compared with paclitaxel showed that the higher concentrations of paclitaxel delivered by nanoalbumin produced a slightly higher level of peripheral neurotoxicity in those patients compared with systemic paclitaxel. Nab, therefore, does not utilize tumor-specific drug delivery. Hence, methods to target nanoalbumin to radiation-inducible receptors within cancer could improve the targeting of radiosensitizing taxanes.

4.2.3.2 Synthetic Nanoparticles

In contrast to natural nanoparticles, the use of synthetic polymers for nanoparticle construction allows for a more specific design that can be tailored towards a particular application. This

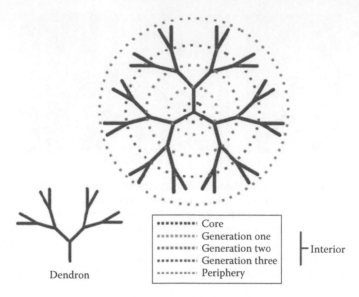

Core
Generation one
Generation two
Generation three
Periphery

Interior

Dendron

FIGURE 4.3 Dendrimers consist of dendron units. The three regions include a core, an interior, and the periphery. Higher generation dendrimers are more branched and have a greater number of end groups. (From Lee, C.C. et al., *Nat. Biotechnol.*, 23, 1517, 2005. With permission.)

flexibility in design uses the different properties of polymers and their combinations to produce individualized properties of nanoparticles. Among the various aspects that can be modified are chain length, molecular weight, particle size, hydrophobicity, surface charge, surface chemistry, and surface morphology. These characteristics can be changed depending on the hydrophobicity of the drugs, the method through which the drugs are administered, and the desired amount of time for sustained release. One of the major drawbacks of polymeric nanoparticles is its lack of site specificity, a problem that can be overcome by the conjugation of specific targeting moieties.

Examples of synthetic nanoparticles include polymeric dendrimers (Figure 4.3).[81] Dendrimers are different from other polymeric nanoparticles in that they have a highly functionalized terminal surface, a narrow molecular weight distribution, specific shape and size characteristics, and a large degree of molecular uniformity. These nanoparticles are useful for drug-delivery because of their well defined size and structure as well as their modifiable surface functionalities.

Polyamidoamine (PAMAM) is a synthetic polymer that is the most common scaffold used in dendrimers. When testing it as a vehicle for methotrexate, the drug showed a markedly decreased toxicity and increased antitumor activity compared with the therapeutic responses of the free drug.[105] Additional advantages of these synthetic nanoparticles are their nonimmunogenic nature and biocompatibility.

Biologically compatible synthetic polymers include polylactic acid (PLA), polyglycolic acid (PGA), their copolymer poly(lactic-*co*-glycolic acid) (PLGA), and polyethylene glycol (PEG). One of the key advantages of using these polymers is their ability to alter the ratio and arrangement of monomers to achieve different physical properties. PLA-PEG and PLGA-PEG nanoparticles have shown prolonged blood circulation.[106] These nanoparticles have been used to carry anticancer drugs such as doxorubicin and paclitaxel.[107] *In vitro* experiments have shown that these nanoparticles can cause cell mortality more than 13 times higher than with drug alone in HT-29 cancer cells.[107] In other experiments, PLGA nanoparticles loaded with doxorubicin targeted cancer cells and sustained drug release at the tumor site.[108] On their own, these molecules have proven to enhance drug delivery. Coupled with a bait against an inducible target in tumors, the targeting efficacy of these molecules may increase even further.

4.3 BIOMARKER DEVELOPMENT USING PHAGE DISPLAY TECHNOLOGY

Optimizing a patient's treatment regimen to a specific malignancy is dependent on a physician's ability to predict the outcome of individual treatments. Glucose analogue fluorine-18 fluorodeoxyglucose (FDG) positron emission tomography (PET)/computed tomography (CT) scans are an example of current technology that point toward how useful this form of assessment can be.[109,110] Yet, many factors still limit the efficacy of this form of FDG/PET, including the inability to detect small tumors,[111] the increase in FDG uptake during endogenously occurring wound repair,[112] and the inability to detect slower-growing cancers.[113] Another form of tumor response prediction includes annexin-V detection using single-photon emission computerized tomography (SPECT) to detect therapy-induced cell apoptosis.[114,115] The limitations of this form of assessment include production under good manufacturing practices (GMP) of the protein and a slow blood clearance resulting in lower-quality images.[116,117]

Here, we discuss using phage-display technology in developing a new means of early, noninvasively assessing tumor response to therapy.

Using phage-display technology, our group has identified the peptide sequence HVGGSSV as a tumor biomarker from a bio-panning process done in both LLC and GL261 gliomas treated with IR.[118] The target molecule for this peptide is currently under investigation. Tumors implanted into the hind limbs of mice were irradiated with 3 Gy radiation. Phage-displayed peptide libraries were administered by intracardiac injection at 4 h following irradiation. The mice were then perfused with 10 mL of phosphate buffered saline (PBS) into the left ventricle that were recovered from the right atrium. Mice were sacrificed and their organs and tumors were removed to quantify plaque-forming units of viruses. The tumors were resected at 6 h after injection of the phage library. The T7 phages were then amplified in bacteria.

Phages that bound the vasculature within irradiated tumors showed enrichment in the tumor relative to other organs. Phages that did not contain the peptide library insert (control phages) did not show enrichment. We found that the recombinant phage showed a background in control organs that was lower than the control phage without DNA insert. Polymerase chain reaction (PCR) was used to amplify the recombinant phage insert coding region directly from the plaques. We sequenced 50 clones following six rounds of selection. We identified sequences that appeared multiple times after six rounds of bio-panning.[118]

These phages were then amplified and administered for several subsequent rounds to mice bearing irradiated tumors. The most predominant peptide (HVGGSSV) was selected for further study. HVGGSSV was found to be the predominant peptide in multiple separate screenings (28% in LLC and 48% in GL261 glioma cells). Of the phage-displayed peptides that have been recovered from irradiated tumors, four of them share the homologous sequence GGSXV-COOH (at the carboxyl-terminus). The probability of this amino acid sequence being present in four different peptides is extremely small. Of these peptides, the HVGGSSV peptide showed the greatest tumor-specific binding.[118]

4.3.1 BIODISTRIBUTION OF RECOVERED PHAGE-BOUND PEPTIDES WITH TUMOR SPECIFICITY

To image the biodistribution of phage-displayed peptides, we utilized near infrared (NIR) imaging of Cy7-labeled peptides on the phages. We compared the tumor-specific binding and the pharmacokinetics of each of a library of phage-displayed peptides. Some of the phages that were recovered from irradiated tumors were compared in order to determine which peptide has the greatest tumor-specific binding. Phages were first labeled with Cy7 to allow NIR imaging. Tumors were implanted into both hind limbs of nude mice. While the mice were given 40 mg/kg of systemic sunitinib (a VEGF receptor tyrosine kinase inhibitor), only the right hind limb tumor was irradiated with 3 Gy radiation. Sunitinib was chosen because it enhances the effects of IR.[119] The left hind limb tumor served as an internal negative control. Cy7-labeled phage was injected into the venous circulation by use of a jugular catheter. The biodistribution of the Cy7-labeled phage was then imaged by NIR imaging each day for a total of nine days. Figure 4.4 shows the NIR imaging

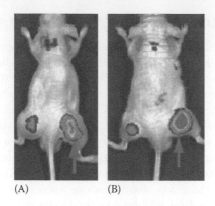

(A)   (B)

FIGURE 4.4   HVGGSSV phage binding to treated tumors. LLC tumors were implanted into both hind limbs of nude mice. The mice were treated systemically with Sunitinib (a receptor tyrosine kinase inhibitor). The tumor in the left hind limb was irradiated with 3 Gy radiation, whereas the right hind limb tumor served as an internal treatment control with drug alone. Cy7-labeled HVGGSSV phage was injected into the circulation through a jugular catheter. Shown are NIR images obtained 48 h after C7-labeled HVGGSSV phage injection into Sunitinib-treated mice bearing LLC tumors (A) or H460 tumors (B). The arrows indicate tumors treated with 3 Gy, whereas tumors in the opposite hind limb received 0 Gy (drug alone). (From Han, Z. et al., *Nat. Med.*, 14, 343, 2008. With permission.)

of the Cy7-labeled phage displaying the HVGGSSV peptide. The phage showed tumor binding at 24 h after irradiation.[118]

4.3.2   PHAGE DISPLAY PEPTIDE BINDING TO HUMAN CANCERS IN MOUSE MODELS

To determine whether the phage display peptide HVGGSSV binding can be used in a variety of human cancers, we studied orthotopic tumors implanted into the brain, lung, and liver as well as heterotopic breast and prostate tumors (Figure 4.5). Biotinylated HVGGSSV was then linked to fluorescent dye, Alexa Fluor 750 conjugated with streptavidin (Figure 4.6). Panel A of Figure 4.5 shows D54 human glioblastoma implanted into the brain of the nude mouse that was treated with 2 Gy radiation. The labeled HVGGSSV-streptavidin was administered by tail vein and imaged by NIR 48 h following administration. Likewise, H460 human lung cancer was implanted into the lung of the nude mouse and HT22 human cancer was implanted into the abdomen and liver of the nude

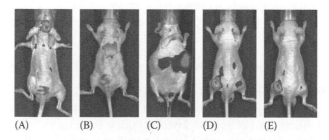

(A)   (B)   (C)   (D)   (E)

FIGURE 4.5   Peptide binding detects response to therapy in all tumor models. (A–E) Tumor development was induced by the following methods: D54 human glioblastoma cells were injected into the cerebra (A); H460 lung cancer cells were injected through the tail vein (to develop pulmonary metastases, B); HT22 human colon cancer cells were injected into the spleen (to develop liver metastases, C); and PC3 prostate cancer cells (D) and MDA-MB-231 breast cancer cells (E) were injected subcutaneously into the hind limbs of nude mice. The tumor-bearing mice were treated with Sunitinib for 1 h before irradiation. Cy7-labeled HVGGSSV peptide was injected intravenously 4 h after radiation treatment. Shown are NIR images obtained 48 h after peptide injection. (From Han, Z. et al., *Nat. Med.*, 14, 343, 2008. With permission.)

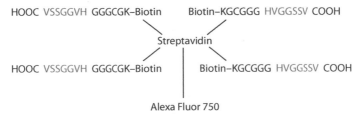

FIGURE 4.6 Conjugated streptavidin-peptide-Alexafluor 750 complex.

mouse (panels B and C). We also studied human prostate cancer line PC3 and breast cancer cell line MDA-MB-231 (panels D and E). All tumors were treated with 2 Gy radiation and peptide was injected 4 h following irradiation.[118]

Peptide bound to the tumor microvasculature of each of these tumor models following irradiation. Moreover, the peptide was cleared from the circulation and appeared in the kidney and urine soon after administration. The peptide remained bound for several days following the treatment of each of the tumor models. These data indicate that the HVGGSSV peptide binds to a wide range of tumor vascular endothelium in response to IR.[118] These mouse models of human cancer can be used to study the efficacy of re-targeted drug delivery to cancer.

4.3.3 TRANSENDOTHELIAL TRANSPORT OF HVGGSSV IN MOUSE MODELS OF CANCER

To determine whether endocytosis occurs in tumor vascular endothelium, we studied HVGGSSV conjugated to nanoalbumin in mouse models of cancer. LLC xenografts in the hind limb of mice were treated with 3 Gy radiation. Nab-HVGGSSV was then administered by tail vein injection at 4 h following irradiation. Tumors were harvested and sections were stained for human albumin using immunohistochemistry. Irradiated control tumors showed no increase in the binding of nanoalbumin, and the scrambled peptide also showed no minimal binding of nanoalbumin. When tumors were pretreated with 2 Gy radiation followed by HVGGSSV conjugated nanoalbumin treatment, nanoalbumin was found within or at the tumor vascular endothelium 24 h after the administration.

To determine the fate of nanoparticles following administration, we studied tumor sections at 7 days following administration. This showed that the nanoparticles entered cancer cells within the tumor. This indicates that the transendothelial transport of HVGGSSV-conjugated nanoalbumin improved the biodistribution of nanoparticles.[120]

In another application of HVGGSSV peptide conjugation, taxol was used as a radiation sensitizing model drug. Abraxane was conjugated with the HVGGSSV peptide using melamine chemistry. HVGGSSV-conjugated nanoalbumin achieved specific binding to tumors and rapidly cleared from the circulation. In comparison, a scrambled peptide conjugated to nanoalbumin showed no increase in binding to irradiated tumors.[121] We also investigated the use of HVGGSSV peptide to deliver nab-paclitaxel specifically to irradiated lung tumors in a mouse model. Lung tumors in the hind limb of nude mice were treated with nab-paclitaxel and radiation, HVGGSSV peptide conjugated nab-paclitaxel and radiation, or scrambled peptide conjugated nab-paclitaxel and radiation. Peptide conjugated nab-paclitaxel showed 25 times higher drug delivery than scrambled peptide conjugated nab-paclitaxel or nab-paclitaxel alone when used in combination with radiation treatment.

4.3.4 IDENTIFICATION AND CHARACTERIZATION OF HVGGSSV
RECOMBINANT PEPTIDE RECEPTOR

We used a phage-displayed peptide library to discover radiation-induced surface proteins in tumor vessels.[68] A GGSS amino acid sequence was found in the binding domain of ligands that bind to endothelial surface receptors.[122–124] In order to identify a potential receptor target, a yeast two hybrid system was used. This system introduces a plasmid coding for the DNA binding domain (DBD), a piece of a transcription factor, conjugated to the recombinant peptide. Additionally, a library of plasmids coding for potential protein targets to HVGGSSV conjugated to the other piece of the aforementioned transcription factor; an activation domain (AD) was introduced into these yeast. An interaction between the HVGGSSV peptide and a binding partner would bring together the AD and DBD components of the transcription factor, leading to the transcription of a reporter gene.

Our two hybrid systems identified the Tax-interacting protein-1 (TIP-1) as a putative receptor for the recombinant HVGGSSV peptide.[125,126] TIP-1 is a membrane-associated protein that binds to the HVGGSSV amino acid sequence at the carboxyl terminus of proteins. The amino acid sequence GGSXV-COOH (carboxyl-terminus) binds to the PDZ domain (normally associated with anchoring transmembrane proteins to the cytoskeleton and holding signal complexes together) within TIP-1[125] and has homology with the recovered HVGGSSV phage peptide (Figure 4.7). In fact, mutation of serine or valine eliminates peptide binding to TIP-1. While TIP-1 has been found to be induced by IR,[126] the role of TIP-1 is still not well understood and is still under investigation.

Homologous sequences

HV|GSSV
RGD|GSSV
H|GSSV
SV|GSRV

FIGURE 4.7 Swiss Pro search for GSSV-COOH PDZ biding proteins. The GSXV portion of the recombinant peptide sequence HVGGSSV shows homology with sequences known to bind to the PDZ domain of TIP-1.

4.4 CASE STUDIES OF STRATEGIES THAT UTILIZE IONIZING RADIATION TO DELIVER THERAPY

4.4.1 TUMOR TARGETING OF LECTINS

Many of the surface proteins and lipids found in cell membranes are glycosylated. By rearranging the combination of a few simple sugars, a broad range of unique chemical structures can be produced. The different cell types in the body express their own sets of glycan arrays, as do diseased and cancerous cells. Lectins are sugar-binding, nonenzymatic proteins that originate from numerous sources in nature and play a role in molecular recognition. They bind to oligosaccharides and proteoglycans in the vascular endothelium in both neoplastic blood and inflamed blood vessels.[127] Lectins normally bind to the O-linked and N-linked glycans that are located on the apical surface of endothelial cells.[127–129] Their specificity opens the doors to the targeting of these molecules to specific cell and tissue types.

Lectins can be combined with other drug delivery vehicles to improve tumor targeting. For example, wheat germ agglutinin (WGA), a lectin that binds to inflamed microvasculature when combined with liposomes, bound to irradiated tumor microvasculature while minimizing binding to organs like the lung and the liver. The WGA combined liposomes were used to deliver cisplatin to irradiated tumor xenografts and produced a significant growth delay when compared with radiation alone.[130]

The liposome incorporates an amphiphilic PEG derivative, *p*-nitrophenylcarbonyl-PEG-1,2-dioleoyl-*sn*-glycero-3-phosphoethanolamine (pNP-PEG-DOPE), which can bind primary-amino group-containing ligands (such as lectin) through the pNP groups that are exposed to water, which forms a nontoxic urethane (carbamate) bond. The molecule was synthesized through a reaction of DOPE with an excess of bis(*p*-nitrophenylcarbonyl)-PEG together in a chloroform/triethylamine mixture (Figure 4.8A). The reaction between the pNP group and the ligand amino group occurs readily at a pH around 8.0, and spontaneous hydrolysis eliminates any free pNP groups[131] (Figure 4.8B).

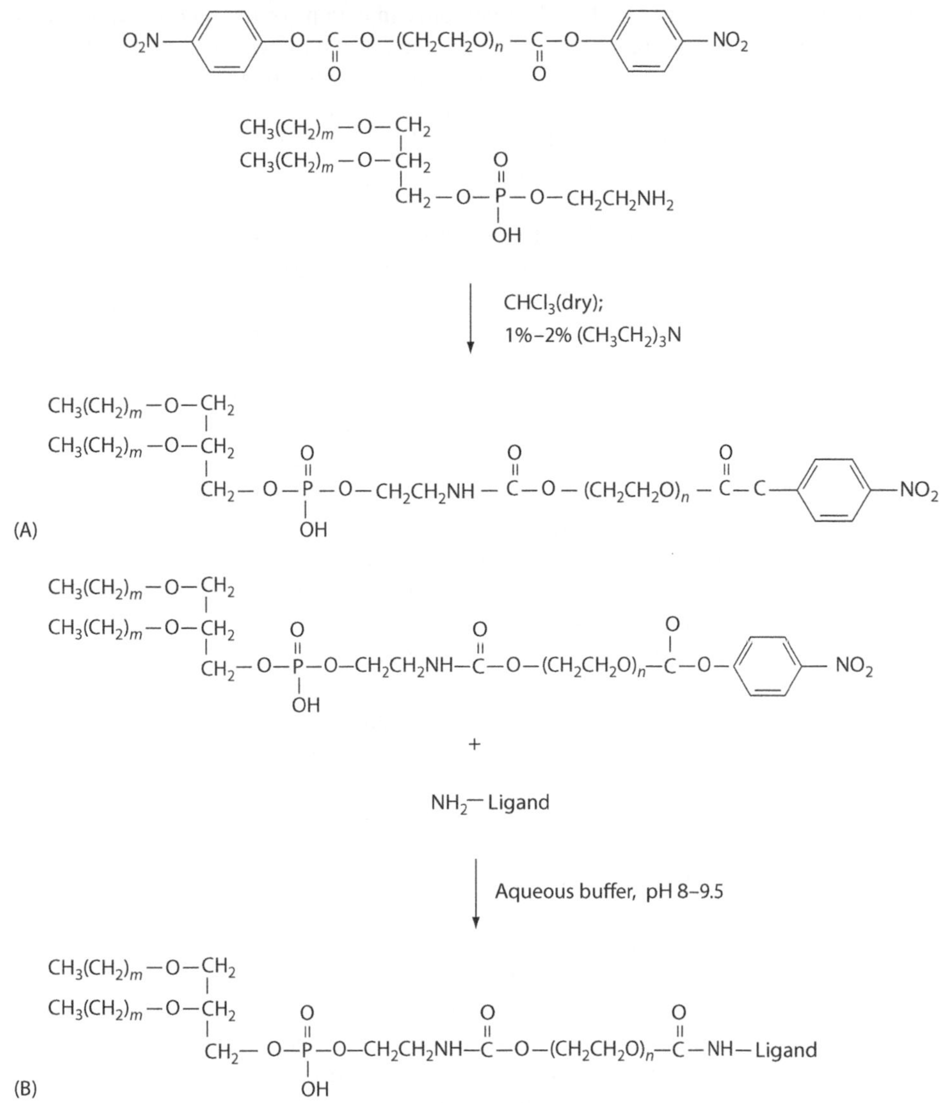

$$O_2N-C_6H_4-O-\overset{O}{\underset{\parallel}{C}}-O-(CH_2CH_2O)_n-\overset{O}{\underset{\parallel}{C}}-O-C_6H_4-NO_2$$

$$CH_3(CH_2)_m-O-CH_2$$
$$CH_3(CH_2)_m-O-\overset{|}{CH_2}$$
$$\overset{|}{CH_2}-O-\overset{O}{\underset{\underset{OH}{|}}{\overset{\parallel}{P}}}-O-CH_2CH_2NH_2$$

$CHCl_3$(dry); 1%–2% $(CH_3CH_2)_3N$

$$CH_3(CH_2)_m-O-CH_2$$
$$CH_3(CH_2)_m-O-\overset{|}{CH_2}$$
$$\overset{|}{CH_2}-O-\overset{O}{\underset{\underset{OH}{|}}{\overset{\parallel}{P}}}-O-CH_2CH_2NH-\overset{O}{\overset{\parallel}{C}}-O-(CH_2CH_2O)_n-\overset{O}{\overset{\parallel}{C}}-C-C_6H_4-NO_2$$

(A)

$$CH_3(CH_2)_m-O-CH_2$$
$$CH_3(CH_2)_m-O-\overset{|}{CH_2}$$
$$\overset{|}{CH_2}-O-\overset{O}{\underset{\underset{OH}{|}}{\overset{\parallel}{P}}}-O-CH_2CH_2NH-\overset{O}{\overset{\parallel}{C}}-O-(CH_2CH_2O)_n-\overset{O}{\overset{\parallel}{C}}-O-C_6H_4-NO_2$$

$+$

NH_2-Ligand

Aqueous buffer, pH 8–9.5

$$CH_3(CH_2)_m-O-CH_2$$
$$CH_3(CH_2)_m-O-\overset{|}{CH_2}$$
$$\overset{|}{CH_2}-O-\overset{O}{\underset{\underset{OH}{|}}{\overset{\parallel}{P}}}-O-CH_2CH_2NH-\overset{O}{\overset{\parallel}{C}}-O-(CH_2CH_2O)_n-\overset{O}{\overset{\parallel}{C}}-NH-Ligand$$

(B)

FIGURE 4.8 (A) Synthesis of pNG-PEG-PE. (B) Attachment of pNP group to the amino group containing ligand. (From Torchilin, V.P. et al., *Biochim. Biophys. Acta*, 1511, 397, 2001. With permission.)

4.4.2 Ionizing Radiation Targeting of Gene Therapy

4.4.2.1 Induction of EGR1 Promoter by Ionizing Radiation

Another strategy that can be used for tumor targeting is to exploit the changes in promoter activity induced by IR. For example, radiation induces the transcription of the early growth response 1 (Egr-1) gene, which is mediated by the activation of a CC(A+T rich)$_6$GG(CArG) motifs in the Egr-1 promoter in HL-525 cells, a human cell line of hematopoietic origin.[132,133] Weichselbaum et al. utilized this inducible promoter by conjugating it to a DNA sequence encoding for human TNF-α, a radiosensitizing cytokine.[134] This linearized construct was transfected into HL525 cells, which were then injected into xenografts of SQ-20B, a radioresistant human squamous cell carcinoma cell line. Female nude mice were subsequently given radiation only in their legs (with lead shields surrounding the rest of their body). Animals given radiation and these recombinant cells exhibited an increase in tumor cures compared with cells given only injections of the recombinant cells or with irradiation alone. In groups only receiving radiation, only 1 of 6 mice were cured. Additionally, no mice were cured in groups receiving only injections of the recombinant cells. However, in groups receiving the recombinant cells and irradiation, 6 of 7 mice were cured. Moreover, there was no increase in systemic or local toxicity in the combined treatment group. The effectiveness of this promoter led researchers to further exploit its benefits using new vehicles.

4.4.2.2 Adenoviral TNF-α Gene Therapy and Radiation Damage

Weichselbaum and colleagues created an adenoviral vector (Ad5) containing DNA sequences of the Egr-1 promoter that was linked to a cDNA encoding the TNF-α gene (Ad.Egr-TNF). This construct was tested on human malignant gliomas (D54) xenografted into nude mice.[135] A total of 71% of the xenografts receiving radiation and Ad.Egr-TNF showed complete tumor regression, in contrast to only 7.4% and 0% of the xenografts treated with radiation or Ad.Egr-TNF alone, respectively. Histopathological analyses of the xenografted glioma treated with Ad.Egr-TNF and radiation showed tumor cell thrombosis by day 4 following treatment and necrosis by day 7. These data suggested that the antitumor effect of combining Ad.Egr-TNF with radiation is, at least in part, mediated by tumor microvasculature destruction.

Since then, significant advances using the construct have been made. One product that has been patented, called TNFerade® (Patent No. 7214,368), has put the construct into a replication deficient adenovirus. In one phase I test study in patients with soft tissue sarcomas in the extremities, 85% of the patients receiving TNFerade and daily fractionated radiation therapy showed objective tumor responses (9 partial, 2 complete recovery).[136] In another phase I study, treatment was given to patients with solid tumors resistant or refractory to standard therapy. Of the 30 patients in the trial, 70% demonstrated objective tumor responses.[137] TNFerade is now entering phase II/III clinical trials.

4.4.2.3 Improving Viral Vehicle Targeting

To improve the targeting efficiency of these viral vehicles,[138] two genetically engineered herpes simplex viruses (R3616, R7020) were tested for their effectiveness in U87 malignant glioma xenografts in nude mice. The R3616 mutant is unique in that it has both copies of its gamma(1)34.5 gene knocked out. The gene normally encodes for the ability for the virus to replicate in the central nervous system and precludes premature shutoff of protein synthesis in human cells triggered by stress associated with the onset of viral DNA synthesis.[139–142] Although these mutants can better discriminate between normal and malignant cells with regard to cytotoxicity, more factors are needed for the complete destruction of tumors in *in vivo* models.[139,143]

Mice that were injected with the R3616 virus and given radiation 1 day later showed a significantly higher reduction in tumor volume in U-87 malignant gliomas when compared with treatment with either radiation or virus alone. Furthermore, *in situ* hybridization (using DNA probes to find the presence or absence of certain sequences in target cells) showed that infected tumors cells were predominant among the irradiated tumor cells. The beneficial effect can be attributed to the enhanced oncolysis in the infection/irradiation groups, which showed two- to fivefold viral replication over the group treated with infection alone.

In a similar experiment, another attenuated HSV recombinant virus (R7020) was also tested for its ability to improve tumor regression. R7020 was originally created for the purpose of prophylactic immunization against infection from HSV-1 and HSV-2.[144,145] Similar to R3616, results showed that IR enhancing R7020 replication in Hep3B xenografts over either infection or irradiation treatments alone.[146] The fact that these two vectors show promise in enhancing tumor regression lends strength to the development of new viral vectors. These may someday include other attenuated replication-competent adenoviruses that have shown promise in enhancing tumor regression with IR.[147,148]

4.4.2.4 Overcoming Viral Limitations with Radiation-Guided Nanoparticles

Generally, adenoviruses are highly efficient in the transduction of targeted cells, but lack gene integration ability.[149] As a result, multiple administrations are required which raises concerns regarding potentially lethal toxicity due to immunological responses to antigens.[149,150] Adeno-associated viruses are less immunogenic but have lower packaging capacity and viral production. Lentiviruses are capable of efficiently and stably transducing cells but are not as selective for *in vivo* delivery and have a risk of producing cancer because of its self-replication potential. Due to the limitations of viral vectors, nonviral vectors are sometimes preferred as vehicles for gene therapy. Compared with viral vectors, previously described liposome and polymer-based particles have been preferred in many clinical trials.[151]

Recently, a liposome vector, called Tf-lipoplex, which complexes with human transferrin (Tf) ligand to the liposomes, was shown to have high tumor-targeting ability due to the high level of expression of Tf receptor (TfR) in pancreas, lung, colon, prostate, and breast cancers.[152–157] Long-term therapeutic efficacy has been achieved with the Tf-lipoplex in p53 gene therapy for head and neck cancer in humans and prostate cancer, without compromising safety.[158–160]

In an experiment by Abela et al., a Tf-lipoplex complex was made that contained plasmid DNA cytomegalovirus-green fluorescent protein (CMV-GFP). Combining Tf-lipoplex therapy with radiation treatment increased the level of transduction (percentage of cells expressing GFP) in LLC1 as well as lung, liver, colon, and prostate cancer cell lines versus nonirradiated groups.[149] *In vivo* studies used a Tf-lipoplex containing plasmid DNA for CMV-LacZ. In these studies, LLC1 xenografts in C57 mice also showed increased LacZ and plasmid content over unirradiated groups. This observation correlated with the increased expression of TfR in tumors. Additionally, the Tf-lipoplex-mediated gene expression was not observed in normal tissues such as liver with radiation treatment. The effectiveness of this treatment provides insight into the further development of ligand-specific lipoplex for delivering gene therapy to malignant cells.

4.4.3 Radiation-Induced Increase in EPR Effect

Radiation was first found to have an effect on the EPR phenomenon seen in tumor tissues in studies of antibodies.[161] In this work, Kalofonos et al. showed that doses of radiation higher than 4 Gy increased both the specific and nonspecific antibody binding within irradiated tumors. This effect was due primarily to increased vascular permeability in tumors at 24 h following irradiation.

Studies of drug delivery systems have focused on liposomal doxyrubicin (Caelyx®).[162] Radiotherapy increased the tumor uptake of doxyrubicin with drug distribution farther from microvasculature in tumor periphery, following irradiation.[162] The mechanisms of radiation-induced increase in vascular permeability are related to changes in cytoskeleton.[163] Radiation causes the activation of RHO kinase and the phosphorylation of downstream myosin light chain resulting in cytoskeletal changes.

The mechanisms by which radiation could induce the enhancement of drug delivery warrant further investigation. In a study of radiation-induced vascular permeability to albumin, pulmonary endothelial cells were grown to confluence on the surface of gelatin-coated polycarbonate filters. It was shown that the amount of albumin transferred from the upper well to the lower well/hour over the period of steady-state clearance increased in monolayers exposed to 15 or 30 Gy radiation.[164] No increase was found in monolayers exposed to 6 Gy.[164] The study shows that IR plays a prominent role in the reversible disorganization of cultured pulmonary endothelial cell monolayers in the absence of serum components or other cell types.

4.4.4 Radiation-Targeted Drug Delivery Using Recombinant Peptides

At present, the nanoalbumin (nab)-paclitaxel drug delivery system (Abraxane) does not achieve tumor-specific drug delivery because it does not reduce the incidence of peripheral neuropathy and other dose-limiting toxicities. Retargeting drug delivery to radiation-inducible receptors within cancer could improve bioavailability and tumor specificity. In this strategy, radiation sensitizing taxanes can be guided to bind within irradiated tissues.

We have identified the peptide ligand HVGGSSV, which binds specifically to irradiated cancers.[118] The HVGGSSV peptide, as an early indicator of tumor response to therapy, was able to bind to responsive tumors within 24 h after treatment.[118] However, its specificity towards treated tumors indicates that it can be used as a ligand for drug delivery vehicles. Recombinant peptides have been conjugated to drug delivery systems including liposomes, nanoalbumin, nanogels, and nanocrystals to target cancer-specific drug delivery.[121,165]

Over the past decade, our laboratory focused on the use of antibodies to guide drug delivery to radiation-inducible antigens in cancer.[46,51] We determined[68] that peptide ligands are more efficient when conjugated to drug delivery systems (Figure 4.9). We found that a fibrinogen-nanoparticle (Fbg-NP) alone achieved no significant growth delay and no tumor regression as compared with untreated control tumors. As compared with untreated control tumors, radiation alone achieved minimal growth delay ($p = 0.11$). Uncoated albumin nanoparticles served as a negative control. Albumin nanoparticles administered with irradiation produced a tumor growth rate that was identical to that of tumors treated with radiation alone. Fbg-NP administered with irradiation resulted in a significant growth delay and tumor regression as compared with tumors treated with irradiation and uncoated albumin nanoparticles (Figure 4.9).

Preclinical studies using these peptides were done using ^{123}I labeled tyrosine at the amino-terminus of the peptide. Results showed a 90-fold increase in nanoparticle binding when prostate tumors were treated with 3 Gy of radiation versus untreated tumors.[166]

Moreover, RGD peptide binding in irradiated tumors has also been studied in clinical trials.[50] Our group utilized ^{99m}Tc-apcitide (Acutect®; Diatide, Inc., Londonderry, New Hampshire), a synthetic

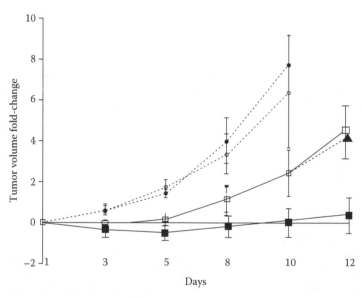

FIGURE 4.9 Radiation-induced activation of the fibrinogen receptor, which can be used as a therapeutic target for vascular embolization. B16F0 tumors implanted into the hind limb of C57BL6 mice. The mice were treated with 10 Gy radiation with or without the indicated (below) nanoparticles. Tumor volumes were measured on the indicated days. Ten mice were entered into each of five groups (untreated control, radiation alone ▲, Fbg-NP alone O, Fbg-NP + radiation ϒ, and albumin nanoparticles + radiation Δ). Uncoated albumin nanoparticles served as a negative control. Fbg-NP administered with irradiation resulted in tumor regression and a significant growth delay as compared to tumors treated with uncoated albumin nanoparticles and irradiation ($p = 0.024$). (From Hallahan, D. et al., *Cancer Cell*, 3, 63, 2003. With permission.)

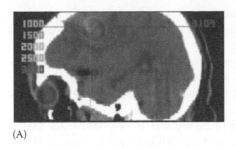 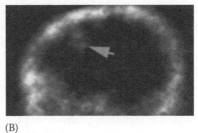

(A)   (B)

FIGURE 4.10   Radiation-guided drug delivery of 99MTc-labeled biapcitide by use of an external radiation beam. (A) [99MTc]-labeled biapcitide binding in a breast cancer brain metastasis after treatment with radiosurgery (single dose of 20 Gy). (B) Dosimetry of the same radiosurgery patient. (From Hallahan, D.E. et al., *J. Control. Release*, 74, 183, 2001. With permission.)

peptide analog of RGD that binds to GP-IIb/IIIa receptors on activated platelets,[47,167] to determine the feasibility of peptide binding in irradiated tumors in patients. We found that the RGD peptidomimetic bound within a metastatic tumor to brains treated with a high dose of radiation in 3/3 patients (Figure 4.10).[50]

4.5   CONCLUSIONS

While radiation has been used to treat cancer for many decades, the identification of radiation-induced molecules has dramatically improved the efficacy of treatment by increasing drug delivery to tumor regions. By looking at the different ways tumors respond to radiation, such as the expression of various proteins such as ICAM-1[54,55] and P-selectin[44] on tumor vasculature in response to the damage caused by IR, molecules can be identified that act as targets. Subsequently, drug delivery vehicles, such as liposomes and dendrimers, can be conjugated to antibodies or ligands that bind to these targets. These various nanoparticles, which on their own have been shown to increase drug delivery to tumor targets, can have significantly increased effectiveness when combined with these targeting agents.[130]

Alternative methods for tumor-toxic payloads have been created that also capitalize on radiation-induced targets. The most notable of these is the use of adenoviruses whose transfection rates increased in the presence of IR.[138] This same technology has led to the creation of the product TNFerade, which is now entering phase II/III clinical trials. Additionally, the efficacy of these viral vectors has led to the identification of another tumor target, Tf, which has been found to be upregulated in response to radiation.[149]

The development of phage display biotechnology has been one of the factors that has helped to push the effort of radiation-induced tumor-targeted therapy forward. This technology allows for rapid screening through billions of different recombinant peptides to find those that are tumor specific.[39] For example, the HVGGSSV peptide was discovered by the use of bacteriophage-displayed peptide libraries in the circulation of mice bearing irradiated tumors.[68,118] HVGGSSV, when conjugated to nanoparticles in the biodistribution and pharmacokinetics studies, showed tumor-specific binding. Fluorescent microscopy showed nanoparticle endocytosis and transendothelial transport of the HVGGSSV-nanoparticles. We also found that that cell surface protein TIP-1 binds to the HVGGSSV peptide. TIP-1 is increased following the irradiation of tumors. Conjugation of HVGGSSV to liposomal doxorubicin and nab-paclitaxel improved tumor-specific drug delivery. We have found that this approach of targeting radiation sensitizing drugs to cancer improves tumor growth delay as compared with nab-paclitaxel with radiation or Cremophor-paclitaxel with radiation.[120]

Further work is needed in the areas of systemic and tumor tissue pharmacokinetics of drugs delivered by targeting peptide ligand conjugation to nanoparticulate carriers. The prospect of using recombinant peptides, such as HVGGSSV or RGD, for targeted delivery of therapies requires the use of sensitive and quantitative imaging techniques to test their efficacy using methods such radioactive isotope-based PET and SPECT imaging.

Nonetheless, the HVGGSSV peptide gives an insight into the range of uses for phage display technology. Not only can the peptide be used to noninvasively assess the tumor response to therapy, it could potentially be used as a targeting agent attached to nanoparticles to guide drug delivery to tumors.

We propose the signaling pathway depicted in Figure 4.11 as responsible for the recombinant peptide binding to receptors on endothelial cell surface. While receptors such as TIP-1 have been

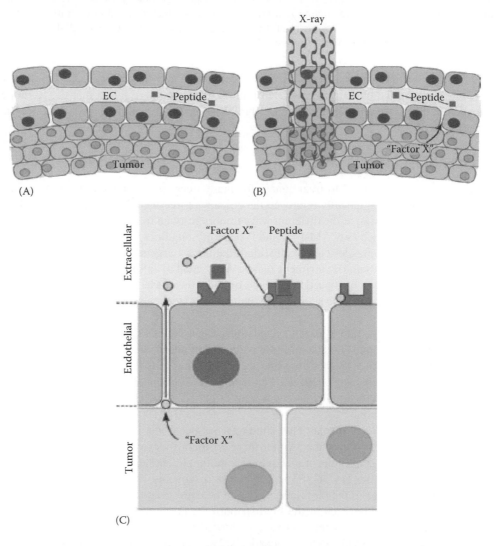

FIGURE 4.11 Possible mechanism of recombinant peptide binding to tumor vasculature in response to IR. (A) Recombinant peptide does not bind to the tumor vasculature when there is no cytotoxic agent. (B) In response to IR, the tumor cell could secrete a cytokine or chemokine ("Factor X"). (C) This factor secreted by the tumor in response to IR could interact with the endothelial cell causing it to manifest an inducible receptor or change the conformation of an existing membrane receptor. Due to the action of the paracrine factor, the recombinant peptide could now bind to the inducible receptor thereby heralding that the cell is dead or dying. (Adapted from Diaz, D. et al., *Expert Rev. Anticancer Ther.*, 8, 1787, 2008. With permission.)

identified, further work needs to be done to find the receptors that can bind to other recombinant peptides. Furthermore, the pathway by which the peptide target receptor is induced is also a point of interest that is still under investigation.

In summary, IR can be used to target chemotherapeutic drugs to tumors by conjugating them with a nanoparticle/recombinant peptide complex. Targeting drugs to tumors that respond to radiotherapy is expected to enhance their biological effect and could reduce systemic toxicity.

> Radiation has been used to treat cancer for many decades. The use of targeted drug delivery in conjunction with radiation has dramatically improved the efficacy of treatment. In addition to active targeting, alternative methods for tumor-toxic payloads have been created, which capitalize on radiation-induced targets. The most notable of these is the use of adenoviruses whose transfection rates increase in the presence of IR. This same technology has led to the creation of the product TNFerade®, which is now entering phase II/III clinical trials.

REFERENCES

1. Cognetti DM, Weber RS, Lai SY. Head and neck cancer: An evolving treatment paradigm. *Cancer* 2008;**113**(7 Suppl):1911–1932.
2. Damascelli B, Patelli GL, Lanocita R, Di Tolla G, Frigerio LF, Marchiano A et al. A novel intraarterial chemotherapy using paclitaxel in albumin nanoparticles to treat advanced squamous cell carcinoma of the tongue: Preliminary findings. *Am J Roentgenol* 2003;**181**(1):253–260.
3. Govindan R, Bogart J, Vokes EE. Locally advanced non-small cell lung cancer: The past, present, and future. *J Thorac Oncol* 2008;**3**(8):917–928.
4. Green MR, Manikhas GM, Orlov S, Afanasyev B, Makhson AM, Bhar P et al. Abraxane, a novel Cremophor-free, albumin-bound particle form of paclitaxel for the treatment of advanced non-small-cell lung cancer. *Ann Oncol* 2006;**17**(8):1263–1268.
5. Ringel I, Horwitz SB. Studies with RP 56976 (taxotere): A semisynthetic analogue of taxol. *J Natl Cancer Inst* 1991;**83**(4):288–291.
6. Choy H. Taxanes in combined-modality therapy for solid tumors. *Oncology* (*Williston Park*) 1999;**13**(10 Suppl 5):23–38.
7. Hainsworth JD. Practical aspects of weekly docetaxel administration schedules. *Oncologist* 2004;**9**(5):538–545.
8. Horwitz SB. Personal recollections on the early development of taxol. *J Nat Prod* 2004;**67**(2):136–138.
9. ten Tije AJ, Verweij J, Loos WJ, Sparreboom A. Pharmacological effects of formulation vehicles: Implications for cancer chemotherapy. *Clin Pharmacokinet* 2003;**42**(7):665–685.
10. Gianni L, Kearns CM, Giani A, Capri G, Vigano L, Lacatelli A et al. Nonlinear pharmacokinetics and metabolism of paclitaxel and its pharmacokinetic/pharmacodynamic relationships in humans. *J Clin Oncol* 1995;**13**(1):180–190.
11. Holmes FA, Madden T, Newman RA, Valero V, Theriault RL, Fraschini G et al. Sequence-dependent alteration of doxorubicin pharmacokinetics by paclitaxel in a phase I study of paclitaxel and doxorubicin in patients with metastatic breast cancer. *J Clin Oncol* 1996;**14**(10):2713–2721.
12. Holmes FA, Rowinsky EK. Pharmacokinetic profiles of doxorubicin in combination with taxanes. *Semin Oncol* 2001;**28**(4 Suppl 12):8–14.
13. Millward MJ, Webster LK, Rischin D, Stokes KH, Toner GC, Bishop JF et al. Phase I trial of cremophor EL with bolus doxorubicin. *Clin Cancer Res* 1998;**4**(10):2321–2329.
14. Authier N, Gillet JP, Fialip J, Eschalier A, Coudore F. Assessment of neurotoxicity following repeated cremophor/ethanol injections in rats. *Neurotox Res* 2001;**3**(3):301–306.
15. Gelderblom H, Verweij J, Nooter K, Sparreboom A. Cremophor EL. The drawbacks and advantages of vehicle selection for drug formulation. *Eur J Cancer* 2001;**37**(13):1590–1598.
16. Lorenz W, Schmal A, Schult H, Lang S, Ohmann C, Weber D et al. Histamine release and hypotensive reactions in dogs by solubilizing agents and fatty acids: Analysis of various components in cremophor El and development of a compound with reduced toxicity. *Agents Actions* 1982;**12**(1–2):64–80.
17. Weiss RB, Donehower RC, Wiernik PH, Ohnuma T, Gralla RJ, Trump DL et al. Hypersensitivity reactions from taxol. *J Clin Oncol* 1990;**8**(7):1263–1268.
18. Windebank AJ, Blexrud MD, de Groen PC. Potential neurotoxicity of the solvent vehicle for cyclosporine. *J Pharmacol Exp Ther* 1994;**268**(2):1051–1056.
19. Di Paolo A, Bocci G. Drug distribution in tumors: Mechanisms, role in drug resistance, and methods for modification. *Curr Oncol Rep* 2007;**9**(2):109–114.

20. Minchinton AI, Tannock IF. Drug penetration in solid tumours. *Nat Rev Cancer* 2006;**6**(8):583–592.
21. Baxter LT, Jain RK. Transport of fluid and macromolecules in tumors. I. Role of interstitial pressure and convection. *Microvasc Res* 1989;**37**(1):77–104.
22. Jain RK, Baxter LT. Mechanisms of heterogeneous distribution of monoclonal antibodies and other macromolecules in tumors: Significance of elevated interstitial pressure. *Cancer Res* 1988;**48**(24 Pt 1):7022–7032.
23. Stohrer M BY, Stangassinger M, Jain RK. Oncotic pressure in solid tumors is elevated. *Cancer Res* 2000;**60**:814–819.
24. DiResta GR, Lee J, Larson SM, Arbit E. Characterization of neuroblastoma xenograft in rat flank. I. Growth, interstitial fluid pressure, and interstitial fluid velocity distribution profiles. *Microvasc Res* 1993;**46**(2):158–177.
25. Jain RK. Physiological barriers to delivery of monoclonal antibodies and other macromolecules in tumors. *Cancer Res* 1990;**50**(3 Suppl):814s–819s.
26. Netti PA, Baxter LT, Boucher Y, Skalak R, Jain RK. Time-dependent behavior of interstitial fluid pressure in solid tumors: Implications for drug delivery. *Cancer Res* 1995;**55**(22):5451–5458.
27. Folkman J. Tumor angiogenesis: Therapeutic implications. *N Engl J Med* 1971;**285**(21):1182–1186.
28. Cox G, Jones JL, Walker RA, Steward WP, O'Byrne KJ. Angiogenesis and non-small cell lung cancer. *Lung Cancer* 2000;**27**(2):81–100.
29. Kim KJ, Li B, Winer J, Armanini M, Gillett N, Phillips HS et al. Inhibition of vascular endothelial growth factor-induced angiogenesis suppresses tumour growth in vivo. *Nature* 1993;**362**(6423):841–844.
30. Witte L, Hicklin DJ, Zhu Z, Pytowski B, Kotanides H, Rockwell P et al. Monoclonal antibodies targeting the VEGF receptor-2 (Flk1/KDR) as an anti-angiogenic therapeutic strategy. *Cancer Metastasis Rev* 1998;**17**(2):155–161.
31. Maliepaard M, Scheffer GL, Faneyte IF, van Gastelen MA, Pijnenborg AC, Schinkel AH et al. Subcellular localization and distribution of the breast cancer resistance protein transporter in normal human tissues. *Cancer Res* 2001;**61**(8):3458–3464.
32. Fetsch PA, Abati A, Litman T, Morisaki K, Honjo Y, Mittal K et al. Localization of the ABCG2 mitoxantrone resistance-associated protein in normal tissues. *Cancer Lett* 2006;**235**(1):84–92.
33. Ross DD, Yang W, Abruzzo LV, Dalton WS, Schneider E, Lage H et al. Atypical multidrug resistance: Breast cancer resistance protein messenger RNA expression in mitoxantrone-selected cell lines. *J Natl Cancer Inst* 1999;**91**(5):429–433.
34. Ding BS, Zhou YJ, Chen XY, Zhang J, Zhang PX, Sun ZY et al. Lung endothelium targeting for pulmonary embolism thrombolysis. *Circulation* 2003;**108**(23):2892–2898.
35. El-Mousawi M, Tchistiakova L, Yurchenko L, Pietrzynski G, Moreno M, Stanimirovic D et al. A vascular endothelial growth factor high affinity receptor 1-specific peptide with antiangiogenic activity identified using a phage display peptide library. *J Biol Chem* 2003;**278**(47):46681–46691.
36. Bockmann M, Drosten M, Putzer BM. Discovery of targeting peptides for selective therapy of medullary thyroid carcinoma. *J Gene Med* 2005;**7**(2):179–188.
37. Bosserhoff AK, Stoll R, Sleeman JP, Bataille F, Buettner R, Holak TA. Active detachment involves inhibition of cell-matrix contacts of malignant melanoma cells by secretion of melanoma inhibitory activity. *Lab Invest* 2003;**83**(11):1583–1594.
38. Saharinen P, Tammela T, Karkkainen MJ, Alitalo K. Lymphatic vasculature: Development, molecular regulation and role in tumor metastasis and inflammation. *Trends Immunol* 2004;**25**(7):387–395.
39. Schluesener HJ, Xianglin T. Selection of recombinant phages binding to pathological endothelial and tumor cells of rat glioblastoma by in-vivo display. *J Neurol Sci* 2004;**224**(1–2):77–82.
40. Wu H, Pancook JD, Beuerlein G, Chilton T, Pecht G, Huse WD et al. Cloning, isolation and characterization of human tumor in situ monoclonal antibodies. *Cancer Immunol Immunother* 2002;**51**(2):79–90.
41. Taguchi E, Nakamura K, Miura T, Shibuya M, Isoe T. Anti-tumor activity and tumor vessel normalization by the vascular endothelial growth factor receptor tyrosine kinase inhibitor KRN951 in a rat peritoneal disseminated tumor model. *Cancer Sci* 2008;**99**(3):623–630.
42. Hallahan D, Clark ET, Kuchibhotla J, Gewertz BL, Collins T. E-selectin gene induction by ionizing radiation is independent of cytokine induction. *Biochem Biophys Res Commun* 1995;**217**(3):784–795.
43. Hallahan D, Kuchibhotla J, Wyble C. Cell adhesion molecules mediate radiation-induced leukocyte adhesion to the vascular endothelium. *Cancer Res* 1996;**56**(22):5150–5155.
44. Hallahan DE, Staba-Hogan MJ, Virudachalam S, Kolchinsky A. X-ray-induced P-selectin localization to the lumen of tumor blood vessels. *Cancer Res* 1998;**58**(22):5216–5220.

45. Cheresh DA. Human endothelial cells synthesize and express an Arg-Gly-Asp-directed adhesion receptor involved in attachment to fibrinogen and von Willebrand factor. *Proc Natl Acad Sci USA* 1987;**84**(18):6471–6475.
46. Hariri G, Zhang Y, Fu A, Han Z, Brechbiel M, Tantawy MN et al. Radiation-guided P-selectin antibody targeted to lung cancer. *Ann Biomed Eng* 2008;**36**(5):821–830.
47. Hawiger J, Timmons S. Binding of fibrinogen and von Willebrand factor to platelet glycoprotein IIb-IIIa complex. *Methods Enzymol* 1992;**215**:228–243.
48. Ruoslahti E. RGD and other recognition sequences for integrins. *Annu Rev Cell Dev Biol* 1996;**12**:697–715.
49. Timmons S, Bednarek MA, Kloczewiak M, Hawiger J. Antiplatelet "hybrid" peptides analogous to receptor recognition domains on gamma and alpha chains of human fibrinogen. *Biochemistry* 1989;**28**(7):2919–2923.
50. Hallahan DE, Geng L, Cmelak AJ, Chakravarthy AB, Martin W, Scarfone C et al. Targeting drug delivery to radiation-induced neoantigens in tumor microvasculature. *J Control Release* 2001;**74**(1–3):183–191.
51. Hallahan DE, Qu S, Geng L, Cmelak A, Chakravarthy A, Martin W et al. Radiation-mediated control of drug delivery. *Am J Clin Oncol* 2001;**24**(5):473–480.
52. Hallahan DE. Radiation-mediated gene expression in the pathogenesis of the clinical radiation response. *Semin Radiat Oncol* 1996;**6**(4):250–267.
53. Walther M, Kaffenberger W, Van Beuningen D. Influence of clinically used antioxidants on radiation-induced expression of intercellular cell adhesion molecule-1 on HUVEC. *Int J Radiat Biol* 1999;**75**(10):1317–1325.
54. Baeuml H, Behrends U, Peter RU, Mueller S, Kammerbauer C, Caughman SW et al. Ionizing radiation induces, via generation of reactive oxygen intermediates, intercellular adhesion molecule-1 (ICAM-1) gene transcription and NF kappa B-like binding activity in the ICAM-1 transcriptional regulatory region. *Free Radic Res* 1997;**27**(2):127–142.
55. Heckmann M, Douwes K, Peter R, Degitz K. Vascular activation of adhesion molecule mRNA and cell surface expression by ionizing radiation. *Exp Cell Res* 1998;**238**(1):148–154.
56. Kyrkanides S, Olschowka JA, Williams JP, Hansen JT, O'Banion MK. TNF alpha and IL-1beta mediate intercellular adhesion molecule-1 induction via microglia-astrocyte interaction in CNS radiation injury. *J Neuroimmunol* 1999;**95**(1–2):95–106.
57. Hong JH, Chiang CS, Campbell IL, Sun JR, Withers HR, McBride WH. Induction of acute phase gene expression by brain irradiation. *Int J Radiat Oncol Biol Phys* 1995;**33**(3):619–626.
58. Hallahan DE, Virudachalam S. Accumulation of P-selectin in the lumen of irradiated blood vessels. *Radiat Res* 1999;**152**(1):6–13.
59. Kneuer C, Ehrhardt C, Radomski MW, Bakowsky U. Selectins—Potential pharmacological targets? *Drug Discov Today* 2006;**11**(21–22):1034–1040.
60. McEver RP. Selectins. *Curr Opin Immunol* 1994;**6**(1):75–84.
61. McEver RP. Regulation of function and expression of P-selectin. *Agents Actions Suppl* 1995;**47**:117–119.
62. Dole VS, Bergmeier W, Mitchell HA, Eichenberger SC, Wagner DD. Activated platelets induce Weibel-Palade-body secretion and leukocyte rolling in vivo: Role of P-selectin. *Blood* 2005;**106**(7):2334–2339.
63. Lin MZ, Teitell MA, Schiller GJ. The evolution of antibodies into versatile tumor-targeting agents. *Clin Cancer Res* 2005;**11**(1):129–138.
64. Wu AM, Senter PD. Arming antibodies: Prospects and challenges for immunoconjugates. *Nat Biotechnol* 2005;**23**(9):1137–1146.
65. Carter P. Improving the efficacy of antibody-based cancer therapies. *Nat Rev Cancer* 2001;**1**(2):118–129.
66. Fang J, Jin HB, Song JD. Construction, expression and tumor targeting of a single-chain Fv against human colorectal carcinoma. *World J Gastroenterol* 2003;**9**(4):726–730.
67. Onoda JM, Piechocki MP, Honn KV. Radiation-induced increase in expression of the alpha IIb beta 3 integrin in melanoma cells: Effects on metastatic potential. *Radiat Res* 1992;**130**(3):281–288.
68. Hallahan D, Geng L, Qu S, Scarfone C, Giorgio T, Donnelly E et al. Integrin-mediated targeting of drug delivery to irradiated tumor blood vessels. *Cancer Cell* 2003;**3**(1):63–74.
69. Forrer P, Jung S, Pluckthun A. Beyond binding: Using phage display to select for structure, folding and enzymatic activity in proteins. *Curr Opin Struct Biol* 1999;**9**(4):514–520.
70. Smith GP, Petrenko VA. Phage display. *Chem Rev* 1997;**97**(2):391–410.

71. Zwick MB, Shen J, Scott JK. Phage-displayed peptide libraries. *Curr Opin Biotechnol* 1998;**9**(4):427–436.

72. Smith GP, Scott JK. Libraries of peptides and proteins displayed on filamentous phage. *Methods Enzymol* 1993;**217**:228–257.

73. Scott JK, Smith GP. Searching for peptide ligands with an epitope library. *Science* 1990;**249**(4967):386–390.

74. Greenwood J, Hunter GJ, Perham RN. Regulation of filamentous bacteriophage length by modification of electrostatic interactions between coat protein and DNA. *J Mol Biol* 1991;**217**(2):223–227.

75. Arap W, Pasqualini R, Ruoslahti E. Cancer treatment by targeted drug delivery to tumor vasculature in a mouse model. *Science* 1998;**279**(5349):377–380.

76. Pasqualini R, Ruoslahti E. Organ targeting in vivo using phage display peptide libraries. *Nature* 1996;**380**(6572):364–366.

77. Koivunen E, Arap W, Rajotte D, Lahdenranta J, Pasqualini R. Identification of receptor ligands with phage display peptide libraries. *J Nucl Med* 1999;**40**(5):883–888.

78. Cesareni G, Castagnoli L, Cestra G. Phage displayed peptide libraries. *Comb Chem High Throughput Screen* 1999;**2**(1):1–17.

79. Frankel A, Li S, Starck SR, Roberts RW. Unnatural RNA display libraries. *Curr Opin Struct Biol* 2003;**13**(4):506–512.

80. Ferrari M. Cancer nanotechnology: Opportunities and challenges. *Nat Rev Cancer* 2005;**5**(3):161–171.

81. Lee CC, MacKay JA, Frechet JM, Szoka FC. Designing dendrimers for biological applications. *Nat Biotechnol* 2005;**23**(12):1517–1526.

82. McNeil SE. Nanotechnology for the biologist. *J Leukoc Biol* 2005;**78**(3):585–594.

83. Vinogradov SV, Batrakova EV, Kabanov AV. Nanogels for oligonucleotide delivery to the brain. *Bioconjug Chem* 2004;**15**(1):50–60.

84. Moghimi SM, Hunter AC, Murray JC. Long-circulating and target-specific nanoparticles: Theory to practice. *Pharmacol Rev* 2001;**53**(2):283–318.

85. Brannon-Peppas L, Blanchette JO. Nanoparticle and targeted systems for cancer therapy. *Adv Drug Deliv Rev* 2004;**56**(11):1649–1659.

86. Duncan R, Coatsworth JK, Burtles S. Preclinical toxicology of a novel polymeric antitumour agent: HPMA copolymer-doxorubicin (PK1). *Hum Exp Toxicol* 1998;**17**(2):93–104.

87. Matsumura Y, Maeda H. A new concept for macromolecular therapeutics in cancer chemotherapy: Mechanism of tumoritropic accumulation of proteins and the antitumor agent smancs. *Cancer Res* 1986;**46**(12 Pt 1):6387–6392.

88. Vasey PA, Kaye SB, Morrison R, Twelves C, Wilson P, Duncan R et al. Phase I clinical and pharmacokinetic study of PK1 [N-(2-hydroxypropyl)methacrylamide copolymer doxorubicin]: First member of a new class of chemotherapeutic agents-drug-polymer conjugates. Cancer Research Campaign Phase I/II Committee. *Clin Cancer Res* 1999;**5**(1):83–94.

89. Maeda H, Fang J, Inutsuka T, Kitamoto Y. Vascular permeability enhancement in solid tumor: Various factors, mechanisms involved and its implications. *Int Immunopharmacol* 2003;**3**(3):319–328.

90. Kripp M, Hofheinz RD. Treatment of lymphomatous and leukemic meningitis with liposomal encapsulated cytarabine. *Int J Nanomed* 2008;**3**(4):397–401.

91. Batist G, Ramakrishnan G, Rao CS, Chandrasekharan A, Gutheil J, Guthrie T et al. Reduced cardiotoxicity and preserved antitumor efficacy of liposome-encapsulated doxorubicin and cyclophosphamide compared with conventional doxorubicin and cyclophosphamide in a randomized, multicenter trial of metastatic breast cancer. *J Clin Oncol* 2001;**19**(5):1444–1454.

92. Emerson DL, Bendele R, Brown E, Chiang S, Desjardins JP, Dihel LC et al. Antitumor efficacy, pharmacokinetics, and biodistribution of NX 211: A low-clearance liposomal formulation of lurtotecan. *Clin Cancer Res* 2000;**6**(7):2903–2912.

93. Krishna R, Webb MS, St Onge G, Mayer LD. Liposomal and nonliposomal drug pharmacokinetics after administration of liposome-encapsulated vincristine and their contribution to drug tissue distribution properties. *J Pharmacol Exp Ther* 2001;**298**(3):1206–1212.

94. Hofheinz RD, Gnad-Vogt SU, Beyer U, Hochhaus A. Liposomal encapsulated anti-cancer drugs. *Anticancer Drugs* 2005;**16**(7):691–707.

95. Northfelt DW, Martin FJ, Working P, Volberding PA, Russell J, Newman M et al. Doxorubicin encapsulated in liposomes containing surface-bound polyethylene glycol: Pharmacokinetics, tumor localization, and safety in patients with AIDS-related Kaposi's sarcoma. *J Clin Pharmacol* 1996;**36**(1):55–63.

96. Mitra S, Gaur U, Ghosh PC, Maitra AN. Tumour targeted delivery of encapsulated dextran-doxorubicin conjugate using chitosan nanoparticles as carrier. *J Control Release* 2001;**74**(1–3):317–323.

97. Paal K, Muller J, Hegedus L. High affinity binding of paclitaxel to human serum albumin. *Eur J Biochem* 2001;**268**(7):2187–2191.

98. Purcell M, Neault JF, Tajmir-Riahi HA. Interaction of taxol with human serum albumin. *Biochim Biophys Acta* 2000;**1478**(1):61–68.

99. Desai N, Trieu V, Yao Z, Louie L, Ci S, Yang A et al. Increased antitumor activity, intratumor paclitaxel concentrations, and endothelial cell transport of cremophor-free, albumin-bound paclitaxel, ABI-007, compared with cremophor-based paclitaxel. *Clin Cancer Res* 2006;**12**(4):1317–1324.

100. John TA, Vogel SM, Tiruppathi C, Malik AB, Minshall RD. Quantitative analysis of albumin uptake and transport in the rat microvessel endothelial monolayer. *Am J Physiol Lung Cell Mol Physiol* 2003;**284**(1):L187–L196.

101. Minshall RD, Tiruppathi C, Vogel SM, Niles WD, Gilchrist A, Hamm HE et al. Endothelial cell-surface gp60 activates vesicle formation and trafficking via G(i)-coupled Src kinase signaling pathway. *J Cell Biol* 2000;**150**(5):1057–1070.

102. Vogel SM, Minshall RD, Pilipovic M, Tiruppathi C, Malik AB. Albumin uptake and transcytosis in endothelial cells in vivo induced by albumin-binding protein. *Am J Physiol Lung Cell Mol Physiol* 2001;**281**(6):L1512–L1522.

103. Gradishar W, Vishalpura T, Franklin M, Bramley T. Cost-effectiveness of nanoparticle albumin-bound paclitaxel versus docetaxel in the treatment of metastatic breast cancer. *Breast Cancer Res Treat* 2005;**94**:S220–S221.

104. Gradishar WJ, Tjulandin S, Davidson N, Shaw H, Desai N, Bhar P et al. Phase III trial of nanoparticle albumin-bound paclitaxel compared with polyethylated castor oil-based paclitaxel in women with breast cancer. *J Clin Oncol* 2005;**23**(31):7794–7803.

105. Kukowska-Latallo JF, Candido KA, Cao Z, Nigavekar SS, Majoros IJ, Thomas TP et al. Nanoparticle targeting of anticancer drug improves therapeutic response in animal model of human epithelial cancer. *Cancer Res* 2005;**65**(12):5317–5324.

106. Avgoustakis K. Pegylated poly(lactide) and poly(lactide-*co*-glycolide) nanoparticles: Preparation, properties and possible applications in drug delivery. *Curr Drug Deliv* 2004;**1**(4):321–333.

107. Feng SS, Mu L, Win KY, Huang G. Nanoparticles of biodegradable polymers for clinical administration of paclitaxel. *Curr Med Chem* 2004;**11**(4):413–424.

108. Chittasupho C, Xie SX, Baoum A, Yakovleva T, Siahaan TJ, Berkland CJ. ICAM-1 targeting of doxorubicin-loaded PLGA nanoparticles to lung epithelial cells. *Eur J Pharm Sci* 2009;**37**(2):141–150.

109. Cullinane C, Dorow DS, Kansara M, Conus N, Binns D, Hicks RJ et al. An in vivo tumor model exploiting metabolic response as a biomarker for targeted drug development. *Cancer Res* 2005;**65**(21):9633–9636.

110. Gatenby RA, Gillies RJ. Why do cancers have high aerobic glycolysis? *Nat Rev Cancer* 2004;**4**(11):891–899.

111. Kumar R, Chauhan A, Zhuang H, Chandra P, Schnall M, Alavi A. Clinicopathologic factors associated with false negative FDG-PET in primary breast cancer. *Breast Cancer Res Treat* 2006;**98**(3):267–274.

112. Bakheet SM, Powe J, Kandil A, Ezzat A, Rostom A, Amartey J. F-18 FDG uptake in breast infection and inflammation. *Clin Nucl Med* 2000;**25**(2):100–103.

113. Avril N, Dose J, Janicke F, Bense S, Ziegler S, Laubenbacher C et al. Metabolic characterization of breast tumors with positron emission tomography using F-18 fluorodeoxyglucose. *J Clin Oncol* 1996;**14**(6):1848–1857.

114. Kolodgie FD, Petrov A, Virmani R, Narula N, Verjans JW, Weber DK et al. Targeting of apoptotic macrophages and experimental atheroma with radiolabeled annexin V: A technique with potential for noninvasive imaging of vulnerable plaque. *Circulation* 2003;**108**(25):3134–3139.

115. Narula J, Acio ER, Narula N, Samuels LE, Fyfe B, Wood D et al. Annexin-V imaging for noninvasive detection of cardiac allograft rejection. *Nat Med* 2001;**7**(12):1347–1352.

116. Belhocine T, Steinmetz N, Hustinx R, Bartsch P, Jerusalem G, Seidel L et al. Increased uptake of the apoptosis-imaging agent (99m)Tc recombinant human Annexin V in human tumors after one course of chemotherapy as a predictor of tumor response and patient prognosis. *Clin Cancer Res* 2002;**8**(9):2766–2774.

117. Lahorte CM, van de Wiele C, Bacher K, van den Bossche B, Thierens H, van Belle S et al. Biodistribution and dosimetry study of 123I-rh-annexin V in mice and humans. *Nucl Med Commun* 2003;**24**(8):871–880.

118. Han Z, Fu A, Wang H, Diaz R, Geng L, Onishko H et al. Noninvasive assessment of cancer response to therapy. *Nat Med* 2008;**14**(3):343–349.

119. Schueneman AJ, Himmelfarb E, Geng L, Tan J, Donnelly E, Mendel D et al. SU11248 maintenance therapy prevents tumor regrowth after fractionated irradiation of murine tumor models. *Cancer Res* 2003;**63**(14):4009–4016.

120. Hariri G, Croce T, Harth E, Han Z, Tantawy N, Peterson T et al. Radiation guided peptide targeting to tumor microvasculature using nanoparticle carriers. *Int J Radiat Oncol Biol Phys* 2007;**69**(3):S151–S152.

121. Hariri G, Han Z, Hallahan D. Radiation-guided drug delivery of nanoparticle albumin-bound paclitaxel to lung cancer. *Int J Radiat Oncol Biol Phys* 2008;**72**(1):S705–S706.

122. Calvo J, Places L, Padilla O, Vila JM, Vives J, Bowen MA et al. Interaction of recombinant and natural soluble CD5 forms with an alternative cell surface ligand. *Eur J Immunol* 1999;**29**(7):2119–2129.

123. Fett JW, Strydom DJ, Lobb RR, Alderman EM, Vallee BL, Artymiuk PJ et al. Lysozyme: A major secretory product of a human colon carcinoma cell line. *Biochemistry* 1985;**24**(4):965–975.

124. Papageorgiou AC, Shapiro R, Acharya KR. Molecular recognition of human angiogenin by placental ribonuclease inhibitor—An X-ray crystallographic study at 2.0 A resolution. *EMBO J* 1997;**16**(17):5162–5177.

125. Alewine C, Olsen O, Wade JB, Welling PA. TIP-1 has PDZ scaffold antagonist activity. *Mol Biol Cell* 2006;**17**(10):4200–4211.

126. Wang H, Fu A, Han Z, Hallahan D. Tax interacting protein (TIP-1): A potential radiation inducible receptor within cancer. *Int J Radiat Oncol Biol Phys* 2007;**69**(3):S590–S591.

127. Debbage PL, Griebel J, Ried M, Gneiting T, DeVries A, Hutzler P. Lectin intravital perfusion studies in tumor-bearing mice: Micrometer-resolution, wide-area mapping of microvascular labeling, distinguishing efficiently and inefficiently perfused microregions in the tumor. *J Histochem Cytochem* 1998;**46**(5):627–639.

128. Alroy J, Goyal V, Skutelsky E. Lectin histochemistry of mammalian endothelium. *Histochemistry* 1987;**86**(6):603–607.

129. Simionescu M, Simionescu N, Palade GE. Differentiated microdomains on the luminal surface of capillary endothelium: Distribution of lectin receptors. *J Cell Biol* 1982;**94**(2):406–413.

130. Geng L, Osusky K, Konjeti S, Fu A, Hallahan D. Radiation-guided drug delivery to tumor blood vessels results in improved tumor growth delay. *J Control Release* 2004;**99**(3):369–381.

131. Torchilin VP, Levchenko TS, Lukyanov AN, Khaw BA, Klibanov AL, Rammohan R et al. p-Nitrophenylcarbonyl-PEG-PE-liposomes: Fast and simple attachment of specific ligands, including monoclonal antibodies, to distal ends of PEG chains via p-nitrophenylcarbonyl groups. *Biochim Biophys Acta* 2001;**1511**(2):397–411.

132. Datta R, Rubin E, Sukhatme V, Qureshi S, Hallahan D, Weichselbaum RR et al. Ionizing radiation activates transcription of the EGR1 gene via CArG elements. *Proc Natl Acad Sci USA* 1992;**89**(21):10149–10153.

133. Datta R, Taneja N, Sukhatme VP, Qureshi SA, Weichselbaum R, Kufe DW. Reactive oxygen intermediates target CC(A/T)6GG sequences to mediate activation of the early growth response 1 transcription factor gene by ionizing radiation. *Proc Natl Acad Sci USA* 1993;**90**(6):2419–2422.

134. Weichselbaum RR, Hallahan DE, Beckett MA, Mauceri HJ, Lee H, Sukhatme VP et al. Gene therapy targeted by radiation preferentially radiosensitizes tumor cells. *Cancer Res* 1994;**54**(16):4266–4269.

135. Staba MJ, Mauceri HJ, Kufe DW, Hallahan DE, Weichselbaum RR. Adenoviral TNF-alpha gene therapy and radiation damage tumor vasculature in a human malignant glioma xenograft. *Gene Ther* 1998;**5**(3):293–300.

136. Mundt AJ, Vijayakumar S, Nemunaitis J, Sandler A, Schwartz H, Hanna N et al. A Phase I trial of TNFerade biologic in patients with soft tissue sarcoma in the extremities. *Clin Cancer Res* 2004;**10**(17):5747–5753.

137. Senzer N, Mani S, Rosemurgy A, Nemunaitis J, Cunningham C, Guha C et al. TNFerade biologic, an adenovector with a radiation-inducible promoter, carrying the human tumor necrosis factor alpha gene: A phase I study in patients with solid tumors. *J Clin Oncol* 2004;**22**(4):592–601.

138. Advani SJ, Sibley GS, Song PY, Hallahan DE, Kataoka Y, Roizman B et al. Enhancement of replication of genetically engineered herpes simplex viruses by ionizing radiation: A new paradigm for destruction of therapeutically intractable tumors. *Gene Ther* 1998;**5**(2):160–165.

139. Chou J, Kern ER, Whitley RJ, Roizman B. Mapping of herpes simplex virus-1 neurovirulence to gamma 134.5, a gene nonessential for growth in culture. *Science* 1990;**250**(4985):1262–1266.

140. Chou J, Roizman B. The gamma 1(34.5) gene of herpes simplex virus 1 precludes neuroblastoma cells from triggering total shutoff of protein synthesis characteristic of programed cell death in neuronal cells. *Proc Natl Acad Sci USA* 1992;**89**(8):3266–3270.

141. Chou J, Roizman B. Herpes simplex virus 1 gamma(1)34.5 gene function, which blocks the host response to infection, maps in the homologous domain of the genes expressed during growth arrest and DNA damage. *Proc Natl Acad Sci USA* 1994;**91**(12):5247–5251.

142. Chou J, Chen JJ, Gross M, Roizman B. Association of a M(r) 90,000 phosphoprotein with protein kinase PKR in cells exhibiting enhanced phosphorylation of translation initiation factor eIF-2 alpha and premature shutoff of protein synthesis after infection with gamma 134.5-mutants of herpes simplex virus 1. *Proc Natl Acad Sci USA* 1995;**92**(23):10516–10520.

143. Markovitz NS, Baunoch D, Roizman B. The range and distribution of murine central nervous system cells infected with the gamma(1)34.5-mutant of herpes simplex virus 1. *J Virol* 1997;**71**(7):5560–5569.

144. Meignier B, Longnecker R, Roizman B. In vivo behavior of genetically engineered herpes simplex viruses R7017 and R7020: Construction and evaluation in rodents. *J Infect Dis* 1988;**158**(3):602–614.

145. Meignier B, Martin B, Whitley RJ, Roizman B. In vivo behavior of genetically engineered herpes simplex viruses R7017 and R7020. II. Studies in immunocompetent and immunosuppressed owl monkeys (*Aotus trivirgatus*). *J Infect Dis* 1990;**162**(2):313–321.

146. Chung SM, Advani SJ, Bradley JD, Kataoka Y, Vashistha K, Yan SY et al. The use of a genetically engineered herpes simplex virus (R7020) with ionizing radiation for experimental hepatoma. *Gene Ther* 2002;**9**(1):75–80.

147. Advani SJ, Chung SM, Yan SY, Gillespie GY, Markert JM, Whitley RJ et al. Replication-competent, nonneuroinvasive genetically engineered herpes virus is highly effective in the treatment of therapy-resistant experimental human tumors. *Cancer Res* 1999;**59**(9):2055–2058.

148. Bradley JD, Kataoka Y, Advani S, Chung SM, Arani RB, Gillespie GY et al. Ionizing radiation improves survival in mice bearing intracranial high-grade gliomas injected with genetically modified herpes simplex virus. *Clin Cancer Res* 1999;**5**(6):1517–1522.

149. Abela RA, Qian J, Xu L, Lawrence TS, Zhang M. Radiation improves gene delivery by a novel transferrin-lipoplex nanoparticle selectively in cancer cells. *Cancer Gene Ther* 2008;**15**(8):496–507.

150. Muruve DA. The innate immune response to adenovirus vectors. *Hum Gene Ther* 2004;**15**(12):1157–1166.

151. Pirollo KF, Xu L, Chang EH. Non-viral gene delivery for p53. *Curr Opin Mol Ther* 2000;**2**(2):168–175.

152. Elliott RL, Elliott MC, Wang F, Head JF. Breast carcinoma and the role of iron metabolism. A cytochemical, tissue culture, and ultrastructural study. *Ann NY Acad Sci* 1993;**698**:159–166.

153. Inoue T, Cavanaugh PG, Steck PA, Brunner N, Nicolson GL. Differences in transferrin response and numbers of transferrin receptors in rat and human mammary carcinoma lines of different metastatic potentials. *J Cell Physiol* 1993;**156**(1):212–217.

154. Ishida O, Maruyama K, Tanahashi H, Iwatsuru M, Sasaki K, Eriguchi M et al. Liposomes bearing polyethyleneglycol-coupled transferrin with intracellular targeting property to the solid tumors in vivo. *Pharm Res* 2001;**18**(7):1042–1048.

155. Joshee N, Bastola DR, Cheng PW. Transferrin-facilitated lipofection gene delivery strategy: Characterization of the transfection complexes and intracellular trafficking. *Hum Gene Ther* 2002;**13**(16):1991–2004.

156. Keer HN, Kozlowski JM, Tsai YC, Lee C, McEwan RN, Grayhack JT. Elevated transferrin receptor content in human prostate cancer cell lines assessed in vitro and in vivo. *J Urol* 1990;**143**(2):381–385.

157. Yanagihara K, Cheng H, Cheng PW. Effects of epidermal growth factor, transferrin, and insulin on lipofection efficiency in human lung carcinoma cells. *Cancer Gene Ther* 2000;**7**(1):59–65.

158. Xu L, Pirollo KF, Chang EH. Transferrin-liposome-mediated p53 sensitization of squamous cell carcinoma of the head and neck to radiation in vitro. *Hum Gene Ther* 1997;**8**(4):467–475.

159. Xu L, Pirollo KF, Chang EH. Tumor-targeted p53-gene therapy enhances the efficacy of conventional chemo/radiotherapy. *J Control Release* 2001;**74**(1–3):115–128.

160. Xu L, Pirollo KF, Tang WH, Rait A, Chang EH. Transferrin-liposome-mediated systemic p53 gene therapy in combination with radiation results in regression of human head and neck cancer xenografts. *Hum Gene Ther* 1999;**10**(18):2941–2952.

161. Kalofonos H, Rowlinson G, Epenetos AA. Enhancement of monoclonal-antibody uptake in human-colon tumor xenografts following irradiation. *Cancer Res* 1990;**50**(1):159–163.

162. Davies Cde L, Lundstrom LM, Frengen J, Eikenes L, Bruland SO, Kaalhus O et al. Radiation improves the distribution and uptake of liposomal doxorubicin (caelyx) in human osteosarcoma xenografts. *Cancer Res* 2004;**64**(2):547–553.

163. Gabrys D, Greco O, Patel G, Prise KM, Tozer GM, Kanthou C. Radiation effects on the cytoskeleton of endothelial cells and endothelial monolayer permeability. *Int J Radiat Oncol Biol Phys* 2007;**69**(5):1553–1562.

164. Friedman M, Ryan US, Davenport WC, Chaney EL, Strickland DL, Kwock L. Reversible alterations in cultured pulmonary artery endothelial cell monolayer morphology and albumin permeability induced by ionizing radiation. *J Cell Physiol* 1986;**129**(2):237–249.

165. Diaz R, Hariri G, Passarella RJ, Wu H, Fu A, Hallahan DE. Radiation-guided platinum drug delivery using recombinant peptides. *Int J Radiat Oncol Biol Phys* 2008;**72**(1):S1.
166. Jaboin JI, Fu A, Hariri G, Han Z, Hallahan D. Novel radiation-guided nanoparticle drug delivery system for prostate cancer. *Int J Radiat Oncol Biol Phys* 2007;**69**(3):S111.
167. Hawiger J, Kloczewiak M, Bednarek MA, Timmons S. Platelet receptor recognition domains on the alpha chain of human fibrinogen: Structure-function analysis. *Biochemistry* 1989;**28**(7):2909–2914.
168. Niessen HW, Krijnen PA, Visser CA, Meijer CJ, Hack CE. Intercellular adhesion molecule-1 in the heart. *Ann N Y Acad Sci* 2002;**973**:573–585.
169. Diaz R, Passarella RJ, Hallahan DE. Determining glioma response to radiation therapy using recombinant peptides. *Expert Rev Anticancer Ther* 2008;**8**(11):1787–1796.

Part II

Nucleic Acid Delivery and Targeting

5 Recent Advances in Gene Expression and Delivery Systems

Ravikiran Panakanti and Ram I. Mahato

CONTENTS

5.1   INTRODUCTION

The potential use of genes as therapeutics has attracted great attention to treat severe and debilitating diseases. Gene therapy is the method of treating diseases using genes so that the patient's somatic cells can produce the specific proteins that are lacking. This will prevent the limitations concerning the administration of therapeutic proteins. It is an approach for treating diseases, or ultimately preventing a disease, by replacing defective genes, introducing new genes, or changing the endogenous expression of genes.

Gene therapy uses viral or nonviral vectors to deliver genes to synthesize specific therapeutic proteins. Viral vectors are derived from retroviruses, lentiviruses, adenoviruses (Adv), adeno-associated viruses (AAV), herpes viruses, and pox viruses.[1] The development of vectors for cell-specific gene expression is the major goal of any gene therapeutic strategy. Significant progress has been made in the construction of gene expression vectors that combine different functions required for efficient gene transfer.[2]

Gene medicine usually contains an expression system that controls the transcription of a gene within the target cell and a specific delivery system that controls the biodistribution of these vectors to specific locations in the body. Cationic liposomes, peptides, and polymers are commonly used as transfection reagents for gene expression plasmids, while viral vectors usually do not require any of these transfection reagents.

> Immune activation by viral vectors is a major concern as many of the vectors with high therapeutic activity *in vitro* fail *in vivo*.[3] Furthermore, scale-up of their production could be challenging. Gene expression plasmids offer multiple advantages over viral gene therapy vectors, including large packaging capacity, stability without integration into the host genome, and lower toxicity. However, their level of expression is often lower and shorter than the viral vectors.

Viral vectors have shown much promise in the field of gene therapy, but there are safety issues and they may also be limited in terms of their DNA-loading capacities.[2] Immune activation by viral vectors is a major concern as many of the vectors with high therapeutic activity *in vitro* fail to do so *in vivo*.[3] Moreover, increasing their yield can be quite difficult. To minimize their immunogenicity, the surface of the viral vectors is often modified by conjugating to poly(ethylene glycol) (PEG).[4]

Gene expression plasmids offer many advantages over viral vectors, including large packaging capacity, no integration into the host genome, and lower toxicity. However, their level of gene expression is often lower and shorter than that of the viral vectors. Recent advances in gene expression systems have shown great improvement in the transfection levels of nonviral vectors. Plasmid vectors can also be used to silence a gene, thereby causing the inhibition of an abnormal protein production in the body.[5] Plasmids have also been shown to play a role in the formation of viral vectors, e.g., two plasmid rescue systems were used to construct an adenoviral vector.

In this chapter, we discuss the recent advances in the development of gene expression and delivery systems, some of the underlying problems involving their use, and approaches to address these issues.

5.2   GENE EXPRESSION SYSTEMS

Gene expression systems are broadly classified into plasmid and viral vectors. Basically, these vectors have the machinery in them to facilitate the production of target proteins in the host upon transfection or transduction.

5.2.1   BASIC COMPONENTS OF PLASMID VECTORS

A gene expression plasmid contains a complementary DNA (cDNA) sequence coding for either a full gene or a minigene, and several other genetic elements including promoters, introns, polyadenylation (polyA) sequences, and transcript stabilizers to control the transcription, translation, and protein stability and/or secretion from the host cell.[6]

The transcription unit comprises of 5' enhancers–promoters upstream of the gene, encoding a therapeutic protein and polyA signal downstream of the gene. An intron is also assembled into an either 5' or 3' untranslated region (UTR), leading to the elevation of mRNA levels. Plasmid vectors can be designed to express two genes simultaneously driven by different promoters or a single promoter or by insertion of an internal ribosome entry site (IRES). IRES was first discovered in picornaviruses, encephalomyocarditis virus (ECMV) and poliovirus.[7,8] They have the ability to translate two open reading frames (ORF) from a single mRNA transcript. Usually the IRES is inserted between two transgenes to be expressed. IRES confers the unequal expression of genes, and usually the expression of the downstream gene is relatively higher than the upstream gene, which may confirm the internal ribosome entry.[8] However, recent studies have shown that this may not be always true. The production of low levels of monocistronic RNAs is putatively due to the splicing of the bicistronic transcript due to the presence of 3' splice site (ss), which can show an increased expression of the downstream gene.[9] This warrants for a careful RNA structural analysis to confirm the functionality of IRES.

We have constructed a bicistronic plasmid vector (phVEGF-hIL-1Ra) encoding human vascular endothelial growth factor (hVEGF) and human interleukin-1 receptor antagonist (hIL-1Ra) driven by cytomegalovirus (CMV) and elongation factor-1α (EF-1α) promoters, respectively in the pBudCE4.1 vector.[10] There was a dose- and time-dependent expression of hVEGF and hIL-1Ra genes when they were transfected to human islets. However, the expression levels of these two genes were not sufficient enough to decrease the blood glucose levels of diabetic mice following transplantation with phVEGF-hIL-1Ra transfected islets. Not only the expression, but the extent of the expression of genes was also low for this bicistronic plasmid.

5.2.1.1 Bacterial Elements

Plasmids encode two features that are important for their propagation in bacteria. One is the bacterial origin of replication (Ori), which is a specific DNA sequence that binds to factors that regulate the replication of plasmids and in turn control the number of copies of plasmids per bacterium. The second required element is a selectable marker, usually a gene that confers resistance to an antibiotic. The marker helps in the selection of bacteria that have the gene expression plasmid of interest. *Escherichia coli* (*E. coli*) are commonly used bacteria for propagating plasmids. It has the property to transfer DNA either by bacterial conjugation, transduction, or transformation. The extensive knowledge about *E. coli*'s physiology and genetics accounts for its preferential use as a host for gene expression. Human insulin was the first product to be produced using recombinant DNA technology from *E. coli*.

5.2.1.2 Transcription Regulatory Elements

Gene expressing plasmids contain transcription regulatory elements (TREs) to control transcription. The Jacob and Monad theory postulates that a repressor protein may bind to the operator region downstream of a promoter preventing RNA polymerase from binding to the host DNA.[11] This operator region may overlap with the promoter for the operon being controlled. However, if this repressor is controlled, it may increase gene expression.[12] TREs play a significant role in gene expression and may also impart specificity. The important sequences in the gene that control transcription are the cis-acting sequences that are situated in the immediate vicinity of the gene and they together constitute the functional unit or domain.[13]

Heterologous TREs can be included in the adenoviral genome to allow replication only in the cells in which TREs are functional, resulting in cell specificity.[14] The addition of new TREs in an expression vector can alter the transcription of the target gene. These new elements can mimic the action of the genomic TREs of the target genes resulting in an alteration in transcription. These elements can be added to either increase or decrease transcription depending on the requirement.

In diseases like cancer, the expression of target genes can be altered by this method.[15] For example, homeodomain-containing transcription factor pancreatic duodenal homeobox-1 (Pdx-1) plays a key role in maintaining the function of the pancreas and is also known to have a prominent role in beta cell development.[16] When this Pdx-1 was introduced into an adenoviral vector and expressed in hepatocytes, they were transformed into pancreatic endocrine hormone–producing cells.[17] Modulating the expression vector with TREs can be done to increase the gene expression.

5.2.1.3   Enhancer

An enhancer is a short region of DNA that can bind trans-acting factors, much like a set of transcription factors, to enhance transcription levels of genes in a gene-cluster. Usually, in the bound, proteins facilitate promoter-binding proteins to interact with the promoter.[18] An enhancer does not need to be particularly close to the genes it acts on, and need not be located on the same chromosome. An enhancer does not need to bind close to the transcription initiation site to affect its transcription, as some have been found to bind several hundred thousand base pairs upstream or downstream of the start site.[19] Enhancers can also be found within introns. An enhancer's orientation may even be reversed without affecting its function. Furthermore, an enhancer may be excised and inserted elsewhere in the chromosome, and still affect gene transcription.[20] That is the reason why intron polymorphisms are important, even though they are not transcribed and translated. Enhancer–promoter interaction also plays a major role in immune reaction following the *in vivo* administration of plasmid vectors. An epo enhancer when inserted into the plasmid expressing vascular endothelial growth factor (VEGF) showed an expression of VEGF in hypoxia conditions, whereas the plasmid without the epo enhancer showed no expression of VEGF.[21]

5.2.1.4   Promoter

A promoter is a DNA sequence that enables a gene to be transcribed. The promoter is recognized by RNA polymerase, which binds it and then initiates transcription. Promoters regulate protein synthesis indirectly by having an active role in demarcating genes to be used for mRNA synthesis. The promoter region is usually the beginning of an operon, which is a collection of neighboring genes, and controls the region transcribed into the same mRNA molecule.[22] Therefore, DNA transcription begins after RNA polymerase has bound downstream of the therapeutic gene. This effect is seen as DNA unwinding into single strands. Therefore, any mutation in this region will prevent RNA polymerase from binding. Transcription begins at the first base of the target gene+1 position, which is the TATAA sequence or TATA box, 5′TATA (A/T) A (A/T)-3′. This region ensures that transcription starts at the proper point and binds the RNA polymerase II complex.[23] Another transcription start site is the CCAAT box (consensus sequences 5′-GGTC-CAATCT-3′) located upstream of the TATA box.

Promoter sequences play an important role not only in initializing gene transcription, but also in immunostimulation.[24] The promoter type governs the strength and duration of transgene expression. Viral promoter elements are first known to be used in an expression vector to express proteins for gene therapy. The CMV, Rous sarcoma virus (RSV), and Simian virus 40 (SV40) are some of the strongest known viral promoters. However, there are some drawbacks with the use of viral promoters such as a lack of specificity and immunostimulation that results in inactivation. For example, a CMV promoter shows expression in most cell types, however, its activity decreases over a period of 3–4 weeks.[25] This is possibly due to the inhibition by cytokines, methylation, or inactivation by repressor proteins. This is also true for other viral promoters like SV40 and RSV.[26] Because of these reasons, there is an urgent need to develop promoters based on nonviral cellular regulatory elements.

Sustained gene expression is quite difficult to achieve. However, some promoters have been reported to confer sustained gene expression from plasmid DNA *in vivo*. These promoters include β-actin, EF-1α, or ubiquitin. The activity of these promoters is usually lower than that of viral promoters, but can be increased by the addition of viral or cellular enhancer components.[27] The CMV early enhancer/chicken β actin (CAG) is a promoter of this kind. It consists of a CMV enhancer and first intron of chicken (or human skeletal) β-actin. It shows activity similar to or more than the CMV promoter.[28,29] It shows a greater activity in viral vectors, but its expression profile needs to be established for use in plasmid vectors.[26]

The EF 1-α promoter has been reported to confer sustained gene expression compared with the CMV promoter, but its expression is 10-fold lower than the CMV promoter.[30] Promoters from three of the known human ubiquitin genes UBA, UBC, and UBB have been incorporated in plasmid vectors. Luciferase gene expression was measurable up to 6 months when the plasmid contained UBC promoter.[30] This clearly suggests that if proper promoters are incorporated into the gene expression system, it is possible to attain sustained gene expression.

5.2.1.5 Untranslated Region

The 5′ untranslated region (5′-UTR) is the region of the mRNA transcript that is located between the capsite and the initiation codon. The linkage between the methylated G residue and the 5′ to 5′ triphosphate bridge is known as the cap structure, which is essential for the efficient initiation of protein synthesis. The 5′-UTR is known to influence mRNA translation efficiency. In eukaryotic cells, initiation factors first interact with the 5′ cap structure and prepare the mRNA by unwinding its secondary structure. An efficient 5′-UTR is usually moderate in length, devoid of a secondary structure, and upstream from initiation codons. It has AUG with an optimal context. Any of the following features that influence the accessibility of the 5′ cap structure to initiation factors will influence the mRNA translability.[31,32]

Initiation codon AUG appears to be the best recognized when it is in the context of the sequence CCRCCAUGG with purine (R) at −3 and/or guanidine (G) at +4 (A of AUG is numbered +1). If an AUG occurs alone or an AUG in conjunction with a short ORF is located between the cap site and the genuine AUG, translation will be inhibited. Secondary structures of the UTRs inhibit translation. 5′-UTR lengths that are greater than 32, but less than 100 nucleotides permit efficient recognition of the first AUG. Most naturally occurring 5′-UTRs are 50–100 nucleotides in length.

The 3′UTR comprises the mRNA sequence following the termination codon. It plays an important role in mRNA stability.[22] AU rich motifs are commonly found in the 3′UTR of mRNA of cytokines, growth factors, and oncogenes. These are mRNA instability elements and should be removed for maximal gene expression. This is achieved when the standard 3′UTR sequence is used in place of the one found in cDNA. Another way is to minimize the length of the 3′UTR by placing the hexanucleotide of the poly A signal immediately downstream of the stop codon.[33]

5.2.1.6 Polyadenylation Signal

The efficiency of poly A is important for gene expression, as transcripts that failed to be cleaved and polyadenylated are rapidly degraded in the nuclear compartment.[34] The poly A signal is a recognition site consisting of the AAUAAA hexamer positioned 10–30 nucleotides upstream of the 5′ end and a GU or U rich element located maximally 30 nucleotides downstream of the 3′ end.[22] The poly A signal is needed for the formation of the 3′ end of most eukaryotic mRNA. It directs two RNA-processing reactions: the site-specific endonucleolytic cleavage of the RNA transcript and the stepwise addition of adenylates to the newly generated 3′ end to form the poly A tail.

5.2.1.7 Intron

The protein coding region in the gene is often interrupted by stretches of noncoding DNA called intron. Transcripts from intronless genes are rapidly degraded in the nuclear compartment, leading to lower gene expression.[35] Therefore, for maximal gene expression in eukaryotic cells, at least one intron should be included within the transcription unit. Introns also promote mRNA export from the nucleus. The addition of intron A or B to the plasmid encoding ICAM-2 promoter and subsequent expression in HUVEC or PsCAM cells increased the expression of the transgene.[28] Introns thus can affect gene expression and if used in a proper way can enhance the expression of transgenes.

5.2.1.8 Stop Signal

Stop signal is the DNA sequence at which RNA polymerase II is halted and detached from the DNA, thereby a stop or nonsense codon stops translation. However, poly A occurs at the 5′ AAUAAA 3′ sequence in the mRNA. The poly A polymerase cleaves after the U residue and adds 50–250 adenylate residues. The stop signal not only plays an important role in gene regulation at the translational level allowing for rapid changes in specific protein levels, but also provides an opportunity to alter codon specificity.

5.2.1.9 Multiple Cloning Sites

A multiple cloning site (MCS), also known as a polylinker, is a short segment of DNA that contains many restriction sites. Restriction sites within an MCS are unique and occur only once within a particular plasmid. MCSs are commonly used for the cloning of single or multiple cDNAs due to its unique restriction endonuclease recognition sites identified with ease. The recombinant plasmid can be altered in such a way that the desired gene can be inserted into the plasmid and expressed. If there is no particular restriction site for a particular transgene, the restriction site can also be inserted into the MCS and can clone the gene.

5.2.1.10 Fusion Tags

Fusion tags are inserted in expression systems so that the DNA location and site specificity can be known. A variety of protein tags have been used to allow recombinant fusion protein to be detected and purified without the use of an antibody or other protein specific assays. Short epitope tags and fluorescent protein tags are commonly used for gene function studies. Epitope tags such as His/C-term, xpress, V5, FLAG, HA, and c-myc circumvent the requirement for specific antibodies against target proteins. Fluorescent protein tags, such as green fluorescent protein (GFP), provides information on the cellular location of the fusion proteins. Since the addition of any amino acid residues may alter the properties of the target proteins, special consideration should be given to the intended use of the protein and on minimizing the adverse effects when picking a tag. Typically, a specific protease cleavage site is introduced in the tag and the target protein to facilitate tag removal if desired. Fusion tags can be incorporated into the plasmid vectors to enhance the protein expression and solubility of the expressed protein.[36] Fusion tags can be classified into two types based on their application: affinity tags and solubility-enhancing tags. Affinity tags help in the purification of recombinant protein, whereas the solubility-enhancing tags can be used to improve the solubility of proteins. Usually the solubility-enhancing tags are either large peptides or proteins. Fusion tags like glutathione *S*-transferase (GST) and maltose binding protein (MBP) show both affinity and solubility-enhancing properties.[37,38]

5.2.2 Persistence of Gene Expression

The regulation of gene expression and having a sustained expression is the key for many diseases. Plasmid-based systems usually confer transient gene expression with less than 20% of the peak level at day 3.[39] This warrants the need for expression of transgene over a period of time. This is especially important in diseases like cancer where the cells divide continuously. An ideal nonviral vector should be able to provide persistent expression of the transgenes without affecting the host cells. Persistent gene expression can be achieved either by the prevention of promoter attenuation, use of replicating plasmid, modulation of immune response, attachment of matrix/scaffold regions, or optimizing plasmid size.

5.2.2.1 Prevention of Promoter Attenuation

The major drawback of nonviral vectors is the lack of sustained gene expression. Transient gene expression *in vivo* is partly due to promoter shutdown.[26] This is especially true for viral promoters, such as CMV and SV40 promoters. The methylation of plasmid DNA is involved in promoter inactivation, which can be prevented by removing the methylation sites (CpG motifs) from the plasmid construct. Transient gene expression is also due to the destruction of the transfected cells by the immune system.[40] Viral promoters are sensitive to cytokines, which may explain the decline of their activity *in vivo*.[26] Promoter inactivation has also been attributed to specific tissue types. For example, smooth muscle gamma actin (SMGA) and flk-1 promoters show their activity specifically in smooth muscles and endothelium, respectively.[2]

5.2.2.2 Use of Replicating Plasmids

Extrachromosomally replicating vectors have great potential for use in gene therapy due to their high transfection levels and sustained expression of transgenes. The use of replicating plasmids results in sustained gene expression without the integration of genes into the host genome. This also reduces the risk of insertional mutagenesis. Replication elements, usually from viral DNA, are inserted into the expression systems that enable the plasmid to replicate extra chromosomally. This can be done by the introduction of a mammalian Ori[41] sequence into the plasmid. The best characterized Oris in mammalian cells are from viral sources, such as SV40, the BK virus (BKV), the bovine papilloma virus (BPV), and the Epstein Barr virus (EBV).[42] Modeling the bacterial power and efficiency of self-replication would greatly increase therapeutic protein expression.

Since the plasmids do not integrate into the host genome, they reside outside as episomes. They have several advantages over integrating systems: (1) the transgene is not interrupted or subjected to regulatory constraints that often occur from integration into cellular DNA, (2) they have higher transfection efficiency, (3) episomes show a low mutation rate and tend not to rearrange, and (4) they have the ability to transfer large amounts of DNA.[2]

Plasmids can replicate in both prokaryotic and eukaryotic cells provided they have certain elements that allow them to do that, e.g., EBV viral elements.[43,44] Several viral constructs including EBV, BKV, SV40, and BPV have been used in constructing replicating plasmid vectors. Trans-acting factors are needed for the formation of episomal vectors, but there is a risk of transformation following their use. This is especially seen in the case of polyomaviruses (BKV, SV40), which contain a T-antigen (Tag) as a trans-acting factor. Tag purportedly binds to tumor suppressor gene p53 causing chromosomal aberrations and alters the gene expression.[45] Considering this, EBV viral elements are safer as they have a low mutation frequency and can easily incorporate large amounts of DNA.[45] EBV nuclear antigen 1 (EBNA1) and oriP constitute the EBV viral elements that impart stability to the viral DNA in the host cells.[43,45] EBNA1 dimer/oriP complex controls the replication and transcription of the plasmid vector. EBNA facilitates the binding of the plasmid vector to the nuclear matrix. EBV-based vectors showed a higher expression of transgenes compared with conventional vectors when they were studied *in vivo*. However, EBV-based vectors are associated with certain drawbacks including integration into the host genome and oncogenicity.[45] Ehrhardt et al. replaced the CMV promoter with a cellular promoter to minimize the silencing effects attributed to nonmammalian sequences.[46] However, if the problems associated with the use of viral elements can be solved, they can be far superior than the conventional vectors.

5.2.2.3 Modulation of Immune Response

One of the major drawbacks of gene therapy is the interaction of the gene expression vectors with the host immune system. Although nonviral vectors produce less immune response compared with viral vectors, their effect should not be overlooked. CpG motifs are unmethylated with an ability to stimulate B cell proliferation, macrophage activation, and the maturation of dendritic cells. The bacterial and viral DNA contain a large amount of unmethylated CpG motifs. Plasmid vectors usually contain bacterial or viral elements with a large number of CpG motifs, which lead to the acute inflammatory response commonly seen in nonviral vectors. The sequence GTCGTT is the most active stimulatory CpG motif in humans leading to the activation of immune pathways. Following activation of the immune system by the CpG motifs, gene expression is decreased due to cytokine mediated promoter shutdown and apoptosis of expressing cells.

> The second generation of adenoviral vectors are less immunogenic, since some of the genes of the adenoviral genome were deleted. However, their expression was not longer than 20–40 days. Following this, gutless vectors were generated in which all the adenoviral genes were deleted. They showed expression for about 84 days.

When constructing plasmid vectors, the immunostimulation of the CpG motifs can be reduced by the methylation of the CpG motifs using neutralizing CpG motifs or by the elimination of CpG motifs. Plasmid vectors containing a significantly lower amount of CpG motifs showed less immunostimulation compared with the ones with more CpG motifs.[47] The presence of a single unmethylated CpG has been shown to elicit an inflammatory response when delivered to the lung.

However, CpG free vectors showed no inflammatory response and increased the duration of transgene expression in the lung.[30]

5.2.2.4 Matrix/Scaffold Attachment Regions

Matrix/scaffold attachment regions (MARs) govern the architecture of the nucleus by establishing protein boundaries. Several proteins bind to MARs and these proteins are known as MAR binding proteins. MAR binding proteins are very significant as they regulate transcription, replication, repair, and combination.[48] Thus, the incorporation of MARs in the plasmid construct may be helpful in maintaining episomal plasmid for extended periods. The potentially immunostimulatory and transforming properties of viral protein used in episomes and other components of the expression system impede the application of these systems for gene therapy. Alternatively, MARs can be incorporated into circular plasmids to replace transacting viral gene products. MARs have been characterized as AT rich sequences generally composed of 4–6 bp motifs such as ATTA, ATTTA, or ATTTTA.[49] These sequences are commonly used with gene enhancers and the Ori. Incorporation of these sequences has been used to enhance the transcriptional activity of integrated transgenes.[49]

MARs are often situated in proximity to promoters, replication origins, and other important regions in the genome. MARs have been known to play a role in several biological activities due to their affinity to the nuclear matrix. They have been known to play a role in the initiation of transcription, promote long-term expression of the transcript by counteracting the effects of DNA methylation, protect transgenes from the negative effects of the genomic surroundings and promote histone acetylation, act as an enhancer, and promote replication.[50] MARs have been incorporated in episomally replicating plasmids to impart stability to the vector and increase the longevity of transgene expression. MARs are used to replace the viral elements from these vectors to minimize the immunostimulatory effects from them. An episomal vector was developed by replacing the Tag protein with MARs from the human β-interferon gene while retaining the SV40 Ori sequence. This vector replicated episomally in CHO cells and showed stable expression for more than 100 divisions. Argyros et al.[51] demonstrated persistent transgene expression in the liver after hydrodynamic injection of the plasmid containing MARs driven by the human liver specific promoter α1-anti-trypsin (AAT). MARs protected the AAT promoter by inhibiting the methylation of CpG motifs, resulting in a sustained expression of luciferase,[51] while the plasmid containing MARs and CMV promoter did not show persistent luciferase expression. This signifies that even though MARs impart extra-chromosomal stability, the duration of gene expression also depends on the choice of promoter used.

5.2.2.5 Plasmid Size

Plasmid stability is dependent on its size. Most gene therapy studies use plasmids of less than 10 kb. To prolong gene expression, bacterial artificial chromosomes (BACs) have been used in nondividing cultures.[52] A BAC-plasmid vector encoding a 185 kb DNA insert of the human beta globin gene and EBV orip and EBNA-1 transactivator showed persistent gene expression indicating the usefulness of plasmid size.[53] An episomal BAC vector encoding the entire genomic human low-density lipoprotein receptor (LDLR) and LacZ showed high transfection and persistent gene expression of LDLR and LacZ.[54]

Bacterial components in the plasmid vector are known to elicit immunostimulation. Therefore, several research groups are investigating the possible use of minicircle plasmids, which do not have bacterial Ori or antibiotic resistance markers. These are generated in *E. coli* by site-specific recombinations. Following an injection of minicircle plasmid encoding $VEGF_{165}$ into the Balb/c mouse heart and skeletal muscle, $VEGF_{165}$ gene expression levels were similar or higher to that observed with conventional plasmid vectors encoding $VEGF_{165}$.[55] In another study, a minicircle-mediated delivery of Interferon-γ (IFN-γ) was more efficient in inducing antiproliferative and anti-tumor effects in human nasopharyngeal cancer cell lines than conventional vectors due to its sustained expression of IFN-γ levels.[56] This suggests that minicircle plasmids may be a viable alternative to conventional plasmids vectors.

5.2.3 SITE-SPECIFIC GENE EXPRESSION

The targeting of gene medicines to specific cells is often required to prevent toxicity to healthy cells and to decrease the required dose. Differential gene expression among cell types is possible because different genes are driven by different sets of promoters and enhancer sequences, and each of these regulatory binding sequences contain binding sites for multiple transcription factors. Changing the set of transcription factors will lead to the activation of a different set of genes, leading to a change in the cell's protein expression profile. The selective expression of transgenes in specific cells or tissues can be achieved by constructing DNA expression cassettes that contain gene regulatory regions that are recognized by transcription factors specially present in or selectively expressed by the target cell population. This targeting is based on tissue specificity where transcription is directed specifically among healthy tissues or is tumor specific by using elements that are active in tumor cells due to aberrant gene expression or tumor biology.

There are various well characterized regulatory elements controlling cell type specific expression, with target tissues including the pancreas, breasts, bones, brain, kidney, bladder, lungs, and liver. Tissue-specific promoters display a natural activity in normal tissues without discriminating the diseased cells from the healthy ones. Therefore, for toxic protein expression, the use of tissue-specific promoters is limited to dispensable tissues such as melanocytes, prostate, breasts, endocrine, and exocrine tissues.[4,57,58] Combining tissue-specific promoters with additional targeting moieties can further increase their utility. For example, a combination of tumor- and tissue-specific promoters may enable the targeting of specific cells/malignancies within nondispensable tissues. Cellular regulatory elements often have low activity, which can be addressed by the inclusion of a strong promoter element from a viral or cellular origin. For example, Pujal and colleagues have shown the specificity of the keratin 7 promoter, which is expressed in pancreatic ductal cells predominantly rather than in acinar cells that depend on the krt 7–234 bp sequence. This sequence is included in a plasmid or viral vector and exhibits the same specificity as the krt7 promoter and may help in targeting pancreatic ductal adenocarcinoma cells *in vitro* and *in vivo*.[59] Targeting expression to a particular organ, tissue, and cell greatly reduces the antibody response to a foreign protein and results in sustained expression.[60]

Most composite promoters contain one or two enhancer elements fused to a heterologous promoter sequence. This concept has been used to create promoters with combinations of regulatory sequences. Li et al. randomly assembled muscle-specific elements from four different muscle-specific promoters and then screened these novel promoters for activity.[61] One sequence showed 8-times the activity of natural muscle promoters. However, this was done *in vitro*. It is more challenging to develop a promoter with greater expression *in vivo*.

5.2.4 PULSATILE GENE EXPRESSION

A gene switch is introduced into an expression system to make use of the circadian rhythm by extraneously administering a compound to control the production of therapeutic proteins by turning on or off the transcription of an administered gene. Gene switches are incorporated into the vector for gene regulation. This feedback control may prevent overexpression and possible deleterious protein production. In this system, the target gene is inactive until the administration of an exogenous compound or ligand.[62,63] Progesterone antagonists, tetracycline, ecdysone, and rapamycin are used as inducing agents to turn on the gene regulation of the expression vector.

5.3 VIRAL VECTORS

Recombinant viruses are unique in being naturally evolved vehicles that efficiently transfer their genes into host cells. Viral vectors are composed of either an RNA or a DNA core, or process different genomic structure and host ranges. However, they often have risks such as toxicity, immunogenicity, and/or potential for viral recombination. The novel developments of viral vectors mainly aim at the reduction of immunogenicity and improved vector production. Several kinds of viruses including retrovirus, Adv, AAV, and herpes simplex virus (HSV) have been manipulated for gene transfer. These viral vectors have their own unique advantages and disadvantages as discussed below.

5.3.1 RETROVIRAL VECTORS

Retroviruses are enveloped single-stranded RNA viruses. Retroviruses have a genome of about 7–10 kb, composed of gag, pol, and env genes flanked by elements called long terminal repeats (LTRs). These are essential for integration into the host genome and signify the beginning and the end of the viral genome. The LTRs control the expression of viral genes, hence they act as enhancer–promoters. The final element of the genome, the packaging signal (ψ), helps in differentiating the viral RNA from the host RNA.[64] Gag proteins are major components of the viral capsid. Pol proteins are involved in the synthesis of viral DNA and the integration into the host DNA, whereas env proteins play a role in the association and entry of viral particles into the host cell.

The viral genome can be manipulated and viral genes can be replaced by inserting transgenes. The transgenes can be controlled by the LTRs or alternate enhancer–promoter sequences can be engineered within the transgene. The chimeric genome is then introduced into packaging cell lines, which produce all the viral genes but these have been separated from the LTRs and the packaging sequence. So, the chimeric viral genomes are assembled to produce the retroviral vector. The culture medium containing the packaging cells that produce the retroviral vector is used directly to infect target cells for gene transfer.

Retroviral vectors have several advantages including the stable transduction of dividing cells and less immunogenic and persistent transgene expression. However, there are several disadvantages of these vectors. These include random insertion into the host genome, limited DNA insertion capacity (8 kb), low titers, inactivation by complement systems, and the inability to transduce nondividing cells.

5.3.2 LENTIVIRAL VECTORS

Although lentiviral vectors belong to the retroviral family, they have the ability to infect both dividing and nondividing cells.[65] The human immunodeficiency virus (HIV) is the best known lentivirus.[66] The HIV lentiviral vector is very efficient as it has the ability to infect and express genes in human helper T cells and macrophages. Apart from the genes gag, pol, and env, the HIV has six accessory proteins tat, rev, vpr, vpu, nef, and vif. These proteins regulate the synthesis and processing of viral RNA and other replicative functions. The accessory proteins can also be removed without affecting the production efficiency of the virus. The env gene from the HIV-based vectors allows the infection of cells that express protein CD4+, so in these vectors, this is substituted with other env genes from other RNA viruses that have a broader infection spectrum.

The significance of lentiviral vectors lies in the fact that they can efficiently transduce nondividing cells or terminally differentiated cells such as neurons, macrophages, hematopoietic stem cells, muscle and liver cells, and other cell types for which gene therapy methods could not be used. These vectors, when injected into the rodent brain, liver, muscle, or pancreatic islet cells show a sustained gene expression for over 6 months.[67] These vectors do not show any immune response and show no potent antibody response; thus, they can be ideal for *in vivo* gene delivery.

Magnetic nanoparticles have been used for the delivery of lentiviral vectors to the endothelial cells. This method provides the direct targeting of the lentiviral vectors to endothelial cells even in perfused blood vessels apart from increasing the transduction efficiency.[68] However, one problem with the lentiviral vector is the random integration with genomic DNA. This integration, although desirable, can be problematic as it can cause differential gene expression in the cells and most importantly insertational mutagenesis resulting in malignant transformation. To alleviate this effect, nonintegrating lentiviral vectors are developed by point mutations into chromosome binding sites and viral DNA-binding sites of the viral integrase.[69]

5.3.3 ADENOVIRAL VECTORS

Adenoviruses are nonenveloped double-stranded DNA viruses and can infect both dividing and nondividing cells. Natural adenoviruses cause benign respiratory tract infection in humans. Their genome contains many genes and they do not integrate into the host DNA. Replication-deficient adenoviruses can be generated by removing the E-1 genes necessary for viral replication and replacing it with the gene of interest (for example, hepatocyte growth factor [HGF]) and a promoter sequence.[70] These recombinant viruses are replicated in cells that express the product of the E-1 gene and are generated in high concentrations.[71]

> MARs are segments of chromatin prepared to delineate the transcriptional portions of expressed genes. Such transcriptionally active domains are flanked by DNA sequences that specifically associate with the nuclear matrix. Incorporation of MARs in the plasmid constructs results in enhanced retention of the plasmids in the nucleus.

Cells infected with recombinant adenoviruses can express the therapeutic gene, but they cannot replicate as the genes needed for replication are absent. These vectors efficiently transduce cells, and gene expression lasts for about 5–10 days. Therefore, Adv vectors are suitable for transient gene expression unlike retroviral vectors, which show long-term expression. Adv vectors show an extended duration of expression when given to nude mice or with an immunosuppressant indicating that the immune system may be responsible for the short duration of expression.[72]

The immune reaction elicits both cell killing "cellular response" and antibody-producing "humoral response." A cellular response results in the killing of infected cells with T-lymphocytes, whereas the humoral response results in the production of antibodies to Adv proteins, resulting in a diminished transgene expression following subsequent infections.[72,73] Moreover, most human beings are likely to have antibodies to Adv from previous infections as it is a commonly found virus infecting the human population. To address this problem, a second generation of Adv vectors were produced where the other genes of the Adv genome were deleted like the E-3 gene required for eliciting an immune response. However, their expression was not longer than 20–40 days.[74]

Gutless Adv vectors are also generated in which all Adv genes are deleted. The viral DNA contains the start and end of the viral genome along with the viral packaging sequence. They showed expression for about 84 days.[75] However, the production of these gutless Adv vectors is somewhat difficult. Furthermore, they still have immunological problems that need to be overcome for their *in vivo* applications. One way of getting around this problem is to develop strategies to target the viral particles to the required cells, tissues, or organs. The targeting of vectors can ideally lead to less immunological responses, and fewer amounts of viral particles are needed to get the desired therapeutic effect. However, Adv vectors transduce cells more efficiently only in the presence of coxsackievirus and adenovirus receptors (CAR).[76,77] An immune response from Adv vectors can further be attenuated by deleting E4 or a part of the E4 region.

To target the Adv vector to a specific cell or tissue, usually Adv capsid, such as its fiber, protein IX (pIX), or hexon is altered. Of these, fiber proteins are the most studied. These proteins consist of a tail, shaft, and knob.[78] The C-terminal knob is responsible for binding with CAR receptors.[66,79] Targeting was achieved by incorporating an RGD peptide or a stretch of lysine residues (KKKKKKK [K7] peptide), in the fiber knob or hexon. These capsid modified Adv will efficiently infect CAR negative cells via interaction between cellular αV integrin/heparan sulfate proteoglycans present on the cell surface.[80–82] pIX can also be altered to achieve the targeted delivery using an Adv vector.[83] pIX is a structural protein that sustains the structural integrity of the viral particles. Kurachi et al. reported the enhanced transduction efficiency of Adv vectors containing an RGD peptide in the c-terminus of pIX with α-helical spacer.[78] Also, modification of hexon containing RGD peptides (DCRGDCF) at the HVR 5 region in the Ad vector can render them infective via the αv-integrin receptor without any affinity to the CAR receptor.[84] Therefore, modifications in the Adv capsid at pIX or hexon containing heterologous peptides render them more selective as compared with that at the fiber in the capsid.

Biermann et al. have also shown that the modification of high-capacity Adv vectors by incorporating either 6X-His epitope or RGD peptide into the HI loop of the fiber knob rendered the vectors more effective and allowed efficient targeting toward different cell types.[85] Targeting can also be achieved by the affinity immobilization of Adv particles to the surfaces of biodegradable nanoparticles resulting in improved transduction through uncoupling cellular uptake from the CAR receptor.[86] The Adv nanoparticles containing inducible nitric oxide synthase (iNOS) inhibited the growth of culture smooth muscle cells compared with the Adv encoding reporter gene GFP without any therapeutic activity (Ad^GFP) or Adv without any genes (Ad free vector).

Islets are nonreplicating cells that secrete insulin following an increase in blood glucose levels in the body. When there is a death of islets due to genetic or immune mediated defects, one of the major alternatives is the transplantation of islets. However, due to inadequate vascularization and subsequent immune attacks, islet transplantation did not achieve the success to which it was entitled. We have shown that hVEGF expression promotes new blood vessel formation and improves the outcome of islet transplantation.[87] To enhance hVEGF gene expression, we transduced human islets with bipartite Adv vectors encoding hVEGF and hIL-1Ra to promote revascularization and protect the human islets from apoptosis (Figure 5.1).[88] A bipartite vector results in simplifying the amplification and purification of Adv vectors but also minimizes the Adv backbone for transduction, thereby lessening the immunogenic effects of the vector. There was a dose-dependent increase in the expression of hVEGF and hIL-1Ra from islets transduced with AdvhVEGF-hIL-1Ra (Figure 5.2). We confirmed whether the Adv vector was causing any detrimental effects to the islets by measuring the stimulation index of islets following transduction by the Adv vector. Islets transduced by the Adv vectors were as functional as untransduced islets. There was a decrease in the caspase-3 levels in the Adv-transduced islets as compared with the untransduced islets when they were incubated with inflammatory cytokines. The expression was several times higher than the bicistronic plasmid vector phVEGF-hIL-1Ra. Following transplantation of AdvhVEGF-hIL-1Ra-transduced islets in nonobese diabetic severe combined immunodeficient (NOD-SCID) mice, there was a decrease in blood glucose levels and an increase in insulin and c-peptide levels (Figure 5.3).

The overexpression of hVEGF can be detrimental to islets and surrounding tissues and can lead to the development of tumors.[89,90] On the other hand, HGF is a potent mitogen of human islets and is known to promote β-cell proliferation and is also anti-apoptotic.[91] Therefore, we constructed a

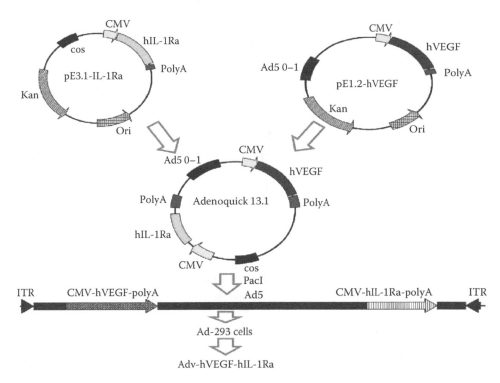

FIGURE 5.1 Construction of E1 and E3 deleted bipartite adenoviral vector by cloning hVEGF and hIL-1Ra into the MCS of shuttle plasmid pE3.1 and pE1.2. These expression cassettes were cloned into Adenoquick plasmid to generate a cosmid containing the entire sequence of recombinant Adv. After transfection into 293 cells, Adv-hVEGF-hIL-1Ra was produced. (Reproduced from Panakanti, R. and Mahato, R.I., *Mol. Pharm.*, 6, 274, 2009. With permission.)

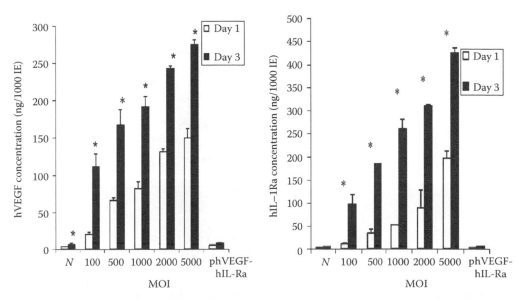

FIGURE 5.2 Expression of hVEGF and hIL-1Ra from human islets following transduction with Adv-hVEGF-IL-1Ra and plasmid vector phVEGF-IL-1Ra at days 1 and 3, respectively. (Reproduced from Panakanti, R. and Mahato, R.I., *Mol. Pharm.*, 6, 274, 2009. With permission.)

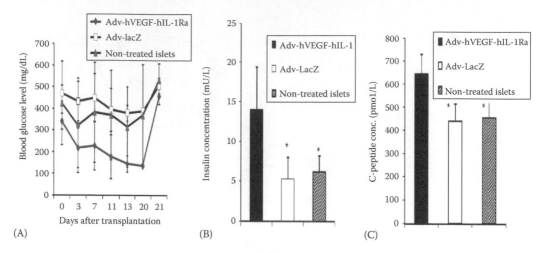

(A) (B) (C)

FIGURE 5.3 Effect of Adv-hVEGF-hIL-1Ra-transduced islets on the outcome of islet transplantation. (A) The non-fasting blood glucose levels in mice transplanted with human islets transduced with Adv-hVEGF-hIL-1Ra, Adv LacZ and nontreated islets. (B) Serum insulin and (C) C-peptide levels in mice measured at day 20 post transplantation. (Reproduced from Panakanti, R. and Mahato, R.I., *Mol. Pharm.*, 6, 274, 2009. With permission.)

bipartite Adv vector encoding hHGF and hIL-1Ra (AdvhHGF-hIL-1Ra) driven under a separate CMV promoter.[88] The vector showed an increase in the hHGF and hIL-1Ra genes with an increase in the multiplicity of infection (MOI) and duration. It did not affect the function of the islets and it showed decreased caspase-3 levels compared with the untransduced islets. Transduction of islets with AdvhHGF-hIL-1Ra enhanced the level of Bcl-2 protein and inhibited the levels of Bax protein demonstrating the protective effect of hHGF and hIL-1Ra co-expression (Figure 5.4). There was also a decrease in the blood glucose levels and an increase in the insulin and c-peptide levels in NOD-SCID mice transplanted with AdvhHGF-hIL-1Ra-transduced islets. Immunohistochemical staining of islet bearing kidney sections revealed stronger positive staining for human insulin, hHGF, and hvWF suggesting more efficient blood vessel formation in AdvhHGF-hIL-1Ra-transduced islets. This shows that Adv vectors can be utilized for efficient and high expression of transgenes with less immunogenic effects compared with nonviral vectors. However, these vectors can still elicit

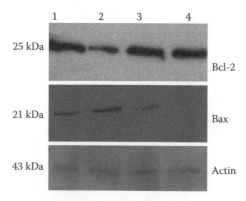

FIGURE 5.4 Effect of hHGF and hIL-1Ra co-expression on Bcl-2 and Bax protein levels. Bcl-2 and Bax was determined at day 3 post-transduction by Western blot analysis. Lane 1, non-transduced islets; lane 2, non-transduced islets with cytokine treatment; lane 3, islets transduced with Adv-hHGF-hIL-1Ra at 500 MOI with cytokine treatment; and lane 4, islets transduced with Adv-hHGF-hIL-1Ra at 1,000 MOI with cytokine treatment. (Reproduced from Panakanti, R. and Mahato, R.I., *Pharm. Res.*, 26, 587, 2009. With permission.)

immune responses, more so in the *in vivo* setting. Therefore, by removing the E4 or part of the E4 genome of the Adv vectors and by selectively targeting the Adv vector to a specific organ or tissue by attaching a ligand (Gal-PEG) to it can further enhance the prospects of Adv vectors in gene therapy.

5.3.4 ADENO-ASSOCIATED VIRAL VECTOR

The AAV is a simple nonpathogenic single-stranded DNA virus and is a member of the parvoviridae family. AAV is composed of two ORF, rep, cap, and two inverted terminal repeats (ITRs) that define the start and end of the viral genome and packaging sequence,[92] whereas the cap gene encodes viral capsid (coat) proteins and the rep gene is for replication and integration. AAV requires additional genes to replicate, which are usually provided by an Adv or an HSV. The AAV vector is produced by replacing the rep and cap genes with the transgene. Only one out of 100–1000 viral particles is infectious. Apart from the production of the AAV vector being laborious, these vectors also have the drawback of limited packaging capacity for the transgene (4.7 kb). Furthermore, there are no packaging cells which can express all the proteins of the virus. Since rAAVs are deleted of viral genes, these vectors are less immunogenic. However, specific circulating bodies to rAAVs have been detected, limiting their potential administration.[93]

5.3.5 OTHER VECTORS

HSV, which infects the cells of the nervous system, is being developed as a vector. This virus contains 80 genes, of which one can be replaced to produce the vector.[41] The use of recombinant baculoviruses containing mammalian regulatory elements for efficient transient and stable transduction of different mammalian cell types is being explored.[94] Alpha viruses are being used in the development of vaccines.[95,96]

5.4 GENE DELIVERY SYSTEMS

Gene delivery systems help in controlling the location of a gene within the body by regulating the biodistribution of a gene expression system. They aid in protecting the gene expression systems from premature degradation in extracellular milieu and allowing nonspecific or cell-specific targeting of the expression system. Some delivery systems are designed for specific targeting to a receptor or aid in intracellular trafficking of the gene expression system. Some of the common gene delivery systems used are discussed below.

5.4.1 LIPOSOMES

Plasmids are generally complexed with cationic liposomes to protect them from *in vivo* degradation and to enhance intracellular delivery. Cationic lipids are composed of a hydrophobic lipid anchor group, linker group, and a positively charged head group. Cationic lipids present in the liposome interact electrostatically with the negatively charged phosphate backbone of the DNA, thereby condensing the DNA into a more compact structure. These are the most commonly used synthetic carriers for the delivery of oligonucleotides, siRNAs, and plasmid DNA. The degree of transfection by cationic liposomes mainly depends on the extent of DNA condensation, cellular uptake by interaction with biological surfaces, and membrane fusion via transient membrane destabilization for cytoplasmic delivery avoiding lysosomal degradation.

pH-sensitive liposomes encapsulate DNA and can be conjugated to a ligand for delivery into ascitic tumors. However, low entrapment efficiency and high serum sensitivity limits their usage. The scenario changed with the introduction of the first cationic lipid, 2,3-dioleyloxypropyl-1-trimethyl ammonium bromide (DOTMA).

Although pH-sensitive liposomes can be used to encapsulate DNA, low entrapment efficiency and high serum sensitivity limits their usage. This scenario changed with the introduction of the first cationic lipid DOTMA.[97] Most of the research is being done to increase the transfection efficiency through the modification of the functional headgroups. Also, enhancing the transgene expression has become the focus of many studies. New cationic lipids were developed by modifying the headgroups of DOTMA, resulting in increased transfection efficiency. (±)-N-(2-hydroxyethyl)-N, N-dimethyl-2,3-bis(tetradecyloxy)-1-propanaminim bromide (DMRIE), which was synthesized by modifying DOTMA showed an increase in transfection efficiency and transgene expression. (3β (N-(N',N'-dimethylaminoethane) carbamoyl) cholesterol (DC–Chol) was the first cholesterol-based cationic lipid.[98] Its structure was further modified by conjugating polyamino groups resulting in more positive charges.[99] Spermine and spermidine were conjugated into cholesterol reduced cytotoxicity and increased the delivery of antisense oligonucloetides.[50] Changing spermine or spermidine into a secondary amine showed better transfection efficiency both *in vitro* and *in vivo*.[100] Some of the cationic lipids such as DC-Chol, DMRIE, and GL-67 have been used in early clinical trials, but the results were not encouraging. Heterocyclic cationic lipids have also been studied for gene delivery. Some of these compounds showed better transfection abilities and lower cytotoxicity compared with cationic lipids with linear primary amines or polyamines as head groups.[98]

Pyridinium-based cationic lipids have been shown to have similar or higher transfection efficiency compared with commercially available cationic lipid formulations. Pyridinium lipids displayed higher transduction efficiency in cells that are not easily transfected by other cationic lipids like lipofectin, and transfect relatively a large group of cells.[101] Zhu et al. have synthesized a series of pyridinium lipids containing a heterocyclic ring and a nitrogen atom and prepared liposomes with co-lipid L-α dioleoylphosphatidylethanolamine (DOPE) and cholesterol (Chol) by sonication.[102] Pyridinium lipids with an amide linker showed significantly higher transfection efficiency compared with their ester counterparts. Liposomes prepared at a 1:1 molar ratio of pyridinium lipid and a colipid showed higher transfection efficiency when either DOPE or cholesterol was used as a colipid to prepare liposomes (Figure 5.5). The pyridinium lipids with a trans-configuration of the double bond in the fatty acid chain showed higher transfection efficiency than its counterparts with cis-configuration at the same fatty acid chain length. In the presence of serum, C16:0 and lipofectamine significantly decreased their transfection efficiencies, which were completely lost at

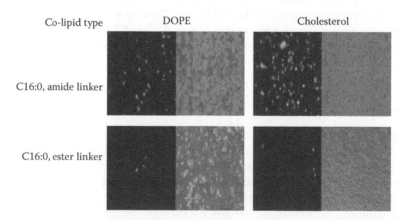

FIGURE 5.5 Comparison of gene expression between amide and ester linker. Lipid 5 (C16:0, amide linker) and lipid 16 (C16:0) were used to prepare liposomes with co-lipid DOPE and cholesterol at the molar ratio of 1:1. Lipoplexes were formed by mixing with luciferase plasmid at the charge ratio of 3:1 (+/−). GFP gene expression was observed 48 h after transfection under fluorescence microscope and normal light as control. The dose of p CMS-EGFP plasmid was 0.4 μg/well for 4×10^4 cells. (Reproduced from Zhu, L. et al., *Bioconjug. Chem.*, 19, 2499, 2008. With permission.)

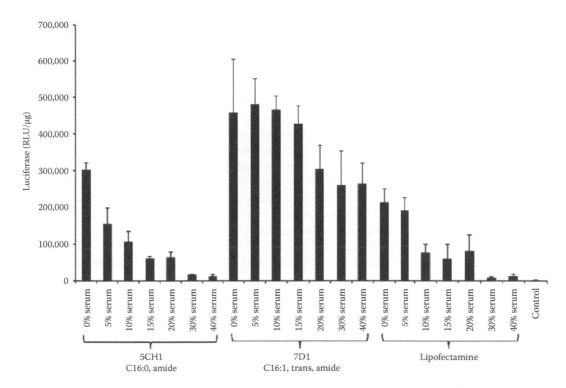

FIGURE 5.6 Influence of serum on transfection of cationic liposomes. The compound C16:1 trans, amide containing DOPE and Chol as co lipids at molar ratio 1:1 showed high transfection efficiency compared with lipofectamine at different serum concentrations. Lipoplexes were formed using luciferase plasmid at charge ratio 3:1. (Reproduced from Zhu, L. et al., *Bioconjug. Chem.*, 19, 2499, 2008. With permission.)

a serum concentration of 30% and higher, while the C16:1 trans-isomer still had high transfection efficiency under these conditions (Figure 5.6).

The liposomal vector interacts with extracellular components in the serum after *in vivo* administration. This often causes failure of the liposomal vector to reach the target cells. To have a targeted liposomal vector system, a ligand is required to bind to the receptor of the target cells. Nasopharyngeal epidermal carcinoma cells that express an excess of folate receptors were targeted by liposome-entrapped polycation-condensed DNA (LPDII) anionic liposome encapsulating polylysine condensed DNA tagged with folate.[103] Lys_2Gal_3, an aminogalactoside, was used to target hepatoma *in vitro*,[104] which is a cationic formulation consisting of lipopolymaine, DOPE (helper lipid), and a galactolipid (DPPE-Lys_2Gal_3).

5.4.2 CATIONIC PEPTIDES

Major difficulties in the nonviral delivery are the ability of the vectors to condense the DNA, targeting the specific cells; disrupt the endosomal membrane; and deliver it to the nucleus. Peptide-based vectors can be successfully employed to overcome these barriers. Cationic peptides condense DNA by interacting with its negatively charged phosphate backbone.

Poly(L-lysine) (PLL) is one of the first cationic peptides to deliver genes. However, an increase in the length of PLL leads to cytotoxicity. It shows less transfection efficiency and needs another fusogenic peptide to facilitate plasmid release into the cytoplasm. Since PLL cannot escape from the endosome without the addition of an endosomolytic agent such as chloroquine, Midoux and Monsingy have constructed a histidine-substituted polylysine, since histidine protonates at acidic pH 8 in the endosome. Cationic peptides can be linked to cell-specific ligands and bound to plasmids through electrostatic interaction. These complexes can interact specifically with target cell receptors leading to the internalization of the complex into the cells.

Synthetic peptides that are conjugated to lipids usually show better binding ability to DNA. For example, the inclusion of dialkyl or diacyl chains in the cationic peptides improves their ability to bind to DNA and reduces the aggregation of complexes in the ionic media.[1,22,105] Synthetic peptides derived from the N-terminus of the influenza virus hemagglutinin and the rhinovirus VP-1 protein[106] or artificial amphipathic peptides were used.[22] These peptides may have specificity for endosomal pH due to acidic residues (glutamic and aspartic acids) aligning on one side of an amphipathic helix. At a neutral pH level, the negatively charged carboxylic groups destabilize the alpha-helical structure resulting in the multimerization of peptides and/or membrane interaction. The pH specificity can be enhanced by introducing additional glutamic acids into the peptide sequence.[107] The enhancement of gene expression is strongly dependent on the peptide sequence. The activity of cationic lipid/DNA complexes has been enhanced with a mixture of Sendai virus envelopes. This approach and related systems utilizing neutral lipids and liposome-like reconstituted envelopes ("virosomes") based on the Sendai virus or the influenza viruses have been found to be effective for gene delivery.[108]

Amphipathic cationic peptides, such as gramicidin S, are incorporated into a DOPE lipid/DNA composition to facilitate gene delivery. The incorporation of gramicidin S and DNA into asialofetuin-labeled liposomes was used for receptor-mediated gene delivery into primary hepatocytes.[109] The influence of influenza virus-based peptides on cationic lipid-based transfection was studied.[110] Wagner et al. showed that the use of positively charged lipospermine/DNA complexes resulted in a 3- to 30-fold enhancement in gene expression by association with peptides.[111] Kamata et al. also showed that influenza-derived peptides can increase the level of gene expression of a lipofectin formulation by up to fivefold.[112] Thus, escape from endocytic vesicles does not seem to be a major barrier for optimized, positively charged DNA/lipospermine or lipofectin complexes. However, for less positively charged lipospermine complexes, gene transfer efficiency was found to be increased by a factor of 50–1000 by synthetic peptides INF6 (influenza virus derived sequence) and INF10 (artificial sequence).[111] Wilke et al. generated novel DNA complexes containing a palmitoyl-modified DNA-binding peptide showing enhanced transfection activity. Gene transfer was found to be restricted to mitotic cells.[113]

Membrane-modifying peptides are able to enhance both lipofection and polyfection. The transfection efficiency of cationic peptide-based systems are strongly dependent on the presence of endosomolytic peptides or related agents (like glycerol, viral particles), which enhance cytoplasmic delivery.[106] Transfection efficiencies can be improved up to more than 1000-fold by endosomolytic compounds.[111]

It is important to determine (1) whether membrane-modulating peptides and DNA carriers can influence other intracellular steps besides endosomal escape or cell membrane fusion, such as the transport of the DNA into the nucleus of the cell and (2) whether the results obtained with membrane-active peptides in cell culture can also be exploited for *in vivo* gene transfer.[108]

5.4.3 CATIONIC POLYMERS AND LIPOPOLYMERS

Polyethyleneimine (PEI), polypropylenimine, and polyamidoamine dendrimers have been employed for gene delivery. PEI[114] is a branched cationic polymer widely used in gene delivery. It condenses the plasmids into colloidal particles that effectively transfect genes into a variety of cells *in vitro*.[115] PEI contains several secondary amines that get protonated in the acidic environment of the endosome. This leads to endosomal swelling and subsequent membrane disruption leading to the release of the vector into the cytosol. However, PEI with a high molecular weight (>25 kDa) shows cytotoxicity and PEI/plasmid vector complexes under aggregation on storage, resulting in less gene expression. The chemical modification of low molecular weight PEIs may improve transfection and reduce cytotoxicity.

Mahato and associates synthesized a water soluble lipopolymer by conjugating cholesteryl chloroformate to branched PEI of 1800 Da through primary and secondary amines.[116] This polymer was nontoxic to CT-26 colon carcinoma cells and did not cause any aggregation compared with PEI/DNA complexes. Cholesterol will promote both micellar formation and hydrophobic interaction with plasmid and cellular membrane while PEI will condense DNA via electrostatic interaction.

5.4.4 Hybrid Vectors

Both viral and nonviral vectors have their own advantages and disadvantages. There is a lot of ongoing research to develop new ways of better utilizing these vectors for gene expression and delivery. One such approach is to overcome the limitations of individual vectors by combining them. These vectors are called hybrid vectors. For example, the adenovirus hexon protein enhances the nuclear translocation and increases the transgene expression of PEI/pDNA complexes.[117] PEG has been widely used for conjugating with the adenoviral vector to prolong its circulation half-life, enhance transgene expression, and prevent immune activation.[118]

Cationic lipids and polymers may help in improving the transduction efficiencies of viral vectors. These are particularly useful in cells that do not have specific viral receptors. The cationic nature of these molecules may promote binding to the negatively charged viral capsid, altering the cell surface and allowing internalization of the viral particles. This can also elicit less immunostimulation. For example, cationic liposomes promote the delivery of Adv vectors into target cells that lack the CAR receptors and αv-integrin receptors, improving transgene expression.[119] Diamond and his colleagues have shown that the delivery of Adv vectors associated with dexamethasone-spermine (DS) conjugate to the lung enhanced targeting to the conducting airway epithelium and reduced immune response.[120] Furthermore, the formulation of Adv encoding LacZ with DS/DOPE allowed the re-administration of the Adv vector, with little loss of the transgene expression.

The Adv vector can also be coated with polymers bearing side chains containing positively charged quaternary amines and carbonyl thiazolidine-2 thione groups to prevent the binding of the Adv vector to plasma protein and consequently prolonging the blood circulation half-life and more deposition of the vector at diseased sites.[121]

5.4.5 Receptor-Mediated Gene Transfer

Targeting ligands have been incorporated into DNA complexes for site- or cell-specific gene delivery.[108] By attaching the DNA to a domain that can bind to a cell surface receptor, such as asialoglycoprotein, transferrin, and folate-receptors, the efficient cellular process of receptor-mediated endocytosis can be utilized. Conjugates with polylysine, protamines, histones, PEI, cationic lipids, and other polycations have been generated and tested for receptor-mediated endocytosis. Hong and his colleagues used hydroxycamptothecin (HCPT)-loaded PEG niosomes attached with transferrin to the terminal group of PEG. This system showed high antitumor activity compared with nontransferrin bound niosomes.[114] To enhance the uptake and specificity, Wu and Wu generated a polylysine-based, asialoglycoprotein receptor-specific gene delivery system by incorporation of asialoorosomucoid–polylysine conjugates into DNA complexes.[122,123] Complexes could be efficiently delivered into endosomes or other internal vesicles of cells, but they were still separated from the cytoplasm by a membrane. This accumulation of complexes in internal vesicles strongly reduced the efficiency of the gene transfer. Receptor-mediated delivery into a hepatocyte cell line resulted in the uptake of DNA into practically all cells, but only a few cells expressed the delivered gene.[124]

5.5 CONCLUDING REMARKS

Although significant progress has been made to employ gene therapy in the clinic to treat various severe and debilitating diseases, there are still no FDA approved products in the market. This can be attributed to the lack of proper gene expression and delivery systems. While viral vectors efficiently transduce cells and have shown promise in their clinical trials, there are still some safety concerns, especially immunostimulation and integration within the host. Although nonviral vectors are relatively safe, transgene expression is very low and transient and thus many vectors have failed to perform well in the clinical trials. Therefore, efforts are being made to generate hybrid systems by combining the beneficial effects of nonviral and viral vectors. This has led to a significant enhancement in gene expression, with minimal toxicity and immunogenicity. Furthermore, the use of cellular promoters offers targeting of the vector to specific target tissues rendering the vector safe and efficacious. There is a definite need to develop targeting strategies for nonviral vectors that can compensate for the inefficient gene transfer.

ACKNOWLEDGMENT

We would like to thank the National Institute of Health (NIH) for financial support (Grant # R O1 DK69968, and R O1 EB003922).

REFERENCES

1. Mahato RI, Rolland A, Tomlinson E. Cationic lipid-based gene delivery systems: Pharmaceutical perspectives. *Pharm Res* 1997; **14**: 853–859.
2. van Gaal EV, Hennink WE, Crommelin DJ, Mastrobattista E. Plasmid engineering for controlled and sustained gene expression for nonviral gene therapy. *Pharm Res* 2006; **23**: 1053–1074.
3. Calcedo R et al. Host immune responses to chronic adenovirus infections in human and nonhuman primates. *J Virol* 2009; **83**: 2623–2631.
4. Sangro B, Herraiz M, Prieto J. Gene therapy of neoplastic liver diseases. *Int J Biochem Cell Biol* 2003; **35**: 135–148.
5. Cheng K, Yang N, Mahato RI. TGF-beta1 gene silencing for treating liver fibrosis. *Mol Pharm* 2009; **6**: 772–779.
6. Brown T. *Gene Cloning: An Introduction*. Chapman & Hall: London, U.K., 1990.
7. Jang SK et al. A segment of the 5′ nontranslated region of encephalomyocarditis virus RNA directs internal entry of ribosomes during in vitro translation. *J Virol* 1988; **62**: 2636–2643.
8. Pelletier J, Sonenberg N. Internal initiation of translation of eukaryotic mRNA directed by a sequence derived from poliovirus RNA. *Nature* 1988; **334**: 320–325.
9. Baranick BT et al. Splicing mediates the activity of four putative cellular internal ribosome entry sites. *Proc Natl Acad Sci USA* 2008; **105**: 4733–4738.
10. Jia X, Cheng K, Mahato RI. Coexpression of vascular endothelial growth factor and interleukin-1 receptor antagonist for improved human islet survival and function. *Mol Pharm* 2007; **4**: 199–207.
11. Voorhees JJ, Duell EA, Chambers DA, Marcelo CL. Regulation of cell cycles. *J Invest Dermatol* 1976; **67**: 15–19.
12. Lund J et al. Transcriptional regulation of the bovine CYP17 gene by cAMP. *Steroids* 1997; **62**: 43–45.
13. Dillon N. Gene regulation and large-scale chromatin organization in the nucleus. *Chromosome Res* 2006; **14**: 117–126.
14. Hoffmann D, Wildner O. Efficient generation of double heterologous promoter controlled oncolytic adenovirus vectors by a single homologous recombination step in *Escherichia coli. BMC Biotechnol* 2006; **6**: 36.
15. Gambari R. New trends in the development of transcription factor decoy (TFD) pharmacotherapy. *Curr Drug Targets* 2004; **5**: 419–430.
16. Melloul D, Marshak S, Cerasi E. Regulation of pdx-1 gene expression. *Diabetes* 2002; **51**(Suppl 3): S320–S325.
17. Kawasaki H et al. In vitro transformation of adult rat hepatic progenitor cells into pancreatic endocrine hormone-producing cells. *J Hepatobiliary Pancreat Surg* 2008; **15**: 310–317.

18. Walther W, Stein U. Cell type specific and inducible promoters for vectors in gene therapy as an approach for cell targeting. *J Mol Med* 1996; **74**: 379–392.
19. Spilianakis CG et al. Interchromosomal associations between alternatively expressed loci. *Nature* 2005; **435**: 637–645.
20. Arnosti DN, Kulkarni MM. Transcriptional enhancers: Intelligent enhanceosomes or flexible billboards? *J Cell Biochem* 2005; **94**: 890–898.
21. Choi UH et al. Hypoxia-inducible expression of vascular endothelial growth factor for the treatment of spinal cord injury in a rat model. *J Neurosurg Spine* 2007; **7**: 54–60.
22. Mahato RI, Smith LC, Rolland A. Pharmaceutical perspectives of nonviral gene therapy. *Adv Genet* 1999; **41**: 95–156.
23. Smale ST, Kadonaga JT. The RNA polymerase II core promoter. *Annu Rev Biochem* 2003; **72**: 449–479.
24. Qin L et al. Promoter attenuation in gene therapy: Interferon-gamma and tumor necrosis factor-alpha inhibit transgene expression. *Hum Gene Ther* 1997; **8**: 2019–2029.
25. Lubansu A et al. Recombinant AAV viral vectors serotype 1, 2, and 5 mediate differential gene transfer efficiency in rat striatal fetal grafts. *Cell Transplant* 2008; **16**: 1013–1020.
26. Yew NS. Controlling the kinetics of transgene expression by plasmid design. *Adv Drug Deliv Rev* 2005; **57**: 769–780.
27. Tenenbaum L et al. Recombinant AAV-mediated gene delivery to the central nervous system. *J Gene Med* 2004; **6**(Suppl 1): S212–S222.
28. Alexopoulou AN, Couchman JR, Whiteford JR. The CMV early enhancer/chicken beta actin (CAG) promoter can be used to drive transgene expression during the differentiation of murine embryonic stem cells into vascular progenitors. *BMC Cell Biol* 2008; **9**: 2.
29. Huang J et al. Myocardial injection of CA promoter-based plasmid mediates efficient transgene expression in rat heart. *J Gene Med* 2003; **5**: 900–908.
30. Gill DR et al. Increased persistence of lung gene expression using plasmids containing the ubiquitin C or elongation factor 1alpha promoter. *Gene Ther* 2001; **8**: 1539–1546.
31. Kozak M. Structural features in eukaryotic mRNAs that modulate the initiation of translation. *J Biol Chem* 1991; **266**: 19867–19870.
32. Kozak M. Regulation of translation in eukaryotic systems. *Annu Rev Cell Biol* 1992; **8**: 197–225.
33. Hartikka J et al. An improved plasmid DNA expression vector for direct injection into skeletal muscle. *Hum Gene Ther* 1996; **7**: 1205–1217.
34. Gregor PD, Kobrin BJ, Milcarek C, Morrison SL. Sequences 3′ of immunoglobulin heavy chain genes influence their expression. *Immunol Rev* 1986; **89**: 31–48.
35. Ryu WS, Mertz JE. Simian virus 40 late transcripts lacking excisable intervening sequences are defective in both stability in the nucleus and transport to the cytoplasm. *J Virol* 1989; **63**: 4386–4394.
36. Esposito D, Chatterjee DK. Enhancement of soluble protein expression through the use of fusion tags. *Curr Opin Biotechnol* 2006; **17**: 353–358.
37. Niiranen L et al. Comparative expression study to increase the solubility of cold adapted Vibrio proteins in *Escherichia coli*. *Protein Expr Purif* 2007; **52**: 210–218.
38. Shih YP et al. High-throughput screening of soluble recombinant proteins. *Protein Sci* 2002; **11**: 1714–1719.
39. Mahato RI et al. Biodistribution and gene expression of lipid/plasmid complexes after systemic administration. *Hum Gene Ther* 1998; **9**: 2083–2099.
40. Ma X, Riemann H, Gri G, Trinchieri G. Positive and negative regulation of interleukin-12 gene expression. *Eur Cytokine Netw* 1998; **9**: 54–64.
41. Fink DJ, DeLuca NA, Goins WF, Glorioso JC. Gene transfer to neurons using herpes simplex virus-based vectors. *Annu Rev Neurosci* 1996; **19**: 265–287.
42. Snowden BW, Blair ED, Wagner EK. Transcriptional activation with concurrent or nonconcurrent template replication has differential effects on transient expression from herpes simplex virus promoters. *Virus Genes* 1989; **2**: 129–145.
43. Black J, Vos JM. Establishment of an oriP/EBNA1-based episomal vector transcribing human genomic beta-globin in cultured murine fibroblasts. *Gene Ther* 2002; **9**: 1447–1454.
44. Kolb AF et al. Site-directed genome modification: Nucleic acid and protein modules for targeted integration and gene correction. *Trends Biotechnol* 2005; **23**: 399–406.
45. Van Craenenbroeck K, Vanhoenacker P, Haegeman G. Episomal vectors for gene expression in mammalian cells. *Eur J Biochem* 2000; **267**: 5665–5678.

46. Ehrhardt A et al. Optimization of cis-acting elements for gene expression from nonviral vectors in vivo. *Hum Gene Ther* 2003; **14**: 215–225.

47. Zhao H et al. Contribution of Toll-like receptor 9 signaling to the acute inflammatory response to nonviral vectors. *Mol Ther* 2004; **9**: 241–248.

48. Chattopadhyay S, Pavithra L. MARs and MARBPs: Key modulators of gene regulation and disease manifestation. *Subcell Biochem* 2007; **41**: 213–230.

49. Boulikas T. Homeotic protein binding sites, origins of replication, and nuclear matrix anchorage sites share the ATTA and ATTTA motifs. *J Cell Biochem* 1992; **50**: 111–123.

50. Guy-Caffey JK et al. Novel polyaminolipids enhance the cellular uptake of oligonucleotides. *J Biol Chem* 1995; **270**: 31391–31396.

51. Argyros O et al. Persistent episomal transgene expression in liver following delivery of a scaffold/matrix attachment region containing non-viral vector. *Gene Ther* 2008; **15**: 1593–1605.

52. Baker A, Cotten M. Delivery of bacterial artificial chromosomes into mammalian cells with psoralen-inactivated adenovirus carrier. *Nucleic Acids Res* 1997; **25**: 1950–1956.

53. Westphal EM et al. A system for shuttling 200-kb BAC/PAC clones into human cells: Stable extrachromosomal persistence and long-term ectopic gene activation. *Hum Gene Ther* 1998; **9**: 1863–1873.

54. Hibbitt OC et al. Delivery and long-term expression of a 135 kb LDLR genomic DNA locus in vivo by hydrodynamic tail vein injection. *J Gene Med* 2007; **9**: 488–497.

55. Stenler S et al. Gene transfer to mouse heart and skeletal muscles using a minicircle expressing human vascular endothelial growth factor. *J Cardiovasc Pharmacol* 2009; **53**: 18–23.

56. Wu J et al. Minicircle-IFNgamma induces antiproliferative and antitumoral effects in human nasopharyngeal carcinoma. *Clin Cancer Res* 2006; **12**: 4702–4713.

57. Greco O et al. Novel chimeric gene promoters responsive to hypoxia and ionizing radiation. *Gene Ther* 2002; **9**: 1403–1411.

58. Bauerschmitz GJ et al. Tissue-specific promoters active in CD44+CD24−/low breast cancer cells. *Cancer Res* 2008; **68**: 5533–5539.

59. Pujal J et al. Keratin 7 promoter selectively targets transgene expression to normal and neoplastic pancreatic ductal cells in vitro and in vivo. *FASEB J* 2009; **23**: 1366–1375.

60. Pastore L et al. Use of a liver-specific promoter reduces immune response to the transgene in adenoviral vectors. *Hum Gene Ther* 1999; **10**: 1773–1781.

61. Li X, Eastman EM, Schwartz RJ, Draghia-Akli R. Synthetic muscle promoters: Activities exceeding naturally occurring regulatory sequences. *Nat Biotechnol* 1999; **17**: 241–245.

62. Wang Y et al. Positive and negative regulation of gene expression in eukaryotic cells with an inducible transcriptional regulator. *Gene Ther* 1997; **4**: 432–441.

63. Gossen M et al. Transcriptional activation by tetracyclines in mammalian cells. *Science* 1995; **268**: 1766–1769.

64. Verma IM. Gene therapy. *Sci Am* 1990; **263**: 68–72, 81–64.

65. Lewis P, Hensel M, Emerman M. Human immunodeficiency virus infection of cells arrested in the cell cycle. *Embo J* 1992; **11**: 3053–3058.

66. Bergelson JM et al. Isolation of a common receptor for Coxsackie B viruses and adenoviruses 2 and 5. *Science* 1997; **275**: 1320–1323.

67. Miyoshi H, Takahashi M, Gage FH, Verma IM. Stable and efficient gene transfer into the retina using an HIV-based lentiviral vector. *Proc Natl Acad Sci USA* 1997; **94**: 10319–10323.

68. Hofmann A et al. Combined targeting of lentiviral vectors and positioning of transduced cells by magnetic nanoparticles. *Proc Natl Acad Sci USA* 2009; **106**: 44–49.

69. Apolonia L et al. Stable gene transfer to muscle using non-integrating lentiviral vectors. *Mol Ther* 2007; **15**: 1947–1954.

70. Guo YH et al. Hepatocyte growth factor and granulocyte colony-stimulating factor form a combined neovasculogenic therapy for ischemic cardiomyopathy. *Cytotherapy* 2008; **10**: 857–867.

71. Yeh P, Perricaudet M. Advances in adenoviral vectors: From genetic engineering to their biology. *FASEB J* 1997; **11**: 615–623.

72. Dai Y et al. Cellular and humoral immune responses to adenoviral vectors containing factor IX gene: Tolerization of factor IX and vector antigens allows for long-term expression. *Proc Natl Acad Sci USA* 1995; **92**: 1401–1405.

73. Yang Y, Ertl HC, Wilson JM. MHC class I-restricted cytotoxic T lymphocytes to viral antigens destroy hepatocytes in mice infected with E1-deleted recombinant adenoviruses. *Immunity* 1994; **1**: 433–442.

74. Engelhardt JF, Ye X, Doranz B, Wilson JM. Ablation of E2A in recombinant adenoviruses improves transgene persistence and decreases inflammatory response in mouse liver. *Proc Natl Acad Sci USA* 1994; **91**: 6196–6200.

75. Chen HH et al. Persistence in muscle of an adenoviral vector that lacks all viral genes. *Proc Natl Acad Sci USA* 1997; **94**: 1645–1650.

76. Wickham TJ. Targeting adenovirus. *Gene Ther* 2000; **7**: 110–114.

77. Mizuguchi H, Hayakawa T. Targeted adenovirus vectors. *Hum Gene Ther* 2004; **15**: 1034–1044.

78. Kurachi S et al. Characterization of capsid-modified adenovirus vectors containing heterologous peptides in the fiber knob, protein IX, or hexon. *Gene Ther* 2007; **14**: 266–274.

79. Tomko RP, Xu R, Philipson L. HCAR and MCAR: The human and mouse cellular receptors for subgroup C adenoviruses and group B coxsackieviruses. *Proc Natl Acad Sci USA* 1997; **94**: 3352–3356.

80. Staba MJ, Wickham TJ, Kovesdi I, Hallahan DE. Modifications of the fiber in adenovirus vectors increase tropism for malignant glioma models. *Cancer Gene Ther* 2000; **7**: 13–19.

81. Dmitriev I et al. An adenovirus vector with genetically modified fibers demonstrates expanded tropism via utilization of a coxsackievirus and adenovirus receptor-independent cell entry mechanism. *J Virol* 1998; **72**: 9706–9713.

82. Koizumi N et al. Generation of fiber-modified adenovirus vectors containing heterologous peptides in both the HI loop and C terminus of the fiber knob. *J Gene Med* 2003; **5**: 267–276.

83. Dmitriev IP, Kashentseva EA, Curiel DT. Engineering of adenovirus vectors containing heterologous peptide sequences in the C terminus of capsid protein IX. *J Virol* 2002; **76**: 6893–6899.

84. Vigne E et al. RGD inclusion in the hexon monomer provides adenovirus type 5-based vectors with a fiber knob-independent pathway for infection. *J Virol* 1999; **73**: 5156–5161.

85. Biermann V et al. Targeting of high-capacity adenoviral vectors. *Hum Gene Ther* 2001; **12**: 1757–1769.

86. Chorny M et al. Adenoviral gene vector tethering to nanoparticle surfaces results in receptor-independent cell entry and increased transgene expression. *Mol Ther* 2006; **14**: 382–391.

87. Cheng K et al. Adenovirus-based vascular endothelial growth factor gene delivery to human pancreatic islets. *Gene Ther* 2004; **11**: 1105–1116.

88. Panakanti R, Mahato RI. Bipartite vector encoding hVEGF and hIL-1Ra for ex vivo transduction into human islets. *Mol Pharm* 2008; **6**: 274–284.

89. Christofori G, Naik P, Hanahan D. Vascular endothelial growth factor and its receptors, flt-1 and flk-1, are expressed in normal pancreatic islets and throughout islet cell tumorigenesis. *Mol Endocrinol* 1995; **9**: 1760–1770.

90. Gannon G et al. Overexpression of vascular endothelial growth factor-A165 enhances tumor angiogenesis but not metastasis during beta-cell carcinogenesis. *Cancer Res* 2002; **62**: 603–608.

91. Beattie GM et al. A novel approach to increase human islet cell mass while preserving beta-cell function. *Diabetes* 2002; **51**: 3435–3439.

92. Muzyczka N. Use of adeno-associated virus as a general transduction vector for mammalian cells. *Curr Top Microbiol Immunol* 1992; **158**: 97–129.

93. Verma IM, Somia N. Gene therapy—promises, problems and prospects. *Nature* 1997; **389**: 239–242.

94. Dukkipati A et al. BacMam system for high-level expression of recombinant soluble and membrane glycoproteins for structural studies. *Protein Expr Purif* 2008; **62**: 160–170.

95. Schlesinger S, Dubensky TW. Alphavirus vectors for gene expression and vaccines. *Curr Opin Biotechnol* 1999; **10**: 434–439.

96. Schlesinger S. Alphavirus vectors: Development and potential therapeutic applications. *Expert Opin Biol Ther* 2001; **1**: 177–191.

97. Felgner PL et al. Lipofection: A highly efficient, lipid-mediated DNA-transfection procedure. *Proc Natl Acad Sci USA* 1987; **84**: 7413–7417.

98. Gao X, Huang L. A novel cationic liposome reagent for efficient transfection of mammalian cells. *Biochem Biophys Res Commun* 1991; **179**: 280–285.

99. Gao X, Huang L. Potentiation of cationic liposome-mediated gene delivery by polycations. *Biochemistry* 1996; **35**: 1027–1036.

100. Lee ER et al. Detailed analysis of structures and formulations of cationic lipids for efficient gene transfer to the lung. *Hum Gene Ther* 1996; **7**: 1701–1717.

101. van der Woude I et al. Novel pyridinium surfactants for efficient, nontoxic in vitro gene delivery. *Proc Natl Acad Sci USA* 1997; **94**: 1160–1165.

102. Zhu L, Lu Y, Miller DD, Mahato RI. Structural and formulation factors influencing pyridinium lipid-based gene transfer. *Bioconjug Chem* 2008; **19**: 2499–2512.

103. Lee RJ, Huang L. Folate-targeted, anionic liposome-entrapped polylysine-condensed DNA for tumor cell-specific gene transfer. *J Biol Chem* 1996; **271**: 8481–8487.

104. Remy JS et al. Targeted gene transfer into hepatoma cells with lipopolyamine-condensed DNA particles presenting galactose ligands: A stage toward artificial viruses. *Proc Natl Acad Sci USA* 1995; **92**: 1744–1748.

105. Wadhwa MS et al. Peptide-mediated gene delivery: Influence of peptide structure on gene expression. *Bioconjug Chem* 1997; **8**: 81–88.

106. Zauner W et al. Glycerol and polylysine synergize in their ability to rupture vesicular membranes: A mechanism for increased transferrin-polylysine-mediated gene transfer. *Exp Cell Res* 1997; **232**: 137–145.

107. Haider M, Megeed Z, Ghandehari H. Genetically engineered polymers: Status and prospects for controlled release. *J Control Release* 2004; **95**: 1–26.

108. Wagner E. Application of membrane-active peptides for nonviral gene delivery. *Adv Drug Deliv Rev* 1999; **38**: 279–289.

109. Hara T et al. Effects of fusogenic and DNA-binding amphiphilic compounds on the receptor-mediated gene transfer into hepatic cells by asialofetuin-labeled liposomes. *Biochim Biophys Acta* 1996; **1278**: 51–58.

110. Esbjorner EK et al. Membrane binding of pH-sensitive influenza fusion peptides. Positioning, configuration, and induced leakage in a lipid vesicle model. *Biochemistry* 2007; **46**: 13490–13504.

111. Kichler A, Mechtler K, Behr JP, Wagner E. Influence of membrane-active peptides on lipospermine/DNA complex mediated gene transfer. *Bioconjug Chem* 1997; **8**: 213–221.

112. Kamata H, Yagisawa H, Takahashi S, Hirata H. Amphiphilic peptides enhance the efficiency of liposome-mediated DNA transfection. *Nucleic Acids Res* 1994; **22**: 536–537.

113. Wilke M et al. Efficacy of a peptide-based gene delivery system depends on mitotic activity. *Gene Ther* 1996; **3**: 1133–1142.

114. Hong M et al. Efficient tumor targeting of hydroxycamptothecin loaded PEGylated niosomes modified with transferrin. *J Control Release* 2009; **133**: 96–102.

115. Boussif O et al. A versatile vector for gene and oligonucleotide transfer into cells in culture and in vivo: Polyethylenimine. *Proc Natl Acad Sci USA* 1995; **92**: 7297–7301.

116. Wang DA et al. Novel branched poly(ethylenimine)-cholesterol water-soluble lipopolymers for gene delivery. *Biomacromolecules* 2002; **3**: 1197–1207.

117. Carlisle RC et al. Adenovirus hexon protein enhances nuclear delivery and increases transgene expression of polyethylenimine/plasmid DNA vectors. *Mol Ther* 2001; **4**: 473–483.

118. Croyle MA et al. PEGylated helper-dependent adenoviral vectors: Highly efficient vectors with an enhanced safety profile. *Gene Ther* 2005; **12**: 579–587.

119. Yotnda P et al. Bilamellar cationic liposomes protect adenovectors from preexisting humoral immune responses. *Mol Ther* 2002; **5**: 233–241.

120. Price AR, Limberis MP, Wilson JM, Diamond SL. Pulmonary delivery of adenovirus vector formulated with dexamethasone-spermine facilitates homologous vector re-administration. *Gene Ther* 2007; **14**: 1594–1604.

121. Subr V et al. Coating of adenovirus type 5 with polymers containing quaternary amines prevents binding to blood components. *J Control Release* 2009; **135**: 152–158.

122. Wu GY, Wu CH. Evidence for targeted gene delivery to Hep G2 hepatoma cells in vitro. *Biochemistry* 1988; **27**: 887–892.

123. Wu GY, Wu CH. Receptor-mediated gene delivery and expression in vivo. *J Biol Chem* 1988; **263**: 14621–14624.

124. Zatloukal K et al. Transferrinfection: A highly efficient way to express gene constructs in eukaryotic cells. *Ann NY Acad Sci* 1992; **660**: 136–153.

6 Cellular Barriers for Nucleic Acid Delivery and Targeting

Arto Urtti

CONTENTS

6.1 INTRODUCTION

Gene transfer is the key technology in the genetic modification of organisms for experimental and therapeutic purposes. Gene therapy holds great promise in medicine, since the exploration of the human genome and post-genomic biology continues to reveal new mechanisms and intervention strategies about the diseases. This approach is a new paradigm in pharmaceutical therapy, since it avoids the extensive search for new pharmacologically active molecules against a target. In the case of gene therapy, the information about the mechanism of the disease reveals the endogenous drug (i.e., the under-expressed or inappropriate gene) in the disease state. The expression can be replenished by providing extra genetic material by gene transfer. For example, the vascular endothelial growth factor (VEGF) gene can be used to induce neo-vessel formation, neurotrophic growth factor genes to revive degenerated neural tissue, and the tyrosin kinase "suicide" genes for rendering the cancer cells susceptible to anticancer drugs.

Gene technology is a versatile method, since it is possible to clone virtually any gene into an expression vector, produce the DNA in cells (bacterial or eukaryotic), and transfer to human cells for treatment. The ultimate goal is not only the gene transfer, but its efficient long-term expression. The expressed protein is the pharmacologically active component that matters. In another form of gene therapy, the transgene is used to express shRNA or siRNA species in the cell. This approach can be used to silence the expression of the target proteins selectively.

There are several gene transfer technologies that are currently used. Most therapeutic approaches are based on the use of viral vectors. Viruses have evolved during hundreds of millions of years to transfer their genetic cargo to the host cells. The viruses are not homogenous groups of organisms—they are rather diverse in many respects.[1]

In general, the viral vectors have a higher efficiency of gene transfer than the nonviral systems. However, the viral systems have their own shortcomings. Some of them cause immune response that leads to decreasing gene transfer efficacy during repeated administration (e.g., adenoviruses), some transfect only dividing cells (e.g., retroviruses), some may have integration related uncertainties (e.g., lentiviruses), and some vectors have limited DNA cargo capacity (e.g., adeno-associated viruses). Despite these problems, it is likely that the first gene therapy products will be based on viral vectors. So far, one gene therapy product has been launched. The interleukin-2 expressing adenoviral gene therapy product was introduced in China a few years ago for the treatment of head and neck cancer. However, this product has not been accepted for clinical use in Europe or in the United States. One antisense oligonucleotide product, fomivirsen, has received marketing authorization in the United States. This product is used to treat retinitis caused by the cytomegalo virus in AIDS patients.

Nonviral DNA delivery systems are based on chemical carriers (e.g., peptides, lipids, and polymers), or physical methods (e.g., electric pulses and ultrasound) that deliver the anionic DNA molecules (e.g., plasmids and oligonucleotides). Typical chemical carrier systems are based on cationic molecules that bind DNA and condense it to nanoparticulates, thereby protecting DNA from enzymatic degradation and increasing cellular uptake.[2] Physical systems are based on signals that open up the cell membranes temporarily and help gene transfer into the cells.

DNA is rapidly degraded after its administration. For example, plasmid DNA is degraded by the nucleases in a few minutes after intravenous administration. Nanoparticle-bound DNA is mostly distributed to the reticuloendothelial system (i.e., the spleen and liver) after adherence of the protein on their surface in plasma. These factors are not relevant in local gene delivery to the muscle, eye, or blood vessel wall from a stent.

This chapter focuses on the steps and mechanisms of gene transfer at the cellular level. The problems at the cellular level are relevant regardless of the route of DNA administration. From the forthcoming discussion, it is evident that the nanoparticle-mediated gene transfer is still showing weak efficacy when compared with the viral vectors. New strategies are needed in this field because the current approaches have not led to breakthroughs. Understanding the rate-determining steps is essential for the rational development of new gene delivery systems.[2–4]

This concise review is focused on the steps of gene delivery in the cells and this chapter addresses the selected open questions in the field.

6.2   STEPS OF NONVIRAL GENE DELIVERY

Nanoparticulate-based DNA delivery systems are based on cationic peptides, lipids, or polymers. These carriers bind and condense DNA based on the interaction of their positive charges with the negative charges on the phosphate backbone of the nucleotides. Usually, the zeta-potential of the nanoparticulates becomes positive at ± ratios above 1.0. At high charge ratios, the particles cannot accommodate excess carriers, which stay free in solution and may contribute to the cytotoxicity of the system.[5]

At the cellular level, the following steps are involved in DNA delivery with chemical nanoparticulate carriers: (1) binding on the cell surface, (2) internalization, (3) endocytosis, (4) endosomal escape, (5) cytoplasmic diffusion, (6) nuclear entry, and (7) gene expression. At some point during this process, DNA is released from the carrier. The carrier protects DNA from premature enzymatic degradation. These steps are schematically shown in Figure 6.1.

After DNA complexation into the nanoparticles, it is bound on the cell surface normally by electrostatic interactions with the negatively charged cell surface. The nanoparticles are then internalized by the endocytic process. The more exact type of endocytosis depends on the cell type and properties of the particles. The endocytosed nanoparticles cannot deliver DNA unless it is released from the endosomes. Otherwise, it would be trafficked to the lysosomes where DNA is enzymatically degraded. DNA or DNA nanoparticles must be able to diffuse in the cytoplasm to the nucleus for activity. Cytoplasmic diffusion is not self-evident because plasmid DNA is a large molecule and cytoplasm is a highly viscous medium. After reaching the nuclear wall, the DNA or DNA nanoparticles must be able to permeate into the nucleus, either by active transport or passive permeation during mitosis.

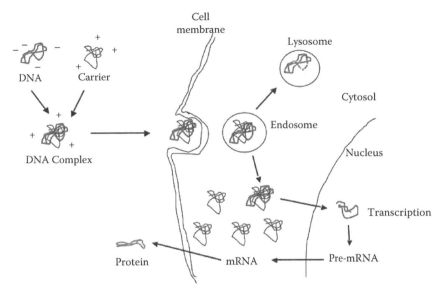

FIGURE 6.1 Steps of efficient trans- and intra-cellular DNA transfer with a nanoparticulate nonviral DNA delivery system. Particles are formed by electrostatic interactions of the cationic carrier with the anionic DNA molecule. They bind on the cell surface and are endocytosed. The nanoparticulates with or without DNA escapes from the endosome before it converts to lysosome, thus avoiding DNA degradation. The escaped nanoparticles transfer to the nuclear surface and are internalized across the nuclear membrane. DNA is released from the carrier at one of these stages, latest in the nucleus. DNA is appropriately localized within the nucleus for transcription. The resulting mRNA is translated to the protein. The role of the free carrier either during the delivery phase or after transcription is one of the open questions in the field.

There are several open questions, discrepancies, and concerns in the literature of DNA delivery. For example, naked DNA produces some transfection *in vivo* in many cases, but virtually never *in vitro* in cell culture.[6]

In general, the transfection *in vivo* with nanocarriers is lower than the levels achieved with cultured cells. Usually, the promising systems from cell culture systems do not transfect well *in vivo*.

> Naked DNA produces some transfection *in vivo* in many cases, but virtually never *in vitro* in cell culture. The transfection *in vivo* with nanocarriers is lower than the levels achieved with cultured cells. Usually, the promising systems from cell culture studies do not transfect well *in vivo*.

One of the reasons could be that the *in vitro* experiments are in most cases done at positive carrier/DNA ratios. In some rare cases, charge ratios of even 200 have been used.[7] Such high charge ratios are not practical *in vivo*. The high excess of free cationic carriers may increase the toxicity. In addition, intravenous administration is very different from the static cell culture plate.

Another concern relates to the methodology. DNA nanoparticles are usually investigated by transfection experiments with marker genes. This method gives the quantification of the protein, but does not tell us about the steps of DNA delivery prior to the expression, transcription, and translation.

Transfection experiments often have limited value in terms of mechanistic understanding. Unfortunately, several steps of gene transfer are difficult to study quantitatively. Confocal microscopy of fluorescently labeled DNA is a useful method for studying the cellular internalization and intracellular translocation, but it gives only qualitative information. In many cases, the resolution is not adequate either to resolve the localization of the transgene in the nucleus or the organization of the DNA nanoparticulates and their conformational changes. New high-resolution quantitative methods are needed to understand the physical and biological behavior of the DNA nanoparticulates.

6.3   CELLULAR UPTAKE

The cellular uptake of the DNA nanoparticulates is not a limiting factor in cell culture conditions. Zabner et al.[8] showed in their early work that approximately 10^4–10^5 copies of plasmid DNA are delivered per cell. The values depend on the cell type; but, in general, the total number of delivered plasmids is not a limiting factor.

The efficient uptake of cationic DNA nanoparticulates is not surprising, because the cell surface is covered by negatively charged proteoglycans.[9] The negatively charged glycosaminoglycan (GAG) chains avidly bind positively charged nanoparticulates. However, GAG chains are not indispensable for cellular uptake.[10] This was shown with mutant cells that are devoid of GAG chains on the surface. In these cells, the cellular uptake was higher than in the wild-type chicken hamster ovary (CHO) cells.[10] Thus, normal cationic DNA nanoparticles can use several mechanisms of cell entry. Probably, their mechanisms are nonspecific due to the strong electrostatic binding of the particles on the cell surface.

More specific binding can be achieved with neutral or negatively charged nanoparticulates that specifically recognize cell surface receptors. Interestingly, DNA nanoparticles coated with hyaluronic acid could be internalized via CD44 receptors.[11] The condensed cationic DNA nanoparticulates can be coated with neutral or negatively charged lipid bilayers to hide the cationic charge but express cell surface receptor recognition molecules. Also, PEGylated lipids can be used to provide "stealth" coating to repel plasma proteins and other polyanionic components in the extracellular space.[12]

The size of the DNA complexes is another important aspect. Typically, the DNA nanoparticles have diameters below 200 nm. Only phagocytosing cells can engulf large micrometer size particles. The smaller particles have the advantage of faster diffusion and penetration to a greater volume of body fluids. On the other hand, larger particles carry a higher DNA dose. Thus, most of the dose may be localized in a minority of the particles in the case of large particle DNA delivery systems. In this respect, monodispersity provides the basis for the best possible reproducibility.

6.4   INTRACELLULAR KINETICS

DNA nanoparticulates are taken up into the cells by endocytic mechanisms.[2] However, there are several types of endocytic mechanisms, like clathrin-coated pits and caveolin-mediated endocytosis.[13] It is not very clear which type of endocytosis should be optimal. Targeting to the specific endosome type is not easy. This field involves mostly qualitative research.

The major difference between caveolae and other endocytic vesicles involves the acidification process. Most endocytic vesicles are acidified by the proton pump on the endosome wall. The acidification is used by some viruses and toxins for activation.[14] This process does not take place in the caveolae. In fact, most of the endocytosed material is shuttled to the lysosomes.[8] This is not a desired situation in DNA delivery because DNA is degraded in the acidic environment.

There are many strategies by which the endocytosed DNA may be liberated into the cytoplasm before acidification and degradation (endosomal escape). For example, pH sensitive fusogenic peptides, polymers with endosomal buffering capacity, and fusogenic lipids can be used to augment DNA escape from the endosomes.[14] However, despite these approaches, only a small fraction of DNA reaches the cytoplasm.[8]

Diffusion of plasmid DNA and DNA nanoparticles is slow in highly viscous gel-like cytoplasm.[15] Thus, all of the released DNA may not reach the nuclear surface. Enzymatic degradation in the cytoplasm could further reduce the amount of DNA that reaches the nuclear membrane. Nanoparticles would protect DNA from the enzymes in the cytoplasm, but, on the other hand, DNA release should be efficient for it to be transcribed. At the moment, it is not known if plasmid DNA should be released early at the level of the endosomal to cytoplasmic transition (like oligonucleotides are released from cationic lipids) or in the nucleus.

DNA release is likely mediated by the competition of the intracellular polyanions, such as glycosaminoglycans, RNAs, anionic lipid membranes of the cell organelles, and proteins for the cationic carrier. In principle, this can lead to different scenarios. First, the cationic nanoparticles may become coated with the polyanion. This could be an uncontrolled random process due to the multiple polyanions available in the cell. Second, the polyanionic cell material may displace DNA from the cationic carrier and thereby release DNA.[5] This would depend on the competition and the relative affinities. Some DNA carriers, such as dioleylglycerylspermine (DOGS) and polyethylene imine (PEI), release DNA easier than some other carriers like poly-L-lysine (PLL).[16] Recently, Ruponen et al. introduced a polymerase chain reaction (PCR) method for quantification of the free and complexed DNA in the cells,[17] which did not show the correlation between DNA release and expression. This lack of correlation could be due to the complexity of many factors contributing to the transfection efficacy.

Some carriers (like PEI) release DNA relatively easily due to weaker binding or degradation of the carrier within the cells.[3,18,19] The results have been positive for such DNA-releasing nanoparticles.

Vuorimaa et al. used fluorescence spectroscopy to analyze the state of the DNA in the complexes.[20] The authors concluded that the DNA in PEI exists in tight and loose states, while only tight components are seen in PLL. Therefore, PEI complexes could release DNA more easily than the PLL complexes.

The final step in the DNA delivery is its access to the nucleus. Nuclear entry is easier in the proliferating cells because the nuclear envelope disappears during certain phases of cell division. The transfection efficiency is reduced by orders of magnitude when the cells stop proliferation and differentiate. This was shown recently with the human corneal epithelial cell line.[21] Nuclear division may also slow down DNA removal from the nucleus. Sometimes the duration of gene expression is longer in differentiated cells, but much shorter in proliferating cells.[22]

Nuclear delivery may be enhanced by attaching the nuclear localizing peptide sequences to the DNA nanoparticulates.[2] However, this approach has not solved the problems even though some positive results were seen.

Two recent studies question the overall importance of the cellular and nuclear delivery of the transgene. Hama et al. showed that plasmid/Lipofectamine® complexes and adenoviruses showed equivalent DNA delivery into the nucleus, but the expression of protein per DNA copy in the nucleus was 8000 times higher in the case of adenovirus.[23] It was shown recently[24] that PLL and PEI delivered approximately equal numbers of DNA copies to the nucleus, but there was about a 100 times higher level of gene expression after PEI delivery as compared with PLL. These could be due to (1) inadequate DNA release by some vectors since bound DNA cannot be transcribed and/or (2) more favorable subnuclear localization of the transgenes by the adenoviruses than the nanoparticulates.[25] These questions remain unanswered as of now.

6.5 TRANSGENE EXPRESSION

Research in nonviral gene delivery has been strongly focused on the steps of DNA delivery in the cells (e.g., cellular uptake and intracellular kinetics). Little attention has been directed toward the complexity of the transgene expression process. There is no information in the literature about the fate of the carrier materials in the cells after the delivery. The carrier materials are polycationic and highly reactive in the cellular environment. Therefore, the possible adverse effects of these carriers cannot be ruled out.

There is growing evidence that the free carrier material within the cell may impair gene expression at sub-toxic doses. Recently, Wen et al. showed that a rapidly degrading version of PEI was more efficient.[18] Presumably, this material released DNA more effectively and the metabolic small molecular degradation products interfered less with the cell functions than the full-length PEI.

Posttranscriptional factors may also have a significant influence on transgene expression.[26] The freed cationic carrier reduced transgene expression effectively. The inhibition seems to take place at the level of translation by the RNA binding of the cationic carriers. It is interesting that some cationic carriers require an excess of cationic charges (and therefore free cationic carrier) in order to exert optimal gene expression. Therefore, the role of free carriers requires further studies.

6.6 CONCLUDING REMARKS

The main focus in the field of nonviral gene delivery has been on the structure and the properties of cationic carriers, and such issues like DNA condensation, cellular uptake, endosomal escape, and nuclear entry. However, many important questions should be addressed in the design of the DNA delivery systems. These questions include efficient and controlled DNA release from the carrier intracellularly, the subnuclear location of the released DNA, and the minimization of carrier interference with gene translation. Additionally, there may be cellular defense mechanisms that silence the transgene (such as miRNA and siRNA systems).

REFERENCES

1. Crystal RG. Transfer of genes to humans: Early lessons and obstacles to success. *Science* 1995, 270(5235), 404–410.
2. Wolff JA, Rozema DB. Breaking the bonds: Non-viral vectors become chemically dynamic. *Mol Ther* 2008, 16(1), 8–15.
3. Luten J, van Nostrum CF, De Smedt SC, Hennink WE. Biodegradable polymers as non-viral carriers for plasmid DNA delivery. *J Control Release* 2008, 126(2), 97–110.
4. Zaldumbide A, Hoeben RC. How not to be seen: Immune-evasion strategies in gene therapy. *Gene Ther* 2008, 15(4), 239–246.
5. Xu Y, Hui SW, Frederik P, Szoka FC Jr. Physicochemical characterization and purification of cationic lipoplexes. *Biophys J*. 1999, 77(1), 341–353.
6. Herweijer H, Wolff JA. Gene therapy progress and prospects: Hydrodynamic gene delivery. *Gene Ther* 2007, 14(2), 99–107.
7. Rahbek UL, Howard KA, Oupicky D, Manickam DS, Dong M, Nielsen AF, Hansen TB, Besenbacher F, Kjems J. Intracellular siRNA and precursor miRNA trafficking using bioresponsive copolypeptides. *J Gene Med* 2008, 10(1), 81–93.
8. Zabner J, Fasbender AJ, Moninger T, Poellinger KA, Welsh MJ. Cellular and molecular barriers to gene transfer by a cationic lipid. *J Biol Chem* 1995, 270(32), 18997–19007.
9. Mislick KA, Baldeschwieler JD. Evidence for the role of proteoglycans in cation-mediated gene transfer. *Proc Natl Acad Sci USA* 1996, 93(22), 12349–12354.
10. Ruponen M, Honkakoski P, Tammi M, Urtti A: Cell surface glycosaminoglycans inhibit cation-mediated gene transfer. *J Gene Med* 2004, 6, 405–414.
11. Hornof M, Fuente M, Hallikainen M, Tammi R, Urtti A. Low molecular weight hyaluronan shielding of DNA/PEI polyplexes facilitates CD44 receptor mediated uptake in human corneal epithelial cells. *J Gene Med* 2008, 10, 70–80.
12. Lehtinen J, Hyvönen Z, Bunjes H, Subrizi A, Urtti A. Glycosaminoglycan resistant and pH-sensitive lipid-coated DNA-complexes produced by detergent dialysis method. *J Control Release* 2008, 131, 145–149.
13. Belting M, Wittrup A. Developments in macromolecular drug delivery. *Methods Mol Biol* 2009, 480, 1–10.
14. Hoekstra D, Rejman J, Wasungu L, Shi F, Zuhorn I. Gene delivery by cationic lipids: in and out of an endosome. *Biochem Soc Trans* 2007, 35, 68–71.
15. Dauty E, Verkman AS. Actin cytoskeleton as the principal determinant of size-dependent DNA mobility in cytoplasm: A new barrier for non-viral gene delivery. *J Biol Chem* 2005, 280(9), 7823–7828.
16. Ruponen M, Ylä-Herttuala S, Urtti A. Interactions of polymeric and liposomal gene delivery systems with extracellular glycosaminoglycans: Physicochemical and transfection studies. *Biochem Biophys Acta* 1999, 1415, 331–341.

17. Ruponen M, Arkko S, Urtti A, Reinisalo M, Ranta VP. Intracellular DNA release and elimination correlate poorly with transgene expression after non-viral transfection. *J Control Release* 2009, 136, 226–231.
18. Wen Y, Pan S, Luo X, Zhang X, Zhang W, Feng M. A biodegradable low molecular weight polyethylenimine derivative as low toxicity and efficient gene vector. *Bioconjug Chem* 2009, 20, 322–332.
19. Arote RB, Hwang SK, Yoo MK, Jere D, Jiang HL, Kim YK, Choi YJ, Nah JW, Cho MH, Cho CS. Biodegradable poly(ester amine) based on glycerol dimethacrylate and polyethylenimine as a gene carrier. *J Gene Med* 2008, 10(11), 1223–1235.
20. Vuorimaa E, Urtti A, Seppänen R, Lemmetyinen H, Yliperttula M. Time-resolved fluorescence spectroscopy reveals differences in structural organisation of cationic polymer–DNA complexes. *J Am Chem Soc* 2008, 130, 11695–11700.
21. Toropainen E, Hornof M, Kaarniranta K, Urtti A. Corneal epithelium as a platform for secretion of transgene products after transfection with liposomal gene eyedrops. *J Gene Med* 2007, 9, 208–216.
22. Mannermaa E, Rönkkö S, Urtti A. Non-invasive kinetic analysis of transgene expression in differentiated cultured retinal pigment epithelial cells. *Curr Eye Res* 2005, 30, 345–353.
23. Hama S, Akita H, Ito R, Mizuguchi H, Hayakawa T, Harashima H. Quantitative comparison of intracellular trafficking and nuclear transcription between adenoviral and lipoplex systems. *Mol Ther* 2006, 13(4), 786–794.
24. Männistö M, Reinisalo M, Ruponen M, Honkakoski P, Tammi M, Urtti A. Polyplex-mediated gene transfer and cell cycle: Effect of carrier on cellular uptake and intracellular kinetics, and significance of glycosaminoglycans. *J Gene Med* 2007, 9, 479–486.
25. Ochiai H, Harashima H, Kamiya H. Intranuclear disposition of exogenous DNA in vivo. Silending, methylation and fragmentation. *FEBS Lett* 2006, 580, 918–923.
26. Hama S, Akita H, Iida S, Mizuguchi H, Harashima H. Quantitative and mechanism-based investigation of post-nuclear delivery events between adenovirus and lipoplex. *Nucleic Acids Res* 2007, 35(5), 1533–1543.

7 Targeted Delivery Systems of Nonviral Nucleic Acid–Based Therapeutics

*Ga Yong Shim, Eun-Joong Kim, Rae Sung Chang,
Han Young Lee, and Yu-Kyoung Oh*

CONTENTS

7.1 INTRODUCTION

7.1.1 OVERVIEW

Recently, various nucleic acid–based therapeutics have emerged as new classes of innovative medicines. One of the central tenets of cell biology is the fact that DNA or RNA nucleotides can modulate the protein expression of cells and tissues in a specific manner. DNA-based modalities include plasmid DNA (pDNA), antisense oligonucleotides (AS-ON), and DNA aptamers. RNA-based entities include ribozymes, small interfering RNAs (siRNAs), and RNA aptamers.

The mechanisms by which nucleic acid–based molecules exert therapeutic activities depend on the nature of the activity. After introduction into the cells, pDNAs encoding specific proteins are transcribed and translated, resulting in therapeutic effects by the expressed proteins. Aptamers are short (15–40 nucleotides long), synthetic, single-stranded ON (ssDNA or ssRNA) capable of binding targets like proteins, carbohydrates, and other small molecules.[1] Because of their specific three-dimensional secondary structure, DNA or RNA aptamers are capable of binding to target molecules with high affinity and specificity. The complex molecular shapes resulting from the intramolecular interactions of aptamers usually provide a tight binding affinity to functional domains, substrate binding sites, or allosteric sites of target proteins. This tight binding allows the aptamer to mediate the regulation of the biological functions.[2]

AS-ONs and siRNAs block the expression of target genes via the specific breakdown of target mRNA. Specifically, AS-ONs inhibit the expression of target mRNA by RNase H. The formation of an AS-ON and mRNA heteroduplex triggers the active endonuclease RNase H to cleave the complementary mRNA, which eventually prevents the synthesis of the target protein.[3] To enhance the activity of antisense drugs, AS-ONs have been chemically stabilized by various modification methods, including phosphothioate modification of the phosphodiester backbone and 2′-OH modification. Locked nucleic acids (LNAs), peptide nucleic acids (PNAs), and morpholino have been developed to improve the cellular uptake and biodistribution of AS-ONs.[4] However, most of the chemically modified AS-ONs do not efficiently activate RNase H. Cellular mechanisms other than the RNase H-mediated degradation pathway are involved in the down-regulation of the target gene expression, either by alternative splicing or by translation arrest.[5]

Compared with AS-ON, siRNAs have a much shorter history of pharmaceutical applications. In 1998, Andrew Z. Fire and Craig C. Mello discovered the RNA interference (RNAi) phenomenon where the expression of a certain gene with a homologous sequence of double-stranded RNA (dsRNA) was specifically down-regulated after introducing the dsRNA into the cells of *Caenorhabditis elegans*.[6] Shortly after this discovery, the molecular mechanisms of RNAi were studied in mammalian cells, igniting the interest of pharmaceutical companies. In mammalian cell cytoplasm, an enzyme known as Dicer initiates RNA silencing by breaking down long dsRNA, thus generating siRNAs with a length of 21–25 nucleotides. The resulting siRNAs are incorporated into the RNA-induced silencing complex (RISC) and unwound into ssRNA, followed by the degradation of sense strand ssRNA.[7] When the RISC containing an antisense strand of ssRNA binds to complementary mRNA, it induces the degradation of the mRNA. The target-specific and potent inhibition mechanisms by siRNA made it possible to develop therapeutic drugs based on entirely new concepts. The identification of highly selective and inhibitory siRNA sequences is much faster than the discovery of new chemicals. Moreover, the drug potential of siRNAs could be enhanced by relatively easy synthesis and large-scale manufacture.[8]

Because of the different functions of nucleic acid–based molecules, the cellular target sites differ among the molecules. In pDNA-based gene therapy, pDNA should be delivered into the nucleus so that RNA polymerases may copy the information of pDNA to mRNA. Following endocytosis, pDNA should thus escape the endosomal barrier and enter through the nuclear pore complex. Unlike pDNA, siRNA must be delivered only to cytoplasm, possibly after endosomal escape. Similar to antibodies, most therapeutic aptamers have been designed to bind to the target molecules on the cell surfaces.

Although these nucleic acid–based molecules differ in their molecular structures, functions, and intracellular targets as summarized in Table 7.1, they all suffer from common problems, namely, limited cellular uptake and *in vivo* instability. Because of their phosphate groups, nucleic acids are anionic, hydrophilic, and unable to enter cells by passive diffusion. Moreover, delivering the nucleic acid–based molecules to target disease sites *in vivo* remains a challenge due to the enzymatic

TABLE 7.1

Comparison of Nonviral Nucleotide-Based Medicines

	pDNA	AS-ON	siRNA	Aptamer
Molecular structure	Circular and double-helix DNA, various nucleotide length, containing functional ORF	ssON, 15–20 nucleotides. Containing complementary sequence to target mRNA	Duplex RNA, 21–23 nucleotides. Containing complementary sequence to target mRNA	ssDNA or ssRNA, 12–30 nucleotides
Function	Expression of therapeutic protein	Suppression of target mRNA expression by RNase H activity	Suppression of target mRNA expression by RISC	Binding to target molecules by its three-dimensional structures
Therapeutic targets	Various therapeutic genes (tumor suppressor genes, biological function enhancer)	Various oncogenes, anti-apoptotic genes, viral genes	Various oncogenes, anti-apoptotic genes, viral genes	Regulation of biological function of target molecules, targeting moiety
Disadvantages	Relatively low efficacy	Relatively low efficacy, low stability	Systemic delivery concerns, off target limit, immune response, high cost	Low efficiency of screening, low stability
Advantages	Low cost, well understood, easy to screen targets	Low cost, specificity, easy to handle	High therapeutic effect, low side effects by biological mechanisms	Highly specificity, low cost
Marketed products	Gendicine, Oncorin (marketed in China)	Vitravene	—	Macugen

Note: ORF, open reading frame; RISC, RNA-induced silencing complex.

digestion of nucleic acids in plasma.[8] To overcome these difficulties, targeted delivery systems are being developed for various nucleic acid–based molecules. This chapter addresses the strategies for delivering these molecules to disease sites, with an emphasis on targeting moieties.

> Gene expression plasmids must enter the nuclei to confer functionality, while AS-ON and siRNA do not need to enter the nucleus for gene silencing.

7.1.2 CURRENT STATUS

For over 20 years, researchers have been developing nucleic acid–based molecules as therapeutic substances. Although progress and clinical outcomes vary among the classes of nucleotide drugs, several products are either on the market or in phase III trials, indicating a bright future for nucleic acid–based molecules as innovative medicines.

Among nucleic acid–based therapeutics, pDNAs have received the most extensive attention worldwide, with two products currently on the market. The first human gene therapy trial started in 1989,[9] and currently there are 1309 clinical trials in progress in 28 countries.[10] The majority of clinical trials focus on cancers (66.5%) as target diseases using viral vector systems (over 67%) for *in vivo* delivery. In gene therapy clinical trials, viral vectors have been predominantly used over nonviral vectors to introduce functional genetic materials *in vivo*. Viral vectors in clinical trials include retroviruses, adenoviruses, adeno-associated viruses, and lentiviruses. Although there are no gene medicines approved by the Food and Drug Administration (FDA) in the United States, two products are on the market in China. China's State Food and Drug Administration (SFDA) approved

Currently, there are 1309 gene therapy clinical trials in progress in 28 countries. The majority of clinical trials focus on cancers (66.5%) as target diseases, using viral vector systems (over 67%) for *in vivo* delivery.

Gendicine® in 2003, a recombinant human adenovirus encoding a wild-type p53 for the treatment of patients with head and neck squamous cell carcinoma[11] and Oncorine®, a genetically modified anticancer adenovirus for killing tumor cells with the mutated *p53* genes, in 2005.[12] These commercially available cancer gene therapy products demonstrated significant effectiveness in a number of patients in China.[13] The long-term safety and efficacy issues still remain to be answered in post-surveillance studies.

Despite the absence of approved gene medicine products in the United States, an AS-ON-based drug, Vitravene®, developed by ISIS Pharmaceuticals, was first approved for human use in the United States and Europe in 1998 and 1999, respectively. This product was approved for the treatment of rhinitis caused by cytomegalovirus infection, an activity based on specific binding to the complementary mRNA sequence of the cytomegalovirus in patients with acquired immune deficiency syndrome (AIDS).[14]

Because AS-ONs can reduce the synthesis of harmful proteins involved in the pathogenesis of various diseases, most anticancer AS-ONs in clinical trials have been designed to inhibit the synthesis of target proteins responsible for anti-apoptotic signaling or malignant proliferation of cancer cells. Prominent AS-ONs in clinical trials include Genasense® (oblimersen sodium, G3139), which targets Bcl-2 oncoprotein, and Affinitak® (aprinocarsen, ISIS 3521, LY900003), which targets the protein kinase C-α. The anticancer efficacies of these AS-ON drugs have been evaluated in combination with various chemotherapeutic agents. Given the completion of clinical trials of these two products, the addition of approved AS-ON drugs may be a reality in the near future.[15]

Although the RNAi phenomenon was first discovered in 1998, remarkable progress has been made with unprecedented speed in the development of siRNAs as pharmaceutical products.[16] The first generations of RNAi therapeutics used local routes to deliver siRNAs, thus avoiding the instability issues following systemic administration. The forerunner in the siRNA field is Cand5® (bevasiranib), developed by Opko Health, which targets vascular endothelial growth factor (VEGF). Cand5 (bevasiranib) is administered by intravitreal injection, and the drug is in phase III clinical trials for the treatment of neovascular age-related macular degeneration (AMD). Sirna Therapeutics' Sirna-027 (termed AGN211745), a chemically modified siRNA targeting VEGF receptor 1, is in phase II clinical trials for the treatment of AMD. ALN-RSV01, developed by Alnylam Pharmaceuticals, is the first antiviral siRNA to be used in a clinical trial. ALN-RSV01 works against the mRNA of the respiratory syncytial virus (RSV) and is being administered intranasally in the clinical trial.[17]

Formulated products are being studied for the systemic administration of siRNAs. CALAA-01, from Calando Pharmaceuticals, is the first systemic and targeted delivery system–based siRNA product in a clinical trial. CALAA-01 is a cyclodextrin-based polymeric nanoparticle containing an siRNA that targets the M2 subunit of ribonucleotide reductase in a variety of tumors. This nanoparticle attached to transferrin (Tf) is capable of targeting tumor cells by preferential binding to the transferrin receptors (TfR). Recently, there has been a huge effort, both in academia and in industry, to develop *in vivo* delivery systems for siRNAs.[18] Given the fervor of research into siRNA-based products, the list of siRNAs in clinical trials is expected to grow substantially in the near future.

Aptamers have been developed as versatile tools in pharmaceutical fields such as target validation, high-throughput screening, diagnostics, and therapeutic agents.[2] The specific binding affinities of the aptamers to targets led to the development of new therapeutic modalities. The first aptamer drug, Macugen® (pegaptanib sodium), targeting VEGF was approved by the U.S. FDA in 2004[1] for the treatment of AMD. More recently, AS1411, which binds to a nucleolin protein on the surface of cancer cells, entered phase II clinical trials for the treatment of acute myeloid leukemia and renal cancer. ARC 1779, an injectable form of a polyethylene glycol (PEG)-linked aptamer that inhibits the function of von Willebrand factor, entered a phase II clinical trial in March 2008.

As listed in Table 7.2, nucleic acid–based drugs have been studied in clinical trials for decades. Although the number of products available on the market is limited, several candidates are in line

TABLE 7.2
Examples of Nonviral Nucleic Acid–Based Medicines in Clinical Trials

Nucleic Acids	Product Name	Developer/ Company	Target	Disease	Status
pDNA	Gendicine	SiBiono GeneTech Co.	p53	Cancer	Approved in China
	H101 (Oncorine)	Sunway Biotech Co.	p53	Cancer	Approved in China
	DTA-H19	BioCancell Therapeutics	Diphtheria toxin A chain	Bladder cancer	II
	pVGI.1	Corautus Genetics	VEGF2	Angina pectoris	II
	Leuvectin	Vical, Inc.	IL-2	Prostate cancer	II
AS-ON	Vitravene (Fomivirsen)	ISIS/Novatis	CMV IE	CMV retinitis	Marked
	Genasense (Oblimersen/G3139)	Genta	Bcl-2	Cancer	III/NDA
	Affinitak (Aprinocarsen/ ISIS3521)	ISIS/Lilly	PKC-α	Cancer	III
	Alicaforsen (ISIS 2302)	ISIS/Atlantic Healthcare	ICAM-1	Crohn's disease	III
	ISIS 2503	ISIS	H-Ras	Cancer	II
	ISIS 5132	ISIS	c-Raf	Cancer	II
	GTI-2501	Lorus Therapeutics	Ribonucleotide reductase R1	Cancer	II
siRNA	Bevasirnanib (Cand 5)	Opko Health	VEGF	AMD	III
				DME	II
	AGN211745 (sirna-027)	Allergan	VEGF receptor	AMD	II
	ALN-RSV01	Alnylam Pharmaceuticals	RSV	RSV infection	II
Aptamer	Macugen (pegaptanib sodium)	Pfizer/Eyetech Pharmaceuticals	VEGF	AMD	Marked
	ARC1779	Archemix Corp.	vWF	TTP	II
	AS1411	Antisoma/ Archemix Corp.	Nucleolin	AML, renal cancer	II

Note: VEGF, vascular endothelial growth factor; IL-2, interleukin-2; CMV, cytomegalovirus; PKC, protein kinase C; ICAM-1, inter-cellular adhesion molecule 1; AMD, age-related macular degeneration; DME, diabetic macular edema; RSV, respiratory syncytial virus; vWF, von Willebrand factor; TTP, thrombotic thrombocytopenic purpura; AML, acute myelocytic leukemia.

for approval. The increase in promising research outcomes at the laboratory level is expected to lead to a long pipeline of nucleic acid–based products in clinical trials, with some possibly reaching the market in the near future.

7.1.3 DELIVERY SYSTEMS

Although nucleic acid–based molecules have achieved significant progress as a new class of therapeutics, several hurdles must be overcome. One hurdle is the limited efficiency of nucleic acid delivery to target cells or tissues. Usually, the delivery systems can be divided into two categories: viral and nonviral. In viral vectors, genes coding proteins or functional RNAs, such as short hairpin RNAs (shRNAs), are inserted into viral genes, and these enter into the host cells by receptor-mediated endocytosis. Nonviral vectors include chemical delivery systems, nanoparticles, and cell vehicles.

7.1.3.1   Viral Vectors

About 68% of gene therapy clinical trials have employed viral vectors as gene delivery systems. For *in vitro* and *in vivo* gene delivery, viral vectors have shown relatively higher transfection efficiency than nonviral vectors (http://www.wiley.co.uk/genetherapy/clinical/). Adenoviruses and retroviruses account for more than 50% of the viral vectors in clinical trials. Their transfection efficiencies are higher than those of nonviral vectors because of the natural tropisms of viruses into specific cells or tissues. However, natural tropisms of viruses often do not match the therapeutic purpose and desired biodistribution patterns.

To redirect the therapeutic gene-encoding viruses to target cells, several studies have involved pseudotyping, adaptor systems, or genetic systems. Pseudotyping designs a viral vector to use a viral attachment protein from a different virus strain or family to target certain cells.[19] In adaptor systems, a molecule that binds to both the viral vector and the target cell receptor is used to facilitate the transduction.[20] For example, adaptor systems include specific interaction between the receptor and the ligand, such as avidin and biotin, or the antigen and the antibody. In genetic systems, a polypeptide, which is a targeting moiety, is incorporated into the vector by genetic means.[21] In addition to these targeting strategies, oncolytic adenoviruses exclusively lyse cancer cells based on the differential replication of the oncolytic viruses, which occurs in cancer cells but not in normal cells. Thus, when the oncolytic viruses deliver therapeutic genes into a tumor, the combined effects of the oncolysis and gene therapy can be observed.[22]

Despite the high efficiencies of gene transfer, viral vectors have suffered from several drawbacks, such as immunogenicity, pathogenicity, the possible onset of leukemia, and design complexity.[23] Jesse Gelsinger was the first patient to die in a clinical trial for gene therapy in 1999. Gelsinger suffered from ornithine transcarbamylase deficiency, an X-linked genetic non-life-threatening disease of the liver. After injections of adenovirus carrying the corrected genes, the patient died of massive immune response. The tragedy subdued the passion for viral vector–based gene therapy and emphasized the need for safer delivery systems.

7.1.3.2   Nonviral Vectors

Recently, nonviral vectors are gaining more attention and researchers are extensively studying their potential to deliver various nucleic acid–based molecules. Compared with viral vectors, nonviral vectors have relatively low immunogenicity and pathogenicity. Chemical, nonviral delivery systems can be generally divided into systems that operate via lipid- and polymer-mediated transfection. Lipofection is the process of transfection mediated by lipid-based systems, such as liposomes, micelles, emulsions, and solid lipid nanoparticles. These lipid-based chemical delivery systems accounted for 7.6% of the clinical gene therapy trials in 2008 (http://www.wiley.co.uk/genetherapy/clinical/). Polymer-based delivery systems have also been actively studied.[24] In general, cationic polymers are employed to deliver nucleic acids that form electrostatic complexes between the positively charged delivery systems and the negatively charged genetic materials. Polyethylenimine (PEI), poly(2-dimethylaminoethyl methacrylate), and poly-L-lysine are frequently used examples of cationic polymers. In addition to high transfection efficiency, biocompatibility and biodegradability are desirable properties for these nonviral delivery systems.

7.2   TARGETING STRATEGIES

To reduce undesirable side effects and enhance therapeutic effects, the design of a targeted delivery system is crucial. Especially for drugs with a narrow therapeutic index, well controlled delivery of therapeutic entities to disease sites is desirable. In cancer therapy, the leaky blood vessels of tumor tissues allow for preferential penetration and retention of nanoparticles as compared with normal blood vessels. This is termed the enhanced permeability and retention (EPR) effect. Because of the EPR effect, nanoparticles with mean sizes less than 400 nm can accumulate in tumor tissue. Such EPR-mediated targeting of delivery systems carrying anticancer drugs is called "passive" targeting.[25] However, this passive targeting strategy is not applicable to all cancer types, and it is not effective enough to treat cancers.

Hence, active targeting systems, in which the delivery of nucleic acid therapeutics could be intelligently directed, are needed. For active targeting, most delivery systems have been modified with target ligands. In addition to the ligand-modified delivery systems, both biological cell-based systems and stimuli-activated systems have recently been studied as new classes of active targeting systems of nucleic acid–based therapeutics. With regard to targeting ligands, various molecules have been used including antibodies, carbohydrates, proteins, peptides, vitamins, small chemicals, and, more recently, targeting aptamers. These target ligands should be able to specifically bind to target cells that selectively overexpress their receptors on surfaces. After targeting ligands recognize the receptors, endocytosis must occur to initiate the intracellular delivery of nucleic acid–based molecules. When targeting ligands bind to their receptor, some ligand–receptor complexes are internalized by "receptor-mediated endocytosis." Because most nucleic acid–based molecules must be delivered to cytoplasms, the internalization capability of receptors should be considered. One of the limiting factors for successful receptor-mediated gene transfer is the endosomal release of nucleic acids after intracellular uptake. Several membrane rupture peptides, such as Influenza HA2, listeriolysin, or mellitin can cause an endosomal escape of nucleic acids to cytoplasms.[26–28] Current examples of active targeting ligands and delivery systems are discussed in the following sections.

7.2.1 Monoclonal Antibody

A monoclonal antibody that binds to specific antigens on target cells has been considered to be one of the most attractive targeting ligands. Due to the specificity of antigen binding, monoclonal antibodies have been extensively used to target the desired cells and deliver therapeutic genes and nucleic acids (Table 7.3). Cancer, the disease most frequently targeted by monoclonal antibodies, may overexpress some receptors or cell surface proteins compared with normal cells. These overexpressed molecules on cancer cells serve as good targets of monoclonal antibodies to actively direct delivery systems carrying nucleic acid–based therapeutics to the cancer cells.

Antibodies can be used either in their native form or in their modified form. Natural antibodies, usually immunoglobulin G (IgG), have two light and two heavy chains. They form the Fab (fragment, antigen binding) region and the Fc (fragment, crystallizable) region. The Fab region is located in the tip of the Y shape of the antibodies and has a binding affinity to a specific antigen. The Fc region, located at the base of the Y-shape antibodies, determines the type of immunoglobulin. Native whole antibodies are more stable than their fragments and can be stored for relatively long periods. However, whole antibodies may bind to some proteins or Fc receptors on immune cells, which may cause immune responses. To avoid the undesired immune responses by the Fc regions of monoclonal antibodies, some fragments of monoclonal antibodies, such as dimers of antigen-binding fragments (F(ab')$_2$) and single-chain fragment variables (scFv), have been developed. Although these engineered fragments are relatively unstable in comparison with whole antibodies, they have low immunogenicity because they lack Fc regions, while maintaining antigen-binding affinity.[29]

Before RNAi was discovered in 1998, pDNA was a major therapeutic genetic material for gene therapy. Numerous studies have thus focused on the targeted delivery of pDNA using monoclonal antibodies as targeting moieties. Monoclonal antibodies were chemically linked to surfaces of cationic liposomes or polymers. Yu and colleagues[30] modified cationic liposomes with anti-transferrin receptor single-chain antibody fragment (TfRscFv) for the targeted delivery of pDNA. The TfRscFv-modified cationic immunoliposomes were complexed with pDNA encoding p53 and were intravenously administered to mice xenografted with prostate cancer cells. The TfRscFv-modified immunoliposomes provided an improved distribution of pDNA to tumor tissues compared with

TABLE 7.3

Examples of Monoclonal Antibody-Mediated Targeting

Nucleic Acids	Antibody	Cargo Genes/ Target Genes	Vehicle	Target Cells	Reference
pDNA	TfRscFv	p53	PEG-liposome	Prostate cancer	[30]
	Anti-PSMA mAb	p53	PEI	Prostate cancer	[33]
	Anti-TAG-72 Fab fragment	Angiostatin K1/3, endostatin and saxatilin	PEG-liposome	Colon cancer	[32]
	TfRscFv	RB94	Liposome	Bladder carcinoma	[31]
siRNA	Anti-HIV-1 envelope Fab fragment, anti-ErbB2 scFv	gag, c-myc, MDM2 and VEGF	Fusion protein (antibody-protamine)	HIV, melanoma	[34]
	Anti-LFA-1 scFv	Ku70, CD4, CCR5, Cyclin D1	Fusion protein (antibody-protamine)	Lymphocytes	[29]
	Anti-HBsAg scFv	HBV genes	Fusion protein (antibody-protamine)	HBV infection	[36]
	Anti-integrin β7 mAb	Cyclin D1	Hyaluronan-liposome, protamine	Leukocytes	[35]
	Anti-CD7 scFv	HIV genes, CCR5	Antibody-oligo-arginine	HIV infection	[37]

Note: PEG, poly(ethylene glycol); PSMA, prostate specific membrane antigen; PEI, poly(ethylenimine); RB94, Retinoblastoma 94; HIV, human immunodeficiency virus; ErbB2, erythroblastic leukemia viral oncogene homolog 2; MDM2, murine double minute 2; LFA-1, leukocyte function-associated antigen 1; Ku70, 70 K subunit of Ku antigen; CCR5, chemokine (C-C motif) receptor 5; HBV, hepatitis B virus.

unmodified liposome carriers. Moreover, the additional use of PEG on the surface of liposomes stabilized the systems, enhancing the delivery of pDNA to tumors. The presence of PEG is thought to prevent the nonspecific binding of undesirable serum proteins, reducing the clearance of the liposome and pDNA complexes by the immune systems, such as the reticuloendothelial system, and allowing the prolonged circulation of lipoplexes in the blood stream.

TfRscFv-modified cationic immunoliposomes were also used to deliver pDNA encoding RB94 to tumor tissues. RB94, a truncated protein of RB110, has tumor suppression activity against several tumors including bladder carcinoma. Pirollo and colleagues utilized the TfRscFv-modified cationic immunoliposomes for the targeted delivery of pDNA encoding RB94 to bladder carcinoma.[31] Following intravenous administration, the complexes of TfRscFv-modified cationic immunoliposomes and pDNA inhibited the growth of tumors in mouse models. Moreover, the administration of immunoliposome and pDNA complexes sensitized the chemotherapeutic effect of gemcitabine in HTB-9 xenograft tumors.

Antitumor-associated glycoprotein (TAG)-72 immunoliposomes were formulated by the conjugation of Fab fragments of recombinant humanized monoclonal antibody to sterically stabilized PEG liposomes.[32] These anti-TAG-72 immunoliposome/pDNA complexes could bind to TAG-72 overexpressing LS174T human colon cancer cells more than plain liposomes *in vitro*. In LS174T tumor mouse models, anti-TAG-72 immunoliposomes efficiently accumulated in tumor tissue after intravenous injection, whereas nontargeted liposomes did not. Moreover, when these anti-TAG-72 immunoliposomes contained pDNA encoding antiangiogenic proteins, such as angiostatin K1/3, endostatin, and saxatilin, they demonstrated significant tumor growth inhibition.

Monoclonal antibodies were linked to cationic polymers for the targeted delivery of nucleic acid–based therapeutics. One of the most widely studied cationic polymers is PEI. A monoclonal antibody binding to a prostate-specific membrane antigen (PSMA) was tagged to PEI and used to deliver pDNA.[33] The anti-PSMA monoclonal antibody-modified PEI showed up to a 20-fold increase in delivery of pDNA compared with unmodified PEI in nude mice bearing orthotopic prostate cancer. Interestingly, this study applied the strong interaction between phenyl(di)borocin acid and salicylhydroxamic acid to attach the anti-PSMA monoclonal antibody to PEI. These two small chemicals have high binding affinities similar to that of an antibody–antigen complex, and they did not induce an immune response *in vivo*.

Starting in the early 2000s, siRNAs gained attention as a new generation of nucleic acid–based therapeutics. As in pDNA gene therapy, the issue of delivering siRNAs to target cells remains a key hurdle for the development of siRNAs as therapeutics. Therefore, numerous investigations into *in vivo* siRNA delivery are in progress. Monoclonal antibodies *per se* have been studied as a major tool for siRNA delivery. To provide cationic properties to a monoclonal antibody, positively charged protamine was fused to the heavy chain Fab fragment of a human immunodeficiency virus (HIV)-1 envelope antibody. The protamine-fused Fab antibody (F105-P) was then used to deliver siRNA to HIV-infected or envelope-transfected cells.[34] Following delivery via F105-P, siRNA silencing of the HIV-1 capsid gene *gag* inhibited the replication of HIV in primary T cells infected with HIV *in vitro*. Intratumoral or intravenous injection of siRNA targeting *c-myc*, *MDM2*, and *VEGF* complexed with F105-P inhibited the growth of the HIV envelope-expressing subcutaneous B16 tumors. Another fusion protein of the ErbB2 single-chain antibody fragment with protamine could provide the targeted delivery of siRNAs to ErbB2-expressing cancer cells. This study suggests the potential of a single-chain antibody fragment as a delivery system of siRNA. However, to deliver siRNA in therapeutically effective doses, the amount of siRNA that can be carried by a single antibody may need to be increased.

Single chain antibody fragments targeting the human integrin lymphocyte function-associated antigen-1(LFA-1) were genetically fused to protamine for the specific delivery of siRNA to primary lymphocytes, monocytes, and dendritic cells.[35] In nude mice inoculated with K562 cells expressing LFA-1, the intravenous injection of the fusion protein and Ku70-specific siRNA complexes silenced the Ku70 protein only in the cells expressing LFA-1 on their surfaces.

The targeted delivery of siRNA using antibodies was also achieved in the hepatitis B virus (HBV) in transgenic mice.[36] Fluorescent siRNA or HBV-specific siRNA was complexed to a fusion protein composed of a single chain of the human variable fragment against the hepatitis B surface antigen, a constant region of the human κ chain, and truncated protamine. After HBV transgenic mice were intravenously dosed with the complexes of fluorescent siRNA and the fusion protein, fluorescence was primarily observed in hepatitis B surface antigen-positive hepatocytes. The systemic administration of siRNAs specific for HBV and the fusion protein complexes effectively suppressed both the gene expression and the replication of HBV in transgenic mice. Moreover, the antibody fusion protein provided targeted delivery of HBV-specific siRNA-producing plasmid in HBV transgenic mice.

Given that β7 integrins are highly expressed in gut mononuclear leukocytes, a monoclonal antibody to β7 integrin was used for targeted delivery of siRNAs to leukocytes involved in gut inflammation.[35] As cargo, neutral liposomes were first prepared using a covalent conjugate of a neutral lipid dipalmitoylphosphatidylethanolamine and hyaluronan. Next, the hyaluronan on the surface of liposomes was covalently modified with a monoclonal antibody against β7 integrin and lyophilized. In this system, cyclin D1-specific siRNA was condensed with protamine and encapsulated in liposomes during the rehydration of prelyophilized liposomes. After intravenous injection into mice with colitis, the immunoliposomes preferentially distributed to the gut. Moreover, the intravenous administration of cyclin D1-specific siRNA (2.5 mg/kg) entrapped in the β7 integrin-tagged immunoliposomes reduced intestinal inflammation in a colitis mouse model.

In addition to the targeted delivery, the β7 integrin-tagged immunoliposomes were notable for their increased capacity to carry siRNA. These liposomes were reported to carry about 4000 siRNA molecules per particle and about 100 siRNA molecules per targeting antibody molecule. Thus, this system significantly improved the delivery capacity of its previous system, integrin-targeted single-chain antibody protamine fusion protein, which could carry only five siRNA molecules per fusion protein.[29]

Instead of protamine, a nine-arginine oligomer was used as a cationic moiety in the antibody-mediated delivery of siRNA. A chemical conjugate of the nine-arginine oligomer to anti-CD7 single-chain antibody fragments (scFvCD7-9R) was designed to deliver siRNAs targeting the viral coreceptor CCR5 and conserved genes of HIV.[37] scFvCD7-9R could specifically deliver antiviral siRNAs to naive T cells in humanized mice reconstituted with CD34+ hematopoietic stem cells, and it effectively suppressed viremia in infected mice. Using an elaborately designed fusion antibody as a T cell-targeted delivery system, this study first suggested the potential of siRNA as anti-HIV therapeutics in a preclinical animal model.

As discussed above, monoclonal antibodies may play a role as targeting ligands for delivering nucleic acid–based therapeutics because of their specific binding affinity to antigens highly expressed on target cells. In addition to the specific binding, the monoclonal antibodies should induce efficient endocytosis following the cell surface binding for intracellular processing or expression of nucleic acid–based therapeutics. Even though the monoclonal antibodies provide specific binding and endocytosis, there still remain several limitations for the successful application of monoclonal antibodies. First, due to the relatively large size of monoclonal antibodies, the biodistribution of monoclonal antibodies to poorly vascularized tissues or central nervous systems protected by blood–brain barriers could be limited. To resolve this size issue, smaller sizes of antibody-mimetic peptides or proteins may be studied as targeting ligands. Second, the Fc portion of monoclonal antibodies has been known to elicit immune responses after repeated use. Although Fab fragments or single-chain antibody fragments have been studied to reduce the immunogenicity, the large-scale production of single-chain antibody fragments is difficult and costly.[38] Third, the limited capacity of monoclonal antibodies to carry therapeutically sufficient amounts of nucleic acid–based therapeutics should be resolved. The tagging of monoclonal antibodies to high capacity nanoparticles entrapping nucleic acid–based therapeutics would be one approach that can improve the cargo capacity of antibodies. Despite these challenging limitations, monoclonal antibodies and their fragments are still attractive targeting systems for nucleic acid–based therapeutics, and they offer huge potential for clinical applications in the near future.

7.2.2 TRANSFERRIN

Tf is a plasma protein that binds and delivers iron to the spleen, liver, and bone marrow through Tf receptors. This glycoprotein has a molecular weight of about 80 kDa and contains two subunits, N-lobe and C-lobe, linked by a short spacer.[39] The Tf monomer can transport one or two iron atoms bound to each lobe. Apo-Tf denotes a Tf molecule without iron, and monoferric or diferric Tf indicates a one- or two-iron-bound Tf, respectively. Tf plays an important role in preventing the circulation of free Fe^{3+}, which may produce free radicals and exert a toxic effect on cells. Therefore, the interaction between Tf and its receptor is very important for the iron homeostasis of the body.[40]

The Tf receptor (CD71), a type II transmembrane glycoprotein, mediates the intracellular delivery of ferric iron through endocytosis and returns to the cell surface in the form of an apo-Tf and receptor complex (Figure 7.1A). In normal cells, the Tf receptor is expressed in low levels. It is expressed at a very high level in actively dividing cells in the tissues, such as the basal epidermis and intestinal epithelium. Moreover, Tf receptors are overexpressed in malignant cancer cells compared with benign cells. Therefore, Tf as a tumor targeting ligand has been extensively employed due to its receptor's overexpression in cancer cells, receptor-mediated internalization, endosomal release, and receptor recycle.[41]

As a targeting ligand, Tf has been associated or covalently conjugated to nonviral delivery systems of nucleic acid–based therapeutics such as pDNA, AS-ON, and siRNA. In the early stages of this strategy, Tf was simply mixed with lipoplex or polyplex to enhance cellular uptake or targeting

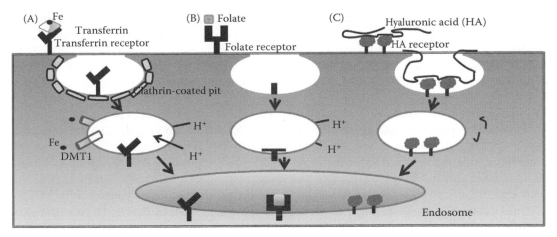

FIGURE 7.1   Receptor-mediated endocytosis pathways. (A) TfR-mediated endocytosis pathway. When Tf binds to TfR on the cell surface, the complex is internalized by receptor-mediated endocytosis through clathrin-coated pits, forming endosomes. Iron is released from Tf and transported out of acidified endosomes via DMT1 (divalent metal transporter 1) transporter. Tf and TfR return to the cell surface, where both participate in another round cycle. (B) FR-mediated endocytosis pathway. After binding of folate to glycosylphosphatidylinositol-anchored FR, the complex is internalized. Folate is released from its receptor in acidified endosomes and FR go back to the cell surface for recycling. (C) HA and receptor-mediated endocytosis pathway. HA can bind to CD44 or its homolog receptors (RHAMM, receptor for hyaluronate-mediated motility; LYVE-1, lymphatic vessel endothelial receptor 1) on cell surface. After internalization, HA is fragmented in endosomes by hyaluronidases and the fragments are released into cytoplasm.

efficiency. Following the incubation of Tf and cationic liposomes, the resulting Tf-associated cationic liposomes were used to form electrostatic complexes with negatively charged nucleic acid–based molecules for targeted delivery to various cancers, such as glioblastoma, hepatocarcinoma, and neuronal cancers.[42]

> As a targeting ligand, Tf has been associated or covalently conjugated to nonviral delivery systems of nucleic acid–based therapeutics such as pDNA, AS-ON, and siRNA.

For example, Tf-associated cationic liposomes were used for the targeted delivery of pDNA encoding human p53. Because the increased expression of wild-type p53 might lead to p53-mediated apoptosis in cancer cells, the pDNA encoding p53 was delivered to cancer cells by cationic liposomes associated with Tf. Cationic liposomes composed of 1,2-dioleoyl-3-trimethylammoniumpropane and dioleoylphosphatidylethanolamine were incubated with iron-saturated holo-Tf. The intravenous administration of Tf-attached cationic liposome/pDNA encoding p53 enhanced the sensitivity of tumors to radiotherapy. The antitumor effects were prolonged, showing no tumor recurrence 6 months after treatment in the head and neck cancer xenograft model.[43]

Tf-associated cationic liposomes were also used to deliver pDNA encoding p53 in osteosarcoma-xenografted mice.[44] Cationic liposomes were prepared using dioleoyl trimethylammonium propane and dioleoyl phosphatidylethanolamine. The complexes of Tf/liposome/pDNA were formed by incubating the cationic liposomes with Tf and then with pDNA. Six treatments of intratumoral injection of the complexes (10 μg of pDNA per dose) resulted in a significant reduction of tumor growth rates.

Tf-associated cationic liposomes were also developed for the aerosol delivery of pDNA encoding endostatin.[45] Cationic liposomes were formulated with stearylamine, phosphatidyl choline, and cholesterol and were mixed with Tf and pDNA. After the aerosol treatment of the tumor-bearing mice with aerosols of Tf/liposome/pDNA complexes (50–500 mg/kg per dose), the increased expression of endostatin was observed in lung tissues. A pDNA dose-dependent reduction in tumor growth was reported.

Cationic polymers were also modified with Tf to confer the targeting capacity to tumor cells. The complexes of the poly-L-lysine polymer and the pDNA encoding β-galactosidase were covalently modified with a multivalent hydrophilic polymer, poly-[N-(2-hydroxypropyl)methacrylamide], to reduce the serum protein binding and were associated with Tf for targeted delivery to leukemia cells. Tf-targeted and hydrophilic polymer-coated complexes provided a 15-fold increase in the transfection activity of β-galactosidase over either simple poly-L-lysine and pDNA complexes or hydrophilic polymer-coated poly-L-lysine and pDNA complexes in K562 leukemia cells.[46]

Tf-cationic liposomes were also applied to deliver AS-ON to cancer cells. Phosphorothioated AS-ON against the human α isoform folate receptor (FR) was complexed to Tf-associated cationic liposomes and delivered to breast cancer cells.[47] The complexes of AS-ON against Bcl-2 and Tf-associated cationic liposomes reduced the expression of Bcl-2 in human leukemia cells and increased the sensitivity of the leukemia cells to the chemotherapeutic agent daunorubicin.[48]

Unlike cationic liposomes, where Tf was typically physically associated, cationic polymers were modified with Tf via covalent binding. Recently, Tf and PEG-conjugated oligoethylenimine were studied for the systemic delivery of siRNA specific to Ran. Three intravenous injections of Tf–PEG–oligoethylenimine and siRNA complexes (2.5 mg siRNA/kg/dose) in neuroblastoma-bearing mice resulted in a more than 80% reduction of the target protein (Ran) and reduced tumor growth.[49]

Tf-linked cyclodextrin polycation nanoparticles were formulated for Tf receptor-expressing tumor targeted delivery of siRNA.[50] siRNA against the EWS-FLI1 was carried by Tf-linked cyclodextrin polycations. The cyclodextrin-containing polycations were first self-assembled with siRNA to form colloidal particles. The colloidal particles were then stabilized with adamantane-linked PEG via the inclusion of adamantane inside the cyclodextrins, and they were conferred with a Tf-based targeting moiety via further inclusion of an adamantane–PEG–Tf conjugate. In tumor-bearing mice, the intravenous administration of Tf nanoparticles carrying anti-EWS-FLI1 siRNA (2.5 mg/kg dose) reduced the expression of EWS-FLI1 in tumor tissues.

As shown in Table 7.4, these studies demonstrated that Tf-attached liposomes or Tf-conjugated cationic polymers may serve as promising targeted delivery systems.[51] However, some problems still remain. In the blood stream, the interaction of Tf-conjugated vectors with serum proteins may occur. This may cause limited access to Tf receptors and other side effects. To solve this problem, further modification of Tf-conjugated carriers should be performed, such as conjugation with PEG. Tf will have higher potential as a targeting agent only if Tf can gain easy access to its receptors through optimization.[52] Once the nucleic acid–based therapeutics were taken up by the cells by Tf receptor-mediated endocytosis, another barrier is the escape for nucleic acids from endosomes to the cytoplasm. The design of pH-sensitive delivery systems which may destabilize in the acidic endosomes and trigger the cytoplasmic delivery of nucleic acid–based therapeutics would be beneficial

TABLE 7.4
Targeted Delivery of Nucleic Acids Using Tf Ligand

Nucleic Acids	Cargo Genes	Vehicle	Target Cells	Reference
pDNA	β-Gal	Polymer-modified poly-L-lysine	Leukemia	[46]
	RAN, luciferase	OEI	Neuroblastoma	[49]
	p53	Liposome	Head and neck cancer	[43]
	p54	Liposome	Osteosarcoma	[44]
	Endostatin	Liposome	Liver cancer	[45]
siRNA	GFP, luciferase, c-JUN	Liposome	Glioblastoma, hepatocarcinoma, neuronal cells	[42]

Note: OEI, oligoethyleneimine; GFP, green fluorescence protein.

to solve the limitation. Alternatively, the co-delivery of Tf-conjugated vectors with pH-sensitive fusogenic peptides might be another feasible approach to enhance the cytoplasmic delivery.

7.2.3 RGD Peptide

Integrins play important roles in multicellular organisms, including angiogenesis, oncogenesis, and other physiological and pathological processes. Integrin, a cell adhesion molecule, binds extracellular matrix and cell-surface ligands. Integrin is composed of heterodimeric receptors that contain large α and small β subunits not homologous to each other. There are at least 18 α and 8 β subunits in humans. Each transmembrane heterodimer interacts with specific ligands.[53] Because integrin is overexpressed in tumor cells and tumor vasculature,[54] the ligands specifically recognized by integrin can be developed as targeting moieties to deliver nucleic acid–based therapeutics to tumors.

RGD (Arg-Gly-Asp) is a well known motif recognized by integrins. The interaction between integrins and RGD-based ligands has been studied both to understand cell-adhesion diseases and for applications to tumor-targeted delivery.[55] Given the importance of angiogenesis in tumor growth and the differential expression of $\alpha_v\beta_3$-integrin on actively angiogenic endothelial cells and not on resting cells, RGD-mediated delivery has been regarded as a promising targeting approach to tumor vasculature. At first, small-molecule drugs or peptide-based drugs were directly conjugated to RGD peptides for targeted drug delivery. Later, polymers, liposomes, and proteins that can load more RGD peptides than single small-molecule drugs were utilized because of the correlation of RGD-mediated cellular uptake to the amount of RGD peptides per carrier.[56]

The enhanced transfer of a pDNA/cationic polymer was shown after the addition of RGD peptides. A four-branched cationic polymer of poly N,N-dimethylaminopropylacrylamide was synthesized for gene delivery in endothelial cells.[57] In the study, they added RGD-containing peptides, GRGDNP, to the polyplex, thus enhancing delivery via the integrin. Due to the surface coating effect of polyplex, the addition of RGD containing peptides protected the polyplexes from aggregation. When pDNA encoding luciferase was delivered by an RGD-linked cationic polymer, luciferase activity was increased in the RGD-containing peptide in a dose-dependent manner. Interestingly, cyclic RGD peptides, RGDFV, provided an eightfold increased delivery effect over the plain polyplex without RGD.[57]

A phosphorothioate sequence of splice-switching ON was conjugated to a maleimide bivalent cyclic RGD peptide for high-affinity binding to $\alpha_v\beta_3$-integrin-positive melanoma cells.[58] To test the delivery of the ON to the nucleus, the $2'$-O-Me phosphorothioate ON was designed to correct the splicing of an aberrant intron inserted into the luciferase reporter gene. Thus, increased expression of luciferase may indicate the nuclear distribution of the splice-correcting ON. When melanoma cells expressing $\alpha_v\beta_3$-integrin were treated with bicyclic RGD and oligodeoxynucleotide (ODN) complexes, luciferase expression was upregulated. In contrast, the treatment of cells with free ODN did not affect the luciferase level.

RGD peptides were conjugated to self-assembling nanoparticles for the delivery of siRNA.[59] The nanoparticles consisted of RGD–PEG–PEI conjugates. RGD peptides were attached to the distal end of PEG and linked with PEI. Vascular endothelial growth factor receptor 2 (VEGFR 2)-specific siRNA was loaded onto the nanoparticles to target tumor neovasculature-expressing integrins. In human umbilical vein endothelial cells (HUVEC) and murine neuroblastoma N2A cells, the specific cellular uptake of siRNA via RGD peptides was demonstrated through competition with free RGD peptides. In tumor-bearing mice, an intravenous injection of the polyplex showed a tumor-specific reduced expression of the target protein and inhibited tumor growth and angiogenesis.

The use of the RGD–PEG–PEI polymer has also been attempted to deliver VEGF-specific siRNA by other groups.[60] siRNAs targeting VEGFA, VEGFR1, or VEGFR2 were complexed to the RGD–PEG–PEI polymer (TargeTran®) and the complexes were intravenously administered to mice infected with the herpes simplex virus-1 at a dose of 40 μg siRNA. The use of the RGD–PEG–PEI polymer as the systemic delivery vehicle enhanced the therapeutic control of VEGF-specific siRNAs against ocular neovascularization.

Unlike other targeting ligands such as sugar and Tf lacking therapeutic efficacy, RGD can serve as a targeting ligand to tumor tissues and an anti-angiogenic molecule as well by antagonizing $\alpha_v\beta_3$-integrin. There have been numerous studies using RGD peptides alone for the anti-angiogenesis treatment of tumors. Indeed, Cilengitide®, a cyclic RGD peptide, is currently in clinical trials for anti-angiogenic cancer therapy.[61] Moreover, recent studies have suggested that RGD peptides can increase the sensitivity of tumors to radiotherapy in breast cancer models.[62] Thus, RGD may provide multifaceted beneficial effects when it is used for the targeted delivery of nucleic acid–based anti-cancer therapeutics.

> Unlike other targeting ligands such as sugar and Tf that lack therapeutic efficacy, the tripeptide RGD can serve as a targeting ligand to tumor tissues and an anti-angiogenic molecule by antagonizing the $\alpha_v\beta_3$-integrin. RGD peptides alone have been used for the anti-angiogenesis treatment of tumors. Indeed, Cilengitide, a cyclic RGD peptide, is currently in clinical trials for anti-angiogenic cancer therapy.

Although several groups reported promising applications of RGD-modified systems for the targeted delivery of nucleic acid–based therapeutics to cancers (Table 7.5), RGD-mediated targeted delivery systems still face some hurdles. For example, expression of the $\alpha_v\beta_3$-integrin is not homogeneous in tumor cells. However, the heterogeneity of integrin levels could be overcome by combination with another ligand targeting other receptors.[56]

7.2.4 FOLATE

Folate, the water-soluble vitamin B_9, is involved in the biosynthesis of nucleotides.[63] This vitamin plays important roles in the synthesis of DNA and RNA. A lack of folate might impair nerve development in premature infants. The cellular uptake of folate is performed by receptor-mediated endocytosis (Figure 7.1B). Two isoforms of FR, known as FR-a and FR-b, have high affinities for folate.[64] FR is overexpressed in tumors, such as ovarian carcinoma, and expressed on limited areas of normal tissue, such as the placenta, lung, and kidney.

Thus, an FR-mediated targeting strategy using folate has been widely studied for the targeted delivery of toxins, chemical drugs, and nucleic acid–based molecules.[65,66] Table 7.6 shows the examples of targeted delivery systems of nucleic acid–based molecules using folate as a targeting ligand. Folate has some advantages as a targeting ligand, such as its small size, which can reduce immunogenicity; an economic benefit; a relatively simple conjugation approach; high binding affinity to its receptor; and induction of internalization into cells.[67]

Chan et al. reported folate-mediated gene delivery using PEGylated chitosan. Folate was conjugated to PEGylated chitosan, which has increased the solubility of chitosan by PEGylation. Folate-linked PEGylated chitosan was synthesized and characterized for the tumor-targeted delivery of

TABLE 7.5
Targeted Delivery of Nucleic Acids Using RGD Peptides

Nucleic Acids	Cargo Genes	Vehicle	Target Cells	Reference
pDNA	Luciferase	Poly(N,N-dimethyl aminopropyl acrylamide)	Endothelial cells	[57]
AS-ON	α FR	Liposome	Breast cancer	[47]
	Bcl-2	Liposome	Leukemia	[48]
	Luciferase	Bivalent RGD-peptide	Melanoma	[58]
siRNA	VEGFR2	RGD-PEG-PEI	HUVEC, neuroblastoma	[59]
	VEGF, VEGFR1, VEGFR2	RGD-PEG-PEI	HSV-1 infection	[60]

Note: HUVEC, human umbilical vein endothelial cell; HSV, herpes simplex virus.

TABLE 7.6
Targeted Delivery of Nucleic Acids Using Folate or Aptamer

Targeting Ligand	Nucleic Acids	Cargo Genes	Vehicle	Target Cells	Reference
Folate	pDNA	Luciferase	PEG-Chitosan	HEK 293 cells	[68]
	AS-ON	GFP	Lipofectamine, PEI, PLL	KB cells	[69]
	siRNA	α_V integrin, survivin	Folate-conjugated ODN	HUVEC, KB cells	[70]
PSMA aptamer	siRNA	Lamin A/C	Aptmar-siRNA conjugates	Prostate cancer	[95]
		PLK1, Bcl-2	Aptmar-siRNA chimera	Prostate cancer	[96]
Anti-gp120 aptamer	siRNA	tat/rev	Aptmar-siRNA chimera	HIV-1 infection	[97]

Note: AS-ON, antisense oligonucleotide; HEK 293, human embryonic kidney cell line; PEI, polyethylenimine; PLL, poly-L-lysine; ODN, oligodeoxynucleotide; PLK 1, polo-like kinase 1.

pDNA.[68] Folate was introduced to the distal end of PEGylated AS-ON targeting green fluorescent protein.[69] This conjugate forms polyelectrolyte complex micelles (PECMs) by using cationic condensing agents like Lipofectamine, PEI, and poly-L-lysine. In human epidermal carcinoma KB, a cell line that overexpresses FR, folate-positive PECMs exhibited a dose-dependent reduction of green fluorescent protein and lower reduction by PECMs without folate was observed. In contrast, FR-negative lung carcinoma A549 cells showed a decreased expression of green fluorescent protein, at a similar level in both PECMs, regardless of folate.

Zhang et al. proposed a new strategy for cell-specific siRNA delivery using folate.[70] Through the base-paired interaction of siRNA to folate-conjugated ODN, tethered siRNA was produced in lengths of 17 nucleotides. FR-expressing cells HUVEC and KB were used to confirm specific cellular uptake and gene silencing, whereas MDA-MB-435S was used as a negative control cell line. The fluorescent-labeled folate accumulated in two of the folate-positive cells, but not in negative cells. siRNA against α_V integrin and survivin silenced the target proteins in FR-overexpressing cells.

Although folate has numerous advantages, such as small molecular size, relatively inexpensive cost, stability, and lower immunogenicity as compared with macromolecular and costly targeting ligands like monoclonal antibodies, there remain hurdles for the successful application of folate as targeting ligands. First, the toxicity of folate conjugates should be optimized. The high binding affinity between folate and FR may cause some problems in targeted delivery. Because of the high affinity, some folate conjugate might be released too late from FR after endocytosis.[71] Recently, hydrolyzable linkers were introduced for easy release of folate. Folate conjugates containing large cargo, such as liposomes, could affect the binding affinity to the FR. Therefore, folate conjugates should be carefully designed to remove undesirable interruptions to FR binding.[72] Second, the linker between the folate and the cargo delivery system should be designed to retain the binding capability of the folate to its receptor, and to release the nucleic acid-carrying delivery systems after uptake into the target cells.

7.2.5 SUGAR

A specifically targeted delivery system is essential for successful gene therapy by nonviral vector. Nonviral vectors including lipids, polymers, and peptides have the advantages of low immunogenicity, unlimited cargo size, and low cost. However, usage of nonviral carriers is still limited by their nonspecific biodistribution and low stability in serum.[73] When siRNAs or pDNAs are injected systemically, they are rapidly degraded by a number of nuclease enzymes. To avoid this degradation in blood, the carriers of nucleic acid–based molecules must be taken up quickly into target tissues and cells.

Certain types of cells overexpress sugar-binding receptors. Sugars bound to the receptors are internalized by receptor-mediated endocytosis. This receptor-mediated endocytosis increases the efficiency of therapeutic gene delivery into specific target cells. Sugar receptor targeting is a possible approach to cell-specific delivery after systemic administration because sugar receptors are found on hepatocytes, macrophages, dendritic cells, and sinusoidal liver cells.

In gene delivery, one of the first successful targetings with sugar moiety was achieved through the asialoglycoprotein receptor (ASGP-R) present on hepatocytes. In the first studies, poly-L-lysine– DNA complexes containing the entire ligand (asialooromucosoid) had a problem related to their large particle size. Recently, small synthetic oligosaccharides have mainly been used as ligands. Glycosylated poly-L-lysine or PEI complexed with pDNA revealed ASGP-R -mediated delivery.[74–76] Several sugars have been studied for sugar receptor targeting (Table 7.7).

7.2.5.1 Mannose

Mannose was used to target mannose receptors, which are especially overexpressed on dendritic cells and macrophages. Mannose-modified cationic lipids and polymers have been designed to enhance the cellular uptake of siRNA and pDNA after systemic administration. Macrophages are hard-to-transfect by the nonviral vector technique, but mannosylated cationic liposomes complexed with pDNA enhanced the gene transfer into macrophages via mannose receptor-mediated endocytosis.[77] Park et al. examined the ability of mesoporous silica nanoparticles coupled with mannosylated PEI to transfect pDNA. In this study, the nanoparticles exhibited a high transfection efficiency of pDNA to macrophages by receptor-mediated endocytosis via mannose receptors.[78]

Given the expression of the mannose receptor on the surface of antigen-presenting cells, mannosylated cationic liposomes were studied for antigen-presenting cell-targeted delivery of DNA vaccines.[79] A mannose-linked cholesterol derivative, cholesten-5-yloxy-N-(4-((1-imino-2-D-thio-mannosyl-ethyl)amino)butyl) formamide, was used to formulate cationic liposomes. Three intraperitoneal injections of pDNA encoding melanoma-associated antigen (50 μg/dose) at 2-week intervals revealed the importance of delivery systems for inducing cellular immune responses. When pDNA-vaccinated mice were challenged with B16BL6 melanoma cells, only the group treated with the complexes of mannosylated cationic liposomes and DNA vaccines exhibited significant antitumor effects and prolonged survival.

TABLE 7.7
Sugar and Polysaccharide-Mediated Targeting

Targeting Ligand	Nucleic Acids	Cargo Genes	Vehicle	Target Cells	Reference
Mannose	pDNA	Luciferase	Liposome	Macrophage, liver	[77]
		Luciferase	Mesoporous silica nanoparticle, PEI	Macrophage	[78]
		Ub-M	Liposome	Antigen presenting cells, melanoma	[79]
Galactose	pDNA	GFP	PEI	Liver	[80]
	siRNA	Ubc13	Liposome	Liver	[82]
HA	pDNA	GFP	Chitosan nanoparticle	Ocular disease	[85]
	siRNA	GFP	Nanogel	HCT-116 cells	[86]

Note: Ub-M, ubiquitinated murine melanoma gp100 and TRP-2 peptide epitopes; HA, hyaluronic acid; HCT-116, human colorectal carcinoma cell line.

7.2.5.2 Galactose

Galactose is a promising targeting moiety to cells that possess high levels of ASGP-R. Parenchymal liver cells such as hepatocytes have a large number of the ASGP-R and recognize galactose residues on the oligosaccharide chains of glycoprotein or on the chemically modified galatosylated carriers. Although the binding affinity of a carbohydrate ligand to ASGP-R is highly influenced by the number and orientation of the sugar residues, the terminal galactose residue is the most important moiety.

Galactosylated PEI-graft-PEG polymers have been used for the hepatocyte-targeted delivery of pDNA encoding green fluorescent protein.[80] The complexes of pDNA and galactosylated PEI-graft-PEG polymers formed nanoparticles, and they showed a higher expression of green fluorescent protein in HepG2 hepatoma cells than did HeLa cervical cancer cells *in vitro*. In this study, the *in vivo* fate of galactosylated polymer and pDNA complexes was traced by radiolabeling the polymer with ^{99m}Tc. Intravenously injected pDNA (15 μg/dose) complexed to the radiolabeled galactosylated polymer showed preferential distribution to the heart and liver in mice. Two days postinjection, an expression of green fluorescent protein was observed in the liver tissue.

Mahato and colleagues used galactosylated PEG for the hepatocyte-specific delivery of ON.[81] In the study, galactosylated PEG was linked to ON via an acid-labile beta-thiopropionate. Using 33P-radiolabed ON as a marker, they studied the effect of galactosylated PEG on the biodistribution. Following intravenous administration of ON (0.2 mg/kg) in a galactosylated PEG conjugate form to rats, 60.2% of the injected dose was found to accumulate in the liver at 30 min. In addition to the higher liver distribution, galactosylated PEG conjugated affected the hepatic cellular localization of ON. Galactosylated PEG-conjugated ON was preferentially distributed to hepatocytes, whereas ON alone revealed higher distribution to nonparenchymal cells.

Galactosylated cationic liposomes were studied for the liver parenchymal cell-selective delivery of siRNA.[82] The galactosylated cationic liposomes were composed of a galactosylated cholesterol derivative, cholesten-5-yloxy-*N*-(4-((1-imino-2-D-thiogalactosylethyl)amino)alkyl)formamide, and a neutral lipid, dioleoylphosphatidylethanolamine. After intravenous administration using the galactosylated cationic liposomes as a carrier, fluorescent siRNA was mainly distributed to the liver and lung tissues. When endogenous Ubc 13-specific siRNA (0.29 nmol/g) was intravenously administered using cationic liposomes with or without the galactose moiety, the 80% reduction of Ubc 13 mRNA expression in liver tissues was observed only in galactosylated cationic liposomes, but it was not seen in plain cationic liposomes.

Since liver parenchymal cells are known to be abundant in ASGP-R recognizing galactose, lactose, or *N*-acetylglucosamine, galactose-tagged carriers might be applied for liver-targeted delivery of nucleic acids. However, the existence of ASGP-R both in normal liver parenchymal cells and pathogenic hepatoma cells may make it difficult for achieving hepatoma-specific targeted delivery via galactose moieties. To improve the preferential delivery to pathogenic cells, the structural modification of sugars providing a higher affinity to the target cell receptor might be considered. Moreover, given that the extent of galactosylation of plasmid delivery systems affected the transfection efficiency,[83] the optimization of galactose density per delivery system needs to be done for maximized delivery efficiency of diverse nucleic acids such as plasmids and siRNAs.

7.2.6 HYALURONIC ACID

Hyaluronic acid (hyaluronan, HA) is a high-molecular-weight glycosaminoglycan, which is a component of the extracellular matrix that is essential for cell growth, structural organ stability, and tissue organization. The chemical structure of HA was determined in the 1950s in the laboratory of Karl Meyer. HA is a polymer of repeating disaccharide units of D-glucuronic acid and (1-b-3) *N*-acetyl-D-glucosamine. The amount of HA in a tissue depends on HA synthesis by HA synthases, internalization by cell surface receptors, and extracellular degradation by hyaluronidases.

HA has a binding affinity to specific cell surface receptors such as CD44, a receptor for hyaluronic acid-mediated motility (RHAMM) and lymphatic vessel endothelial hyaluronan receptor-1 (LYVE-1). The principal receptor of HA is known as CD44, which can regulate cell proliferation and movement. After internalization into the cells, HA is fragmented into endosomes, and the fragments of HA are released into the cytoplasm (Figure 7.1C). Several downstream pathways after the activation of CD44 by HA are deregulated in cancer, and some of these pathways lead to tumor growth, progression, and metastasis. Alterations in both CD44 and HA expression have been widely observed in tumors from cancer patients and in animal models of tumors. During carcinogenesis, the expression of the standard form of CD44 is up-regulated in certain cancers.[84]

HA-chitosan nanoparticles were designed for topical ocular delivery of genes.[85] HA has been commonly used in ophthalmology due to its biocompatible, biodegradable, and mucoadhesive properties. Moreover, the localization of CD44 has been observed in ocular tissues. HA-chitosan nanoparticles were prepared by a ionotropic gelation technique and loaded with pDNA encoding enhanced green fluorescent protein. Following the topical ocular treatment of a rabbit eye at a dose of 50 µg pDNA per eye, pDNA-loaded HA-chitosan nanoparticles expressed green fluorescent proteins at the corneal epithelium.

Park and colleagues developed HA-based nanogels encapsulating siRNA for specific delivery to CD44 overexpressing cells.[86] A thiol group-functionalized HA solution was emulsified and ultrasonically cross-linked to form an HA nanogel networked with disulfide linkages. For encapsulation of siRNA in the nanogel, siRNA was added to the thiol-conjugated HA emulsion before the disulfide cross-linking step. Rhodamine-labeled HA nanogels were efficiently taken up by CD44 overexpressing HCT-116 cells, but not by CD44-deficient NIH-3T3 cells. When HA nanogel-loaded siRNA was delivered to HCT-116 cells, they silenced the siRNA target protein in a dose-dependent manner.

HA-conjugated PEI was recently designed to enhance the delivery of siRNA.[87] The electrostatic interaction between the negatively charged siRNA and the cationic PEI of HA–PEI conjugates may have allowed the formation of nanoparticles. HA–PEI conjugates provided a higher uptake of fluorescent siRNA to B16F1 cells expressing LYVE-1, one of the HA receptors, in comparison with LYVE-1-deficient HEK-293 cells.

A recent study reported a correlation between CD44 expression and the invasiveness of breast cancer cells.[88] Other studies suggested that the molecular sizes of HA fragments play a role in the downstream pathways of HA-responsive cells. Depending on its size, HA exerted differential regulations on the wound-healing process of fibroblasts.[89] Given these observations, HA-mediated targeted delivery systems of nucleic acid–based therapeutic moieties need to account for the molecular sizes of HA and different expression levels of HA receptors depending on the progression stage of the cancer.

HA-mediated tumor targeting systems may need to exploit the leaky vasculature of tumor tissues. Although CD44 expression is known to be upregulated in many cancers of epithelial origin, CD44 is also present on normal epithelial cells. Extravasation to the tumor tissues might be a prerequisite of expecting the tumor-targeting of nucleic acids by HA-linked delivery systems. One of the limitations in the use of HA as a tumor-targeted delivery of anticancer nucleic acid would be the distribution of HA-linked systems to skin tissues where the expression level of CD44 is high. Indeed, a dose-limiting toxicity was observed after administration of the CD44 antibody and anticancer chemical drug conjugate, due to notable distribution to the skin.[84] Since nucleic acids can be more specifically designed and interact with intracellular targets, such nonspecific side effects due to the skin distribution might be possibly avoided by a careful design of nucleic acid cargo molecules.

7.2.7 Aptamer

The term aptamer originated from the Latin *aptus*, which means fitted. An aptamer is a molecule composed of nucleic acid or peptide that binds a target molecule specifically. Aptamers are generally produced by a systemic evolution of ligands by exponential enrichment (SELEX), a method that selects the optimized "best aptamer" by cycling target-interacted molecules in a nucleic acid library including random sequences. The target of the aptamer might be small molecules, proteins, nucleic acids, or even cells.[90]

There are many advantages to using aptamers as targeting moieties. First, aptamers can specifically interact with a variety of target molecules. Futhermore, aptamers have an economic benefit because of the feasibility of chemical synthesis and modification. Nucleic acid–based aptamers can provide reversible conformational change under various pH levels or temperatures, whereas proteins are irreversibly denatured at high temperatures. Moreover, nucleic acid–based aptamers have lower immunogenicity than antibodies *in vivo*, suggesting the future use of aptamers as a substitute for antibodies.[91]

The first successful RNA aptamer was designed for PSMA. A PSMA is a type II transmembrane glycoprotein overexpressed in prostate cancer. PSMAs can be used for evaluating targeted delivery systems using PSMA-positive LNCaP cells and PSMA-negative PC3 cells.[92] The PSMA-specific RNA aptamer has been widely used in the targeted delivery of chemotherapeutic drugs such as hydrophobic docetaxel or hydrophilic doxorubicin-encapsulated polymeric nanoparticles.[93,94]

Recently, aptamer-mediated targeted delivery was extended to nucleic acid–based therapeutics. Aptamer-mediated siRNA delivery was developed using the PSMA aptamer as a targeting moiety. The biotinylated aptamer was coupled to biotinylated siRNA via a streptavidin bridge. Lamin A/C-specific siRNA was used for aptamer conjugation. The aptamer–streptavidin–siRNA conjugate was taken up by PSMA-expressing LNCaP cells and exerted an RNAi effect against Lamin A/C for 3 days.[95]

For the cell-specific delivery of siRNA, the PSMA aptamer was genetically linked to siRNA.[96] The chimera of the PSMA aptamer-siRNA was generated by *in vitro* transcription. This chimera contains siRNA against polo-like kinase 1 (PLK1) or Bcl2, which is highly expressed in tumors. When applied to LNCaP cells expressing PSMA, these aptamer–siRNA chimeras were internalized and processed by Dicer enzymes, resulting in the depletion of the siRNA target proteins and cell death. The intratumoral administration of the PSMA aptamer–siRNA inhibited the growth of LNCaP tumors, but it did not inhibit the growth of PC3 tumors in nude mice. This result suggests the potential cell-specific delivery of aptamer–siRNA conjugates. However, further studies using intravenous injection must be performed for clinical application.

An anti-gp120-specific aptamer was recently designed for cell-specific delivery of antiviral siRNA targeting HIV type 1 tat/rev.[97] To form an aptamer–siRNA chimera, covalent binding and complementary base pairing were utilized. Sense strands of siRNA were covalently linked to an RNA aptamer by a four-nucleotide linker (CUCU). Antisense strands of siRNA formed a double-stranded siRNA by complementary base pairing with the aptamer-linked sense strand portion of the siRNA. The resulting chimera was bound to gp120 on the surface of HIV-infected cells and internalized, inhibiting the replication of HIV.

This series of approaches demonstrates the possibility of the aptamer-mediated cell-specific delivery of siRNAs. Although aptamers are expected to replace antibodies as a targeting moiety, there remain some challenges for successful delivery. In the case of the siRNA–aptamer chimera, the low stability in the blood stream still exists because of the nucleic acid nature of the delivery vehicle, an aptamer. Chemical modification of the aptamer or the additional use of second carriers should be accomplished to increase stability for *in vivo* application.

7.2.8 SMALL-SIZE CHEMICALS

Recently, small-molecule chemicals have been used for the targeted delivery of nucleic acid–based therapeutics. The small chemicals may have advantages over macromolecular targeting moieties such as Tf and monoclonal antibodies in terms of large-scale production, convenience of handling, physical stability, and costs. Prostaglandin E2 was recently studied as a targeting moiety for the delivery of Fas siRNA to cardiomyocytes.[98] Prostaglandin E2 was conjugated to the amine-terminated end of the siRNA sense strand. The reducible cationic copolymer, synthesized via the Michael-type polyaddition of 1,6-diaminohexane and cystamine bis-acrylamide (poly(DAH/CBA)), tightly condensed the prostaglandin E2-siRNA conjugate to form nanosize polyplexes. The resulting polyplexes were efficiently taken up by rat cardiomyocytes (H9C2 cells) by prostaglandin E2 receptor-mediated endocytosis, which reduced the expression of the target protein Fas, a key regulator of ischemia-induced apoptosis.

Anisamide, a ligand for sigma receptors, was used for the targeted delivery of siRNA to sigma receptor-expressing tumor cells.[99,100] Self-assembled nanoparticles were formulated by mixing carrier DNA, siRNA, protamine, and lipids. The nanoparticles were modified by 1,2-distearoyl-sn-glycero-3-phosphoethanolamine-PEG-anisamide conjugate by a post-insertion method to confer stability and targeting capability. Epidermal growth factor receptor-specific siRNAs were used as nucleic acid therapeutics. Four hours after intravenous administration of the anisamide-tagged nanoparticles to mice xenografted with an aggressive lung cancer cell line, NCI-H460, 70%–80% siRNA accumulation was seen in the tumor tissues. Three daily injections (1.2 mg/kg) of siRNA formulated in the anisamide-targeted nanoparticles silenced the epidermal growth factor receptor in the tumor, and this resulted in a 40% inhibition of tumor growth.[99]

Although small-size chemicals have merit in large-scale productions, such as relatively low cost, physical stability, and convenience in chemical modification, they still suffer from lower specificity as targeting molecules as compared with antibodies or peptides. For a successful application of small sized chemicals, the elucidation and understanding of the biology of target receptors should be done in parallel. Ideal receptors for small-sized chemicals may exist as a high density on the target cell surface and may allow the rapid cellular internalization of delivery systems after recognition. Moreover, the rapid recycling of the receptors to the target cell surfaces may increase the intracellular delivery efficiency of nucleic acid–based therapeutics. The future study of small-sized chemicals whose receptors are specifically and highly expressed in target tissues may promote the wide use of chemicals as intelligent targeting moieties.

> Although small-size chemicals have relative advantage in large-scale production, such as relatively low cost, physical stability, and convenience in chemical modification, they suffer from lower specificity as targeting molecules as compared with antibodies or peptides.

7.2.9 CELL-MEDIATED TARGETING

Cell vehicle–based targeting might be a new field of delivery strategies, but it is a field with great potential. Cell vehicles used for gene delivery can be categorized as prokaryotes and eukaryotes. Among prokaryotic cells, anaerobic bacteria have been genetically engineered to target therapeutic genes to the hypoxic tumor sites.[101] These specialized anaerobic prokaryotic delivery vehicles have the following characteristics: (1) they target the hypoxic tumor microenvironment after systemic administration and (2) they enhance the active immune response to prevent metastasis or suppress the proliferation of tumor tissues.[102]

Anaerobic and attenuated *Salmonella choleraesuis* was exploited as a vector for the targeted delivery of the endostatin gene to tumor tissues.[103] The expression of endostatin persisted for at least 10 days after the administration of the gene-carrying bacteria to mice. When systemically administered into mice bearing melanomas or bladder tumors, *S. choleraesuis* carrying the eukaryotic pDNA encoding endostatin significantly inhibited tumor growth by 40%–70% and prolonged the survival of the mice with anti-angiogenic effects. Host immune responses and hypoxia of tumor tissues may affect the tumor-targeting potential of *S. choleraesuis*. The biggest challenge facing the use of anaerobic bacteria as hypoxic tumor-targeting vehicles is the safety issue from a regulatory aspect.

Macrophages and erythrocytes have been used as eukaryotic cell vehicles. Macrophages have an inherent ability to recognize and accumulate in pathological sites, such as tumors and inflammatory tissues. Therefore, this natural targeting by macrophages may provide therapeutic effects without toxicity and immunogenic response.[104]

Recently, macrophages genetically modified with NK4 pDNA showed the *in vivo* antitumor effect in a tumor-bearing mouse model.[105] Mouse peritoneal macrophages were introduced with pDNA encoding hepatocyte growth factor antagonist NK4 by a cationic dextran-mediated reverse transfection technique. The NK4 protein was secreted from the genetically engineered macrophages at a higher amount and for a longer time compared with the macrophages transfected with pDNA encoding NK by the conventional transfection method. Following the intravenous injection in tumor-bearing mice, the genetically engineered macrophages accumulated in the tumor tissue and showed significant antitumor activity.

Other than macrophages, erythrocyte ghosts were used as cell vehicles for the blood-targeted delivery of pDNA.[106] Erythrocytes are one of the most safe and effective delivery vehicles and they provide long circulation properties.[107] Nucleic acids can be introduced into erythrocyte ghosts through transient membrane pores formed by hypotonic osmotic shock (Figure 7.2). The membrane pores of erythrocyte ghosts are then resealed in the isotonic condition. Oh and colleagues encapsulated pDNA in erythrocyte ghosts by electroporation in hypotonic conditions.[106] After intravenous administration in mice, the level of pDNA in the blood was orders of magnitude higher following the erythrocyte ghost-mediated delivery compared with the injection of the naked form. Moreover, pDNA-loaded erythrocyte ghosts showed gene expression targeted to the blood cells. At 3 days post-dose, substantial expression levels of pDNA delivered in erythrocyte ghosts were observed only in the blood and not in other organs. This result highlights the potential of erythrocyte ghosts as a safe, prolonged, and blood-targeted delivery system of therapeutic genes.

Smooth muscle cells were studied as a pulmonary vasculature delivery vehicle of pDNA encoding VEGF.[108] The pulmonary artery smooth muscle cells were transfected with pDNA by a commercially available transfection agent, and 500,000 of these were injected into the jugular vein of rats. Four weeks postinjection, the plasmid VEGF transcript was detected in the pulmonary tissue of animals injected with pVEGF-transfected cells, demonstrating survival of the transfected cells and persistent transgene expression.

Skin fibroblast cells were used as a vehicle for transferring the angiopoietin-1 gene to acute lung injury.[109] Angiopoietin-1, a ligand for the endothelial Tie2 receptor, is an endothelial survival and vascular stabilization factor that reduces endothelial permeability and inhibits leukocyte–endothelium interactions. Skin fibroblast cells isolated from rats were transfected with pDNA encoding human angiopoietin-1 and injected into the pulmonary circulation. The *in vivo* transfer of the angiopoietin

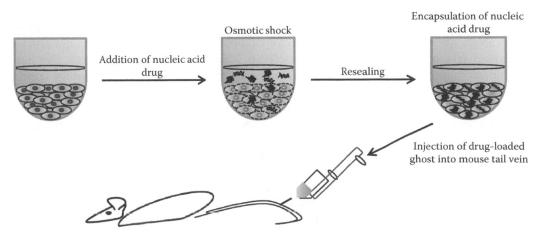

FIGURE 7.2 Entrapment of nucleic acids in erythrocyte ghosts. Red blood cell suspensions are added with nucleic acids, and placed in hypotonic conditions to create transient pores in the cell membrane. During the osmotic shock, reddish heme proteins leak out and the nucleic acids move into erythrocyte ghosts through the pores. At the isotonic condition, the pores are resealed and the nucleic acids are entrapped inside the erythrocyte ghosts.

gene by cell-based vehicles improved the morphologic, biochemical, and molecular indices of lung injury and inflammation.

Mesenchymal stem cells were exploited as a delivery vehicle of pDNA encoding angiopoietin 1.[110] Syngeneic mesenchymal stem cells were transfected with pDNA encoding angiopoietin 1 and injected into the jugular vein of mice induced with lung injury. The administration of mesenchymal stem cells transfected with pDNA encoding angiopoietin 1 almost completely reversed the lipopolysaccharide-induced increases in lung permeability. Fluorescently tagged mesenchymal stem cells were detected in the lung tissues for up to 3 days.

For cell-based targeted gene delivery, cells were generally introduced with pDNA encoding specific genes *ex vivo* and were administered to the body. When introducing such genetically modified cells systemically, several problems still remain. Unanswered questions remain about the efficiency of cell distribution to the target tissues, the retention of the cells in the tissues after delivery, and the exact amount of therapeutic proteins that may be expressed from the genetically engineered cells.

7.2.10 STIMULUS-TRIGGERED TARGETING

Stimulus-triggered delivery strategies control the drug action in the intended target sites by localized application of external stimuli such as electric pulse, ultrasound, light, heat, or magnetic fields. The external stimuli can selectively activate drugs in the target sites and/or improve the localized delivery of drugs across mechanical and physiological barriers. Recently, stimulus-triggered delivery has been studied as one of targeting technologies for nucleic acid–based therapeutics. Electrical pulse, ultrasound, and magnetic fields have been shown to guide the localized delivery of nucleic acid–based therapeutics in a target area.

7.2.10.1 Electroporation

Electroporation is a physical method of delivering nucleic acid and its derivatives directly into the cytoplasm through the pores transiently created in the cell membrane by electrical pulses.[111] Electroporation was used for the *in vitro* transfer of genes into mouse lyoma cells in 1982.[112] Since then, electroporation has been widely used for the *in vitro* or *ex vivo* transfer of pDNAs to target cells, due to relatively high transfection efficiency and convenient experimental protocol. Nowadays, the *in vivo* applications of electroporation for gene delivery have been reported in a variety of tissues including skeletal muscle, tumors, kidney, liver, and skin.[113] Following intramuscular electroporation, the gene expression in muscle increased about 100-fold as compared with plasmid injection alone.[114] *In vivo* electroporation was attempted for enhanced intradermal delivery of pDNA via the cutaneous application of electrodes.[115] Electroporation was also implemented for intra-articular targeted delivery of pDNA encoding tumor necrosis factor receptor in the joint area. The intra-articular electrotransfer of pDNAs encoding therapeutic proteins would be useful for the targeted therapy of inflammatory articular joint disorders such as rheumatoid arthritis.[116] The first clinical study using electroporation-based pDNA delivery was initiated in 2004. In this phase I study, human interleukin-12-encoding pDNA was intralesionally electroporated for gene delivery against metastatic melanoma.[117]

Electroporation has been commonly used as an alternative to viral gene delivery systems for the introduction of therapeutic genes into different tissues, including muscle, skin, liver, and solid tumors, for the treatment of various diseases such as cancer, arthritis, multiple sclerosis, and inflammation. Further improvements of device, the lack of toxicity due to electric pulse, and the reduction of costs should be considered for the clinical application of this technology for targeted delivery of nucleic acid–based therapeutics.

7.2.10.2 Ultrasound-Triggered Delivery

Similar to electroporation, sonoporation is a method of introducing drugs and nucleic acid–based molecules into the cells by the formation of temporary pores.[118] Unlike electroporation, sonoporation utilizes ultrasound waves to perturb the cell membrane. Ultrasound has long been used in medicine, and is known to allow easy focusing and penetration deep into the body. Broad ranges of frequency waves by ultrasound make very small holes in cell membranes and allow the penetration of macromolecules like pDNA into living cells of target sites. Microbubbles are known to enhance the ultrasound-mediated transfer of genes into cells.[119] Currently, several microbubble products are commercially available. Optison®, one of the commonly used microbubbles, is a human serum albumin microsphere encapsulating perflutren gas as a contrast agent.

Several studies reported that microbubble contrast agents could enhance the ultrasound-triggered gene delivery to target tissues *in vivo*. In mice, the efficiency of ultrasound-mediated pDNA delivery in skeletal muscle was enhanced by the intramuscular injection of a microbubble contrast agent.[120] The ultrasound-mediated lung delivery of naked pDNA was shown to be dependent on the co-treatment with microbubbles in mice.[121] The transfection of pDNA encoding Smad7 in the peritoneal cavity was shown to be efficient after intraperitoneal administration of a mixture containing pDNA and microbubble followed by abdominal ultrasound application.[122] Coupled with microbubbles, ultrasound pulsed at 1 MHz enhanced the expression of intraportally injected pDNA in the liver tissue.[123]

Another approach in ultrasound-mediated nucleic acid delivery is the use of bubble liposomes that entrap an ultrasound imaging gas. Bubble liposomes containing perfluoropropane gas were shown to introduce pDNA encoding luciferase into solid tumor tissues more effectively than cationic lipid–based delivery systems. The combination of bubble liposomes and ultrasound was suggested for the application of *in vivo* tumor-specific cancer gene therapy.[124]

Recently, ultrasound-triggered siRNA targeting was attempted by using cationic nanoliposomes as delivery vectors of siRNA.[125] In this study, cationic nanoliposomes composed of 1,2-dioleoyl-3-trimethylammonium-propane, 1,2-dioleoyl-*sn*-glycero-3-phosphoethanolamine, and 1,2-distearoyl-*sn*-glycero-3-phosphoethanolamine-*N*-[amino(polyethylene glycol)2000] were complexed to siRNAs specific for B-Raf or Akt3. Low frequency (20 kHz) ultrasound treatment followed by the topical application of siRNA and cationic nanoliposomal complexes provided the inhibition of cutaneous melanoma growth in mice.

Being noninvasive and relatively less expensive, ultrasound has been used in diagnostic fields of medicine for a long time. This technique has recently been recognized as a promising tool for facilitating targeted gene transfer to near-skin tissues as a targeted delivery technology. The optimization of ultrasound parameters for the efficient transfer of nucleic acid–based molecules, the development of convenient and economic ultrasound-generating devices, and the reduction of toxicity should be studied further.

7.2.10.3 Magnetic Field–Guided Delivery

Magnetofection is a method that uses magnetic fields to introduce magnetic nanoparticles containing nucleic acids into the target cells (Figure 7.3).[111] Nanoparticles consisted of superparamagnetic iron oxide were generally used as a core component for responsiveness to magnetic fields. Cationic moiety-modified magnetic nanoparticles have been used for the delivery of negatively charged nucleic acid–based molecules after the formation of complexes by electrostatic interactions. With appropriate magnetic field application, magnetofection was shown to be effective for the delivery of nucleic acids to hard-to-transfect cells, such as suspension cells[126] and mouse embryonic stem cells.[127]

PEI-coated magnetic nanoparticles were used for the intracellular delivery of siRNA.[128] The magnetic nanoparticles formed complexes with siRNA against enhanced green fluorescent protein. For magnetic field–guided siRNA delivery, the culture plates containing the complexes of siRNA and magnetic nanoparticles were placed on a magnet for 15 min. The cells exhibited a reduction of the target protein in the stable expression cell line.

Even though most magnetofection studies have been done *in vitro* for the cellular delivery of genetic materials *in vitro* or *ex vivo*, the feasibility of magnetic force–guided gene delivery was

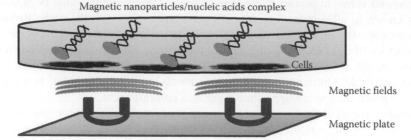

FIGURE 7.3 Magnetic field–guided delivery of nucleic acids. The complexes of magnetic nanoparticles and nucleic acids are added to cell culture medium, and rapidly introduced into cells after application of magnetic fields. Magnetic fields can be applied to *ex vivo* delivery of nucleic acids to target cells or *in vivo* local application near target tissues.

recently demonstrated *in vivo*. In this study, a cationic PEI-coated superparamagnetic particle was coupled with a cationic lipid and pDNA complexes and administered into the nasal cavity of a mouse. The external application of a magnetic rod onto the nostril resulted in the enhanced gene transfer in the airway epithelium,[129] suggesting the possibility of remotely controlled targeting *in vivo*.

Given the potential and recent successes of magnetofection in hard-to-transfect cells as well as *in vivo*, it is expected that more studies will be done for the targeted delivery of siRNAs and ON by magnetic forces. For advances in magnetically guided nucleic acid delivery, interdisciplinary studies may need to be done for the optimization of parameters such as the chemical compositions of magnetic particles, strengths of magnetic field, and formulations.

7.3 FUTURE PROSPECTS

Nucleic acid–based molecules are regarded as the next generation of innovative medicines. The successful development of nucleic acid–based therapeutics requires the development of intelligent and targeted delivery systems. Although EPR effects have been achieved for tumor tissues undergoing active angiogenesis with passive targeting, cell-type-specific active targeting delivery systems should be developed to maximize the therapeutic effect while minimizing the undesirable off-target effects.

For the targeted delivery of nucleic acid–based therapeutics, various approaches have exploited targeting moieties such as antibodies, peptides, Tf, folate, small chemicals, aptamers, and cells. Each targeted delivery system has its advantages and limitations (Table 7.8). The nucleic acid type-dependent optimization of the formulations is also necessary. For example, in pDNA delivery, the capability of the delivery systems to provide nuclear transport is important, whereas the delivery systems of siRNA only require cytoplasmic delivery. Such differences should be taken into account before applying the appropriate targeting strategies for each type of nucleic acid.

In most studies, the outcome of the targeted delivery was focused on the therapeutic efficacy. The physicochemical stability of the nucleic acid–based molecules during storage as well as the issue of scale-up should also be considered after optimization of the targeted delivery formulations. More quantitative information on the pharmacokinetics and dose-dependent pharmacodynamic aspects of targeted delivery systems should be investigated.

In summary, nonviral delivery systems using target-specific, safe, and effective moieties for gene delivery remain an ongoing challenge. Specific cell- and tissue-targeted delivery methods for nucleic acid delivery are currently under investigation. Their ultimate success will depend on many relevant parameters, including transfection efficacy, toxicity, an absence of nonspecific effects, and the ability of the transfer vectors to overcome numerous biological barriers after systemic or local administration to reach their target tissue/organ.

TABLE 7.8
Summary of Targeting Strategies

Category	Targeting Strategies	Principle	Advantages	Disadvantages
Biological	Monoclonal antibody	Binding to specific antigens on cancer cells	Specific antigen binding affinity	Limited numbers of administration or use of engineered antibody fragments due to immune responses
	Tf	Transport of iron ion to TfR	TfR-mediated delivery to cancer cells	Nonspecific binding to serum proteins in blood stream
	RGD peptide	Arg-Gly-Asp motif recognized by integrins	Overexpression of integrin in tumor vasculature, small size, anti-angiogenesis effects of RGD alone	Heterogeneity of integrin levels in various tumor cells
	Folate	Water-soluble vitamin B9 involved in the biosynthesis of nucleotides	Specific delivery to cancer cells overexpressing FR, small size, stability, low cost	Delayed escape from endosome due to high affinity of folate and FR
	HA	Binding to specific cell surface receptors (CD44, RHAMM, LYVE-1, etc.)	Overexpression of CD44 on tumor cells, prolonged circulation in blood stream	High distribution to the skin tissues with high levels of CD44
	Aptamer	Binding to specific target molecules by three-dimensional structure	High binding affinity. Relatively low cost, low immunogenicity	Hard to screen the candidates. Low stability *in vivo*
Cell-mediated	Macrophage	Natural homing mobility to pathological sites	Ability to recognize and accumulate in tumors and inflammatory tissues	Relatively hard to be genetically engineered
	Erythrocyte ghost	Introduction of nucleic acid drugs in erythrocyte by transient pore formation	Protected from enzymatic degradation and prolonged circulation, biocompatible, biodegradable	Relatively low encapsulation efficiency, limitation of target tissues
	Stem cell	Natural homing capability of stem cells	Potential application to various diseases	Possibility of side effects due to unregulated growth *in vivo*. Relatively hard to be genetically engineered
Physical	Electroporation	Introduction of nucleic acid by electrically created pores in cell membrane	High transfection efficiency. *Ex vivo* delivery of nucleic acid to target cells	Relatively high cytotoxicity due to electric stimulus. Need to improve the device. Limitation of *in vivo* target sites
	Ultrasound	Delivery by formation of temporary pores by ultrasound waves	Noninvasive approach. Currently used in the diagnostic imaging	Limitation of target sites. Low transfection efficiency. Requirements for microbubbles
	Magnetofection	Magnetic field–guided delivery of nucleic acids using magnetic nanoparticles	Rapid rate of transfection, application to hard-to-transfect cells	Low biocompatibility of magnetic particles

REFERENCES

1. Ireson CR, Kelland LR. Discovery and development of anticancer aptamers. *Mol Cancer Ther* 2006; **5**: 2957–2962.
2. Proske D, Blank M, Buhmann R, Resch A. Aptamers—Basic research, drug development, and clinical applications. *Appl Microbiol Biotechnol* 2005; **69**: 367–374.
3. Juliano R, Alam MR, Dixit V, Kang H. Mechanisms and strategies for effective delivery of antisense and siRNA oligonucleotides. *Nucleic Acids Res* 2008; **36**: 4158–4171.
4. Manoharan M. Oligonucleotide conjugates as potential antisense drugs with improved uptake, biodistribution, targeted delivery, and mechanism of action. *Antisense Nucleic Acid Drug Dev* 2002; **12**: 103–128.
5. Crooke ST. Molecular mechanisms of action of antisense drugs. *Biochim Biophys Acta* 1999; **1489**: 31–43.
6. Fire A, Xu S, Montgomery MK, Kostas SA, Driver SE, Mello CC. Potent and specific genetic interference by double-stranded RNA in *Caenorhabditis elegans*. *Nature* 1998; **391**: 806–811.
7. Doi N, Zenno S, Ueda R, Ohki-Hamazaki H, Ui-Tei K, Saigo K. Short-interfering-RNA-mediated gene silencing in mammalian cells requires Dicer and eIF2C translation initiation factors. *Curr Biol* 2003; **13**: 41–46.
8. Bumcrot D, Manoharan M, Koteliansky V, Sah DW. RNAi therapeutics: A potential new class of pharmaceutical drugs. *Nat Chem Biol* 2006; **2**: 711–719.
9. Rosenberg SA, Aebersold P, Cornetta K, Kasid A, Morgan RA, Moen R, Karson EM, Lotze MT, Yang JC, Topalian SL, Merino M, Culver K, Miller AD, Blaese RM, Anderson WF. Gene transfer into humans-immunotherapy of patients with advanced melanoma, using tumor-infiltrating lymphocytes modified by retroviral gene transduction. *N Engl J Med* 1990; **323**: 570–578.
10. Edelstein ML, Abedi MR, Wixon J. Gene therapy clinical trials worldwide to 2007—An update. *J Gene Med* 2007; **9**: 833–842.
11. Peng Z. Current status of gendicine in China: Recombinant Ad-p53 agent for treatment of cancers. *Hum Gene Ther* 2005; **16**:1016–1027.
12. Wilson JM. Gendicine: The first commercial gene therapy product. *Hum Gene Ther* 2005; **16**: 1014–1015.
13. Peng Z, Yu Q, Bao L. The application of gene therapy in China. *IDrugs* 2008; **11**: 346–350.
14. Opalinska JB, Gewirtz AM. Nucleic-acid therapeutics: Basic principles and recent applications. *Nat Rev Drug Discov* 2002; **1**: 503–514.
15. Rayburn ER, Zhang R. Antisense, RNAi, and gene silencing strategies for therapy: Mission possible or impossible? *Drug Discov Today* 2008; **13**: 513–521.
16. Melnikova I. RNA-based therapies. *Nat Rev Drug Dis* 2007; **6**: 863–864.
17. DeVincenzo J, Cehelsky JE, Alvarez R, Elbashir S, Harborth J, Toudjarska I, Nechev L, Murugaiah V, Van Vliet A, Vaishnaw AK, Meyers R. Evaluation of the safety, tolerability and pharmacokinetics of ALN-RSV01, a novel RNAi antiviral therapeutic directed against respiratory syncytial virus (RSV). *Antiviral Res* 2008; **77**: 225–231.
18. Behlke MA. Progress towards *in vivo* use of siRNAs. *Mol Ther* 2006; **13**: 644–670.
19. Kwon I, Schaffer DV. Designer gene delivery vectors: Molecular engineering and evolution of adeno-associated viral vectors for enhanced gene transfer. *Pharm Res* 2008; **25**: 489–499.
20. Wu H, Curiel DT. Fiber-modified adenoviruses for targeted gene therapy. *Methods Mol Biol* 2008; **434**: 113–132.
21. Waehler R, Russell SJ, Curiel DT. Engineering targeted viral vectors for gene therapy. *Nat Rev Genet* 2007; **8**: 573–587.
22. Yoo JY, Kim JH, Kwon YG, Kim EC, Kim NK, Choi HJ, Yun CO. VEGF-specific short hairpin RNA-expressing oncolytic adenovirus elicits potent inhibition of angiogenesis and tumor growth. *Mol Ther* 2007; **15**: 295–302.
23. Lundstrom K. Latest development in viral vectors for gene therapy. *Trends Biotechnol* 2003; **21**: 117–122.
24. Luten J, van Nostrum CF, De Smedt SC, Hennink WE. Biodegradable polymers as non-viral carriers for plasmid DNA delivery. *J Control Release* 2008; **126**: 97–110.
25. Peer D, Karp JM, Hong S, Farokhzad OC, Margalit R, Langer R. Nanocarriers as an emerging platform for cancer therapy. *Nat Nanotechnol* 2007; **2**: 751–760.
26. Ogris M, Carlisle RC, Bettinger T, Seymour LW. Melittin enables efficient vesicular escape and enhanced nuclear access of nonviral gene delivery vectors. *J Biol Chem* 2001; **276**: 47550–47555.

27. Saito G, Amidon GL, Lee KD. Enhanced cytosolic delivery of plasmid DNA by a sulfhydryl-activatable listeriolysin O/protamine conjugate utilizing cellular reducing potential. *Gene Ther* 2003; **10**: 72–83.

28. Boeckle S, Fahrmeir J, Roedl W, Ogris M, Wagner E. Melittin analogs with high lytic activity at endosomal pH enhance transfection with purified targeted PEI polyplexes. *J Control Release* 2006; **112**: 240–248.

29. Peer D, Zhu P, Carman CV, Lieberman J, Shimaoka M. Selective gene silencing in activated leukocytes by targeting siRNAs to the integrin lymphocyte function-associated antigen-1. *Proc Natl Acad Sci USA* 2007; **104**: 4095–4100.

30. Yu W, Pirollo KF, Rait A, Yu B, Xiang LM, Huang WQ, Zhou Q, Ertem G, Chang EH. A sterically stabilized immunolipoplex for systemic administration of a therapeutic gene. *Gene Ther* 2004; **11**: 1434–1440.

31. Pirollo KF, Rait A, Zhou Q, Zhang XQ, Zhou J, Kim CS, Benedict WF, Chang EH. Tumor-targeting nanocomplex delivery of novel tumor suppressor RB94 chemosensitizes bladder carcinoma cells *in vitro* and *in vivo*. *Clin Cancer Res* 2008; **14**: 2190–2198.

32. Kim KS, Lee YK, Kim JS, Koo KH, Hong HJ, Park YS. Targeted gene therapy of LS174 T human colon carcinoma by anti-TAG-72 immunoliposomes. *Cancer Gene Ther* 2008; **15**: 331–340.

33. Moffatt S, Papasakelariou C, Wiehle S, Cristiano R. Successful *in vivo* tumor targeting of prostate-specific membrane antigen with a highly efficient J591/PEI/DNA molecular conjugate. *Gene Ther* 2006; **13**: 761–772.

34. Song E, Zhu P, Lee SK, Chowdhury D, Kussman S, Dykxhoorn DM, Feng Y, Palliser D, Weiner DB, Shankar P, Marasco WA, Lieberman J. Antibody mediated *in vivo* delivery of small interfering RNAs *via* cell-surface receptors. *Nat Biotechnol* 2005; **23**: 709–717.

35. Peer D, Park EJ, Morishita Y, Carman CV, Shimaoka M. Systemic leukocyte-directed siRNA delivery revealing cyclin D1 as an anti-inflammatory target. *Science* 2008; **319**: 627–630.

36. Wen WH, Liu JY, Qin WJ, Zhao J, Wang T, Jia LT, Meng YL, Gao H, Xue CF, Jin BQ, Yao LB, Chen SY, Yang AG. Targeted inhibition of HBV gene expression by single-chain antibody mediated small interfering RNA delivery. *Hepatology* 2007; **46**: 84–94.

37. Kumar P, Ban HS, Kim SS, Wu H, Pearson T, Greiner DL, Laouar A, Yao J, Haridas V, Habiro K, Yang YG, Jeong JH, Lee KY, Kim YH, Kim SW, Peipp M, Fey GH, Manjunath N, Shultz LD, Lee SK, Shankar P. T cell-specific siRNA delivery suppresses HIV-1 infection in humanized mice. *Cell* 2008; **134**: 577–586.

38. Balmain A, Gray J, Ponder B. The genetics and genomics of cancer. *Nat Genet* 2003; **33**: 238–244.

39. Daniels TR, Delgado T, Rodriguez JA, Helguera G, Penichet ML. The transferrin receptor part I: Biology and targeting with cytotoxic antibodies for the treatment of cancer. *Clin Immunol* 2006; **121**: 144–158.

40. Gomme PT, McCann KB. Transferrin: Structure, function and potential therapeutic actions. *Drug Discov Today* 2005; **10**: 267–273.

41. Aqarwal A, Saraf S, Asthana A, Gupta U, Gajbhiye V, Jain NK. Ligand based dendritic systems for tumor targeting. *Int J Pharm* 2008; **350**: 3–13.

42. Cardoso ALC, Simoes S, de Almeida LP, Pelisek J, Culmsee C, Wagner E, Pedroso de Lima MC. siRNA delivery by a transferrin-associated lipid-based vector: A non-viral strategy to mediate gene silencing. *J Gene Med* 2007; **9**: 170–183.

43. Xu L, Pirollo KF, Tang WH, Rait A, Chang EH. Transferrin-liposome mediated systemic p53 gene therapy in combination with radiation in regression of human head and neck cancer xenografts. *Hum Gene Ther* 1999; **10**: 2941–2952.

44. Nakase M, Inui M, Okumura K, Kamei T, Nakamura S, Tagawa T. p53 gene therapy of human osteosarcoma using a transferrin-modified cationic liposome. *Mol Cancer Ther* 2005; **4**: 625–631.

45. Li X, Fu GF, Fan YR, Shi CF, Liu XJ, Xu GX, Wang JJ. Potent inhibition of angiogenesis and liver tumor growth by administration of an aerosol containing a transferrin-liposome-endostatin complex. *World J Gastroenterol* 2003; **9**: 262–266.

46. Dash PR, Read ML, Fisher KD, Howard KA, Wolfert M, Oupicky D, Subr V, Strohalm J, Ulbrich K, Seymour LW. Decreased binding to proteins and cells of polymeric gene delivery vectors surface modified with a multivalent hydrophilic polymer and retargeting through attachment of transferrin. *J Biol Chem* 2000; **275**: 3793–3802.

47. Jhaveri MS, Rait AS, Chung KN, Trepel, JB, Chang EH. Antisense oligonucleotides targeted to the human alpha folate receptor inhibit breast cancer cell growth and sensitize the cells to doxorubicin treatment. *Mol Cancer Ther* 2004; **3**: 1505–1512.

48. Chiu SJ, Liu S, Perrotti D, Marcucci G, Lee RJ. Efficient delivery of a Bcl-2-specific antisense oligode-oxyribonucleotide (G3139) via transferrin receptor-targeted liposomes. *J Control Release* 2006; **112**: 199–207.

49. Tietze N, Pelisek J, Philipp A, Roedl W, Merdan T, Tarcha P, Ogris M, Wagner E. Induction of apoptosis in murine neuroblastoma by systemic delivery of transferrin-shielded siRNA polyplexes for downregulation of Ran. *Oligonucleotides* 2008; **18**: 161–174.

50. Hu-lieskovan S, Heidel JD, Bartlett DW, Davis ME, Triche TJ. Sequence-specific knockdown of EWS-FLI1 by targeted, nonviral delivery of small interfering RNA inhibits tumor growth in a murine model of metastatic Ewing's sarcoma. *Cancer Res* 2005; **65**: 8984–8992.

51. Daniels TR, Delgado T, Helguera G, Penichet ML. The transferrin receptor part II: Targeted delivery of therapeutic agents into cancer cells. *Clin Immunol* 2006b; **121**: 159–176.

52. Qian ZM, Li H, Sun H, Ho K. Targeted drug delivery *via* the transferrin receptor-mediated endocytosis pathway. *Pharmacol Rev* 2002; **54**: 561–587.

53. Takada Y, Ye X, Simon S. The integrins. *Genome Biol* 2007; **8**: 215.

54. Nemeth JA, Nakada MT, Trikha M, Lang Z, Gordon MS, Jayson GC, Corringham R, Prabhakar U, Davis HM, Beckman RA. Alpha-v integrins as therapeutic targets in oncology. *Cancer Invest* 2007; **25**: 632–646.

55. Huveneers S, Truong H, Danen HJ. Integrins: Signaling, disease, and therapy. *Int J Radiat Biol* 2007; **83**: 743–751.

56. Temming K, Schiffelers RM, Molema G, Kok RJ. RGD-based strategies for selective delivery of thera-peutics and imaging agents to the tumour vasculature. *Drug Resist Updat* 2005; **8**: 381–402.

57. Ishikawa A, Zhou YM, Kambe N, Nakayama Y. Enhancement of star vector-based gene delivery to endothelial cells by addition of RGD-peptide. *Bioconjug Chem* 2008; **19**: 558–561.

58. Alam MR, Dixit V, Kang H, Li ZB, Chen X, Trejo J, Fisher M, Juliano RL. Intracellular delivery of an anionic antisense oligonucleotide *via* receptor-mediated endocytosis. *Nucleic Acids Res* 2008; **36**: 2764–2776.

59. Schiffelers RM, Ansari A, Xu J, Zhou Q, Tang Q, Storm G, Molema G, Lu PY, Scaria PV, Woodle MC. Cancer siRNA therapy by tumor selective delivery with ligand-targeted sterically stabilized nanoparticle. *Nucleic Acids Res* 2004; **32**: e149.

60. Kim B, Tang Q, Biswas PS, Xu J, Schiffelers RM, Xie FY, Ansari AM, Scaria PV, Woodle MC, Lu P, Rouse BT. Inhibition of ocular angiogenesis by siRNA targeting vascular endothelial growth factor path-way genes: Therapeutic strategy for herpetic stromal keratitis. *Am J Pathol* 2004; **165**: 2177–2185.

61. Cai W, Chen X. Anti-angiogenic cancer therapy based on integrin alphavbeta3 antagonism. *Anticancer Agents Med Chem* 2006; **6**:407–428.

62. Burke PA, DeNardo SJ, Miers LA, Lamborn KR, Matzku S, DeNardo GL. Cilengitide targeting of alpha(v)beta(3) integrin receptor synergizes with radioimmunotherapy to increase efficacy and apoptosis in breast cancer xenografts. *Cancer Res* 2002; **62**: 4263–4272.

63. Low PS, Lu Y. Folate-mediated delivery of macromolecular anticancer therapeutic agents. *Adv Drug Deliv Rev* 2002; **54**: 675–693.

64. Low PS, Henne WA, Doorneweerd DD. Discovery and development of folic-acid-based receptor target-ing for imaging and therapy of cancer and inflammatory diseases. *Acc Chem Res* 2008; **41**: 120–129.

65. Jaracz S, Chen J, Kuznetsova LV, Ojima I. Recent advances in tumor-targeting anticancer drug conju-gates. *Bioorg Med Chem* 2005; **13**: 5043–5054.

66. Salazar MD, Ratnam M. The folate receptor: What does it promise in tissue-targeted therapeutics? *Cancer Metastasis Rev* 2007; **26**: 141–152.

67. Sudimack J, Lee RJ. Targeted drug delivery via the folate receptor. *Adv Drug Deliv Rev* 2000; **41**: 147–162.

68. Chan P, Kurisawa M, Chung JE, Yang YY. Synthesis and characterization of chitosan-g-poly(ethylene glycol)-folate as a non-viral carrier for tumor-targeted gene delivery. *Biomaterials* 2007; **28**: 540–549.

69. Kim SH, Jeong JH, Mok H, Lee SH, Kim SW, Park TG. Folate receptor targeted delivery of polyelec-trolyte complex micelles prepared from ODN-PEG-folate conjugate and cationic lipids. *Biotechnol Prog* 2007; **23**: 232–237.

70. Zhang K, Wang Q, Xie Y, Mor G, Sega E, Low PS, Huang Y. Receptor-mediated delivery of siRNAs by tethered nucleic acid base-paired interactions. *RNA* 2008; **14**: 577–583.

71. Hilgenbrink AR, Low PS. Folate receptor-mediated drug targeting: From therapeutics to diagnostics. *J Pharm Sci* 2005; **94**: 2135–2146.

72. Low PS, Antony AC. Folate receptor-targeted drugs for cancer and inflammatory diseases. *Adv Drug Deliv Rev* 2004; **56**: 1055–1058.

73. Plank C, Mechtler K, Szoka FC Jr, Wagner E. Activation of the complement system by synthetic DNA complexes: A potential barrier for intravenous gene delivery. *Hum Gene Ther* 1996; **7**: 1437–1446.
74. Plank C, Zatloukal K, Cotten M, Mechtler K, Wagner E. Gene transfer into hepatocytes using asialoglycoprotein receptor mediated endocytosis of DNA complexed with an artificial tetra-antennary galactose-ligand. *Bioconjug Chem* 1992; **13**: 533–539.
75. Zanta MA, Boussif O, Adib A, Behr JP. *In vitro* gene delivery to hepatocytes with galactosylated polyethylenimine. *Bioconjug Chem* 1997; **8**: 839–844.
76. Midoux P, Monsigny M. Efficient gene transfer by histidylated polylysine/pDNA complexes. *Bioconjug Chem* 1999; **10**: 406–411.
77. Kawakami S, Sato A, Nishikawa M, Yamashita F, Hashida M. Mannose receptor-mediated gene transfer into macrophages using novel mannosylated cationic liposomes. *Gene Ther* 2000; **7**: 292–299.
78. Park IY, Kim IY, Yoo MK, Choi YJ, Cho MH, Cho CS. Mannosylated polyethylenimine coupled mesoporous silica nanoparticles for receptor-mediated gene delivery. *Int J Pharm* 2008; **359**: 280–287.
79. Lu Y, Kawakami S, Yamashita F, Hashida M. Development of an antigen-presenting cell-targeted DNA vaccine against melanoma by mannosylated liposomes. *Biomaterials* 2007; **28**: 3255–3262.
80. Kim EM, Jeong HJ, Park IK. Asialoglycoprotein receptor targeted gene delivery using galactosylated polyethylenimine-graft-poly(ethylene glycol): *In vitro* and *in vivo* studies. *J Control Release* 2005; **28**: 557–567.
81. Zhu L, Ye Z, Cheng K, Miller DD, Mahato RI. Site-specific delivery of oligonucleotides to hepatocytes after systemic administration. *Bioconjug Chem* 2008; **19**: 290–298.
82. Sato A, Takagi M, Shimamoto A, Kawakami S, Hashida M. Small interfering RNA delivery to the liver by intravenous administration of galactosylated cationic liposomes in mice. *Biomaterials* 2007; **28**: 1434–1442.
83. Kunath K, von Harpe A, Fischer D, Kissel T. Galactose-PEI-DNA complexes for targeted gene delivery: Degree of substitution affects complex size and transfection efficiency. *J Control Release* 2003; **88**:159–172.
84. Platt VM, Szoka FC Jr. Anticancer therapeutics: Targeting macromolecules and nanocarriers to hyaluronan or CD44, a hyaluronan receptor. *Mol Pharm* 2008; **5**: 474–486.
85. de la Fuente M, Seijo B, Alonso MJ. Bioadhesive hyaluronan-chitosan nanoparticles can transport genes across the ocular mucosa and transfect ocular tissue. *Gene Ther* 2008; **15**: 668–676.
86. Lee H, Mok H, Lee S, Oh YK, Park TG. Target-specific intracellular delivery of siRNA using degradable hyaluronic acid nanogels. *J Control Release* 2007; **119**: 245–252.
87. Jiang G, Park K, Kim J, Kim KS, Oh EJ, Kang H, Han SE, Oh YK, Park TG, Kwang Hahn S. Hyaluronic acid-polyethyleneimine conjugate for target specific intracellular delivery of siRNA. *Biopolymers* 2008; **89**: 635–642.
88. Udabage L, Brownlee GR, Nilsson SK, Brown TJ. The over-expression of HAS2, Hyal-2 and CD44 is implicated in the invasiveness of breast cancer. *Exp Cell Res* 2005; **310**: 205–217.
89. David-Raoudi M, Tranchepain F, Deschrevel B, Vincent JC, Bogdanowicz P, Boumediene K, Pujol JP. Differential effects of hyaluronan and its fragments on fibroblasts: Relation to wound healing. *Wound Repair Regen* 2008; **16**: 274–287.
90. Mairal T, Ozalp VC, Lozano Sánchez P, Mir M, Katakis I, O'Sullivan CK. Aptamers: Molecular tools for analytical applications. *Anal Bioanal Chem* 2008; **390**: 989–1007.
91. Bunka DHJ, Stockley PG. Aptamers come of age—At last. *Nat Rev Microbiol* 2006; **4**: 588–596.
92. Lupold SE, Hicke BJ, Lin Y, Coffey DS. Identification and characterization of nuclease-stabilized RNA molecules that bind human prostate cancer cells *via* the prostate-specific membrane antigen. *Cancer Res* 2002; **62**: 4029–4033.
93. Farokhzad OC, Cheng J, Teply BA, Sherifi I, Jon S, Kantoff PW, Richie JP, Langer R. Targeted nanoparticle-aptamer bioconjugates for cancer chemotherapy *in vivo*. *Proc Natl Acad Sci USA* 2006; **103**: 6315–6320.
94. Zhang L, Radovic-Moreno AF, Alexis F. Co-delivery of hydrophobic and hydrophilic drugs from nanoparticle-aptamer bioconjugates. *Chem Med Chem* 2007; **2**: 1268–1271.
95. Chu TC, Twu KY, Ellington AD, Levy M. Aptamer mediated siRNA delivery. *Nucleic Acids Res* 2006; **34**: e73.
96. McNamara JO 2nd, Andrechek ER, Wang Y, Viles KD, Rempel RE, Gilboa E, Sullenger BA, Giangrande PH. Cell type-specific delivery of siRNAs with aptamer-siRNA chimeras. *Nat Biotechnol* 2006; **24**: 1005–1015.
97. Zhou J, Li H, Li S, Zaia J, Rossi JJ. Novel dual inhibitory function aptamer-siRNA delivery system for HIV-1 therapy. *Mol Ther* 2008; **16**: 1481–1489.

98. Kim SH, Jeong JH, Ou M, Yockman JW, Kim SW, Bull DA. Cardiomyocyte-targeted siRNA delivery by prostaglandin E(2)-Fas siRNA polyplexes formulated with reducible poly(amido amine) for preventing cardiomyocyte apoptosis. *Biomaterials* 2008; **29**: 4439–4446.

99. Li SD, Chen YC, Hackett MJ, Huang L. Tumor-targeted delivery of siRNA by self-assembled nanoparticles. *Mol Ther* 2008; **16**: 163–169.

100. Chono S, Li SD, Conwell CC, Huang L. An efficient and low immunostimulatory nanoparticle formulation for systemic siRNA delivery to the tumor. *J Control Release* 2008; **131**: 64–69.

101. Ryan RM, Green J, Lewis CE. Use of bacteria in anti-cancer therapies. *Bioessays* 2006; **28**: 84–84.

102. Wei MQ, Mengesha A, Good D, Anné J. Bacterial targeted tumour therapy-dawn of a new era. *Cancer Lett* 2008; **259**: 16–27.

103. Lee CH, Wu CL, Shiau AL. Endostatin gene therapy delivered by *Salmonella choleraesuis* in murine tumor models. *J Gene Med* 2004; **6**: 1382–1383.

104. Burke B. Macrophages as novel cellular vehicles for gene therapy. *Expert Opin Biol Ther* 2003; **3**: 919–924.

105. Okasora T, Jo JI, Tabata Y. Augmented anti-tumor therapy through natural targetability of macrophages genetically engineered by NK4 plasmid DNA. *Gene Ther* 2008; **15**: 524–530.

106. Byun HM, Suh D, Yoon H, Kim JM, Choi HG, Kim WK, Ko JJ, Oh YK. Erythrocyte ghost-mediated gene delivery for prolonged and blood-targeted expression. *Gene Ther* 2004; **11**: 492–496.

107. Magnani M, Rossi L, Fraternale A, Bianchi M, Antonelli A, Crinelli R, Chiarantini L. Erythrocyte-mediated delivery of drugs, peptides and modified oligonucleotides. *Gene Ther* 2002; **9**: 749–751.

108. Campbell AI, Zhao Y, Sandhu R, Stewart DJ. Cell-based gene transfer of vascular endothelial growth factor attenuates monocrotaline-induced pulmonary hypertension. *Circulation* 2001; **104**: 2242–2248.

109. McCarter SD, Mei SH, Lai PF, Zhang QW, Parker CH, Suen RS, Hood RD, Zhao YD, Deng Y, Han RN, Dumont DJ, Stewart DJ. Cell-based angiopoietin-1 gene therapy for acute lung injury. *Am J Respir Crit Care Med* 2007; **175**: 1014–1026.

110. Mei SH, McCarter SD, Deng Y, Parker CH, Liles WC, Stewart DJ. Prevention of LPS-induced acute lung injury in mice by mesenchymal stem cells overexpressing angiopoietin 1. *PLoS Med* 2007; **4**: e269.

111. Russ V, Wagner E. Cell and tissue targeting of nucleic acids for cancer gene therapy. *Pharm Res* 2007; **24**: 1047–1057.

112. Neumann E, Schaefer-Ridder M, Wang Y, Hofschneider PH. Gene transfer into mouse lyoma cells by electroporation in high electric fields. *EMBO J* 1982; **1**: 841–845.

113. Isaka Y, Imai E. Electroporation-mediated gene therapy. *Expert Opin Drug Deliv* 2007; 4: 561–571.

114. Aihara H, Miyazaki J. Gene transfer into muscle by electroporation *in vivo*. *Nat Biotechnol* 1998; **16**: 867–870.

115. Heller LC, Jaroszeski MJ, Coppola D. Optimization of cutaneous electrically mediated plasmid DNA delivery using novel electrode. *Gene Ther* 2007; **14**: 275–280.

116. Bloquel C, Denys A, Boissier MC, Apparailly F, Bigey P, Scherman D, Bessis N. Intra-articular electrotransfer of plasmid encoding soluble TNF receptor variants in normal and arthritic mice. *J Gene Med* 2007; **9**: 986–993.

117. Heller LC, Heller R. In vivo electroporation for gene therapy. *Hum Gene Ther* 2006; **17**: 890–897.

118. Kim HJ, Greenleaf JF, Kinnick RR, Bronk JT, Bolander ME. Ultrasound-mediated transfection of mammalian cells. *Hum Gene Ther* 1996; **7**: 1339–1346.

119. Liu Y, Miyoshi H, Nakamura M. Encapsulated ultrasound microbubbles: Therapeutic application in drug/gene delivery. *J Control Release* 2006; **114**: 89–99.

120. Wang X, Liang HD, Dong B, Lu QL, Blomley MJ. Gene transfer with microbubble ultrasound and plasmid DNA into skeletal muscle of mice: Comparison between commercially available microbubble contrast agents. *Radiology* 2005; **237**: 224–229.

121. Xenariou S, Griesenbach U, Liang HD, Zhu J, Farley R, Somerton L, Singh C, Jeffery PK, Ferrari S, Scheule RK, Cheng SH, Geddes DM, Blomley M, Alton EW. Use of ultrasound to enhance nonviral lung gene transfer *in vivo*. *Gene Ther* 2007; **14**: 768–774.

122. Guo H, Leung JC, Chan LY, Tsang AW, Lam MF, Lan HY, Lai KN. Ultrasound-contrast agent mediated naked gene delivery in the peritoneal cavity of adult rat. *Gene Ther* 2007; **14**: 1712–1720.

123. Shen ZP, Brayman AA, Chen L, Miao CH. Ultrasound with microbubbles enhances gene expression of plasmid DNA in the liver via intraportal delivery. *Gene Ther* 2008; **15**: 1147–1155.

124. Suzuki R, Takizawa T, Negishi Y, Utoguchi N, Sawamura K, Tanaka K, Namai E, Oda Y, Matsumura Y, Maruyama K. Tumor specific ultrasound enhanced gene transfer in vivo with novel liposomal bubbles. *J Control Release* 2008; **125**: 137–144.

125. Tran MA, Gowda R, Sharma A, Park EJ, Adair J, Kester M, Smith NB, Robertson GP. Targeting V600EB-Raf and Akt3 using nanoliposomal-small interfering RNA inhibits cutaneous melanocytic lesion development. *Cancer Res* 2008; **68**: 7638–7649.

126. Mykhaylyk O, Zelphati O, Rosenecker J, Plank C. siRNA delivery by magnetofection. *Curr Opin Mol Ther* 2008; **10**: 493–505.

127. Lee CH, Kim EY, Jeon K, Tae JC, Lee KS, Kim YO, Jeong MY, Yun CW, Jeong DK, Cho SK, Kim JH, Lee HY, Riu KZ, Cho SG, Park SP. Simple, efficient, and reproducible gene transfection of mouse embryonic stem cells by magnetofection. *Stem Cells Dev* 2008; **17**:133–141.

128. Plank C, Anton M, Rudolph C, Rosenecker J, Krötz F. Enhancing and targeting nucleic acid delivery by magnetic force. *Expert Opin Biol Ther* 2003; **3**: 745–758.

129. Xenariou S, Griesenbach U, Ferrari S. Using magnetic forces to enhance non-viral gene transfer to airway epithelium *in vivo*. *Gene Ther* 2006; **13**: 1545–1552.

8 Delivery and Targeting of Oligonucleotides and siRNA

Ningning Yang and Ram I. Mahato

CONTENTS

8.1 INTRODUCTION

Oligodeoxynucleotides (ODNs) are increasingly being recognized as potential therapeutic agents to modulate aberrant gene expression for treating various diseases, including cancers[1–3] and viral infections.[4,5] Concerted efforts have made significant progress in turning these nucleic acids into therapeutics. Apart from immune-stimulation and enzymatic cleavage, the most important feature of ODNs is their ability to block mRNA function by sequence-specific hybridization with target mRNA.[6] Theoretically, the antisense strategy can be used to target any gene in the body, which allows these nucleic acids to achieve broader therapeutic potential than small molecules.

Antisense therapeutic strategies for inhibiting aberrant protein expression have been developed a lot and some of them have already been in clinical trials.[7] In 2005, the first antisense ODN drug, Vitravene (Fomivirsen), was approved by the United States Food and Drug Administration (FDA).[8] After this approval, more and more clinical trials are being conducted not only for ODNs, but also for other nucleic acid drugs, which are discussed in detail in this chapter.

Because of their large molecular weight and negative charge, the delivery of gene drugs is still a big challenge to scientists. For the most popularly used two therapeutic nucleotides, single-stranded antisense oligodeoxyribonucleotides (AS-ODNs) and double-stranded small interfering RNAs (siRNAs), the molecular weight is at least 6 and 13 kDa, respectively. The size of other ODNs is also very big. Their large molecular weight prevents them from passing the endothelium smoothly, which is the most important physiological barrier for systemic administration. For many organs and tissues, systemic administration is the only way to be reached by the therapeutic agents in bloodstream. Phosphodiester ODNs are degraded by endo- and exo-nucleases after systemic and local administration. Besides big size and poor biostability, the toxicity induced by these nucleic acids is another big barrier to their therapeutic application. How to achieve efficient gene silencing at a nontoxic dose is the most important issue for the success of ODN and siRNA delivery. Various polymer and lipid carriers have been synthesized for their delivery and targeting. In addition, chemical and backbone modifications are used to increase the stability of ODNs.

This chapter discusses the mode of action, stability, and delivery considerations of ODNs and siRNAs as well as ways to overcome their biological barriers.

8.2 SINGLE-STRANDED OLIGONUCLEOTIDES

8.2.1 ANTISENSE OLIGODEOXYRIBONUCLEOTIDES

An AS-ODN is a short single-stranded nucleic acid that binds to specific mRNA and forms a short double-stranded hybrid. The length of AS-ODNs is about 13–25 bases. AS-ODNs can inhibit the translation of mRNA by binding to the mRNA molecules.[9] The term "antisense" ODNs is commonly used because their sequences are complementary to target mRNA, which is called the "sense" sequence. The binding affinity and sequence specificity determine the ability of an AS-ODN to form a hybrid with a target mRNA. The binding affinity depends on the number of hydrogen bonds formed between the AS-ODN and the target mRNA sequence. The affinity can be determined by measuring the melting temperature (T_m), at which half of the double-stranded hybrid is dissociated into single strands. Binding affinity is also determined by the concentration of AS-ODNs and the ionic strength of the solvent in which hybridization occurs.[10]

Most antisense ODNs follow the two major mechanisms of action (Figure 8.1): the RNase-H-dependent degradation of mRNA[11,12] and the steric-hindrance of the translational machinery.[13] The RNase-H-dependent cleavage of mRNA is the most effective and frequently used mechanism for antisense knockdown. RNase-H is a ribonuclease that can recognize the RNA–DNA hybrid duplex and cleave a 3′-O–P-bond of the mRNA strand in the mRNA-ODN complex. This endonuclease catalyzes the cleavage of RNA via a hydrolytic mechanism with assistance from an enzyme-bound divalent metal ion. Once the mRNA is cleaved, the AS-ODN dissociates from the duplex and induces another round of RNase-H-dependent degradation. Thus, it can be looked upon as a catalytic process because this procedure decreases the required concentration of AS-ODNs. Nevertheless, RNase-H recognition is limited to only a few compounds. Some chemically modified AS-ODNs, which have higher stability than unmodified ODNs, cannot be recognized by RNase-H.

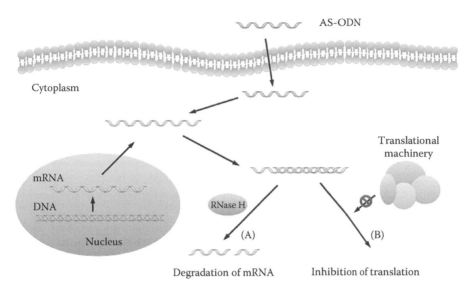

AS-ODN

Cytoplasm

Translational
machinery

mRNA

DNA

RNase H

Nucleus

(A)

(B)

Degradation of mRNA   Inhibition of translation

FIGURE 8.1 Mechanisms of action of AS-ODNs. (A) RNase-H dependent degradation of mRNA. In this strategy, RNase-H recognizes RNA-DNA hybrid duplex and cleaves 3′-O-P-bond of the mRNA strand in the mRNA-ODN complex. (B) Steric-hindrance of the translational machinery. In this strategy, an AS-ODN binds to the single-stranded mRNA by Watson–Crick base pairing strength and forbids the translational machine to move forward.

The steric hindrance mechanism is also termed "translational arrest," in which an AS-ODN binds to the single-stranded mRNA by Watson–Crick base pairing. This hybrid formation can sterically stop the translation of target mRNA. During the process, the binding of the translational related factors to mRNA may be blocked sterically.

8.2.2 TRIPLEX-FORMING OLIGONUCLEOTIDES

Triplex forming oligonucleotides (TFOs) show a different strategy of gene silencing compared with AS-ODNs. TFOs, around 10–30 nt in length, can form a triplex with the specific genomic DNA sequences to interfere with transcription, replication, repair, and recombination.[14] TFOs bind to the major groove of duplex DNA, which have runs of purines on one strand and pyrimidines on the other. TFOs are composed of either polypurine or polypyrimidine, but bind only to the purine-rich strand of their target DNA duplex.[15] According to their base composition, TFOs containing C and T nucleotides bind in a parallel orientation to the target strand, and TFOs containing G and A or T nucleotides bind in an antiparallel orientation to the target strand, respectively.[16,17] After binding, the transcription of the target gene is blocked.

Transcriptional inhibition gives TFOs several advantages over other gene silencing technologies.[18,19] Since there are only two copies (two alleles) of a target gene in the genomic DNA, their blockage means that there will be no transcription of the DNA into the RNA. Since there may be thousands of copies of an mRNA for a specific gene, antisense may not block all these mRNAs. Furthermore, specific mRNAs are continuously transcribed from genomic DNA in the nucleus, even though those in the cytoplasm have been silenced. Therefore, the inhibition of gene transcription might decrease the mRNA level in a more efficient way, at least in some cases.

> Transcriptional inhibition gives TFOs several advantages over antisense ODNs. Since there are only two copies (two alleles) of a target gene in the genomic DNA, their blockage would completely prevent the transcription of DNA into RNA.

8.2.3 Immunomodulatory Oligonucleotides

Bacterial DNA can stimulate the proliferation of B cells and the production of inflammatory cytokines by monocytes and other cells, while vertebrate DNA cannot.[20] Several studies have found that the unmethylated CpG dinucleotide sequence in DNA is required for this immune-stimulatory activity.[21,22] Furthermore, single-stranded ODNs containing unmethylated CpG motifs, which are derived from bacterial DNA, are also immunostimulatory, especially with a nuclease-resistant phosphorothioate (PS) backbone.[21] CpG ODN, 18 to 24 bp in length, binds to the endosomal toll-like receptor 9 (TLR9) and is taken up by the cells via endocytosis. Once TLR9 is triggered, it may activate numerous signaling transduction pathways and lead to the release of many cytokines, such as IFN-γ, IL-12, and IL-18. The released cytokines directly stimulate B-lymphocytes, dendritic cells, and natural killer (NK) cells, resulting in innate immunity and antibody-dependent cell cytotoxicity. The signaling pathways activated by CpG DNA in B cells drive them to secrete IL-6, IL-10, and immunoglobulin,[23,24] and to proliferate in a polyclonal T-cell independent manner.[25] A CpG ODN can also indirectly modulate T-cell responses by increased levels of costimulatory molecules from dendritic cells after the application of CpG ODN.[26]

The activation of Th1-dominant immune responses by CpG ODN results in the production of several cytokines and CpG ODNs are promising candidates for treating cancer and allergic diseases as vaccine adjuvants and as immune therapeutics. A therapeutic application for CpG ODN is an adjuvant for cancer treatment. Current ongoing clinical trials combine CpG ODN with chemotherapy or vaccines to treat tumors because CpG ODN can induce protective immune responses against a lethal tumor challenge.[27,28] Another important utility of CpG ODN is the treatment of allergic diseases such as asthma. Due to the favorable Th1-based response induced by CpG ODN, it will redirect the undesirable Th2 responses of allergic disease.[22,29] Ongoing clinical trials will give us a complete evaluation of this immunomodulatory ODN.

8.2.4 Ribozyme and DNAzymes

A ribozyme, also called RNA enzyme or catalytic RNA, is an RNA molecule that specifically cleaves RNA sequences of choice. Natural ribozymes can form and dissolve covalent bonds by transesterification, hydrolysis, and peptidyl transfer.[30] They catalyze not only either the hydrolysis of one of their own phosphodiester bonds or that of bonds in other RNAs, but also the aminotransferase activity of the ribosome. Natural ribozymes can be put into three distinct categories: the self-splicing introns (groups I and II), ribonuclease P (RNase P), and the small catalytic ribozymes.[30–32] Groups I and II introns and RNase P belong to the larger, more complicated ribozymes with hundreds of nucleotides in length. The small ribozymes include hammerhead and hairpin ribozymes, which contain 50–70 nt and are commonly used in molecular biology research.[33]

For each category, the specificity of ribozymes for a particular cleavage site is determined by different mechanisms. For the hammerheads, hairpins, or group I introns, it is determined by base-pairing between the ribozyme and its RNA target. For the RNase P category, it is determined by the pairing of a guide RNA with the RNA target. For group II introns, it is determined by the pairing of the ribozyme to its DNA target. For all categories, the target length is another important key.

The ability to engineer small ribozymes that can cleave heterologous RNAs in a sequence-specific manner has enabled the extensive application of hammerhead and hairpin ribozymes as gene knockdown tools and potential therapeutic agents to treat AIDS and cancer patients.[34] Actually, ribozymes have been investigated to inactivate specific genes for the last two decades and have been used as functional genomic study tools, especially in the pre-RNAi era.[33] Phase I clinical trials using ribozyme to treat AIDS patients have been conducted and demonstrated initial success. However, some aspects require further investigation, such as ribozyme stability, ribozyme-substrate colocalization, and tissue-specific delivery.[35]

DNAzymes (or deoxyribozymes) are RNA-cleaving analogues of ribozymes. DNAzymes are composed of a catalytic domain flanked by a target-recognition complementary domain. DNAzymes are more stable than ribozymes due to their DNA backbones.

8.2.5 Nucleic Acid Aptamer

Aptamers are ODNs or peptides that can bind to their specific targets, ranging from small molecules,[36] peptides,[37] and amino acids[38] to proteins.[39] A nucleic acid aptamer is a linear sequence of nucleotides, typically 15–40 nt long. Mostly, when we talk about aptamers, we are referring to nucleic acid aptamers. The intramolecular interaction folds the chain of nucleotides to a complex three-dimensional shape. The shape of the aptamer allows it to bind tightly against the surface of its target. Since some aptamers have tight interaction with their targets, they are also chosen as target ligands for site-specific drug delivery. These aptamers are selected according to a predefined equilibrium (K_d), rate constants (k_{off}, k_{on}), and thermodynamic parameters (ΔH, ΔS) of aptamer-target interaction. Kinetic capillary electrophoresis technology is used for the selection of these smart aptamers. Nucleic acid aptamers are usually created by isolating them from synthetic combinatorial nucleic acid libraries by *in vitro* selection, systematic evolution of ligands by exponential enrichment (SELEX). The first aptamer-based drug, called Macugen and discovered by OSI Pharmaceuticals, has been approved by the FDA for treating age-related macular degeneration (AMD).

The discovery of the RNA switches led to more investigation of the nucleic acid aptamers.[40–42] RNA switches (commonly known as riboswitches) are also capable of binding to small molecule ligands and can control gene expression. Riboswitches are found in the untranslated regions (5′-UTR) of mRNA and therefore belong to the noncoding part of the mRNA. Many riboswitches consist of an aptamer domain or a sensor region, which is responsible for ligand binding. Riboswitches modulate gene expression at the level of transcription or translation. Since there are similar properties between riboswitches and aptamers, many natural aptamers were found to exist in riboswitches.

8.3 DOUBLE-STRANDED THERAPEUTIC OLIGONUCLEOTIDES

Double-stranded therapeutic ODNs can be classified into two groups: decoy oligodeoxynucleotides and siRNAs.

8.3.1 Decoy Oligodeoxynucleotides

Decoy ODNs are double-stranded DNA sequences that interact with proteins based on Watson–Crick base pairing and prevent the targeting transcription factors from their natural interaction partners. Therefore, transcription factors will be removed from their endogenous cis-elements. Decoy ODNs against positive transcription factors can inhibit the expression of activated genes, and those against negative transcription factors can enhance the expression of suppressed genes.[43] After the first artificial 14mer E2F decoy ODN, targeted to E2F transcription factor (E2F TF), was synthesized by Morishita et al. in 1995,[44] other decoy ODNs to target different proteins such as creb, NF-kB, STAT-1, and AP-1 have also been found.[45–47] Decoy ODNs have been applied to treat cancer, renal diseases, viral diseases, or cardiovascular diseases because many of these diseases are due to the deregulation of different transcription factors. The decoy ODN strategy may not only offer a powerful target-based gene therapy method but also provides a genetic tool for studying the cellular regulatory processes including upstream transcription regulation and downstream production.[43,48] In 1996, the FDA approved the clinical application of decoy ODN against E2F to treat neointimal hyperplasia in vein bypass grafts.[26]

8.3.2 Small Interfering RNA

siRNAs are a class of double-stranded RNA (dsRNA) sequences, which are 21 nt long. Since the discovery of siRNAs in 1998, more and more investigations have been focused on this RNA interference (RNAi) technology.[49] RNAi can be initiated not only by siRNA, but also by long dsRNA, plasmid or virus-based short hairpin RNA (shRNA), and microRNA (miRNA). Long dsRNA, shRNA, and pre-miRNA are processed by Dicer into 21–23 nt siRNA duplexes with symmetric 2 or 3 nt 3′-overhangs and 5′-phosphate groups. The processed siRNA is incorporated into a protein complex called the RNA-induced silencing complex (RISC). Dicer also plays an important role in the early steps of RISC formation.[50] Argonaute 2, the catalytic component contained within RISC, unwinds siRNA and cleaves the sense strand, which is also called the passenger strand.[51] The activated RISC selectively degrades the sequence-specific mRNA with the assistance from the antisense strand of the siRNA still remaining.[52] After RISC cleaves the target mRNA, the antisense strand siRNA is not affected. Thus, the RISC can undergo numerous cycles of mRNA cleavage, which further propagates gene silencing.[53]

8.4 BARRIERS TO OLIGONUCLEOTIDE-BASED THERAPEUTICS

Although ODNs and siRNAs have shown great therapeutic potential in treating various diseases, their *in vivo* applications still face several barriers, such as bio-instability, toxicity, and distribution to nontarget cells.

8.4.1 Instability of ODNs and siRNAs

Native ODNs and siRNAs are rapidly degraded by serum and cellular proteins, and their stability is greatly affected by physiological pH environments. Clinical applications of these nucleic acids require increasing their stability while retaining their capacity to inhibit aberrant protein expression. One approach is the chemical modification of ODNs and siRNAs. Figure 8.2 illustrates different structural modifications. These include modifications at backbones, PSs and boranophosphates, or riboses, 2′ position of ribose modification, to enhance their stability without losing their bioactivity.

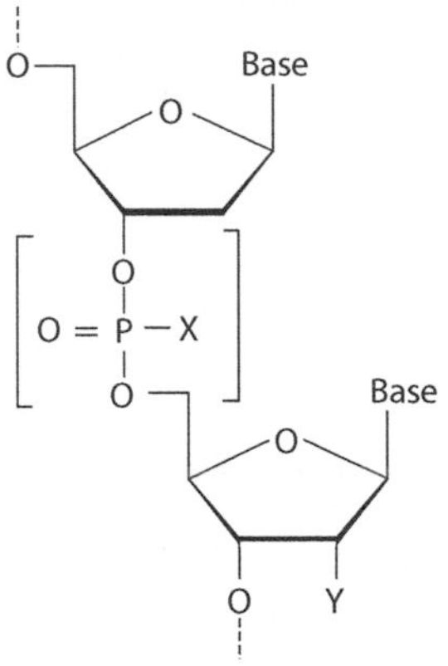

8.4.1.1 Phosphorothioates and Boranophosphate Modification

Since native phosphodiester ODNs are quite unstable, the ODN backbone is often modified not only to improve the stability of ODNs and siRNAs, but also to help them cross the highly impermeable lipid bilayer of the cell membrane.[54] PS or boranophosphate modifications of inter-nucleoside linkage are the two types that improve the stability of ODNs and siRNAs.

PSs are a variant of natural ODNs in which one of the nonbridging oxygens is replaced by a sulfur atom. This modification lowers the melting temperature (T_m) of the mRNA and hybridization efficiency with target mRNA compared with their phosphodiester counterparts. Fortunately, the modified AS-ODN can still be a substrate for RNase-H to trigger the RNase-H dependent mRNA degradation process. Nevertheless, the main drawback of the PS modification is that modified nucleotides may induce undesirable effects by binding to plasma proteins.[55,56]

FIGURE 8.2 Backbone and ribose modifications of ODNs and siRNAs. X means backbone modification. X=−S is PS, X=−BH₃ is boranophosphate. Y means 2′-position of ribose modification. Including 2′-O-methyl (Y=−CH₃), 2′-O-methoxyethyl (Y=−O−CH₂−CH₂−OCH₃), 2′-fluoro (Y=−F). In case of locked nucleic acid (LNA), ribose ring is "locked" by a methylene bridge connecting the 2′-O atom (Y=−O) and the 4′-C atom.

Thioate linkages do not always enhance siRNA stability, because PS may reduce the affinity between the two strands of the siRNA duplexes as compared with unmodified RNA.[57] One interesting study showed that only PS modified siRNAs reduced the inhibition ability to enhanced green fluorescent protein (EGFP) mRNA.[58] In this study, the PS linkages were incorporated into the sense strand of siRNA and led to 62% unmodified siRNA induced inhibition, whereas PS linkages in either the antisense or both strands of the siRNAs led to just less than 50% inhibition of that observed using unmodified siRNA. However, modification involving both 2′-position and PS in the antisense strand showed lower levels of EGFP gene silencing.

PS modification can be easily placed in the nucleic acid sequences at any desired position by two major routes. The first one is the sulfurization in a solution of elemental sulfur in carbon disulfide on a hydrogen phosphonate.[59] However, the toxicity of carbon disulfide is a barrier for clinical application. The second synthetic method avoids the problem of elemental sulfur's insolubility in most organic solvents and the toxicity of carbon disulfide. This method sulfurizes phosphite triesters with either tetraethylthiuram disulfide (TETD) or 3H-1,2-bensodithiol-3-one 1,1-dioxide (BDTD), and can yield higher purity PSs than before.[60]

An alternate backbone modification to increase the biological stability of ODNs and siRNAs is the boranophosphate linkage. In boranophosphate ODNs and siRNAs, the nonbridging phosphodiester oxygen is replaced with an isoelectronic borane ($-BH_3$) moiety. Boranophosphates have many of the same advantages as phosporothioates. Boranophosphates maintain the ability to make a base pair with high specificity and affinity to targets as the unmodified gene drugs. They can also be readily incorporated into DNA and RNA molecules by DNA and RNA polymerases to synthesize stereoregular boranophosphate DNA and RNA.[61–63] Other additional properties of boranophosphates make them more suitable for clinical use than PSs.[64] Since each boranophosphate linkage has a negative charge, the charge distribution of boranophosphates differs from that of normal phosphates and PSs, and thus increases their hydrophobicity, which facilitates their efficient internalization into the cells. Furthermore, boranophosphate ODNs are minimally toxic to rodents and humans.[65]

Unfortunately, boranophosphate-modified RNAs cannot easily be manufactured using standard chemical synthesis methods. Boranophosphate bases are incorporated into RNA by *in vitro* transcription,[66] which makes specific site selective incorporation of this modification very difficult.

> Thioate linkages do not always enhance siRNA stability, because PS may reduce the affinity between the two strands of the siRNA duplexes as compared with unmodified RNA.

8.4.1.2   2′ Ribose Modification

The sugar moiety of ODNs and siRNAs can be modified at the 2′ position of the ribose, replacing the nonbridging oxygen by 2′-O-methyl (2′-OMe), 2′-O-methoxy-ethyl (2′-MOE), or 2′-fluoro (2′-F).

2′-O-Methyl and 2′-O-methoxy-ethyl modifications are the most important members of this class. The DNA/RNA hybrid by AS-ODNs made of these building blocks is very stable. Furthermore, these AS-ODNs are less toxic than PSs ODNs and even have a slightly enhanced affinity towards their complementary RNAs.[67] The 2′-O-methyl and 2′-O-methoxy-ethyl modified ODNs are also called second-generation ODNs, while PSs are called first-generation ODNs. For siRNA, 2′-OMe and 2′-F modified siRNAs have enhanced not only their plasma stability but also their *in vivo* potency.[68]

2′-O-Alkyl AS-ODNs cannot trigger the RNase-H-dependent cleavage of the target mRNA because the correct width of the minor groove of the DNA/RNA hybrid is necessary for substrate recognition by RNase-H. The absence or change of the 2′-OH function in the DNA/RNA hybrid duplex in the minor groove might alter the interactions between the duplex and the outer sphere Mg^{2+}–water complex in RNase-H.[69] Thus, 2′-O-alkyl AS-ODNs can only take their antisense effect due to a steric block of translation.[67,70]

In contrast to the typical role of AS-ODNs in inhibiting protein expression, blocking of a splice site in an mRNA by an ODN can increase the expression of a specific protein. For example, in one form of β-thalassemia, a genetic blood disorder, a mutation in intron 2 of the β-globin gene causes aberrant splicing of β-globin pre-mRNA and leads to β-globin deficiency. When 2′-O-methyl ODNs with or without PS were targeted to the aberrant splice site, correct splicing was restored generating correct β-globin mRNA and protein in different mammalian cell lines.[71]

Another interesting study related to 2′-position modified siRNAs has shown that 2′-F modified siRNAs may not be more potent than unmodified siRNAs in animals. Even though the modified siRNAs have greatly increased resistance to nuclease degradation in plasma, this increase in stability did not translate into enhanced or prolonged silencing of a target gene in mice after tail vein injection.[72] In this study, siRNAs modified with 2′-F pyrimidines were functional in cell culture and had greatly increased the stability and prolonged half-life in human plasma, compared with unmodified siRNAs. Although the 2′-F modified siRNAs inhibited the expression of the target gene in mice, the inhibitory ability of modified siRNAs was not better than that of the unmodified ones. The reason may be that 2′-F modified siRNAs and unmodified siRNAs have different nonspecific binding tendency *in vivo*.

Locked nucleic acid (LNA), also referred to as inaccessible RNA, is a family of conformationally locked nucleotide analogs in which the ribose ring is "locked" by a methylene bridge connecting the 2′-O of the ribose with the 4′-C atom. LNA nucleotides can be mixed with DNA or RNA bases in the ODNs and siRNAs whenever desired. LNA ODNs showed an enhanced stability against nucleolytic degradation[73] and high target affinity. However, LNA appears to show hepato-toxicity as indicated by serum transaminases concentration, organ weight, and body weight.[74] LNA were also compatible with siRNA intracellular machinery, increased nuclease resistance, and furthermore, reduced sequence-related off-target effects.[57,75]

8.4.2   Nonspecific Binding and Toxicity

Nonspecific binding (commonly known as the off-target effect) of ODNs has troubled scientists since the beginning, even though one off-target effect initiated by CpG-ODNs is now being investigated for therapeutic purposes. An off-target reaction with unintended sequences is also adversely affecting the progress of RNAi technology. These off-target effects come from the binding not only to nontarget sequences, but also to the plasma proteins.

A high concentration of ODNs and siRNAs increases their interaction with nontarget sequences, leading to toxic side effects. Off-target effects of AS-ODN usually occur if the concentration is higher than 200 nM.[76] Semizarov et al. also found similar results for siRNAs that the specificity of siRNAs is concentration-dependent.[77] When the concentrations of siRNA reached 100 nM, siRNA nonspecifically stimulated a significant number of apoptosis-related nontarget genes. This evidence suggests that gene silencing experiments should be designed under the concentration threshold. Since an siRNA recognizes its targets by sequence complementarity, potential off-target effects of siRNAs could also be decreased by the proper selection of siRNA sequences within 100 nt from the 5′ termini of the target mRNA.[78] Off-target effects of siRNA can also be minimized by using smart pools of siRNAs, which means the mixture of siRNAs target different regions of mRNA of the same gene and reduce the off-target effect induced by only one siRNA in the same total concentration, but that is higher than the single one in the pool. Moreover, 2′-MOE modification was also reported to reduce the "off-target" effect,[79] suggesting that proper chemical modifications can reduce the off-target effects.

The binding to plasma protein also affects the target specificity and gene silencing efficiencies of ODNs and siRNAs. Even though PS modification increases the stability of ODNs and siRNAs, it promotes their binding to plasma proteins. To minimize the binding to plasma proteins, while still maintaining high stability, ODNs are often partially phosphorothioated. Since the main reason for the degradation of ODNs and siRNAs is exonuclease attack, the entire sequence can be protected by a few PS linkages at the terminals. The incorporation of several central PS residues in a potent

AS-ODN, which is termed "gapmers," can still activate RNase-H-dependent cleavage but retain many of the valuable properties of the unmodified nucleic acid sequence.[80]

Besides off-target effects, the systemic administration of siRNA duplexes may lead to an innate immune-response,[81] inducing a high level of inflammatory cytokines, such as tumor necrosis factor-alpha (TNF-α), interleukin-6 (IL-6), and interferons (IFNs) and innate immunity, which can be mediated by toll-like receptors (TLRs).[81] The innate immunity of siRNAs can also be triggered by non-TLR-mediated pathways, such as siRNA binding to retinoic acid inducible gene 1 (RIG1) in the cytoplasm. 2′-OMe modified siRNAs have been shown to prevent recognition by the innate immune system.[82] Combined with the ability of reducing off-target effects of siRNA, 2′-OMe modification of ribose does reduce the toxicity of synthetic siRNAs.

> To minimize binding to plasma proteins, while still maintaining high stability, ODNs are often partially phosphorothioated. Since the main reason for the degradation of ODNs and siRNAs is exonuclease attack, the entire sequence can be protected by a few PS linkages at the terminals. The incorporation of several central PS residues in a potent AS-ODN, which is termed "gapmers," can still activate RNase-H-dependent cleavage but retain many of the valuable properties of the unmodified nucleic acid sequence.

8.4.3 Physiological Barriers

Different physiological structures prevent the nucleotides from being delivered to the target successfully. The most important three physiological barriers are capillary endothelia, endosome/lysosome membranes, and nuclear membranes (Figure 8.3).

8.4.3.1 Capillary Endothelium

The most important physiological barrier to ODN and siRNA delivery is the capillary endothelium, which is a thin monolayer of cells that line the interior surface of blood vessels with or without

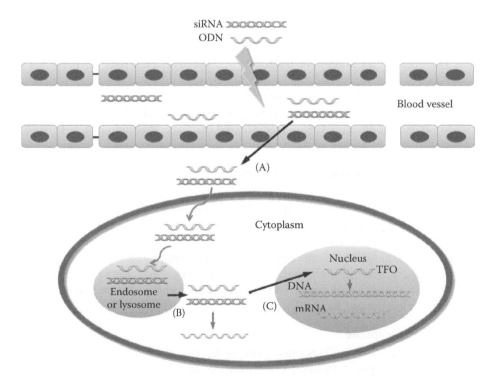

FIGURE 8.3 Physiological barriers of ODNs and siRNA. (A) Capillary endothelium. (B) Endosomal and lysosomal membranes. (C) Nuclear membranes.

special basement membranes. Although the endothelial cells are also the therapeutic targets in some diseases, for example, high blood pressure, in most situations ODNs and siRNAs have to extravasate the endothelium to reach tissue parenchymal cells.

The capillary endothelia in various organs and tissues have different extravasation properties according to the morphology and continuity of the endothelial layer and the basement membrane.[83] The capillary endothelia, found in cardiac, smooth muscles, lung, skin, subcutaneous, and mucous membranes, have little fenestrations because these endothelial cells are joined by tight junctions and continuous subendothelial basement membranes.[84] Therefore, the particles larger than 2.0 nm are very hard to be extravasated. In some organs, the endothelial cells with tight junctions make a unique structure for self-protection and filter function, such as the blood–brain barrier (BBB). The capillary endothelia, found in the kidney, small intestine, and salivary glands, are composed of fenestrated endothelial cells and a continuous basement membrane.[85] Except the glomerular capillaries in the kidney, these types of capillaries allow the extravasation of particles less than 11 nm in diameter. For the glomerular capillaries, the effective permeation is allowed for particles smaller than 30 nm. Moreover, due to the negative charges on the glomerular capillary walls, the extravasation is also affected by the molecular charge of ODNs and siRNAs or their formulated complexes. The capillary endothelia, found in the liver, spleen, and bone marrow, have fenestrations up to 150 nm.[84] In addition, the basement membrane is absent in the liver and discontinuous in the spleen and bone marrow. All of these properties allow the ODNs and siRNAs to pass through the sinusoidal gaps of the liver to reach the hepatocytes.

Inflammation, tumor formation, and fibrosis lead to changes in endothelial barriers. Inflammation facilitates the distribution of ODNs and siRNAs to the interstitial spaces, not only due to the increased fenestration between endothelial cells,[86] but also due to the increased permeability of the endothelial cells themselves.[87] In the case of solid tumors, many newly formed tumor vessel endothelial cells are poorly aligned with wide fenestrations, lacking a smooth muscle layer. Combined with other factors, such as noneffective lymphatic drainage, solid tumor tissues have an enhanced permeability and retention (EPR) effect, which will allow the efficient distribution of ODNs and siRNAs to the tumor cells. In these tissues, low molecular weight drugs are cleared with short plasma half-lives with little distribution to the tumor, whereas high molecular weight drugs or nanoparticles accumulate in inflammatory and tumor tissues eventually.[88] However, for liver fibrosis it is a different case. After fibrosis, sinusoidal gaps, which are up to 150 nm in width under nonpathological conditions, are almost closed leading to a decreased free exchange flow between hepatocytes and sinusoidal blood. This change makes the delivery of ODNs and siRNAs formulated in large size nanoparticles much more difficult. Cheng et al. showed that the accumulation of TFO in fibrotic rat livers decreased from 44% to 34% of the total IV injection compared with a normal liver.[89]

8.4.3.2 Endosomal and Lysosomal Membranes

Other barriers are the endosomal and lysosomal membranes. Endocytosis appears to be the major pathway for the cellular uptake of ODNs and siRNAs.[90] After endocytosis, ODNs and siRNAs have to escape from the endosome and lysosome before being degraded. There are several strategies for ODNs and siRNAs to escape into the cytoplasm, including the destabilization of the endosomal compartment,[91] an exchange of cationic lipids with anionic phospholipids in the cytoplasm-facing membrane monolayer,[92] and endosomolysis by osmotic swelling.[93] For cationic liposome formulated ODNs and siRNAs, the choice of proper co-lipids, which can disrupt the endosomal or lysosomal membrane, help them to escape more efficiently.

8.4.3.3 Nuclear Membrane

Unlike AS-ODNs and siRNAs, TFOs must enter the nucleus to form a triple helix with genomic DNA to inhibit transcription. Although particles smaller than 30 kD can pass through the nuclear pore complex by passive diffusion, the intra-nuclear concentration of TFOs must be high enough to compete with the transcriptional factors at the same genome gene site. Fortunately, many sorting signals, such as nuclear localization signal (NLS) peptides, have been discovered[94] that can facilitate the nuclear translocation of proteins and RNAs.

8.5 SYNTHETIC CARRIERS FOR NUCLEIC ACID DELIVERY

ODNs and siRNAs are polyanoins that are fairly unstable *in vivo* and widely distributed to most peripheral tissues after systemic administration. Therefore, synthetic carriers, such as lipids and polymers are commonly used for enhancing their stability and controlling their biodistribution after systemic or local administration.

8.5.1 COMPLEX FORMATION

8.5.1.1 Cationic Lipids

Cationic lipids are by far the most commonly used transfection agents for ODNs and siRNAs. Cationic liposomes can be used to either encapsulate these nucleic acids or form lipid/nucleic acid lipoplexes. Cationic liposomes have been used for nucleic acid delivery for more than 20 years. In 1987, the efficiency of the cationic lipid *N*-[1-(2,3-dioleyloxy)propyl]-*N,N,N*-trimethyl ammonium chloride (DOTMA) to deliver both DNA and RNA into mouse, rat, and human cell lines was first investigated.[95] However, many of the cationic lipids used in early clinical trials, such as 3β-[*N*-(*N',N'*-dimethylaminoethane)-carbamoyl] cholesterol (DC-Chol), 1,2-dimyristyloxypropyl-3-dimethyl-hydroxy ethyl ammonium bromide (DMRIE), and GL-67, did not show high efficiency *in vivo*. Therefore, more and more cationic lipids were synthesized and tested for nucleic acid delivery.

Recently, for *in vivo* siRNA studies, Morrissey and colleagues reported the inhibition of hepatitis B virus (HBV) replication in mice after the systemic administration of stable nucleic acid/lipid particles (SNALPs) that targeted HBV mRNA (HBV263M).[4] A dose-dependent reduction in serum HBV DNA levels was observed 7 days after three daily intravenous injections of anti-HBV siRNA SNALP at a dose of 3 mg/kg/day. Furthermore, a similar reduction in HBV replication had been maintained for more than 6 weeks. Zimmerman and colleagues also encapsulated ApoB-specific siRNAs in SNALP and injected it intravenously into cynomolgus monkeys at doses of 1 or 2.5 mg/kg.[96] A single siRNA injection resulted in the dose-dependent silencing of ApoB mRNA expression in the liver 48 h after administration, with gene silencing of more than 90%. The silencing effect persisted for 11 days at the highest administered dose of 2.5 mg/kg.

In our laboratory, Zhu et al. synthesized a series of pyridinium lipids with a heterocyclic positively charged ring linked to different types of fatty acids via ester or amide spacers.[97] These lipids showed enhanced *in vitro* transfection efficiency for both plasmid and siRNAs. The transfection efficiency of these pyridinium lipids was dependent on the hydrophobic chain lengths used. A length beyond 16 C decreased the transfection efficiency. An increase in the aliphatic chain length of amphipathic compounds is known to increase both the phase transition temperature and bilayer stiffness of the resulting vesicles, and having a stiff bi-layer is unsuitable for membrane fusion.[98]

The transfection efficiency of cationic liposomes can also be improved by conjugation to targeting ligands. When vitamin-A-coupled liposomes were used for the delivery of anti-gp46 siRNA dimethylnitrosamine (DMN) induced in liver fibrotic rats,[99] there was prolonged survival of liver fibrotic rats in a dose-dependent manner. Rats were almost cured of liver fibrosis after administration.

Lipidoids are another class of lipid-like material for the delivery of siRNAs to the liver after systemic administration.[100] The basic synthesis idea is to conjugate alkyl-acrylates or alkyl-acrylamides to primary or secondary amines. Among the huge library of lipidoids, 98N$_{12}$-5 (5-tail) was found to be optimal for *in vivo* delivery of siRNA compared with other similar compounds (Figure 8.4). Almost 80% of the injected dose was distributed to the liver and could induce persistent

Among various dendritic polymers, polyamidoamine (PAMAM) dendrimers have recently attracted interest for nucleic acid delivery because of their well-defined surface functionality, low polydispersity, good water solubility, and nontoxicity.

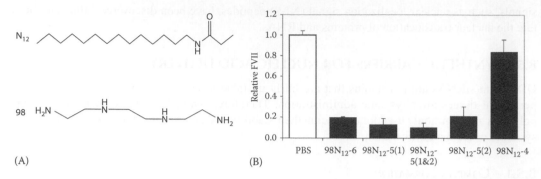

(A)   (B)

FIGURE 8.4 *In vivo* efficacy of siRNA formulated with lipidoid 98N12 with different tail numbers. (A) Structure of N_{12} and 98 lipidoids; (B) transfection efficiency of different $98N_{12}$ compounds. From left to right are blank control, the 6-tail compound ($98N_{12}$-6), one isomer of the 5-tail compound, mixture of the two 5-tail isomers, another isomer of the 5-tail compound and the 4-tail compound. Factor VII-targeting siRNA was formulated using these compounds and administered to C57BL6 mice at 2.5 mg/kg via single IV bolus injection. Twenty-four hours after administration, serum Factor VII protein levels were quantified.

gene silencing without loss of activity following repeated administration. The lipidoids showed high safety and efficiency in all the three animal models: mice, rats and nonhuman primates.

8.5.1.2 Cationic Polymers

Various cationic polymers including polyethyleneimine (PEI),[101] poly(L-lysine) (PLL),[102] PAMAM dendrimer,[103] polyallylamine,[104] and methacrylate/methacrylamide polymers[105] have been synthesized for nucleic acid delivery and targeting. Polymeric carriers hold promise due to their versatile chemistries, targetability, and low toxicity, but they usually have poor transfection efficiency.

Among various cationic polymers, PEI remains very popular, which has either a branched or linear form. PEI is available in a broad molecular weight ranging from <1 kDa to 1.6×10^3 kDa, but PEI of 5–25 kDa are widely used for gene transfer since high molecular weight PEI is cytotoxic to the cells.[106,107] Low molecular weight PEI, by contrast, has shown low toxicity in cell culture studies.[108,109] Forrest et al. has combined the low toxicity properties of low molecular weight PEI with the high transfection efficiency of high molecular weight PEI by coupling low molecular weight PEIs (800 Da) together to form conjugates of 14–30 kDa using short diacrylate cross-linkers.[110] These degradable polymers have similar DNA-binding properties to commercially available 25 kDa PEI, but exhibit 2- to 16-fold higher transfection efficiency and are essentially nontoxic. Other strategies to reduce the toxicity and improve the stability are synthesizing PEI with graft copolymers such as linear poly(ethylene glycol) (PEG)[111,112] or glycosylated.[113] Petersen et al. have synthesized two series of polyethylenimine-graft-poly(ethylene glycol) (PEI-g-PEG) block copolymers[112] by grafting PEI (25 kDa) to PEG (5 kDa) or a series of PEG of 550 Da–20 kDa. The size and morphology of resulting polyplexes were drastically changed. PEG (5 kDa) significantly reduced the diameter of complexes from 142 ± 59 to 61 ± 28 nm. Copolymers with PEG (20 kDa) yielded small, compact complexes with DNA while copolymers with PEG (550 Da) resulted in large and diffuse structures. The zeta-potential of complexes was reduced with an increasing degree of PEG grafting if molecular weight was more than 5 kDa. The cytotoxicity was independent of PEG molecular weight but was affected by the degree of PEG substitution. The copolymers with more than six PEG blocks formed DNA complexes of low toxicity.

Dendrimers consist of a central core molecule as roots, from which some treelike branches originate in an ordered way. This unique architecture gives dendrimers various distinctive properties. The intrinsic viscosity of the dendrimer solution does not increase linearly with mass,[114] which makes the application of the formulation by polymer dendrimers much easier. Furthermore, the treelike structure can maximize the exposed surface area, which facilitates the interaction between dendrimers and nucleic acids. The multiple surface groups of dendrimer allow conjugation of various targeting ligands and other moieties to confer site-specificity and reduced toxicity.

Among various dendritic polymers, PAMAM dendrimers have recently attracted interest for nucleic acid delivery because of their well defined surface functionality, low polydispersity, good water solubility, and nontoxicity. Bielinska et al. transfected ODN/PAMAM complexes into D5 mouse melanoma and Rat2 embryonal fibroblast cell lines *in vitro*.[115] The ODN/dendrimer complexes showed a good silencing effect with very little cytotoxicity compared with lipofectamine and DEAE dextran complexes. PAMAM dendrimers also showed strong binding affinity for siRNA molecules.[116] These nondegraded dendrimers condensed siRNAs into nanoscale particles and protected them from enzymatic degradation, leading to gene silencing.

8.5.2 BIOCONJUGATION

Most cationic lipids and polymers used as transfection agents are toxic, which limits their clinical applications. To avoid the use of polycations, Rajur et al. conjugated ODNs to asialoglycoprotein (ASGP) using sulfosuccinimidyl 6-[3'-(pyridyldithio)propionamido] hexanoate (sulfo-LC-SPDP0).[117] Direct conjugation of molecules to the ODNs often tends to disturb the bio-ability of the ODNs, which is essential for errant protein knocking down. Therefore, ODNs were covalently conjugated to carbohydrate clusters for specific delivery to the hepatocytes[118] and other cells.

Various carriers are also utilized for the conjugation of siRNAs, including cholesterol, VE, and PEG. The site for conjugation is crucial for siRNAs. The integrity of the 5'-terminus of the antisense strand of siRNA, which is complementary to the target mRNA and incorporated into RISC to initiate the mRNA cleavage, is crucial for the initiation of RNAi.[119] Therefore, the 5'-terminus cannot be used for conjugation. Either the 3'- or 5'-terminus of the sense strand is generally used for conjugation. Moreover, the linkages between carriers and siRNAs should be acid- or enzyme-sensitive to allow a complex formation between RISC and siRNA in the cytoplasm. Since matrix metalloproteinase 1 (MMP1) is upregulated in liver fibrosis, a special six amino acid peptide, substrate for MMP1, is used as an enzyme-sensitive linker.

Then, how do we decrease the toxicity and increase the target efficiency of therapeutic ODNs? The most important strategy is the addition of targeting ligands. Many diseases change the physiology of cells, such as special-receptor upregulation. For example, liver fibrosis leads to the activation of hepatic stellate cells (HSCs), which affects the liver architecture and eventually liver function. Since Mannose-6-phosphate (M6P) receptors of HSCs get upregulated upon HSC activation, Mahato's laboratory synthesized M6P-bovine serum albumin (M6P-BSA) and conjugated the TFOs via a disulfide bond for enhanced TFO delivery to the HSCs.[120] They also checked the influence of the M6P number per conjugate molecule on the biodistribution and hepatic uptake of M6P-BSA-TFO.[121] The molar ratio of M6P: BSA to 21 and 27 resulted in an increased liver accumulation to 52.6% and 67.4%, respectively, whereas free TFO showed a liver accumulation of about 45%.

Since the treatment of liver fibrosis may require repeated injections of TFO at high doses, high molecular weight globular BSA (MW=67,000) may not be a suitable carrier for TFO delivery to the HSCs due to the possible immune reaction. *N*-(2-Hydroxypropyl) methacrylamide (HPMA) copolymer has shown great potential for the delivery of small molecular drugs.[122] Therefore, Yang et al. synthesized M6P-GFLG-HPMA-GFLG-ONP and conjugated it to TFO via a GFLG linker, which is a lysosomally degradable tetrapeptide linker and is known to be cleaved by lysosomal enzymes, allowing TFO release of the cytoplasm after cellular uptake. The HPMA copolymer (MW=40,000 Da) conjugate of TFOs increased the liver accumulation of the TFO to 80% of the total injected dose, which is quite high compared with free TFO (45%) (Figure 8.5).[123]

PEGylation is known to significantly enhance the ODN stability against exonuclease and reduce renal clearance compared with unmodified ODNs.[124] The conjugation of PEG to ODNs can decrease the RES clearance of administered nucleotides and prolong their circulating time in blood.[125,126] Zhu et al. conjugated Gal-PEG to ODNs via an acid-labile linker. The conjugation of PEG prolonged

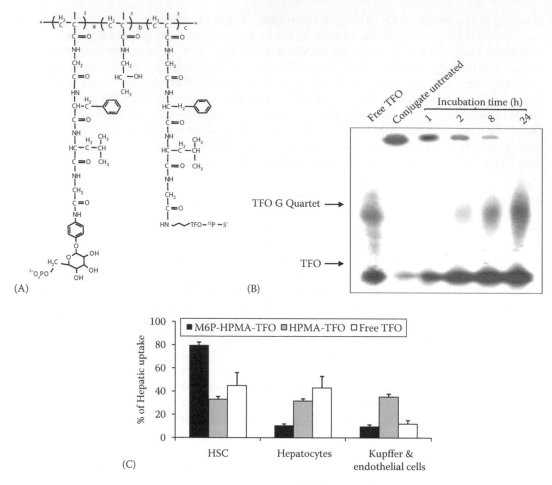

(A)   (B)

(C)

FIGURE 8.5 Delivery efficiency of M6P-GFLG-HPMA-GFLG-^{32}P-TFO. (A) Structure of M6P-GFLG-HPMA-GFLG-^{32}P-TFO. (B) Enzymatic dissociation of ^{32}P-TFO from M6P-GFLG-HPMA-GFLG-^{32}P-TFO by papain. (C) Intrahepatic distribution of M6P-GFLG-HPMA-GFLG-^{32}P-TFO in fibrotic rats. Cells were isolated at 30 min postinjection of M6P-GFLG-HPMA-GFLG-^{32}P-TFO, HPMA-GFLG-^{32}P-TFO or ^{32}P-TFO at dose of 0.2 mg TFO/kg of body weight. The associated radioactivity was measured. The contribution of each liver cell type was exposed as the percentage of total liver uptake. Results are expressed as the mean ± SD ($n=3$).

the circulation time, but also decreased the binding of ODNs, which were G-rich PS ODNs, to the serum protein. With the assistance of galactose as the ligands, Gal-PEG-ODNs were delivered to the hepatocytes (Figure 8.6). After endocytosis, the low pH level in the endosome made the β-thiopropionate linkage cleaved and ODNs were released from the conjugates gradually. After conjugation with PEG, the elimination half-life of the ODNs increased from 34 to 118 min.[89,125]

In 2004, cholesterol was covalently linked to the 3'-terminus of the sense strand of siRNAs, which contained selective stabilizing modification and were designed to target the apolipoprotein B (apoB) mRNA.[127] In this case, Soutschek and his colleagues used a pyrrolidone linkage that is not bio-cleavable. The cholesterol-siRNA conjugate (Chol-siRNA) showed not only significantly higher cellular uptake but also enhanced gene silencing compared with the un-conjugated siRNA. Following intravenous injection into mice, the Chol-siRNA conjugates are taken up by several tissues including the liver, jejunum, heart, kidneys, lungs, and fat tissue. Significant silencing of the apoB gene was observed at mRNA and protein levels in the liver and the jejunum. Furthermore, this reduction resulted in a decreased plasma apoB protein level and a consequent decreased level

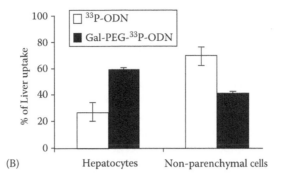

FIGURE 8.6   Delivery efficiency of Gal-PEG-^{33}P-ODN. (A) Structure of Gal-PEG-^{33}P-ODN. (B) Intrahepatic distribution of ^{33}P-ODN and Gal-PEG-^{33}P-ODNs after systemic administration in rats. Liver cells were isolated at 30 min postinjection of ^{33}P-ODN or Gal-PEG-^{33}P-ODN by liver perfusion. The associated radioactivity was measured. Results are expressed as the mean ± SD ($n=4$).

of blood cholesterol. However, the siRNA dose (50 mg/kg) in animal experiments is too high for clinical applications. The cholesterol conjugate was also applied to deliver ODNs.[128] Cheng et al. conjugated cholesterol to ODNs by a disulfide bond and showed high cellular uptake, because the cholesterol conjugation increased hydrophobicity and cellular association.

In addition to the Chol-siRNA conjugate, a series of siRNAs have been conjugated with lipid-like carriers, including α-tocopherol (vitamin E), steroids, and lipids.[96,129,130] Lipoproteins may facilitate the cellular uptake of these conjugates. A critical factor determining the affinity of fatty acid–conjugated siRNAs to lipoprotein particles is the length of the alkyl chain, a major determinant of lipophilicity.[96] So far, only lipophilic siRNAs showed lipid-metabolism-related-gene silencing, Apo B. Therefore, this raises the question: Does the lipid-like-molecule-siRNA conjugate only silence lipid-metabolism-related genes? More research is needed to clarify this question.

8.6   PHARMACOKINETICS AND BIODISTRIBUTION

ODNs are accumulated in most peripheral tissues after systemic administration, particularly the kidney and liver, but with little distribution to the central nervous system. The biphasic plasma half-lives of ODNs are several minutes, while PS ODNs showed distribution half-lives ranging from many minutes to hours.[131–134] The major route of ODN elimination is the kidneys, even though PS ODNs efficiently bind to plasma proteins. These highly protein bound ODNs usually have a longer circulation time than would be expected of a simple phosphodiester ODN.

Pharmacokinetic profiles of various chemically modified ODNs, especially for the 2′-MEO AS-ODNs, have been determined and found to be similar to those of PS ODNs.[133,135] The *in vivo* fate of 2′-MEO modified ODNs were also studied and compared in rodents, monkeys, and humans.[136] In this study, the plasma pharmacokinetics of 2′-MOE partially modified AS-ODNs was similar in mice, rats, dogs, monkeys, and humans. After intravenous administration, the plasma concentration–time profiles were polyphasic as characterized by a rapid distribution phase (half-lives in hours) and were followed by a slower elimination phase with half-lives, but longer in the study of humans, from 5 to 31 days. The plasma clearance of monkeys and humans was similar, about one tenth of the mice. An allometric comparison of the clearance estimated at similar doses across all species was done. From mouse to man, a linear relationship based on body weight alone was shown.

The pharmacokinetic profile of LNA ODNs in rodents is similar to that of PS ODNs, except that there was high urinary excretion of intact LNA ODNs compared with PS ODNs.[137] This is possibly due to the extensive binding of PS ODNs to serum proteins leading to poor renal clearance, while LNA ODNs do not bind to serum proteins and thus are easily filtered out of the kidney.[138] Even though this property of LNA ODNs reduces nonspecific interaction, it also makes the clearance of LNA ODNs faster. Furthermore, chimeric DNA/LNA ODNs are more stable than isosequential PS ODNs, which have half-lives of more than 10 h. Peptide nucleic acids (PNAs) did not show any increase in the distribution half-life.[139]

Native siRNAs had an elimination half-life of 6 min only,[127] shorter than that of ODNs. The shorter half-life may be partly due to the higher instability of siRNAs compared with ODNs. The biodistribution of radiolabeled siRNAs in mice showed an accumulation primarily in the liver and kidneys, which is similar to that of ODNs.[140] They were also detected in the heart, spleen, and lung. Actually, the high renal uptake facilitates the target delivery of siRNA to this tissue.[141]

The conjugation of cholesterol,[127] tocopherol,[130] or other lipid moieties[142] enhances the binding of ODNs to serum lipoproteins and/or albumin. This results in enhanced circulation time and, more importantly, hepatic uptake via the low-density lipoprotein receptor. Other conjugation with macro molecular materials also changed the pharmacokinetic profiles of ODNs and siRNAs.

Bioimaging allows a real time analysis of the ODN and the siRNA.[143] Micro SPECT or other radioimaging techniques can provide detailed information on the distribution of ODNs and siRNAs. However, there are several underlying issues. One is how to separate the label from the molecule being studied, which is a common problem for almost all radiolabeling methods. More importantly, there may be a discrepancy between the physical biodistribution and the functional biodistribution of ODNs and siRNAs. For example, in a study, LNA ODNs were designed to cause an alteration in mRNA splicing. The major effects were observed in the liver, colon, and small intestine; however, the major site of accumulation of the LNA was the kidney.[144] Therefore, one should be careful in predicting pharmacological effects when using radiolabeling data although it represents the pharmacokinetics and biodistribution of gene drugs.

8.7 CLINICAL TRIALS

Several companies initiated clinical trials of ODNs in the early 1990s. The most intensively studied ODNs are PS ODNs, which are well absorbed and distributed widely to most peripheral tissues, but poorly distributed to the brain.[145] Other modified ODNs also proceeded to clinical trials. Table 8.1 shows a universal applicability of antisense strategies to treat a broad range of diseases including viral infections, cancer, and inflammatory diseases. In 1998, the first antisense drug, Vitravene (Fomivirsen), was approved by the FDA for treating cytomegalovirus (CMV)-induced retinitis in patients with AIDS.[8] However, it is the only ODN drug approved by the FDA so far, even though several PS ODNs have been in Phase III trials, such as Affinitac (ISIS 3521) and Alicaforsen (ISIS 2302). However, Alicaforsen failed to show significant efficacy in a Phase III study for treating Crohn's disease[146] and is now being investigated in a restructured Phase III trial. Many other ODNs have reached the stage of clinical trials. ISIS 104838 against TNF-α is being tested for treating inflammatory diseases such as rheumatoid arthritis and psoriasis.[135]

A retrovirally expressed ribozyme that targets the HIV tat and rev exons entered clinical testing in late 1996 and is currently in Phase II testing for patients with AIDS-related lymphoma. Ribozyme Pharmaceuticals (Boulder, Colorado) performs clinical trials on Angiozyme (Table 8.1). Angiozyme is a stabilized hammerhead ribozyme that is targeted against the vascular endothelial growth factor (VEGF) receptor. It is designed to reduce tumor growth by inhibiting angiogenesis. Heptazyme, a ribozyme targeting the 5′-UTR of the hepatitis C virus (HCV) RNA genome, has recently completed a Phase I/II clinical trial in patients with chronic hepatitis C.

TABLE 8.1
Current Clinical Trials for ODNs and siRNA

Products	Nucleic Acids	Disease	Status
Genasense	AS-ODN	Cancer	Phase II, III
AP 12009	AS-ODN	Astrocytoma, glioblastoma	Phase IIb, III
AEG35156	AS-ODN	Cancer	Phase I/II
OGX-427	AS-ODN	Bladder neoplasm	Phase I
SPC2996	AS-ODN	Chronic lymphocytic leukemia	Phase I/II
G4460	AS-ODN	Chronic myelogenous leukemia	Phase II
Alicaforsen (ISIS 2302)	AS-ODN	Crohn's disease	Phase III
Angiozyme	Ribozyme	Metastatic colorectal cancer	Phase II
Herzyme	Ribozyme	Cancer	Phase I
Angiozyme	Aptamer	Cancer	Phase II
Herzyme	Aptamer	Cancer	Phase I
AGN211745	siRNA	AMD	Phase II
DOTAP:Chol-fus1	siRNA	Non-small-cell lung cancer	Phase I
I5NP	siRNA	AKI	Phase I
Cand5	siRNA	Diabetic macular edema	Phase II
AVI-4658 (PMO)	Other	Becker's muscular dystrophy	Phase I/II

Acuity Pharmaceuticals performed the first clinical trial for siRNA therapy for AMD in 2004. After the successful Phase II trials reported that all doses were well tolerated without adverse systemic effects, testing was moved into Phase III trials. The siRNA treatment for AMD was also performed by Allergan in a Phase II trial. The trials related to various diseases, such as solid tumor cancer and acute kidney injury (AKI), are in good progress. The active trials so far are listed in Table 8.1. However, another interesting report is about a Phase II clinical trial by OPKO Health on the treatment of diabetic macular edema, which is the swelling of the retina in diabetes mellitus due to the leakage of fluid from blood vessels within the macula. It was shown that anti-VEGF siRNA efficacy in the eye is not due to specific gene silencing but because of the nonspecific stimulation of the TLR3 pathway,[147] which can reduce angiogenesis, but the therapeutic effects observed in other applications of siRNA are still encouraging.

> Acuity Pharmaceuticals performed the first clinical trial for siRNA therapy for the treatment of AMD in 2004. After the successful Phase II trials reported that all doses were well tolerated without adverse systemic effects, testing was moved into Phase III trials.

8.8 CONCLUDING REMARKS

Despite many hurdles, ODN and siRNA-based strategies for inhibiting aberrant protein expression offers great hope for treating many severe and debilitating diseases. Although significant improvements have been made by chemical modifications of ODNs and siRNAs to decrease the degradation of ODNs and siRNAs, some modifications also lead to many unwanted effects, including nonspecific protein binding to toxicity to nontarget cells. Therefore, a delicate act is needed for optimal therapeutic effects, with little toxicity. This can be achieved with a proper charge ratio, limited chemical modification, and conjugation to some targeting moieties.

The incorporation of tissue-specific ligands into the therapeutic particles makes target-specific delivery possible. The chemical modification of ODNs and siRNAs themselves enhances their biostability and reduces the off-target effects in some cases. Other methods are also applied to prevent the nucleic acids from being cleared by the immune system before they take proper effect.

ACKNOWLEDGMENT

This work was supported by R01 EB003922 and DK69968 from the National Institute of Health.

REFERENCES

1. Kim SH et al. Local and systemic delivery of VEGF siRNA using polyelectrolyte complex micelles for effective treatment of cancer. *J Control Release* 2008; **129**: 107–116.
2. Ptasznik A et al. Short interfering RNA (siRNA) targeting the Lyn kinase induces apoptosis in primary, and drug-resistant, BCR-ABL1(+) leukemia cells. *Nat Med* 2004; **10**: 1187–1189.
3. Xia CF et al. Intravenous siRNA of brain cancer with receptor targeting and avidin-biotin technology. *Pharm Res* 2007; **24**: 2309–2316.
4. Morrissey DV et al. Potent and persistent in vivo anti-HBV activity of chemically modified siRNAs. *Nat Biotechnol* 2005; **23**: 1002–1007.
5. Okumura A, Pitha PM, Harty RN. ISG15 inhibits Ebola VP40 VLP budding in an L-domain-dependent manner by blocking Nedd4 ligase activity. *Proc Natl Acad Sci USA* 2008; **105**: 3974–3979.
6. Sharma HW, Narayanan R. The therapeutic potential of antisense oligonucleotides. *Bioessays* 1995; **17**: 1055–1063.
7. Orr RM. Technology evaluation: Fomivirsen, Isis Pharmaceuticals Inc/CIBA vision. *Curr Opin Mol Ther* 2001; **3**: 288–294.
8. Marwick C. First "antisense" drug will treat CMV retinitis. *JAMA* 1998; **280**: 871.
9. Loke SL et al. Characterization of oligonucleotide transport into living cells. *Proc Natl Acad Sci USA* 1989; **86**: 3474–3478.
10. Breslauer KJ, Frank R, Blocker H, Marky LA. Predicting DNA duplex stability from the base sequence. *Proc Natl Acad Sci USA* 1986; **83**: 3746–3750.
11. Walder RY, Walder JA. Role of RNase H in hybrid-arrested translation by antisense oligonucleotides. *Proc Natl Acad Sci USA* 1988; **85**: 5011–5015.
12. Boiziau C et al. Inhibition of translation initiation by antisense oligonucleotides via an RNase-H independent mechanism. *Nucleic Acids Res* 1991; **19**: 1113–1119.
13. Bonham MA et al. An assessment of the antisense properties of RNase H-competent and steric-blocking oligomers. *Nucleic Acids Res* 1995; **23**: 1197–1203.
14. Rogers FA, Lloyd JA, Glazer PM. Triplex-forming oligonucleotides as potential tools for modulation of gene expression. *Curr Med Chem Anticancer Agents* 2005; **5**: 319–326.
15. Casey BP, Glazer PM. Gene targeting via triple-helix formation. *Prog Nucleic Acid Res Mol Biol* 2001; **67**: 163–192.
16. Letai AG et al. Specificity in formation of triple-stranded nucleic acid helical complexes: Studies with agarose-linked polyribonucleotide affinity columns. *Biochemistry* 1988; **27**: 9108–9112.
17. Ye Z, Guntaka RV, Mahato RI. Sequence-specific triple helix formation with genomic DNA. *Biochemistry* 2007; **46**: 11240–11252.
18. Maher LJ, III. Prospects for the therapeutic use of antigene oligonucleotides. *Cancer Invest* 1996; **14**: 66–82.
19. Praseuth D, Guieysse AL, Helene C. Triple helix formation and the antigene strategy for sequence-specific control of gene expression. *Biochim Biophys Acta* 1999; **1489**: 181–206.
20. Yamamoto S et al. DNA from bacteria, but not from vertebrates, induces interferons, activates natural killer cells and inhibits tumor growth. *Microbiol Immunol* 1992; **36**: 983–997.
21. Krieg AM. Lymphocyte activation by CpG dinucleotide motifs in prokaryotic DNA. *Trends Microbiol* 1996; **4**: 73–76.
22. Krieg AM. Immune effects and mechanisms of action of CpG motifs. *Vaccine* 2000; **19**: 618–622.
23. Redford TW, Yi AK, Ward CT, Krieg AM. Cyclosporin A enhances IL-12 production by CpG motifs in bacterial DNA and synthetic oligodeoxynucleotides. *J Immunol* 1998; **161**: 3930–3935.
24. Yi AK et al. Rapid immune activation by CpG motifs in bacterial DNA. Systemic induction of IL-6 transcription through an antioxidant-sensitive pathway. *J Immunol* 1996; **157**: 5394–5402.
25. Krieg AM et al. CpG motifs in bacterial DNA trigger direct B-cell activation. *Nature* 1995; **374**: 546–549.
26. Hartmann G, Weiner GJ, Krieg AM. CpG DNA: A potent signal for growth, activation, and maturation of human dendritic cells. *Proc Natl Acad Sci USA* 1999; **96**: 9305–9310.
27. Barchet W, Wimmenauer V, Schlee M, Hartmann G. Accessing the therapeutic potential of immunostimulatory nucleic acids. *Curr Opin Immunol* 2008; **20**: 389–395.

28. Kanzler H, Barrat FJ, Hessel EM, Coffman RL. Therapeutic targeting of innate immunity with Toll-like receptor agonists and antagonists. *Nat Med* 2007; **13**: 552–559.

29. Fonseca DE, Kline JN. Use of CpG oligonucleotides in treatment of asthma and allergic disease. *Adv Drug Deliv Rev* 2009; **61**: 256–262.

30. Doudna JA, Cech TR. The chemical repertoire of natural ribozymes. *Nature* 2002; **418**: 222–228.

31. Doherty EA, Doudna JA. Ribozyme structures and mechanisms. *Annu Rev Biophys Biomol Struct* 2001; **30**: 457–475.

32. Puerta-Fernandez E, Romero-Lopez C, Barroso-delJesus A, Berzal-Herranz A. Ribozymes: Recent advances in the development of RNA tools. *FEMS Microbiol Rev* 2003; **27**: 75–97.

33. Li QX, Tan P, Ke N, Wong-Staal F. Ribozyme technology for cancer gene target identification and validation. *Adv Cancer Res* 2007; **96**: 103–143.

34. Akashi H, Matsumoto S, Taira K. Gene discovery by ribozyme and siRNA libraries. *Nat Rev Mol Cell Biol* 2005; **6**: 413–422.

35. Khan AU. Ribozyme: A clinical tool. *Clin Chim Acta* 2006; **367**: 20–27.

36. Mannironi C, Di Nardo A, Fruscoloni P, Tocchini-Valentini GP. In vitro selection of dopamine RNA ligands. *Biochemistry* 1997; **36**: 9726–9734.

37. Nieuwlandt D, Wecker M, Gold L. In vitro selection of RNA ligands to substance P. *Biochemistry* 1995; **34**: 5651–5659.

38. Geiger A et al. RNA aptamers that bind L-arginine with sub-micromolar dissociation constants and high enantioselectivity. *Nucleic Acids Res* 1996; **24**: 1029–1036.

39. Lupold SE, Hicke BJ, Lin Y, Coffey DS. Identification and characterization of nuclease-stabilized RNA molecules that bind human prostate cancer cells via the prostate-specific membrane antigen. *Cancer Res* 2002; **62**: 4029–4033.

40. Nahvi A et al. Genetic control by a metabolite binding mRNA. *Chem Biol* 2002; **9**: 1043.

41. Winkler W, Nahvi A, Breaker RR. Thiamine derivatives bind messenger RNAs directly to regulate bacterial gene expression. *Nature* 2002; **419**: 952–956.

42. Winkler WC, Cohen-Chalamish S, Breaker RR. An mRNA structure that controls gene expression by binding FMN. *Proc Natl Acad Sci USA* 2002; **99**: 15908–15913.

43. Tomita N, Kashihara N, Morishita R. Transcription factor decoy oligonucleotide-based therapeutic strategy for renal disease. *Clin Exp Nephrol* 2007; **11**: 7–17.

44. Morishita R et al. A gene therapy strategy using a transcription factor decoy of the E2F binding site inhibits smooth muscle proliferation in vivo. *Proc Natl Acad Sci USA* 1995; **92**: 5855–5859.

45. Romanelli A et al. Molecular interactions with nuclear factor kappaB (NF-kappaB) transcription factors of a PNA-DNA chimera mimicking NF-kappaB binding sites. *Eur J Biochem* 2001; **268**: 6066–6075.

46. Stojanovic T et al. STAT-1 decoy oligodeoxynucleotide inhibition of acute rejection in mouse heart transplants. *Basic Res Cardiol* 2009; **104**: 719–729.

47. De Croos JN, Pilliar RM, Kandel RA. AP-1 DNA binding activity regulates the cartilage tissue remodeling process following cyclic compression in vitro. *Biorheology* 2008; **45**: 459–469.

48. Cho-Chung YS. CRE-enhancer DNA decoy: A tumor target-based genetic tool. *Ann NY Acad Sci* 2003; **1002**: 124–133.

49. Pontes O et al. The Arabidopsis chromatin-modifying nuclear siRNA pathway involves a nucleolar RNA processing center. *Cell* 2006; **126**: 79–92.

50. Lee YS et al. Distinct roles for *Drosophila* Dicer-1 and Dicer-2 in the siRNA/miRNA silencing pathways. *Cell* 2004; **117**: 69–81.

51. Matranga C et al. Passenger-strand cleavage facilitates assembly of siRNA into Ago2-containing RNAi enzyme complexes. *Cell* 2005; **123**: 607–620.

52. Ameres SL, Martinez J, Schroeder R. Molecular basis for target RNA recognition and cleavage by human RISC. *Cell* 2007; **130**: 101–112.

53. Hutvagner G, Zamore PD. A microRNA in a multiple-turnover RNAi enzyme complex. *Science* 2002; **297**: 2056–2060.

54. Overhoff M, Sczakiel G. Phosphorothioate-stimulated uptake of short interfering RNA by human cells. *EMBO Rep* 2005; **6**: 1176–1181.

55. Stein CA. Phosphorothioate antisense oligodeoxynucleotides: Questions of specificity. *Trends Biotechnol* 1996; **14**: 147–149.

56. Amarzguioui M, Holen T, Babaie E, Prydz H. Tolerance for mutations and chemical modifications in a siRNA. *Nucleic Acids Res* 2003; **31**: 589–595.

57. Braasch DA et al. RNA interference in mammalian cells by chemically-modified RNA. *Biochemistry* 2003; **42**: 7967–7975.

58. Chiu YL, Rana TM. siRNA function in RNAi: A chemical modification analysis. *RNA* 2003; **9**: 1034–1048.

59. Connolly BA, Eckstein F, Grotjahn L. Direct mass spectroscopic method for determination of oxygen isotope position in adenosine 5′-O-(1-thiotriphosphate). Determination of the stereochemical course of the yeast phenylalanyl-tRNA synthetase reaction. *Biochemistry* 1984; **23**: 2026–2031.

60. Cain K, Partis MD, Griffiths DE. Dibutylchloromethyltin chloride, a covalent inhibitor of the adenosine triphosphate synthase complex. *Biochem J* 1977; **166**: 593–602.

61. Porter KW, Briley JD, Shaw BR. Direct PCR sequencing with boronated nucleotides. *Nucleic Acids Res* 1997; **25**: 1611–1617.

62. Shaw BR et al. Reading, writing, and modulating genetic information with boranophosphate mimics of nucleotides, DNA, and RNA. *Ann NY Acad Sci* 2003; **1002**: 12–29.

63. Lato SM et al. Boron-containing aptamers to ATP. *Nucleic Acids Res* 2002; **30**: 1401–1407.

64. Summers JS, Shaw BR. Boranophosphates as mimics of natural phosphodiesters in DNA. *Curr Med Chem* 2001; **8**: 1147–1155.

65. Hall IH et al. Hypolipidemic activity of boronated nucleosides and nucleotides in rodents. *Biomed Pharmacother* 1993; **47**: 79–87.

66. Hall AH et al. RNA interference using boranophosphate siRNAs: Structure–activity relationships. *Nucleic Acids Res* 2004; **32**: 5991–6000.

67. Kurreck J, Wyszko E, Gillen C, Erdmann VA. Design of antisense oligonucleotides stabilized by locked nucleic acids. *Nucleic Acids Res* 2002; **30**: 1911–1918.

68. Allerson CR et al. Fully 2′-modified oligonucleotide duplexes with improved in vitro potency and stability compared to unmodified small interfering RNA. *J Med Chem* 2005; **48**: 901–904.

69. Nishizaki T, Iwai S, Ohtsuka E, Nakamura H. Solution structure of an RNA.2′-O-methylated RNA hybrid duplex containing an RNA.DNA hybrid segment at the center. *Biochemistry* 1997; **36**: 2577–2585.

70. Urban E, Noe CR. Structural modifications of antisense oligonucleotides. *Farmaco* 2003; **58**: 243–258.

71. Sierakowska H, Sambade MJ, Agrawal S, Kole R. Repair of thalassemic human beta-globin mRNA in mammalian cells by antisense oligonucleotides. *Proc Natl Acad Sci USA* 1996; **93**: 12840–12844.

72. Layzer JM et al. In vivo activity of nuclease-resistant siRNAs. *RNA* 2004; **10**: 766–771.

73. Wahlestedt C et al. Potent and nontoxic antisense oligonucleotides containing locked nucleic acids. *Proc Natl Acad Sci USA* 2000; **97**: 5633–5638.

74. Swayze EE et al. Antisense oligonucleotides containing locked nucleic acid improve potency but cause significant hepatotoxicity in animals. *Nucleic Acids Res* 2007; **35**: 687–700.

75. Elmen J et al. Locked nucleic acid (LNA) mediated improvements in siRNA stability and functionality. *Nucleic Acids Res* 2005; **33**: 439–447.

76. Miyagishi M, Hayashi M, Taira K. Comparison of the suppressive effects of antisense oligonucleotides and siRNAs directed against the same targets in mammalian cells. *Antisense Nucleic Acid Drug Dev* 2003; **13**: 1–7.

77. Semizarov D et al. Specificity of short interfering RNA determined through gene expression signatures. *Proc Natl Acad Sci USA* 2003; **100**: 6347–6352.

78. Qiu S, Adema CM, Lane T. A computational study of off-target effects of RNA interference. *Nucleic Acids Res* 2005; **33**: 1834–1847.

79. Davis S, Lollo B, Freier S, Esau C. Improved targeting of miRNA with antisense oligonucleotides. *Nucleic Acids Res* 2006; **34**: 2294–2304.

80. Yu D et al. Stereo-enriched phosphorothioate oligodeoxynucleotides: Synthesis, biophysical and biological properties. *Bioorg Med Chem* 2000; **8**: 275–284.

81. Robbins M, Judge A. MacLachlan I. siRNA and innate immunity. *Oligonucleotides* 2009; **19**: 89–102.

82. Cekaite L, Furset G, Hovig E, Sioud M. Gene expression analysis in blood cells in response to unmodified and 2′-modified siRNAs reveals TLR-dependent and independent effects. *J Mol Biol* 2007; **365**: 90–108.

83. Takakura Y, Mahato RI, Hashida M. Extravasation of macromolecules. *Adv Drug Deliv Rev* 1998; **34**: 93–108.

84. Seymour LW. Passive tumor targeting of soluble macromolecules and drug conjugates. *Crit Rev Ther Drug Carrier Syst* 1992; **9**: 135–187.

85. Karnovsky MJ. The ultrastructural basis of capillary permeability studied with peroxidase as a tracer. *J Cell Biol* 1967; **35**: 213–236.

86. Schnittler HJ et al. Role of actin and myosin in the control of paracellular permeability in pig, rat and human vascular endothelium. *J Physiol* 1990; **431**: 379–401.

87. Brett J et al. Tumor necrosis factor/cachectin increases permeability of endothelial cell monolayers by a mechanism involving regulatory G proteins. *J Exp Med* 1989; **169**: 1977–1991.
88. Fang J, Seki T, Maeda H. Therapeutic strategies by modulating oxygen stress in cancer and inflammation. *Adv Drug Deliv Rev* 2009; **61**: 290–302.
89. Cheng K, Ye Z, Guntaka RV, Mahato RI. Biodistribution and hepatic uptake of triplex-forming oligonucleotides against type alpha1(I) collagen gene promoter in normal and fibrotic rats. *Mol Pharm* 2005; **2**: 206–217.
90. Lebedeva I, Benimetskaya L, Stein CA, Vilenchik M. Cellular delivery of antisense oligonucleotides. *Eur J Pharm Biopharm* 2000; **50**: 101–119.
91. Farhood H, Serbina N, Huang L. The role of dioleoyl phosphatidylethanolamine in cationic liposome mediated gene transfer. *Biochim Biophys Acta* 1995; **1235**: 289–295.
92. Xu Y, Szoka FC, Jr. Mechanism of DNA release from cationic liposome/DNA complexes used in cell transfection. *Biochemistry* 1996; **35**: 5616–5623.
93. Boussif O et al. A versatile vector for gene and oligonucleotide transfer into cells in culture and in vivo: Polyethylenimine. *Proc Natl Acad Sci USA* 1995; **92**: 7297–7301.
94. Macara IG. Transport into and out of the nucleus. *Microbiol Mol Biol Rev* 2001; **65**: 570–594, table of contents.
95. Felgner PL et al. Lipofection: A highly efficient, lipid-mediated DNA-transfection procedure. *Proc Natl Acad Sci USA* 1987; **84**: 7413–7417.
96. Zimmermann TS et al. RNAi-mediated gene silencing in non-human primates. *Nature* 2006; **441**: 111–114.
97. Zhu L, Lu Y, Miller DD, Mahato RI. Structural and formulation factors influencing pyridinium lipid-based gene transfer. *Bioconjug Chem* 2008; **19**: 2499–2512.
98. Morille M et al. Progress in developing cationic vectors for non-viral systemic gene therapy against cancer. *Biomaterials* 2008; **29**: 3477–3496.
99. Sato Y et al. Resolution of liver cirrhosis using vitamin A-coupled liposomes to deliver siRNA against a collagen-specific chaperone. *Nat Biotechnol* 2008; **26**: 431–442.
100. Akinc A et al. A combinatorial library of lipid-like materials for delivery of RNAi therapeutics. *Nat Biotechnol* 2008; **26**: 561–569.
101. Godbey WT, Wu KK, Mikos AG. Poly(ethylenimine) and its role in gene delivery. *J Control Release* 1999; **60**: 149–160.
102. Wagner E, Ogris M, Zauner W. Polylysine-based transfection systems utilizing receptor-mediated delivery. *Adv Drug Deliv Rev* 1998; **30**: 97–113.
103. Haensler J, Szoka FC Jr. Polyamidoamine cascade polymers mediate efficient transfection of cells in culture. *Bioconjug Chem* 1993; **4**: 372–379.
104. Boussif O et al. Synthesis of polyallylamine derivatives and their use as gene transfer vectors in vitro. *Bioconjug Chem* 1999; **10**: 877–883.
105. van de Wetering P et al. Structure–activity relationships of water-soluble cationic methacrylate/methacrylamide polymers for nonviral gene delivery. *Bioconjug Chem* 1999; **10**: 589–597.
106. Fischer D et al. In vitro cytotoxicity testing of polycations: Influence of polymer structure on cell viability and hemolysis. *Biomaterials* 2003; **24**: 1121–1131.
107. Fischer D et al. A novel non-viral vector for DNA delivery based on low molecular weight, branched polyethylenimine: Effect of molecular weight on transfection efficiency and cytotoxicity. *Pharm Res* 1999; **16**: 1273–1279.
108. Funhoff AM et al. Endosomal escape of polymeric gene delivery complexes is not always enhanced by polymers buffering at low pH. *Biomacromolecules* 2004; **5**: 32–39.
109. Godbey WT et al. Poly(ethylenimine)-mediated transfection: A new paradigm for gene delivery. *J Biomed Mater Res* 2000; **51**: 321–328.
110. Forrest ML, Koerber JT, Pack DW. A degradable polyethylenimine derivative with low toxicity for highly efficient gene delivery. *Bioconjug Chem* 2003; **14**: 934–940.
111. Vinogradov SV, Bronich TK, Kabanov AV. Self-assembly of polyamine-poly(ethylene glycol) copolymers with phosphorothioate oligonucleotides. *Bioconjug Chem* 1998; **9**: 805–812.
112. Petersen H et al. Polyethylenimine-graft-poly(ethylene glycol) copolymers: Influence of copolymer block structure on DNA complexation and biological activities as gene delivery system. *Bioconjug Chem* 2002; **13**: 845–854.
113. Leclercq F et al. Synthesis of glycosylated polyethylenimine with reduced toxicity and high transfecting efficiency. *Bioorg Med Chem Lett* 2000; **10**: 1233–1235.

114. Bosman AW, Janssen HM, Meijer EW. About dendrimers: Structure, physical properties, and applications. *Chem Rev* 1999; **99**: 1665–1688.

115. Bielinska A et al. Regulation of in vitro gene expression using antisense oligonucleotides or antisense expression plasmids transfected using starburst PAMAM dendrimers. *Nucleic Acids Res* 1996; **24**: 2176–2182.

116. Zhou J et al. PAMAM dendrimers for efficient siRNA delivery and potent gene silencing. *Chem Commun (Camb)* 2006: 2362–2364.

117. Rajur SB, Roth CM, Morgan JR, Yarmush ML. Covalent protein-oligonucleotide conjugates for efficient delivery of antisense molecules. *Bioconjug Chem* 1997; **8**: 935–940.

118. Maier MA et al. Synthesis of antisense oligonucleotides conjugated to a multivalent carbohydrate cluster for cellular targeting. *Bioconjug Chem* 2003; **14**: 18–29.

119. Jeong JH, Mok H, Oh YK, Park TG. siRNA conjugate delivery systems. *Bioconjug Chem* 2009; **20**: 5–14.

120. Ye Z, Cheng K, Guntaka RV, Mahato RI. Targeted delivery of a triplex-forming oligonucleotide to hepatic stellate cells. *Biochemistry* 2005; **44**: 4466–4476.

121. Ye Z, Cheng K, Guntaka RV, Mahato RI. Receptor-mediated hepatic uptake of M6P-BSA-conjugated triplex-forming oligonucleotides in rats. *Bioconjug Chem* 2006; **17**: 823–830.

122. Kopecek J, Kopeckova P, Minko T, Lu Z. HPMA copolymer-anticancer drug conjugates: Design, activity, and mechanism of action. *Eur J Pharm Biopharm* 2000; **50**: 61–81.

123. Yang N, Ye Z, Li F, Mahato RI. HPMA polymer-based site-specific delivery of oligonucleotides to hepatic stellate cells. *Bioconjug Chem* 2009; **20**: 213–221.

124. Zhao H et al. A new platform for oligonucleotide delivery utilizing the PEG prodrug approach. *Bioconjug Chem* 2005; **16**: 758–766.

125. Zhu L et al. Site-specific delivery of oligonucleotides to hepatocytes after systemic administration. *Bioconjug Chem* 2008; **19**: 290–298.

126. Kim SH et al. PEG conjugated VEGF siRNA for anti-angiogenic gene therapy. *J Control Release* 2006; **116**: 123–129.

127. Soutschek J et al. Therapeutic silencing of an endogenous gene by systemic administration of modified siRNAs. *Nature* 2004; **432**: 173–178.

128. Cheng K, Ye Z, Guntaka RV, Mahato RI. Enhanced hepatic uptake and bioactivity of type alpha1(I) collagen gene promoter-specific triplex-forming oligonucleotides after conjugation with cholesterol. *J Pharmacol Exp Ther* 2006; **317**: 797–805.

129. Lorenz C et al. Steroid and lipid conjugates of siRNAs to enhance cellular uptake and gene silencing in liver cells. *Bioorg Med Chem Lett* 2004; **14**: 4975–4977.

130. Nishina K et al. Efficient in vivo delivery of siRNA to the liver by conjugation of alpha-tocopherol. *Mol Ther* 2008; **16**: 734–740.

131. Agrawal S, Temsamani J, Tang JY. Pharmacokinetics, biodistribution, and stability of oligodeoxynucleotide phosphorothioates in mice. *Proc Natl Acad Sci USA* 1991; **88**: 7595–7599.

132. Cossum PA et al. Disposition of the 14C-labeled phosphorothioate oligonucleotide ISIS 2105 after intravenous administration to rats. *J Pharmacol Exp Ther* 1993; **267**: 1181–1190.

133. Geary RS et al. Pharmacokinetic properties of 2′-O-(2-methoxyethyl)-modified oligonucleotide analogs in rats. *J Pharmacol Exp Ther* 2001; **296**: 890–897.

134. Zhang R et al. Pharmacokinetics and tissue distribution in rats of an oligodeoxynucleotide phosphorothioate (GEM 91) developed as a therapeutic agent for human immunodeficiency virus type-1. *Biochem Pharmacol* 1995; **49**: 929–939.

135. Sewell KL et al. Phase I trial of ISIS 104838, a 2′-methoxyethyl modified antisense oligonucleotide targeting tumor necrosis factor-alpha. *J Pharmacol Exp Ther* 2002; **303**: 1334–1343.

136. Yu RZ et al. Cross-species pharmacokinetic comparison from mouse to man of a second-generation antisense oligonucleotide, ISIS 301012, targeting human apolipoprotein B-100. *Drug Metab Dispos* 2007; **35**: 460–468.

137. Fluiter K et al. In vivo tumor growth inhibition and biodistribution studies of locked nucleic acid (LNA) antisense oligonucleotides. *Nucleic Acids Res* 2003; **31**: 953–962.

138. Yang CJ et al. Synthesis and investigation of deoxyribonucleic acid/locked nucleic acid chimeric molecular beacons. *Nucleic Acids Res* 2007; **35**: 4030–4041.

139. McMahon BM et al. Pharmacokinetics and tissue distribution of a peptide nucleic acid after intravenous administration. *Antisense Nucleic Acid Drug Dev* 2002; **12**: 65–70.

140. Braasch DA et al. Biodistribution of phosphodiester and phosphorothioate siRNA. *Bioorg Med Chem Lett* 2004; **14**: 1139–1143.

141. van de Water FM et al. Intravenously administered short interfering RNA accumulates in the kidney and selectively suppresses gene function in renal proximal tubules. *Drug Metab Dispos* 2006; **34**: 1393–1397.

142. Wolfrum C et al. Mechanisms and optimization of in vivo delivery of lipophilic siRNAs. *Nat Biotechnol* 2007; **25**: 1149–1157.

143. Merkel OM et al. In vivo SPECT and real-time gamma camera imaging of biodistribution and pharmacokinetics of siRNA delivery using an optimized radiolabeling and purification procedure. *Bioconjug Chem* 2009; **20**: 174–182.

144. Roberts J et al. Efficient and persistent splice switching by systemically delivered LNA oligonucleotides in mice. *Mol Ther* 2006; **14**: 471–475.

145. Crooke ST. Progress in antisense technology: The end of the beginning. *Methods Enzymol* 2000; **313**: 3–45.

146. Dove A. Isis and antisense face crucial test without Novartis. *Nat Biotechnol* 2000; **18**: 19.

147. Kleinman ME et al. Sequence- and target-independent angiogenesis suppression by siRNA via TLR3. *Nature* 2008; **452**: 591–597.

9 Liposomes for Nonviral Gene Delivery

Jiasheng Tu, Yan Shen, Hui Pang, and Yubing Yu

CONTENTS

9.1 INTRODUCTION

In the past 20 years, more than 400 clinical studies in gene therapy have been initiated.[1] Gene therapy can be used to introduce exogenous genetic material (such as DNA, small interfering RNA [siRNA], and oligonucleotides) into cells or tissues to cure a disease or to improve associated symptoms. Gene therapy starts with the choice of a therapeutic gene, but most critical is the success in gene transfer to the target tissues. The delivery of naked nucleic acids (NAs) is not effective as they are degraded very quickly by nucleases and do not passively diffuse across plasma membranes due to their large hydrodynamic size and negative charge.

Historically, three approaches have primarily been used for gene delivery. The first approach consists of the use of free NAs. The direct injection of free DNA to the tumor site produces high levels of gene expression. The simplicity of this approach led to its use in a number of experimental protocols.[2,3] This strategy appears to be limited to tissues that are easily accessible by direct injection, such as the skin and muscles,[4] but is not suitable for systemic delivery due to the presence of serum nucleases. The second approach involves using genetically altered viruses. Viral vectors are biological systems derived from naturally evolved viruses capable of transferring their genetic materials into the host cells. Many viruses including the retrovirus, adenovirus, herpes simplex virus (HSV), and adeno-associated virus (AAV) have been modified to eliminate their toxicity and maintain their high capacity for gene transfer.[5–8] Viral vectors effectively transduce cells, leading to high levels of gene expression (Table 9.1). However, the limitations associated with viral vectors, in terms of safety, immunogenicity, low transgene size, and high cost, have encouraged researchers to focus on alternative systems. The third approach is to use synthetic carriers, such as cationic liposomes,[9] polymers,[10,11] and peptides. The advantages associated with these gene carriers include their reproducible and relatively cost-effective large-scale manufacture, low immunogenic response, feasibility of selective modifications, and the capacity to carry large inserts (up to 52 kb).[12,13]

While the transfection efficiency of nonviral vectors is still lower than that of their viral counterparts, a number of adjustments (e.g., ligand attachment) can improve these carriers—which are, thus far, believed to be the most promising of gene delivery systems. Nonetheless, this class of vectors has to be modified to make systemic delivery possible. To date, their systemic administration has resulted in toxic responses attributed to the positive charge, which is unacceptable for the proposed clinical applications. Currently, the main objective in gene therapy via a systemic pathway is the development of a stable and nontoxic nonviral vector that can encapsulate and deliver foreign genetic materials into specific cell types, such as cancerous cells, with the transfection efficiency of viral vectors. In the case of cationic liposomes, both membrane fusion and endocytosis have been proposed as mechanisms for the DNA or oligonucleotide uptake into the cells.[14] The pathway followed by the cationic carriers, from the exterior of the cell to the nucleus, is not yet fully understood,

TABLE 9.1
The Major Viral Vectors Used by Scientists in Gene Therapy

Vector	Insert Size (kb)	Integrate	Titer	Transduction Efficiency	Major Advantage(s)	Major Obstacle(s)
MMLV	≤8	Yes	10^6	High	Stable transfection of dividing cells	Infects only rapidly dividing cells
Adeno	≤7.5	No	10^{12}	High	Transfects nearly all cell types dividing or nondividing	Transient expression triggers immune response, common human virus
AAV	≤4	Yes (?)	10^6	High	Stable transfection	Small insert size, integration poorly understood
HSV	≤20	No	10^{10}	Low	Large insert size; Neuron specificity	Transient expression, potential to generate infectious HSV in humans
Vaccinia	≤25	No	N/A	High	Infects a variety of cells effectively	Limited to non-small pox vaccinated or immunocompromised individuals

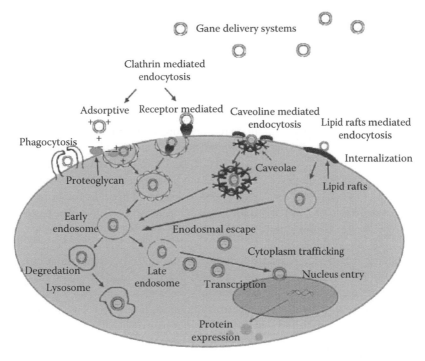

FIGURE 9.1 The pathway and mechanisms of gene delivery in tumor tissues.

but the fusion of the vesicles with the plasma membrane is perceived as a better route, since it avoids the endolysosomal compartment (with its acidic environment resulting in DNA/RNA degradation). However, studies of electron and fluorescence microscopy have shown that lipoplexes can be detected in intracellular vesicles beneath the cell membrane, suggesting that they enter the cells by endocytosis and will thus be directed toward the endolysosomal compartment. There are a multitude of endocytic pathways that can be processed by the carrier systems: clathrin-mediated endocytosis via coated pits (adsorptive or receptor mediated), lipid-raft-mediated endocytosis (caveolae mediated or not), phagocytosis, and macropinocytosis (Figure 9.1).

Liposomes are micro- or nano-particulate vesicles formed by the self-assembly of natural (e.g., phospholipids, cholesterol, etc.) or synthetic cationic amphiphiles in an aqueous environment. Liposomes are one of the most widely used nonviral vectors in human gene therapy studies.[15–18] The ability of cationic liposomes to mediate transfection was attributed to the intrinsic properties of these systems. For example, spontaneous electrostatic interaction between the positively charged vesicles and the negatively charged pDNA (and oligonucleotides) ensures the efficient condensation of the NAs. By modifying the lipid composition, the liposomes/NA complex can be designed to exhibit an appropriate charge that enhances cellular uptake.

9.2 LIPOSOME-BASED SYSTEMS AS NONVIRAL VECTORS

Liposomes are formed by lipid bilayer(s) surrounding aqueous compartment(s). First described by Bangham[19] on the basis of size, liposomes could be small unilamellar vesicles (SUV; i.e., having a single lipid bilayer 20–100 nm in diameter), large unilamellar vesicles (LUV; 50–400 nm), and multilamellar vesicles (MLV; 400–5000 nm). Frequently prepared using nontoxic phospholipids and cholesterol, they are biodegradable, biocompatible, and nonimmunogenic.[20] Considering the nature of the drug and the liposomal composition, both hydrophilic and hydrophobic compounds can interact with liposomes in different ways—they can be incorporated into the bilayer membrane, adsorbed on the surface, anchored at the polar head group region, or entrapped in the aqueous core.[21] In gene therapy applications, negatively charged DNA neutralizes cationic liposomes resulting in aggregation and continuous fusion with time, while DNA gets entrapped during this process.[5] Liposomes have proven to be useful tools for the delivery of genetic materials into cells.[22,23]

9.2.1 Cationic Liposomes

Cationic lipids are positively charged amphiphilic molecules made of a cationic polar head group (usually amino groups), a hydrophobic domain (comprising alkyl chains or cholesterol), and a linker connecting the polar head group with the nonpolar tail (Figure 9.2). Lipoplexes (Figure 9.3), also known as cationic liposomes, are capable of delivering DNA or RNA, including both plasmids encoding shRNA and siRNA duplexes, through the cellular membrane, and achieving high RNA inference (RNAi).[24–26] They have recently emerged as leading nonviral vectors in worldwide gene therapy clinical trials (Table 9.2). In particular, Lipofectamine® 2000 is frequently used for the delivery of siRNA.[27,28] The morphology and size of lipoplexes may vary due the lipidic composition of vesicles, the manner in which the complexes are formed, the lipid: NA ratio, the size of the NA construct, batch-to-batch variation in reagents, and the technique used to treat and visualize these complexes.[29,30] Hydrophobic interactions are also believed to aid complex formation between lipids and NAs.[31] Hence, depending on the positive (cationic lipid) to negative (phosphate group on NA) charge ratio,[32] lipoplexes may enter cells through electrostatic interaction with such charged residues at the cell surface as sialic acid moieties, or by hydrophobic interaction with the hydrophobic regions of the plasma membrane. In addition, both mechanisms may be at play with every lipofection.

Despite the successes using lipoplexes, these agents allow for little control over the process of their interaction with NAs. NA/liposome complexes of excessive size, low stability, and/or with incomplete encapsulation of NA molecules may expose NAs to potential enzymatic or physical degradation prior to delivery to the cells. The complexes are usually unstable in serum. Therefore, optimal transfection is usually performed *in vitro* using serum-free conditions, which has obvious shortcomings for potential *in vivo* applications. In addition, such complexes do not work efficiently with many cell types, and are toxic to cells and experimental animals.[33]

> NA/liposome complexes of excessive size, low stability, and/or with incomplete encapsulation of NA molecules may expose NAs to potential enzymatic or physical degradation prior to delivery to the cells. The complexes are usually unstable in serum. In addition, such complexes do not efficiently transfect many cell types, and are toxic to cells and experimental animals.

9.2.2 Polycation Liposomes

Sugiyama[34] developed the polycation liposomes (PCLs) as a synthetic carrier that possesses the advantages of both cationic liposomes and polycations for gene delivery.[35,36] PCLs are prepared by the modification of the liposomal surface with cetylated polyethylenimine (PEI) of an average molecular weight 600–1800 (Figure 9.4). PCL showed various advantageous properties such as high efficiency of gene transfer, low cytotoxicity, applicability for *in vivo* use, and enhanced efficacy of gene transfer in the presence of serum. The mechanism of the PCL-mediated gene transfer is a fusion with an endosomal membrane or destabilization of the membrane by PCLs, leading to the cytosolic delivery of DNA. Due to the incorporation of polycations (such as PEI) in PCL, unlike cationic liposomes, the DNA is released into the cytoplasm from endosomes, due to the proton-sponge effect of PEI that induces the massive proton accumulation and passive chloride influx into the newly formed endosomes. Rapid osmotic swelling resulting in endosomal rupture allows for the translocation of DNA into the nucleus without any degradation. The DNA may be further delivered to the nucleus by the polycation.[37,38]

In addition, liposome (LP)-mediated gene transfer can be augmented by the addition of natural polycations such as protamine sulfate (PS), poly-L-lysine (PLL), and spermine.[39,40] These polycations form complexes with DNA and condense DNA from an extended conformation to a highly

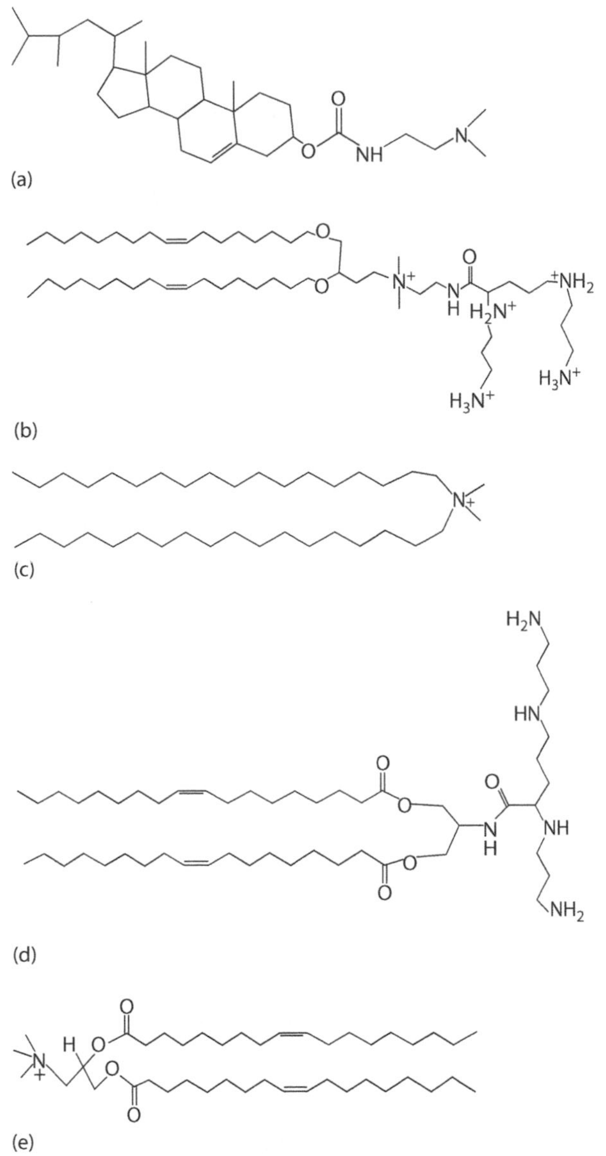

(a)

(b)

(c)

(d)

(e)

FIGURE 9.2 Structures of several cationic lipids. CCS, *N*-palmitoyl-D-erythro-sphingosyl carbamoyl-spermine; DC-Chol, 3β-[*N*-(*N'*,*N'*-dimethylaminoethane)-carbamoyl] cholesterol hydrochloride; diC14-amidine, *N*-*t*-butyl-*N'*-tetradecyl-3-tetradecylamin-opropionamidine; DOEPC, 1,2-dipalmitoyl-*sn*-glycero-3-ethylphosphocholine, respectively; DMKD, *O,O'*-dimyristyl-*N*-lysyl glutamate; DMKE, *O,O'*-dimyristyl-*N*-lysyl aspartate; DOTAP, 1,2-dioleoyl-3-trimethylammoniumpr opane, respectively; DODAB (DDAB), dioctadecyldimethylammonium bromide; DODAP, 1,2-dioleoyl-3-dimethylammoniumpropane; DOGS, dioctadecylamidoglycylspermine; DOSPA, 1,3-dioleoyloxy-*N*-[2-(sperminecarboxamido)ethyl]-*N,N*-dimethyl-1-propanaminium trifluoroacetate; DOSPER, 1,3-dioleoyloxy-2-(6-carboxyspermyl)-propylamide; DOTIM, octadecenolyoxy [ethyl-2-heptadecenyl-3 hydroxyethyl] imidazolinium chloride; DOTMA, *N*-[1-(2,3-dioleyloxy)propyl]-*N,N,N*-trimethyl-ammonium chloride.

(continued)

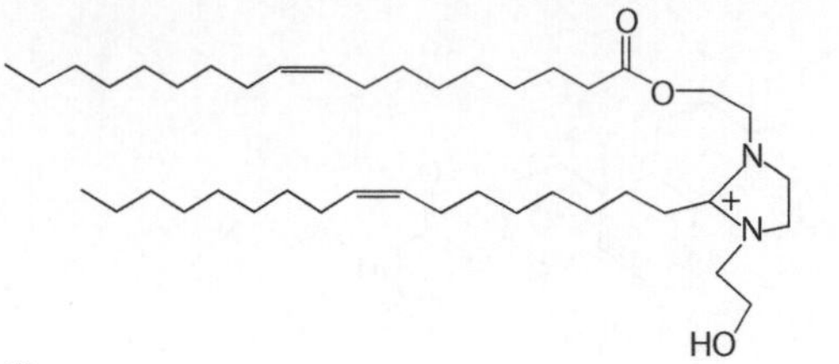

(f)

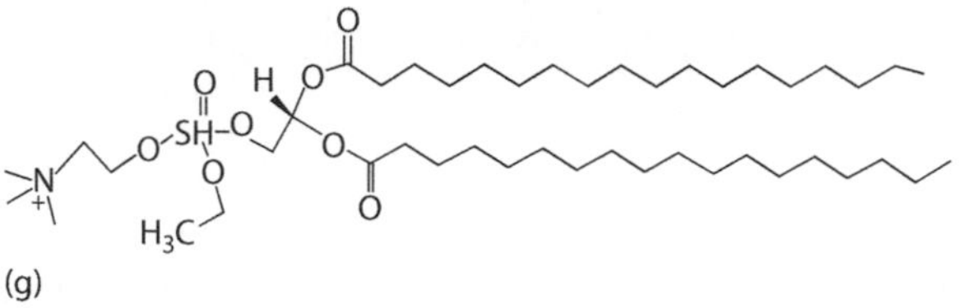

(g)

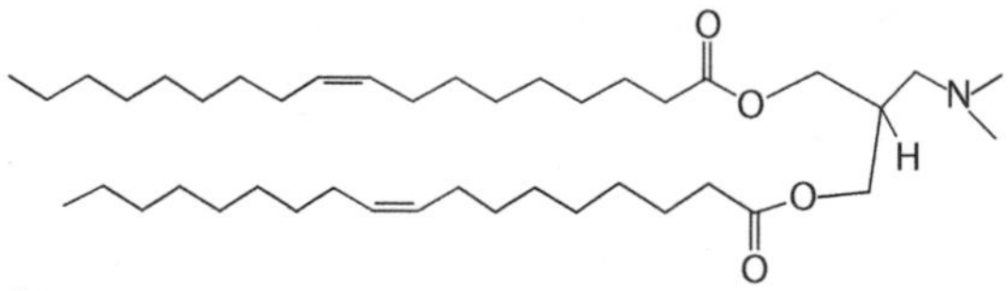

(h)

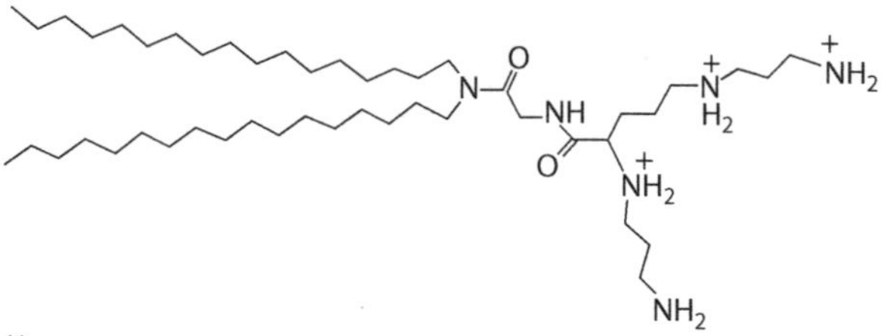

(i)

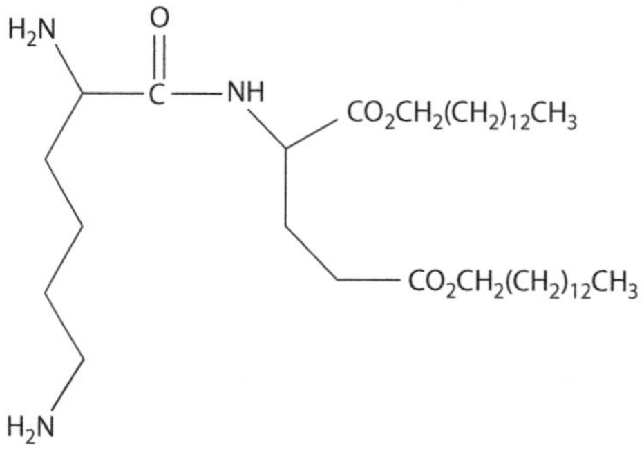

(j)

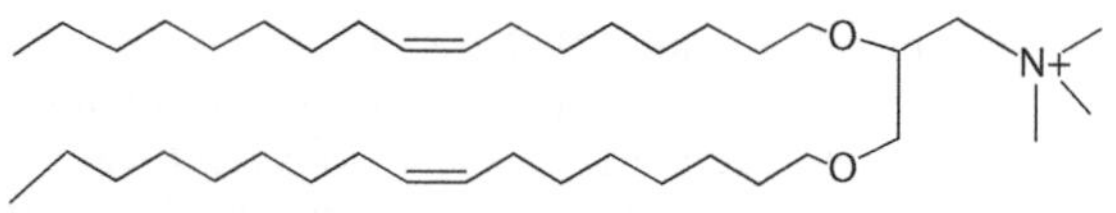

(k)

FIGURE 9.2 (continued)

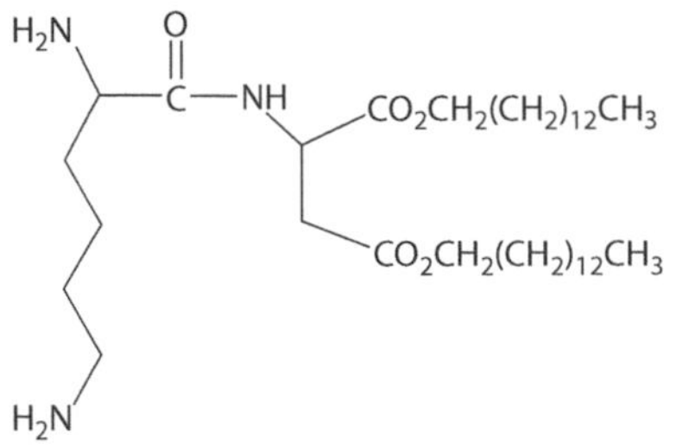

H₂N
(l)

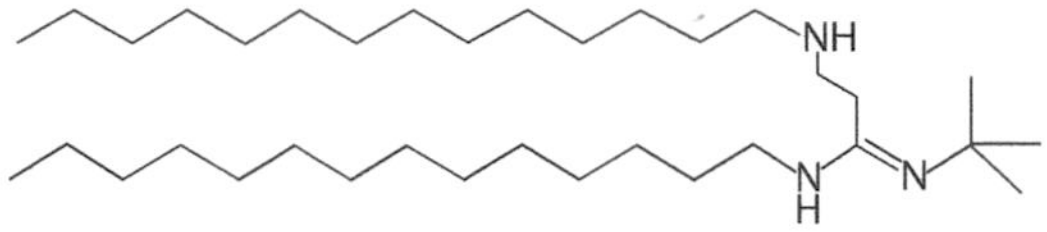

(m)

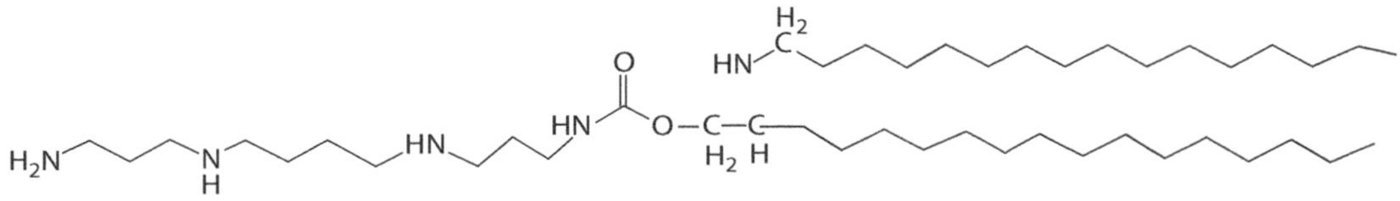

(n)

FIGURE 9.2 (continued)

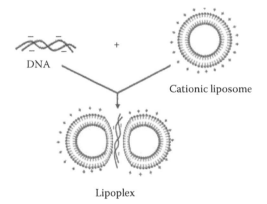

DNA

+

Cationic liposome

Lipoplex

FIGURE 9.3 One of the hypothesized structures of a lipoplex.

compact structure of 30–100 nm in size. Although these polycations by themselves mediate DNA delivery, they exhibit a synergistic effect when combined with cationic LPs. Polycations condense DNA into ternary complexes such as LP/polycation/DNA complexes. These particles showed an enhanced gene expression over that seen with LP/DNA binary complexes. This enhancement could be due to a highly compacted complex, which may assist cellular uptake and/or for the protection of DNA against enzymatic digestion. Also, PS has a peptide functional moiety that can act as a nuclear localization signal (NLS). The NLS can help DNA translocation to the nucleus. In case of spermine, once these particles enter the nucleus, it may dissociate more readily and help DNA to bind with transcription machinery.[41] NLS is an amino acid sequence that acts like a "tag" on the exposed surface of a protein. This sequence is used to target the protein to the cell nucleus through the nuclear pore complex and to direct a newly synthesized protein into the nucleus via its recognition by cytosolic nuclear transport receptors. Typically, this signal consists of one or more short sequences of positively charged lysines or arginines. Different nuclear localized proteins may share the same NLS.

TABLE 9.2
Some of the Cationic Lipids Used for Gene Delivery

	Commercial Name	Lipid	Molar Ratio	Available from
1	DMRIE-C	DMRIEZ:Cholesterol	1:1	GibcoBRL
2	Lipofectin	DOTMA:DOPE	1:0.9	GibcoBRL
3	Lipofectamine	DOSPA:DOPE	1:0.65	GibcoBRL
4	DC-Chol	DC-Chol:DOPE	1:0.67	Sigma
5	LipofectASE	DDAB:DOPE	1:2.1	GibcoBRL
6	TransfectASE	DDAB:DOPE	1:3	GibcoBRL
7	Transfectam	DOGS	—	Promega
8	DOTAP	DOTAP	—	Avanti
9	Tfx-50	Tfx-50:DOPE	1:1	Primega
10	Cellfectin	TM-TPS:DOPE	1:1.5	GibcoBRL
11	GL67	Lipid67:DOPE	1:2	Genzyme

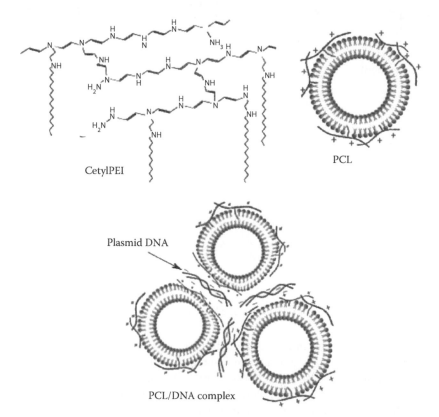

CetylPEI

PCL

Plasmid DNA

PCL/DNA complex

FIGURE 9.4   The structure of "PCL."

9.2.3   WRAPPED LIPOSOMES

The practical application of liposomes comprised of neutral lipids is limited because the NA encapsulation efficiency is low.[42,43] The encapsulation efficiency is significantly higher in cationic liposomes. Furthermore, the presence of cationic lipid facilitates uptake by cells *in vitro*.[31,44] However, cationic liposomes are unstable in plasma and are eliminated rapidly from the blood after intravenous administration. Consequently, cationic liposomes do not deliver genes efficiently to target sites.[45] Previously, we described the preparation and pharmaceutical properties of a novel formulation of liposomes that were covered with neutral lipids composed of egg phosphatidylcholine (EPC) and 1,2-distearoyl-*sn*-glycero-3-phosphoethanolamine-*N*-methoxy(polyethylene glycol) 2000 (PEG-DSPE); Yamauchi[46] adopted the term "wrapped liposomes" (WLs) to describe this formulation.

Novel WLs comprised of polyanion drug or gene and cationic lipid complexes wrapped with neutral lipids were prepared using an efficient, innovative procedure (Figure 9.5). The initial studies were conducted with dextran, fluorescein, 10,000 molecular weight, anionic (DFA) (Molecular Probes (Invitrogen), Eugene, Oregon) as a model of a polyanionic drug.[46] WLs, which were prepared with a high encapsulation efficiency and were of a small diameter, were more stable in fetal bovine serum (FBS) than naked (i.e., not wrapped with neutral lipids) DFA/cationic lipid complexes. Furthermore, Yamauchi et al. demonstrated that the intravenous administration of the WL to rats generated high blood levels of DFA that were maintained for several hours. This was in marked contrast to the high clearance of DFA observed when it was administered in free form or in naked complexes. These results suggest that WL-based formulations could offer important advantages for the administration of different NA drugs including antisense oligonucleotide (asODN), plasmids, and siRNAs, which may lead to their improved therapeutic effectiveness. The preparation method of WLs is expected to be adaptable to a large manufacturing scale.[47]

The improved drug delivery properties of the WLs relative to other formulations suggested that this technology could offer important advantages for the administration of other polyanionic drugs, including antisense oligodeoxynucleotides (ODNs). In the present study, Yamauchi et al.[46] investigated the value of WLs for formulating fluorescence-labeled phosphorothioated ODN (F-ODN).

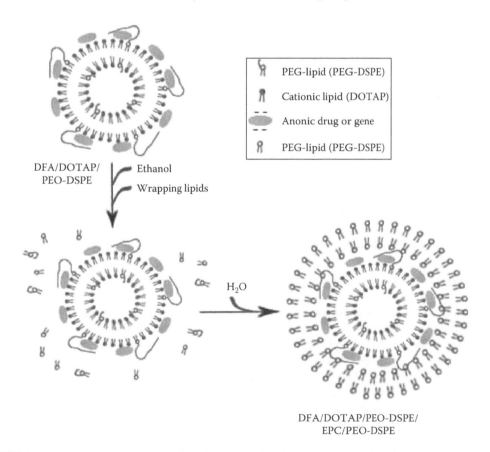

FIGURE 9.5 Procedure for the preparation of wrapped liposomes.

WLs encapsulating F-ODN/cationic lipid complexes were prepared efficiently using a similar methodology to that used in our earlier study. Studies confirmed that these WLs were stable *in vitro*. Following intravenous administration to mice, free F-ODN and naked F-ODN/cationic lipid complexes were rapidly eliminated whereas the administration of the WLs resulted in high blood concentrations of drug that were maintained for several hours. Additional studies were conducted in mice that were inoculated with tumor cells (Caki-1 xenograft model, human kidney); in these experiments, the intravenous administration of WLs delivered 13 times more F-ODN to the tumor site than what was achieved after an injection of free F-ODN.

9.2.4 Fusogenic Liposomes

Fusogenic liposomes (FLs) can potentially facilitate the intracellular delivery of encapsulated drugs by fusing with the target cell. A variety of approaches can be envisioned for constructing FLs. Examples include the inclusion of lipids that are able to form nonbilayer phases, such as 1,2-dioleoyl-*sn*-glycero-3-phosphatidylethanolamine (DOPE), which can promote the destabilization of the bilayer, inducing fusion events.[48] Furthermore, alterations in the lipid composition can render liposomes pH sensitive, leading to enhanced fusogenic tendencies in low pH compartments such as endosomes.[39,49–51] Nonphospholipid FLs composed primarily of dioxyethylene acyl ethers and cholesterol fuse with plasma membranes of erythrocytes and fibroblasts.[52] Alternatively, efficient FLs can be achieved by incorporating fusogenic proteins into the liposome membrane,[53–55] or entrapping them within liposomes.[56]

Viral coat proteins, such as hemagglutinin of the influenza virus and the glycoprotein complex of the Semliki Forest virus, are believed to facilitate the fusion of virion particles with the plasma membrane of the host cells (Figure 9.6). The acidic environment of the endosomal compartment induces conformational changes in the viral coat protein, leading to a fusion of the viral coat protein with the endosomal membrane, destabilization and disruption of the endosomal membrane, and transfer of genetic material into the cytosol of the host cells. Similarly, the Sendai virus also exploits its coat proteins to fuse with the plasma membrane of the target cells to inject its genetic material. This system can achieve the delivery of soluble drugs into the cytoplasm[57–60] and protect NA drugs from hydrolytic and enzymatic degradation.

Kunisawa et al.[57] developed FLs with Sendai virus envelope glycoproteins on the surface. These FLs could efficiently introduce encapsulated nucleotides and/or proteins into the cytoplasm by direct fusion with the plasma membrane without significant cytotoxicity.[61] Mizuguchi et al.[62–67] also demonstrated an application of FLs for gene therapy, cancer chemotherapy, and vaccine development. They established a protocol for encapsulating nanoparticles into liposomes. When nanoparticles were encapsulated in conventional liposomes, an endocytosis-mediated uptake of nanoparticles was observed. In contrast, a significant amount of nanoparticles were delivered into the cytoplasm without any cytotoxicity when the particles were encapsulated in FLs. Additionally, FLs could deliver nanoparticles containing DNA oligonucleotides into the cytoplasm. These results indicate that this combinatorial nanotechnology using FLs and nanoparticles could be a valuable platform for regulating the intracellular pharmacokinetics of gene-based drugs.[68]

Sakaguchi et al.[69] developed complexes of liposomes containing 3-(*N*-(*N*,*N*-dimethylaminoethane) carbamoyl) cholesterol (DC-chol) and succinylated poly(glycidol) (SucPG), which become fusogenic under weakly acidic conditions. Three types of cationic lipids with different polar groups were used for preparing lipoplexes: DC-chol, *N*-[1-(2,3-dioleoyloxy)propyl]-*N*,*N*,*N*-trimethylammonium methylsulfate (DOTAP), and 3,5-dipentadecyloxybenzamidine (TRX-20) with dimethylamino, trimethylammonium, and benzamidine groups, respectively. Complexation with the SucPG-modified transferrin-bearing liposomes affected the transfection activity of these lipoplexes differently. The TRX-20 lipoplexes exhibited the most marked enhancement of the transfection activity upon complexation with the SucPG-modified liposomes among these lipoplexes. The cationic lipid/DNA charge ratio of the lipoplex and the amount of the transferrin-bearing

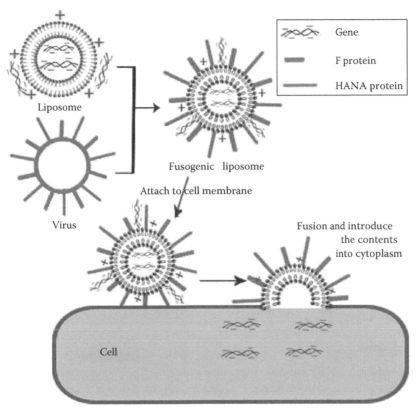

FIGURE 9.6 Schematic showing the steps and hypothesized intermediate structures of fusogentic liposomes.

SucPG-modified liposomes associated to the lipoplex also affected the transfection activity of the resultant complexes. Highly potent gene vectors were obtained by adjusting these factors.

9.2.5 ANIONIC LIPOPLEXES

To reduce the lipofection-associated cytotoxicity, we have recently developed an anionic lipoplex system composed of naturally occurring membrane lipids.[70] An anionic lipoplex formation was achieved by complexation between the pDNA and anionic liposomes using divalent Ca^{2+} ion bridges (Figure 9.7).[70] Although there have been a few previous attempts[52,71] to use anionic lipids for gene transfer, not much is known about anionic liposome entrapment and/or complex formation with DNA molecules or the process of forming anionic lipoplexes or complexes between anionic lipids and DNA using divalent Ca^{2+} cations.

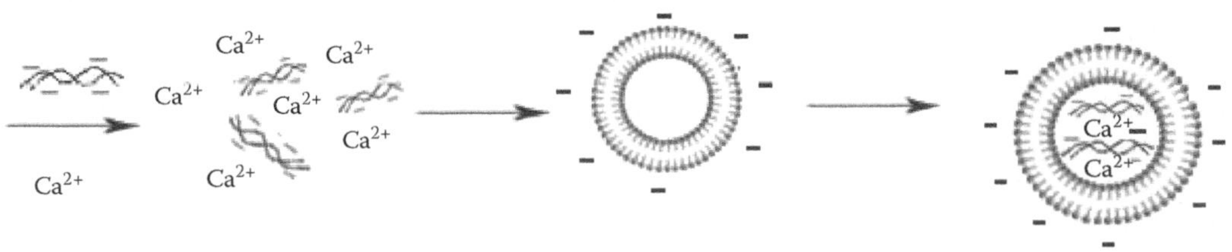

FIGURE 9.7 Schematic showing the steps and hypothesized intermediate structures of anionic lipoplex.

Patil et al.[72] have recently reported a novel anionic lipoplex DNA delivery system composed of a ternary complex of endogenous nontoxic anionic lipids, Ca^{2+} cations, and pDNA encoding a gene of interest. They reported high transfection efficiency and low toxicity. In this work, they investigated the electrochemical and structural properties of anionic lipoplexes and compared them with those of the Ca^{2+}–DNA complexes. A biophysical characterization was used to explain the transfection efficiency of anionic lipoplexes in mammalian CHO-K_1 cells. Circular dichroism and fluorescence spectroscopy showed that the pDNA underwent a conformational transition from native B-DNA (the right-handed typical form of double helix DNA in which the chains twist up and to the right around the front of the axis of the helix and that usually has 10 base pairs in each helical turn and two grooves on the external surface) to Z-DNA (Z-DNA is one of the many possible double helical structures of DNA). It is a left-handed double helical structure in which the double helix winds to the left in a zigzag pattern (instead of to the right, like the more common B-DNA form) due to the compaction and condensation upon the Ca^{2+}-mediated complex formation with anionic liposomes. The Ca^{2+} interaction with pDNA during the formation of lipoplexes also led to an increased association of supercoiled pDNA with the lipoplexes, leading to charge neutralization—which is expected to facilitate transfection. However, up to 10-fold higher concentrations of Ca^{2+} alone (in the absence of the anionic liposomes) were unable to induce these changes in pDNA molecules. This indicated that the DNA was indeed complexing with anionic lipids and that this complexation was facilitated by Ca^{2+} ions.

9.2.6 FLUIDOSOMES

To overcome antibiotic resistance, fluid liposomes, named fluidosomes, were developed. These are negatively charged liposomes without cholesterol that are made of a combination of dipalmitoylphosphatidylcholine (DPPC) and dimyristoylphosphatidylglycerol (DMPG) phospholipids (at a molar ratio from 5:1 to 18:1). These liposomes have an overall low gel–liquid crystalline transition temperature (T_C, $\leq 37°C$).[73] They were conceived as a delivery vehicle to enhance drug penetration through bacterial membranes.[74,75] Fluidosomes have shown a marked improvement of bactericidal activity against *in vitro* and *in vivo* extracellular infections, even when initiated with resistant strains. Recently, it was demonstrated that the superior bactericidal effect of fluidosomes results from its ability to interact directly with the bacterial outer membrane, which leads to the increased penetration of the drug in parallel with the incorporation of the liposomal membranes in the bacterial cells.

The fluid liposome-encapsulated antibiotics succeed in eradicating *Pseudomonas aeruginosa* in an animal model of chronic pulmonary infection.[75] Recently, the superior efficiency of fluid liposome-encapsulated aminoglycoside antibiotics in an animal model of bacterial infection was reported by an independent group.[76] We have demonstrated that the enhanced bactericidal activity of fluid liposomes results from an enhanced rate of fusion between the liposomes and the bacterial membranes.[77] Previous studies analyzing the innocuousness of fluid liposomes have demonstrated that they do not induce an immune response following repeated intraperitoneal and intratracheal administrations to mice,[78] and that they do not fuse with human lung epithelial cells.[79]

Antisense therapy for treating bacterial infections is an attractive alternative to overcoming drug resistance problems. However, the penetration of asODN into bacterial cells is a major hurdle that has delayed research and application in this field. Fillion et al.[52] defined the efficient conditions for encapsulating pDNA and asODN in a fluid, negatively-charged liposome. Subsequently, they evaluated the potential of liposome-encapsulated asODN to penetrate the bacterial outer membrane and to inhibit gene expression in bacteria. They found that $48.9\% \pm 12\%$ and $43.5\% \pm 4\%$ of the purified pDNA and asODN, respectively were encapsulated in the liposomes. A fluorescence-activated cell sorting (FACS) analysis showed that about 57% of bacterial cells had internalized the encapsulated asODN, whereas free asODN were negligible. The uptake of encapsulated anti-lacZ asODN resulted in a 42% reduction of beta-galactosidase—compared with 9% and 6% for the encapsulated mismatch as ODN and the free asODN, respectively. This work shows that it is possible to encapsulate relatively large amounts of negatively charged molecules in negatively charged fluid liposomes. It further suggests that fluid liposomes could be used to deliver NAs to bacteria to inhibit essential bacterial genes.

> Fluid liposomes, named fluidosomes, are negatively charged liposomes without cholesterol. They are made of a combination of DPPC and DMPG phospholipids (at a molar ratio from 5:1 to 18:1). These liposomes have an overall low gel-liquid crystalline transition temperature (T_C, ≤37°C). They may be used as a delivery vehicle to enhance drug penetration through bacterial membranes.

9.3 TARGETING STRATEGIES FOR LIPOSOME-BASED GENE DELIVERY

Most of the transfection studies have been done with cells *ex vivo* or by injection at the target site of action. However, targeted delivery is required if these routes cannot be used. Although the efficacy of these approaches has been established in several *in vitro* and *in vivo* models,[80,81] the clinical use of genes is impaired due to a number of chemical and biological barriers.

Liposomes have several advantages for site-specific gene delivery. To facilitate their use as drug delivery vehicles, we will discuss three components of liposome design: (1) the identification of candidate cell surface receptors for targeting, (2) the identification of ligands that maintain binding specificity and affinity, and (3) increasing liposome circulating times and preventing rapid nonspecific clearance of liposomes into the reticuloendothelial organs.

9.3.1 INTRODUCTION

There are three main strategies for homing particulate carrier systems to target sites: (1) the physicochemical approaches based on the complex formation between a homing device and a surface-exposed molecule at the target site; (2) the use of stimuli-responsive systems, used as "smart" delivery systems; and (3) physical drug targeting strategies.

With physicochemical approaches, homing devices, which are the molecules that recognize or are recognized by the target cells due to the preferential affinity of target cell surface expressed molecules, are attached to the carrier surface (Figure 9.8). These homing devices are designed such

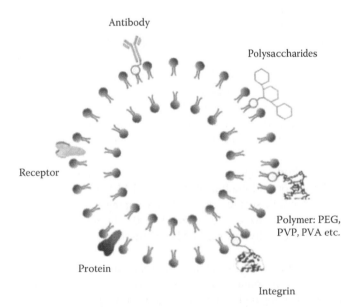

FIGURE 9.8 Approaches based on specific surface structures on the target sites.

that they only recognize and interact with specific structures on the surface of target cells or tissues. This type of interaction is based on hydrophobic interactions, hydrogen bonding, and/or salt bridges between homing device and specific surface structures on the target sites. Antibody antigen interactions are examples of this approach.

The use of stimuli-responsive systems makes the delivery system an active participant, rather than a passive vehicle, in the optimization of therapy. Several families of molecular assemblies can be employed as stimuli-responsive liposomes for either passive or active targeting. The composition of these molecular assemblies can be manipulated to obtain liposomes of desired stimuli-responsive property. The benefit of stimuli-responsive liposomes is especially important when the stimuli are unique to disease pathology, allowing the liposomes to respond specifically to the pathological "triggers." Examples of biological stimuli include pH, temperature, and the redox microenvironment (Table 9.3).

Physical drug targeting strategies are designed to accumulate carrier-associated drug at target sites by physical means. Some examples are the use of local magnetic fields or ultrasound. Over the years, the physicochemical approach has received much attention. We will discuss these strategies in detail below.

> Stimuli-responsive liposomes allow drug release in response to biological stimuli including pH, temperature, and the redox microenvironment.

9.3.2 COMMON TARGETING LIGANDS AND AGENTS

Potential methods for liposome targeting include coupling to antibodies[82–85] and the inclusion of ligands that bind proteins expressed, for example, on cancer cell membranes or endothelial cells lining the newly generated blood vessels in the tumor. Examples of such proteins include the folate receptor (FR). It is induced on the surface of actively growing tumor cells, possibly due to increased requirements for DNA synthesis.[86–88] Another example is the integrin surface receptor,[89,90] which is expressed on the endothelial cells in the neovasculature of growing tumors. Other examples include galactolipids, which target the ASGPR of the human hepatoma HepG2 cells.[91,92]

9.3.2.1 Antibody Targeting

Antibody-coated liposomes (liposomes that have antibodies covalently attached to their surface), known as immunoliposomes, have been extensively studied. The antibodies are attached either with the liposome phospholipid headgroup[93] or to the terminus of the PEGylated lipid. The latter approach has proven to be more successful, due to better accessibility of the antibody to its target.[94]

Pan and Lee[95] prepared anti-epidermal growth factor receptor (EGFR) immunoliposomes using folate–folate binding protein (FBP) affinity. An anti-EGFR antibody (cetuximab or C_{225}) was covalently linked to FBP via a thioether bond. The immunoliposomes were evaluated for uptake and cytotoxicity in EGFR-overexpressing U87 human glioblastoma cells. These immunoliposomes exhibited excellent stability under the physiological pH and quickly released the bound FBP-C_{225} at a low pH value of 3.5. Flow cytometry and fluorescence microscopy showed similar receptor-specific binding and internalization of both folate-FBP affinity-coupled and covalently coupled C_{225}-immunoliposomes, but not for the nontargeted IgG-immunoliposomes.

Marty et al.[96] developed a target for anti-angiogenic tumor therapy using phage display technology. A single chain antibody fragment (scFv-CM_6) was isolated that specifically binds to the extracellular part of the tumor endothelial marker 1 (TEM_1). TEM_1 is a protein predominantly expressed on the endothelial cell surface in newly developing blood vessels and on tumor cells. ScFv-CM_6 was further functionalized and coupled to the liposomes. These immunoliposomes showed an increased binding affinity toward TEM1-expressing IMR-32 tumor cells compared with control liposomes.

Brignole et al.[97] described a novel therapeutic approach for neuroblastoma based on anti-GD_2 (a tumor-associated antigen) liposomal systems that deliver asODN to cancer cells to modulate oncogene expression. The disialoganglioside GD_2 is a promising tumor-associated antigen since it is expressed at high levels on human neuroblastoma cells, but is detected only in normal cerebellum

TABLE 9.3
Stimuli That Can Be Utilized to Control the Behavior and Properties of Drug Delivery Systems

Stimuli		Stimuli Origin	Stimuli-Responsive Polymer or Lipid	Benefit
pH	Internal	Decreased pH in pathological areas, such as tumors, infarcts, and inflammations, because of hypoxia and massive cell death; decreased pH in cell cytoplasm, endosomes, and lysosomes	Anionic liposomes containing phosphatidylethanolamine (PE); Histidine-modified galactosylated cholesterol derivative-cationic liposome; dioleoylpho-sphatidylethanolamine liposomes with PEG via disulfide linkage; transferrin-modified liposomes (T_f-L) with a pH-sensitive fusogenic peptide (GALA)	Drug release was faster at low pH and able to target intracellularly; cytoplasmic delivery; at low pH it allows fusion of endosomal membranes and destabilization of the endosomes
Redox	Internal	Increased concentration of glutathione inside many pathological cells compared to its extracellular concentration	Cationic lipoic acid; poly(ethylene glycol)-modified thiolated gelatin nanoparticles	DNA release depends on the redox state which increased several fold of transgene expression; intracellular DNA delivery in response to glutathione redox environment
Temperature	Internal	Hyperthermia associated with inflammation	Dioleoylphosphatidylethanolamine vesicles bearing poly (*N*-isopropylacrylamide); poloxamer F127 containing liposomes; thiopolycation PESC;	Thiopolyplexes releases DNA in reductive environment; efficient gene transfection
	External	Can be caused inside target tissues by locally applied ultrasound or by locally applied high frequency causing the oscillation of target accumulated magneto-sensitive nanoparticles with heat release		
Magnetic field	External	Magnetic field of different gradients and profiles applied to the body can concentrate magneto-sensitive DDS in required areas	Magnetic polyacrylamide particles containing nanosize magnetic iron oxide namely magnemite (γ-Fe_2O_3) or magnetite (Fe_3O_4); Superparamagnetic iron oxide nanoparticles (SPIONs)	Magnetic targeting or guiding magnetically susceptible particles toward the intended pathology site under the influence of external magnets; directly kill tumors or make them more susceptible in combination with radiation or chemotherapy

(continued)

TABLE 9.3 (continued)
Stimuli That Can Be Utilized to Control the Behavior and Properties of Drug Delivery Systems

Stimuli		Stimuli Origin	Stimuli-Responsive Polymer or Lipid	Benefit
Ultrasound	External	Sonication can be applied to the body to get a diagnostic signal from echogenic contrast agents and can also facilitate DDS penetration into cells and drug/gene release from ultrasound-sensitive DDS	Acoustically active liposomes, containing a small quantity of a certain gas (air) or perfluorated hydrocarbon and initially developed as ultrasound contrast agent	Accumulation in required areas can be made leaky by the locally applied external ultrasound. Focused ultrasound in combination with MRI and ultrasound imaging has great potential to bring ultrasound triggered drug release to the clinic, while employing pressure and temperature sensitive delivery vehicles.

Source: Torchilin, V., *Eur. J. Pharm. Biopharm.*, 71, 431, 2009. With permission.

and peripheral nerves. Furthermore, asODN have attracted much interest because of their ability to stimulate immune responses.[98]

Pardridge et al.[98] have prepared PEGylated immunoliposomes (PIL) carrying short hairpin RNA (shRNA) expression plasmids to target human EGFR expression. EGFR plays an oncogenic role in solid cancer, including brain primary and metastatic cancers. The PIL is comprised of a mixture of lipids containing PEG, which stabilizes the PIL structure *in vivo*. The target specificity of PILs is ensured by the conjugation of approximately 1% of PEG residues to monoclonal antibodies (mAbs) that bind to specific endogenous receptors, i.e., insulin and transferrin receptors (T_fR) located in the vascular endothelium of the blood brain barrier (BBB) and brain cellular membranes, respectively. The treatment of an experimental human brain tumor in severe combined immunodeficient (SCID) mice with weekly intravenous RNAi therapy caused a reduced tumor expression of EGFR and an 88% increase in survival.

Gosk et al.[99] prepared PIL directed against the vascular cell adhesion molecule-1 (VCAM-1), a surface receptor overexpressed on tumor vessels. They investigated liposomal targeting both *in vitro* and *in vivo*. Anti-VCAM-1 liposomes displayed specific binding to activated endothelial cells under static as well as under simulated blood flow conditions. The *in vivo* targeting of immunoliposomes was analyzed in mice bearing human Colo 677 tumor xenografts 30 min and 24 h post intravenous injection. Whereas biodistribution studies using [^{3}H]-labeled liposomes displayed only marginal tumor accumulation of VCAM-1 targeted versus nonspecific immunoliposomes, VCAM-1 targeted immunoliposomes accumulated in tumor vessels with increasing intensities from 30 min to 24 h.

Volker et al.[100] generated immunoliposomes targeting proliferating endothelial cells by chemically coupling a single-chain Fv fragment (scFv A5) directed against human endoglin to the liposomal surface. The immunoliposomes (ILA5) showed rapid and strong binding to human endoglin-expressing endothelial cells (HUVEC, HDMEC), while no binding was observed with various endoglin-negative cell lines and blood lymphocytes.

Wang and Huang[49] and Akhtar et al.[101] reported that pH-sensitive immunoliposomes could mediate the target-specific delivery of pDNA to lymphoma cells grown in a nude mouse model. Gene delivery was more efficient by pH-insensitive immunoliposomes. These pH-sensitive immunoliposomes also reduce the degradation of the NAs by lysosomes.

Ma and Wei[102] have estimated the efficiency of pH-sensitive liposomes and immunoliposomes to deliver asODN into human leukemia cells *in vitro*. The cellular uptake of a 18mer anti-myb oligonucleotide encapsulated in liposomes was three- to fivefold higher than that of ^{32}P-oligonucleotides alone.

9.3.2.2 Integrin Targeting

Integrins are receptors expressed in the neo-vasculature during tumor angiogenesis. Hölig et al.[103] investigated the targeting of small peptides toward integrins by phage display library selection of peptides targeting tumor blood vessels. The peptide sequence showing the most efficient binding to the $\alpha_v\beta_3$-integrin receptor was the Arg-Gly-Asp (RGD) tripeptide. This peptide was inserted in the CDCRGDCFC-peptide motif and coupled to free drugs.

Hood et al.[90] synthesized a cationic polymerized liposome, with encapsulated DNA, bearing ligand targeting $\alpha_v\beta_3$-integrins of the M_{21}-melanoma xenograft tumors. Gene expression was very high in the tumor compared with the nonangiogenic tissue. The delivery of a mutant Raf gene, blocking endothelial cell signaling and angiogenesis, caused sustained tumor regression after a single systemic administration. Based on this work on integrin targeting, the strategy to target neo-endothelial cells instead of the tumor cells themselves seems to be a promising approach for cancer treatment.

Townsend et al.[104] showed the anti-adhesive potential of an antisense ODN approach designed to suppress the cellular function of the α_V-integrin subunit in breast cancer cells. The α_V integrins play a major role in breast cancer metastasis. In this study, they inhibited α_V subunit synthesis in the human breast carcinoma cell line, MDA-MB231, by a partially phosphorothioated antisense ODN (5543-ODN). The α_V antisense 5543-ODN reduced α_V, but not actin, mRNA transcription, and protein expression by 55% and 65%, respectively. The control sense and mismatch sequences were inactive. The asODN-treated cells also showed an increase in apoptotic cell death.

Partlow et al.[105] defined the delivery mechanisms of fluorescently-labeled nanoparticles (comprising a lipid/surfactant monolayer surrounding a dense lipophobic, hydrophobic perfluorocarbon [PFC] core) complexed with $\alpha_v\beta_3$-integrin targeting ligands by incubating with $\alpha_v\beta_3$-integrin expressing cells (C32 melanoma). There were specific nanoparticle-to-cell interactions, predominantly via lipid mixing and subsequent intracellular trafficking through lipid raft-dependent processes.

The immunohistochemical staining of irradiated tumors showed an accumulation of $\alpha_{(2b)}\beta_{(3)}$ integrin, which is a fibrinogen receptor. Hallahan et al.[106] studied the tumor targeting efficiency of ligands to radiation-induced $\alpha_{(2b)}\beta_{(3)}$. Radiopharmaceuticals were localized to irradiated tumors by use of $\alpha_{(2b)}\beta_{(3)}$ ligands conjugated to nanoparticles and liposomes. Fibrinogen-conjugated nanoparticles bound to the radiation-activated receptor, obliterated tumor blood flow, and significantly increased tumor regression. Radiation-guided drug delivery to the tumor blood vessels is a novel paradigm for targeted drug delivery.

Parkhouse et al.[107] reported two new methods for inhibiting gene expression. The Poly(ethylene glycol)bis(N-methyl-2-(methylamino)ethylcarbamate)-block-polyamidoamine [N,N'-dimethylethylenediamine-alt-N,N'-methylenebisacrylamide)-N-propionamidomethyl-acrylamide-block-poly(ethylene glycol)bis(N-methyl-2-(methylamino)ethyl carbamate: DMEDA-PEG-DMEDA-(MBA-DMEDA)$_{(n+1)}$-PEG-DMEDA] was modified to contain an integrin-binding peptide ligand "RGDSPASSKP." The conjugation of the ligand was achieved either before or after complex formation. A comparison of the two systems showed that the postcomplexation strategy led to small and discrete toroidal nanoparticles, while the precomplexation particles showed loose complexes. The targeted particles showed an increased uptake into cells compared with unmodified complexes. However, no significant increase in transfection was seen.

Giancotti[108] has found that integrin β_4 is a laminin receptor upregulated in tumor cells and angiogenic endothelial cells. Biochemical studies have indicated that β_4 combines with and enhances the signaling function of multiple receptor tyrosine kinases, including $ErbB_2$, EGF-R, and Met. Genetic studies revealed that β_4 signaling promotes both angiogenesis and tumorigenesis.[109] The author discussed the hypothesis that β_4 promotes both processes by amplifying receptor-tyrosine-kinase signaling. Therefore, the author proposed that a simultaneous blockade of β_4 and receptor-tyrosine-kinase signaling represents a rational approach to cancer and anti-angiogenic therapy.

Schneider et al.[110] have investigated the usefulness of two small synthetic peptides comprising either a linear or a cyclic PLAEIDGIELTY (a synthetic peptide) domain and a DNA-binding moiety of 16 lysine residues to mediate gene transfer selectively into $\alpha_9\beta_1$-integrin-displaying cells. Such specific gene delivery could only be achieved with the peptide containing the cyclic PLAEIDGIELTY domain. However, inclusion of the cationic liposome Lipofectamine into peptide/DNA complexes resulted in an efficient gene transfer for both peptides with significant targeting specificity. The $\alpha_9\beta_1$-integrin is present only in a few highly specialized tissues, but is abundant throughout the human airway epithelia *in vivo*. Targeting gene vectors to this integrin, therefore, appears to be a useful approach to gene therapy of lung diseases such as cystic fibrosis. As the integrin $\alpha_9\beta_1$ is associated with tissue differentiation during fetal development and may cause a resurgence of the fetal phenotype in colon cancers, such vectors may also be applicable for prenatal and cancer gene therapy.

9.3.2.3 Receptor Targeting

Over the past decade, there has been an increasing interest in using nanotechnology for cancer therapy. The development of smart targeted delivery systems (such as liposome, micelles) that can deliver drugs at a sustained rate directly to cancer cells may provide better efficacy and lower toxicity for treating primary and advanced metastatic tumors. We highlight some of the promising classes of targeting molecules that are under development for the delivery systems.

9.3.2.3.1 Folate-Receptor Targeting

Folic acid is a vitamin that is essential for the biosynthesis of nucleotides. It is consumed in elevated quantities by proliferating cells and is transported across the plasma membrane using either the membrane-associated reduced folate carrier or the FR. The former is found in virtually all cells, while the latter is found primarily on polarized epithelial cells and activated macrophages.[88] The reduced folate carrier is capable of internalizing the necessary folate in normal cells. However, FR is frequently overexpressed on tumor cells as a consequence of increased folate requirements, and, furthermore, its expression level increases with advancing stage of the disease.[111]

Yoshizawa et al.[112] developed folate-linked nanoparticles (NP-F) for tumor-targeted siRNA delivery. They evaluated the potential of NP-F-mediated tumor gene therapy in human nasopharyngeal KB cells, which overexpress FR. NP-F showed a significantly higher intracellular amount of siRNA and a stronger localization of siRNA in the cytoplasm than nanoparticles. When the siRNA targeting Her-2 gene was transfected into cells by NP-F and the nanoparticles, NP-F significantly inhibited the tumor growth and selectively suppressed Her-2 protein expression more than nanopartices. In *in vivo* gene therapy, an NP-F nanoplex of Her-2 siRNA by intratumoral injection significantly inhibited the tumor growth of KB xenografts compared with control siRNA, but a nontargeting nanoparticle (NP-P) nanoplex did not.

Liang et al.[113] linked folate (FA) on PEG and then grafted the FA-PEG onto hyperbranched PEI 25 kDa. FA-PEG-grafted-hyperbranched-PEI (FA-PEG-PEI) effectively condensed pDNA into nanoparticles with a positive surface charge. When tested in different cell lines (i.e., HEK 293T, glioma C6, and hepatoma HepG2 cells), no significant cytotoxicity of FA-PEG-PEI was found compared with PEG-PEI. More importantly, a significant increase in transfection efficiency was exhibited in FA-targeted cells. A reporter assay showed that FA-PEG-PEI/pDNA complexes had significantly higher transgene activity than that of PEI/pDNA in FR-positive (HEK 293T and C6) cells but not FR-negative (HepG2) cells.

Luten et al.[114] developed a new cationic biodegradable polyphosphazene, bearing both pendant primary and tertiary amine side groups, viz., poly(2-dimethylaminoethylamine-*co*-diaminobutane) phosphazene (poly(DMAEA-*co*-BA)phosphazene). PEG and PEG-folate were coupled to polyplexes based on this polymer, leading to small (size 100 and 120 nm, respectively) and almost neutral particles. *In vitro* tissue culture experiments showed a low cytotoxicity of both uncoated and coated polyplexes. However, PEG-coated polyplexes showed a twofold lower transfection activity in OVCAR-3 cells as compared with uncoated polyplexes. On the other hand, PEG-folate coated polyplexes had a threefold higher transfection than PEG-coated polyplexes. When free folate was added to the transfection medium, only the transfection activity of the targeted polyplexes was reduced, indicating that the internalization of the targeted PEG polyplexes occurred via the FR.

Yang et al.[115] developed a new method of preparing FR-targeted lipid vesicles that were highly efficient in encapsulating ODN inside. The ODNs formulated in these vesicles were efficiently protected from degradation by nucleases compared with free ODNs. Folate efficiently mediated the intracellular delivery of ODN to KB tumor cells that overexpress FR. The delivery of EGFR antisense ODN via FR-targeted lipid vesicles resulted in a significant down-regulation of EGFR expression in KB cells and cell growth inhibition, far more efficient than that with free ODN or ODN encapsulated in ligand-free lipid vesicles.

Mansouri et al.[116] synthesized and characterized FA-chitosan-DNA nanoparticles and evaluated their cytotoxicity *in vitro*. FA-nanoparticles had lower cytoxicity, good DNA condensation, positive zeta potential, and particle size around 118 nm, which makes them a promising candidate as a nonviral gene vector.

Shi et al.[117] designed FR-targeted pH-sensitive liposomes to promote the efficient release of entrapped agents in response to low pH levels. FR-targeted pH-sensitive liposomes produced increased cytosolic release of entrapped calcein and enhanced cytotoxicity of entrapped cytosine-beta-D-arabinofuranoside, as shown by an 11-fold reduction in the $IC_{(50)}$ (the half maximal inhibitory concentration) in KB cells, compared with FR-targeted non-pH-sensitive liposomes. Furthermore, FR-targeted pH-sensitive liposomes combined with polylysine-condensed pDNA, were shown to mediate FR-specific luciferase gene expression into KB cells in the presence of 10% serum. These findings suggest that cationic lipid-containing pH-sensitive liposomes, combined with FR targeting, are effective vehicles for intracellular gene delivery.

Gao et al.[118] designed a new multifunctional nanodevice (MND) for gene delivery. This MND was equipped with folic acid as a ligand, which was conjugated to the terminal amido of poly(aminopoly(ethylene glycol)cyanoacrylate-*co*-hexadecyl cyanoacrylate) (poly(H(2)NPEGCA-*co*-HDCA)) to synthesize poly(folate-HNPEGCA-*co*-HDCA); PS as a DNA condenser and for nuclear transfer; PEG chain from poly(Folate-HNPEGCA-*co*-HDCA) for decreasing macrophage recognition and extending half-life; and DOPE for endosomal escape. The MND showed the highest transfection efficiency (0.66 ng luciferase/mg protein) in KB cells, which was much higher compared with A549 cells or other formulations such as Lipofectamine. In addition, MND also showed good protection of encapsulated pDNA and low cytotoxicity. The authors concluded that MND could be a potent carrier for NA delivery.

9.3.2.3.2 Targeting Carbohydrate Receptors

Receptors for carbohydrates, such as ASGPR on hepatocytes and mannose receptor (MR) on macrophages and liver endothelial cells, produce opportunities for cell-specific gene delivery with liposomal carriers. In their delivery, however, not only the receptor recognition but also the accessibility to the cell surface plays an important role.

9.3.2.3.2.1 Asialoglycoprotein-Receptor Targeting An ASGPR is a well-characterized molecular target expressed on the hepatocyte surface.[119] There are several galactose- or lactose-terminated compounds, such as asialoorosomucoid,[120] galactosylated poly-L-glutamic acid,[121] asialofetuin glycopeptide,[122] and lactosylceramide[123] that can be used as the targeting ligands in the liver-targeting liposomes, polymers, or nanoparticles.[124]

Watanabe et al.[125] designed a lactosylated cationic liposome carrier for siRNA delivery. siR-NAs targeting the hepatitis C virus (HCV) gene were complexed with cationic liposomes containing lactose residues and transfected into hepatocytes *in vitro* and injected *in vivo*. They efficiently suppressed intrahepatic HCV expression in transgenic mice. Furthermore, this system did not activate the interferon (IFN) system. Their results suggest that lactosylated cationic liposomes have the potential to deliver siRNAs for treating liver diseases.

β-Sitosterol-β-D-glucoside (sito-G) is the major component of soybean sterylglucoside (SG), a kind of plant extract mixture with all the components containing one glucose residue.[15] Both SG and sito-G are recognized specifically by ASGPR and the neutral liposomes containing SG or sito-G could target the liver.[126,127] Meanwhile, SG and sito-G are abundant and inexpensive, and, therefore, may be preferred as liver-targeting ligands. Hwang et al.[128] reported the cationic liposomes containing sito-G as the liver targeting gene delivery carrier with enhanced transfection efficiency. Shi et al.[129] reported that the cationic liposomes containing SG targeted the liver.

Zhang et al.[130] developed co-modified liver-targeting cationic liposomes as a gene carrier to deliver asODN into hepatocytes for treating hepatitis B virus (HBV) infection. Liposomes were conjugated with sito-G and the nonionic surfactant, Brij 35. The asODN-encapsulating cationic liposomes exhibited high transfection efficiency and strong gene inhibition in primary rat hepatocytes and HepG cells, respectively. The ligand, sito-G, was confirmed to enhance ASGPR-mediated endocytosis, the nonionic surfactant Brij 35 seemed to facilitate membrane fusion, and co-modification resulted in efficient transfection, but not enhanced cytotoxicity.

9.3.2.3.2.2 Mannose Receptor Targeting The MR is a 175 kDa type I membrane protein expressed by most tissue macrophages and lymphatic and hepatic endothelia. Macrophages are important targets for the gene therapy of diseases such as Gaucher's disease[131] and human immunodeficiency virus (HIV) infection.[132]

Kawakami et al.[133,134] synthesized a mannosylated cholesterol derivative, cholesten-5-yloxy-*N*-(4-((1-imino-2-b-D-thiomannosylethyl)amino)alkyl)formamide (Man-C4-Chol), for gene delivery to macrophages, which express MRs on their surface. The complexes of pDNA and mannosylated cationic liposomes were recognized and taken up by MRs on mouse peritoneal macrophages. After intravenous injection of pDNA–Man-C4-Chol:DOPE (6:4) liposome complexes in mice, enhanced gene expression was observed in the liver compared with that by pDNA/DC-Chol:DOPE (6:4) liposome complexes, which showed marked expression only in the lung (Figure 9.6). In addition, preferential gene expression was observed in the liver nonparenchymal cells with Man-C4-Chol:DOPE (6:4) liposome/pDNA complexes, which was significantly reduced by predosing with mannosylated bovine serum albumin (BSA). These results suggested that pDNA complexed with mannosylated liposomes exhibits high transfection efficiency in liver non parenchymal cells due to recognition by MRs. This may be attributed to liposome uptake by Kupffer cells around the sinusoidal membranes.

Lu et al.[135] developed mannosylated cationic liposomes *N*-[1-(2,3-dioleyloxy)propyl]-*N*,*N*,*N*-trimethyl ammonium chloride (DOTMA)/cholesten-5-yloxy-*N*-(4-((1-imino-2-D-thioman-nosyl-ethyl)amino)butyl) formamide (Man-C_4-Chol)/Chol (Man-liposomes) to study the targeted delivery of pDNA to antigen-presenting cells (APCs). In this study, they used melanoma-associated antigen expressing pDNA (pUb-M) and Man liposomes to create a novel APC-targeted DNA vaccine against melanoma. They examined its potency by measuring the Ub-M mRNA expression in splenic dendritic cells and macrophages, the cytotoxic T lymphocyte (CTL) activity against melanoma B16BL6 cells, and the melanoma B16BL6-specific anti-tumor effect after intraperitoneal administration. The authors demonstrated that Man-liposomes enhanced pUb-M gene delivery approximately five times higher into dendritic cells and macrophages than unmodified lipoplex and naked DNA. They also strongly induced CTL activity against melanoma, inhibited its growth, and prolonged the survival after tumor challenge, compared with unmodified liposomes. These results demonstrated that Man-liposomes efficiently delivered pDNA to APCs to induce the strong immunopotency of a DNA vaccine against melanoma.

Mannnosylerythritol lipid A (MEL-A), a biosurfactant produced by microorganisms, has many biological activities. Igarashi et al.[136] prepared a MEL-liposome (MEL-L) composed of 3β-[N-(N',N'-dimethylaminoethane)-carbamoyl] cholesterol (DC-Chol), DOPE, and MEL-A and investigated its transfection efficiency in human cervix carcinoma Hela cells. MEL-A induced a significantly higher gene expression, compared with commercially available Tfx20® and the liposome without MEL-A.

Park et al.[137] determined the ability of mesoporous silica nanoparticles (MSN) coupled with mannosylated polyethylenimine (MP), abbreviated as MPS, to transfect pDNA *in vitro*. Cytotoxicity studies showed that MPS/DNA complexes had high cell viability compared with PEI 25K. These complexes showed enhanced transfection efficiency in HeLa cells through receptor-mediated endocytosis via MRs. These results indicate that MPS can be employed as a potential gene carrier for mannose-presenting cells.

9.3.2.3.2.3 CD$_{44}$ Receptor Targeting CD$_{44}$ belongs to a family of multifunctional transmembrane glycoproteins expressed in numerous cells and tissues, including tumor cells and carcinoma tissues.[138] CD$_{44}$ is often expressed in a variety of isoforms, products of a single gene generated by alternative splicing of variant exons, inserted into an extracellular membrane (ECM) proximal domain.[139,140] The expression of certain CD$_{44}$ variant (CD$_{44}$v) isoforms is closely associated with tumor progression. CD$_{44}$ is expressed in both normal and tumor stem cells, displaying a unique ability to initiate normal and/or tumor cell-specific properties. CD$_{44}$ has been suggested as one of the important surface markers for both normal stem cells and cancer stem cells.[141]

The principal ligand of the CD$_{44}$ receptor is hyaluronic acid (HA, hyaluronate, hyaluronan), a linear polymer of repeating disaccharide units [D-glucuronic acid (1-β-3) N-acetyl-D-glucosamine (1-β-4)]n. CD$_{44}$ can, however, interact with several additional molecules such as galectin-8,[142] collagen, fibronectin, fibrinogen, laminin, chondroitin sulfate, mucosal vascular addressin, serglycin/gp600, and osteopontin (OPN). The fact that both CD$_{44}$ and HA are overexpressed at sites of tumor attachment and HA binding to CD$_{44}$ stimulates a variety of tumor cell-specific functions and tumor progression suggests that HA–CD$_{44}$ interaction is a critical requirement for tumor progression. HA can be coupled with an active cytotoxic agent directly to form a nontoxic prodrug. Alternatively, a suitable polymer with covalently attached HA and drug can be used as a carrier.

Direct conjugations of a low molecular weight HA to cytotoxic drugs such as butyric acid,[143] paclitaxel,[144] and doxorubicin[145] have been reported. These conjugates are internalized into cancer cells through receptor-mediated endocytosis, followed by the intracellular release of active drugs, thus restoring their original cytotoxicity. Elron–Gross et al.[146] reported diclofenac encapsulated in bioadhesive liposomes (BAL) carrying HA on their surface (HA-BAL). The therapeutic activity of liposomal diclofenac was evaluated in CT-26 cells that possess CD$_{44}$ HA receptors. The cellular affinity of HA-BAL was 40-fold higher than that of regular liposomes.

Lee et al.[147] prepared novel HA nanogels physically encapsulating green fluorescence protein (GFP) siRNA by an inverse water-in-oil emulsion method. HA/siRNA nanogels were readily taken up by HA receptor positive HCT-116. The release rates of siRNA from HA nanogels could be modulated by changing the concentration of glutathione (GSH) in the buffer solution, indicating that the degradation/erosion of disulfide cross-linked HA nanogels, triggered by an intracellular reducing agent, controlled the release pattern of siRNA. When HA nanogels containing GFP siRNA were co-transfected with GFP plasmid/Lipofectamine complexes to HCT-116 cells, significant GFP gene silencing was observed in both serum and nonserum conditions. The gene silencing effect was reduced in the presence of free HA in the transfection medium, revealing that HA nanogels were selectively taken up by HCT-116 cells via receptor-mediated endocytosis.

Jiang et al.[148] developed a novel target-specific siRNA delivery system using the PEI-HA conjugate. Anti-PGL$_3$(luciferase reporter vectors)-Luc siRNA was used as a model system suppressing luciferase gene expression. The cytotoxicity of siRNA/PEI-HA complex to B$_{16}$F$_1$ cells was lower than that of siRNA/PEI complexes. When B$_{16}$F$_1$ and HEK-293 cells were treated with fluorescein isothiocyanate (FITC)-labeled siRNA/PEI-HA complexes, B$_{16}$F$_1$ cells, with a lymphatic vessel endothelial hyaluronan receptor-1 (LYVE-1) showed higher green fluorescent intensity than HEK-293 cells. This indicated an HA receptor-mediated endocytosis of the complex.

9.3.2.4 Growth Factor Receptors

9.3.2.4.1 Vascular Endothelial Growth Factor Receptors and Ligands

The receptors for vascular endothelial growth factor (VEGF) and related ligands have multiple immunoglobulin G-like extracellular domains and intracellular tyrosine kinase activity.[149,150] In the tumor microenvironment, upregulation of both VEGF and its receptors occurs, leading to a high concentration of occupied receptors on the tumor vascular endothelium. VEGF and its receptors are well-characterized pro-angiogenic molecules and are a target for antiangiogenic therapy.

Kim et al.[151] developed a polyelectrolyte complex (PEC) micelle-based siRNA delivery system for anti-angiogenic gene therapy. The interaction between PEG-conjugated VEGF siRNA and PEI led to the spontaneous formation of PEC micelles (VEGF siRNA-PEG/PEI), having a characteristic siRNA/PEI inner core with a surrounding PEG shell layer. Intravenous as well as intratumoral administration of PEC micelles significantly inhibited VEGF expression at the tumor tissue and suppressed tumor growth in a murine tumor model without any detectable inflammatory responses.

Liu et al.[152] investigated the effects of VEGF (C-term) gene transfer for treating lymphedema using plasmid pcDNA3.1-VEGF-C. They produced a surgical model of the secondary lymphedema in the rat hindlimb and treated it with a local intradermal VEGF-C transfection. The results showed a reduction in lymphedema in the treated group as compared with the control group. Histological and immunofluorescent studies showed numerous newly formed lymphatic vessels in the treated group.

Murata et al.[153] studied the preparation of sustained release poly (DL-lactic/glycolic acid) (PLGA) microspheres encapsulating anti-VEGF siRNA with a carrier (arginine or branched PEI) using the w/o/w in-water drying method. Briefly, 0.4% polyvinyl alcohol (PVA) (W$_1$) containing siRNA, carrier (arginine or PEI), and PLGA was dissolved in CH$_2$Cl$_2$ (O) and homogenized to form W$_1$/O emulsion, and the resulting emulsion was homogenized with 0.25% PVA (W$_2$). The resulting W$_1$/O/W$_2$ emulsion was stirred gently to evaporate the organic solvent. The microspheres were passed through a 75-μm sieve to remove large particles and then sedimented by centrifugation. The PLGA microspheres containing siRNA encapsulated with arginine or PEI were collected by centrifugation, rinsed with distilled water three times, and then lyophilized. There was significant regression of the tumor when these microspheres were administered to mice bearing ascitic tumor cells (S-180) tumors. These results indicate that the microspheres carrying anti-VEGF siRNA achieved a higher level of VEGF gene silencing.

9.3.2.4.2 Insulin-Like Growth Factor Receptors

The insulin-like growth factor-I receptor (IGF-IR) is a tyrosine kinase receptor that has 70% homology with the insulin receptor. When activated by the binding of its ligands (IGF-I and IGF-II), IGF-IR plays a crucial role in cell growth, influencing a number of pathways that regulate proliferation, transformation, and cell survival.[154,155] IGF-IR is also an important factor in tumor metastasis.[156] IGF-IR expression apparently protects cancer cells from apoptosis. A decrease in the level of IGF-IR caused massive apoptosis of tumor cells *in vivo*[157,158] resulting in a significant inhibition of tumorigenesis and metastasis.[159,160]

Since IGF-IR is not an absolute requirement for normal growth, but is essential for the conditions that occur in malignancy, cancer cells may be uniquely susceptible to therapeutic approaches that downregulate IGF-IR levels. For almost a decade, researchers used antisense (AS) molecules to interfere with IGF-IR expression in various tumor models, including human glioblastoma, melanoma, breast, and lung carcinomas.[161] More recently, an expression vector producing an anti-IGF-IR mRNA, that down-regulates IGF-IR, was shown to reverse the transformed phenotype of human cervical cancer cells (even human papillomavirus-16 and -18 positive cell lines), inhibiting tumorigenesis in nude mice.[162] In most of these studies, the tumor cells were treated *ex vivo*. The results were significant enough to lead one group to perform an AS IGF-IR pilot study in patients with malignant astrocytoma.[163] These results demonstrate that a reduction of IGF-I receptor expression can inhibit both the *in vitro* and *in vivo* growth of a human rhabdomyosarcoma cell line and suggest a role for the IGF-I receptor in mediating neoplastic growth in this mesenchymally derived tumor.

Insulin-like growth factor-II/mannose-6-phosphate (IGF-II/M6P) receptor is a single transmembrane domain glycoprotein which recognizes, via distinct sites, two classes of ligands: (1) M6P-containing lysosomal enzymes and (2) IGF-II, a mitogenic polypeptide with structural homology to IGF-I and insulin.[164–166] The IGF-II/M6P receptor is widely distributed in various tissues, including the brain. At the cellular level, a subset of the receptor is located at the plasma membrane, where it regulates the internalization of IGF-II and various exogenous M6P-containing ligands for their subsequent clearance or activation. However, a majority of receptors are expressed within endosomal compartments and are involved in the intracellular trafficking of lysosomal enzymes.

Liver fibrosis is characterized by the abnormal accumulation of extracellular matrix (ECM), namely fibrillar collagens in the hepatic stellate cells (HSCs). Ye et al.[167] developed an antigene approach using a type alpha-1(I) collagen gene promoter specific triplex-forming oligonucleotide (TFO) to inhibit collagen gene expression. To enhance the overall delivery of TFOs to the liver and more specifically to HSCs, these authors synthesized mannose 6-phosphate-bovine serum albumin (M6P-BSA) by phosphorylating *p*-nitrophenyl-alpha-D-mannopyranoside, reducing its nitro group and reacting it with thiophosgene to produce *p*-isothiocyanatophenyl-6-phospho-alpha-D-mannopyranoside (itcM6P) for conjugation with BSA. ^{33}P-TFO was conjugated with M6P-BSA via a disulfide bond, and the stability of $(M6P)_{20}$-BSA-TFO conjugate was determined. Following tail vein injection into rats, $(M6P)_{20}$-BSA-^{33}P-TFO rapidly cleared from the circulation and accumulated mainly in the liver. Almost 66% of the injected $(M6P)_{20}$-BSA-^{33}P-TFO accumulated in the liver at 30 min postinjection, which was significantly higher than that deposited after an injection of ^{33}P-TFO.

9.3.2.5 Peptides and Proteins

Protein and nucleic-acid-based therapeutic molecules such as peptide nucleic acids (PNAs) have provided new perspectives for pharmaceutical research.[168] However, their development is limited by their low stability *in vivo*, poor cellular uptake, and inefficient cellular trafficking. To circumvent these problems, efforts have been harnessed to improve the chemistry of these molecules. Moreover, several delivery systems have been recently developed, including promising tools based on peptide sequences that can cross the cellular barriers. Protein receptors such as transferrin and cell-penetrating peptides (CPPs) such as Tat[169] are covalently linked to their cargoes.

9.3.2.5.1 Transferrin Receptor

T_fR (also known as CD71), a type II transmembrane glycoprotein homodimer (180 kDa) on the surface of cells, is a vital protein involved in iron homeostasis and the regulation of cell growth.[170] T_fR is ubiquitously expressed on normal cells and its expression is upregulated in the cells with a high proliferation rate or on the cells that require large amounts of iron.[171] T_fR expression is significantly upregulated in a variety of malignant cells. In many cases, increased T_fR expression correlates with the tumor stage and is associated with poor prognosis.[172]

Therapeutic genes or pieces of DNA can be delivered to malignant cells via T_f targeted liposomes. Delivery of the anti-angiogenic endostatin gene by the aerosol administration of T_f-liposomes to xenogenic mouse liver tumor-bearing mice inhibited the angiogenesis and the growth of these tumors.[173,174]

T_f-liposomes could also deliver Bcl-2 asODN to human K562 cells.[175] Bcl-2 is an antiapoptotic protein frequently overexpressed in tumors. This overexpression is associated with a resistance to chemotherapy, including daunorubicin.[176] Delivery of Bcl-2 antisense ODNs resulted in a decrease in Bcl-2 expression and a 10-fold increase in K562 sensitivity to daunorubicin.[175] These effects were blocked by the addition of free T_f, indicating that targeting was mediated via T_fR. These studies indicate that therapies targeting T_fR can be used in combination with traditional chemotherapeutic drugs as beneficial treatment modalities for human malignancies.

Liposomes targeting T_fR have been studied to deliver the tumor suppressor gene p53. p53 is a transcription factor that is activated upon DNA damage. It has been termed the "guardian of the genome."[177] Malignant cells often have p53 mutations, compromising its function. The reintroduction of the wild type (wt) p53 gene into malignant cells has been an important goal for gene therapy. T_f-liposomes encapsulating wt p53, in combination with radiotherapy, led to the complete regression of human prostate cancer DU145 xenografts in nude mice.[178] T_fR liposomes also decreased the tumor volume of human prostate cancer PC3 xenografts.[179] The expression levels of p53 correlated with growth inhibition and increased the survival of tumor-bearing mice. T_f-liposomes encapsulating p53 gene also blocked the growth of established human osteosarcoma HOSM-1 xenografts in nude mice and decreased the tumor volume to 1/10th that of control mice.[180]

9.3.2.5.2 Low-Density Lipoprotein Receptor and Its Family Members

The low-density lipoprotein (LDL) receptor is an endocytic receptor that transports relevant macromolecules, mainly the cholesterol-rich lipoprotein LDL, into cells through a process called receptor-mediated endocytosis.[181] This process involves the cell surface receptor recognizing an LDL particle from the ECM, internalizing it through clathrin-coated pits, and transporting it intracellularly via a vesicle.[181–183] Subsequently, the vesicle degrades upon fusion with the lysosome, releasing lipids into the cytoplasm for cell use. Meanwhile, the receptor recycles back to the cell surface to bind another LDL particle.[181–183] Much of our current knowledge of receptor-mediated endocytosis originated from the pioneering studies on the LDL receptor pathway conducted by Goldstein and Brown.[183]

Lipid-based formulations, such as liposomes, can interact with lipoproteins, and the LDL receptor may be involved in the cellular uptake of these lipid complexes. Amin et al.[184–186] attempted to elucidate the mechanisms by which anionic liposomes can interact with neoplastic cells for the site-specific drug delivery of anticancer drugs such as methotrexate. *In vitro* studies using three distinct cell lines, CV1-P, CHO wildtype, and CHOldlA7 (a cell line lacking the LDL receptor) revealed that liposomes could be taken up directly by the LDL receptor. Previous work by the authors showed that a 75–100 mol % egg phosphatidylglycerol (EPG) increased the interaction of the incorporated drugs with the CV1-1P and CHO wild type, which express LDL receptors, compared with CHOldlA7, which lacked these receptors.[127] This suggested an LDL-dependent delivery of anionic liposomes and that it may be mediated by the LDL receptor.

In continuum, all three cell lines, including CHOldlA7, transfected with human LDL receptors were incubated in the presence and absence of two different mAbs—one specific to the LDL receptor and another to apoB100 (IgG-C7 and IgG-5E11, respectively). The results revealed that the treatment groups with the mAb showed a significant decrease in the cellular association of 75–100 mol % EPG liposomes in all three cell lines. It provided further evidence of the role of the LDL receptor in the uptake of these liposomes.

Lakkaraju et al.[187] hypothesized that LDL receptor-related protein (LRP) may be playing a role in the endocytosis of anionic liposome encapsulated oligonucleotides in neurons. The authors encapsulated Cy3-labeled oligonucleotides (Cy3ONs), which were antisense to p53 mRNA, in anionic liposomes and examined its uptake in cultured rat hippocampal neurons by confocal microscopy. Each stage in the endocytic pathway was biochemically interfered with specific proteins to determine the role of that protein in the internalization of the liposomes. In addition, treatment with receptor-associated protein (RAP) and anti-LRP antibody inhibited both the binding and internalization of the liposomes. Meanwhile, fibroblasts which lacked LRP did not internalize the liposomes. They concluded that the anionic liposomes utilized constitutive endocytosis of LRP to enter neurons, followed by intracellular transport and processing via the classical endocytic pathway. Furthermore, Rensen et al.[188] formulated an apoE enriched liposome that mimicked LDL. It showed the site-specific delivery of anti-tumor agents to cancer cells via the LDL receptor both *in vivo* and *in vitro*. In addition, *in vitro* studies in B16 melanoma cells showed the binding of liposomes exclusively to the LDL receptor via the apoE moiety with higher affinity than the LDL itself. They concluded that these apoE liposomes were taken up by the LDL receptor both *in vitro* and *in vivo*.[189,190]

9.3.2.5.3 TAT Peptide

TAT peptide, the most frequently used of the CPPs, is derived from the transcriptional activator protein encoded by human immunodeficiency virus type 1 (HIV-1).[191] Most of the CPPs, such as TAT, oligo-Arg, transportan, and penetratin, are used with covalent-linkage to their cargoes. These CPPs are internalized by cells together with their cargo, essentially through an endocytotic pathway.

TAT peptide-liposomes have also been used for gene delivery. For this, TAT peptide-liposomes prepared with the addition of a small quantity of a cationic lipid (DOTAP) were incubated with DNA. The liposomes formed noncovalent complexes with DNA. The TAT peptide-liposome/DNA complexes, when incubated with mouse fibroblast NIH 3T3 cells and cardiac myocytes H9C2, showed substantially higher transfection *in vitro*, with lower cytotoxicity than the commonly used Lipofectin® reagent. Flow cytometry data demonstrated that the treatment of NIH/3T3 cells with TAT peptide-liposome/pEGFP-N1 complexes had high transfection efficiency.[192] Similar results were obtained with all other cell lines tested. Confocal microscopy confirmed the transfection of various cells with TAT peptide-liposome/DNA complexes. From 30% to 50% of both cell types in the field of view show a bright green fluorescence, while lower fluorescence was observed in virtually all other cells.

In vivo, the intratumoral injection of TAT peptide-liposome/DNA complexes also resulted in efficient transfection. Histologically, hematoxylin/eosin stained tumor slices in both control and experimental animals showed a typical pattern of poorly differentiated carcinoma. However, under the fluorescence microscope, samples from control mice (nontreated mice or mice injected with TAT peptide-free liposome/plasmid complexes) showed only a background fluorescence, while slices from tumors injected with TAT peptide-liposome/plasmid complexes contained bright green fluorescence in tumor cells, indicating an efficient TAT peptide-mediated transfection.[192] This study thus revealed the usefulness of TAT peptide-liposomes for *in vitro* and localized *in vivo* gene therapy.

The potential of TAT peptide-modified liposomes to enhance the delivery of the model gene, GFP, using a plasmid vector pEGFP-N1 to human brain tumor U-87 MG cells was investigated *in vitro* and in an intracranial model in nude mice.[193] The size distribution of DNA-loaded TAT peptide-liposomes was narrow (around 250 nm) and the DNA condensation was evident at lipid/DNA (+/−) charge ratios of 5 and higher. TAT peptide-lipoplexes demonstrated the enhanced delivery of pEGFP-N1 to U-87 MG tumor cells *in vitro* at lipid/DNA (+/−) charge ratios of 5 and 10. *In vivo* transfection of intracranial brain tumors by intratumoral injections of TAT peptide-lipoplexes showed the enhanced delivery of pEGFP-N1 selectively to tumor cells and effective transfection, compared with plain plasmid-loaded lipoplexes. No transfection was noted in the normal brain adjacent to the tumor. Thus, TAT peptide-lipoplexes can be used to augment gene delivery to tumor cells when injected intratumorally, without affecting the normal tissues.

Zhang et al.[194] described a novel approach for the delivery of siRNA encapsulated into liposomes that involves arginine octamer (R8) molecules attached to their outer surface (R8-liposomes), which belongs to a large group of CPPs. The R8-liposomal human double minute gene 2 (HDM2)-siRNA complex demonstrated significant stability against degradation in the blood serum (siRNA-loaded R8-liposomes remained intact even after 24 h incubation). They also showed higher transfection efficiency into the three tested lung tumor cell lines. siRNA delivery was efficient in the presence of plasma proteins and nonspecific toxicity was low. SiRNA in R8-liposomes effectively inhibited target gene expression and significantly reduced the proliferation of cancer cells. This approach offers the potential for siRNA delivery for various *in vitro* and *in vivo* applications.

A potential alternative to the use of liposomal transfection agents is the covalent conjugation of a CPP, with the intention of imparting on the oligonucleotide or siRNA an enhanced ability to enter mammalian cells and reach the appropriate RNA target. Turner et al.[195] developed robust methods for the chemical synthesis of disulfide-linked conjugates of oligonucleotide analogues, siRNA, and PNAs, with a range of cationic and other CPPs. They obtained a reduced expression of P38α MAP kinase mRNA in HeLa cells using μM concentrations of penetratin or TAT peptides conjugated to the 3′-end of the sense strand of siRNA. However, the most promising results to date have been with a 16-mer PNA conjugated to the CPP transportan or a double CPP R(6)-penetratin, where they have demonstrated TAT-dependent trans-activation inhibition in HeLa cells. These results suggested the possibility of the development of CPP-PNA conjugates as anti-HIV agents as well as other potential applications involving nuclear cell delivery, such as the redirection of splicing.

9.3.3 INCREASING LIPOSOME CIRCULATING TIME

The ability to generate long circulating liposomal gene delivery systems using PEGylated lipid should prove useful for systemic gene delivery applications. For instance, the ability of long circulating liposomes to accumulate within tumors is expected to be advantageous for cancer gene therapy applications involving tumor suppressor genes or suicide genes. For example, the avoidance of RES uptake, especially by Kupffer cells, the resident macrophages of the liver, could enhance the opportunity for liposomes to deliver genes to hepatocytes, the target cells of several gene therapies for blood protein deficiencies.

Clearly, if the liposome carrier is not sufficiently stable in plasma under physiological conditions, its contents will be lost before it can be delivered to target tissues. Stability against leakage has been promoted by the use of phospholipids that remain in the gel (solid) phase at physiological temperatures. Thus, DPPC and distearoylphosphatidylcholine (DSPC), which have phase transition temperatures of 48°C and 58°C, respectively, have been widely used for this purpose. The presence of cholesterol at about 33–50 mol % is important both for enhancing stability against leakage[196] and in minimizing phospholipid exchange.[197] The lipid exchange with other structures in circulation, such as red blood cells and lipoproteins, can lead to the depletion of the high phase transition temperature lipids and their replacement with less physiologically stable components.

Lipid purity is a key determinant in optimizing *in vivo* liposome circulation times—as even low levels of impurities in the lipid components can adversely affect liposome biodistribution. Under physiological conditions, lipid impurities, including lysophospholipids,[198] lipid hydrolysis products,[199] unsaturated fatty acids,[200] and uneven chain lengths,[201] can weaken membrane bilayers, potentially causing the loss of their entrapped contents. Also, impurities present at the liposome surface may lead to opsonization, destabilization, and/or an increased rate of removal from the circulation.[202] These impurities can be shielded, in part, by the use of lipids with large, relatively inert, hydrophilic head groups. Phospholipid derivatives of Gm$_1$ monosialoganglioside and PEG provide such steric shielding and have demonstrated prolonged circulation times. Both approaches of high purity lipid components and stearic shielding have been used successfully to produce high circulating drug levels and the preferential delivery of entrapped materials to solid tumors *in vivo*.[203]

PEGylated lipids are widely used in liposomal drug delivery to provide a polymer coat that can confer favorable pharmacokinetic characteristics on particles in the circulation. Recently, these lipids were employed in the self-assembly of cationic and neutral lipids with polynucleic acids to form small, stable lipid/DNA complexes that exhibit long circulation times *in vivo* and accumulate at the sites of disease. However, the presence of a steric barrier lipid might inhibit the transfection efficiency of lipid/DNA complexes by reducing particle-membrane contact. In this study, Song et al.[204] examined the effect of varying the size of the hydrophobic anchor and hydrophilic headgroup of

PEGylated lipids on both gene and antisense delivery into cells in culture. Lipid/DNA complexes were made using unilamellar vesicles composed of 5 mol % PEGylated lipids in combination with equimolar DOPE and the cationic lipid dioleyldimethylammonium chloride. Using HeLa and HepG2 cells, they showed that PEG-lipids had a minimal effect on the binding and endocytosis of lipid/DNA complexes, but they severely inhibited gene transfer and the endosomal release of antisense ODNs into the cytoplasm. Decreasing the size of the hydrophobic anchor or the PEG moiety enhanced DNA transfer by the complexes.

Takeuchi et al.[205] evaluated the circulating properties of liposomes coated with modified PVA (PVA-R: PVA derivatives bearing a hydrophobic anchor (CH–S–) at the terminal of the molecule) with different molecular weights of 6,000, 9,000, and 20,000. The circulation of PVA-R coated liposomes was prolonged by increasing the molecular weight of PVA-R. The aggregation and/or fusion of the liposomes in the presence of serum *in vitro* was also decreased by coating the liposomes

> Under physiological conditions, lipid impurities, including lysophospholipids, lipid hydrolysis products, unsaturated fatty acids, and uneven chain lengths, can weaken membrane bilayers, potentially causing the loss of their entrapped contents. Also, impurities present at the liposome surface may lead to opsonization, destabilization, and/or an increased rate of removal from the circulation.

with PVA-R with a higher molecular weight. There was a good correlation between the circulation time and the physical stability of the uncoated and the various PVA-R coated liposomes. The circulation time of PVA-R (molecular weight 20,000) coated liposomes (ca. 1.3 mol % coating) was comparable with that of a stealth liposome (SL) prepared with 8 mol % of DSPE-PEG (molecular weight of PEG 2000).

9.3.4 TRIGGERED RELEASE (STIMULI-RESPONSIVE LIPOSOMES)

Active targeting has not yet been sufficient to obtain a significantly increased efficacy in the treatment of cancer when compared with passively accumulating PEGylated liposomes. This could be due to the destructive uptake of the liposomes by the target cells, possibly attributable to lysosomal degradation.[206] The receptor targeted strategy, directed against the surface of the tumor cells, leads to the internalization of the liposomes by endocytosis. The endosomes transport their cargo to lysosomes, which may result in the degradation of the carried drugs if the drugs do not escape the severe endosomal/lysosomal environment. Consequently, liposomes have to be designed either to escape the endosomes after cell internalization or to release the drugs outside the cell.

The degradation of the carried drugs also depends on their chemical stability, e.g., anthracyclines are very stable in acid and may have a long half-life in endosomes/lysosomes. The chemical and metabolic stability of the drugs is, therefore, very important and should be considered in relation to active targeting and triggering strategies. Several strategies have been proposed to accomplish site-specific triggered drug release in tumor tissue. Liposomes destabilized by acid[207–209] or by small changes in temperature[210–212] and light[213,214] have been shown to be useful for releasing encapsulated drugs. However, liposomes designed with these specific trigger mechanisms have not yet reached the pharmaceutical market. A more recently proposed principle for site-specific drug release is the enzymatically triggered approach.[215,216]

9.3.4.1 Acid-Triggered Release

The original strategy of using the acidic microenvironment characterizing tumors for triggered release has not been very successful. This is because the highest acidity in tumors is distant from the tumor vasculature. As a result, liposomes often fail to reach this tissue. In addition, the pH of the tumor interstitium rarely declines below 6.5, making it technically difficult to design liposomes that are stable in the blood but disrupt in the tumor tissue. A more viable strategy has been to exploit the acidic environment in endosomes and lysosomes, where the pH level is below 5.0. The triggered release of pH-sensitive liposomes is probably the most biocompatible method for releasing drugs directly in the cytoplasm of cells.

When liposomes are internalized to endosomes, they enter a very acidic environment. However, after cell uptake, the liposomes are eventually delivered to lysosomes[215] where both the carrier and the drug are degraded by metabolic enzymes. To prevent the lysosomal degradation of the carried drug, the drug has to escape the endosomes upon cellular internalization. This has been made possible by the use of FLs, which were discussed earlier. After cell internalization, the pH change triggers a liposome morphology change where a lipid bilayer, Lα, to hexagonal, HII, phase transition occurs (Figure 9.9). The most common strategy has been to use diacylphosphatidylethanolamine (DOPE) as a liposome component. DOPE solely does not form liposomes, but can form liposomes with micelle forming lipids, such as PEGylated lipids. Mixtures of these lipids can form stable liposomes. After acid catalyzed cleavage or removal of the PEGylated lipids from the liposomes, they become fusogenic and are expected to fuse with the endosome membrane leading to drug release into the cytoplasm of the cell.[217]

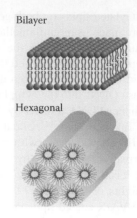

FIGURE 9.9   The phase transition from a lipid bilayer (Lα) to hexagonal.

In the investigation by Tamaddon et al.,[218] a phosphorothioate (PS) ODN was encapsulated in a DODAP-containing cationic liposome by ethanol injection with 73% efficiency. ODN release from endosomes into the cytoplasm was pH-sensitive and was in good agreement with model membrane studies in terms of amount and mechanism. The possible role of acidic pH inside the endosome could be attributed to DODAP, an ionizable amino-lipid, which is neutral at physiologic pH, but becomes cationic at acidic pH of the late endosome. The positive charge facilitates the electrostatic interaction of the liposomes with anionic lipids of the endosomal membrane. This destabilizes the endosomal membrane, leading to the release of ODNs into the cytoplasm from the late endosomal compartment. This process could be diminished by chloroquine-induced pH augmentation. In addition, chloroquine can also act as a calmodulin antagonist and can inhibit late endosome–lysosome interaction.

The triggered release of adsorbed PEG-b-polycation polymers from pH-dependent (PD) liposomes enables protection from immune recognition during circulation (pH 7.4) and the subsequent intracellular delivery of siRNA within the endosome (pH ~ 5.5). Auguste et al.[219] utilized the shift in pH from the bloodstream to the endosome to trigger the release of PEG-b-polycation polymers from PD liposomes. siRNA encapsulation within PEG113 (113 means ethylene glycol repeat units)-DMA31 (31 means DMA repeat units) and PEG113-DMA62 (62 means DMA repeat units) coated PD liposomes resulted in enhanced (up to 10-fold) gene knockdown relative to bare PD and phosphatidylcholine (PC) liposomes.

To enhance the transfection efficiency by promoting the release of lipoplexes from the endosome to the cytoplasm, Shigeta et al.[220] utilized the "proton sponge effect." They synthesized a novel pH-sensitive histidine-modified galactosylated cholesterol derivative (Gal-His-C_4-Chol) for efficient gene delivery to hepatocytes. Since the imidazole group of histidine has a pK_a of 6.0, they expected the Gal-His-C_4-Chol lipoplexes not to have a positively charged imidazole group under neutral conditions. Liposomes containing Gal-His-C_4-Chol showed a 10-fold higher transfection efficiency than conventional Gal-C_4-Chol liposomes in HepG2 cells.

Ponnappa et al.[221] delivered an antisense PS oligonucleotide (S-ODN) targeted against TNF-α mRNA (TJU-2755) using pH-sensitive liposomes. They found that oligonucleotides encapsulated in pH-sensitive liposomes can be used to efficiently deliver oligonucleotides to liver cells. The efficacy of pH-sensitive liposome-encapsulated TJU-2755 was assessed in ethanol-fed animals. Liposomal delivery of TJU-2755 allowed a much lower dose (1.9 mg/kg BW/day for 2 days) of the S-ODN to reduce serum TNF-α (by 54%) and liver injury (by 60%) in ethanol-fed rats. These data indicate that pH-sensitive liposome-encapsulated S-ODNs targeted against TNF-α have therapeutic potential in the treatment of alcoholic liver disease.

9.3.4.2 Light-Triggered Release

Liposomes can be made photosensitive by the use of lipids that either isomerize, fragment, or polymerize upon photoexcitation.[213] Drug release from liposomes by photopolymerization was described by Bondurant et al.[213] They reported a PEG-liposome formulation containing 1,2-bis[10-(20,40-hexadienoyloxy)-decanoyl]-*sn*-glycero-3-phosphocholine (bis-SorbPC), a photosensitive lipid that forms a cross-linked lipid network upon exposure to UV-light. The polymerization causes leakage during the polymerization process due to the formation of defects in the bilayer. However, the use of UV-light is not very suitable for biological applications due to the potential damage to healthy tissue. It is, therefore, desirable to use light with a longer wavelength.

The incorporation of a cyanine dye into the PEG-liposomes made them sensitive to visible light. Collier et al.[222] reported the use of plasmalogen photooxidation as a triggered release strategy. This idea relies on an increase in membrane permeability upon photooxidative cleavage of plasmenyl-choline to single-chain surfactants.

Høgset et al.[223] studied photochemical internalization (PCI) for the light-induced delivery of genes, proteins, and other therapeutic molecules including nonviral and adenoviral vectors. Whereas PCI in general increases the efficiency of transfection with polycations such as polylysine and PEI, its effect on transfection with cationic lipids is much more variable.[224,225] In some cell lines, PCI seems to reduce cationic lipid mediated transfection; while in other cell lines, PCI can have the opposite effect.[226] It also seems that the effect of PCI depends on the type of lipid used for transfection. For example, in HCT 116 cells, PCI can enhance transfection mediated by a haminoethyl-dimyristoyl Rosenthal inhibitor ether (hAE-DMRIE)/DOPE, while hAE-DMRIE-mediated transfection was not affected.[226]

Lipophilic photosensitizers hold the potential for cancer photodynamic therapy. Namiki et al.[227] developed photosensitive stealth liposomes (PSSLs) incorporating a lipophilic photosensitizer into its lipid bilayer. The PSSLs were composed of lipophilic chlorine 6 (Ce6) ester, 2-dilauroyl-*sn*-phosphatidylcholine (DLPC), DOPE, and PEG-2000-DSPE. Its photodynamic effect ($100\,J/cm^2$ of 665 nm diode laser light) was evaluated in gastric cancer cell lines and gastric tumor-bearing nude mice models. In gastric cancer cell lines, the 80% lethal concentration (LC_{80}) of PSSLs was a maximum of 53 times as low as that of Ce6 sodium salt (Ce6-Na). PSSLs completely destroyed all tumors in animal models and tumor recurrence levels were minimal ($1.5\% \pm 0.9\%$). PSSLs achieved greater photodynamic effects in gastric cancer cell lines and in murine models than Ce6-Na. PSSLs hold promise for the photodynamic therapy of gastric cancer.

9.3.4.3 Heat-Triggered Release

In 1978, Yatvin et al.[228] proposed the use of mild local hyperthermia for tumor-specific drug release. Their basic strategy was to design liposomes with the main phase transition just above the physiological temperature and a narrow phase transition region for selective and controlled drug release. Yatvin et al. used DPPC as the main lipid component and added small amounts of DSPC to adjust the main phase transition temperature. In a test system *in vitro*, protein synthesis by *Escherichia coli* was inhibited and killing of the cells was enhanced by heating the neomycin-containing liposomes to their phase transition temperature to maximize drug release. In the presence of serum, the ratio of release at 44°C to that at 37°C can be made greater than 100:1, suggesting possible applications in the treatment of tumors or local infection.

The development of sterically stabilized liposomes led Gaber et al.[229] to design long circulating thermosensitive liposomes that released more than 60% of their contents when heated at 42°C for 30 min *in vitro*. The use of hyperthermia further increases liposome tumor accumulation as a consequence of increased tumor blood flow and increased microvascular permeability. In addition, hyperthermia itself could be cytotoxic.[230]

Various researchers have investigated the modification of liposomes with *N*-isopropyl acrylamide (NIPAAm) copolymers to obtain liposomes with temperature-sensitivity. Han et al.[231]

investigated the surface modification of thermosensitive liposomes using poly(*N*-isopropylacrylam-ide-*co*-acrylamide) (NIPAAm-AAM) and PEG. Drug (doxorubicin) release from NIPAAm-AAM/PEG modified liposomes was increased around the transition temperature of the polymer. In addition, modified liposomes were as stable in the serum as unmodified liposomes. This suggested that NIPAAm-AAM/PEG modified liposomes were suitable for targeted-drug delivery.

Chandaroy et al.[232] studied the temperature-sensitive dioleoylphosphatidylcholine (DOPC) liposomes containing Pluronic® F127 (P-127). P-127 interacts with the liposomal lipid bilayer at an elevated temperature and causes the release of encapsulated fluorescent markers. A concentration of P-127 was critical in destabilizing the liposomal membrane at a precise temperature. The authors further showed that SLs containing PEG 5000-DSPE with P-127 showed similar temperature-dependent drug release.

To achieve a sustained pharmacological activity of ODNs and avoid repeated administrations, Fatal et al.[233] developed a delivery system that combined sustained release and improved intracellular penetration. These systems were designed for the intravitreal delivery of antisense ODNs. They used liposomes dispersed in a thermosensitive gel (poloxamer 407). Both liposomes and microspheres are suitable for the local delivery of ODNs. Thermosensitive gels, such as poloxamer 407, when used alone or in combination with the sterically stabilized liposomes, allow prolonged retention of the ODNs in the vitreous. After intravitreal administration in a rabbit model, liposomes and liposome-gel formulations given 1 day postinjection provided significantly higher drug levels than the control solution of the oligothymidilate pdT16. In addition, there was no significant difference in the amounts of pdT16 found in the vitreous humor between the liposomes and liposome-gel. Nevertheless, because of their better stability in the absence of poloxamer, liposomes alone were allowed to a larger extent to control the delivery of ODNs as compared with the liposome-gel formulations, since 37% of the ODNs were still found in the vitreous 15 days after administration. In addition, the ODNs found in the vitreous humor were protected against degradation by their encapsulation within liposomes.

9.3.4.4 Enzyme-Triggered Release

The use of enzymes that are upregulated in tumor tissue for site-specific drug release is probably the most intriguing trigger principle. Cell-associated proteases have been suggested as possible candidates for the enzymatically triggered drug release from liposomes.[234] Two strategies for the design of lipid conjugates that are activated by proteases were suggested. The first is based on the cleavage of the lipid conjugate, resulting in the generation of fusogenic lipids that destabilize the liposome. The other involves lipid conjugates acting as masking components that protect other fusogenic lipids within the liposome membrane until enzymatic cleavage removes the conjugate.

Davis and Szoka[234] designed liposomes sensitive to alkaline phosphatase. Their liposomes consisted of cholesterol phosphate derivatives and DOPE. It could be induced to collapse upon the phosphatase-catalyzed removal of the phosphate group. This strategy can be used for targeting since the membrane bound forms of phosphatase are overexpressed in tumor tissue.[235] As described under a light-triggered release, Thompson et al. also used enzymes as part of a trigger mechanism. They used phospholipase A2 (PLA2)[236] and transglutaminase[237] for site-specific drug release. Alonso et al.[238,239] used sphingomyelinase and phospholipase C as enzymatic triggers of liposome mixtures of sphingomyelin, PC, phosphatidylethanolamine, and cholesterol to create FLs.

Villar et al.[240,241] suggested that phosphatidylinositol (PI)-specific phospholipase C can be employed for triggered drug release by promoting the site-specific formation of FLs. LUV containing PI, neutral phospholipids, and cholesterol are induced to fuse by the catalytic activity of phosphatidylinositol-specific phospholipase C (PI-PLC). PI cleavage by PI-PLC is followed by vesicle aggregation, intervesicular lipid mixing, and the mixing of vesicular aqueous contents. An average of 2–3 vesicles merge into a large one in the fusion process. Vesicle fusion is accompanied by the leakage of vesicular contents. A novel method has been developed to monitor the mixing of lipids located in the inner monolayers of the vesicles involved in fusion. Using this method, the mixing of inner monolayer lipids and that of vesicular aqueous contents are seen to occur simultaneously, thus giving rise to the fusion pore. Kinetic studies show, for fusing vesicles, second-order dependence of lipid mixing on diacylglycerol concentration in the bilayer. Varying proportions of PI in the liposomal formulation lead to different physical effects of PI-PLC. Specifically, 30–40 mol % of PI lead to vesicle fusion, while with 5–10 mol % PI only hemifusion is detected, i.e., the mixing of outer monolayer lipids without the mixing of aqueous contents. However, when diacylglycerol is included in the bilayers containing 5 mol % PI, PI-PLC activity leads to complete fusion.

Fogged et al.[242] found that long-circulating liposomes, which are sensitive to secretory phospholipase A(2) (sPLA(2)), are feasible delivery systems for the systemic administration of drugs due to their passive targeting to pathological tissue via the enhanced permeability and retention (EPR) effect and their site-specific, enzyme-triggered release of encapsulated drug in response to sPLA(2), which exists locally at elevated levels at, e.g., sites of inflammation. However, recent data suggests that endosomal membrane destabilizing approaches could be used to design sPLA(2)-sensitive liposomes as successful delivery systems for siRNA for systemic administration. Fogged et al.[243] used a double emulsion technique to encapsulate siRNA into SLs designed for the localized, active release of siRNA by sPLA(2). SL siRNA formulation increased the uptake of siRNA into vesicular compartments of HeLa cells in a concentration-dependent manner that could be augmented by exogenous sPLA(2). The authors hypothesized that SL can be used to target siRNAs to inflamed tissues for silencing the cytokine expression in rheumatoid arthritis.

9.3.4.5 Oxidation/Reduction-Triggered Release

A high-redox potential difference (~100- to 1000-fold) exists between the reducing intracellular space and the oxidizing extracellular space. This enables it as a potential stimulus for the delivery of gene therapeutics.[244] Redox-sensitive liposomes rely on the higher intracellular reduction capacity compared with the extracellular milieu.[245] Gene-delivery systems containing disulfide linkages may undergo disulfide cleavage in the lysosomal compartments.[246]

Disulfide (–S–S–) bonds can be used as linkers for targeting conjugates. They can also be used to prepare lipids with disulfide bridges, where the disulfide bond is critical to liposomal stability. Upon reaching intracellular spaces, the thiolated liposomes destabilize in response to glutathione. This destabilizing effect is attributed to the reduction of disulfide bridges of liposomes. As a consequence, the active component encapsulated in liposomes is released intracellularly. Disulfide-mediated redox stimuli-responsive liposomes are prepared using standard phospholipids and a small quantity of lipid whose hydrophobic and hydrophilic parts are linked through a disulfide bond. Such liposomes exhibit stability until they reach a reducing environment that cleaves the disulfide bonds, thus disrupting the liposomal membrane and releasing the liposomal contents.[247]

Thiocholesterol-based cationic lipids (TCL) were synthesized for use in liposomes to encapsulate DNA.[248] The resulting lipoplexes released their content in the presence of low concentrations of reducing agents.[248] TCL can be incorporated into liposomes and used to package DNA into a lipoplex, thereby protecting it from DNase digestion. DNA is rapidly released from the complex in the presence of low concentrations of reducing agents. The lipoplex mediated efficient transfection activity and had low cytotoxicity. To improve the biocompatibility of the cationic lipoplex, TCL were used as a component in the assembly of a nanolipoparticle (NLP). The particle surface was subsequently modified by disulfide exchange to replace the cationic group with a negatively charged (glutathione) or a zwitterionic (cysteine)-reducing agent. A cell-binding ligand (TAT peptide, sequence GRKKRRQRRRGYG) was then incorporated onto the particle surface to enhance the particle-cell recognition. The sequentially assembled cell-binding NLP with a zwitterionic surface gave a larger transfection yield than the cationic NLP at all concentrations tested. At low DNA concentrations, the enhancement was 80-fold. The disulfide cationic lipids and the sequential assembly strategy enable one to tailor the surface charge, hydrophilicity, and recognition elements of a nanosized gene carrier. This results in increased gene transfer activity in a biocompatible particle.

Redox-sensitive liposomes with a long circulation half-life were reported by Kirpotin et al.[249] These liposomes contained detachable disulfide-linked PEG polymer coating.

9.3.5 PHYSICAL METHODS (ULTRASOUND-BASED APPROACHES)

Ultrasound-based approaches increase the transport of the therapeutic agent across the cell membrane or endothelial barriers.[250–253] Using appropriate operating parameters, ultrasound can cause cavitation—a process of nucleation, growth, and oscillation of gaseous cavities. Cavitation involves the rapid growth and collapse of bubbles (inertial cavitation) or sustained oscillatory motion of bubbles (stable cavitation). Both forms of cavitation can produce strong physical–chemical and biological effects in tissues. Most organisms exhibit an innate ability to respond to various environmental insults so as to facilitate robust recovery and minimal long-term effects of the insult. An ultrasound also exerts nonlethal trauma to the biological milieu and can incite a survival response. Biological responses of ultrasounds on cells and tissues have been previously addressed in the literature.[254,255]

Most of these therapies are based on the physical effects of ultrasound on cells and tissues such as the controlled disruption of various biological barriers including cell membranes and tissues for drug and gene delivery.

Ultrasound-enhanced gene delivery has been successfully demonstrated both *in vitro* and *in vivo*.[256] The transfection efficiency of this system is not only influenced by the ultrasonic parameters, the presence of preexistent cavitation nuclei, called ultrasound contrast agents, and the local concentration of pDNA, but also by the transfection agent. Significant enhancement in transfection efficiency was reported in cell culture and *in vivo* using DNA complexes with cationic lipids.[257–259] Ultrasound increased transfection by DNA alone up to 18-fold. PEI complexation of the DNA (polyplex formation) increased transfection up to 90-fold. Most significantly, however, the combination of ultrasound and PEI synergistically increased transfection as much as 200-fold, which resulted in reporter gene expression by 34% of cells.

Kinetic measurements indicated that ultrasound alone acts rapidly, whereas increased transfection by PEI, either alone or in combination with ultrasound, strongly benefited from a 4 h incubation with the DNA plasmid after sonication.[260] Thus, the effect of an ultrasound is expected to be synergistic with a liposome transfection agent, since the ultrasound-enhanced membrane permeability normally occurs at the time of ultrasound application.

The systemic application of naked pDNA in combination with ultrasound was inefficient, probably due to the degradation of the naked DNA by serum nucleases and low DNA concentrations in the environment of sonoporated cells. The combined use of ultrasound with high efficiency transfection agents is a promising direction for ultrasound-enhanced liposomal gene delivery. The newly developed acoustically-active echogenic liposome, in the form of a liposome associated with a gas bubble, provides a platform for such applications. Liposomes composed of PEG, DSPC, and perfluoropropane gas provided a 60% increase in the expression of GFP pDNA in rat eyes when ultrasound (1.2 W/cm^2, 20 s, duty cycle 50%) was applied. The transfection efficiency of such bubble liposomes was 100-fold higher than that of the popular lipofection agent, Lipofectamine 2000.[261,262]

9.4   CONCLUDING REMARKS

The success of gene therapy greatly depends on the delivery vectors, which can be generally categorized as viral and nonviral vectors. Viral vectors have dominated the clinical trials in gene therapy due to their relatively high transduction efficiency. However, after the adverse events in clinical trials (i.e., adenovirus vector caused a patient death in 1999 and retrovirus vector induced a lymphoproliferative disorder in 2002–2003), safety issues of the viral vectors became a major concern.

On the other hand, nonviral vectors are much less immunotoxic. The use of nonviral vectors in clinical trials increased from 23.3% to 26.5% from 2004 to 2007, while that of the viral vector dropped from 70% to 67.4%.[1,263] An ideal gene delivery vector should be effective, specific, long-lasting, and safe. Advances in nonviral gene delivery systems have led to an increased number of products entering into clinical trials.

A full understanding of gene delivery barriers helps the rational design of a more efficient gene carrier.[264] Therefore, intensive mechanistic studies need to be performed to have more insightful information regarding the barriers that prevent the effective transfection of nonviral vectors. We expect to see an increased number of novel materials for overcoming the barriers. The first barrier encounter by the complexes in the course of gene delivery is the outer cell membrane, which serves as a selective size exclusion barrier. The cellular barriers that may be limiting transfection, including endosomal escape and complex unpacking.

Pharmacokinetic studies of the vector allowing the prediction of efficacy and toxicity are expected to become requirements for effective gene delivery. The development of self-assembled nanoparticles dominates the nonviral research because of the manufacturing and stability issues. Significant effort has been put into condensing NAs into particles, whereas the mechanism of unpacking and their release from the carrier requires further studies. Only the released NA is bioavailable. If the payload can be programmed to release only after delivering into the cells, the transfection efficiency can be greatly enhanced.

The rate limiting step for nonviral gene delivery is nuclear translocation. Although there have been extensive studies for improving the nuclear delivery, efficient methods are still limited. Oligonucleotide delivery, including antisense,[265,266] siRNA,[267] and miRNA, is not restricted by this limitation since their site of action is located in the cytoplasm. Additionally, oligonucleotides can be chemically synthesized with high purity and quality, and their stability can be enhanced by chemical modification. It is anticipated that oligonucleotide delivery will be the major focus in the nonviral field. In the meantime, developing a vector that facilitates the nuclear entry of NAs continues to be a major task. For this, investigators may use the experience from the research in viral vectors, which shows great efficiency in nuclear delivery. Finally, more collaboration between nonviral and viral fields should take place, and the communication will provoke novel ideas in the vector design and development.

So what makes for an ideal nanovector? Important for biological function, DNA/siRNA requires protection from enzymatic degradation and cellular uptake without lysosomal compartmentalization; furthermore, convenience and reproducibility of drug production, the ability to target the desired cell type, and a lack of immune response are desirable. The large majority of current nonviral methodologies have relied on nanoparticles or insoluble-complex formation to protect the DNA/siRNA from theDNase/RNase-rich *in vivo* environment as well as help DNA/siRNA cross cellular membranes. Unfortunately, nanoparticle delivery systems have been shown to have limitations *in vivo* due to insufficient biodistribution, low transfection efficiency, rapid plasma clearance, and cellular toxicity. Moreover, multiple nonviral-based delivery methods have been used *in vivo* for delivering siRNA, including hydrodynamic injection, cationic liposome encapsulation, the formation of cationic complexes, and antibody-specific targeting delivery systems.

Most of the current gene therapy approaches make use of viral vectors. Due to the high transduction efficiency for different quiescent and dividing cell types, viral delivery systems require a powerful technique to deliver DNA to cells. High-titer concentrations ($>10^8$ viral particles per milliliter) allow many cells to be infected; however, problems such as the danger of viral toxicity and relatively strong host responses resulting from the activation of the human immune system are to be solved.

There is still no perfect nanoscaled delivery system that achieves all of the requirements. Each of the current methods of gene delivery, whether viral or nonviral, have some limitations, and maybe there will never be a generalized delivery system for all applications; instead, the choice of vector would depend on its use. All of these desired properties exist in various delivery systems, so an ideal vector may have properties from both types of system—viral and nonviral.[268]

REFERENCES

1. Edelstein ML, Abedi MR, Wixon J. Gene therapy clinical trials worldwide to 2007—An update. *J Gene Med* 2007; **9**: 833–842.
2. Shi F, Rakhmilevich AL, Heise CP, Oshikawa K, Sondel PM, Yang N-S, Mahvi DM. Intratumoral injection of interleukin-12 plasmid DNA, either naked or in complex with cationic lipid, results in similar tumor regression in a murine model. *Mol Cancer Ther* 2002; **1**: 949–957.
3. Walther W, Stein U, Voss C, Schmidt T, Schleef M, Schlag PM. Stability analysis for long-term storage of naked DNA: Impact on nonviral in vivo gene transfer. *Anal Biochem* 2003; **318**: 230–235.
4. Mansouri S, Lavigne P, Corsi K, Benderdour M, Beaumont E, Fernandes JC. Chitosan-DNA nanoparticles as non-viral vectors in gene therapy: Strategies to improve transfection efficacy. *Eur J Pharm Biopharm* 2004; **57**: 1–8.
5. El-Aneed A. An overview of current delivery systems in cancer gene therapy. *J Control Release* 2004; **94**: 1–14.
6. Kim KH, Yoon DJ, Moon YA, Kim YS. Expression and localization of human papillomavirus type 16 E6 and E7 open reading frame proteins in human epidermal keratinocyte. *Yonsei Med J* 1994; **35**: 1–9.
7. Varmus H. Retroviruses. *Science* 1988; **240**: 1427–1435.
8. Muzyczka N. Use of adeno-associated virus as a general transduction vector for mammalian cells. *Curr Top Microbiol Immunol* 1992; **158**: 97–129.
9. Akhtar S, Hughes MD, Khan A, Bibby M, Hussain M, Nawaz Q, Double J, Sayyed P. The delivery of antisense therapeutics. *Adv Drug Deliv Rev* 2000; **44**: 3–21.
10. Eliyahu H, Barenholz Y, Domb AJ. Polymers for DNA delivery. *Molecules* 2005; **10**: 34–64.
11. Pack DW, Hoffman AS, Pun S, Stayton PS. Design and development of polymers for gene delivery. *Nat Rev Drug Discov* 2005; **4**: 581–593.
12. Kreiss P, Cameron B, Rangara R, Mailhe P, Aguerre-Charriol O, Airiau M, Scherman D, Crouzet J, Pitard B. Plasmid DNA size does not affect the physicochemical properties of lipoplexes but modulates gene transfer efficiency. *Nucleic Acids Res* 1999; **27**: 3792–3798.
13. Corsi K, Chellat F, Yahia L, Fernandes JC. Mesenchymal stem cells, MG63 and HEK293 transfection using chitosan-DNA nanoparticles. *Biomaterials* 2003; **24**: 1255–1264.
14. Pedroso de Lima MC, Simoes S, Pires P, Faneca H, Duzgunes N. Cationic lipid-DNA complexes in gene delivery: From biophysics to biological applications. *Adv Drug Deliv Rev* 2001; **47**: 277–294.
15. Gao X, Huang L. Cationic liposome-mediated gene transfer. *Gene Ther* 1995; **2**: 710–722.
16. Liu Y, Liggitt D, Zhong W, Tu G, Gaensler K, Debs R. Cationic liposome-mediated intravenous gene delivery. *J Biol Chem* 1995; **270**: 24864–24870.
17. Ramesh R, Saeki T, Templeton NS, Ji L, Stephens LC, Ito I, Wilson DR, Wu Z, Branch CD, Minna JD, Roth JA. Successful treatment of primary and disseminated human lung cancers by systemic delivery of tumor suppressor genes using an improved liposome vector. *Mol Ther* 2001; **3**: 337–350.
18. Dass CR, Walker TL, Decruz EE, Burton MA. Cationic liposomes and gene therapy for solid tumors. *Drug Deliv* 1997; **4**: 151–165.
19. Bangham AD, Standish MM, Watkins JC. Diffusion of univalent ions across the lamellae of swollen phospholipids. *J Mol Biol* 1965; **13**: 238–252.
20. Voinea M, Simionescu M. Designing of 'intelligent' liposomes for efficient delivery of drugs. *J Cell Mol Med* 2002; **6**: 465–474.
21. Grabielle-Madelmont C, Lesieur S, Ollivon M. Characterization of loaded liposomes by size exclusion chromatography. *J Biochem Biophys Methods* 2003; **56**: 189–217.
22. Lebedeva I, Benimetskaya L, Stein CA, Vilenchik M. Cellular delivery of antisense oligonucleotides. *Eur J Pharm Biopharm* 2000; **50**: 101–119.
23. Simoes S, Slepushkin V, Gaspar R, de Lima MC, Duzgunes N. Gene delivery by negatively charged ternary complexes of DNA, cationic liposomes and transferrin or fusigenic peptides. *Gene Ther* 1998; **5**: 955–964.
24. Ma Z, Li J, He F, Wilson A, Pitt B, Li S. Cationic lipids enhance siRNA-mediated interferon response in mice. *Biochem Biophys Res Commun* 2005; **330**: 755–759.

25. Spagnou S, Miller AD, Keller M. Lipidic carriers of siRNA: Differences in the formulation, cellular uptake, and delivery with plasmid DNA. *Biochemistry* 2004; **43**: 13348–13356.
26. Sioud M, Sorensen DR. Cationic liposome-mediated delivery of siRNAs in adult mice. *Biochem Biophys Res Commun* 2003; **312**: 1220–1225.
27. Dalby B, Cates S, Harris A, Ohki EC, Tilkins ML, Price PJ, Ciccarone VC. Advanced transfection with Lipofectamine 2000 reagent: Primary neurons, siRNA, and high-throughput applications. *Methods* 2004; **33**: 95–103.
28. Brazas RM, Hagstrom JE. Delivery of small interfering RNA to mammalian cells in culture by using cationic lipid/polymer-based transfection reagents. *Methods Enzymol* 2005; **392**: 112–124.
29. Dass CR, Su T. Delivery of lipoplexes for genotherapy of solid tumours: Role of vascular endothelial cells. *J Pharm Pharmacol* 2000; **52**: 1301–1317.
30. Dass CR, Saravolac EG, Li Y, Sun LQ. Cellular uptake, distribution, and stability of 10–23 deoxyribozymes. *Antisense Nucleic Acid Drug Dev* 2002; **12**: 289–299.
31. Wong FM, Reimer DL, Bally MB. Cationic lipid binding to DNA: Characterization of complex formation. *Biochemistry* 1996; **35**: 5756–5763.
32. Liu F, Huang L. Development of non-viral vectors for systemic gene delivery. *J Control Release* 2002; **78**: 259–266.
33. Ohki EC, Tilkins ML, Ciccarone VC, Price PJ. Improving the transfection efficiency of post-mitotic neurons. *J Neurosci Methods* 2001; **112**: 95–99.
34. Sugiyama M, Matsuura M, Takeuchi Y, Kosaka J, Nango M, Oku N. Possible mechanism of polycation liposome (PCL)-mediated gene transfer. *Biochim Biophys Acta* 2004; **1660**: 24–30.
35. Yamazaki Y, Nango M, Matsuura M, Hasegawa Y, Hasegawa M, Oku N. Polycation liposomes, a novel nonviral gene transfer system, constructed from cetylated polyethylenimine. *Gene Ther* 2000; **7**: 1148–1155.
36. Oku N, Yamazaki Y, Matsuura M, Sugiyama M, Hasegawa M, Nango M. A novel non-viral gene transfer system, polycation liposomes. *Adv Drug Deliv Rev* 2001; **52**: 209–218.
37. Pollard H, Remy JS, Loussouarn G, Demolombe S, Behr JP, Escande D. Polyethylenimine but not cationic lipids promotes transgene delivery to the nucleus in mammalian cells. *J Biol Chem* 1998; **273**: 7507–7511.
38. Kircheis R, Kichler A, Wallner G, Kursa M, Ogris M, Felzmann T, Buchberger M, Wagner E. Coupling of cell-binding ligands to polyethylenimine for targeted gene delivery. *Gene Ther* 1997; **4**: 409–418.
39. Gao X, Huang L. Potentiation of cationic liposome-mediated gene delivery by polycations. *Biochemistry* 1996; **35**: 1027–1036.
40. Li S, Huang L. In vivo gene transfer via intravenous administration of cationic lipid-protamine-DNA (LPD) complexes. *Gene Ther* 1997; **4**: 891–900.
41. Ibanez M, Gariglio P, Chavez P, Santiago R, Wong C, Baeza I. Spermidine-condensed DNA and cone-shaped lipids improve delivery and expression of exogenous DNA transfer by liposomes. *Biochem Cell Biol* 1996; **74**: 633–643.
42. Yu RZ, Geary RS, Leeds JM, Watanabe T, Fitchett JR, Matson JE, Mehta R, Hardee GR, Templin MV, Huang K, Newman MS, Quinn Y, Uster P, Zhu G, Working PK, Horner M, Nelson J, Levin AA. Pharmacokinetics and tissue disposition in monkeys of an antisense oligonucleotide inhibitor of Ha-ras encapsulated in stealth liposomes. *Pharm Res* 1999; **16**: 1309–1315.
43. Hu Y, Jin Y, Xia Y. The characterization of cationic fusogenic liposomes mediated antisense oligonucleotides into HeLa cells. *Drug Dev Ind Pharm* 2004; **30**: 135–141.
44. Meyer O, Kirpotin D, Hong K, Sternberg B, Park JW, Woodle MC, Papahadjopoulos D. Cationic liposomes coated with polyethylene glycol as carriers for oligonucleotides. *J Biol Chem* 1998; **273**: 15621–15627.
45. Litzinger DC, Brown JM, Wala I, Kaufman SA, Van GY, Farrell CL, Collins D. Fate of cationic liposomes and their complex with oligonucleotide in vivo. *Biochim Biophys Acta* 1996; **1281**: 139–149.
46. Yamauchi M, Kusano H, Saito E, Iwata T, Nakakura M, Kato Y, Uochi T, Akinaga S, Aoki N. Improved formulations of antisense oligodeoxynucleotides using wrapped liposomes. *J Control Release* 2006; **114**: 268–275.
47. Yamauchi M, Kusano H, Saito E, Iwata T, Nakakura M, Kato Y, Aoki N. Development of wrapped liposomes: Novel liposomes comprised of polyanion drug and cationic lipid complexes wrapped with neutral lipids. *Biochim Biophys Acta* 2006; **1758**: 90–97.
48. Ellens H, Bentz J, Szoka FC. Fusion of phosphatidylethanolamine-containing liposomes and mechanism of the L alpha-HII phase transition. *Biochemistry* 1986; **25**: 4141–4147.

49. Wang CY, Huang L. Highly efficient DNA delivery mediated by pH-sensitive immunoliposomes. *Biochemistry* 1989; **28**: 9508–9514.

50. El Baraka M, Pecheur EI, Wallach DF, Philippot JR. Non-phospholipid fusogenic liposomes. *Biochim Biophys Acta* 1996; **1280**: 107–114.

51. Tari AM, Zhou F, Huang L. Two types of pH-sensitive immunoliposomes, in *Liposome Technology*, G. Gregoriadis, Ed., 1993, CRC Press: Boca Raton, FL, pp. 289–300.

52. Fillion P, Desjardins A, Sayasith K, Lagace J. Encapsulation of DNA in negatively charged liposomes and inhibition of bacterial gene expression with fluid liposome-encapsulated antisense oligonucleotides. *Biochim Biophys Acta* 2001; **1515**: 44–54.

53. Compagnon B, Milhaud P, Bienvenue A, Philippot JR. Targeting of poly(rI)-poly(rC) by fusogenic (F protein) immunoliposomes. *Exp Cell Res* 1992; **200**: 333–338.

54. de Fiebre CM, Bryant SO, Notabartolo D, Wu P, Meyer EM. Fusogenic properties of Sendai virosome envelopes in rat brain preparations. *Neurochem Res* 1993; **18**: 1089–1094.

55. Bron R, Ortiz A, Wilschut J. Cellular cytoplasmic delivery of a polypeptide toxin by reconstituted influenza virus envelopes (virosomes). *Biochemistry* 1994; **33**: 9110–9117.

56. Glushakova SE, Omelyanenko VG, Lukashevitch IS, Bogdanov AA Jr., Moshnikova AB, Kozytch AT, Torchilin VP. The fusion of artificial lipid membranes induced by the synthetic arenavirus 'fusion peptide'. *Biochim Biophys Acta* 1992; **1110**: 202–208.

57. Kunisawa J, Nakagawa S, Mayumi T. Pharmacotherapy by intracellular delivery of drugs using fusogenic liposomes: Application to vaccine development. *Adv Drug Deliv Rev* 2001; **52**: 177–186.

58. Murthy N, Xu M, Schuck S, Kunisawa J, Shastri N, Frechet JM. A macromolecular delivery vehicle for protein-based vaccines: Acid-degradable protein-loaded microgels. *Proc Natl Acad Sci USA* 2003; **100**: 4995–5000.

59. Morris MC, Depollier J, Mery J, Heitz F, Divita G. A peptide carrier for the delivery of biologically active proteins into mammalian cells. *Nat Biotechnol* 2001; **19**: 1173–1176.

60. Mathew E, Hardee GE, Bennett CF, Lee KD. Cytosolic delivery of antisense oligonucleotides by listeriolysin O-containing liposomes. *Gene Ther* 2003; **10**: 1105–1115.

61. Mizuguchi H, Nakagawa T, Nakanishi M, Imazu S, Nakagawa S, Mayumi T. Efficient gene transfer into mammalian cells using fusogenic liposome. *Biochem Biophys Res Commun* 1996; **218**: 402–407.

62. Mizuguchi H, Nakagawa T, Toyosawa S, Nakanishi M, Imazu S, Nakanishi T, Tsutsumi Y, Nakagawa S, Hayakawa T, Ijuhin N, Mayumi T. Tumor necrosis factor alpha-mediated tumor regression by the in vivo transfer of genes into the artery that leads to tumors. *Cancer Res* 1998; **58**: 5725–5730.

63. Mizuguchi H, Nakanishi M, Nakanishi T, Nakagawa T, Nakagawa S, Mayumi T. Application of fusogenic liposomes containing fragment A of diphtheria toxin to cancer therapy. *Br J Cancer* 1996; **73**: 472–476.

64. Nakanishi T, Hayashi A, Kunisawa J, Tsutsumi Y, Tanaka K, Yashiro-Ohtani Y, Nakanishi M, Fujiwara H, Hamaoka T, Mayumi T. Fusogenic liposomes efficiently deliver exogenous antigen through the cytoplasm into the MHC class I processing pathway. *Eur J Immunol* 2000; **30**: 1740–1747.

65. Hayashi A, Nakanishi T, Kunisawa J, Kondoh M, Imazu S, Tsutsumi Y, Tanaka K, Fujiwara H, Hamaoka T, Mayumi T. A novel vaccine delivery system using immunopotentiating fusogenic liposomes. *Biochem Biophys Res Commun* 1999; **261**: 824–828.

66. Kunisawa J, Nakanishi T, Takahashi I, Okudaira A, Tsutsumi Y, Katayama K, Nakagawa S, Kiyono H, Mayumi T. Sendai virus fusion protein mediates simultaneous induction of MHC class I/II-dependent mucosal and systemic immune responses via the nasopharyngeal-associated lymphoreticular tissue immune system. *J Immunol* 2001; **167**: 1406–1412.

67. Sakaue G, Hiroi T, Nakagawa Y, Someya K, Iwatani K, Sawa Y, Takahashi H, Honda M, Kunisawa J, Kiyono H. HIV mucosal vaccine: Nasal immunization with gp160-encapsulated hemagglutinating virus of Japan-liposome induces antigen-specific CTLs and neutralizing antibody responses. *J Immunol* 2003; **170**: 495–502.

68. Kunisawa J, Masuda T, Katayama K, Yoshikawa T, Tsutsumi Y, Akashi M, Mayumi T, Nakagawa S. Fusogenic liposome delivers encapsulated nanoparticles for cytosolic controlled gene release. *J Control Release* 2005; **105**: 344–353.

69. Sakaguchi N, Kojima C, Harada A, Koiwai K, Shimizu K, Emi N, Kono K. Enhancement of transfection activity of lipoplexes by complexation with transferrin-bearing fusogenic polymer-modified liposomes. *Int J Pharm* 2006; **325**: 186–190.

70. Patil SD, Rhodes DG, Burgess DJ. Anionic liposomal delivery system for DNA transfection. *AAPS J* 2004; **6**: e29.

71. Lakkaraju A, Dubinsky JM, Low WC, Rahman YE. Neurons are protected from excitotoxic death by p53 antisense oligonucleotides delivered in anionic liposomes. *J Biol Chem* 2001; **276**: 32000–32007.

72. Patil SD, Rhodes DG, Burgess DJ. Biophysical characterization of anionic lipoplexes. *Biochim Biophys Acta* 2005; **1711**: 1–11.

73. Beaulac C, Clement-Major S, Hawari J, Lagace J. Eradication of mucoid *Pseudomonas aeruginosa* with fluid liposome-encapsulated tobramycin in an animal model of chronic pulmonary infection. *Antimicrob Agents Chemother* 1996; **40**: 665–669.

74. Schiffelers RM, Storm G, ten Kate MT, Bakker-Woudenberg IA. Therapeutic efficacy of liposome-encapsulated gentamicin in rat *Klebsiella pneumoniae* pneumonia in relation to impaired host defense and low bacterial susceptibility to gentamicin. *Antimicrob Agents Chemother* 2001; **45**: 464–470.

75. Beaulac C, Clement-Major S, Hawari J, Lagace J. In vitro kinetics of drug release and pulmonary retention of microencapsulated antibiotic in liposomal formulations in relation to the lipid composition. *J Microencapsul* 1997; **14**: 335–348.

76. Sachetelli S, Khalil H, Chen T, Beaulac C, Senechal S, Lagace J. Demonstration of a fusion mechanism between a fluid bactericidal liposomal formulation and bacterial cells. *Biochim Biophys Acta* 2000; **1463**: 254–266.

77. Sachetelli S, Beaulac C, Riffon R, Lagace J. Evaluation of the pulmonary and systemic immunogenicity of Fluidosomes, a fluid liposomal-tobramycin formulation for the treatment of chronic infections in lungs. *Biochim Biophys Acta* 1999; **1428**: 334–340.

78. Desjardins A, Chen T, Khalil H, Sayasith K, Lagace J. Differential behaviour of fluid liposomes toward mammalian epithelial cells and bacteria: Restriction of fusion to bacteria. *J Drug Target* 2002; **10**: 47–54.

79. Larsen HJ, Bentin T, Nielsen PE. Antisense properties of peptide nucleic acid. *Biochim Biophys Acta* 1999; **1489**: 159–166.

80. Wang S, Lee RJ, Cauchon G, Gorenstein DG, Low PS. Delivery of antisense oligodeoxyribonucleotides against the human epidermal growth factor receptor into cultured KB cells with liposomes conjugated to folate via polyethylene glycol. *Proc Natl Acad Sci USA* 1995; **92**: 3318–3322.

81. Leonetti C, Biroccio A, Benassi B, Stringaro A, Stoppacciaro A, Semple SC, Zupi G. Encapsulation of c-myc antisense oligodeoxynucleotides in lipid particles improves antitumoral efficacy in vivo in a human melanoma line. *Cancer Gene Ther* 2001; **8**: 459–468.

82. Torchilin V. Multifunctional and stimuli-sensitive pharmaceutical nanocarriers. *Eur J Pharm Biopharm* 2009; **71**: 431–444.

83. Park JW, Kirpotin DB, Hong K, Shalaby R, Shao Y, Nielsen UB, Marks JD, Papahadjopoulos D, Benz CC. Tumor targeting using anti-her2 immunoliposomes. *J Control Release* 2001; **74**: 95–113.

84. Park JW, Hong K, Kirpotin DB, Colbern G, Shalaby R, Baselga J, Shao Y, Nielsen UB, Marks JD, Moore D, Papahadjopoulos D, Benz CC. Anti-HER2 immunoliposomes: Enhanced efficacy attributable to targeted delivery. *Clin Cancer Res* 2002; **8**: 1172–1181.

85. Sapra P, Allen TM. Ligand-targeted liposomal anticancer drugs. *Prog Lipid Res* 2003; **42**: 439–462.

86. Lu Y, Low PS. Folate-mediated delivery of macromolecular anticancer therapeutic agents. *Adv Drug Deliv Rev* 2002; **54**: 675–693.

87. Aronov O, Horowitz AT, Gabizon A, Gibson D. Folate-targeted PEG as a potential carrier for carboplatin analogs. Synthesis and in vitro studies. *Bioconjug Chem* 2003; **14**: 563–574.

88. Lu Y, Low PS. Immunotherapy of folate receptor-expressing tumors: Review of recent advances and future prospects. *J Control Release* 2003; **91**: 17–29.

89. Arap W, Pasqualini R, Ruoslahti E. Cancer treatment by targeted drug delivery to tumor vasculature in a mouse model. *Science* 1998; **279**: 377–380.

90. Hood JD, Bednarski M, Frausto R, Guccione S, Reisfeld RA, Xiang R, Cheresh DA. Tumor regression by targeted gene delivery to the neovasculature. *Science* 2002; **296**: 2404–2407.

91. Remy JS, Kichler A, Mordvinov V, Schuber F, Behr JP. Targeted gene transfer into hepatoma cells with lipopolyamine-condensed DNA particles presenting galactose ligands: A stage toward artificial viruses. *Proc Natl Acad Sci USA* 1995; **92**: 1744–1748.

92. Zanta MA, Boussif O, Adib A, Behr JP. In vitro gene delivery to hepatocytes with galactosylated polyethylenimine. *Bioconjug Chem* 1997; **8**: 839–844.

93. Koning GA, Morselt HW, Gorter A, Allen TM, Zalipsky S, Scherphof GL, Kamps JA. Interaction of differently designed immunoliposomes with colon cancer cells and Kupffer cells. An in vitro comparison. *Pharm Res* 2003; **20**: 1249–1257.

94. Maruyama K, Ishida O, Takizawa T, Moribe K. Possibility of active targeting to tumor tissues with liposomes. *Adv Drug Deliv Rev* 1999; **40**: 89–102.

95. Pan X, Lee RJ. Construction of anti-EGFR immunoliposomes via folate-folate binding protein affinity. *Int J Pharm* 2007; **336**: 276–283.

96. Marty C, Langer-Machova Z, Sigrist S, Schott H, Schwendener RA, Ballmer-Hofer K. Isolation and characterization of a scFv antibody specific for tumor endothelial marker 1 (TEM1), a new reagent for targeted tumor therapy. *Cancer Lett* 2006; **235**: 298–308.

97. Brignole C, Marimpietri D, Pagnan G, Di Paolo D, Zancolli M, Pistoia V, Ponzoni M, Pastorino F. Neuroblastoma targeting by c-myb-selective antisense oligonucleotides entrapped in anti-GD2 immuno-liposome: Immune cell-mediated anti-tumor activities. *Cancer Lett* 2005; **228**: 181–186.

98. Zhang Y, Zhang YF, Bryant J, Charles A, Boado RJ, Pardridge WM. Intravenous RNA interference gene therapy targeting the human epidermal growth factor receptor prolongs survival in intracranial brain cancer. *Clin Cancer Res* 2004; **10**: 3667–3677.

99. Gosk S, Moos T, Gottstein C, Bendas G. VCAM-1 directed immunoliposomes selectively target tumor vasculature in vivo. *Biochim Biophys Acta* 2008; **1778**: 854–863.

100. Völkel T, Hölig P, Merdan T, Müller R, Kontermann RE. Targeting of immunoliposomes to endothelial cells using a single-chain Fv fragment directed against human endoglin (CD105). *Biochim Biophys Acta* 2004; **1663**: 158–166.

101. Akhtar S, Basu S, Wickstrom E, Juliano RL. Interactions of antisense DNA oligonucleotide analogs with phospholipid membranes (liposomes). *Nucleic Acids Res* 1991; **19**: 5551–5559.

102. Ma DD, Wei AQ. Enhanced delivery of synthetic oligonucleotides to human leukaemic cells by lipo-somes and immunoliposomes. *Leuk Res* 1996; **20**: 925–930.

103. Hölig P, Bach M, Völkel T, Nahde T, Hoffmann S, Müller R, Kontermann RE. Novel RGD lipopeptides for the targeting of liposomes to integrin-expressing endothelial and melanoma cells. *Protein Eng Des Sel* 2004; **17**: 433–441.

104. Townsend PA, Villanova I, Uhlmann E, Peyman A, Knolle J, Baron R, Teti A, Horton MA. An antisense oligonucleotide targeting the alphaV integrin gene inhibits adhesion and induces apoptosis in breast cancer cells. *Eur J Cancer* 2000; **36**: 397–409.

105. Partlow KC, Lanza GM, Wickline SA. Exploiting lipid raft transport with membrane targeted nanopar-ticles: A strategy for cytosolic drug delivery. *Biomaterials* 2008; **29**: 3367–3375.

106. Hallahan D, Geng L, Qu S, Scarfone C, Giorgio T, Donnelly E, Gao X, Clanton J. Integrin-mediated targeting of drug delivery to irradiated tumor blood vessels. *Cancer Cell* 2003; **3**: 63–74.

107. Parkhouse SM, Garnett MC, Chan WC. Targeting of polyamidoamine-DNA nanoparticles using the Staudinger ligation: Attachment of an RGD motif either before or after complexation. *Bioorg Med Chem* 2008; **16**: 6641–6650.

108. Giancotti FG. Targeting integrin beta4 for cancer and anti-angiogenic therapy. *Trends Pharmacol Sci* 2007; **28**: 506–511.

109. Nikolopoulos SN, Blaikie P, Yoshioka T, Guo W, Giancotti FG. Integrin beta4 signaling promotes tumor angiogenesis. *Cancer Cell* 2004; **6**: 471–483.

110. Schneider H, Harbottle RP, Yokosaki Y, Jost P, Coutelle C. Targeted gene delivery into alpha9beta1-integrin-displaying cells by a synthetic peptide. *FEBS Lett* 1999; **458**: 329–332.

111. Toffoli G, Cernigoi C, Russo A, Gallo A, Bagnoli M, Boiocchi M. Overexpression of folate binding protein in ovarian cancers. *Int J Cancer* 1997; **74**: 193–198.

112. Yoshizawa T, Hattori Y, Hakoshima M, Koga K, Maitani Y. Folate-linked lipid-based nanoparticles for synthetic siRNA delivery in KB tumor xenografts. *Eur J Pharm Biopharm* 2008; **70**: 718–725.

113. Liang B, He ML, Xiao ZP, Li Y, Chan CY, Kung HF, Shuai XT, Peng Y. Synthesis and characterization of folate-PEG-grafted-hyperbranched-PEI for tumor-targeted gene delivery. *Biochem Biophys Res Commun* 2008; **367**: 874–880.

114. Luten J, van Steenbergen MJ, Lok MC, de Graaff AM, van Nostrum CF, Talsma H, Hennink WE. Degradable PEG-folate coated poly(DMAEA-*co*-BA)phosphazene-based polyplexes exhibit receptor-specific gene expression. *Eur J Pharm Sci* 2008; **33**: 241–251.

115. Yang L, Li J, Zhou W, Yuan X, Li S. Targeted delivery of antisense oligodeoxynucleotides to folate receptor-overexpressing tumor cells. *J Control Release* 2004; **95**: 321–331.

116. Mansouri S, Cuie Y, Winnik F, Shi Q, Lavigne P, Benderdour M, Beaumont E, Fernandes JC. Characterization of folate-chitosan-DNA nanoparticles for gene therapy. *Biomaterials* 2006; **27**: 2060–2065.

117. Shi G, Guo W, Stephenson SM, Lee RJ. Efficient intracellular drug and gene delivery using folate receptor-targeted pH-sensitive liposomes composed of cationic/anionic lipid combinations. *J Control Release* 2002; **80**: 309–319.

118. Gao Y, Gu W, Chen L, Xu Z, Li Y. A multifunctional nano device as non-viral vector for gene delivery: In vitro characteristics and transfection. *J Control Release* 2007; **118**: 381–388.

119. Kim KS, Lei Y, Stolz DB, Liu D. Bifunctional compounds for targeted hepatic gene delivery. *Gene Ther* 2007; **14**: 704–708.

120. Singh M, Ariatti M. Targeted gene delivery into HepG2 cells using complexes containing DNA, cationized asialoorosomucoid and activated cationic liposomes. *J Control Release* 2003; **92**: 383–394.

121. Hirabayashi H, Nishikawa M, Takakura Y, Hashida M. Development and pharmacokinetics of galactosylated poly-L-glutamic acid as a biodegradable carrier for liver-specific drug delivery. *Pharm Res* 1996; **13**: 880–884.

122. Kallinteri P, Liao WY, Antimisiaris SG, Hwang KH. Characterization, stability and in-vivo distribution of asialofetuin glycopeptide incorporating DSPC/CHOL liposomes prepared by mild cholate incubation. *J Drug Target* 2001; **9**: 155–168.

123. Spanjer HH, Scherphof GL. Targeting of lactosylceramide-containing liposomes to hepatocytes in vivo. *Biochim Biophys Acta* 1983; **734**: 40–47.

124. Popielarski SR, Hu-Lieskovan S, French SW, Triche TJ, Davis ME. A nanoparticle-based model delivery system to guide the rational design of gene delivery to the liver. 2. In vitro and in vivo uptake results. *Bioconjug Chem* 2005; **16**: 1071–1080.

125. Watanabe T, Umehara T, Yasui F, Nakagawa S, Yano J, Ohgi T, Sonoke S, Satoh K, Inoue K, Yoshiba M, Kohara M. Liver target delivery of small interfering RNA to the HCV gene by lactosylated cationic liposome. *J Hepatol* 2007; **47**: 744–750.

126. Shimizu K, Qi XR, Maitani Y, Yoshii M, Kawano K, Takayama K, Nagai T. Targeting of soybean-derived sterylglucoside liposomes to liver tumors in rat and mouse models. *Biol Pharm Bull* 1998; **21**: 741–746.

127. Kawano K, Nakamura K, Hayashi K, Nagai T, Takayama K, Maitani Y. Liver targeting liposomes containing beta-sitosterol glucoside with regard to penetration-enhancing effect on HepG2 cells. *Biol Pharm Bull* 2002; **25**: 766–770.

128. Hwang SH, Hayashi K, Takayama K, Maitani Y. Liver-targeted gene transfer into a human hepatoblastoma cell line and in vivo by sterylglucoside-containing cationic liposomes. *Gene Ther* 2001; **8**: 1276–1280.

129. Shi J, Yan WW, Qi XR, Maitani Y, Nagai T. Characteristics and biodistribution of soybean sterylglucoside and polyethylene glycol-modified cationic liposomes and their complexes with antisense oligodeoxynucleotide. *Drug Deliv* 2005; **12**: 349–356.

130. Zhang Y, Rong QX, Gao Y, Wei L, Maitani Y, Nagai T. Mechanisms of co-modified liver-targeting liposomes as gene delivery carriers based on cellular uptake and antigens inhibition effect. *J Control Release* 2007; **117**: 281–290.

131. Ohashi T, Boggs S, Robbins P, Bahnson A, Patrene K, Wei FS, Wei JF, Li J, Lucht L, Fei Y, et al. Efficient transfer and sustained high expression of the human glucocerebrosidase gene in mice and their functional macrophages following transplantation of bone marrow transduced by a retroviral vector. *Proc Natl Acad Sci USA* 1992; **89**: 11332–113326.

132. Kohn DB, Sarver N. Gene therapy for HIV-1 infection. *Adv Exp Med Biol* 1996; **394**: 421–428.

133. Kawakami S, Sato A, Nishikawa M, Yamashita F, Hashida M. Mannose receptor-mediated gene transfer into macrophages using novel mannosylated cationic liposomes. *Gene Ther* 2000; **7**: 292–299.

134. Sato A, Kawakami S, Yamada M, Yamashita F, Hashida M. Enhanced gene transfection in macrophages using mannosylated cationic liposome-polyethylenimine-plasmid DNA complexes. *J Drug Target* 2001; **9**: 201–207.

135. Lu Y, Kawakami S, Yamashita F, Hashida M. Development of an antigen-presenting cell-targeted DNA vaccine against melanoma by mannosylated liposomes. *Biomaterials* 2007; **28**: 3255–3262.

136. Igarashi S, Hattori Y, Maitani Y. Biosurfactant MEL-A enhances cellular association and gene transfection by cationic liposome. *J Control Release* 2006; **112**: 362–368.

137. Park IY, Kim IY, Yoo MK, Choi YJ, Cho MH, Cho CS. Mannosylated polyethylenimine coupled mesoporous silica nanoparticles for receptor-mediated gene delivery. *Int J Pharm* 2008; **359**: 280–287.

138. Bourguignon LY, Singleton PA, Zhu H, Zhou B. Hyaluronan promotes signaling interaction between CD44 and the transforming growth factor beta receptor I in metastatic breast tumor cells. *J Biol Chem* 2002; **277**: 39703–39712.

139. Screaton GR, Bell MV, Jackson DG, Cornelis FB, Gerth U, Bell JI. Genomic structure of DNA encoding the lymphocyte homing receptor CD44 reveals at least 12 alternatively spliced exons. *Proc Natl Acad Sci USA* 1992; **89**: 12160–12164.

140. Screaton GR, Bell MV, Bell JI, Jackson DG. The identification of a new alternative exon with highly restricted tissue expression in transcripts encoding the mouse Pgp-1 (CD44) homing receptor. Comparison of all 10 variable exons between mouse, human, and rat. *J Biol Chem* 1993; **268**: 12235–12238.

141. Al-Hajj M, Wicha MS, Benito-Hernandez A, Morrison SJ, Clarke MF. Prospective identification of tumorigenic breast cancer cells. *Proc Natl Acad Sci USA* 2003; **100**: 3983–3988.

142. Eshkar SL, Ronen D, Levartovsky D, Elkayam O, Caspi D, Aamar S, Amital H, Rubinow A, Golan I, Naor D, Zick Y, Golan I. The involvement of CD44 and its novel ligand galectin-8 in apoptotic regulation of autoimmune inflammation. *J Immunol* 2007; **179**: 1225–1235.

143. Coradini D, Pellizzaro C, Miglierini G, Daidone MG, Perbellini A. Hyaluronic acid as drug delivery for sodium butyrate: Improvement of the anti-proliferative activity on a breast-cancer cell line. *Int J Cancer* 1999; **81**: 411–416.

144. Luo Y, Ziebell MR, Prestwich GD. A hyaluronic acid-taxol antitumor bioconjugate targeted to cancer cells. *Biomacromolecules* 2000; **1**: 208–218.

145. Luo Y, Bernshaw NJ, Lu ZR, Kopecek J, Prestwich GD. Targeted delivery of doxorubicin by HPMA copolymer-hyaluronan bioconjugates. *Pharm Res* 2002; **19**: 396–402.

146. Elron-Gross I, Glucksam Y, Melikhov D, Margalit R. Cyclooxygenase inhibition by diclofenac formulated in bioadhesive carriers. *Biochim Biophys Acta* 2008; **1778**: 931–936.

147. Lee H, Mok H, Lee S, Oh YK, Park TG. Target-specific intracellular delivery of siRNA using degradable hyaluronic acid nanogels. *J Control Release* 2007; **119**: 245–252.

148. Jiang G, Park K, Kim J, Kim KS, Oh EJ, Kang H, Han SE, Oh YK, Park TG, Kwang HS. Hyaluronic acid-polyethyleneimine conjugate for target specific intracellular delivery of siRNA. *Biopolymers* 2008; **89**: 635–642.

149. Fuh G, Li B, Crowley C, Cunningham B, Wells JA. Requirements for binding and signaling of the kinase domain receptor for vascular endothelial growth factor. *J Biol Chem* 1998; **273**: 11197–11204.

150. Keyt BA, Nguyen HV, Berleau LT, Duarte CM, Park J, Chen H, Ferrara N. Identification of vascular endothelial growth factor determinants for binding KDR and FLT-1 receptors. Generation of receptor-selective VEGF variants by site-directed mutagenesis. *J Biol Chem* 1996; **271**: 5638–5646.

151. Kim SH, Jeong JH, Lee SH, Kim SW, Park TG. Local and systemic delivery of VEGF siRNA using polyelectrolyte complex micelles for effective treatment of cancer. *J Control Release* 2008; **129**: 107–116.

152. Liu Y, Fang Y, Dong P, Gao J, Liu R, Hhahbaz M, Bi Y, Ding Z, Tian H, Liu Z. Effect of vascular endothelial growth factor C (VEGF-C) gene transfer in rat model of secondary lymphedema. *Vascul Pharmacol* 2008; **48**: 150–156.

153. Murata N, Takashima Y, Toyoshima K, Yamamoto M, Okada H. Anti-tumor effects of anti-VEGF siRNA encapsulated with PLGA microspheres in mice. *J Control Release* 2008; **126**: 246–254.

154. Baserga R. Controlling IGF-receptor function: A possible strategy for tumor therapy. *Trends Biotechnol* 1996; **14**: 150–152.

155. Baserga R. The IGF-I receptor in cancer research. *Exp Cell Res* 1999; **253**: 1–6.

156. Brodt P, Samani A, Navab R. Inhibition of the type I insulin-like growth factor receptor expression and signaling: Novel strategies for antimetastatic therapy. *Biochem Pharmacol* 2000; **60**: 1101–1107.

157. Resnicoff M, Abraham D, Yutanawiboonchai W, Rotman HL, Kajstura J, Rubin R, Zoltick P, Baserga R. The insulin-like growth factor I receptor protects tumor cells from apoptosis in vivo. *Cancer Res* 1995; **55**: 2463–2469.

158. Resnicoff M, Burgaud JL, Rotman HL, Abraham D, Baserga R. Correlation between apoptosis, tumorigenesis, and levels of insulin-like growth factor I receptors. *Cancer Res* 1995; **55**: 3739–3741.

159. D'Ambrosio C, Ferber A, Resnicoff M, Baserga R. A soluble insulin-like growth factor I receptor that induces apoptosis of tumor cells in vivo and inhibits tumorigenesis. *Cancer Res* 1996; **56**: 4013–4020.

160. Resnicoff M, Sell C, Rubini M, Coppola D, Ambrose D, Baserga R, Rubin R. Rat glioblastoma cells expressing an antisense RNA to the insulin-like growth factor-1 (IGF-1) receptor are nontumorigenic and induce regression of wild-type tumors. *Cancer Res* 1994; **54**: 2218–2222.

161. Bianco R, Troiani T, Tortora G, Ciardiello F. Intrinsic and acquired resistance to EGFR inhibitors in human cancer therapy. *Endocr Relat Cancer* 2005; **12**(Suppl 1): S159–S171.

162. Nakamura K, Hongo A, Kodama J, Miyagi Y, Yoshinouchi M, Kudo T. Down-regulation of the insulin-like growth factor I receptor by antisense RNA can reverse the transformed phenotype of human cervical cancer cell lines. *Cancer Res* 2000; **60**: 760–765.

163. Andrews DW, Resnicoff M, Flanders AE, Kenyon L, Curtis M, Merli G, Baserga R, Iliakis G, Aiken RD. Results of a pilot study involving the use of an antisense oligodeoxynucleotide directed against the insulin-like growth factor type I receptor in malignant astrocytomas. *J Clin Oncol* 2001; **19**: 2189–2200.

164. Dahms NM, Hancock MK. P-type lectins. *Biochim Biophys Acta* 2002; **1572**: 317–340.
165. Ghosh P, Dahms NM, Kornfeld S. Mannose 6-phosphate receptors: New twists in the tale. *Nat Rev Mol Cell Biol* 2003; **4**: 202–212.
166. Hawkes C, Kar S. The insulin-like growth factor-II/mannose-6-phosphate receptor: Structure, distribution and function in the central nervous system. *Brain Res Brain Res Rev* 2004; **44**: 117–140.
167. Ye Z, Cheng K, Guntaka RV, Mahato RI. Targeted delivery of a triplex-forming oligonucleotide to hepatic stellate cells. *Biochemistry* 2005; **44**: 4466–4476.
168. Morris MC, Deshayes S, Simeoni F, Aldrian-Herrada GF, Heitz GD. A noncovalent peptide-based strategy for peptide and short interfering RNA delivery, in *Cell-Penetrating Peptides*, Ü. Langel, Ed., 2007, Taylor & Francis: Boca Raton, FL, pp. 387–408.
169. Fawell S, Seery J, Daikh Y, Moore C, Chen LL, Pepinsky B, Barsoum J. Tat-mediated delivery of heterologous proteins into cells. *Proc Natl Acad Sci USA* 1994; **91**: 664–668.
170. Daniels TR, Delgado T, Rodriguez JA, Helguera G, Penichet ML. The transferrin receptor part I: Biology and targeting with cytotoxic antibodies for the treatment of cancer. *Clin Immunol* 2006; **121**: 144–158.
171. Trinder D, Baker E. Transferrin receptor 2: A new molecule in iron metabolism. *Int J Biochem Cell Biol* 2003; **35**: 292–296.
172. Kawabata H, Yang R, Hirama T, Vuong PT, Kawano S, Gombart AF, Koeffler HP. Molecular cloning of transferrin receptor 2. A new member of the transferrin receptor-like family. *J Biol Chem* 1999; **274**: 20826–20832.
173. Gomme PT, McCann KB, Bertolini J. Transferrin: Structure, function and potential therapeutic actions. *Drug Discov Today* 2005; **10**: 267–273.
174. Li X, Fu GF, Fan YR, Shi CF, Liu XJ, Xu GX, Wang JJ. Potent inhibition of angiogenesis and liver tumor growth by administration of an aerosol containing a transferrin-liposome-endostatin complex. *World J Gastroenterol* 2003; **9**: 262–266.
175. Chiu SJ, Liu S, Perrotti D, Marcucci G, Lee RJ. Efficient delivery of a Bcl-2-specific antisense oligodeoxyribonucleotide (G3139) via transferrin receptor-targeted liposomes. *J Control Release* 2006; **112**: 199–207.
176. Kostanova-Poliakova D, Sabova L. Anti-apoptotic proteins-targets for chemosensitization of tumor cells and cancer treatment. *Neoplasma* 2005; **52**: 441–449.
177. Smith ND, Rubenstein JN, Eggener SE, Kozlowski JM. The p53 tumor suppressor gene and nuclear protein: Basic science review and relevance in the management of bladder cancer. *J Urol* 2003; **169**: 1219–1228.
178. Xu L, Frederik P, Pirollo KF, Tang WH, Rait A, Xiang LM, Huang W, Cruz I, Yin Y, Chang EH. Self-assembly of a virus-mimicking nanostructure system for efficient tumor-targeted gene delivery. *Hum Gene Ther* 2002; **13**: 469–481.
179. Seki M, Iwakawa J, Cheng H, Cheng PW. p53 and PTEN/MMAC1/TEP1 gene therapy of human prostate PC-3 carcinoma xenograft, using transferrin-facilitated lipofection gene delivery strategy. *Hum Gene Ther* 2002; **13**: 761–773.
180. Nakase M, Inui M, Okumura K, Kamei T, Nakamura S, Tagawa T. p53 gene therapy of human osteosarcoma using a transferrin-modified cationic liposome. *Mol Cancer Ther* 2005; **4**: 625–631.
181. Nykjaer A, Willnow TE. The low-density lipoprotein receptor gene family: A cellular Swiss army knife? *Trends Cell Biol* 2002; **12**: 273–280.
182. Willnow TE, Nykjaer A, Herz J. Lipoprotein receptors: New roles for ancient proteins. *Nat Cell Biol* 1999; **1**: E157–E162.
183. Brown MS, Goldstein JL. A receptor-mediated pathway for cholesterol homeostasis. *Science* 1986; **232**: 34–47.
184. Amin K, Wasan KM, Albrecht RM, Heath TD. Cell association of liposomes with high fluid anionic phospholipid content is mediated specifically by LDL and its receptor, LDLr. *J Pharm Sci* 2002; **91**: 1233–1244.
185. Amin K, Ng KY, Brown CS, Bruno MS, Heath TD. LDL induced association of anionic liposomes with cells and delivery of contents as shown by the increase in potency of liposome dependent drugs. *Pharm Res* 2001; **18**: 914–921.
186. Amin K, Heath TD. LDL-induced association of anionic liposomes with cells and delivery of contents. II. Interaction of liposomes with cells in serum-containing medium. *J Control Release* 2001; **73**: 49–57.
187. Lakkaraju A, Rahman YE, Dubinsky JM. Low-density lipoprotein receptor-related protein mediates the endocytosis of anionic liposomes in neurons. *J Biol Chem* 2002; **277**: 15085–15092.

188. Rensen PC, Schiffelers RM, Versluis AJ, Bijsterbosch MK, Van Kuijk-Meuwissen ME, Van Berkel TJ. Human recombinant apolipoprotein E-enriched liposomes can mimic low-density lipoproteins as carriers for the site-specific delivery of antitumor agents. *Mol Pharmacol* 1997; **52**: 445–455.

189. Versluis AJ, Rensen PC, Rump ET, Van Berkel TJ, Bijsterbosch MK. Low-density lipoprotein receptor-mediated delivery of a lipophilic daunorubicin derivative to B16 tumours in mice using apolipoprotein E-enriched liposomes. *Br J Cancer* 1998; **78**: 1607–1614.

190. Versluis AJ, Rump ET, Rensen PC, van Berkel TJ, Bijsterbosch MK. Stable incorporation of a lipophilic daunorubicin prodrug into apolipoprotein E-exposing liposomes induces uptake of prodrug via low-density lipoprotein receptor in vivo. *J Pharmacol Exp Ther* 1999; **289**: 1–7.

191. Jeang KT, Xiao H, Rich EA. Multifaceted activities of the HIV-1 transactivator of transcription, Tat. *J Biol Chem* 1999; **274**: 28837–28840.

192. Torchilin VP, Levchenko TS, Rammohan R, Volodina N, Papahadjopoulos-Sternberg B, D'Souza GG. Cell transfection in vitro and in vivo with nontoxic TAT peptide-liposome-DNA complexes. *Proc Natl Acad Sci USA* 2003; **100**: 1972–1977.

193. Gupta B, Levchenko TS, Torchilin VP. TAT peptide-modified liposomes provide enhanced gene delivery to intracranial human brain tumor xenografts in nude mice. *Oncol Res* 2007; **16**: 351–359.

194. Zhang C, Tang N, Liu X, Liang W, Xu W, Torchilin VP. siRNA-containing liposomes modified with polyarginine effectively silence the targeted gene. *J Control Release* 2006; **112**: 229–239.

195. Turner JJ, Jones S, Fabani MM, Ivanova G, Arzumanov AA, Gait MJ. RNA targeting with peptide conjugates of oligonucleotides, siRNA and PNA. *Blood Cells Mol Dis* 2007; **38**: 1–7.

196. Gregoriadis G, Davis C. Stability of liposomes in vivo and in vitro is promoted by their cholesterol content and the presence of blood cells. *Biochem Biophys Res Commun* 1979; **89**: 1287–1293.

197. Kirby C, Clarke J, Gregoriadis G. Cholesterol content of small unilamellar liposomes controls phospholipid loss to high density lipoproteins in the presence of serum. *FEBS Lett* 1980; **111**: 324–328.

198. Zuidam NJ, Gouw HK, Barenholz Y, Crommelin DJ. Physical (in) stability of liposomes upon chemical hydrolysis: The role of lysophospholipids and fatty acids. *Biochim Biophys Acta* 1995; **1240**: 101–110.

199. Eriksson O, Saris NE. The phospholipase A2-induced increase in the permeability of phospholipid membranes to Ca^{2+} and H^+ ions. *Biol Chem Hoppe Seyler* 1989; **370**: 1315–1320.

200. Almog R, Forward R, Samsonoff C. Stability of sonicated aqueous suspensions of phospholipids under air. *Chem Phys Lipids* 1991; **60**: 93–99.

201. Mattai J, Sripada PK, Shipley GG. Mixed-chain phosphatidylcholine bilayers: Structure and properties. *Biochemistry* 1987; **26**: 3287–3297.

202. Patel HM. Serum opsonins and liposomes: Their interaction and opsonophagocytosis. *Crit Rev Ther Drug Carrier Syst* 1992; **9**: 39–90.

203. Gabizon A, Papahadjopoulos D. Liposome formulations with prolonged circulation time in blood and enhanced uptake by tumors. *Proc Natl Acad Sci USA* 1988; **85**: 6949–6953.

204. Song LY, Ahkong QF, Rong Q, Wang Z, Ansell S, Hope MJ, Mui B. Characterization of the inhibitory effect of PEG-lipid conjugates on the intracellular delivery of plasmid and antisense DNA mediated by cationic lipid liposomes. *Biochim Biophys Acta* 2002; **1558**: 1–13.

205. Takeuchi H, Kojima H, Yamamoto H, Kawashima Y. Evaluation of circulation profiles of liposomes coated with hydrophilic polymers having different molecular weights in rats. *J Control Release* 2001; **75**: 83–91.

206. Gerasimov OV, Boomer JA, Qualls MM, Thompson DH. Cytosolic drug delivery using pH- and light-sensitive liposomes. *Adv Drug Deliv Rev* 1999; **38**: 317–338.

207. Ishida T, Kirchmeier MJ, Moase EH, Zalipsky S, Allen TM. Targeted delivery and triggered release of liposomal doxorubicin enhances cytotoxicity against human B lymphoma cells. *Biochim Biophys Acta* 2001; **1515**: 144–158.

208. Drummond DC, Zignani M, Leroux J. Current status of pH-sensitive liposomes in drug delivery. *Prog Lipid Res* 2000; **39**: 409–460.

209. Shin J, Shum P, Thompson DH. Acid-triggered release via dePEGylation of DOPE liposomes containing acid-labile vinyl ether PEG-lipids. *J Control Release* 2003; **91**: 187–200.

210. Kong G, Anyarambhatla G, Petros WP, Braun RD, Colvin OM, Needham D, Dewhirst MW. Efficacy of liposomes and hyperthermia in a human tumor xenograft model: Importance of triggered drug release. *Cancer Res* 2000; **60**: 6950–6957.

211. Kono K. Thermosensitive polymer-modified liposomes. *Adv Drug Deliv Rev* 2001; **53**: 307–319.

212. Needham D, Dewhirst MW. The development and testing of a new temperature-sensitive drug delivery system for the treatment of solid tumors. *Adv Drug Deliv Rev* 2001; **53**: 285–305.

213. Bondurant B, Mueller A, O'Brien DF. Photoinitiated destabilization of sterically stabilized liposomes. *Biochim Biophys Acta* 2001; **1511**: 113–122.
214. Shum P, Kim JM, Thompson DH. Phototriggering of liposomal drug delivery systems. *Adv Drug Deliv Rev* 2001; **53**: 273–284.
215. Davidsen J, Jorgensen K, Andresen TL, Mouritsen OG. Secreted phospholipase A(2) as a new enzymatic trigger mechanism for localised liposomal drug release and absorption in diseased tissue. *Biochim Biophys Acta* 2003; **1609**: 95–101.
216. Meers P. Enzyme-activated targeting of liposomes. *Adv Drug Deliv Rev* 2001; **53**: 265–272.
217. Ohkuma S, Poole B. Fluorescence probe measurement of the intralysosomal pH in living cells and the perturbation of pH by various agents. *Proc Natl Acad Sci USA* 1978; **75**: 3327–3331.
218. Tamaddon AM, Shirazi FH, Moghimi HR. Modeling cytoplasmic release of encapsulated oligonucleotides from cationic liposomes. *Int J Pharm* 2007; **336**: 174–182.
219. Auguste DT, Furman K, Wong A, Fuller J, Armes SP, Deming TJ, Langer R. Triggered release of siRNA from poly(ethylene glycol)-protected, pH-dependent liposomes. *J Control Release* 2008; **130**: 266–274.
220. Shigeta K, Kawakami S, Higuchi Y, Okuda T, Yagi H, Yamashita F, Hashida M. Novel histidine-conjugated galactosylated cationic liposomes for efficient hepatocyte-selective gene transfer in human hepatoma HepG2 cells. *J Control Release* 2007; **118**: 262–270.
221. Ponnappa BC, Dey I, Tu GC, Zhou F, Aini M, Cao QN, Israel Y. In vivo delivery of antisense oligonucleotides in pH-sensitive liposomes inhibits lipopolysaccharide-induced production of tumor necrosis factor-alpha in rats. *J Pharmacol Exp Ther* 2001; **297**: 1129–1136.
222. Collier JH, Hu BH, Ruberti JW, Zhang J, Shum P, Thompson DH, Messersmith PB. Thermally and photochemically triggered self-assembly of peptide hydrogels. *J Am Chem Soc* 2001; **123**: 9463–9464.
223. Hogset A, Prasmickaite L, Engesaeter BO, Hellum M, Selbo PK, Olsen VM, Maelandsmo GM, Berg K. Light directed gene transfer by photochemical internalisation. *Curr Gene Ther* 2003; **3**: 89–112.
224. Prasmickaite L, Hogset A, Berg K. Evaluation of different photosensitizers for use in photochemical gene transfection. *Photochem Photobiol* 2001; **73**: 388–395.
225. Hogset A, Prasmickaite L, Hellum M, Engesaeter BO, Olsen VM, Tjelle TE, Wheeler CJ, Berg K. Photochemical transfection: A technology for efficient light-directed gene delivery. *Somat Cell Mol Genet* 2002; **27**: 97–113.
226. Hellum M, Hogset A, Engesaeter BO, Prasmickaite L, Stokke T, Wheeler C, Berg K. Photochemically enhanced gene delivery with cationic lipid formulations. *Photochem Photobiol Sci* 2003; **2**: 407–411.
227. Namiki Y, Namiki T, Date M, Yanagihara K, Yashiro M, Takahashi H. Enhanced photodynamic antitumor effect on gastric cancer by a novel photosensitive stealth liposome. *Pharmacol Res* 2004; **50**: 65–76.
228. Yatvin MB, Weinstein JN, Dennis WH, Blumenthal R. Design of liposomes for enhanced local release of drugs by hyperthermia. *Science* 1978; **202**: 1290–1293.
229. Gaber MH, Wu NZ, Hong K, Huang SK, Dewhirst MW, Papahadjopoulos D. Thermosensitive liposomes: Extravasation and release of contents in tumor microvascular networks. *Int J Radiat Oncol Biol Phys* 1996; **36**: 1177–1187.
230. Dewhirst MW, Prosnitz L, Thrall D, Prescott D, Clegg S, Charles C, MacFall J, Rosner G, Samulski T, Gillette E, LaRue S. Hyperthermic treatment of malignant diseases: Current status and a view toward the future. *Semin Oncol* 1997; **24**: 616–625.
231. Han HD, Shin BC, Choi HS. Doxorubicin-encapsulated thermosensitive liposomes modified with poly(*N*-isopropylacrylamide-*co*-acrylamide): Drug release behavior and stability in the presence of serum. *Eur J Pharm Biopharm* 2006; **62**: 110–116.
232. Chandaroy P, Sen A, Hui SW. Temperature-controlled content release from liposomes encapsulating Pluronic F127. *J Control Release* 2001; **76**: 27–37.
233. Fattal E, De Rosa G, Bochot A. Gel and solid matrix systems for the controlled delivery of drug carrier-associated nucleic acids. *Int J Pharm* 2004; **277**: 25–30.
234. Davis SC, Szoka FC, Jr. Cholesterol phosphate derivatives: Synthesis and incorporation into a phosphatase and calcium-sensitive triggered release liposome. *Bioconjug Chem* 1998; **9**: 783–792.
235. Millan JL, Fishman WH. Biology of human alkaline phosphatases with special reference to cancer. *Crit Rev Clin Lab Sci* 1995; **32**: 1–39.
236. Wymer NJ, Gerasimov OV, Thompson DH. Cascade liposomal triggering: Light-induced Ca^{2+} release from diplasmenylcholine liposomes triggers PLA2-catalyzed hydrolysis and contents leakage from DPPC liposomes. *Bioconjug Chem* 1998; **9**: 305–308.

237. Zhang ZY, Shum P, Yates M, Messersmith PB, Thompson DH. Formation of fibrinogen-based hydrogels using phototriggerable diplasmalogen liposomes. *Bioconjug Chem* 2002; **13**: 640–646.

238. Ruiz-Arguello MB, Goni FM, Alonso A. Vesicle membrane fusion induced by the concerted activities of sphingomyelinase and phospholipase C. *J Biol Chem* 1998; **273**: 22977–22982.

239. Goni FM, Alonso A. Membrane fusion induced by phospholipase C and sphingomyelinases. *Biosci Rep* 2000; **20**: 443–463.

240. Villar AV, Alonso A, Goni FM. Leaky vesicle fusion induced by phosphatidylinositol-specific phospholipase C: Observation of mixing of vesicular inner monolayers. *Biochemistry* 2000; **39**: 14012–14018.

241. Villar AV, Goni FM, Alonso A. Diacylglycerol effects on phosphatidylinositol-specific phospholipase C activity and vesicle fusion. *FEBS Lett* 2001; **494**: 117–120.

242. Foged C, Nielsen HM, Frokjaer S. Phospholipase A2 sensitive liposomes for delivery of small interfering RNA (siRNA). *J Liposome Res* 2007; **17**: 191–196.

243. Foged C, Nielsen HM, Frokjaer S. Liposomes for phospholipase A2 triggered siRNA release: Preparation and in vitro test. *Int J Pharm* 2007; **331**: 160–166.

244. Saito G, Swanson JA, Lee KD. Drug delivery strategy utilizing conjugation via reversible disulfide linkages: Role and site of cellular reducing activities. *Adv Drug Deliv Rev* 2003; **55**: 199–215.

245. Schafer FQ, Buettner GR. Redox environment of the cell as viewed through the redox state of the glutathione disulfide/glutathione couple. *Free Radic Biol Med* 2001; **30**: 1191–1212.

246. Collins DS, Unanue ER, Harding CV. Reduction of disulfide bonds within lysosomes is a key step in antigen processing. *J Immunol* 1991; **147**: 4054–4059.

247. West KR, Otto S. Reversible covalent chemistry in drug delivery. *Curr Drug Discov Technol* 2005; **2**: 123–160.

248. Huang Z, Li W, MacKay JA, Szoka FC, Jr. Thiocholesterol-based lipids for ordered assembly of bioresponsive gene carriers. *Mol Ther* 2005; **11**: 409–417.

249. Kirpotin D, Hong K, Mullah N, Papahadjopoulos D, Zalipsky S. Liposomes with detachable polymer coating: Destabilization and fusion of dioleoylphosphatidylethanolamine vesicles triggered by cleavage of surface-grafted poly(ethylene glycol). *FEBS Lett* 1996; **388**: 115–118.

250. Mitragotri S. Healing sound: The use of ultrasound in drug delivery and other therapeutic applications. *Nat Rev Drug Discov* 2005; **4**: 255–260.

251. ter Haar G. Therapeutic applications of ultrasound. *Prog Biophys Mol Biol* 2007; **93**: 111–129.

252. Duvshani-Eshet M, Machluf M. Efficient transfection of tumors facilitated by long-term therapeutic ultrasound in combination with contrast agent: From in vitro to in vivo setting. *Cancer Gene Ther* 2007; **14**: 306–315.

253. Duvshani-Eshet M, Benny O, Morgenstern A, Machluf M. Therapeutic ultrasound facilitates antiangiogenic gene delivery and inhibits prostate tumor growth. *Mol Cancer Ther* 2007; **6**: 2371–2382.

254. Baker ML, Dalrymple GV. Biological effects of diagnostic ultrasound: A review. *Radiology* 1978; **126**: 479–483.

255. Barnett SB, ter Haar GR, Ziskin MC, Nyborg WL, Maeda K, Bang J. Current status of research on biophysical effects of ultrasound. *Ultrasound Med Biol* 1994; **20**: 205–218.

256. Newman CM, Bettinger T. Gene therapy progress and prospects: Ultrasound for gene transfer. *Gene Ther* 2007; **14**: 465–475.

257. Anwer K, Kao G, Proctor B, Anscombe I, Florack V, Earls R, Wilson E, McCreery T, Unger E, Rolland A, Sullivan SM. Ultrasound enhancement of cationic lipid-mediated gene transfer to primary tumors following systemic administration. *Gene Ther* 2000; **7**: 1833–1839.

258. Greenleaf WJ, Bolander ME, Sarkar G, Goldring MB, Greenleaf JF. Artificial cavitation nuclei significantly enhance acoustically induced cell transfection. *Ultrasound Med Biol* 1998; **24**: 587–595.

259. Huang SL, McPherson DD, MacDonald RC. Ultrasound in conjunction with an ultrasonic-reflective transfection agent enhances gene delivery to cells. *J Am Coll Cardiol* 2002; **39**: 228A–229A.

260. Deshpande MC, Prausnitz MR. Synergistic effect of ultrasound and PEI on DNA transfection in vitro. *J Control Release* 2007; **118**: 126–135.

261. Suzuki R, Takizawa T, Negishi Y, Hagisawa K, Tanaka K, Sawamura K, Utoguchi N, Nishioka T, Maruyama K. Gene delivery by combination of novel liposomal bubbles with perfluoropropane and ultrasound. *J Control Release* 2007; **117**: 130–136.

262. Huang SL. Liposomes in ultrasonic drug and gene delivery. *Adv Drug Deliv Rev* 2008; **60**: 1167–1176.

263. Edelstein ML, Abedi MR, Wixon J, Edelstein RM. Gene therapy clinical trials worldwide 1989–2004—an overview. *J Gene Med* 2004; **6**: 597–602.

264. Remaut K, Lucas B, Raemdonck K, Braeckmans K, Demeester J, De Smedt SC. Can we better understand the intracellular behavior of DNA nanoparticles by fluorescence correlation spectroscopy? *J Control Release* 2007; **121**: 49–63.

265. Fujita M, Lee BS, Khazenzon NM, Penichet ML, Wawrowsky KA, Patil R, Ding H, Holler E, Black KL, Ljubimova JY. Brain tumor tandem targeting using a combination of monoclonal antibodies attached to biopoly(beta-L-malic acid). *J Control Release* 2007; **122**: 356–363.

266. Palma E, Cho MJ. Improved systemic pharmacokinetics, biodistribution, and antitumor activity of CpG oligodeoxynucleotides complexed to endogenous antibodies in vivo. *J Control Release* 2007; **120**: 95–103.

267. Sato A, Choi SW, Hirai M, Yamayoshi A, Moriyama R, Yamano T, Takagi M, Kano A, Shimamoto A, Maruyama A. Polymer brush-stabilized polyplex for a siRNA carrier with long circulatory half-life. *J Control Release* 2007; **122**: 209–216.

268. Reischl D, Zimmer A. Drug delivery of siRNA therapeutics: Potentials and limits of nanosystems. *Nanomedicine* 2009; **5**: 8–20.

Part III

Intracellular/Organelle-Specific Strategies

10 Delivering the Bullet to the Right Intracellular Target: A Cellular Perspective on Drug Delivery

Maria Teresa Tarragó-Trani and Brian Storrie

CONTENTS

10.1 INTRODUCTION

With the advent of genome sequencing and the tremendous success of reductionist approaches in molecular cell biology aimed at understanding the nature of complex systems in terms of interactions of their components, we now have gained immensely detailed knowledge of membrane trafficking, i.e., the flux of vesicular carriers and their contents between subcellular compartments such as the endoplasmic reticulum (ER), Golgi apparatus (GA), endosomes, and the plasma membrane. Much is known about the role of individual proteins and the importance of their domains in the functioning and stability of these proteins.[1–9] In this chapter, we highlight the possible clinical applications of the knowledge of membrane trafficking as exemplified by two systems: (1) the generation of peptides involved in Alzheimer's disease (AD) and their possible control and (2) the use of a declawed protein toxin fragment as a delivery vehicle and an imaging tool.

10.2 RATIONAL INTRACELLULAR DRUG DELIVERY KNOWING THE INDIVIDUAL SYSTEM

10.2.1 Preventing Alzheimer's Disease

10.2.1.1 Enzymology of β-Amyloid Peptide Generation

AD is a neurodegenerative disorder associated with aging. The main clinical manifestations of AD are the progressive loss of memory and cognitive abilities. Pathologically, AD is characterized by the extracellular accumulation of β-amyloid peptide (Aβ) aggregates (better known as amyloid plaque) in the brain, and intraneuronal deposits of neurofibrillary tangles composed of aberrantly phosphorylated forms of tau protein, a microtubule-binding protein.[10–13] Aβ peptide is produced by the sequential proteolytic cleavage of amyloid precursor protein (APP) by the enzymes β- and γ-secretases, probably in endosomes. The Aβ peptide plays a critical role in the pathological development of AD. The exact physiological function of the Aβ peptide and APP remains to be elucidated.

APP is a type I transmembrane protein, which is synthesized in the ER and transported to the cell membrane through the GA, where it acquires several post-translational modifications such as glycosylation, phosphorylation, and sulfation.[14,15] At steady state, approximately 10% of total cellular APP resides at the plasma membrane. The rest is distributed among the *trans*-Golgi network (TGN) and endosomes. APP can be cleaved in one of two alternate ways. At the cell surface, APP can be proteolytically cleaved by α-secretases, releasing a large soluble amino terminal (N-terminal) fragment, APPα ectodomain (sAPPα), into the extracellular space. The α-secretase cleavage site is within the Aβ domain of APP, 83 amino acids from the carboxy terminus (C-terminus), and prevents the release of a discrete Aβ peptide (Figure 10.1). The C-terminal fragment (CTFα) remains in the membrane and it is subsequently cleaved by γ-secretase to yield a small N-terminal fragment designated as p3 and a cytoplasmic polypeptide termed APP intracellular domain or AICD.[11,14] This APP-processing pathway is referred as the non-amyloidogenic APP-processing pathway.

Alternatively, APP may be processed first by β-secretase and subsequently by γ-secretase. β-Secretase, also known as the β-site APP-cleaving enzyme (BACE), is a type I transmembrane protein of the pepsin family of aspartyl proteases.[11,16,17] It cleaves APP at 99 amino acids from the C-terminus, producing the sAPPβ fragment. This fragment is released into the luminal/extracellular space. The C-terminal fragment (CTFβ) remains embedded in the membrane (Figure 10.1). CTFβ is in turn cleaved within the membrane by γ-secretase. γ-Secretase cleaves CTFβ between residues 38 and 43 (from the newly formed N-terminus), generating the Aβ peptide and AICD. The Aβ peptide occurs as 40- and 42-residue long isoforms (Aβ40 and Aβ42), with most of the Aβ peptides being Aβ40, and the Aβ42 variant being a minor fraction. The Aβ42 variant is more hydrophobic and susceptible to aggregation than Aβ40. It is also the isoform predominantly found in the AD amyloid plaques.[10] We note that γ-secretase is a multimeric protein complex composed of the integral membrane proteins presenilin 1 (PS1), presenilin 2 (PS2), nicastrin, APH1, PEN2, and possibly TMP21.[12,18]

The APP gene has been mapped to chromosome 21. Mutations in this gene, within or adjacent to the Aβ region, can cause early-onset AD.[12] Additional copies of the chromosome produce the

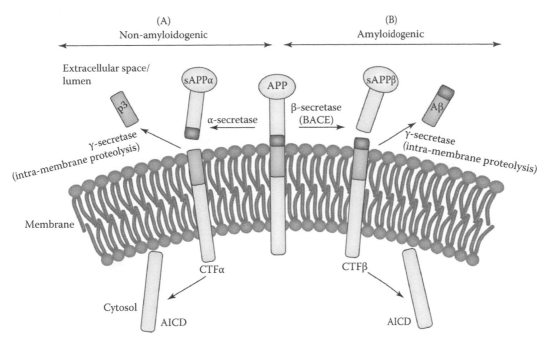

FIGURE 10.1 Proteolysis of APP. APP can be proteolytically processed in two alternate pathways. (A) Non-amyloidogenic pathway, APP is likely cleaved at the cell surface by α-secretase to produce a large soluble fragment released into the extracellular space, sAPPα, and a C-terminal fragment, CTFα that remains in the membrane. CTFα is then cleaved by γ-secretase within the Aβ domain to yield p3 and AICD. (B) Amyloidogenic pathway, APP is presumed to be cleaved by β-secretase (BACE) in endosomal compartments, producing sAPPβ and CTFβ which is in turn cleaved by γ-secretase, releasing Aβ peptide and AICD. APP, amyloid precursor protein; CTF, C-terminal fragment; AICD, APP intracellular domain.

same effect. Furthermore, mutations in the genes of PS1 and PS2, protein subunits that form part of the multimeric γ-secretase complex, can lead to early-onset AD. Interestingly, all these mutations affect APP processing and Aβ peptide metabolism.[11,12] On the other hand, in late-onset AD, defects in APP or secretase genes have not been observed. Therefore, dysfunction in other components of the system that regulate the production of Aβ peptide are probably involved. APP, BACE, and γ-secretase are transmembrane proteins that are transported and sorted through the secretory and endocytic pathways. They, therefore, must pass transitorily through most membrane compartments of these pathways.

10.2.1.2 Protein Location and Regulation of Amyloid Protein Generation

To generate the Aβ peptide, at some point, enzymes and substrates must converge in space and time (see Figure 10.2 for a schematic depiction of intra-cellular geography and Table 10.1 for a summary of the components involved in AD). Hence, abnormalities in the membrane traffic and dynamics of these proteins have long been suspected as a potential source of anomalous Aβ peptide formation.[12] The majority of mature BACE distributes to the endosomes. Lower levels have been observed in the TGN and the plasma membrane, indicating that the protein cycles between these membrane compartments, with a longer stay in the endosomes. The intracellular distribution and trafficking of γ-secretase is not as clear. This enzyme is active in the endosomal compartments.[19]

Several studies show that endosomes are the site of APP cleavage by BACE (Figure 10.2). Hence, the proposal that the maintenance of APP at the plasma membrane may then increase the

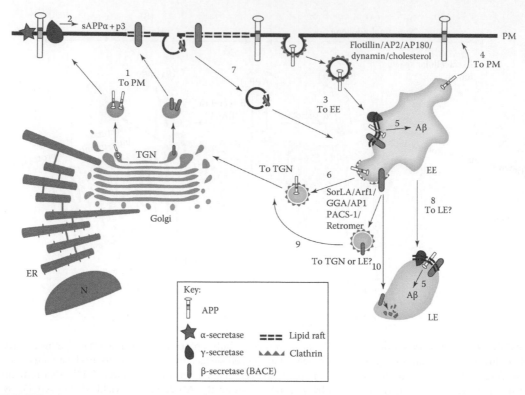

FIGURE 10.2 Intracellular geography, APP trafficking, and production of Aβ peptide. APP, α-secretase, BACE, and γ-secretase are delivered to the plasma membrane through the secretory/biosynthetic pathway (1). A fraction of APP undergoes non-amyloidogenic proteolytic processing at the cell surface (2), whereas the rest of APP molecules are internalized, presumably by flotillin, clathrin coats, AP2, AP180 and other adaptor proteins, into EE and/or recycling endosomes (3). In the endosomal system, APP can be shuttled back to the cell surface (4) or retrieved by the receptor sorLA in association with Arf1, GGA, PACS-1, AP1, clathrin and/or elements of the retromer complex and shuttled to the TGN (6). Presumably BACE (7) and γ-secretase are also subject to recycling through the plasma membrane and endosomal system. Based on available data, it is hypothesized that in AD neurons the receptor sorLA is downregulated resulting in failure to sort APP out of endosomes, and increased contact time of APP with BACE and γ-secretase which leads to amyloidogenic processing (5) of APP and subsequent Aβ formation in EE [but LE are a likely site of Aβ formation too (8)]. Other causes of amyloidogenic processing of APP in endosomes should be considered such as failure to retrieve BACE out of endosomes and either shuttle it to TGN (9) or to LE/lysosomes (10) for degradation. APP, amyloid precursor protein; BACE, β-site APP cleaving enzyme or β-secretase; EE, early endosomes; ER, endoplasmic reticulum; LE, late endosomes; N, nucleus; PM, plasma membrane; TGN, *trans*-Golgi network.

probability of APP processing by the non-amyloidogenic pathway through avoidance of BACE activity. In brief, a block in endocytosis results in the diminished production of Aβ peptide.[20,21] In addition, BACE enzymatic activity is optimal at acidic pH, which is the pH of endosomes. Recent studies indicate that most of the β-cleavage of APP occurs in the early endosomes (EE). In one study, sAPPβ colocalized with early endosomal antigen-1 (EEA-1) and Rab5 (small GTPase of the Rab family), markers of this cellular compartment.[21] Also, fluorescence resonance energy transfer (FRET) measurements located the conditions for optimal molecular interaction between APP and BACE in EE.[22] In agreement with these findings,[23] showed that increased neuronal activity, and hence enhanced endocytosis and recycling of cell surface receptors at synaptic endings, increases the secretion of Aβ peptide in transgenic mice expressing Swedish APP mutation. Results from this

TABLE 10.1
AD Protein Components

Name	Localization	Role
APP	Plasma membrane, TGN, endosomes	Type I transmembrane protein, alternatively processed into the non-amyloidogenic pathway by α-secretase followed by γ-secretase; or into the amyloidogenic pathway by BACE and γ-secretase producing Aβ peptide involved in AD pathogenesis.
α-Secretase	Plasma membrane	Type I transmembrane protein of pepsin family of aspartyl proteases. Cleaves APP within Aβ site, 89 amino acids from C-terminus, producing soluble N-terminal fragment sAPPα and C-terminal fragment (CTFα).
β-Secretase (BACE)	Endosomes, TGN	Cleaves APP, 99 amino acids from C-terminus producing N-terminal fragment, sAPPβ and C-terminal fragment, CTFβ.
γ-Secretase	Endosomes, plasma membrane	Multimeric protein complex composed of at least five integral membrane subunits, which functions as an intramembrane protease. It cleaves CTFα to produce small N-terminal fragment, p3, and the cytoplasmic polypeptide, AICD. It cleaves CTFβ generating N-terminal Aβ peptide and AICD.
Aβ peptide	Peptide aggregates accumulate extracellularly	Product of sequential proteolytic cleavage of BACE and γ-secretase. Peptides can range in size from 38 to 43 amino acids long. Aggregates of Aβ accumulate in neurons of AD brains.
Sortilin family of receptors (sortilin, sorLA, sorCS)	Endosomes, TGN, plasma membrane	Type 1 transmembrane protein that interacts with APP and may be involved in recycling of APP from endosomes to TGN mediated by elements of the retromer complex, and/or clathrin and clathrin adaptor proteins (AP1, GGA).
Retromer complex	Cytoplasmic phase of endosomal membranes and cytoplasm	Complex of five peripheral membrane protein subunits, arranged into two subcomplexes, a trimer (Vps26p, Vps29p, Vps35p) and a dimer (Vps5p, Vps17 in yeast; SNX1, SNX2 in mammals). It functions as a protein coat that mediates retrograde transport of transmembrane proteins from endosomes to TGN (e.g., lysosomal enzyme receptors, Vps10, MPR; sortilin receptors).
Flotillins	Cytoplasmic phase of plasma membrane	Peripheral membrane proteins that may regulate endocytosis of APP.

study also indicate that endogenous Aβ peptide may perform a physiological role in the depression of synaptic transmission.

Both APP and BACE contain clathrin sorting signals in their cytoplasmic domains. This is typical of transmembrane proteins that transit from the plasma membrane to EE, or from the TGN to EE in clathrin-coated vesicles. BACE contains a dileucine-based clathrin sorting motif

DXXLL, using single letter amino acid codes with X being nonspecific. This motif, in general, has been associated with clathrin-coated vesicles that are formed in the TGN and are destined to fuse with EE. APP has a tyrosine-based clathrin sorting signal (NPXY). This signal is usually found in clathrin-coated vesicles produced at the plasma membrane and transported to EE.[24] The presence of these clathrin sorting signals in APP and BACE strongly support the dynamic nature of their sorting pathways at the interface of the TGN and the endosomal membrane system.

10.2.1.3 Sortilin Family Proteins as Receptors in APP and BACE Trafficking

APP and BACE traffic from TGN to endosomes in neuronal cells.[25] This transport is regulated by the sortilin family of receptors, which includes sortilin, sorLA, and sorCS. These receptors are type 1 transmembrane proteins with luminal/extracellular multi-ligand-binding domains. Among the binding domains displayed by sortilin receptors relevant to AD pathogenesis are a domain structurally related to the low-density lipoprotein receptor (LDLR) family and a luminal domain homologous to that of the yeast vacuolar protein sorting 10 protein (Vps10p).

Vps10p is a receptor for lysosomal enzymes in yeast, with a function equivalent to that of the mannose-6-phosphate receptor (MPR) in higher eukaryotes. Vps10p binds lysosomal enzymes in the TGN and transports them to the EE. Once the lysosomal enzymes dissociate in the acidic pH of the EE, the empty Vps10p receptors are shuttled back to the TGN to be reused. Specifically in yeast, Vps10s is transported in retrograde fashion (inward flow or movement towards the cell body) from the EE to the TGN by the retromer complex. The yeast retromer complex is composed of five protein subunits, viz., Vps5p, Vps17p, Vps26p, Vps29p, and Vps35p, which are arranged into two subcomplexes. The trimer (consisting of Vps26p, Vps29p, and Vps35p) is thought to participate in cargo selection through the interaction of Vps35p with the cytosolic tails of cargo proteins, and the dimer (composed of Vps5p and Vps17p) is involved in promoting the vesicle/tubule formation.[26,27] Both Vps5p and Vps17p contain a PX (phox) domain that mediates binding to phosphoinositides in the target membrane, and a BAR domain, a banana-shaped domain, that binds to the membrane through its concave side. The BAR domain may be involved in sensing and inducing membrane curvature.[26,27] The components of the yeast retromer are conserved in higher eukaryotes, and all have homologs in mammalian cells, except for Vps17p. The mammalian homologs of Vps5p are sorting nexin-1 (SNX1) and sorting nexin-2 (SNX2); both isoforms are believed to compose the mammalian dimer sub-complex. The mammalian homologs of Vps26p, Vps29p, and Vps35p retain the same names as in yeast. Similar to the role of the yeast retromer complex in recycling a lysosomal hydrolase receptor (Vps10p) from endosomes to TGN, the mammalian retromer complex is implicated in recycling MPR from endosomes to TGN.

The components of the retromer complex are highly expressed in the normal human brain. Reduced expression of these components has been reported in brain tissue from individuals with AD. The initial gene expression profiling of brain cells or lymphoblasts harvested from individuals with AD indicated that Vps35p, Vps26p, and sorLA levels are downregulated as compared with control cells.[28,29] A recent multi-cohort genetic study found that some inherited variations in the sorLA gene are associated with late-onset AD.[30] The link between sorLA expression, intracellular transport, and the processing of APP in neurons has been investigated. Several studies indicate that sorLA and APP colocalize in endosomal and GA compartments where they interact via their luminal and cytoplasmic domains. Overexpression of sorLA promotes the redistribution of APP to the TGN and decreased processing to Aβ.[31–35] On the other hand, the loss of sorLA in knock-out mouse models or the suppression of sorLA by short interfering RNA (siRNA) leads to increased levels of Aβ.[30,31] Given all these results and the fact that sorLA shares homology with the yeast sorting receptor Vps10p, sorLA may act as a sorting receptor for APP. It may (1) control APP transport along the TGN, endosome, and plasma membrane route,

(2) limit the exposure of APP with BACE and γ-secretase in early/late endosomal compartments, and (3) favor the non-amyloidogenic processing of APP.[31,33,34] SorLA contains, in its cytoplasmic domain, a Golgi-localized, gamma-ear-containing ADP ribosylation factor (Arf)-binding protein (GGA) motif and an acidic cluster-dileucine-like motif, which is recognized by the clathrin adaptor protein, AP1.

Both GGA and AP1 are required for sorLA transport from TGN to endosomes, indicating that sorLA distributes, at least transiently, in endosomal compartments.[32,34] Most of sorLA is localized intracellularly, while roughly 5%–10% of sorLA is present at the plasma membrane. From the plasma membrane, it undergoes endocytosis mediated by the clathrin adaptor protein, AP2, and possibly by the phosphofurin acidic cluster-sorting protein-1 (PACS-1).[32,34] After internalization, sorLA accumulates in EE where it seems to be recycled to the TGN by GGA, AP1, PACS-1, and components of the retromer complex, SNX1 and Vps35p.[32,34] SNX1 and Vps35p suppression by siRNA decreased sorLA levels, apparently caused by the redistribution of sorLA to lysosomes leading to its degradation.[32]

Whether all the components of the retromer complex are involved in the retrograde transport of sorLA to TGN is not clear. A recent study shows that sortilin colocalizes to the same transport vesicles and intracellular compartments as MPR, and as MPR, it is retracted from EE by SNX1.[36] These results suggest a mechanism by which sorLA may restrict the stay of APP in the endosomal compartments, where APP is likely processed by BACE and γ-secretase to generate Aβ peptide. SorLA may retrieve APP from endosomes and transport it back to TGN, possibly mediated by elements of the retromer complex. The function of sorLA in the selective sorting of APP into a retromer-based recycling pathway, and its significance in APP processing, has been demonstrated in experiments in which siRNA inhibition of sorLA, Vps26Ap,[30] or Vps35p[29] expression led to increased Aβ peptide production. In addition, overexpression of sorLA[29,31,33] or Vps35p[29] resulted in the downregulation of Aβ peptide formation.

In summary, genetic, biochemical, and cellular studies provide strong evidence for the involvement of sorLA and some constituents of the retromer complex in regulating the transit of APP through the endosomal compartments, where most of APP amyloidogenic processing takes place. SorLA and components of the retromer complex may well be considered as potential targets for future AD therapies.

> AD is characterized by the extracellular accumulation of Aβ aggregates (better known as amyloid plaque) in the brain. The Aβ peptide is produced by the sequential proteolytic cleavage of APP by the enzymes β- and γ-secretases, probably in endosomes. Both APP and BACE contain clathrin sorting signals in their cytoplasmic domains. They traffic from the TGN to the endosomes in the neuronal cells. This transport is regulated by the sortilin family of receptors, which includes sortilin, sorLA, and sorCS.

10.2.1.4 Flotillin Isoforms Regulate APP Endocytosis into a Specialized Clathrin-Dependent Pathway That Promotes β-Amyloid Formation

Another membrane protein that has been implicated in regulating APP endocytosis is flotillin. Flotillins are highly conserved in nature and expressed in almost every organism. They exist in two isoforms: flotillin 1 and flotillin 2. Flotillins are peripheral membrane proteins anchored to the cytoplasmic membrane bilayer through palmitoyl and myristoyl chains, where they form a loop structure. Both their N- and C-terminal domains face the cytosol and a hydrophobic internal domain (next to the N-terminus) interacts with the membrane.[37,38] The configuration of flotillin at the plasma membrane resembles that of caveolin, although the proteins do not share sequence homology. Flotillin is found primarily at the plasma membrane where it is assembled into stable and relatively uniform clusters consisting of homo- and hetero-oligomeric complexes of flotillin 1 and 2.[38] In addition, flotillin can be found in recycling endosomes, lysosomes, and multivesicular bodies (MVBs).

Flotillins have been proposed to regulate a novel clathrin- and caveolin-independent endocytic pathway. For a detailed review of endocytosis, we refer the reader to recent reviews by Doherty and McMahon[39] and Mayor and Pagano[5] and to Figure 10.3. As reviewed by Doherty and McMahon,[39] flotillin is part of 1 of at least 10 different, major pathways of endocytosis in cells. By immuno-fluorescence techniques,[40] Glebov et al. observed flotillin 1 in punctate structures associated with

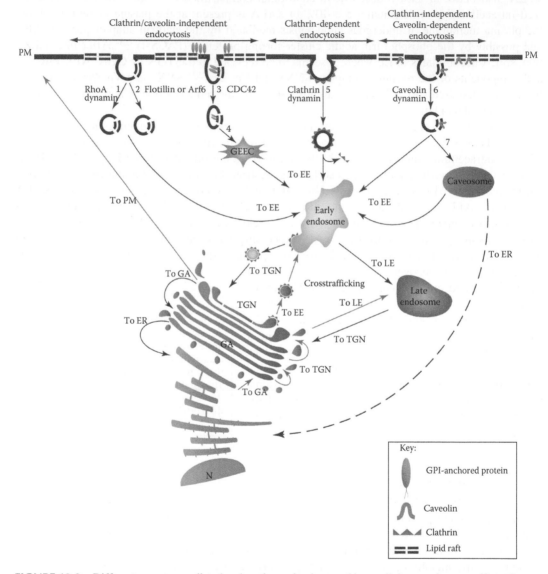

FIGURE 10.3 Different receptor-mediated endocytic mechanisms and intracellular membrane traffic pathways. Different endocytic pathways can coexist in a cell. Clathrin-dependent pathway (5) is characterized by clathrin-coated vesicles and it is dependent on dynamin. Clathrin-independent pathways can be caveolin-dependent (6), or caveolin-independent (1, 2, 3). Clathrin-independent, caveolin-independent pathways (1, 2, 3) can be subdivided according to dynamin-dependent: e.g., RhoA-regulated pathway (1); dynamin-independent: e.g., flotillin-dependent pathway, and Arf6-regulated pathway (2), or CDC42-regulated pathway (3). Most internalized cargo is delivered to the EE or to intermediate compartments such as the GEEC (4) or to the caveosome (7). Black arrows correspond to the endocytic and retrograde pathways, and gray arrows correspond to the secretory/biosynthetic pathways. EE, early endosomes; ER, endoplasmic reticulum; GA, Golgi apparatus; GPI, glycosylphosphatidylinositol-anchored proteins; LE, late endosomes; N, nucleus; PM, plasma membrane; TGN, *trans*-Golgi network.

the plasma membrane in Hela and COS-7 cells. It was also found in distinct endocytic intermediates that colocalized with glycosylphosphatidyl-inositol-linked proteins (GPI-linked proteins) and cholera toxin subunit B (CTB), but not with transferrin or caveolin-1. The silencing of flotillin 1 by siRNA inhibited the endocytosis of CTB and a GPI-linked protein. Both the receptor for CTB (the ganglioside GM1) and GPI-anchored proteins are markers of lipid rafts. Lipid rafts are plasma membrane microdomains with a highly ordered structure distinct from the surrounding membrane area. They are rich in cholesterol, glycosphingolipids, and saturated lipids.[41] Flotillins are found in association with lipid rafts. Furthermore, the flotillin 1-mediated uptake of CTB and GPI-linked proteins was not inhibited by the overexpression of a dominant-negative dynamin mutant,[40] indicating that internalization did not appear to require dynamin.

Several studies show that flotillins accumulate in endosomes of AD neurons and in the multivesicular bodies (MVBs) of transgenic mice neurons overexpressing human APP and PS1.[42] Furthermore, amyloid deposits in the brains of AD patients contain flotillins, as determined by immunostaining.[43] A recent study by Schneider et al. indicates that flotillins may have a role in regulating the endocytosis of APP.[44] Using mouse neuroblastoma cells and neurons, they showed that flotillins and cholesterol promote the clustering of APP at the cell surface and stimulate the endocytosis of APP into a specialized clathrin-dependent pathway that favors Aβ peptide production. When flotillin 2 was downregulated by siRNA, there was a reduction in APP endocytosis, accompanied by a decrease in Aβ peptide production. The flotillin- and clathrin-dependent endocytosis of APP requires AP2, AP180, dynamin, and cholesterol, but not epsin 1. In contrast to the results obtained by Glebov et al.,[40] these results reveal a separate endocytic pathway mediated by flotillins, but with many of the attributes of classic clathrin-dependent endocytosis. In addition, Schneider et al.[44] highlight a role for flotillins and cholesterol, both associated with lipid rafts, in the amyloidogenic processing of APP.

10.2.1.5 The Role of Lipid Rafts in Amyloid Generation

Lipid rafts have been implicated as the sites where amyloidogenic processing of APP occurs.[45] Lipid rafts were originally characterized as plasma membrane fractions insoluble in cold Triton X-100, a non-ionic detergent, and sensitive to cholesterol depleting agents.[41,46–48] Proteins found in these detergent-insoluble membranes, besides GPI-anchored proteins, include many acylated signaling proteins (e.g., Src family kinases, growth factor receptors, G-proteins, nitric oxide synthase, integrins, and cholesterol-binding proteins such as caveolin). Signaling lipids such as $PI(4,5)P_2$, arachidonic acid, and phosphatidylserine are also present in the lipid rafts.[49] Lipid rafts may have a role in the segregation of signaling proteins and lipids within a membrane microdomain to increase the proximity, efficiency, specificity, and regulation of signaling cascades.[50]

BACE contains several palmitoyl groups, a feature typical of proteins associated with lipid rafts. Both BACE and γ-secretase have been found to be associated with lipid raft microdomains.[15,51] Ehehalt et al.[52] demonstrated that the depletion of cholesterol in mouse neuroblastoma cells markedly reduced Aβ peptide generation. In addition, when APP and BACE were cross-linked with antibodies at the cell surface, they copatched with each other and with a GPI-anchored raft-associated protein. The copatching was inhibited by cholesterol removal. They also showed that Aβ peptide is generated within the endocytic system, whereas α-secretase processing of APP (non-amyloidogenic pathway) occurs at the plasma membrane.

In vitro studies using purified, recombinant BACE reconstituted into unilamellar vesicles of different lipid compositions showed that BACE activity is stimulated by cerebrosides and cholesterol, representative raft lipids.[53] Furthermore, ganglioside GM1 (another raft-associated lipid) and cholesterol bind Aβ and act as nucleation seeds for Aβ aggregation. So, overall, there seems to be a relationship between lipid rafts, total cellular cholesterol levels, and Aβ peptide production.

Polymorphisms in apolipoprotein E (ApoE), the major cholesterol transport protein expressed in the brain, are associated with the late-onset of AD. Specifically, allele APOE4 is a genetic risk factor for AD.[54] The cholesterol-lowering drugs simvastatin and lovastatin decrease the intracellular and extracellular levels of Aβ peptide in cultured neurons.[55] Epidemiological studies show a reduced incidence of AD in patients treated with cholesterol-lowering statins.[56,57] In fact, clinical trials to assess the efficacy of statins in controlling the progression of AD are currently in progress.[12,58]

In conclusion, several lines of evidence point to cholesterol and lipid rafts as factors involved in the process of Aβ peptide formation and the development of AD, however, the cellular and molecular mechanisms implicated in this process are for the most part unknown.

> Lipid rafts are characterized as plasma membrane fractions and are sensitive to cholesterol depleting agents. Lipid rafts have been implicated as the sites where amyloidogenic processing of APP occurs. Lipid rafts may have a role in the segregation of signaling proteins and lipids within a membrane microdomain to increase the proximity, efficiency, specificity, and regulation of signaling cascades.

10.2.1.6   Therapeutics: Membrane Delivery of a BACE Inhibitor

Both BACE and γ-secretase have been chosen as therapeutic targets for AD, based on the critical role they play in Aβ formation. γ-Secretase inhibitors have been tested in clinical trials (see reviews by Fleisher et al.[59] and Roberson and Mucke[60]). They have had limited success due to the fact that γ-secretase cleaves other substrates necessary for normal cellular functions, such as the Notch receptor. γ-secretase modulators may be more promising.[61–63] BACE, with a more restricted repertoire of substrates, is the more appealing target. Many peptide-based as well as nonpeptide-based BACE inhibitors have been developed in recent years. We direct the reader to such excellent reviews on the diversity of BACE inhibitors as those by Ghosh et al.,[64] Hills and Vacca,[65] Silvestri,[66] Tung et al.,[67] and Wolfe.[68] Here, we concentrate on the question of optimal delivery route.

Rajendran et al.[69] took an innovative approach to target BACE using a lipid-anchored inhibitor. This work illustrates the value of delivering a drug to the corresponding intracellular location of the target. They found that a nonpermeable transition state peptide inhibitor of BACE[67] that was effective in blocking BACE activity in *in vitro* enzymatic assays was unsuccessful in inhibiting BACE in cellular assays. Based on these results and the fact that BACE cleavage seems to occur in endocytic compartments (see above), they designed a lipid-linked derivative of the soluble peptide inhibitor. They expected this derivative to insert itself into the membrane, more specifically into lipid rafts, and thus be capable of sustaining endocytosis and facilitating its delivery to endosomes.

The peptide inhibitor was coupled by its C-terminus, using a polyethylene glycol (PEG) linker, to a sterol (dihydrocholesterol). When tested in Hela cells or neuroblastoma cells expressing the Swiss APP mutant gene (swAPP), the sterol-anchored inhibitor was indeed severalfold more efficient at blocking Aβ peptide formation than the free inhibitor. Using a fluorescent derivative of the sterol-linked inhibitor (with equivalent inhibitory capacity as the nonfluorescent sterol derivative), they demonstrated that the sterol-linked inhibitor was rapidly internalized and accumulated in endosomes that also carried BACE and APP. The inhibition of endocytosis by expressing a dominant negative mutant of dynamin resulted in the diminished internalization of lipid-linked inhibitor. The internalization of the lipid-linked inhibitor correlated with the reduced BACE cleavage of APP and increased α-secretase cleavage of APP. The free inhibitor was poorly internalized and failed to inhibit the BACE cleavage of APP. Therefore, the sterol anchor was efficient at targeting the inhibitor to the endosomes—where BACE cleavage of APP occurs. Importantly, the sterol-linked inhibitor also proved to be effective *in vivo*, by reducing Aβ peptide production in a transgenic fly model and in transgenic mice over-expressing human wild type or mutant APP, presenilin, and/or wild type BACE.

As BACE seems to be associated in the membrane with lipid rafts (see above), the authors[69] predicted that the sterol anchor may induce the localization of the sterol-linked inhibitor in the membrane within lipid raft microdomains. To test this hypothesis, they attached different lipid anchors (palmityl, myristyl, and oleyl chains) to the inhibitor with varied affinity for lipid rafts and determined their ability to inhibit BACE as compared with the sterol-linked inhibitor. Of all three fatty acyl chain derivatives, the most active against BACE was the palmitoyl-linked inhibitor, followed by the myristyl-linked derivative. Also the sterol- and palmitoyl-linked inhibitor preferentially partitioned into the raft-like liquid ordered phase of artificial lipid bilayers. This phase contained both raft-like liquid ordered and nonraft-like disordered phases, as determined by fluorescence correlation spectroscopy and avalanche photodiode imaging.

In summary, the attachment of a sterol moiety to an impermeable, soluble, transition state peptide inhibitor promoted the anchoring of the inhibitor into the plasma membrane, forcing the inhibitor to enter the endocytic pathway and to localize to endocytic compartments where BACE, a membrane protein, is known to be active. Consequently, the effectiveness of the inhibitor was maximized by means of confining the inhibitor not only to the same intracellular compartment, but also to the membrane microdomain (lipid rafts) where BACE concentrates. In addition, by anchoring the inhibitor to the lipid bilayer, it decreased the dimensionality of inhibitor diffusion to two dimensions, thus enhancing contact between the inhibitor and the enzyme. In conclusion, the principles illustrated here can be applied to target other membrane proteins and intracellular compartments.

> The attachment of a sterol moiety to an impermeable state peptide inhibitor promoted the anchoring of the inhibitor into the plasma membrane, forcing the inhibitor to enter the endocytic compartments where BACE, a membrane protein, is known to be active. Consequently, the effectiveness of the inhibitor was maximized by means of confining the inhibitor not only to the same intracellular compartment, but also to the membrane microdomain (lipid rafts) where BACE concentrates.

10.2.2   A DECLAWED PROTEIN TOXIN SUBUNIT AS A CARRIER FOR ANTIGENIC PEPTIDES, DRUGS, AND IMAGING AGENTS

Next, we highlight the retrograde trafficking pathway(s) as defined by research on Shiga toxins (ST) and Shiga-like toxins (SLT) and the potential role of declawed toxin subunits as carriers of drugs, antigens, and imaging agents into the cell. For a recent general review on retrograde trafficking pathways in cells, the reader is referred to an excellent article by Johannes and Popoff.[70]

Endocytosis is the starting point for the internalization of proteins and lipids into cells and, therefore, a potential portal into the cell.[5,39] Research on the trafficking of bacterial or plant A/B-type toxins, such as ST and SLT (described in greater detail in the following section), has revealed retrograde trafficking pathways between endosomes and the ER[70] that can be exploited for the targeted delivery of drugs, bypassing the acid hydrolytic environment of the lysosome.[71] In these pathways, the GA is frequently central.

In the A/B-type toxins, the B-subunit is the targeting subunit (Figure 10.4). It can be expressed independently of the A or catalytic subunit, which confers cytotoxic properties on the protein. Hence, targeted carriers can be readily created. We use these examples to illustrate principles that are applicable to a wide range of carriers that fall into the B-class targeting subunit.

10.2.2.1   Endocytosis and Endocytic Pathways (Figure 10.3)

Endocytosis is a vital process in all eukaryotic cells, which mediates the internalization of material from the extracellular space (nutrients, hormones, fluids, particles) into the cell that otherwise would not be able to cross the hydrophobic lipid bilayer of the plasma membrane. Endocytosis is essential for sustaining necessary cellular functions, such as cell-signaling, nutrient and fluid uptake, cell-adhesion, cell-migration, receptor down-regulation, membrane recycling, cell growth, and differentiation, just to name a few.

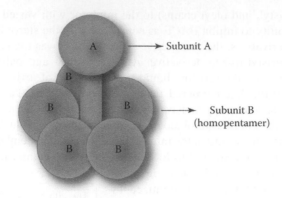

FIGURE 10.4 Structure of ST/SLT. ST/STL is composed of two polypeptide subunits, designated as A and B. The toxic A subunit, a 32 kDa polypeptide, is an *N*-glycosidase that cleaves a unique adenine residue in the 28S rRNA of the 60S ribosomal subunit, which results in inactivation of protein synthesis and ultimately leads cell death. The B subunit, which is nontoxic and confers binding specificity, consists of a complex of five identical B subunits monomers, 8 kDa in size each, arranged in the shape of a toroid. Stoichiometrically, one subunit A associates noncovalently with a subunit B pentamer to give the holotoxin.

Endocytosis is the starting point for the transport of ligands from the plasma membrane to EE. From there, internalized proteins and lipids can take several paths: (1) proteins and lipids to be reused are salvaged in recycling endosomes and returned to the plasma membrane; (2) some proteins and lipids are transported from EE to late endosomes (LE) and in turn to lysosomes where they are degraded; or (3) a fraction of proteins and lipids move directly from EE to the GA, sidestepping the LE/lysosomal path and hence avoiding degradation.

In general, any endocytic pathway occurs in three steps[5]: (1) cargo is selected at the cell surface; (2) selected cargo is packaged into a vesicle that requires the formation and detachment of the vesicle from the cytosolic side of the plasma membrane; and (3) the delivery of the vesicle to the earliest acceptor compartment, which in most cases is the EE. Several pathways for the internalization of ligand/receptor complexes at the plasma membrane have been described.[5,39] The best-studied endocytic mechanism involves the formation of clathrin-coated vesicles. More recently discovered clathrin-independent mechanisms have been described and are less well understood. The clathrin-independent pathways include endocytic mechanisms initialized within lipid-rich microdomains at the plasma membrane, represented by lipid rafts- and caveolae-dependent uptake. These endocytic mechanisms are illustrated in Figure 10.3. Macropinocytosis and phagocytosis are also clathrin-independent pathways.[39]

In this section, we briefly go through the general characteristics of the different endocytic pathways described to date. This section is not intended to be a comprehensive description of endocytic pathways but just a brief section to give enough basic information to help the reader understand succeeding sections. For comprehensive publications on this subject, the following reviews are highly recommended: Doherty and McMahon,[39] Mayor and Pagano,[5] Mousavi et al.,[72] Rodemar and Haucke,[73] and Sandvig et al.[74]

10.2.2.1.1 Clathrin-Dependent Endocytosis

Clathrin-dependent uptake is the best-defined endocytic mechanism. Clathrin is a cytosolic fibrous protein with the shape of a three-limbed triskelion that has the ability to self-polymerize into a basket-like structure, typical of the ones observed in clathrin-coated vesicles.[72] The biogenesis of clathrin-coated vesicles starts with the recognition of specific targeting sequences in the cytosolic domain of plasma membrane receptors by cytosolic adaptor proteins. The most common endocytic signals encompass tyrosine-based and leucine-based tetrapeptide sequences that interact with several cytosolic adaptor proteins, principally AP2 (adaptor/assembly protein 2), AP180, Eps 15, and Epsin.[6,75,76] Adaptor proteins are involved in the location of clathrin assembly on the plasma membrane and the promotion of clathrin polymerization. Initially, adaptor proteins Epsin and AP2, besides interacting with the receptor signal motifs, bind regions of the inner leaflet of the plasma membrane rich in phosphatidyl inositol, 4,5 bisphosphate [PI(4,5) P_2] with the subsequent recruitment of other adaptor proteins, clathrin, and the assembly of the clathrin coat.[77,78] Recruited clathrin molecules assemble within the plasma membrane into a planar lattice that further develops into the cage/basket-like structure with the concomitant formation of a deeply invaginated clathrin-coated pit that leads to the release of the clathrin-coated vesicle.[79,80] The curvature of the clathrin-like basket structure provides the driving force for the formation and release of the vesicle from the plasma membrane, together with dynamin.[72,81] Dynamin is a large GTPase that arranges into a helical polymer that surrounds the nascent vesicle neck which after GTP hydrolysis induces the fission of the vesicle from the plasma membrane.[39] Interestingly, it has been shown that dynamin is involved in actin filament assembly; dynamin and actin are also recruited sequentially at sites of endocytosis.[82,83] Cholesterol may also contribute to membrane invagination since cells depleted of cholesterol with sterol-binding agents show numerous flat clathrin-coated patches at the plasma membrane and very little deeply invaginated coated pits.[72,84,85]

10.2.2.1.2 Clathrin-Independent Endocytosis

Endocytic pathways that do not require clathrin have been more recently described and are not as well understood as the clathrin-dependent pathway. Essentially, the clathrin-independent pathways have been classified based on their requirement of dynamin, caveolin, flotillin, various small GTPases, cholesterol, and other raft-associated lipids.[5,39]

Caveolin-dependent (or caveolae-dependent) endocytosis is probably the most studied clathrin-independent pathway. Caveolae are 50–80 nm uncoated cell surface invaginations initially observed by electron microscopy by Palade[86] and Yamada.[87] Caveolae are abundant in some cell types such as muscle, endothelia, and adipocytes corresponding to about 35% of the cell surface; in contrast they are absent in lymphocytes and neurons.[41] Caveolae are characterized by the presence of the protein caveolin and similar lipid and protein content as lipid rafts.[88–92] Caveolae thus colocalize with detergent-insoluble membrane fractions, are sensitive to cholesterol depletion, and share many of the molecular markers present in lipid rafts.[93,94] Caveolin is a 21 kDa integral membrane protein, with 3 covalently attached palmitoyl groups, that binds cholesterol and glycolipids.[41,95] Caveolin has an atypical topology in the plasma membrane as it forms an intra-membrane hairpin loop, with both N- and C-terminal domains in the cytosol.[96] Three isoforms of caveolin have been described. Caveolin-1 and caveolin-2 are present in all cells with caveolae and caveolin-3 is found only in muscle cells. Caveolin-1 monomers oligomerize to form complexes at the plasma membrane, which may have a role in affecting the membrane curvature and thus caveolae formation.[97] Several studies indicate that in caveolae-containing cells, only a minor pool of caveolae is engaged in active endocytosis. In fluorescence recovery experiments after photobleaching (FRAP)[98] in cells expressing chimeric caveolin-1-green fluorescent protein (GFP), they found that caveolae labeled with the caveolin-1-GFP remained static. The integrity of caveolae has been shown to be dependent on cholesterol as treatment with cholesterol-depleting agents causes the disappearance of caveolae structures and the redistribution of caveolin-1 along the plasma membrane. Likewise, depolymerization of the actin cytoskeleton results in the clustering of caveolae at the plasma membrane, indicating a role of actin in the stabilization of caveolae at the plasma membrane.[98,99] Other lines of evidence have shown that filamin, an actin-binding protein, is a ligand for caveolin-1, and the activation of Rho, which causes the reorganization of actin cytoskeleton, also affects the redistribution of caveolae.[100] In addition, the treatment of cells with phosphatase inhibitors stimulates caveolae-dependent endocytosis whereas genistein, a Src-family kinase inhibitor, prevents caveolar endocytosis, indicating that reversible phosphorylation may play a role in caveola formation and budding.[94,101] Other studies have shown that the overexpression of caveolin-1 in transformed NIH-3T3 cells decreases the rate of endocytosis of the autocrine motility factor receptor (AMF-R), a transmembrane protein with steady-state residency in caveolae at the plasma membrane and the smooth ER, indicating that caveolin-1 may actually be a negative regulator of caveolae-dependent endocytosis.[102] Consistent with this is the fact that transformed NIH-3T3 with a low-level expression of caveolin-1 showed greater caveolar-dependent endocytosis compared with the cells overexpressing caveolin-1. As in clathrin-dependent endocytosis, caveolae-dependent endocytosis relies on the GTPase dynamin (see above), which may function to regulate the budding of caveolae from the plasma membrane.[102]

Extensive studies on cholera toxin (CT) and simian virus 40 (SV40) internalization have demonstrated the involvement of caveolae in their endocytosis. SV40 infects cells through binding to major histocompatibility complex class I (MHC-I) antigens at the cell surface. Pelkmans et al.[103] observed that in CV-1 cells (African green monkey kidney fibroblast cell line), SV40 associates with caveolae at the plasma membrane and moves from the plasma membrane in small caveolin-1-positive vesicles into caveosomes, a neutral pH compartment that does not contain markers of endosomes, lysosomes, ER, or GA. SV40 is transported from caveosomes directly to smooth ER using caveolin-1-free tubular vesicles that move along microtubules. Additionally, SV40 binding to its receptor in caveolae induces actin cytoskeleton reorganization and recruitment of dynamin.[104] SV40 infection is also dependent on cholesterol and the activation of tyrosine kinases in caveolae. The pathway of entry of SV40 is unusual in that it initially enters the caveosomes, an organelle biochemically distinct from endosomes, thus bypassing endosomes and GA to reach the smooth ER. Surprisingly, in a recent study, it was found that SV40 can infect cells that do not express caveolin-1, initially transferring to neutral pH caveosome-like structures devoid of caveolin-1 and then transferring to the ER via microtubule-dependent vesicular carriers.[105] This alternative pathway is independent of caveolae, clathrin, dynamin, and Arf6 (small GTPase), but dependent on cholesterol and tyrosine kinases activation.[106] The AMF-R (see above), a cellular protein in NIH-3T3 cells, upon binding to AMF is internalized via caveolae-, dynamin- and cholesterol-dependent endocytosis and is subsequently taken directly to the smooth ER by vesicular/tubular transport, in a fashion similar to SV40,[102] suggesting that the SV40 intracellular route to the ER may actually be a normal membrane trafficking pathway.

Clathrin- and caveolin-independent pathways have been sub-classified by their reliance on the small GTPases (RhoA, Arf6, CdC42), dynamin,[5] and flotillin (covered in Section 10.2.1.4). For example, the internalization of the interleukin-2-receptor (IL-2) in lymphocytes[107] is regulated by the small GTPase RhoA, requires dynamin, and occurs in association with detergent-resistant membrane domains (lipid rafts). Clathrin-caveolin and dynamin-independent pathways regulated by the small GTPase CDC42 are responsible for much of the fluid-phase uptake in many cells,[108] the non-caveolar entry of CTx, and the internalization of GPI-anchored proteins.[109] The CDC42-regulated internalization of GPI-anchored proteins originates in the detergent-resistant membrane domains and takes place in morphologically distinctive tubular carriers. GPI-anchored proteins as well as fluid-phase markers accumulate in a separate tubular-vesicular acidic intracellular compartment different from EE, designated as the GPI-anchored protein-enriched early endosomal compartment (GEEC[5]). In addition, a clathrin- and caveolin-independent endocytic pathway regulated by Arf6 has been implicated in the uptake of the MHC-I complex proteins and some GPI-anchored proteins without any dynamin requirement.[5,39]

In conclusion, besides the well-characterized clathrin-dependent endocytic pathway, a number of other clathrin-independent pathways have been unraveled. These clathrin-independent pathways have been subclassified by their requirement for caveolin, flotillin, dynamin, and small GTPases.

The outline below and Figure 10.3 give an overall classification of these different endocytic pathways.

1. Clathrin-dependent (requires dynamin)
2. Clathrin-independent:
   a. Caveolin/caveolae-dependent (requires dynamin)
   b. Caveolin/caveolae-independent:
      i. Flotillin-dependent (dynamin may be required)
      ii. RhoA-regulated (requires dynamin)
      iii. CDC42-regulated (dynamin-independent)
      iv. Arf6-regulated (dynamin-independent)

10.2.2.2 Biology of Shiga Toxins and Shiga-Like Toxins

Shiga toxins (STs) are a group of toxins produced by *Shigella dysenteriae* type 1 and by some *Escherichia coli* strains.[110–113] These toxins cause severe illnesses, such as hemolytic colitis and hemolytic uremic syndrome, especially in young children. STs are composed of two polypeptide subunits, designated as A and B. The toxic A subunit, a 32 kDa polypeptide, is an *N*-glycosidase that cleaves a unique adenine residue in the 28S rRNA of the 60S ribosomal subunit, which results in the inactivation of protein synthesis and ultimately leads to cell death. The B subunit, which is nontoxic and confers binding specificity, consists of a complex of five identical B subunit monomers, each 8 kDa in size, arranged in the shape of a toroid. Stoichiometrically, one subunit A associates noncovalently with a subunit B pentamer to provide the holotoxin (Figure 10.4). Given that the *E. coli* related STs have a similar structure and biological activity to ST, they have been classified as Shiga-like toxins (SLT).[111,114]

The B subunit of STs and SLTs (STB and SLTB) recognizes and binds to the cell surface glycosphingolipid, globotriaosylceramide, or Gb$_3$ (galactose-α-1,4-galactose-β-1,4-glucose ceramide), inducing the receptor-mediated internalization of the holotoxin. STB and SLTB exhibit a high affinity for Gb$_3$, with a dissociation constant (K_d) in the range of 10^{-17} to 10^{-12} M[115] and about three binding sites per B subunit monomer.[116] ST/SLT is synthesized as a nontoxic proprotein, which is activated shortly after endocytosis by proteolytic cleavage of the A subunit by furin in EE.[113] The cleavage of the A subunit by furin produces two fragments (A1 and A2) that are held together by an internal disulfide bond. ST/SLT travels in retrograde fashion to the ER, where the enzyme protein disulfide isomerase releases A1 from the rest of the molecule (A2 and subunit B remain associated). A1, which retains the toxic enzymatic activity, translocates then to the cytosol from the ER, allegedly using the cellular ER-associated protein degradation (ERAD) machinery.[113] In the cytosol, A1 modifies 28S rRNA, subsequently inhibiting protein synthesis and ultimately causing cell death.

> STs cause severe illnesses, such as hemolytic colitis and hemolytic uremic syndrome, especially in young children. STs are composed of two polypeptide subunits, designated as A and B. The toxic A subunit causes the inactivation of protein synthesis and ultimately leads to cell death. The B subunit is nontoxic and confers binding specificity. Stoichiometrically, one subunit A associates noncovalently with a subunit B pentamer to provide the holotoxin.

10.2.2.3 ST/SLT Entry and the Path to the Endoplasmic Reticulum*

10.2.2.3.1 Endocytosis

The first step for the entry of a ST/SLT into cells is the binding of its B subunit (STB/SLTB) to the glycolipid receptor, Gb$_3$, in the plasma membrane of target cells. Then, ST/SLT is internalized via clathrin-dependent and independent mechanisms.[113,117–120] The particular endocytic mechanism used by STs/SLTs may well be cell-specific, but both clathrin-dependent and

---

* See Table 10.2 for a summary of the different steps taken by ST/SLT to reach the ER.

TABLE 10.2
Steps in ST/SLT Transport from Cell Surface to ER and Cytosol

Step	Mechanism	Requirements
Endocytosis	Clathrin-dependent	Clathrin coat
		Clathrin adaptors: epsin, eps15
		Dynamin (large GTP-binding protein involved in vesicle fission from membrane)
		Cholesterol
	Clathrin-independent	Lipid rafts/cholesterol
		Dynamin may/may not be required
		Binding Gb_3 (receptor) can induce own ST/SLT internalization
Endosome to TGN	Clathrin-dependent	Clathrin coat
		Clathrin adaptors: epsinR
		Dynamin
		Small GTPases: rab6A′ (targeting and fusion of vesicles with TGN)
		Vesicle and target membrane tethering and fusion factors. v-SNARES: VAMP3/cellubrevin; VAMP4. t-SNARES: syntaxin 6/syntaxin 16/Vtu1A; syntaxin 5/GS28/Ytk6/GS15. Golgin-97, golgin-245
		Cholesterol, calcium
	Retromer complex	Retromer coat: dimer, SNX1/SNX2; trimer, Vps26p/Vps29p/Vps35p. Dimer binds curved membranes through phosphoinositides and recruits trimer. Trimer functions in cargo selection
		It is undetermined whether the retromer complex and clathrin sorting system function in parallel in redundant pathways or sequentially in the same pathway
TGN/Golgi to ER	COP-I independent	Rab6
ER to Cytosol	Retro-translocation of subunit A (toxic) through ERAD machinery	ERAD (Sec61 translocon)

independent pathways can also coexist in a cell. For example, Nichols et al. show in COS-7 cells that when clathrin-dependent internalization was disrupted by expressing dominant negative mutants of the clathrin adaptors (epsin and eps15), the endocytosis of lipid raft markers (GPI-anchored proteins), CTB, and STB was unaffected.[121] Nonetheless, as compared with untreated cells, transferrin uptake was significantly decreased. The total uptake of STB and CTB from the cell surface was reduced in cells where clathrin-coat formation was inhibited, consistent with STB (and CTB) using both clathrin-dependent and independent endocytic pathways in these cells. Similarly, STB uptake still occurred in cells in which either clathrin, clathrin adaptors (epsinR and AP1), or dynamin expression was blocked. This was in agreement with the clathrin-independent uptake of STB.[118,119] Clathrin-independent pathways are generally poorly understood, but in the case of STs/SLTs, they appear to be mediated by the association of Gb_3 with lipid rafts.

The clathrin-independent uptake of STs/SLTs is severely impaired when lipid raft microdomains are destabilized by cellular cholesterol depletion,[121,122] further supporting lipid raft involvement. On the other hand, a recent study shows that STB promotes the formation of cell surface tubular membrane invaginations upon binding to Gb_3 in Hela cells or model membranes.[123] Dynamin or actin inhibition, cholesterol extraction, or energy depletion in Hela cells increased the number of STB-induced cell surface tubular invaginations. This indicated that STB binding to the membrane itself, without the aid of cellular proteins or energy, was causing the membrane invaginations. The number of invaginations increased because the lack of dynamin function impeded tubule scission. The binding of a monoclonal antibody against Gb_3 or a mutant STB with decreased binding capacity failed to induce membrane invaginations in cells and model membranes, demonstrating that just binding to Gb_3 does not promote invaginations.

The authors propose a model in which STB binding causes lipid reorganization, probably due to the segregation of Gb_3 at STB binding sites ($\approx 15\,Gb_3$ molecules/1 STB molecule). This energetically favors the regions of negative curvature (invagination) in the membrane and leads to the formation of high-density STB clusters. In summary, high-capacity/affinity-STB binding to its receptor at the cell surface, a biophysical process, can provide the driving force to induce membrane invagination.

10.2.2.3.2 Endosome to TGN Transport

Subsequent to the uptake by clathrin-dependent or independent pathways, STs/SLTs initially localize to EE,[124] as demonstrated by the colocalization with markers of this compartment, e.g., transferrin receptor and EEA1. Unlike ST/SLT, some A/B family toxins, such as Diphtheria, *Clostridium*, and *Anthrax* toxins, continue transport to the more acidic late endosomes (LE) where their toxic A subunit can translocate into the cytosol (Cabiaux,[125] Watson and Spooner[126] for reviews). On the other hand, ST/SLT, CT, *E. coli* heat labile toxin (HLE), *Pseudomonas* exotoxin (PE), and ricin translocate into the cytosol from the ER. In order to reach the ER, they bypass the LE/lysosomal path and, hence, avoid degradation.

This retrograde route was discovered and delineated by studies done primarily with STs/SLTs.[124,127,128] The initial assumption was that the ST/SLT, once in EE, would move to LE and move along one of the paths taken by the MPR to recycle back to the GA. The MPR binds lysosomal enzymes in TGN and targets them to the lysosomes via endosomes.[129] MPR is retrieved from early and LE back to the TGN and reused to deliver more lysosomal enzymes to lysosomes. The transport of MPR from LE to GA is regulated by the small GTPase, Rab9, and its effector protein, tail-interactin protein of 47 kDa molecular weight (called TIP47).[130,131] The expression of inducible Rab9 dominant negative mutant in cells inhibits the transport of MPR to TGN. However, it does not inhibit the localization of ST/SLT and ricin to TGN. This indicates that STs/SLTs and ricin do not transit along with MPR to TGN along the late endosomal retrieval path.[132–134]

Interestingly, recent studies indicate that ST/SLT may be sorted and transported from EE to TGN with the aid of the clathrin coat machinery, and even the retromer complex might be involved.[118,119,135,136] Saint-Pol et al. reported that ST was effectively internalized by HeLa cells, even when clathrin expression was inhibited by siRNA.[119] Nonetheless, the inhibition of clathrin or epsinR, but not AP1, blocked the retrograde transport of ST from EE to TGN. In a related study, Lauvrak et al. confirm that clathrin is necessary for ST traffic from EE to TGN, and further demonstrates that dynamin is also required.[118] Collectively, these studies provide evidence that clathrin, epsinR, and dynamin have a functional role in the EE to TGN retrograde transport of ST.

Furthermore, the retromer complex has been implicated in the transport of STs from EE to TGN. The siRNA suppression of SNX1 or Vps26p expression in HeLa cells halted the transfer of STs from EE to TGN. It remains unclear whether the retromer complex and the clathrin sorting system work in parallel in redundant pathways, or sequentially in the same pathway. Popoff et al. present preliminary evidence that argues in favor of clathrin and the retromer acting sequentially in a single pathway. They propose a model where clathrin functions first to induce membrane curvature, tubule formation, and the sorting of STs. This is followed by the retromer complex carrying out ST transport to TGN.[136] Further studies are necessary to determine the individual functions of clathrin and the retromer complex in EE to TGN transport and how their functions are synchronized in this process.

Targeting and fusion of EE-derived vesicles carrying ST to TGN is mediated by a range of molecules that include Rab6A′ [118,119,124,137–141] and the following soluble *N*-ethylmaleimide-sensitive fusion factor attachment protein receptors (SNARE): v-SNAREs (VAMP3/cellubrevin and VAMP4) and the t-SNAREs (syntaxin 6, syntaxin 16, and Vti1A),[137,141] syntaxin 5, GS28, Ykt6, and GS15.[142]

10.2.2.3.3   TGN/Golgi to ER Transport

ST/SLT, as well as other A/B protein toxins such as CT, HLE, PE, and ricin traffic from the TGN to the GA and to the ER in retrograde fashion, using a pathway that is independent of the well-known COPI-retrograde transport used to salvage ER resident proteins that escape to the GA. COPI is a coat complex with a function similar to that of the clathrin coat.[2,6,8,9,143–145] COPI-coated vesicles are involved in anterograde vesicle traffic within the GA and in retrograde traffic from GA to ER, to retrieve ER resident proteins that escape the ER into the GA. COPI coat components recognize a tetrapeptide sequence (KKXX or RRXX) in the cytosolic domain of ER resident proteins. These signals act as retrieval signals.[6,9,144] The ER luminal proteins that escape to GA are retrieved by the KDEL receptor, which recognizes the KDEL amino acid sequence in luminal proteins. The KDEL receptor, in turn, is recognized by the COPI coat. The KDEL receptor system actively operates in the GA and ER/GA intermediate compartments to sort out and capture the escaped ER resident proteins. The retrograde transport of these toxins may be mediated by the KDEL receptor system.

However, ST/SLT does not have a KDEL signal. Moreover, the addition of a KDEL signal to STB does not improve its rate of retrograde transport to ER.[146] CT has a KDEL sequence in the catalytic A subunit. CTB, by itself, is able to reach the ER without the A subunit.[147] HLE has a KDEL-like signal in the toxic A subunit (RDEL), that likewise is not absolutely necessary for transport to the ER.[147] PE has a KDEL-like signal, RDELK, that itself does not bind to the KDEL receptor. However, the last lysine is removed during internalization, thereby creating the RDEL sequence that binds the KDEL receptor.[148] The RDEL sequence seems to be necessary for PE to reach the ER. Recent studies indicate that PE may be able to use more than one pathway to reach the ER.[149]

How do these toxins reach the ER?

GA resident enzymes constantly cycle from the GA to ER and back. This continuous cycling of GA resident enzymes has been demonstrated by experiments in which treatment with brefeldin A (BFA) causes the re-localization of GA resident proteins to the ER, and practically the collapse of the GA into the ER.[8,143,150,151] BFA is a fungal macrolide that inhibits Arf1, a small GTPase necessary in the recruitment of COPI coat component proteins to GA membranes. Thus, it blocks COPI-dependent anterograde and retrograde transport from GA to ER. Given that retrograde traffic from GA to ER continues, independent of COPI, the outcome of BFA treatment is the relocation of GA lipids and resident proteins to the ER and the dispersal of the GA. Similarly, the expression of the dominant-negative mutants of Arf1 or the components of the COPI coat complex,[152–154] as well as the expression of dominant-negative mutants of other small GTPases involved in ER to Golgi membrane traffic (such as Sar1p, a small GTPase required for the recruitment of COPII coat proteins to the ER membranes,[153,155–159] Rab6,[152,160–162] Rab33b,[163,164] and other Rab proteins), all cause the same effect as that of BFA treatment, viz., the redistribution of GA proteins and lipids to ER.

Girod et al.[152] reported that the microinjection of the anti-COPI coat antibodies or the expression of Arf1 mutants does not interfere with GA to ER transport of STs/SLTs or with the apparent recycling to the ER of GA resident proteins. In contrast, overexpression of a negative dominant mutant of Rab6 (Rab6-GDP), a small GTPase involved in intra GA transport, blocks transport to the ER of STs/SLTs and GA glycosylation enzymes, but not the KDEL receptor or PE, a toxin containing a KDEL-like retrieval signal. This evidence supports the existence of an alternate transport pathway from GA to ER, independent of COPI but dependent on Rab6, which normally operates in the cycling of GA enzymes and is exploited by toxins to reach the ER.

The transfer of the toxic catalytic A subunit of these toxins from the ER to the cytosol is thought to occur through the ERAD machinery. The ERAD machinery translocates misfolded proteins into the cytosol through the Sec61p translocon. These misfolded proteins are then ubiquitinated and subsequently degraded by the proteasome. CT, ricin, PE, and ST/SLT interact with Sec61p translocon components. This indicates that these toxins take over the cellular ERAD machinery for retrotranslocation from ER into the cytosol.[165–168]

Not surprisingly, some cellular proteins seem to use the EE to TGN pathway. One of these is TGN38/46, a protein that resides in the TGN but cycles from the cell surface to EE to TGN.[169,170] No known function has been associated with TGN38/46. However, it is commonly used as a marker for TGN. Other proteins, such as GPP130 and GP73, reside in the cis GA, which are the Golgi cisternae at which material from the ER enters the Golgi stack. Upon treatment of cells with agents that increase the internal pH of GA and endosomes, these two proteins relocalize to EE. When GPP130 is overexpressed, part of it redistributes to EE.[171–173] Moreover, GPP130 is sialylated and phosphorylated, two post-translational modifications that occur in later GA compartments. These observations suggest the cycling of these two proteins from cis GA to the plasma membrane, endosomes, TGN, and back to the cis GA.

Recent kinetic studies[174] have shown that the accumulation of GPP130 in EE in response to the increase in pH is attributable to a three- to fourfold decrease in the rate of endosome to GA transport, resulting in an increased time of stay of GPP130 in endosomes. Similarly, the transport of SLTB in the presence of pH elevator agents slows down the rate of the exit of SLTB from EE to TGN, which results in the accumulation of SLTB in EE. These suggest that SLTB and GPP130 may either share the same transport system out of endosomes to TGN, or that GPP130 is necessary for the transport of proteins from the endosomes to the GA.[172,174]

The inhibition of GPP130 expression by siRNA results in the blocked exit of SLTB from endosomes to TGN. It also results in the accumulation of cellular proteins that cycle via this route (GP73 and TGN46) in endosomes. Therefore, GPP130 may actually have a functional role in the traffic from endosomes to the GA.[172] Together, these examples establish a major nondegradative/nonlysosomal pathway for drug delivery within cells.

10.2.2.4 Presentation of Major Histocompatibility Complex Class-I (MHC-I) Antigens via Carrier Proteins

ST/SLT has been sought as a vector to deliver antigens to the MHC-I pathway of antigen presenting cells (APC). This is due to the unique trafficking pathway of ST and SLT, discussed above, and the expression of Gb_3 in APC, such as dendritic cells and some B cells.[175,176]

In the classical MHC-I antigen presentation pathway, endogenously synthesized defective cellular proteins and viral proteins are degraded in the cytosol by the proteasome and then loaded into MHC-I molecules in the ER.[177] The antigenic peptides generated in the cytosol by the proteasome are translocated into the ER by specialized ATP-dependent ABC-type transmembrane transporters in the ER membrane associated with antigen processing and presentation (TAP). Once in the ER, antigenic peptides are loaded into newly synthesized MHC-I molecules, thus forming MHC-I/peptide complexes. These complexes are delivered to the plasma membrane via the secretory pathway.

On the other hand, exogenous antigens enter the endocytic pathway, eventually reaching the late endosomal/lysosomal compartments, where they are fragmented into peptides by resident proteases.

These peptides are loaded on MHC-II molecules and transported to the plasma membrane via the same endosomal system. Even though there is a clear distinction between the presentation of endogenous antigens by MHC-I molecules and exogenous antigens by MHC-II molecules, exogenous antigens can be presented by MHC-I molecules and intracellular antigens can be presented by MHC-II molecules. Some APCs, such as dendritic cells, present peptides derived from exogenous antigens in both MHC-II and MHC-I molecules. This process is called cross-presentation.[177,178] For a simple diagrammatic overview of antigen processing, the reader is directed to Figure 1 of the article by Kim et al.[179]

Exogenous antigens can be loaded on to MHC-I molecules following endocytosis. However, how the antigens enter the cytosol from LE/lysosomes is still uncertain. It has been suggested that the antigens leak into the cytosol either by a transitory rupture of the late endosomal/lysosomal membrane or by as yet uncharacterized specific transmembrane channels in the endosomes/lysosomes. Another possibility is that the internalized exogenous antigens may use the retrograde pathway from endosomes to the GA and then to the ER as STs/SLTs; or they can move directly from endosomes to ER as SV40 does.[103] They may subsequently egress from the ER lumen into the cytosol by making use of the ERAD machinery. Alternatively, there is evidence indicating that exogenously derived peptide antigens may be loaded on MHC-I molecules (possibly recycled MHC-I molecules from the plasma membrane) by the endocytic pathway in a TAP-independent manner and therefore, may not require transport to the cytosol.

APC bearing MHC-I/peptide complexes are recognized by $CD8^+$ cytotoxic T lymphocytes (CTL), initiating a primary immune response that leads to the maturation of CTL, the recognition by mature CTLs of the MHC-I presented antigens in diseased cells that may either be virally infected or sustain genetic abnormalities such as, for example, cancer cells; and the subsequent destruction of the diseased cells by activated CTL. Similarly, APC presenting MHC-II/peptide complexes are recognized by $CD4^+$ helper T lymphocytes (T_H1), leading to the activation of T_H1, which in turn secrete the cytokine, IL-2. IL-2 promotes the growth, differentiation, and activation of CTL. Some APC present exogenous antigens in MHC-I and MHC-II molecules, therefore they are able to produce the activation of CTL and induce the cell-mediated and humoral immune responses necessary to eliminate virus infected and cancer cells. Several strategies have been designed to artificially stimulate APC to present exogenous antigens through the MHC-I pathway to induce immune protection towards viral infections and tumors. One innovative approach is the use of STB as a vector to deliver exogenous antigens to the MHC-I pathway of APC, devised by the group of Johannes and Tartour.[175,180–182] In initial studies, Lee et al.[181] showed that recombinant fusion proteins composed of STB and a model tumor antigen, Mage 1, were internalized by peripheral blood mononuclear lymphocytes (PBML) and presented in the MHC-I pathway to Mage 1-specific CTL. This was independent of carrying an active or inactive ER retrieval signal (KDEL and KDELGL). Epstein-Barr virus (EBV) transformed-B cells (EBV-B cells) and dendritic cells pulsed with STB-Mage 1 fusion protein were also able to present this antigen in an MHC-1-restricted pathway to Mage 1-specific CTL.

In contrast, T cells, which do not express Gb_3, when pulsed with STB-Mage 1 could not present STB-Mage 1-derived antigens. The treatment of EBV-B cells with BFA, which negatively affects STB transport to the ER and transport of MHC-I/peptide complexes to the plasma membrane, inhibited the presentation of STB-Mage 1 in the MHC-I pathway and failed to activate Mage 1-specific CTL. These indicate that the internalization of STB-Mage 1 is necessary for MHC-I antigen presentation. Also, immunofluorescent analysis showed that STB-Mage 1 accumulated in ER and GA of EBV-B cells and did not colocalize with compartments labeled with lysosomal markers. These initial findings revealed that indeed STB could be used as a nonliving, nontoxic vaccine vector.

In related studies, Haicheur et al.[175] reported that STB fused to a tumor peptide derived from mouse mastocytoma P815 induces specific CTL response in mice without the need for adjuvant. They also showed *in vitro* that STB fused to other exogenous antigenic peptides targets them to the MHC-I pathway of mouse dendritic cells. This process is dependent on internalization via receptor-mediated endocytosis since antibodies against STB as well as the inhibition of Gb_3 synthesis prevented antigen presentation. STB delivery of exogenous antigens to the MHC-I pathway in mouse dendritic cells is blocked by treatment with BFA and with lactacystin, a specific proteasome inhibitor, indicating that STB targets exogenous antigens to the classic MHC-I presentation pathway. Also, mouse dendritic cells deficient in TAP failed to present STB-delivered antigens confirming the latter results. Interestingly, in another study, Haicheur et al.[180] found that chemically coupling STB to ovalbumin (OVA) (STB–OVA) delivered OVA-derived peptides into both MHC-I and MHC-II antigen presentation pathways in mouse dendritic cells.

When the STB trafficking pathway in mouse dendritic cells was investigated, it was found that not all internalized STB followed the retrograde transport pathway to the ER. A portion of STB colocalized with late endosomal/lysosomal compartments. This indicated how STB targets exogenous antigens to the MHC-II pathway. However, these results do not establish the mechanisms by which STB delivers exogenous antigens to the MHC-I pathway. A fraction of STB–OVA that follows retrograde transit to ER may translocate to the cytosol from this site. However, there is no evidence that STB itself transfers to the cytosol from ER. When ST holotoxin reaches the ER, only the catalytic ST A subunit translocates to the cytosol. There is also the possibility that STB in mouse dendritic cells may enter the cytosol by translocating from the LE/lysosomes. In human monocyte dendritic cells, STB does not use the retrograde route to ER, as it does in HeLa cells and it accumulates in LE/lysosomes.[138] It seems that the localization of STB in LE/lysosomes of human dendritic cells was related to the fact that Gb_3 is not organized in detergent-resistant microdomains (lipid rafts) in the plasma membrane of these cells, as compared with HeLa cells.[138]

Mice vaccinated with STB–OVA produced a specific anti-OVA CTL response as well as an anti-OVA humoral immune response without the use of adjuvants.[180,182] Splenocytes and T_H1 cells from SLTB–OVA-immunized mice secreted higher levels of gamma interferon (IFN-γ) and anti-OVA IgG2a-type antibodies as compared with mice immunized with OVA only.[180] In addition, OVA-specific CD8$^+$ T cells (CTL) were detected *ex vivo* in mice immunized with STB–OVA. These cells were long lasting as they could be detected up to 91 days after the last vaccination.[182] Mice depleted of dendritic cells failed to exhibit an OVA-specific CTL immune response upon STB–OVA injection. This indicated that dendritic cells are required in this process.

Also, mice immunized with STB coupled to a tumor antigen (E7) protected the mice against a challenge with tumor cells expressing the E7 antigen.[182] STB, when used as a vector to deliver exogenous antigens to mice, resulted in the stimulation of strong and durable CTL and humoral immune responses and tumor protection. Similar results are expected in humans since Gb_3 is expressed in both mice and human dendritic cells. These point to the potential of STB to be used as a nonlive, nontoxic vaccine delivery system for prophylaxis and therapy for cancer and infectious diseases. Current antiviral and antitumor vaccine strategies are aimed at the design of vaccines that preferably elicit both antibody and cell-mediated immune responses, which involve concomitant antigen presentation in MHC-I and MHC-II pathways. Vaccines based on attenuated recombinant live viral or bacterial vectors, as well as naked plasmid DNA encoding protein antigens have been successful in inducing both humoral and cell-mediated immunity. Nonetheless, attenuated recombinant live vectors may be potentially unsafe, particularly in immune-deficient individuals, and naked plasmid DNA vaccines need improvement in gene transfer and expression efficiency. To this extent, STB encompasses a set of characteristics that favor its role as a vaccine vector:

> The B subunit of Shiga toxin (STB), when used as a vector to deliver exogenous antigens to mice, caused the stimulation of strong and prolonged CTL, humoral immune responses, and tumor protection. These point to the potential of STB to be used as a vaccine delivery system for prophylaxis and therapy for cancer and infectious diseases.

- STB specifically targets dendritic cells
- STB has been shown to deliver antigens in both MHC-I and MHC-II antigen presentation pathways

- STB is nonreplicative and nontoxic
- STB can be produced in large quantities as a recombinant protein

10.2.2.5 Targeted Cancer Therapy and Diagnostic Imaging

The expression and metabolism of cell-surface glycolipids and glycoproteins is altered during oncogenic transformation. Consequently, numerous tumor-associated antigens correspond to glycosyl structures.[183] The expression of globotriaosylceramide or Gb_3 (also known as CD77 and P^k antigen), the receptor for STs/SLTs, is enhanced in various cancers, such as ovarian carcinoma,[184–186] lymphomas, myelomas, breast cancer cells,[176] astrocytoma cells,[187] malignant meningiomas,[188] colon cancer,[189] and testicular cancer.[190,191] Furthermore, Gb_3 is expressed in metastatic tumors originating from ovarian,[184,185] breast,[176] and colon carcinomas.[189]

On the other hand, Gb_3 is expressed in several normal tissues throughout the body,[192–194] including the kidney epithelium and endothelial cells, in addition to being found in human milk.[195] Gb_3 is also expressed in subsets of dendritic cells and CD77 positive germinal center B-lymphocytes.[175,176,196,197] Gb_3 is strongly expressed in red blood cell membranes of P^k blood type individuals (0.01% of the population), while only traces are found in red blood cell membranes of most of the population.[198]

The specific binding of STs/SLTs to Gb_3, coupled with the increased levels of Gb_3 found in particular cancers, have led to the development of strategies that utilize STs/SLTs to target these cancerous tissues. In initial studies conducted by Lingwood's group, SLT1 holotoxin was used to kill several human ovarian-derived tumor cells, including multidrug resistant variants.[185] They reported that SLT1 was effective in killing ovarian tumor cells with LD_{50}s ranging from 0.001 to 100 ng/mL of SLT1 depending on the level of Gb_3 expression of individual cell lines. Interestingly, they found that the multidrug-resistant ovarian tumor cell variants, which contained higher Gb_3 levels, were more sensitive to SLT1 than the drug-sensitive parental cell line that expressed less Gb_3. Additionally, SLT1 prevented the growth of metastatic tumors to the lung in a murine metastatic fibrosarcoma model, and the SLT1 effect was abrogated in mice immunized with SLTB1. Other significant observations were made in this study, for instance, surgically removed primary ovarian tumors contained increased levels of Gb_3 relative to normal ovaries and ovarian metastases showed considerably high levels of Gb_3. Furthermore, Gb_3 was present in both the tumor-like gland tissue and the tumor vasculature,[185] suggesting a potential role for SLT1 as an antiangiogenic agent.[199] Supplementary studies by Arab et al.[187] on the expression of Gb_3 in ovarian hyperplasias demonstrated that Gb_3 was present in both benign and malignant tumors, and the highest Gb_3 content was observed in secondary ovarian metastases and tumors refractory to chemotherapy. In addition, they reported high Gb_3 expression in undifferentiated neoplastic ovarian tissue, not only in the tumor mass, but also in blood vessels adjacent to and within the tumor. Other studies have shown that SLT1, at a concentration of 50 ng/mL, caused apoptosis to astrocytoma cells derived from primary human brain tumors.[187] Apparently, STB binding and internalization alone was able to cause apoptosis in astrocytoma cells.[187] Other brain tumors such as malignant meningiomas are sensitive to SLT1 cytotoxicity, both *in vitro* and *in vivo*.[188]

Further applications of SLT in cancer therapy are illustrated by the work of Gariepy and colleagues, who have applied SLT1 in the *ex vivo* purging of malignant cells (expressing Gb_3) from autologous stem cell grafts of breast cancer, lymphoma, and myeloma patients.[176,200] LaCasse et al.[176] reported expression of Gb_3 in 13 out of 18 breast cancer cell lines tested, including cell lines derived from breast cancer metastasis. Sensitivity to the toxin was correlated, although not linearly, with the level of Gb_3 expression in the breast cancer cell lines, with LD_{50}s ranging from as low as 0.01 to 40 ng/mL. Also, 8 out of 10 primary breast cancer biopsies screened showed Gb_3 expression. In the 134 tumor samples obtained from hematological cancers, Gb_3 was expressed in several types of lymphomas and myelomas. *Ex vivo* SLT-1 treatment of various lymphoma and myeloma samples resulted in the depletion of malignant B cells by 3- to 28-fold, whereas normal hematopoietic progenitor cells, which are Gb_3 negative, were unaffected by SLT1 and remained functionally intact. These results clearly indicate that SLT1 may be useful as an *ex vivo* purging agent to eliminate malignant cells from autologous stem cell grafts.

Kovbasnjuk et al.[189] have reported that Gb_3 is significantly expressed in the primary lesions of metastatic colon cancer and in liver metastases while Gb_3 is absent in normal colonic epithelium. Furthermore, in human colon cell lines, they identified a subpopulation of cells expressing high levels of Gb_3 that at the same time displayed invasive characteristics. Normal polarized epithelial cells devoid of endogenous Gb_3 were transfected with Gb_3 synthase, which resulted in Gb3 expression and induction of cell invasiveness. Similarly, the inhibition of Gb_3 synthesis in colon cancer epithelial cells by treatment with siRNA blocked cell invasiveness, suggesting that subpopulations of Gb_3-expressing cells may be involved in the process of tumor cell invasion and metastasis in colon cancer. In addition, treatment of human colon cancer cells with STB selectively killed Gb_3-positive cells by apoptosis. The STB treatment of nude mice bearing colon cancer cell grafts inhibited tumor growth while tumor grafts in STB-untreated nude mice continued to grow.

This group of studies using the complete holotoxin clearly shows that the ST/SLT is effective at killing cells that express the Gb_3 receptor. Nonetheless, cancer therapies based on the holotoxin may pose major risks, and the fact that the nontoxic subunit STB/SLTB without the toxic fragment (subunit A) can be produced functionally intact as a recombinant protein, render STB/SLTB as a drug delivery vehicle, a more logical approach.

In fact, SLTB has been tested as a carrier to deliver the photosensitizers and drugs to target cells.

For example:

- SLTB coupled to the photosensitizer Chlorin e6 (Ce6) was significantly more phototoxic than free Ce6 to cells expressing Gb_3 (Vero cells).[201]
- STB coupled to a glycoporphyrin photosensitizer was phototoxic to HeLa cells. The phototoxicity was almost null in cells where Gb_3 biosynthesis was inhibited.[202]
- The pro-apoptotic drug benzodiazepine RO5-4864, which targets mitochondrial peripheral benzodiazepine receptors, was coupled to STB to increase water solubility and to deliver the drug to cancer cells. This conjugate was cytotoxic to cancer cells expressing Gb_3.[203]
- A conjugate of STB and a topoisomerase I inhibitor prodrug was designed by covalent linking through a disulfide bond.[204] This bond is slowly cleaved along the retrograde route, releasing active prodrug. This STB/topoisomerase I inhibitor conjugate was cytotoxic to cultured colorectal carcinoma cells expressing Gb_3. The Gb_3 negative control cells did not show sensitivity to the conjugate.

SLTB was tested as a carrier to deliver the photosensitizer Chlorin e6 (Ce6) to cells expressing Gb_3 (Vero cells) as a multilevel approach to achieve selective cell killing. SLTB targeting provides one level of selection while the confined activation of the photosensitizer by local illumination, provides a second.[201] Ce6 was chosen both for its phototoxic properties and its potential for covalent conjugation to SLTB. However, as other molecules structurally related to porphyrins, Ce6 tends to self-aggregate in aqueous solutions due to its hydrophobicity and planar structure and can associate nonspecifically to hydrophobic regions of proteins. As a result, when Ce6 was covalently coupled to SLTB, the Ce6-SLTB conjugate contained 10% noncovalently associated Ce6, even after several cleanup steps, including affinity chromatography. The Ce6-SLTB conjugate provided a mixed delivery system in Vero cells in which Ce6 accumulated in the GA and ER, reflecting a typical intracellular distribution of SLTB, and in mitochondria and other cellular membranes representing the distribution of free Ce6. Importantly, the Ce6-SLTB conjugate enhanced the delivery of Ce6 to Vero cells by one order of magnitude as compared with free Ce6, and delivery was receptor-dependent as demonstrated by competitive inhibition studies, indicating that Ce6-SLTB behaved as a vehicle to effectively deliver Ce6 to Vero cells. Furthermore, improved intracellular Ce6 delivery by Ce6-SLTB paralleled Ce6-SLTB-mediated cell phototoxicity, as Ce6-SLTB was 12-fold more photodynamically toxic than free Ce6, displaying an LD_{50} of about $0.1\,\mu M$ Ce6-SLTB expressed as Ce6 content ($\approx 4\,\mu g/mL$ SLTB) (see Figure 10.5). Being Ce6 a fluorescent molecule and based on average measured Ce6 fluorescence per cell, cell killing appeared to be proportional to Ce6 fluorescence accumulation in cells, irrespective of whether Ce6 was delivered via SLTB or as free Ce6. Therefore, it was concluded that there was little enhancement or detriment to cell killing from having Ce6 delivered to multiple subcellular sites as is the case with Ce6-SLTB versus free Ce6 delivery. Much of the cell killing

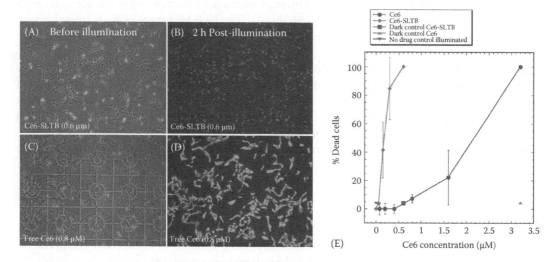

FIGURE 10.5 Photosensitizer delivery via SLTB greatly increases the efficiency of photodynamic cell killing. Vero cells were incubated for 4h in the dark with free Ce6 ($0.8\,\mu M$) or Ce6-SLTB ($0.6\,\mu M$ Ce6). Cells were washed three times, followed by irradiation with a 100W halogen lamp (fluence rate of $18.6\,mW/cm^2$ and a light dose of $4.5\,J/cm^2$). Following irradiation, cells were incubated in the same media for 2h. Phase-contrast pictures of the cells before and after illumination were taken with an Axiovert S100TV inverted microscope (Zeiss, Jena, Germany), equipped with Plan-Neofluar 10×/0.3 numerical aperture objective (Zeiss, Jena, Germany). Focusing, positioning and image capture before illumination was done with very low halogen light intensity and the use of two optical density filters of 3% and 15% light transmission. Live and dead cells were assessed using the fluorescent probes calcein AM and ethidium homodimer-1 (Molecular Probes, Eugene, OR). Calcein AM itself is nonfluorescent and permeable to membranes; it becomes fluorescent when hydrolyzed by esterases in live cells. It accumulates within the cell and fills the cell profile with dye as shown for the live cells in D (green fluorescence in the real world). With cell death, it lost from the cytoplasm as shown in B. Ethidium homodimer-1 is nonpermeable to live cells, but penetrates the damaged membranes of dead cells accumulating in the nucleus, where its fluorescence is enhanced by DNA binding. In dead cells, only the nucleus lights up as shown in B (red fluorescence in the real world). In brief, after 2h, irradiated dishes were washed 3× with warm CO_2-independent media. Followed by incubation with a solution containing $2\,\mu M$ calcein AM and $4\,\mu M$ ethidiumhomodimer-1 in the same media, for 35–45 min at room temperature. Fluorescence was visualized with a Zeiss 103W 100W mercury arc lamp and excitation and emission wavelengths were selected with narrow, band-pass filter sets. Panel A, phase contrast image of cells treated with Ce6-SLTB before light exposure; panel B, nuclei light up in cells treated with Ce6-SLTB, 2h post-illumination; panel C, phase contrast image of cells treated with free Ce6 before light exposure; panel D, cytoplasm lights up in cells treated with free Ce6, 2h post-illumination. Panel E, % dead cells ([cell number before illumination-live cell number post-illumination]×100/cell number before illumination) was plotted versus concentration.

in either case was presumably due to delivery to mitochondria. Whether photosensitizer delivery to strictly GA and ER can produce similar levels of cell killing remains to be elucidated and it will require further studies with more hydrophilic and less planar photosensitizers, with reduced tendency to be absorbed to proteins and to self-aggregate. The ER as a major calcium store within cells is a potential source of apoptotic cell killing. Recent evidence has implicated the GA in apoptosis.[205] Despite the uncertainty of whether delivery of Ce6 by Ce6-SLTB to multiple subcellular sites is preferable to a single site, this study shows that the Ce6-SLTB delivery of Ce6 increased cell-killing efficacy relative to free Ce6; this study also highlights a prospective function for SLTB (or STB) as a vehicle for delivering not only photosensitizers but other therapeutic drugs to target cells.

In a similar study,[202] a glycosylated porphyrin photosensitizer, [TPP(p-O-β-D-GluOH)$_3$], linked to STB has been tested in HeLa cells. A recombinant STB variant with a cysteine residue added to the C-terminus was used to covalently couple to the glycosylated porphyrin. When tested in HeLa cells, this conjugate was five times more phototoxic than the free porphyrin, with an LD$_{50}$ of 0.6 μM expressed as molar concentration of TPP(p-O-β-D-GluOH)$_3$. They show that the phototoxic effect was specific for cells expressing the Gb$_3$ receptor, since in HeLa cells in which Gb3 expression was inhibited using a 1-phenyl-2-hexadecanoyl-amino-3-morphorpholin-1-propanol (PPMP), the phototoxicity to the conjugate was significantly reduced as compared with control HeLa cells. In contrast, the phototoxicity of the free photosensitizer was equivalent in both PPMP-treated and control cells. Furthermore, in HeLa cells treated with BFA, which halts STB transport to Golgi/ER and in turn causes accumulation of STB in endosomal compartments, the conjugate was less phototoxic as compared with HeLa cells in which the conjugate accumulated in the GA/ER compartments. These results indicate that cell killing was more effective at the level of the GA/ER compartments than in endosomes; these results also show that STB provides a route to deliver drugs to ER/GA compartments that bypass the late endosomal compartments where drugs may be degraded, thus limiting their action.

Other examples of the capability of STB as a vector to specifically and effectively deliver anticancer agents intracellularly include the covalent association of STB with the pro-apoptotic drug benzodiazepine RO5-4864, which targets mitochondrial peripheral benzodiazepine receptors.[203] The RO5-4864-STB conjugate was designed to increase the water solubility of RO5-4864 thereby facilitating its delivery. The conjugate contained a linker arm that was stable in serum but cleaved intracellularly. This conjugate was cytotoxic to cancer cells expressing Gb$_3$,[203] as to where the release of the drug from the conjugate occurred was not determined in this study. Similarly, a conjugate of STB and a topoisomerase I inhibitor prodrug was designed by covalent linking through a disulfide bond.[204] This bond is slowly cleaved along the retrograde route, releasing active prodrug. This STB/topoisomerase I inhibitor conjugate was cytotoxic to cultured colorectal carcinoma cells expressing Gb$_3$, whereas Gb$_3$ negative control cells were not sensitive to the conjugate.

A role for STB/SLTB in tumor imaging has been proposed.[206] Visualizing agents that may be chemically attached to STB/SLTB include radioactive isotopes (e.g., technetium-99, iodine-125, thallium-201, and fluor-18), paramagnetic contrast agents (e.g., gadolinium and iron oxides), and fluorescent dyes (e.g., Cy3 and fluorescein). Moreover, STB/SLTB can be genetically altered to include amino acids with side chains suitable for covalent linkage to other molecules[180] as well as to make chimeric proteins containing, for instance, a green fluorescent protein (GFP) for visualization.

A recent study[207] explores the use of STB in the targeted imaging of digestive tumors. This study used transgenic mice carrying oncogenes that are associated with spontaneous digestive tumorigenesis. Mouse spontaneous intestinal adenocarcinomas were found to express Gb$_3$. They were visualized *in situ* by confocal laser endoscopy in conjunction with oral administration of fluorophore-labeled STB. The fluorophore-labeled STB strongly accumulated in the tumor lesions of affected mice. This accumulation was STB-dependent, as was demonstrated by immunocytochemistry.

Control experiments with wild-type mice demonstrated that only isolated single cells, corresponding to enteroendocrine cells, were visible in the intestinal epithelium.

In other studies, fluor-18-labeled STB was used in whole body PET imaging of transgenic and control mice. STB-targeted PET imaging showed that the majority of radioactivity accumulated in the urinary tract of both transgenic and wild-type mice. Lower levels of radioactivity were observed in the spleen, lungs, and liver. In wild-type mice, no radioactivity was associated with the intestinal tract. In a transgenic mouse, two areas of the digestive tract showed strong labeling. These were Gb_3-positive colon adenocarcinoma tumors. The intracellular transport of STB was analyzed in primary cell cultures established from mouse colon adenocarcinoma tumors. In these cells, STB followed the retrograde transport pathway to GA and ER. This indicated that tumor visualization reflected the specific and stable association of STB with the tumor cells.

In a related study, Viel et al.[208] evaluated a fluorophore-labeled STB derivative for its potential as a cell-specific imaging agent in two models of human colorectal carcinoma. They used optical imaging to show the *in vivo* localization of fluorophore-labeled STB in nude mice bearing colorectal carcinoma xenografts expressing Gb_3. STB differentially accumulated in the xenografted area, including the tumor cells; the surrounding epithelial cells of neovascularization; and in monocytes and macrophages. The fluorophore-labeled STB was slowly eliminated by renal excretion over the course of several days. At the cellular level, confocal microscopy of tumor sections corroborated that STB accumulated in tumor cells expressing Gb_3. These results indicated the capability of STB to deliver the fluorophore to target cells.

In conclusion, STB/SLTB can be used as a vector to deliver drugs and imaging agents to target tissues. This opens a broad window of applications for STB/SLTB, for example, as an aid in the detection of metastases, selection of tumor sites to perform biopsies, and mapping of tumor areas to be surgically removed. At the same time, as part of the process of identifying STB/SLTB as a therapeutic and diagnostic tool, an in-depth investigation of the short- and long-term side effects of STB/SLTB to humans and animals is essential.

10.3 CONCLUDING REMARKS

In this chapter, the principles of targeted intracellular delivery were illustrated through two case studies. In the first case of AD, it was demonstrated that the knowledge of lipid rafts and the ability to target a drug to a lipid raft can result in a more efficient inhibition within the endosomes of BACE activity, resulting in decreased amyloid peptide generation. In the second case, the use of a recombinant protein toxin subunit as a carrier for antigenic peptides, drugs, and imaging reagents was demonstrated. It highlighted how detailed knowledge of trafficking pathways can be used to maximize the efficient intracellular delivery via a carrier protein.

In summary, recent progress in molecular cell biology has generated immense knowledge of membrane trafficking pathways. Effective intracellular drug delivery requires a thorough understanding of the physiological and pathological processes. Progress in the use of this knowledge requires a creative application of this knowledge.

ABBREVIATIONS

Aβ	amyloid-β peptide
AD	Alzheimer's disease
AICD	APP intracellular domain
APC	antigen presenting cells
APP	amyloid precursor protein
BACE	β-site APP cleaving enzyme or β-secretase
CT	cholera toxin

CTF	C-terminal fragment
CTL	cytotoxic T lymphocytes
EE	early endosomes
EEA1	early endosome antigen 1
ER	endoplasmic reticulum
ERAD	ER-associated protein degradation
GA	Golgi apparatus
Gb$_3$	globotriaosylceramide
GEEC	GPI-anchored protein enriched early endosomal compartment
GFP	green fluorescent protein
GGA	Golgi-localized, gamma-ear-containing ADP ribosylation factor (Arf)-binding protein
GM1	ganglioside GM1
GPI-linked protein	glycosylphosphatidyl-inositol-linked protein
HLE	*E. coli* heat labile toxin
IL-2	interleukin-2
LE	late endosomes
MHC	major histocompatibility complex
MPR	mannose-6-phosphate receptor
PACS-1	phosphofurin acidic cluster-sorting protein-1
PE	*Pseudomonas* exotoxin
PS1/2	presenilin 1 and presenilin 2
siRNA	small interfering RNA
SLT	Shiga-like toxin
SNX	sorting nexin
ST	Shiga toxin
STB/SLTB	Shiga toxin subunit B/Shiga-like toxin subunit B
T$_H$1	helper T lymphocytes
TGN	*trans*-Golgi network

REFERENCES

1. Behnia R, Munro S. Organelle identity and the signposts for membrane traffic. *Nature* 2005; **438**: 597–604.
2. De Matteis MA, Luini A. Exiting the Golgi complex. *Nat Rev Mol Biol* 2008; **7**: 273–284.
3. Grosshans BL, Ortiz D, Novick P. Rabs and their effectors: Achieving specificity in membrane traffic. *Proc Natl Acad Sci USA* 2006; **103**: 11821–11827.
4. Lowenthal, MS, Howell, KE, Wu, CC. Proteomic analysis of the stacked Golgi complex. *Methods Mol Biol* 2008; **432**: 37–49.
5. Mayor S, Pagano R. Pathways of clathrin-independent endocytosis. *Nat Rev Mol Cell Biol* 2007; **8**: 603–612.
6. Mellman I, Warren G. The road taken: Past and future foundations of membrane traffic. *Cell* 2000; **100**: 99–112.
7. Seaman MN. Endosome protein sorting: Motifs and machinery. *Cell Mol Life Sci* 2008; **65**: 2842–2858.
8. Storrie B. Maintenance of Golgi apparatus structure in the face of continuous protein recycling to the endoplasmic reticulum: Making ends meet. *Int Rev Cytol* 2005; **244**: 69–94.
9. van Vliet C, Thomas EC, Merino-Trigo A, Teasdale RD, Gleeson PA. Intracellular sorting and transport of proteins. *Prog Biophys Mol Biol* 2003; **83**: 1–45.
10. Haass C, Selkoe DJ. Soluble protein oligomers in neurodegeneration: Lessons from the Alzheimer's amyloid β-peptide. *Nat Rev Mol Cell Biol* 2007; **8**: 101–112.
11. LaFerla FM, Green KN, Oddo S. Intracellular amyloid-β in Alzheimer's disease. *Nat Rev Neurosci* 2007; **8**: 499–509.

12. Small SA, Gandy S. Sorting through the cell biology of Alzheimer's disease: Intracellular pathways to pathogenesis. *Neuron* 2006; **52**: 15–31.
13. Zhang YW, Xu H. Molecular and cellular mechanisms for Alzheimer's disease: Understanding APP metabolism. *Curr Mol Med* 2007; **7**: 687–698.
14. Thinakaran G, Koo EH. Amyloid precursor protein trafficking, processing and function. *J Biol Chem* 2008; **283**: 29615–29619.
15. Vetrivel K, Thinakaran G. Amyloidogenic processing of β-amyloid precursor protein in intracellular compartments. *Neurology* 2006; **66**(Suppl 1): S69–S73.
16. Cole SL, Vassar R. The role of amyloid precursor protein processing by BACE1, the β-secretase, in Alzheimer disease pathophysiology. *J Biol Chem* 2008; **283**: 29621–29625.
17. Vassar R, Bennett BD, Babu-Khan S, Kahn S, Mendiaz EA, Denis P, Teplow DB, Ross S, Amarante P, Loeloff R, Luo Y, Fisher S, Fuller J, Edenson S, Lile J, Jarosinski MA, Biere AL, Curran E, Burgess T, Louis JC, Collins F, Treanor J, Rogers G, Citron M. Beta-secretase cleavage of Alzheirmer's amyloid precursor protein by the transmembrane aspartic protease BACE. *Science* 1999; **286**: 735–741.
18. Steiner H, Fluhrer R, Haass C. Intramembrane proteolysis by γ-secretase. *J Biol Chem* 2008; **283**: 29627–29631.
19. Lah JJ, Levey AI. Endogenous presenilin-1 targets to endocytic rather than biosynthetic compartments. *Mol Cell Neurosci* 2000; **16**: 111–126.
20. Carey RM, Balcz BA, Lopez-Coviella I, Slack BE. Inhibition of dynamin-dependent endocytosis increases shedding of the amyloid precursor protein ectodomain and reduces generation of amyloid beta protein. *BMC Cell Biol* 2005; **6**: 30.
21. Rajendran L, Honsho M, Zahn TR, Keller P, Geiger KD, Verkade P, Simons K. Alzheimer's disease β-amyloid peptides are released in association with exosomes. *Proc Natl Acad Sci USA* 2006; **103**: 11172–11177.
22. Kinoshita A, Fukumoto H, Shah T, Whelan CM, Irizarry MC, Hyman BT. Demonstration by FRET of BACE interaction with the amyloid precursor protein at the cell surface and in early endosomes. *J Cell Sci* 2003; **116**(Pt 16): 3339–3346.
23. Kamenetz F, Tomita T, Hsieh H, Seabrook G, Borchelt D, Iwatsubo T, Sisodia S, Malinow R. APP processing and synaptic function. *Neuron* 2003; **37**: 925–937.
24. Bonifacino JS, Traub LM. Signals for sorting of transmembrane proteins to endosomes and lysosomes. *Annu Rev Biochem* 2003; **72**: 395–447.
25. Small SA. Retromer sorting: A pathogenic pathway in late-onset Alzheimer's disease. *Arch Neurol* 2008; **65**: 323–328.
26. Bonifacino JS, Hurley JH. Retromer. *Curr Op Cell Biol* 2008; **20**: 427–436.
27. Seaman MN. Recycle your receptors with retromer. *Trends Cell Biol* 2005; **15**: 68–75.
28. Scherzer CR, Offe K, Gearing M, Rees HD, Fang G, Heilman CJ, Schaller C, Bujo H, Levey AI, Lah JJ. Loss of apoliprotein E receptor LR11 in Alzheimer's disease. *Arch Neurol* 2004; **61**: 1200–1205.
29. Small SA, Kent K, Pierce A, Leung C, Kang MS, Okada H, Honig L, Vonsattel JP, Kim TW. Model-guided microarray implicates the retromer complex in Alzheimer's disease. *Ann Neurol* 2005; **58**: 909–919.
30. Rogaeva E, Meng Y, Lee JH, Gu Y, Kawarai T, Zou F, Katayama T, Baldwin CT, Cheng R, Hasegawa H, Chen F, Shibata N, Lunetta KL, Pardossi-Piquard R, Bohm C, Wakutani Y, Cupples LA, Cuenco KT, Green RC, Pinessi L, Rainero I, Sorbi S, Bruni A, Duara R, Friedland RP, Inzelberg R, Hampe W, Bujo H, Song YQ, Andersen OM, Willnow TE, Graff-Radford N, Petersen RC, Dickson D, Der SD, Fraser PE, Schmitt-Ulms G, Younkin S, Mayeux R, Farrer LA, St George-Hyslop P. The neuronal sortilin-related receptor SORL1 is genetically associated with Alzheimer's disease. *Nat Genet* 2007; **39**: 168–177.
31. Andersen OM, Reiche J, Schmidt V, Gotthardt M, Spoelgen R, Behlke J, von Arnim CAF, Breiderhoff T, Jansen P, Wu X, Bales KR, Cappai R, Masters CL, Gliemann J, Mufson EJ, Hyman BT, Paul SM, Nykjaer A, Willnow T. Neuronal sorting protein-related receptor sorLA LR11 regulates processing of the amyloid precursor protein. *Proc Natl Acad Sci USA* 2005; **102**: 13461–13466.
32. Nielsen MS, Gustafsen C, Madsen P, Nyengaard JR, Hermey G, Bakke O, Mari M, Schu P, Pohlmann R, Dennes A, Petersen CM. Sorting by the cytoplasmic domain of the amyloid precursor protein binding receptor SorLA. *Mol Cell Biol* 2007; **27**: 6842–6851.
33. Offe K, Dodoson SE, Shoemaker T, Fritz JJ, Gearing M, Levey A, Lah J. The lipoprotein receptor LR11 regulates amyloid production and amyloid precursor traffic in endosomal compartments. *J Neurosci* 2006; **26**: 1596–1603.
34. Schmidt V, Sporbert A, Rohe M, Reimer T, Rehm A, Andersen OM, Willnow T. SorLA/LR11 regulates processing of amyloid precursor protein via interaction with adaptors GGA and PACS-1. *J Biol Chem* 2007; **282**: 32956–32964.

35. Spolgen R, von Arnim CAF, Thomas AV, Peltan ID, Koker M, Deng A, Irizarry MC, Andersen OM, Willnow TE, Hyman BT. Interaction of the cytosolic domains of sorLA/LR11 with the amyloid precursor protein (APP) and β-secretase β-site APP-cleaving enzyme. *J Neurosci* 2006; **26**: 418–428.

36. Mari M, Bujny MV, Zeuschner D, Geerts WJC, Griffith J, Petersen CM, Cullen PJ, Klumperman J, Geuze HJ. SNX1 defines an early endosomal recycling exit for sortilin and mannose-6-phosphate receptors. *Traffic* 2008; **9**: 380–393.

37. Babuke T, Tikkanen R. Dissecting the molecular function of reggie/flotillin proteins. *Eur J Cell Biol* 2007; **86**: 525–532.

38. Langhorst MF, Reuter A, Stuermer CAO. Scaffolding microdomains and beyond: The function of reggie/flotillin proteins. *Cell Mol Life Sci* 2005; **62**: 2228–2240.

39. Doherty GJ, McMahon HT. Mechanisms of endocytosis. *Annu Rev Biochem* 2009; **78**: 857–902.

40. Glebov OO, Bright NA, Nichols BJ. Flotillin-1 defines a clathrin-independent endocytic pathway in mammalian cells. *Nat Cell Biol* 2006; **8**: 46–54.

41. Laude AJ, Prior IA. Plasma membrane microdomains: Organization, function and trafficking. *Mol Memb Biol* 2004; **21**: 193–205.

42. Langui D, Girardot N, Hachimi KH, Allinquant B, Blanchard V, Pradier L, Duyckaerts C. Subcellular topography of neuronal Aβ peptide in APPxPS1 transgenic mice. *Am J Pathol* 2004; **165**: 1465–1477.

43. Kokubo H, Lemere CA, Yamaguchi H. Localization of flotillins in human brain and their accumulation with the progression of Alzheimer's disease pathology. *Neurosci Lett* 2000; **290**: 93–96.

44. Schneider A, Rajendran L, Honsho M, Gralle N, Donnert G, Wouters F, Hell SW, Simons M. Flotillin-dependent clustering of the amyloid precursor protein regulates its endocytosis and amyloidogenic processing in neurons. *J Neurosci* 2008; **28**: 2874–2882.

45. Cordy JM, Hooper NM, Turner AJ. The involvement of lipid rafts in Alzheimer's disease. *Mol Membr Biol* 2006; **23**: 111–122.

46. Garcia-Marcos M, Pochet S, Tandel S, Fontanils U, Astigarraga E, Fernandez-Gonzalez JA, Kumps A, Marino A, Dehaye JP. Characterization and comparison of raft-like membranes isolated by two different methods from rat submandibular gland cells. *Biochim Biophys Acta* 2006; **1758**: 796–806.

47. Pike LJ. Lipid rafts: Bringing order to chaos. *J Lipid Res* 2003; **44**: 655–667.

48. Simons K, Ikonen E. Functional rafts in cell membranes. *Nature* 1997; **387**: 569–572.

49. Foster LJ, De Hoog CL, Mann M. Unbiased quantitative proteomics of lipid rafts reveals high specificity for signaling factors. *Proc Natl Acad Sci USA* 2003; **100**: 5813–5818.

50. Simons K, Toomre D. Lipid rafts and signal transduction. *Nat Rev Mol Cell Biol* 2000; **1**: 31–39.

51. Benjannet S, Elagoz A, Wickham L, Mamarbachi M, Munzer JS, Basak A, Lazure C, Cromlish JA, Sisodia S, Checler F, Chrétien M, Seidah NG. Post-translational processing of β-secretase (β-amyloid-converting enzyme) and its ectodomain shedding: The pro- and transmembrane/cytosolic domains affect its cellular activity and amyloid-beta production. *J Biol Chem* 2001; **276**: 10879–10877.

52. Ehehalt R, Keller P, Haass C, Thiele C, Simons K. Amyloidogenic processing of the Alzheimer β-amyloid precursor protein depends on lipid rafts. *J Cell Biol* 2003; **160**: 113–123.

53. Kalvodova L, Kahya N, Schwille P, Ehehalt R, Verkade P, Drechsel D, Simons K. Lipids as modulators of proteolytic activity of BACE: Involvement of cholesterol, glycosphingolipids, and anionic phospholipids *in vitro*. *J Biol Chem* 2005; **280**: 36818–36823.

54. Huang Y. Apolipoprotein E and Alzheimer disease. *Neurology* 2006; **66**: S79–S85.

55. Fassbender K, Simons M, Bergmann C, Stroick M, Lutjohann D, Keller P, Runz H, Kuhl S, Bertsch T, von Bergmann K, Hennerici M, Beyreuther K, Hartmann T. Simvastatin strongly reduces levels of Alzheimer's disease beta-amyloid peptides Abeta 42 and Abeta 40 in vitro and in vivo. *Proc Natl Acad Sci USA* 2001; **98**: 5856–5861.

56. Jick H, Zornberg GL, Jick SS, Seshadri S, Drachman DA. Statins and the risk of dementia. *Lancet* 2000; **356**: 1627–1631.

57. Wolozin B, Kellman W, Ruosseau P, Celesia GG, Siegel G. Decreased prevalence of Alzheimer disease associated with 3-hydroxy-3-methylglutaryl coenzyme A reductase inhibitors. *Arch Neurol* 2000; **57**: 1439–1443.

58. Sparks DL, Kryscio RJ, Sabbagh MN, Connor DJ, Sparks, LM, Liebsack C. Reduced risk of incident AD in elective statin use in a clinical trial cohort. *Curr Alzheimer Res* 2008; **5**: 416–421.

59. Fleisher AS, Raman R, Siemers ER, Becerra L, Clark CM, Dean RA, Farlow MR, Galvin JE, Peskind ER, Quinn JF, Sherzai A, Sowell BB, Aisen PS, Thal LJ. Phase 2 safety trial targeting amyloid beta production with a gamma-secretase inhibitor in Alzheimer's disease. *Arch Neurol* 2008; **65**: 1031–1038.

60. Roberson ED, Mucke L. 100 years and counting: Prospects for defeating Alzheimer's disease. *Science* 2006; **314**: 781–784.

61. Evin G. γ-Secretase modulators: Hopes and setbacks for the future of Alzheimer's treatment. *Expert Rev Neurother* 2008; **8**: 1611–1613.

62. Weggen S, Rogers M, Eriksen J. NSAIDs: Small molecules for prevention of Alzheimer's disease or precursors for future drug development. *Trends Pharmacol Sci* 2007; **28**: 536–543.

63. Wolfe MS. Inhibition and modulation of γ-secretase for Alzheimer's disease. *Neurotherapeutics* 2008; **5**: 391–398.

64. Ghosh AK, Gemma S, Tang J. β-Secretase as a therapeutic target for Alzheimer's disease. *Neurotherapeutics* 2008; **5**:399–408.

65. Hills ID, Vacca JP. Progress toward a practical BACE-1 inhibitor. *Curr Opin Drug Discov Dev* 2007; **10**: 383–391.

66. Silvestri R. Boom in the development of non-peptidic β-secretase (BACE1) inhibitors for the treatment of Alzheimer's disease. *Med Res Rev* 2009; **2**: 295–338.

67. Tung JS, Davis DL, Anderson JP, Walker DE, Mamo S, Jewett N, Hom RK, Sinha S, Thorsett ED, John V. Design of substrate-based inhibitors of human β-secretase. *J Med Chem* 2002; **45**: 259–262.

68. Wolfe MS. Selective amyloid-β lowering agents. *BMC Neurosci* 2008; **9**(Suppl 2): S4.

69. Rajendran L, Schneider A, Schlechtingen G, Weidlich S, Ries J, Braxmeier T, Schwille P, Schulz JB, Schroeder C, Simons M, Jennings G, Knolker HJ, Simons K. Efficient inhibition of the Alzheimer's disease β-secretase by membrane targeting. *Science* 2008; **320**: 520–523.

70. Johannes L, Popoff V. Tracing the retrograde route in protein trafficking. *Cell* 2008; **135**: 1175–1187.

71. Tarragó-Trani MT, Storrie B. Alternate routes for drug delivery to the cell interior: Pathways to the Golgi apparatus and endoplasmic reticulum. *Adv Drug Deliv Rev* 2007; **59**: 782–797.

72. Mousavi SA, Malerod L, Berg T, Kjeken R. Clathrin-dependent endocytosis. *Biochem J* 2004; **377**: 1–16.

73. Rodemer C, Haucke V. Clathrin/AP-2-dependent endocytosis: A novel playground for the pharmacological toolbox. *Handb Exp Pharmacol* 2008; **186**: 105–122.

74. Sandvig K, Torgersen ML, Raa HA, van Deurs B. Clathrin-independent endocytosis: From nonexisting to an extreme degree of complexity. *Histochem Cell Biol* 2008; **129**: 267–276.

75. Ohno H, Stewart J, Fournier MC, Bosshart H, Rhee I, Miyatake S, Saito T, Gallusser A, Kirchhausen T, Bonifacino JS. Interaction of tyrosine-based sorting signals with clathrin-associated proteins. *Science* 1995; **269**: 1872–1875.

76. Simonsen A, Bremnes B, Nordeng TW, Bakke O. The leucine-based motif DDQxxLI is recognized both for internalization and basolateral sorting of invariant chain in MDCK cells. *Eur J Cell Biol* 1998; **76**: 25–32.

77. Ford MG, Pearse BM, Higgins MK, Vallis Y, Owen DJ, Gibson A, Hopkins CR, Evans PR, MacMahon HT. Simultaneous binding of PtdIns(4,5)P2 and clathrin by AP180 in the nucleation of clathrin lattices on membranes. *Science* 2001; **291**: 1051–1055.

78. Takei K, Haucke V. Clathrin-mediated endocytosis: Membrane factors pull the trigger. *Trends Cell Biol* 2001; **11**: 385–391.

79. Jin AJ, Nossal R. Topological mechanisms involved in the formation of clathrin-coated vesicles. *Biophys J* 1993; **65**: 1523–1537.

80. Schmidt AA. Membrane transport: The making of a vesicle. *Nature* 2002; **419**: 347–349.

81. Kozlov MM. Fission of biological membranes: Interplay between dynamin and lipids. *Traffic* 2001; **2**: 51–65.

82. Lee E, De Camilli P. Dynamin at actin tails. *Proc Natl Acad Sci USA* 2002; **96**: 161–166.

83. Merrifield CJ, Feldman ME, Wan L, Almers W. Imaging actin and dynamin recruitment during invagination of single clathrin-coated pits. *Nat Cell Biol* 2002; **4**: 691–698.

84. Rodal SK, Skeretting G, Garred O, Vilhardt F, van Deurs B, Sandvig K. Extraction of cholesterol with methyl-beta-cyclodextrin perturbs formation of clathrin-coated endocytic vesicles. *Mol Biol Cell* 1999; **10**: 961–974.

85. Subtil A, Gaidarov I, Kobylarz, K, Lampson MA, Keen JH, McGraw TE. Acute cholesterol depletion inhibits clathrin-coated pit budding. *Proc Natl Acad Sci USA* 1999; **96**: 6775–6780.

86. Palade GE. Fine structure of blood capillaries. *J Appl Phys* 1953; **24**: 1424.

87. Yamada E. The fine structure of the gall bladder epithelium of the mouse. *J Biophys Biochem Cytol* 1955; **1**: 445–458.

88. Couet J, Belanger MM, Roussel E, Drolet MC. Cell biology of caveolae and caveolin. *Adv Drug Del Rev* 2001; **49**: 223–235.

89. Harder T, Simons K. Caveolae, DIGs, and the dynamics of sphingolipid-cholesterol microdomains. *Curr Opin Cell Biol* 1997; **9**: 534–542.

90. Parton RG, Simons K. The multiple faces of caveolae. *Nat Rev Mol Cell Biol* 2007; **8**:185–194.

91. Rothberg KG, Heuser JE, Donzell WC, Ying YS, Genney JR, Anderson RG. Caveolin, a protein component of caveolae membrane coats. *Cell* 1992; **68**:673–678.

92. Sharma DK, Brown JC, Choudhury A, Peterson TE, Holicky E, Marks DL, Simari R, Parton RG, Pagano RE. Selective stimulation of caveolar endocytosis by glycosphingolipids and cholesterol. *Mol Biol Cell* 2004; **15**: 3114–3122.

93. Shajahan AN, Timblin BK, Sandoval R, Tiruppathi C, Malik AB, Minshall RD. Role of Src-induced dynamin-2 phosphorylation in caveolae-mediated endocytosis in endothelial cells. *J Biol Chem* 2004; **279**: 20392–20400.

94. Nichols B. Caveosomes and endocytosis of lipid rafts. *J Cell Sci* 2003; **116**: 4707–4714.

95. Nichols BJ, Lippincott-Schwartz J. Endocytosis without the clathrin coats. *Trends Cell Biol* 2001; **13**: 406–412.

96. Schlegel A, Lisanti MP. A molecular dissection of caveolin-1 membrane attachment and oligomerization. Two separate regions of the caveolin-1 C-terminal domain mediate membrane binding and oligomer/oligomer interaction *in vivo*. *J Biol Chem* 2000; **275**: 21605–21617.

97. Parton RG, Hanzal-Bayer M, Hancock JF. Biogenesis of caveolae: A structural model for caveolin-induced domain formation. *J Cell Sci* 2006; **119**: 787–796.

98. Thomsen P, Roepstorff K, Stahlhut M, van Deurs B. Caveolae are highly immobile plasma membrane microdomains, which are not involved in constitutive endocytic trafficking. *Mol Biol Cell* 2002; **13**: 238–250.

99. Fujimoto T, Miyawaki A, Mikoshiba K. Inositol 1,4,5-trisphosphate receptor-like protein in plasmalemmal caveolae is linked to actin filaments. *J Cell Sci* 1995; **108**: 7–15.

100. Stahlhut M, van Deurs B. Identification of filamin as a novel ligand for caveolin-1: Evidence for the organization of caveolin-1-associated membrane domains by the actin cytoskeleton. *Mol Biol Cell* 2000; **11**: 325–337.

101. Parton RG, Joggerst B, Simons K. Regulated internalization of caveolae. *J Cell Biol* 1994; **127**: 1199–1215.

102. Le PU, Guay G, Altschuler Y, Nabi IR. Caveolin-1 is a negative regulator of caveolae-mediated endocytosis to the endoplasmic reticulum. *J Biol Chem* 2002; **277**: 3371–3379.

103. Pelkmans L, Kartenbeck J, Helenius A. Caveolar endocytosis of simian virus 40 reveals a new two-step vesicular transport pathway to the ER. *Nat Cell Biol* 2001; **3**: 473–483.

104. Pelkmans L, Puntener D, Helenius A. Local actin polymerization and dynamin recruitment in SV40-induced internalization of caveolae. *Science* 2002; **296**: 535–539.

105. Torgersen ML, Skretting G, van Deurs B, Sandvig K. Internalization of Cholera toxin by different endocytic mechanisms. *J Cell Sci* 2001; **114**: 3737–3747.

106. Damm EM, Pelkmans L, Kartenbeck J, Mezzacasa A, Kurzchalia T, Helenius A. Clathrin- and caveolin-1-independent endocytosis: Entry of simian virus 40 into cells devoid of caveolae. *J Cell Biol* 2005; **168**: 477–488.

107. Lamaze C, Dujeancourt A, Baba T, Lo CG, Benmerah A, Dautry-Varsat A. Interleukin 2 receptors and detergent-resistant membrane domains define a clathrin-independent endocytic pathway. *Mol Cell* 2001; **7**: 661–671.

108. Kirkham M, Fujita A, Chadda R, Nixon SJ, Kurzchalia TV, Sharma DK, Pagano RE, Hancock JF, Mayor S, Parton RG. Ultrastructural identification of uncoated caveolin-independent early endocytic vehicles. *J Cell Biol* 2005; **168**: 465–476.

109. Sabharanjak S, Sharma P, Parton RG, Mayor S. GPI-anchored proteins are delivered to recycling endosomes via a distinct cdc42-regulated, clathrin-independent pinocytic pathway. *Dev Cell* 2002; **2**: 411–423.

110. Acheson DWK, Calderwood SB, Boyko SA, Lincicome LL, Kane AV, Donohue-Rolfe A, Keusch GT. Comparison of Shiga-like toxin I B-subunit expression and localization in *Escherichia coli* and *Vibrio cholerae* by using *trc* or iron-regulated promoter system. *Infect Immun* 1993; **61**: 1098–1104.

111. Calderwood SB, Auclair F, Dohanue-Rolfe A, Keusch GT, Mekalanos JJ. Nucleotide sequence of the Shiga-like toxin genes of *Escherichia coli*. *Proc Natl Acad Sci USA* 1987; **84**: 4364–4368.

112. O'Brian AD, Tesh VL, Donohue-Rolfe A, Jackson MP, Olsnes S, Sandvig K, Lindberg AA, Keusch GT. Shiga toxin: Biochemistry, genetics, mode of action, and role in pathogenesis. *Curr Top Microbiol Immunol* 1992; **182**: 65–94.

113. Sandvig K. The Shiga toxins: Properties and action on cells. In *The Comprehensive Sourcebook of Bacterial Protein Toxins*, 3rd edn., eds. J.E. Alouf and M.R. Popoff, pp. 310–322. Oxford, England: Academic Press, Elsevier Ltd., 2006.

114. Donohue-Rolfe A, Acheson A, Kane AV, Keusch GT. Purification of Shiga and Shiga-like toxins I and II by receptor analog affinity chromatography with immobilized P1 glycoprotein and the production of cross-reactive monoclonal antibodies. *Infect Immun* 1989; **57**: 3888–3893.

115. Peter MG, Lingwood CA. Apparent cooperativity in multivalent verotoxin-globotriaosyl ceramide binding: Kinetic and saturation binding studies with [^{125}I]verotoxin. *Biochim Biophys Acta* 2000; **1501**: 116–124.

116. Ling H, Boodhoo A, Hazes B, Cummings MD, Armstrong GD, Brunton JL, Read RJ. Structure of the Shiga-like toxin I B-pentamer complexed with an analogue of its receptor Gb$_3$. *Biochemistry* 1998; **37**: 1777–1788.

117. Iversen TG, Skretting G, van Deurs B, Sandvig K. Formation of clathrin-coated pits with long dynamin-wrapped necks upon inducible expression of antisense clathrin. *Proc Natl Acad Sci USA* 2003; **100**: 5175–5180.

118. Lauvrak SU, Togersen ML, Sandvig K. Efficient endosome-to-Golgi transport of Shiga toxin is dependent on dynamin and clathrin. *J Cell Sci* 2004; **117**(Pt 11): 2321–2331.

119. Saint-Pol A, Yélamos B, Amessou M, Mills IG, Dugast M, Tenza D, Schu P, Antony C, McMahon HT, Lamaze C, Johannes L. Clathrin adaptor epsinR is required for retrograde sorting on early endosomal membranes. *Dev Cell* 2004; **6**: 525–538.

120. Sandvig K, Olsnes S, Brown JE, Petersen OW, van Deurs B. Endocytosis from coated pits of Shiga toxin: A glycolipid-binding protein from *Shigella dysenteriae 1*. *J Cell Biol* 1989; **108**: 1331–1343.

121. Nichols BJ, Kenworthy AK, Polishchuk RS, Lodge R, Roberts TH, Hirschberg K, Phair RD, Lippincott-Schwartz J. Rapid cycling of lipid raft markers between the cell surface and Golgi complex. *J Cell Biol* 2001; **153**: 529–541.

122. Kovbasnjuk O, Edidin M, Donowitz M. Role of lipid rafts in Shiga toxin 1 interaction with the apical surface of Caco-2 cells. *J Cell Sci* 2001; **114**(Pt 22): 4025–4031.

123. Römer W, Berland L, Chambon V, Gaus K, Windschiegl B, Tenza, D, Aly MR, Fraisier V, Florent JC, Perrais D, Lamaze C, Raposo, G, Steinem C, Sens P, Bassereau P, Johannes L. Shiga toxin induces tubular membrane invaginations for its uptake into cells. *Nature* 2007; **450**: 670–675.

124. Mallard F, Tenza D, Antony C, Salamero J, Goud B, Johannes L. Direct pathway from early/recycling endosomes to the Golgi apparatus revealed through the study of Shiga toxin-B fragment transport. *J Cell Biol* 1998; **143**: 973–990.

125. Cabiaux V. pH-sensitive toxins: Interactions with membrane bilayers and application to drug delivery. *Ad Drug Del Rev* 2004; **56**: 987–997.

126. Watson P, Spooner RA. Toxin entry and trafficking in mammalian cells. *Ad Drug Del Rev* 2006; **58**: 1581–1596.

127. Sandvig K, Garred O, Prydz K, Kozlov JV, Hansen SH, van Deurs B. Retrograde transport of endocytosed Shiga toxin to the endoplasmic reticulum. *Nature* 1992; **358**: 510–512.

128. Schapiro FB, Lingwood C, Furuya W, Grinstein S. pH-independent retrograde targeting of glycolipids to the Golgi complex. *Am J Physiol* 1998; **274**: C319–C332.

129. Dahms NM, Lobel P, Kornfeld S. Mannose 6-phosphate receptors and lysosomal enzyme targeting. *J Biol Chem* 1989; **264**: 12115–12118.

130. Bonifacino JS, Rojas R. Retrograde transport from endosomes to the trans-Golgi network. *Nat Rev Mol Cell Biol* 2006; **7**: 568–579.

131. Lombardi D, Soldati T, Riederer MA, Goda Y, Zerial M, Pfeffer SR. Rab9 functions in transport between late endosomes and trans Golgi network. *EMBO J* 1993; **12**: 677–682.

132. Iversen TG, Skretting G, Llorente A, Nicoziani P, van Deurs B, Sandvig K. Endosome to Golgi transport of Ricin is independent of clathrin and of the Rab9-Rab11-GTPases. *Mol Biol Cell* 2001; **12**: 2099–2107.

133. Lauvrak S, Llorente A, Iversen TG, Sandvig K. Selective regulation of the Rab9-independent transport of ricin to the Golgi apparatus by calcium. *J Cell Sci* 2002; **115**: 3449–3456.

134. Sandvig K, Grimmer S, Lauvrak SU, Torgersen ML, Skretting G, van Deurs B, Iversen TG. Pathways followed by Ricin and Shiga toxin into cells. *Histochem Cell Biol* 2002; **117**: 131–141.

135. Bujny MV, Popoff V, Johannes L, Cullen PJ. The retromer component sorting nexin-1 is required for efficient retrograde transport of Shiga toxin from early endosome to the trans Golgi network. *J Cell Sci* 2007; **120**: 2010–2021.

136. Popoff V, Mardones GA, Tenza D, Rojas R, Lamaze C, Bonifacino JS, Raposo G, Johannes L. The retromer complex and clathrin define an early endosomal retrograde exit site. *J Cell Sci* 2007; **120**: 2022–2031.

137. Amessou M, Fradagrada A, Falguieres T, Lord JM, Smith DC, Roberts LM, Lamaze C, Johannes L. Syntaxin 16 and syntaxin 5 are required for efficient retrograde transport of several exogenous and endogenous cargo proteins. *J Cell Sci* 2007; **120**: 1457–1468.

138. Falguieres T, Mallard F, Baron C, Hanau D, Lingwood C, Goud B, Salamero J, Johannes L. Targeting of Shiga toxin B-subunit to retrograde transport route in association with detergent-resistant membranes. *Mol Biol Cell* 2001; **12**: 2453–2468.

139. Mallard F, Tang DBL, Galli T, Tenza D, Saint-Pol A, Yue X, Antony C, Hong WJ, Goud B, Johannes L. Early/recycling endosomes-to-TGN transport involves two SNARE complexes and a Rab6 isoform. *J Cell Biol* 2002; **156**: 653–664.

140. Monier S, Jollivet F, Janoueix-Lerosey I, Johannes L, Goud B. Characterization of novel Rab6-interacting proteins involved in endosome-to-TGN transport. *Traffic* 2002; **3**: 289–297.

141. Wilcke M, Johannes L, Galli T, Mayau V, Goud B, Salamero J. Rab11 regulates the compartmentalization of early endosomes required for efficient transport from early endosomes to the trans-Golgi network. *J Cell Biol* 2000; **151**: 1207–1220.

142. Tai G, Lu L, Wang TL, Tang BL, Goud B, Johannes L, Hong W. Participation of the syntaxin 5/Ykt6/GS28/GS15 SNARE complex in transport from early/recycling endosome to the trans-Golgi network. *Mol Biol Cell* 2004; **15**: 4011–4022.

143. Altan-Bonnet N, Sougrat R, Lippincott-Schwartz J. Molecular basis for Golgi maintenance and biogenesis. *Curr Op Cell Biol* 2004; **16**: 363–372.

144. Farquhar MG, Palade GE. The Golgi apparatus: 100 years of progress and controversy. *Trends Cell Biol* 1998; **8**: 2–10.

145. Marsh BJ, Howell KE. The mammalian Golgi-complex debates. *Nat Rev Mol Cell Biol* 2002; **3**: 789–795.

146. Johannes L, Tenza D, Antony C, Goud B. Retrograde transport of KDEL-bearing B-fragment of Shiga Toxin. *J Biol Chem* 1997; **272**: 19554–19561.

147. Fujinaga Y, Wolf AA, Rodighiero C, Wheeler H, Tsai B, Allen L, Jobling MG, Rapoport T, Holmes RK, Lencer WI. Gangliosides that associate with lipid rafts mediate transport of Cholera and related toxins from the plasma membrane to the endoplasmic reticulum. *Mol Biol Cell* 2003; **14**: 4783–4793.

148. Hessler JL, Kreitman RJ. An early step in *Pseudomonas* exotoxin action is removal of the terminal lysine residue, which allows binding to the KDEL receptor. *Biochemistry* 1997; **36**: 14577–14582.

149. Smith DC, Spooner RA, Watson PD, Murray JL, Hodge TW, Amessou M, Johannes L, Lord JM, Roberts LM. Internalized *Pseudomonas* exotoxin A can exploit multiple pathways to reach the endoplasmic reticulum. *Traffic* 2006; **7**: 379–393.

150. Lippincott-Schwartz J, Yuan L, Bonifacino JS, Klausner RD. Rapid redistribution of Golgi proteins into the ER in cells treated with brefeldin A: Evidence for membrane cycling from Golgi to ER. *Cell* 1989; **56**: 801–813.

151. Sciaky N, Presley J, Smith C, Zaal KJ, Cole N, Moreira JE, Terasaki M, Siggia E, Lippincott-Schwartz J. Golgi tubule traffic and the effects of brefeldin A visualized in living cells. *J Cell Biol* 1997; **139**: 1137–1155.

152. Girod A, Storrie B, Simpson JC, Johannes L, Goud B, Roberts LM, Lord JM, Nilsson T, Pepperkok R. Evidence for a COP-I-independent transport route from the Golgi complex to the endoplasmic reticulum. *Nat Cell Biol* 1999; **1**: 423–430.

153. Puri S, Linstedt, AD. Capacity of the Golgi apparatus for biogenesis from the endoplasmic reticulum. *Mol Cell Biol* 2003; **14**: 5011–5018.

154. Ward TH, Polishchuk RS, Caplan S, Hirschberg K, Lippincott-Schwartz J. Maintenance of Golgi structure and function depends on the integrity of ER export. *J Cell Biol* 2001; **155**: 557–570.

155. Miles S, McManus H, Forsten KE, Storrie, B. Evidence that the entire Golgi apparatus cycles in interphase HeLa cells: Sensitivity of Golgi matrix proteins to an ER exit block. *J Cell Biol* 2001; **155**: 543–555.

156. Rhee SW, Starr T, Forsten-Williams K, Storrie B. The steady-state distribution of glycosyltransferases between the Golgi apparatus and the endoplasmic reticulum is approximately 90:10. *Traffic* 2005; **6**: 978–990.

157. Seemann J, Jokitalo E, Pypaert M, Warren G. Matrix proteins can generate the higher order architecture of the Golgi apparatus. *Nature* 2000; **407**: 1022–1026.

158. Storrie B, White J, Rottger S, Stelzer EH, Suganuma T, Nilsson T. Recycling of Golgi-resident glycosyltransferases through the ER reveals a novel pathway and provides explanation for nocodazole-induced Golgi scattering. *J Cell Biol* 1998; **143**: 1505–1521.

159. Stroud WJ, Jiang S, Jack G, Storrie B. Persistence of Golgi matrix distribution exhibits the same dependence on Sar1p activity as a Golgi glycosyltransferase. *Traffic* 2003; **4**: 631–641.

160. del Nery E, Miserey-Lenkei S, Falguieres T, Nizak C, Johannes L, Perez F, Goud B. Rab6A and Rab6A' GTPases play non-overlapping roles in membrane trafficking. *Traffic* 2006; **7**: 394–407.

161. White J, Johannes L, Mallard F, Girod A, Grill S, Reinsch S, Keller P, Tzschaschel B, Echard A, Goud B, Stelzer EHK. Rab6 coordinates a novel Golgi to ER retrograde transport pathway in live cells. *J Cell Biol* 1999; **147**: 743–759.

162. Young J, Stauber T, del Nery E, Vernos I, Pepperkok R, Nilsson T. Regulation of microtubule-dependent recycling at the trans-Golgi network by Rab6A and Rab6A'. *Mol Cell Biol* 2005; **16**: 162–177.

163. Jiang S, Storrie B. Cisternal Rab proteins regulate Golgi apparatus redistribution in response to hypotonic stress. *Mol Cell Biol* 2005; **16**: 2586–2596.

164. Valsdottir R, Hashimoto H, Ashman K, Koda T, Storrie B, Nilsson, T. Identification of rabaptin-5, rabex-5, and GM130 as putative effectors of Rab33b, a regulator of retrograde traffic between Golgi apparatus and ER. *FEBS Lett* 2001; **508**: 201–209.

165. Ackerman AL, Giodini A, Cresswell P. A role for the endoplasmic reticulum protein retrotranslocation machinery during crosspresentation by dendritic cells. *Immunity* 2006; **25**: 607–617.

166. Slominska-Wojewodzka M, Gregers TF, Walchli S, Sandvig S. EDEM is involved in retrotranslocation of Ricin from the endoplasmic reticulum to the cytosol. *Mol Biol Cell* 2006; **17**: 1664–1675.

167. Schmitz A, Herrgen H, Winkeler A, Herzog V. Cholera toxin is exported from microsomes by the Sec61p complex. *J Cell Biol* 2000; **148**: 1203–1212.

168. Yu M, Haslam DB. Shiga toxin is transported from the endoplasmic reticulum following interaction with the luminal chaperone HEDJ/ERdj3. *Infect Immun* 2005; **73**: 2524–2532.

169. Ghosh RN, Mallet WG, Soe TT, McGraw TE, Maxfield FR. An endocytosed TGN38 chimeric protein is delivered to the TGN after trafficking through the endocytic recycling compartment in CHO cells. *J Cell Biol* 1998; **142**: 923–936.

170. Mallet WG, Maxfield FR. Chimeric forms of furin and TGN38 are transported from the plasma membrane to the trans-Golgi network via distinct endosomal pathways. *J Cell Biol* 1999; **146**: 345–359.

171. Bachert C, Lee TH, Linstedt AD. Lumenal endosomal and Golgi-retrieval determinants involved in pH-sensitive targeting of and early Golgi protein. *Mol Biol Cell* 2001; **12**: 3152–3160.

172. Natarajan R, Linstedt AD. A cycling cis-Golgi protein mediates endosome-to-Golgi traffic. *Mol Biol Cell* 2004; **15**: 4798–4806.

173. Puri S, Bachert C, Fimmel CJ, Linstedt AD. Cycling of early Golgi proteins via the cell surface and endosomes upon luminal pH disruption. *Traffic* 2002; **3**: 641–653.

174. Starr T, Forsten-Williams K, Storrie B. Both post-Golgi and intra-Golgi cycling affect the distribution of the Golgi phosphoprotein GPP130. *Traffic* 2007; **8**: 1265–1279.

175. Haicheur N, Bismuth E, Bosset S, Adotevi O, Warnier G, Lacabanne V, Regnault A, Desaymard C, Amiogorena S, Ricciardi-Castagnoli P, Goud B, Fridman WH, Johannes L, Tartour E. The B subunit of Shiga toxin fused to a tumor antigen elicits CTL and targets dendritic cells to allow MHC class I-restricted presentation of peptides derived from exogenous antigens. *J Immunol* 2000; **165**: 3301–3308.

176. LaCasse EC, Bray MR, Patterson B, Lim WM, Perampalam S, Radvanyi LG, Keating A, Stewart AK, Buckstein R, Sandhu JS, Miller N, Banerjee D, Singh D, Belch AR, Pilarski LM, Gariepy J. Shiga-like toxin-1 receptor on human breast cancer, lymphoma, and myeloma, and absence from CD34+ hematopoietic stem cells: Implications of *ex vivo* tumor purging and autologous stem cell transplantation. *Blood* 1999; **94**: 2901–2910.

177. Trombetta ES, Mellman I. Cell biology of antigen processing *in vitro* and *in vivo*. *Annu Rev Immunol* 2005; **23**: 975–1028.

178. Smith DC, Lord JM, Roberts LM, Tartour E, Johannes L. 1st class ticket to class I: Protein toxins as pathfinders for antigen presentation. *Traffic* 2002; **3**: 697–704.

179. Kim Y, Kang K, Kim I, Lee J, Oh C, Ryoo J, Jeong E, Ahn K. Molecular mechanisms of MHC class I-antigen processing: Redox considerations. *Antioxid Redox Signal* 2009; **11**: 908–936.

180. Haicheur N, Benchetrit F, Amessou M, Leclerc C, Falguieres T, Fayolle C, Bismuth E, Fridman WH, Johannes L, Tartour E. The B subunit of Shiga toxin coupled to full-size antigenic protein elicits humoral and cell-mediated immune responses associated with a T_h1-dominant polarization. *Int Immunol* 2003; **15**: 1161–1171.

181. Lee RS, Tartour E, van der Bruggen P, Vantomme V, Joyeux I, Goud B, Fridman WH, Johannes L. Major histocompatibility complex class I presentation of exogenous soluble tumor antigen fused to the B-fragment of Shiga toxin. *Eur J Immunol* 1998; **28**: 2726–2737.

182. Vingert B, Adotevi O, Patin D, Jung S, Shrikant P, Freyburger L, Eppolito C, Sapoznikov A, Amessou M, Quintin-Colonna F, Fridman WH, Johannes L, Tartour E. The Shiga toxin B-subunit targets antigen *in vivo* to dendritic cells and elicits anti-tumor immunity. *Eur J Immunol* 2006; **36**: 1124–1135.

183. Hakomori SI. Glycosylation defining cancer malignancy: New wine in an old bottle. *Proc Natl Acad Sci USA* 2002; **99**: 10231–10233.

184. Arab S, Russel E, Chapman WB, Rosen B, Lingwood CA. Expression of the Verotoxin receptor glycolipid globotriaosylceramide, in ovarian hyperplasias. *Oncol Res* 1997; **9**: 553–563.

185. Farkas-Himsley H, Hill R, Rosen B, Arab S, Lingwood CA. The bacterial colicin active against tumor cells *in vitro* and *in vivo* is Verotoxin 1. *Proc Natl Sci USA* 1995; **92**: 6996–7000.

186. Lingwood CA, Khine AA, Arab S. Globotriaosyl ceramide (Gb$_3$) expression in human tumor cells: Intracellular trafficking defines a new retrograde transport pathway from the cell surface to the nucleus, which correlates with sensitivity to Verotoxin. *Acta Biochim Pol* 1998; **45**: 351–359.

187. Arab S, Murakami M, Dirks P, Boyd B, Habbard SL, Lingwood CA, Rutka JT. Verotoxins inhibit the growth of and induce apoptosis in human astrocytoma cells. *J Neuro-Oncol* 1998; **40**: 137–150.

188. Salhia B, Rutka JT, Lingwood CA, Nutikka A, Van Furth WR. The treatment of malignant meningioma with Verotoxin. *Neoplasia* 2002; **4**: 304–311.

189. Kovbasnjuk O, Mourtazina R, Baibakov B, Wang T, Elowsky C, Choti MA, Kane A, Donowitz M. The glycosphingolipid globotriaosylceramide in metastatic transformation of colon cancer. *Proc Natl Acad Sci USA* 2005; **102**: 19087–19092.

190. Ohyama C, Fukushi Y, Satoh M, Saitoh S, Orikasa S, Nudelman E, Straud M, Hakomori S. Changes in glycolipid expression in human testicular tumor. *Int J Cancer* 1990; **45**: 1040–1044.

191. Ohyama C, Orikasa S, Satoh M, Saito S, Ohtani H, Fukushi Y. Globotriaosyl ceramide glycolipid in seminoma: Its clinicopathological importance in differentiation from testicular malignant lymphoma. *J Urol* 1992; **148**: 72–75.

192. Hughes AK, Ergonul Z, Stricklett PK, Kohan DE. Molecular basis for high renal cell sensitivity to the cytotoxic effects of Shigatoxin-1: Upregulation of globotriaosylceramide expression. *J Am Soc Nephrol* 2002; **13**: 2239–2245.

193. Lingwood CA. Glycolipid receptors for Verotoxin and *Helicobacter pylori*: Role in pathology. *Biochim Biophys Acta* 1999; **1455**: 375–386.

194. Ohmi K, Kiyokawa N, Takeda T, Fujimoto J. Human microvascular endothelial cells are strongly sensitive to Shiga toxins. *Biochem Biophys Res Commun* 1998; **251**: 137–141.

195. Newburg DS, Ashkenazi S, Cleary TG. Human milk contains the Shiga toxin and Shiga-like toxin receptor glycolipid Gb$_3$. *J Infect Dis* 1992; **166**: 832–836.

196. Arbus GS, Grisaru S, Segal O, Dosch M, Pop M, Lala P, Nutikka A, Lingwood CA. Verotoxin targets lymphoma infiltrates of patients with post-transplant lymphoproliferative disease. *Leuk Res* 2000; **24**: 857–864.

197. Butch AW, Nahm MH. Functional properties of human germinal center B cells. *Cell Immunol* 1992; **140**: 331–344.

198. Bitzan M, Richardson S, Huang C, Boyd B, Petric M, Kamali MA. Evidence that Verotoxins (Shiga-like toxins) from *Escherichia coli* bind to P blood group antigens of human erythrocytes *in vitro*. *Infect Immun* 1994; **62**: 3337–3347.

199. Heath-Engel HM, Lingwood CA. Verotoxin sensitivity of ECV304 cells *in vitro* and *in vivo* in xenograft tumor model: VT1 as a tumor neovascular marker. *Angiogenesis* 2003; **6**: 129–141.

200. LaCasse EC, Saleh MT, Patterson B, Minden MD, Gariepy J. Shiga-like toxin purges human lymphoma from bone marrow of severe combined immunodeficient mice. *Blood* 1996; **88**: 1561–1567.

201. Tarragó-Trani MT, Jiang S, Harich KC, Storrie B. Shiga-like toxin subunit B (SLTB)-enhanced delivery of Chlorin e6 (Ce6) improves cell killing. *Photochem Photobiol* 2006; **82**: 527–537.

202. Amessou M, Carrez D, Patin D, Sarr M, Grierson DS, Croisy A, Tedesco AC, Maillard P, Johannes L. Retrograde delivery of photosensitizer (TPPp-O-β-GluOH)$_3$ selectively potentiates its photodynamic activity. *Bioconjug Chem* 2008; **19**: 532–538.

203. El Alaoui A, Schmidt F, Sarr M, Decaudin D, Florent JC, Johannes L. Synthesis and properties of a mitochondrial peripheral benzodiazepine receptor conjugate. *Chem Med Chem* 2008; **3**: 1687–1695.

204. El Alaoui A, Schmidt F, Amessou M, Sarr M, Decaudin D, Florent JC, Johannes L. Shiga toxin-mediated retrograde delivery to a topoisomerase I inhibitor prodrug. *Angew Chem Int Ed Engl* 2007; **46**: 6469–6472.

205. Hicks S, Machamer CE. Golgi structure in stress sensing and apoptosis. *Biochim Biophys Acta* 2005; **1744**: 406–414.

206. Storrie B, Tarragó-Trani MT, English S. B/B-like fragment targeting for the purposes of photodynamic therapy and medical imaging. United States Patent 6,631,283, 2003.
207. Jansen KP, Vignjevic D, Boisgard R, Falguieres T, Bousquet G, Decaudin D, Dolle F, Louvard D, Tavitian B, Robine S, Johannes L. *In vivo* tumor targeting using a novel intestinal pathogen-based delivery approach. *Cancer Res* 2006; **66**: 7230–7236.
208. Viel T, Dransart E, Nemati F, Henry E, Theze B, Decaudin D, Lewandowski D, Boisgard R, Johannes L, Tavitian B. In vivo tumor targeting by the B-subunit of Shiga toxin. *Mol Imaging* 2008; **7**: 239–247.

11 Mitochondria-Targeted Drug Delivery

Volkmar Weissig and Gerard G. M. D'Souza

CONTENTS

11.1 INTRODUCTION

11.1.1 MITOCHONDRIAL RENAISSANCE AT THE END OF THE TWENTIETH CENTURY

The 1990s witnessed an amazing resurgence of mitochondrial research, which symbolically culminated in *Science* featuring on its front cover of the March 5, 1999 issue a textbook image of an isolated mitochondrion. Two main areas of research involving mitochondria were responsible for this "mitochondrial boom" observed during the 1990s.

First, two landmark papers published in 1988 revealed for the first time a causative link between defects in the mitochondrial genome and human diseases. Wallace et al. described an association between a mitochondrial missense mutation and maternally transmitted Leber's hereditary optic neuropathy.[1] Holt et al. showed the presence of mitochondrial DNA deletions in patients with spontaneous mitochondrial encephalomyopathies.[2] Thereafter, during the 1990s, the number of human diseases recognized to be caused by mitochondrial DNA mutations has soared. Over 340 distinct mitochondrial disorders have been identified.[3] It has been estimated that every 15 min a child is born with a mitochondrial disease or who will develop one by 5 years of age.[4] Mitochondrial DNA

A causative link between defects in the mitochondrial genome and human diseases has been discovered for the first time in 1988. As of today, over 360 human mitochondrial DNA diseases have been identified most of which are neuromuscular and neurodegenerative disorders.

diseases and therapeutic strategies for their treatment, however, shall not be the subject of this chapter. The reader is referred to several excellent review papers covering this area.[5–13]

Second, the past decade has revealed an astonishing new function of mitochondria in cell metabolism. In 1990, B cell lymphoma-2 (Bcl-2) protein was found in the mitochondrial membrane, indicating for the first time that mitochondria are implicated in the regulation of mammalian cell apoptosis (or "Programmed Cell Death").[14,15] The following years saw the identification of a variety of mitochondrial proteins capable of triggering apoptosis once they are released from the mitochondrial intermembrane space into the cytosol. Most surprisingly, among those proapoptotic mitochondrial proteins was cytochrome c, which was known for its role in biological oxidation since the early 1920s. When outside mitochondria, cytochrome c forms a complex with two cytosolic proteins, Apaf1 (apoptotic protease-activating factor 1) and pro-caspase 9. The resulting complex, then referred to as apoptosome, auto-catalytically activates caspase 9, which in turn leads to the activation of a cascade of proteolytic enzymes responsible for cellular apoptosis.

The breathtaking revelation of the role of mitochondria in apoptosis could not have been better characterized by Brown, Nicholls, and Cooper, who wrote in 1998 in the preface to a book derived from the Annual Symposium of the Biochemical Society held at Sheffield University: "Who would have believed it?! Mitochondria, the powerhouse of cellular life, are also the motors of cell death. Few would have accepted this even 5 years ago".[16]

11.1.2 MITOCHONDRIA AND CANCER

Apoptosis is a fundamental biological process, which is essential for organ development during embryogenesis as well as for the elimination of cells affected by pathogens or any other damaging events. "Diseased" cells and cells not required anymore essentially commit suicide for the benefit of the whole organism. Apoptosis at the wrong time or the wrong place may lead to degenerative disorders, while resistance to apoptosis may lead to the uncontrolled proliferation and growth of cells.

The avoidance of apoptosis is a prerequisite for malignant cell growth and is considered one of the hallmarks of cancer cells.[17] Limitless replicative potential, self-sufficiency in growth signals, insensitivity to antigrowth signals, sustained angiogenesis, tissue invasion, and metastasis are the other characteristic features of cancer cell physiology.

Considering the recently recognized crucial role that mitochondria play in the complex apoptotic mechanism, the finding that cancer cell mitochondria are involved in conferring apoptosis resistance to transformed cells should not be surprising. Based on his observation that even under aerobic conditions cancer cells keep producing their adenosine triphosphate (ATP) mainly through glycolysis, Otto Warburg hypothesized in 1926 that cancer may be caused by impaired mitochondrial function[18] (referenced in Ref.[19]).

The exact mechanism of how mitochondria are involved in malignant transformation of a cell as well as how mitochondrial metabolism is altered in cancer cells to avoid apoptosis has still to be elucidated. A discussion of these aspects is beyond the scope of this chapter. Guido Kroemer, one of the leading investigators in this field, emphasized recently that the essential hallmarks of cancer are intertwined with an altered cancer cell-intrinsic metabolism, either as a consequence or as a cause.[20] He further suggested that the resistance of cancer cell mitochondria against apoptosis-associated permeabilization and the altered contribution of these organelles to metabolism might be closely related.[20] This bridged Otto Warburg's early work with the most recent revelations about the role mitochondria play in apoptosis.

11.1.3 MITOCHONDRIA AS A TARGET FOR CANCER CHEMOTHERAPY

Mitochondria as a potential target for anticancer drugs were mentioned in the literature for the first time in 1997 and 1998. Guchelaar et al. argued for the exploration of apoptosis by modulating the extrinsic and intrinsic regulators in a positive or negative direction in order to improve the efficacy of anticancer treatment. Decaudin et al.[22] discussed strategies for the development of chemotherapeutic agents acting on mitochondria.

Subsequently, the number of laboratories investigating mitochondria as a target for anticancer drugs has grown significantly. For illustration, Figure 11.1 shows the number of publications referenced in Medline with the terms "cancer" and "mitochondria" appearing in their abstract. Concomitant with this explosion of papers, a flood of patent applications has been filed in this area.[23]

A large variety of small molecules have been identified to trigger apoptosis by directly acting on the mitochondria. Such molecules include clinically approved drugs such as paclitaxel,[24–27] VP-16 (etoposide),[28,29] and vinorelbine,[25] and an increasing number of experimental anticancer drugs such as betulinic acid, lonidamine, CD-437 (synthetic retinoids), and ceramide.[30] Moreover, the number of newly discovered compounds triggering apoptosis by acting on mitochondria keeps growing.[31] Many of these agents induce apoptosis under circumstances in which conventional drugs do not display any pro-apoptotic activity. Reasons for the failure of drugs to trigger apoptosis in cancer cells may lie in the disruption of endogenous apoptosis-inducing pathways, e.g., such as those involving p53, death receptors, or apical caspase activation.

Ralph et al. recently proposed calling this emerging class of drugs "mitocans"—to signify their mitochondrial targeting and anticancer roles.[23] This group of drugs would include hexokinase inhibitors, electron transport chain blockers, activators of the mitochondrial permeability transition pore complex (mPTPC), inhibitors of Bcl-2 anti-apoptotic family proteins, and Bax/Bid pro-apoptotic mimetics.[23]

The mechanism by which mitocans trigger apoptosis depends on the molecular mitochondrial target site. For example, several *in vitro* and *in vivo* studies have demonstrated that the synthetic retinoid CD437 is able to induce apoptosis in a variety of human carcinoma cells including lung, breast, cervical, and ovarian cancer.[30] In intact cells, CD437-dependent caspase activation is preceded by the release of cytochrome c from mitochondria.[32] Moreover, when added to isolated mitochondria, CD437 causes membrane permeabilization. This effect is prevented by inhibitors of the

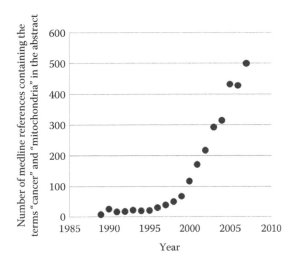

FIGURE 11.1   The number of publications referenced by Medline (as of October 2008), with the terms "cancer" and "mitochondria" appearing in their abstract, has grown significantly since the turn of the century.

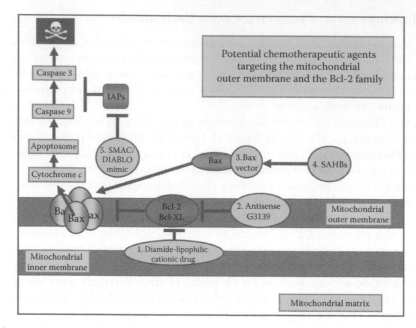

FIGURE 11.2 Potential chemotherapeutic approaches targeting the mitochondrial outer membrane and the Bcl-2 family. Mitochondrial outer membrane permeabilization is regulated by the Bcl-2 family of proteins. Therefore, targeting strategies to induce apoptosis are aimed at either inhibiting Bcl-2 antiapoptotic proteins or inducing Bax-like proapoptotic proteins. Bax vectors have been used to deliver Bax and form a pore in the mitochondrial outer membrane. This pore releases proapoptotic cytochrome c and other factors from the intermembrane space. BH3 stapled peptides (SAHBs) that activate Bax have been employed to induce apoptosis. The caspases are negatively regulated by a family of proteins known as the inhibitors of apoptosis proteins (IAPs), including Xl-linked IAP (XIAP). These themselves are also regulated by the IAP-inhibitor proteins, such as the second mitochondria derived activator of caspase/direct IAP binding protein with low pI (Smac/DIABLO), which serve to restore caspase activity. Smac/DIABLO mimics have recently been used to induce apoptosis. (Reprinted from Armstrong, J.S., *Br. J. Pharmacol.*, 147, 239, 2006. With permission.)

mPTPC, such as cyclosporine A. Therefore, CD437 represents a low-molecular weight compound, which exerts its cytotoxic effect via the mPTPC, i.e., by acting directly at the surface or inside of mitochondria. The variety of molecular mitochondrial targets for potential chemotherapeutic agents (i.e., mitocans) is illustratively summarized in Figures 11.2 and 11.3.

11.2 LEVELS OF DRUG TARGETING

The definition by Ralph et al. of "mitocans" as "mitochondrial targeting" is unfortunately misleading when interpreted in the context of drug delivery. Targeting from the point of view of drug delivery implies an active predisposition for a particular location or in other words the ability of a molecule to "home in" on a particular location. The term mitochondrial targeting applied to mitocans would therefore imply that all mitocans have a predisposition for selective accumulation in the mitochondria. While this may be true for some mitocan molecules, it cannot be applied to all of them. Many mitocans just act on targets located in or on the mitochondrion but have no predisposition for selectively accumulating there. To truly be defined as "mitochondrial targeting," a drug molecule would have to achieve several levels of preferential accumulation as outlined in Figure 11.4.

Following systemic administration, the drug has to reach the tumor mass, which is composed of malignant cells, i.e., tumor cells and the supporting stroma. The stroma, in turn, is made up of connective tissue, blood vessels, and inflammatory cells. Therefore, the selective drug accumulation in a solid tumor is the first step towards selectively killing cancer cells. The drug still has to

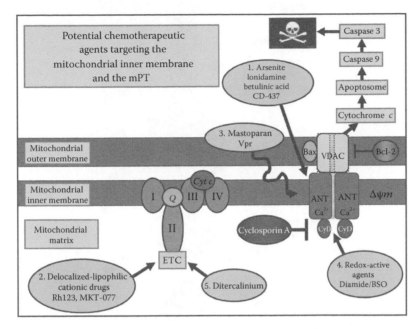

FIGURE 11.3 Potential chemotherapeutic approaches targeting the mitochondrial inner membrane and the mitochondrial PT. Mitochondrial inner membrane permeabilization and the PT is regulated by calcium and oxidative stress. Targeting strategies include activating the PT, inhibiting electron transport and oxidative phosphorylation, and depleting mitochondrial DNA (mtDNA). Agents such as arsenite, lonidamine, betulinic acid, and CD437 target the PT and induce loss of the membrane pontential. Delocalized lipophilic cations accumulate in the mitochondria matrix, leading to the loss of respiration and inhibition of electron transport. Helical peptides such as mastoparan and Vpr permeabilize mitochondrial membranes and induce PT. Redox modulating compound, such as diamide, deplete glutathione (GSH) stores, leading to the oxidation and cross-linking of critical mitochondrial redox-sensitive thiol groups at the matrix surface of the PT. mtDNA depleting agents, such as ditercalinium inhibit respiration, electron transport, and oxidative phosphorylation. (From Armstrong J.S., *Br. J. Pharmacol.*, 147, 239, 2006. With permission.)

home in on the tumor cell and once inside the cell, it has to reach its final subcellular target, for example, mitochondria—in the case of mitocans. Furthermore, to eventually be able to home in on its subcellular target, each drug molecule has to traverse numerous biological membranes, which in essence separate these levels of drug targeting from each other. Currently, the need for drug targeting is well accepted up to the cellular level as evidenced by the large number of approaches being explored to achieve a cell-specific accumulation of drugs. However, there is less acceptance of the need for targeting at a subcellular level based on an argument that once a drug gets inside a cell it will eventually find its way to the subcellular target.

11.2.1 Factors Determining the Intracellular Distribution of Low-Molecular-Weight Drugs

Two major groups of factors determine the fate of a low-molecular-weight drug molecule once it has entered a cell: first, the intracellular environment and second, the nature of the drug itself. Both these groups of factors are tightly intertwined with each other.

Fluid-phase viscosity of the cytoplasm, collisional interactions due to macromolecular crowding, and binding to intracellular components are all factors that prevent the free diffusion of solutes inside a cell.[34,35] Their impact on the cytoplasmic diffusion of a low-molecular-weight compound is measurable and can be expressed as the translational diffusion coefficient. For example, using spot photobleaching, it was possible to measure the movement of DNA fragments of different sizes

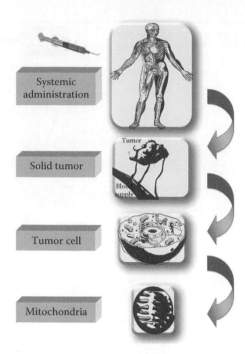

FIGURE 11.4 Three levels of drug targeting. Following its systemic administration, the drug has to reach the site of the solid tumor, then the tumor cells inside the tumor mass, and subsequently the tumor cell mitochondria.

following the microinjection of HeLa cells into the cytoplasm.[34] Not surprisingly, the rate of diffusion decreased with the increasing size of the DNA. Fragments larger than 3 kb actually did not diffuse at all; the implications of this finding for the area of gene therapy are obvious. Most DNA constructs for gene therapy are larger than 3 kb and even if delivered into the cytosol such constructs could not be expected to find their way to the nucleus by diffusion alone.

The extent to which a drug might interact or even bind to subcellular components, like membranes and cell organelles, depends on the physicochemical properties of the drug. Based on the intracellular distribution of a large variety of fluorophores, Richard Horobin has developed a quantitative structure activity relationship (QSAR) model for predicting the cellular uptake and intracellular distribution of low-molecular-weight compounds.[36] Horobin's QSAR approach is based on the calculation of the following parameters for a given chemical structure: Charge (Z), amphiphilic index (AI), conjugated bond number (CBN), partition coefficient (log P), pK_a value, molecular weight, the size of the largest conjugated fragment (LCF), and the ratio of LCF:CBN. Figures 11.5 and 11.6 illustrate Horobin's QSAR decision rules for predicting the membrane permeation and intracellular distribution, respectively of low-molecular-weight compounds. The former figure shows the parameters that the molecule needs to meet in order to cross the cell membrane, and the latter depicts criteria for selected organelle specificities.

11.2.2 MITOCHONDRIOTROPIC MOLECULES

Recently, Horobin's QSAR model was applied to low-molecular-weight compounds known to selectively accumulate in mitochondria, compounds that generally have been referred to as "mitochondriotropics".[37] A dataset of more than 100 such molecules was examined using physicochemical classifications, QSAR models, and the Fick–Nernst–Planck physicochemical model. Using a combination of the latter two models, the mitochondriotropic behavior of >80% of the dataset could

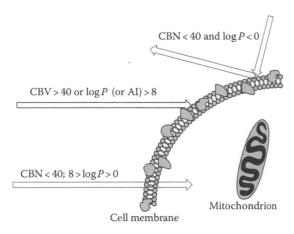

FIGURE 11.5   Richard Horobin's QSAR decision rules for predicting membrane permeation of low-molecular weight compounds (for abbreviations see Figure 11.5). (Courtesy of Richard W. Horobin.)

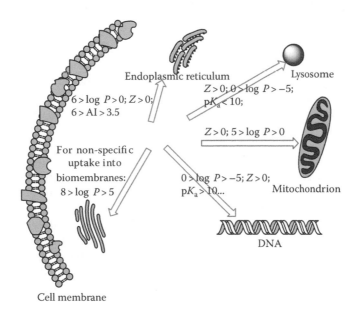

FIGURE 11.6   Richard Horobin's QSAR decision rules for predicting the intracellular distribution of low-molecular weight compounds (for abbreviations see Figure 11.5). (Courtesy of Richard W. Horobin.)

be predicted. This helped form the basis of the detailed guidelines for the design of optimal mitochondriotropic structures.

Consequently, low-molecular-weight compounds that display a high degree of mitochondriotropism can now be designed and synthesized. Such molecules target mitochondria—in the sense of "homing in" on mitochondria. Their selective mitochondrial accumulation involves several mechanisms, like electric potential, ion-trapping, and complex formation with cardiolipin as well as membrane partitioning as a basis for nonspecific accumulation. Such mitochondriotropics do not necessarily have a molecular target at or inside the mitochondria and are consequently different from mitocans. Mitocans do not automatically home in on mitochondria, but once they randomly collide with the organelle, they interact with their molecular target site and trigger a physiological response. Therefore, the question arises of how to find or how to design and synthesize a molecule that displays a high degree of mitochondriotropism, i.e., a molecule able to home in on mitochondria; and which is, at the same time, capable of triggering a specific physiologic response, such as apoptosis via recognizing a specific molecular target.

There are two principal approaches: to screen chemical libraries or to make use of emerging biopharmaceutical nanotechnologies. For example, in 2002, utilizing a cell-based assay for screening a chemical library of 16,000 compounds, a small molecule called F16 was identified as a potent anti-cancer agent.[38,39] This molecule was found to accumulate almost completely in the mitochondrial matrix in response to the elevated mitochondrial membrane potential. The concentration of F16 in the matrix leads to depolarization, opening of the permeability transition (PT) pore, cytochrome c release, cell cycle arrest, and, subsequently, cell death by apoptosis.[39] F16 fulfills Horobin's QSAR criteria for mitochondrial accumulation and displays mitochondria-based cytotoxicity. A screening of large chemical libraries is expected to reveal similar potent drug candidates, which also accumulate at their intracellular site of action.

However, even the perfect molecule combining physiological activity and organelle-specific tropism still needs to be delivered to the diseased tissue, e.g., a solid tumor.

11.3 PHARMACEUTICAL NANO-DRUG DELIVERY SYSTEMS

Many potent drug candidates identified *in vitro* have been shelved due to their poor solubility in aqueous media, which drastically reduces their bioavailability. Likewise, quite soluble compounds have a limited ability to cross lipid membranes, making the cell interior almost inaccessible to them. The general question arises whether it is easier to design a drug that combines all essential physicochemical properties for providing high systemic, tissue, cellular, and subcellular bioavailability with the desired high pharmacological activity or to design a tissue-, cell-, and organelle-specific delivery technology applicable to a wide variety of small pharmacologically active molecules.

With the development of liposome-based drug delivery systems, an important step has been taken. Liposomes, the prototype of all nano-drug delivery systems currently under development, are artificial phospholipid vesicles able to encapsulate water-soluble drugs in their aqueous inner space as well as lipophilic drugs in the phospholipid bilayer membrane. Accidentally discovered by Alex Bangham in the early 1960s[40,41] and proposed by Gregory Gregoriadis in the early 1970s as a potential drug carrier system,[42,43] they found their way into the clinic with the FDA approval of Doxil® and Daunoxome® during the 1990s. The former formulation is a colloidal solution of phospholipid vesicles of 100 nm in diameter with encapsulated doxorubicin hydrochloride; the latter is made up of 45 nm of liposomes with encapsulated daunorubicin. In both formulations, the liposomal surface was modified with polyethylene glycol (PEG) to significantly increase the vesicle's circulation time following their systemic administration. A long circulation time, in turn, results in an increased accumulation of the liposomal drug at sites of vascular damage, such as in solid tumors and at inflamed areas.

The selective accumulation of nanoparticulate drug carriers is known as the enhanced permeability and retention (EPR) effect.[44,45] Having entered the solid tumor, liposomes eventually disintegrate (by a process that is not well understood) and release the free drug into the tumor interstitium. Depending on the drug's physicochemical properties, it may then diffuse into the tumor cell interior and a portion of it might randomly be able to interact with its subcellular target site. Obviously, turning the passive and random nature of the last two steps, i.e., crossing the tumor cell membrane and reaching the subcellular target site, into active and controlled processes should significantly increase any drug's therapeutic efficiency. Hence, greater benefit can be realized by combining the tissue (e.g., solid tumor) specifities of FDA-approved nano-drug delivery technology with the organelle-specific tropisms of small molecules as modeled by Horobin's QSAR approach. Appropriately, subcellular, i.e., organelle-specific, drug delivery is emerging as the new frontier in drug delivery.[46]

11.3.1 DQAsomes as the Prototype for Mitochondria-Specific Pharmaceutical Nanocarriers

11.3.1.1 Self-Assembly of Mitochondriotropic Bolaamphiphiles

An accidental discovery in the mid-1990s has revealed an approach towards developing mitochondria-specific (i.e., subcellular) nano-drug delivery systems. While screening drugs known to accumulate in mitochondria and exploring the ability to interfere with mitochondrial DNA metabolism in the bacteria *P. falciparum*,[47] it was found that dequalinium chloride, a bolaamphiphilic dicationic quinolinium derivative (Figure 11.7A), tends to self-assemble into nanoparticulate structures when sonicated in an aqueous buffer. These nano-assemblies had been called at the time of their discovery "DQAsomes," i.e., dequalinium-derived liposome-like vesicles.[48]

A structure–activity relationship study, though limited to only nine bolaamphiphilic dicationic quinolinium derivatives (examples shown in Figure 11.8), revealed valuable guidelines for the future synthesis of compounds possessing a low critical vesicle concentration (CVC), i.e., a strong tendency to form stable vesicles.[50] The critical vescicle concentration is a parameter of amphiphiles analogous to critical micelle concentration that is defined as the concentration above which the amphiphile forms vesicles. The vesicles may be differentiated from micelles in that the core of the vesicle is an entrapped volume of the dispersion medium. In an aqueous medium, a vesicle has an entrapped aqueous compartment while a micelle would have a nonaqueous or hydrophobic core.

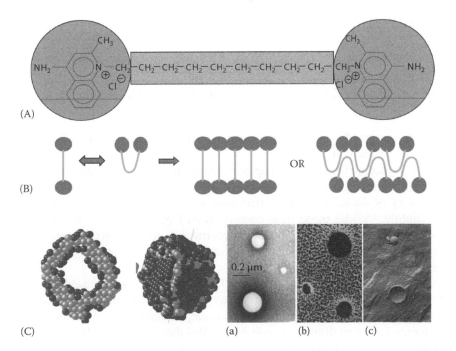

FIGURE 11.7 (A) Chemical structure of dequalinium chloride, with overlaid colors indicating in blue the hydrophilic part and in yellow the hydrophobic part of the molecule. (B) Theoretical possible conformations of dequalinium chloride, i.e., stretched versus horseshoe conformation, leading to either a monolayer or a bilayer membranous structure following the process of self-assembly. (C), left panel: Monte Carlo computer simulations demonstrate the possible self-assembly of dequalinium chloride into vesicles. The first image represents a transverse section of the second image, which represents a complete spherical vesicle. (C), right panel: Electron micrographs of vesicles ("DQAsomes") made from dequalinium chloride; from left to right: negatively stained transmission electron micrograph, rotary shadowed transmission electron micrograph, freeze fracture scanning electron micrograph. (Reprinted from Cheng, S.M. et al., DQAsome as mitochondria-targeted nanocarriers for anti-cancer drugs, in *Nanotechnology for Cancer Therapy*, Amiji, M.M. (ed.), CRC Press, Boca Raton, FL, 2007. With permission.)

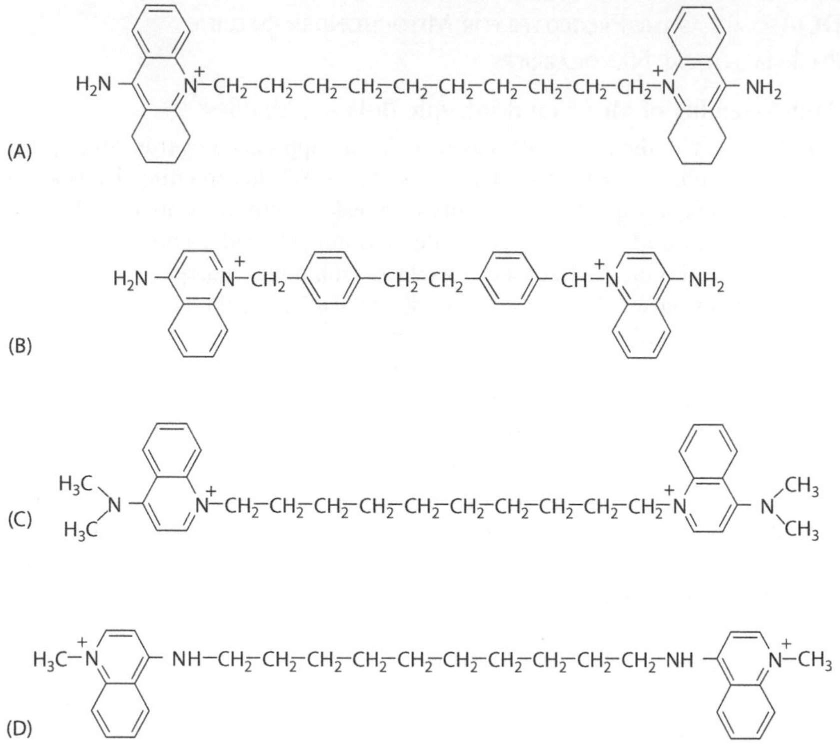

FIGURE 11.8 Chemical structures of dequalinium derivatives tested for their self-assembly behavior and cytotoxicity (these compounds were synthesized and provided by Robin Ganellin from the University College of London).

CVC is easily determined by dynamic light scattering measurements of the colloidal size vesicles that are formed above the CVC.

For example, replacing the methyl group at the aromatic ring in dequalinium chloride (Figure 11.7A) with an aliphatic ring system (Figure 11.8, compound A), which one would expect to increase the hydrophobicity of the heterocycle, confers unexpected superior vesicle-forming properties to this bolaamphiphile. Vesicles made from compound A, Figure 11.8, have, in contrast to vesicles made from dequalinium, with 169 ± 50 nm a very narrow size distribution ("beautisomes"). The size distribution of these vesicles compared with DQAsomes is highly stable, even after storage at room temperature for over 5 months.

In contrast to dequalinium-based vesicles (i.e., DQAsomes), bolasomes made from compound A are also stable upon a 1:10 dilution of the original vesicle preparation. While DQAsomes slowly disintegrate over a period of several hours, vesicles made from compound A do not show any change in size distribution following dilution. In conclusion, this data suggest that bulky aliphatic residues attached to the heterocycle in dequalinium-like bolaamphiphiles favor the self-association of the planar ring system. It was speculated that the bulky group sterically prevents the free rotation of the hydrophilic head of the amphiphile around the CH_2-axis, thus contributing to improved intermolecular interactions between the amphiphilic monomers.[50]

> Upon probe sonication, dequalinium chloride suspended in aqueous medium self-assembles into liposome-like vesicles called DQAsomes.

11.3.1.2 Toxicity of DQAsomes and DQAsome-Like Vesicles

Dequalinium salts are well known for their antiseptic activity.[51–53] They have also been extensively investigated as potential anticancer drugs.[54–57] There is no consensus, however, about their molecular

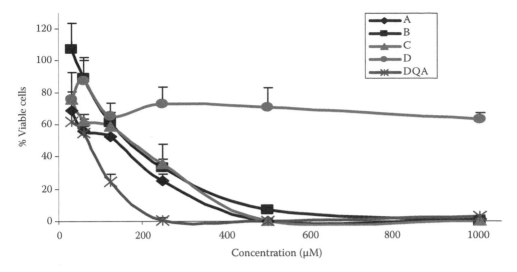

FIGURE 11.9   Cytotoxicity of vesicles made from the dequalinium analogs shown in Figure 11.5 HeLa cells were seeded at 3000 cells/well and treated in triplicate with indicated concentrations of dequalinium or one of its derivatives for 2 h. After the 2 h exposure, cells were washed once with complete media and allowed to grow in fresh complete media for 24 h followed by the measurement of metabolic activity using the commercially available Celltitre 96 reagent (Promega). (From Weissig V. et al., *J. Liposome Res.*, 16, 249, 2006. With permission.)

target, though the small conductance Ca^{2+}-activated K^+ channel, F1-ATPase, calmodulin, and proteinase K all have been suggested.[58–60] Interestingly, dequalinium also displays distinct structural similarities with several neuromuscular blocking agents, like decamethonium or succinylcholine, although related pharmacological activities have not been reported yet.

During the assessment of the cytotoxicity of a few dequalinium derivatives, all of them formed stable vesicles and offered some insights into structural arrangements that might be associated with the toxicity of this group of compounds. For example, compound D displays significantly decreased cytotoxicity in contrast to all other derivatives, including dequalinium itself (Figure 11.9).

Although the testing of only five quinolinium derivatives does not constitute a systematic structure–activity relationship study, two major structural differences between compound D and all other derivatives are apparent. First, only in compound D, both the quinolinium ring systems are linked to the hydrophobic CH_2 chain via a secondary amino group. Second, due to these inserted amino functions, the distance between both quinolinium ring systems in compound D is the largest among the compounds tested. Also, considering that dequalinium and compounds A–C display almost identical levels of cytotoxicity, it was concluded that the substitution pattern at the ring system does not seem to have significant impacts on cytotoxicity in HeLa cells.[61]

11.3.1.3   DQAsomes for Mitochondrial DNA Delivery

Just like cationic liposomes, which have been explored extensively since the early 1990s as a nonviral transfection vector, DQAsomes were found to bind and condense plasmid DNA.[48,62] Yet, unlike cationic liposomes, DQAsomes are composed entirely of molecules known to accumulate selectively inside mitochondria. This raised the question about their potential use as a mitochondria-specific transfection vector.[63–65]

But is there any need for such a vector? There clearly is. Since their first description in 1988,[1,2] the number of human diseases that have been recognized to be caused by mitochondrial DNA mutations has soared during the 1990s. There is no satisfactory treatment for the vast majority of patients due to the fact that any mitochondrial DNA defect affects the respiratory chain, i.e., the final common pathway of oxidative metabolism. Strategies to sidestep this defect by giving alternative metabolic carriers of energy, therefore, only temporarily alleviate clinical symptoms. The only approach towards a permanent cure of mitochondrial DNA diseases would have to involve gene therapeutic approaches. However, by the end of the 1990s, no mitochondria-specific transfection vector had been described. Given this background about mitochondrial DNA diseases and considering the (putative) mitochondriotropism of DQAsomes, these unique nanovesicles have been extensively and successfully tested for their ability to selectively deliver pDNA and oligonucleotides to mitochondria in living mammalian cells.

DQAsomes condense and protect the pDNA from nuclease digestion.[62] DQAsome/pDNA complexes ("DQAplexes") are readily taken up by mammalian cells and are endosomolytically active.[66] A very intriguing feature of DQAsomes as a mitochondria-targeted transfection vector is the ability of DQAsome/pDNA complexes ("DQAplexes") to selectively release the DNA upon contact with mitochondrial, but not plasma, membranes. This unique and highly desirable property was first verified using cell membrane-mimicking liposomal membranes[67] as well as isolated rat liver mitochondria.[68] More importantly, however, employing a new assay for the selective staining of free cytosolic pDNA could also demonstrate that DQAplexes release pDNA upon contact with mitochondrial membranes inside living mammalian cells.[66] The mechanism of this phenomenon has not yet been elucidated. It has been speculated that the selective destabilization of DQAsomes at mitochondrial membranes may either be caused by the difference in the lipid composition between cytoplasmic and mitochondrial membranes, or by the membrane potential driven diffusion of individual dequalinium molecules from the DQAsome/pDNA complex into the mitochondrial matrix leading to the disintegration of the complex.[66]

Direct evidence for the ability of DQAsomes and DQAsome-like vesicles to transport DNA selectively to the site of mitochondria was provided by studying the intracellular distribution of mitochondrial leader sequence peptide–pDNA conjugates in cultured BT20 cells using confocal fluorescence microscopy.[69]

Figure 11.10 shows images of the confocal fluorescence micrographs obtained in this study. In this figure, the mitochondria are stained red, while nucleic acids (pDNA and oligonucleotides, respectively) are labeled with a green fluorophore. In the overlaid images (Figure 11.10c and f), mixed pixels are pseudocolored in white. Both overlaid images show that almost all of the intracellular green

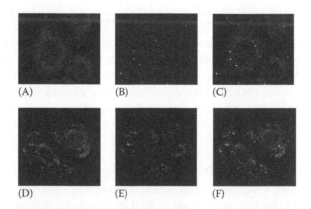

FIGURE 11.10 (A–C) Confocal fluorescence micrographs of BT20 cells stained with Mitotracker® Red CMXRos (red), which selectively stains mitochondrial membranes, after exposure to complexes of DQAsomes with fluorescein labeled oligonucleotide-mitochondrial leader sequence peptide (green); (A) red channel, (B) green channel, (C) overlay of red and green channels with white indicating co-localization of red and green fluorescence. (D–F) Confocal fluorescence micrographs of BT20 cells stained with Mitotracker® Red CMXRos (red) after exposure to linearized fluorescein labeled MLS-pDNA conjugate (green) complexed with cyclohexyl-DQAsomes; (D) green channel, (E) red channel, (F) overlay of red and green channels with white indicating co-localization of red and green fluorescence. For viewing the images in their original color, the reader is referred to the referenced original publication. (From D'Souza, G.G. et al., *Mitochondrion*, 5, 352, 2005. With permission.)

fluorescence co-localizes with the red mitochondrial fluorescence. This observation demonstrates that in addition to mediating the cellular uptake of the DNA conjugate, the use of DQAsomes leads to a definite association of the internalized DNA conjugate with mitochondria. The same study also showed that commercially available DNA delivery vectors like Lipofectin® do not transport nucleic acids to mitochondria. This study also revealed that linear DNA conjugates might be better suited for mitochondria-targeted delivery than circular pDNA conjugates. Moreover, conjugating pDNA with mitochondria leader sequence peptides alone was not sufficient to achieve substantial mitochondrial accumulation of the conjugate.

11.3.2 Mitochondriotropic Liposomes

11.3.2.1 Surface Modification of Liposomes with Mitochondriotropic Ligands

Though the enormous potential of liposomes as a nano-drug delivery system was well established by the beginning of the twenty-first century, their use for subcellular, i.e., organelle-targeted, drug delivery had not been addressed well. In general, liposomes are usually taken up by cells via endocytotic pathways leading to their association with acidic vesicles.[70] Molecules delivered to the endocytic pathway via liposomes can label a variety of intracellular organelles, including dynamic acidic tubular structures.[71,72] A fraction of liposomes, which are able to escape from acidic vesicles, may even interact in a nonspecific way with other cell organelles.

In the mid-1980s, Cudd and Nicolau had demonstrated that a portion of liposomes may even associate with mitochondria.[73–75] Considering the absence of any inherent mitochondriotropism of conventional liposomes, their association with mitochondria is thought to be caused by random interaction. To render liposomes mitochondria-specific, their surface may be modified or coated with mitochondriotropic ligands. A large variety of mitochondriotropic molecules are known,[37] among them methyltriphenylphosphonium (MTPP), which was shown about 40 years ago to be rapidly taken up by mitochondria in living cells.[76] Exploiting the marked mitochondriotropism of MTPP, Murphy and colleagues were able to demonstrate that the conjugation of biologically active molecules to triphenylphosphonium cations (TPP) facilitates their selective accumulation in mammalian mitochondria *in vitro* and *in vivo*.[77–79]

In 2005, Boddapati et al. replaced the methyl group in MTPP with a stearyl residue[80] in order to graft mitochondriotropic TPP cations onto the surface of liposomes.[81] The intracellular distribution of such surface-modified liposomes (stearyl triphenylphosphonium [STPP] liposomes) was studied using confocal fluorescence microscopy using rhodamine-labeled phosphatidylethanolamine (Rh-PE) incorporated in the liposomal membrane. Since the mitochondriotropic TPP residue is positively charged, liposomes made with the cationic lipid dioleoyl timethyl ammonium propane (DOTAP) were used as a control. Both preparations, STPP liposomes and DOTAP liposomes, were designed to bear the same surface charge of +30 ± 12 mV. Flow cytometry revealed that over the time period analyzed, DOTAP and STPP were identical in their effect on the association of liposomes with the cells (Figure 11.11A).

However, the confocal fluorescence microscopy data demonstrated significant differences in the intracellular distribution of STPP versus DOTAP liposomes. While STPP liposomes almost completely associated with mitochondria (Figure 11.11B), DOTAP liposomes showed significantly less mitochondrial association as indicated by the greater amount of red fluorescence still visible in the composite image and much less yellow than that seen for STPP liposomes.

In summary, the data from flow cytometry and confocal fluorescence microscopy demonstrate that while the surface charge of liposomes may mediate cell association, an appropriate targeting ligand on the surface of liposomes is needed for organelle-specific, i.e., mitochondria-specific liposomal targeting.

> Liposomes are rendered mitochondria-specific via surface modification with mitochondriotropic ligands. Methyltriphenylphosphonium is an example of such mitochondriotropic molecules, which are taken up rapidly by mitochondria in living cells mainly in response to the high mitochondrial membrane potential.

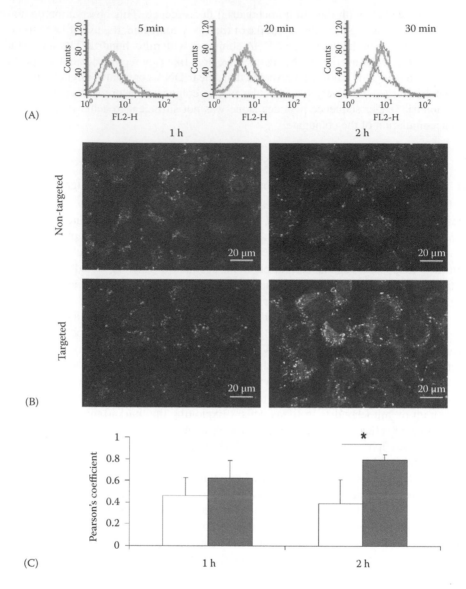

FIGURE 11.11 Interaction of liposome formulations with cells. (A) Flow cytometric analysis of liposome binding to 4T1 mouse mammary carcinoma cells. Liposomes were prepared with rhodamine labeled-phosphatidyl ethanolamine and either 1.5 mol % DOTAP or 1.5 mol % stearyl triphenylphosphonium (STPP) were incubated with 4T1 cells for 5, 20, or 30 min. The amount of cell-associated fluorescence after washing was measured by flow cytometry (y-axis denote cell counts and x-axis denotes fluorescence intensity). Purple line shows unstained cells, red line shows DOTAP liposomes, and green line shows STPP liposomes. (B) Overlaid multichannel confocal fluorescence micrographs. Red channel (excitation wavelength, EX, 548 nm; emission wavelength, EM, 719 nm): Rhodamine labeled-PE. Green channel (EX 505 nm, EM 530 nm): MitoFluor Green stained mitochondria. Blue channel (EX 385 nm, EM 470 nm): Hoechst 33342 stained nuclei. Yellow: colocalization of red and green fluorescence. (C) Analysis of fluorescence colocalization. Pearson correlation coefficient ± standard deviation ($n=6$) for colocalization of rhodamine fluorescence with Mitofluor green fluorescence obtained with ImageJ software. Open bars indicate DOTAP modified nanocarrier, shaded bars indicate STPP modified nanocarrier (* indicates a p-value of <0.005). For viewing the images in their original color, the reader is referred to the referenced original publication. (Reprinted from Boddapati, S.V. et al., *Nano Lett.*, 8, 2559, 2008. With permission.)

11.3.2.2 Mitochondria-Targeted Delivery of Liposomal Ceramide

Ceramide is a sphingolipid signaling molecule that mediates a wide range of biological responses to extracellular stimuli.[83–85] Anticancer drugs cause an increase of the ceramide level in the vicinity of mitochondria.[86] Such an increase is thought to be necessary for the formation of ceramide channels in the mitochondrial membrane, which subsequently lead to the release of cytochrome-c from the mitochondrial intermembrane space.[87,88]

Boddapati et al.[82] incorporated ceramide into STPP liposomes and tested these formulations for their apoptotic activity *in vitro* and *in vivo*. Following the *in vitro* exposure of human colon cancer cells to liposomal ceramide, the authors found that in contrast to all controls and at the low drug concentration used, only the mitochondria-targeted ceramide was able to elicit a strong apoptotic response. For *in vivo* application, STPP liposomes were surface-modified with PEG. Interestingly, the cationic TPP ligand did not significantly change the biodistribution of STPP-PEG5000 liposomes in comparison with the conventional charge-neutral PEG-liposomes. Most notably, the tumor accumulation of STPP-PEG liposomes was almost identical to their noncharged counterparts.

Mice were inoculated by subcutaneous injection with mouse mammary carcinoma cells. Upon the formation of palpable tumors, the mice were divided into three groups for treatment with either buffer, empty STPP-PEG liposomes, or ceramide-loaded STPP-PEG liposomes.

Figure 11.12A shows the tumor volumes measured over the course of the tumor growth inhibition study. In the case of buffer-treated and empty STPP-PEG liposome-treated groups, half of the animals developed necrotic morbidity after 12 days and had to be euthanized. Remarkably, none of the mice treated with ceramide-loaded liposomes showed any morbidity even after 18 days. A statistical analysis of the tumor growth rate at the 12 day time point ($n = 6$) showed that the treatment with ceramide in STPP-PEG liposomes significantly inhibited the tumor growth rate compared with sham treatment (Figure 11.12B).

The demonstrated efficacy of mitochondria-targeted ceramide is in contrast to a previous study in which ceramide was incorporated into nontargeted liposomes. While Stover et al.[89] used ceramide doses of 36 mg/kg up to 72 mg/kg, Boddapati et al.[82] were working with a dose of only 6 mg/kg. Even at this low dose, a significant reduction in tumor growth was observed.

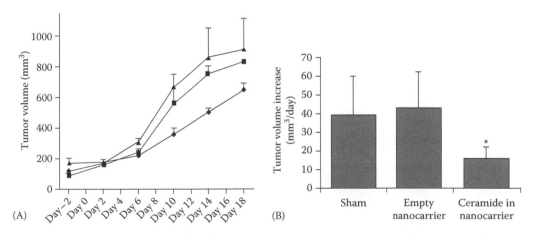

FIGURE 11.12 Tumor growth inhibition. (A) Tumor volume (mm³) measured over time period of treatment in Balb/c mice bearing murine 4T1 mammary carcinoma tumors ($n = 6$); after treatment with buffer (■), empty STPP nanocarrier (▲), and ceramide in STPP nanocarrier (♦). (B) Tumor growth in mm³/day at day 12 ($n = 6$, error bars denote standard deviation) (*indicates a student *t* test *p*-value of <0.05). (Reprinted from Boddapati, S.V. et al., *Nano Lett.*, 8, 2559, 2008. With permission.)

11.4 CONCLUDING REMARKS

During the last decade, it has become increasingly evident that drugs act on targets located on or inside subcellular compartments. Mitochondria have emerged as prime subcellular targets for cancer as well as several other diseases. Not surprisingly, there is increasing interest in understanding the mechanisms of cell uptake and the subsequent subcellular disposition of molecules as well as pharmaceutical nanocarriers in an effort to improve drug action. Emerging strategies like QSAR now offer the potential to design molecules capable of selective accumulation in a subcellular compartment of choice. This combined with the recent demonstration that pharmaceutical nanocarriers can also be targeted to subcellular compartments potentially represents an important milestone on the path to improved drug therapy. Mitochondria-specific drug-loaded nanocarriers have been shown to significantly enhance the therapeutic effect of potential anticancer agents. Such nanocarriers offer a significant benefit because they allow the organelle-specific delivery of low-molecular-weight compounds without the need for their chemical modification. It is anticipated that these advances will lead to the development of nanocarriers bearing suitable ligands for the targeting of a variety of other organelles, such as lysosomes or peroxisomes, thereby offering improved therapy for a number of diseases associated with organelle disfunction.

REFERENCES

1. Wallace DC et al. Mitochondrial DNA mutation associated with Leber's hereditary optic neuropathy. *Science* 1988; 242: 1427–1430.
2. Holt IJ, Harding AE, Morgan-Hughes JA. Deletions of muscle mitochondrial DNA in patients with mitochondrial myopathies. *Nature* 1988; 331: 717–719.
3. Naviaux RK. Developing a systematic approach to the diagnosis and classification of mitochondrial disease. *Mitochondrion* 2004; 4: 351–361.
4. Cohen BH. Incidence and prevalence rates of mitochondrial diseases. *UMDF Mitochondrial News* 2006; 11: 5–16.
5. Chinnery PF, Turnbull DM. Mitochondrial DNA and disease. *Lancet* 1999; 354: SI17–21.
6. Dimauro S, Davidzon G. Mitochondrial DNA and disease. *Ann Med* 2005; 37: 222–232.
7. Druzhyna NM, Wilson GL, LeDoux SP. Mitochondrial DNA repair in aging and disease. *Mech Ageing Dev* 2008; 129: 383–390.
8. D'Souza GG, Boddapati SV, Weissig V. Gene therapy of the other genome: The challenges of treating mitochondrial DNA defects. *Pharm Res* 2007; 24: 228–238.
9. Greaves LC, Taylor RW. Mitochondrial DNA mutations in human disease. *IUBMB Life* 2006; 58: 143–151.
10. Krishnan KJ, Reeve AK, Turnbull DM. Do mitochondrial DNA mutations have a role in neurodegenerative disease? *Biochem Soc Trans* 2007; 35: 1232–1235.
11. Kyriakouli DS et al. Progress and prospects: Gene therapy for mitochondrial DNA disease. *Gene Ther* 2008; 15: 1017–1023.
12. Taylor RW, Turnbull DM. Mitochondrial DNA mutations in human disease. *Nat Rev Genet* 2005; 6: 389–402.
13. Wallace DC. Mitochondrial diseases in man and mouse. *Science* 1999; 283: 1482–1488.
14. Chen-Levy Z, Cleary ML. Membrane topology of the Bcl-2 proto-oncogenic protein demonstrated in vitro. *J Biol Chem* 1990; 265: 4929–4933.
15. Hockenbery D et al. Bcl-2 is an inner mitochondrial membrane protein that blocks programmed cell death. *Nature* 1990; 348: 334–336.
16. Brown GC, Nicholls DG, Cooper CE, eds. *Mitochondria and Cell Death*, 1999; Princeton University Press: Princeton, NJ.
17. Hanahan D, Weinberg RA. The hallmarks of cancer. *Cell* 2000; 100: 57–70.
18. Warburg O. *Ueber den Stoffwechsel der Tumore*, 1930; Springer Verlag: Berlin, Germany.
19. Gogvadze V, Orrenius S, Zhivotovsky B. Mitochondria in cancer cells: What is so special about them? *Trends Cell Biol* 2008; 18: 165–173.
20. Kroemer G, Pouyssegur J. Tumor cell metabolism: Cancer's Achilles' heel. *Cancer Cell* 2008; 13: 472–482.

21. Guchelaar HJ et al. Apoptosis: Molecular mechanisms and implications for cancer chemotherapy. *Pharm World Sci* 1997; 19: 119–125.
22. Decaudin D et al. Mitochondria in chemotherapy-induced apoptosis: A prospective novel target of cancer therapy (review). *Int J Oncol* 1998; 12: 141–152.
23. Ralph SJ et al. Mitocans: Mitochondrial targeted anti-cancer drugs as improved therapies and related patent documents. *Recent Pat Anticancer Drug Discov* 2006; 1: 327–346.
24. Andre N et al. Paclitaxel targets mitochondria upstream of caspase activation in intact human neuroblastoma cells. *FEBS Lett* 2002; 532: 256–260.
25. Andre N et al. Paclitaxel induces release of cytochrome c from mitochondria isolated from human neuroblastoma cells'. *Cancer Res* 2000; 60: 5349–5353.
26. Ferlini C et al. Bcl-2 down-regulation is a novel mechanism of paclitaxel resistance. *Mol Pharmacol* 2003; 64: 51–58.
27. Kidd JF et al. Paclitaxel affects cytosolic calcium signals by opening the mitochondrial permeability transition pore. *J Biol Chem* 2002; 277: 6504–6510.
28. Fujino M et al. Distinct pathways of apoptosis triggered by FTY720, etoposide, and anti-Fas antibody in human T-lymphoma cell line (Jurkat cells). *J Pharmacol Exp Ther* 2002; 300: 939–945.
29. Itoh M et al. Etoposide-mediated sensitization of squamous cell carcinoma cells to tumor necrosis factor-related apoptosis-inducing ligand (TRAIL)-induced loss in mitochondrial membrane potential. *Oral Oncol* 2003; 39: 269–276.
30. Costantini P et al. Mitochondrion as a novel target of anticancer chemotherapy. *J Natl Cancer Inst* 2000; 92: 1042–1053.
31. Armstrong JS. Mitochondrial medicine: Pharmacological targeting of mitochondria in disease. *Br J Pharmacol* 2007; 151: 1154–1165.
32. Marchetti P et al. The novel retinoid 6-[3-(1-adamantyl)-4-hydroxyphenyl]-2-naphtalene carboxylic acid can trigger apoptosis through a mitochondrial pathway independent of the nucleus. *Cancer Res* 1999; 59: 6257–6266.
33. Armstrong JS. Mitochondria: A target for cancer therapy. *Br J Pharmacol* 2006; 147: 239–248.
34. Lukacs GL et al. Size-dependent DNA mobility in cytoplasm and nucleus. *J Biol Chem* 2000; 275: 1625–1629.
35. Seksek O, Biwersi J, Verkman AS. Translational diffusion of macromolecule-sized solutes in cytoplasm and nucleus. *J Cell Biol* 1997; 138: 131–142.
36. Horobin RW. Uptake, distribution and accumulation of dyes and fluorescent probes within living cells: A structure–activity modelling approach. *Adv Colour Sci Technol* 2001; 4: 101–107.
37. Horobin RW, Trapp S, Weissig V. Mitochondriotropics: A review of their mode of action, and their applications for drug and DNA delivery to mammalian mitochondria. *J Control Release* 2007; 121: 125–136.
38. Fantin VR, Leder P. F16, a mitochondriotoxic compound, triggers apoptosis or necrosis depending on the genetic background of the target carcinoma cell. *Cancer Res* 2004; 64: 329–336.
39. Fantin VR et al. A novel mitochondriotoxic small molecule that selectively inhibits tumor cell growth. *Cancer Cell* 2002; 2: 29–42.
40. Bangham AD, Standish MM, Miller N. Cation permeability of phospholipid model membranes: Effect of narcotics. *Nature* 1965; 208: 1295–1297.
41. Bangham AD, Standish MM, Watkins JC. Diffusion of univalent ions across the lamellae of swollen phospholipids. *J Mol Biol* 1965; 13: 238–252.
42. Gregoriadis G. Letter: Enzyme-carrier potential of liposomes in enzyme replacement therapy. *N Engl J Med* 1975; 292: 215.
43. Gregoriadis G et al. Drug-carrier potential of liposomes in cancer chemotherapy. *Lancet* 1974; 1: 1313–1316.
44. Matsumara Y, Oda T, Maeda H. General mechanism of intratumor accumulation of macromolecules: Advantage of macromolecular therapeutics. *Gan To Kagaku Ryoho* 1987; 14: 821–829.
45. Maeda H et al. Tumor vascular permeability and the EPR effect in macromolecular therapeutics: A review. *J Control Release* 2000; 65: 271–284.
46. Lim CS. Organelle-specific targeting in drug delivery and design. *Adv Drug Deliv Rev* 2007; 59: 697.
47. Rowe TC, Weissig V, Lawrence JW. Mitochondrial DNA metabolism targeting drugs. *Adv Drug Deliv Rev* 2001; 49: 175–187.
48. Weissig V et al. DQAsomes: A novel potential drug and gene delivery system made from dequalinium. *Pharm Res* 1998; 15: 334–337.

49. Cheng SM, Boddapati SV, D'Souza GM, Weissig V. DQAsomes as mitochondria-targeted nanocarriers for anti-cancer drugs, in *Nanotechnology for Cancer Therapy*, M.M. Amiji (ed.), 2007, CRC Press: Boca Raton, FL, pp. 787–802.

50. Weissig V, Lizano C, Ganellin CR, Torchilin VP. DNA binding cationic bolasomes with delocalized charge center: A structure–activity relationship study. *STP Pharma Sci* 2001; 11: 91096.

51. D'Auria FD, Simonetti G, Strippoli V. Antimicrobial characteristics of a tincture of dequalinium chloride. *Ann Ig* 1989; 1: 1227–1241.

52. Spangberg L et al. Antimicrobial and toxic effect in vitro of a bisdequalinium acetate solution for endodontic use. *J Endod* 1988; 14: 175–178.

53. Aron MC. Cytotoxic potential of 2 root canal irrigating agents. *Rev Fr Endod* 1986; 5: 13–26.

54. Galeano E et al. Effects of the antitumoural dequalinium on NB4 and K562 human leukemia cell lines. Mitochondrial implication in cell death. *Leuk Res* 2005; 29: 1201–1211.

55. Modica-Napolitano JS et al. The selective in vitro cytotoxicity of carcinoma cells by AZT is enhanced by concurrent treatment with delocalized lipophilic cations. *Cancer Lett* 2003; 198: 59–68.

56. Manetta A et al. Failure to enhance the in vivo killing of human ovarian carcinoma by sequential treatment with dequalinium chloride and tumor necrosis factor. *Gynecol Oncol* 1993; 50: 38–44.

57. Bleday R et al. Inhibition of rat colon tumor isograft growth with dequalinium chloride. *Arch Surg* 1986; 121: 1272–1275.

58. Abdul M, Santo A, Hoosein N. Activity of potassium channel-blockers in breast cancer. *Anticancer Res* 2003; 23: 3347–3351.

59. Rotenberg SA et al. Inhibition of rodent protein kinase C by the anticarcinoma agent dequalinium. *Cancer Res* 1990; 50: 677–685.

60. Hait WN. Targeting calmodulin for the development of novel cancer chemotherapeutic agents. *Anticancer Drug Des* 1987; 2: 139–149.

61. Weissig V et al. Liposomes and liposome-like vesicles for drug and DNA delivery to mitochondria. *J Liposome Res* 2006; 16: 249–264.

62. Lasch J et al. Dequalinium vesicles form stable complexes with plasmid DNA which are protected from DNase attack. *Biol Chem* 1999; 380: 647–652.

63. Weissig V, Torchilin VP. Mitochondriotropic cationic vesicles: A strategy towards mitochondrial gene therapy. *Curr Pharm Biotechnol* 2000; 1: 325–346.

64. Weissig V, Torchilin VP. Towards mitochondrial gene therapy: DQAsomes as a strategy. *J Drug Target* 2001; 9: 1–13.

65. Weissig V, Torchilin VP. Cationic bolasomes with delocalized charge centers as mitochondria-specific DNA delivery systems. *Adv Drug Deliv Rev* 2001; 49: 127–149.

66. D'Souza GG et al. DQAsome-mediated delivery of plasmid DNA toward mitochondria in living cells. *J Control Release* 2003; 92: 189–197.

67. Weissig V, Lizano C, Torchilin VP. Selective DNA release from DQAsome/DNA complexes at mitochondria-like membranes. *Drug Deliv* 2000; 7: 1–5.

68. Weissig V, D'Souza GG, Torchilin VP. DQAsome/DNA complexes release DNA upon contact with isolated mouse liver mitochondria. *J Control Release* 2001; 75: 401–408.

69. D'Souza GG, Boddapati SV, Weissig V. Mitochondrial leader sequence—Plasmid DNA conjugates delivered into mammalian cells by DQAsomes co-localize with mitochondria. *Mitochondrion* 2005; 5: 352–358.

70. Huth U et al. Fourier transformed spectral bio-imaging for studying the intracellular fate of liposomes. *Cytometry A* 2004; 57: 10–21.

71. Straubinger RM, Papahadjopoulos D, Hong KL. Endocytosis and intracellular fate of liposomes using pyranine as a probe. *Biochemistry* 1990; 29: 4929–4939.

72. Straubinger RM et al. Endocytosis of liposomes and intracellular fate of encapsulated molecules: Encounter with a low pH compartment after internalization in coated vesicles. *Cell* 1983; 32: 1069–1079.

73. Cudd A, Nicolau C. Interaction of intravenously injected liposomes with mouse liver mitochondria. A fluorescence and electron microscopy study. *Biochim Biophys Acta* 1986; 860: 201–214.

74. Cudd A, Nicolau C. Intracellular fate of liposome-encapsulated DNA in mouse liver. Analysis using electron microscope autoradiography and subcellular fractionation. *Biochim Biophys Acta* 1985; 845: 477–491.

75. Cudd A et al. Liposomes injected intravenously into mice associate with liver mitochondria. *Biochim Biophys Acta* 1984; 774: 169–180.

76. Liberman EA et al. Mechanism of coupling of oxidative phosphorylation and the membrane potential of mitochondria. *Nature* 1969; 222: 1076–1078.

77. Murphy MP, Smith RA. Targeting antioxidants to mitochondria by conjugation to lipophilic cations. *Annu Rev Pharmacol Toxicol* 2007; 47: 629–656.
78. Ross MF et al. Rapid and extensive uptake and activation of hydrophobic triphenylphosphonium cations within cells. *Biochem J* 2008; 411: 633–645.
79. Smith RA et al. Delivery of bioactive molecules to mitochondria in vivo. *Proc Natl Acad Sci USA* 2003; 100: 5407–5412.
80. Boddapati SV et al. Mitochondriotropic liposomes. *J Liposome Res* 2005; 15: 49–58.
81. Torchilin VP, Weissig V, Martin FJ, Heath TD, New RRC. Surface modification of liposomes, in *Liposomes: A Practical Approach*, V.P. Torchilin, Weissig, V. (eds.), 2003, Oxford University Press: Oxford, U.K.
82. Boddapati SV et al. Organelle-targeted nanocarriers: specific delivery of liposomal ceramide to mitochondria enhances its cytotoxicity in vitro and in vivo. *Nano Lett* 2008; 8: 2559–2563.
83. Struckhoff AP et al. Novel ceramide analogs as potential chemotherapeutic agents in breast cancer. *J Pharmacol Exp Ther* 2004; 309: 523–532.
84. Kolesnick R. The therapeutic potential of modulating the ceramide/sphingomyelin pathway. *J Clin Invest* 2002; 110: 3–8.
85. Birbes H et al. Mitochondria and ceramide: Intertwined roles in regulation of apoptosis. *Adv Enzyme Regul* 2002; 42: 113–129.
86. Kok JW, Sietsma H. Sphingolipid metabolism enzymes as targets for anticancer therapy. *Curr Drug Targets* 2004; 5: 375–382.
87. Siskind LJ et al. Enlargement and contracture of C2-ceramide channels. *Biophys J* 2003; 85: 1560–1575.
88. Siskind LJ, Colombini M. The lipids C2- and C16-ceramide form large stable channels. Implications for apoptosis. *J Biol Chem* 2000; 275: 38640–38644.
89. Stover TC et al. Systemic delivery of liposomal short-chain ceramide limits solid tumor growth in murine models of breast adenocarcinoma. *Clin Cancer Res* 2005; 11: 3465–3474.

Part IV

Prodrug Strategies

Site-Specific Prodrug
Activation Strategies for
Targeted Drug Action

Mark D. Erion

CONTENTS

12.1   INTRODUCTION

The prodrug concept, as first introduced by Albert, defined a prodrug as a biologically inactive agent that is converted *in vivo* through enzymatic and/or chemical reactions to a therapeutically active drug.[1] Traditionally, prodrugs are used in the pharmaceutical industry when the active drug exhibits limitations in either its pharmaceutical properties (e.g., solubility, taste, stability) or its pharmacokinetic profile (e.g., oral bioavailability, half-life).[2] The successful application of prodrug strategies over the past two decades has increased the percentage of drugs gaining approval as prodrugs to 5%–7%[3] and has spurred efforts to discover new strategies.[4,5]

A less well developed application of the prodrug concept entails the use of prodrugs for site-specific drug delivery.[6] Targeting drugs to pathophysiologically relevant sites represents an attractive strategy for simultaneously optimizing the efficacy and safety profiles of drug candidates.[7] Historically, site-specific drug delivery is achieved using local drug administration strategies[8] or drug conjugate strategies, wherein the drug is attached to a macromolecular carrier that recognizes organ-specific markers (e.g., antigens and receptors). In some cases, the markers are expressed on the surface of the vascular endothelium[9,10] and, therefore, require cleavage of the drug conjugate by enzymes circulating in the blood or on the surface of the endothelium prior to distribution of the drug into the target tissue (Figure 12.1, path a). The distribution of the drug into the target tissue requires the uptake to be significantly faster than the rate of drug removal from the local site via the circulation.

Alternatively, drug conjugates can recognize cell surface proteins unique to the target cell that are either noninternalizing, and therefore require the conjugate to cleave prior to drug uptake, or are proteins that undergo receptor-mediated endocytosis (Figure 12.1, path b) and trafficking to the lysosome, where the drug conjugate hydrolyzes. Anatomical constraints (e.g., the extra-cellular matrix or epithelial and endothelial barriers) greatly limit the passage of the conjugate across the

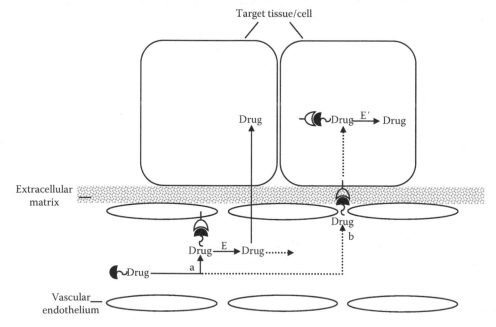

FIGURE 12.1   Site-specific drug delivery using a drug conjugate ⟨∿. Drug conjugates bind to tissue-specific biomarkers ⟨ expressed on the vascular endothelium (path a) or target tissue (path b). The drug conjugate in path a is cleaved by an enzyme (E) present in blood or on the surface of the endothelial cell membrane to produce the drug which is taken up by the tissue or eliminated from the target tissue via the circulation. The drug conjugate in path b crosses the vascular endothelium and extracellular matrix and binds to the target tissue biomarker after which the complex undergoes internalization via endocytosis and the conjugate is cleaved by enzyme E′.

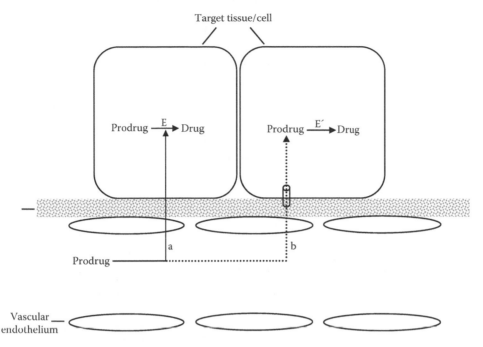

FIGURE 12.2   Site-specific drug delivery using a prodrug strategy. Prodrugs achieve site specific activation either by undergoing uptake and cleavage by an enzyme (E) that is tissue specific (path a) or by undergoing tissue-specific uptake via a transporter or receptor expressed on the membrane of the target tissue followed by cleavage via a nontissue specific enzyme (E′) (path b).

endothelial barrier except in tissues such as the liver,[11] kidney, and spleen, where the endothelium of the microvascular wall exhibits large fenestrations; or in tumors, where the neovasculature is dilated and often leaky due to the resident endothelial cells being poorly aligned and disorganized.[12] Consequently, drug conjugates are unable to deliver high drug levels to most tissues due to the low overall exposure coupled with the slow rates of drug-conjugate uptake and hydrolysis.

Prodrugs offer an alternative drug targeting strategy (Figure 12.2, path a) that differs from drug-conjugate strategies largely because unlike drug conjugates, prodrugs distribute to intracellular sites and are usually less expensive to manufacture, more likely to be orally bioavailable, and less likely to induce an immune reaction. The major challenge facing prodrug strategies is the natural existence of tissue-specific mechanisms for prodrug uptake and/or transformation that enables high tissue targeting.

This chapter focuses on the use of prodrugs for site-specific drug delivery and includes specific examples that highlight the potential of this strategy, the challenges that remain, and the possible solutions to these challenges that provide promise for the future.

> Prodrugs offer an alternative drug targeting strategy that differs from drug-conjugate strategies largely because they efficiently distribute to intracellular sites, are more likely to be orally bioavailable, and are less likely to induce an immune reaction. The major challenge facing prodrug strategies is the natural existence of tissue-specific mechanisms for prodrug uptake and/or transformation that enables high tissue targeting.

12.2   DRUG TARGETING POTENTIAL

The ability of prodrugs to achieve site-specific drug targeting is dependent on numerous factors (Figure 12.3). First, the prodrug needs to remain intact during transit from the site of administration to the target tissue and then undergo efficient uptake by the tissue. Second, targeting is dependent on the mechanism of prodrug cleavage and related organ specificity. Lastly, targeting is also highly

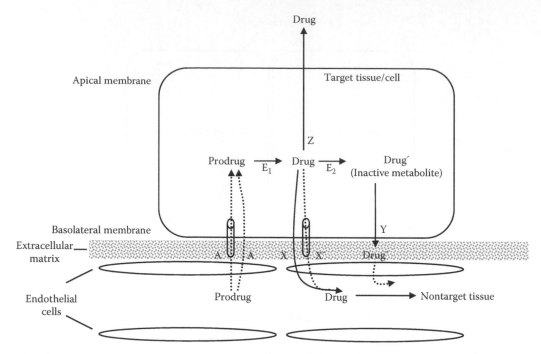

FIGURE 12.3   Prodrug uptake, metabolism and cellular elimination. Prodrug uptake occurs by either passive diffusion (A) or active transport (A'). Intracellular conversion to the drug is catalyzed by enzyme E_1 after which the drug is either eliminated passively (X) or via a transporter (X'). The drug may also be eliminated across the apical membrane (Z); or metabolized to an inactive metabolite (Drug') by enzyme E_2 and eliminated (Y) into the systemic circulation.

dependent on the fate of the active drug produced following prodrug cleavage and pathways governing the metabolism, elimination, and nontarget tissue uptake of the biologically active drug.

12.2.1   CELLULAR UPTAKE

Prodrugs achieve site-specific drug delivery only if the prodrug is (a) absorbed from the site of administration, (b) remains intact during transit to the target cell, and (c) undergoes efficient cellular uptake. As with all drugs, oral absorption is largely determined by physicochemical properties that prodrugs are often used to improve (e.g., enhanced lipophilicity, reduced molecular charge, and/or increased aqueous solubility). Nevertheless, incorporating the prodrug moiety can also impede intestinal absorption as a consequence of the increased molecular weight and, in some cases, diminished solubility and/or an increased number of hydrogen bond donor/acceptor groups.

The premature degradation of the prodrug due to aqueous instability or enzymatic cleavage can also limit prodrug exposure to the target cell. For example, prodrugs that are esters are typically cleaved by esterases (e.g., carboxylesterase, cholinesterases, paraoxonases), which are ubiquitously distributed throughout the body.[13]

Lastly, prodrugs that reach the target cell must be taken up by the cell in order to deliver high intracellular levels of the drug. In some cases, prodrug exposure to the target tissue is limited by physiologic barriers (e.g., blood–brain barrier) that require further optimization of the prodrug's physicochemical properties. Cellular uptake of the prodrug is achieved via either passive diffusion across the cellular membrane, active transport, or receptor-mediated endocytosis. The latter processes require structures and functionality recognized by specific cell membrane proteins. Moreover, the rate of uptake is dependent on their expression in the target tissue and kinetic characteristics (e.g., saturation and the rate of endocytosis).

12.2.2   Prodrug Activation

Site-specific drug delivery using prodrugs generally requires prodrugs that distribute into the target tissue and undergo efficient conversion to the active drug. Typically, this results from an enzyme-catalyzed reaction, although there are examples of nonenzymatic transformations (e.g., the proton pump inhibitor omeprazole,[14] which covalently modifies cysteine residues on the luminal side of H^+/K^+-ATPase following the acid catalyzed prodrug activation). Ideally, the enzyme responsible for cleaving the prodrug is expressed only in the target tissue (Figure 12.2). Alternatively, prodrugs activated by enzymes expressed in multiple tissues can be used for targeting if the prodrug is preferentially distributed to the target tissue using cell-specific receptors or transporters. Less ideal are prodrugs that cleave in the local vicinity of the target cell (either on the cell surface or inside a nearby cell) and then act on the target cell through a "bystander effect."[15] Targeting in this case is dependent on the rate of drug uptake into the target tissue relative to the rate of drug loss from the site.

The challenge facing efforts to utilize prodrugs for site-specific drug delivery is the availability of enzymes that are both tissue specific and are capable of catalyzing reactions exploitable by a prodrug. Unfortunately, most enzymes that are relatively tissue-specific fail to catalyze reactions useful for cleaving prodrugs or are highly substrate specific. High-substrate specificity greatly diminishes the attractiveness of a prodrug-cleaving enzyme since these enzymes are typically unable to tolerate large structural changes without unacceptable decreases in catalytic efficiency. Accordingly, most prodrugs are designed to be activated by esterases, which exhibit broad substrate specificity and high catalytic efficiency but are not expressed in a tissue-specific manner. A few prodrug classes are activated by oxidases, such as cytochrome P450s, which represent potentially attractive prodrug targets not only because they catalyze reactions useful for prodrug cleavage but also because they act on a vast array of structurally diverse substrates.[16] One cytochrome P450 isozyme, CYP3A4, is expressed primarily in the liver (hepatocytes) with appreciable activity found only in one other tissue, namely the small intestine.[17] As described in Section 12.3, prodrugs activated by CYP3A4 are now being explored clinically as a strategy for liver-specific drug delivery.[18]

> Most enzymes that are relatively tissue-specific often fail to catalyze the cleavage of prodrugs or are highly substrate specific. High-substrate specificity greatly diminishes the attractiveness of a prodrug-cleaving enzyme since these enzymes are typically unable to tolerate large structural changes without unacceptable decreases in catalytic efficiency.

12.2.3   Drug Accumulation, Elimination, and Distribution

Site-specific prodrug activation is unlikely to achieve the maximum benefit of targeted drug therapy if the active drug produced inside the cell is rapidly excreted into the systemic circulation and taken up by nontarget tissues. While higher drug concentrations may still be achieved in the target tissue, relative to nontarget tissues (since the drug excreted into the circulation will be diluted by the whole body volume), even greater targeting is possible if either

- The drug that escapes is unable to distribute into nontarget tissues
- Prodrug cleavage results in a drug and/or intermediate that is retained by the target cell due to its physicochemical properties and, therefore, can accumulate to higher intracellular concentrations before undergoing elimination

The anti-cancer prodrugs ifosfamide and cyclophosphamide represent drugs that fail to result in site-specific drug delivery despite being activated by a relatively liver-specific cytochrome P450. As illustrated in Figure 12.4, the activation of cyclophosphamide produces relatively long-lived intermediates that readily diffuse into the systemic circulation. These intermediates distribute throughout the body prior to being converted to the active drug via a slow β-elimination reaction. Consequently, these drugs are used to treat extra-hepatic tumors and are associated with extra-hepatic toxicity (primarily, bladder toxicity).[19]

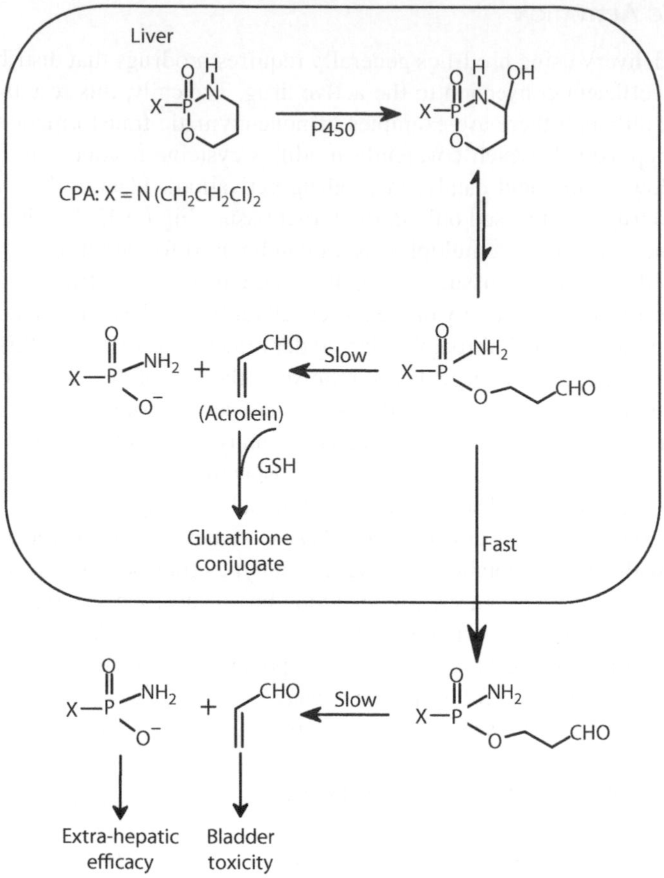

FIGURE 12.4 Cyclophosphamide (CPA) activation and excretion. CPA is oxidized by a cytochrome P450 to intermediates that rapidly escape the hepatocyte and then undergo a slow β-elimination reaction to acrolein and the biologically active nitrogen mustard.

In addition to selecting drugs that are retained inside the cell for a sustained period, targeting can be enhanced by selecting drugs whose elimination and/or distribution properties limit exposure to nontarget tissues. As highlighted in Figure 12.3, one strategy entails the selection of drugs that undergo rapid intracellular degradation to inactive metabolites. A second strategy useful in targeting drugs to the liver or kidney entails the selection of drug candidates that are eliminated from these organs using transport mechanisms present on the apical membrane. This results in high targeting if the drug eliminated into the bile (liver) or proximal tubule (kidney) is not reabsorbed. Another mechanism for enhanced targeting relies on the selection of drugs that, once eliminated into the systemic circulation, are unable to be taken up and/or activated to the biologically active form in nontarget tissues. Limited drug distribution can arise from the physicochemical properties of the active drug or because the drug in circulation requires metabolic activation and the enzymes used in this activation are only present in the target cell (e.g., acyclovir, an antiviral activated only by viral thymidine kinase).

12.2.4 OTHER PRODRUG DESIGN FACTORS

The identification of prodrug strategies suitable for site-selective drug delivery is sometimes complicated by factors unrelated to drug targeting. For example, the by-products generated following prodrug cleavage should be nontoxic, nonimmunogenic, and readily eliminated. Simple ester- and phosphate-based prodrugs (e.g., enalapril and fosphenytoin) typically produce suitable by-products but fail to achieve organ-specific drug delivery. In contrast, by-products derived from alternative prodrug classes are usually less well characterized and in some cases contain functional groups known to be associated with an increased risk of toxicity and/or mutagenicity (e.g., cyclophosphamide).

Other factors include the cost and synthetic feasibility of prodrug manufacturing, as well as the physicochemical properties that affect formulation development. Potential drug development challenges associated with the prodrug target also need to be carefully considered. For example, differences in the expression of proteins involved in the targeting mechanism can result in unacceptable intra- and interpatient variability. Moreover, the risk of significant drug–drug interactions requires analysis, including whether other drugs used to treat the target disease engage the same mechanisms employed by the prodrug for cellular uptake, metabolism, and/or elimination.

12.2.5 Alternative Strategies

The challenges described above are principally related to finding a targeting strategy that enables a prodrug to achieve site-selective drug delivery. Currently, there are a limited number of naturally occurring enzymes that catalyze reactions suitable for cleaving prodrugs. Moreover, the enzymes most commonly used by prodrugs, e.g., esterases and phosphatases, are expressed nonselectively across tissues and, therefore, by themselves are inadequate for drug targeting. In the absence of target enzymes, prodrugs are being designed to be substrates for transporters overexpressed in the target cell (e.g., see Section 12.4.1). Alternatively, prodrug strategies are being used that take advantage of physiologic barriers such as the blood-brain barrier (e.g., see Section 12.4.2).

More recently, advances in gene therapy and antibody research are being coupled with prodrug design to gain site-specific drug delivery.[20] One strategy entails the coupling of antibodies (that recognize target tissue-specific antigens) with enzymes useful for cleaving prodrugs. The strategy, now known as antibody-directed enzyme prodrug therapy (ADEPT), is being used for the treatment of cancer.[21] In some cases, microbial enzymes with substrate specificities different than the human enzyme equivalent are being delivered using viral vectors or antibodies to tissues in order to gain specificity. Examples include yeast cytosine deaminase,[22] bacterial purine nucleoside phosphorylase,[23] and viral thymidine kinase.[24] In other cases, human enzymes are being expressed using one of the above strategies in tissues not normally capable of expressing the associated activity. For example, gene directed prodrug therapy is being used to deliver P450 activity to tumors to enhance the sensitivity of these tumors to chemotherapeutic prodrugs cleaved by certain P450 isozymes.[25,26]

12.3 LIVER-SPECIFIC DRUG DELIVERY USING HEPDIRECT PRODRUGS

To illustrate some of the concepts discussed in Section 12.2, a class of prodrugs called HepDirect prodrugs will be discussed in detail. Results from preclinical and clinical studies on HepDirect prodrugs of drugs from different structural classes targeting different diseases illustrate the prodrug properties required for organ-selective drug delivery, the advantages and challenges of using a P450 for prodrug activation, and the potential therapeutic benefits of liver-specific drug delivery.

12.3.1 HepDirect Prodrug Concept

HepDirect prodrugs are aryl-substituted cyclic prodrugs of phosphates and phosphonates that undergo an oxidative-cleavage reaction in the liver[27,28] (Figure 12.5). Liver targeting is achieved in part because unlike most other phosph(on)ate prodrugs,[4] HepDirect prodrugs are highly stable in aqueous solutions, plasma, and tissues other than the liver; and to a lesser extent in the small intestine. Prodrug stability enables high levels of the prodrug to be delivered to the liver, since the prodrug survives transit through the intestine and absorption into the portal vein. Moreover, prodrug that

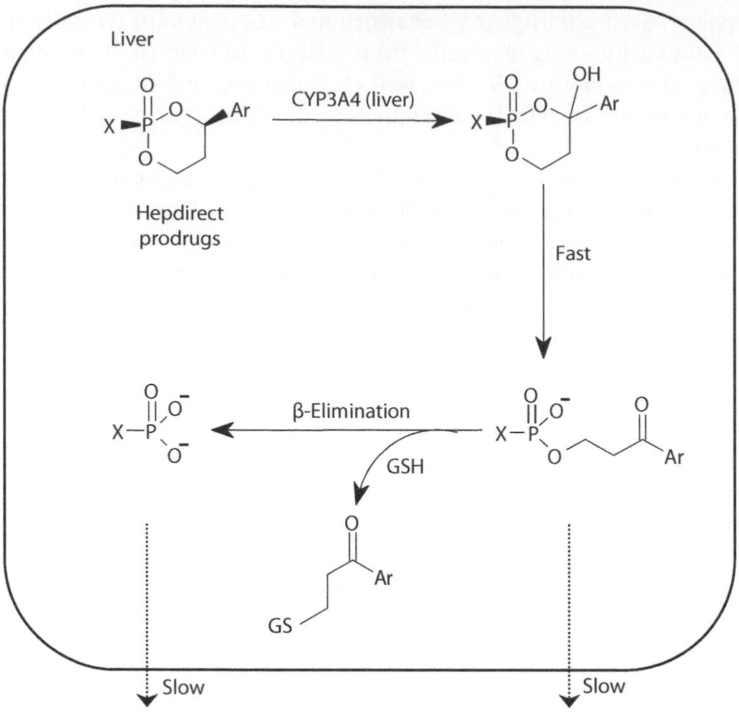

FIGURE 12.5 Mechanism of HepDirect prodrug activation, liver targeting, and by-product capture as a glutathione (GSH) conjugate. The aryl (Ar) substituent enhances CYP oxidation rates. Given the broad substrate specificity of CYP3A, X has few structural limitations. X-PO3 = typically represents the biologically active drug or an intermediate to the active drug. One exception is when X is attached to P via a heteroatom, particularly oxygen. In this case, the dephosphorylated compound may be the biologically active drug.

fails to undergo metabolism in the liver on the first pass is often returned intact to the liver via the systemic circulation as a consequence of the high stability of HepDirect prodrugs in the blood and extra-hepatic tissues.

Liver-targeting is achieved using HepDirect prodrugs in part because the enzyme responsible for prodrug activation, namely CYP3A4, is expressed primarily in the liver. Mechanistic studies indicate that prodrug cleavage begins with a CYP3A4-catalyzed hydroxylation of the C4 methine[27] (Figure 12.5). The hydroxylated intermediate then undergoes rapid and irreversible ring-opening to generate a negatively charged intermediate. This intermediate subsequently undergoes a β-elimination reaction to produce the phosph(on)ate and an aryl vinyl ketone. The latter reacts instantaneously with the high levels of glutathione that exist in hepatocytes[29] to produce a glutathione conjugate. Unlike both cyclophosphamide and ifosfamide (refer to Section 12.2.3), HepDirect prodrug activation results in the rapid intracellular production of a negatively charged intermediate that is retained by hepatocytes. This confines the product as well as the by-product to the target tissue.

As described in the following sections, liver targeting is further enhanced through the selection of active drugs that, after production in hepatocytes, are either

- Eliminated in the bile and not reabsorbed (e.g., pradefovir, see Section 12.3.2)
- Metabolized to inactive metabolites prior to escape into the systemic circulation (e.g., MB07133, see Section 12.5.2.1)
- Poorly distributed to extra-hepatic tissues either due to poor uptake (e.g., MB07811, see Section 12.3.4) or poor conversion to the active drug in these tissues (e.g., see Section 12.3.3)

12.3.1.1   Advantages and Limitations of CYP3A4 as a Prodrug Target

The results in preclinical models and in human clinical trials support CYP3A4[30] as a potential prodrug target. The diversity of drug classes that have demonstrated liver targeting using the HepDirect prodrug concept now encompasses drugs active against hepatitis B, hepatitis C, hepatocellular carcinoma, liver fibrosis, diabetes, and hyperlipidemia. The results from these studies suggest that CYP3A4 is an attractive prodrug target capable of accommodating structurally diverse compounds and still catalyzing the oxidative cleavage of the HepDirect prodrug moiety. Moreover, the results also demonstrate that CYP3A4, despite being a relatively catalytically inefficient enzyme, converts HepDirect prodrugs at rates sufficient to deliver therapeutically active drug levels across multiple species and disease states.

Nevertheless, it is important to recognize that a CYP3A-dependent strategy for liver-specific drug delivery poses several potential drug development challenges. One concern is related to CYP3A expression in the gastrointestinal tract and the potential for prodrug cleavage in the small intestine, resulting in reduced oral bioavailability and/or gastrointestinal (GI) toxicity. Results from animals administered the HepDirect prodrug pradefovir show low levels of the active drug in the intestine, relative to the liver; high oral bioavailability across several species (rats, dogs, and monkeys); and no GI toxicity.[28,31] Moreover, studies conducted in rats and monkeys that evaluated the portal and systemic levels of pradefovir and the product of pradefovir conversion, 9-(2-phosphonyl-methoxyethyl)adenine (PMEA), suggested that the liver, not the small intestine, was responsible for prodrug conversion.[28,31] The low GI extraction exhibited by pradefovir likely reflects both its rapid absorption from the small intestine and the relatively inefficient enzyme, CYP3A4, catalyzing prodrug conversion in the GI. HepDirect prodrugs with longer intestinal residence times, due to structural features that invoke p-glycoprotein (pGp) substrate activity[32] or other mechanisms that limit oral absorption, may exhibit increased GI extraction and, therefore, reduced drug delivery to the liver.[33]

Another potential concern with prodrugs cleaved using a CYP3A-catalyzed reaction is the potential for large intra- and interpatient variability. Most of the variability arises from differences in CYP3A expression in the liver and small intestine, which can vary as much as 40-fold[34] across individuals, although typically the range is 10-fold or less.[35,36] Minimal differences in expression are observed between gender, race, and age. CYP3A activity in humans is comprised largely of CYP3A isoenzymes CYP3A4 and CYP3A5, which exhibit overlapping substrate specificities. The expression of both CYP3A4 and CYP3A5 is altered by diet, hormones, and environmental factors. Only CYP3A5 exhibits functionally important polymorphisms. Interestingly, despite these differences in gene expression, the majority of individuals exhibit only a four- to sixfold difference in CYP3A-dependent clearances. Moreover, CYP3A metabolized drugs with high oral bioavailability are associated with low interpatient variability,[37] whereas drugs with low oral bioavailability often exhibit high variability—possibly because of the variations in the intestinal CYP3A and pGp activities.[38] Consistent with these findings, pradefovir exhibits low interpatient drug variability.[39]

The largest CYP3A-related concern that may hinder the use of HepDirect prodrugs in certain diseases is the potential for significant drug–drug interactions. More than 50% of all marketed drugs are metabolized by CYP3A4.[40] Of particular concern are the interactions with drugs with narrow therapeutic indices, especially if the co-administered drug is commonly used by the target patient population. Potent CYP inhibition generally represents a greater drug–drug interaction concern than CYP induction, since inhibition often results in adverse events produced by higher circulating levels of the co-administered drug, whereas induction leads to diminished efficacy due to increased metabolism to inactive metabolites. Importantly, HepDirect prodrugs, such as pradefovir are neither potent human CYP inhibitors ($IC_{50} > 10 \mu M$) nor inducers[41] and, therefore, are not expected to affect the pharmacokinetics of CYP-metabolized drugs. In contrast, drugs that either inhibit or induce CYP3A4 are expected to affect the conversion of HepDirect prodrugs and, therefore, represent drug combinations that require evaluation in human clinical trials to assess each potential interaction and its clinical significance.

Another potential risk associated with HepDirect prodrugs is related to the aryl vinyl ketone by-product produced following prodrug activation. Vinyl ketones as a compound class are associated with significant toxicity, including both cytotoxicity and genotoxicity.[42] Toxicity is attributed to the alkylation of essential proteins and DNA. Toxicity is low or absent in tissues that express P450s, such as the liver and the intestine, since these tissues contain millimolar intracellular levels of glutathione.[43] Glutathione rapidly reacts with vinyl ketones to form a nontoxic glutathione conjugate. Consequently, drugs that undergo metabolism to a highly reactive vinyl ketone in the liver (e.g., acetaminophen) exhibit good safety as long as glutathione levels remain above 0.5–1 mM (ca. 20% of normal liver levels).[29] Liver toxicity is observed under conditions that cause glutathione depletion such as high dose acetaminophen or when acetaminophen is administered to subjects with low basal levels of glutathione due to poor nutrition and/or alcohol abuse.

Glutathione is present in extra-hepatic tissues and in the blood and is therefore available to capture vinyl ketone that escapes the liver or is produced outside the liver (e.g., via the glutathione conjugate following a reverse Michael reaction). For example, cyclophosphamide is oxidized by the liver and eliminated by the kidneys as the oxidized intermediate, which subsequently accumulates in the bladder and results in bladder toxicity after conversion to acrolein (Figure 12.4). Both acetaminophen and cyclophosphamide are administered to humans at relatively high doses and as such are able to overwhelm the natural protection provided by tissue glutathione. In contrast, drugs that undergo covalent modification but are administered at low human doses are not known to result in toxicity or human cancers presumably because of the presence of an adequate natural defense mechanism.[44]

Studies designed to test the acute safety of HepDirect prodrugs showed that, even at high doses, prodrug turnover produced only modest (~25%) transient reductions in hepatic glutathione levels. Unlike acetaminophen, no evidence of liver toxicity was found, as judged by both serum liver enzyme levels and liver histology.[28] While the lack of liver toxicity may be due to rapid detoxification by intracellular glutathione, it may also arise from differences in the toxicity potential of aryl vinyl ketones relative to other vinyl ketones as suggested by results in glutathione-depleted hepatocytes treated with a HepDirect prodrug[28] and results from an embryotoxicity study with phenyl vinyl ketone.[45] In addition, no by-product-related toxicity has been observed to date in long-term animal toxicology studies as well as in both *in vitro* and *in vivo* genetic toxicology studies.[31]

12.3.2 Pradefovir: HepDirect Prodrug of an Antiviral Nucleotide

HepDirect prodrugs of the antiviral agent 9-(2-phosphonylmethoxyethyl)adenine (PMEA) were studied[46] in an effort to find a drug candidate with improved therapeutic potential relative to the chronic hepatitis B antiviral drug adefovir dipivoxil (Hepsera®, Gilead Sciences, Inc., Foster City, California).[47] Adefovir dipivoxil is the bispivaloyloxymethyl (POM) prodrug of PMEA, which, unlike HepDirect prodrugs, is rapidly metabolized to PMEA by esterases present in the gastro-intestinal tract, blood, and other tissues including the kidney and liver (Figure 12.6). PMEA in circulation distributes primarily to the kidneys where it accumulates and results in kidney toxicity. Dose-limiting kidney toxicity in the phase 3 clinical trials led to the marketing approval of a sub-maximally effective dose of adefovir dipivoxil.[48]

In an effort to achieve greater antiviral activity by targeting PMEA and PMEA-related metabolites preferentially to the liver, HepDirect prodrugs of PMEA were prepared and tested in preclinical models.[28] As shown in Figure 12.7, pradefovir exhibited a 12-fold and an 84-fold increase in the liver-to-kidney and liver-to-intestine ratio, respectively, in rats relative to adefovir dipivoxil. The enhanced liver/intestine ratio is noteworthy given that these are the only two organs that express CYP3A at appreciable levels.[17] This enhancement in liver targeting was attributed in part to the

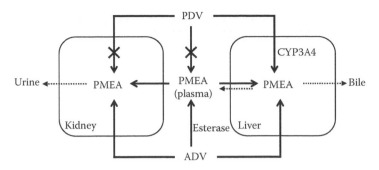

FIGURE 12.6 Pathways for PMEA production, distribution, and elimination from prodrugs adefovir dipivoxil (ADV) and pradefovir (PDV).

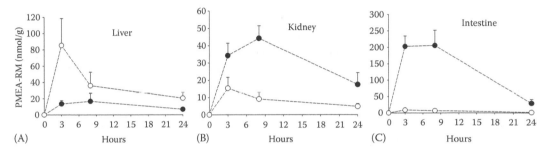

FIGURE 12.7 PMEA-related metabolites (PMEA-RM = PMEA + PMEAp + PMEApp) in liver, kidney, and intestine determined at 3, 8, and 24 h after oral administration of pradefovir (open circles) or adefovir (closed circles) to normal fasted rats at a 30 mg/kg PMEA-equivalent dose. PMEAp and PMEApp are the mono- and diphosphorylated metabolites of PMEA, respectively, which are generated by action of nucleotide kinases that are expressed inside cells.

lower intestinal specific activity of CYP3A relative to esterase activity. Liver targeting was confirmed in subsequent studies in rats using whole body autoradiography and in male cynomolgus monkeys.[31]

The increased liver-to-kidney ratio was postulated to arise from differences in the route of PMEA clearance for PMEA in the circulation relative to PMEA generated in hepatocytes.[28] Anionic compounds undergo both renal and biliary clearance depending on transport efficiencies of the transporters on the basolateral and apical surfaces of hepatocytes and renal tubular cells.[49] Since PMEA administered intravenously (IV) is cleared largely by the kidney, the increase in the liver-to-kidney ratio with pradefovir suggests that PMEA in the circulation has limited ability of entering the liver[50] and PMEA generated in the hepatocyte is effluxed both into the circulation via bi-directional anion transporters on the sinusoidal membrane and into the bile via multidrug resistance proteins (MRPs) on the biliary canalicular membrane. Efflux of PMEA by MRP-4 and MRP-5 is reported to occur in cultured rat microglia.[51] The biliary clearance reduces the systemic exposure to PMEA since the anionic charge of PMEA limits the reabsorption of PMEA transferred to the intestine from the bile.

The advancement of pradefovir into human clinical trials demonstrated for the first time the ability of HepDirect prodrugs to undergo prodrug cleavage in humans.[39] A subsequent phase 2 trial provided evidence for liver targeting based on plasma PMEA exposure vs. change in hepatitis B virus (HBV) DNA levels in patients treated with either pradefovir or adefovir dipivoxil for 24 weeks.[52] As shown in Figure 12.8, the 5 mg pradefovir dose achieved antiviral activity (HBV reduction, defined as the percent of patients with HBV DNA less than 400 copies/mL) similar to the 10 mg adefovir dose, but with significantly reduced (85%) plasma PMEA exposure.[52] Moreover, the highest dose of

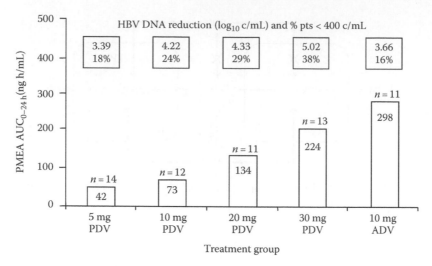

FIGURE 12.8   PMEA exposure (AUC_{0-24h}) and antiviral activity as measured by HBV DNA reduction ($\log_{10}$ copies/mL) and percentage of patients with less than 400 copies/mL after 24 weeks of treatment with once daily administration of pradefovir (PDV) or adefovir dipivoxil (ADV) to patients with chronic hepatitis B.

pradefovir, 30 mg once daily, resulted in significantly greater antiviral activity (~1.5 log reduction in mean HBV DNA levels) and a greater percentage of patients with HBV DNA less than 400 copies/mL than adefovir, which was confirmed at 48 weeks. At this dose, the circulating levels of PMEA remained approximately 25% lower than the levels associated with adefovir. These results, while indirect, suggest that the difference in prodrug moiety between pradefovir and adefovir enables the liver-selective delivery of PMEA.

12.3.3   HepDirect Prodrugs of Nucleoside 5′-Monophosphates

Nucleoside analogues represent a well-studied drug class used primarily as antiviral and anticancer agents. Both activities require the stepwise conversion of the nucleoside to the corresponding 5′-monophosphate by a nucleoside kinase. This is followed by the conversion of the nucleoside 5′-monophosphates (NMP) to the biologically active 5′-triphosphate analogue (nucleoside triphosphate [NTP]) by nucleotide kinases. NTPs prevent DNA, or in some cases RNA, strand elongation through the inhibition of polymerases or through initial incorporation into the strand causing chain termination. Not surprisingly, the production of NTPs in nontarget cells can produce unwanted and significant toxicities through the inhibition of cellular proliferation, the disruption of mitochondrial function, and/or nonselective interactions with proteins that are regulated by nucleotides.[53] Consequently, there have been considerable efforts to discover safer and more effective nucleoside therapies.

Much of the research over the past two decades has been focused on the identification of analogues that, upon conversion to the corresponding NTPs, exhibit greater specificity.[54] The structural modifications used to gain specificity, however, proved to be detrimental to the efficient intracellular activation of the nucleoside to the NTP. Much of the inefficiency stemmed from the poor structural tolerance of the nucleoside kinases catalyzing the first step.[55]

12.3.3.1   Nucleoside Kinase Bypass Strategy

Efforts have been on-going for over three decades to find strategies that deliver the corresponding nucleoside 5′-monophosphate (NMP) in order to bypass the rate-limiting nucleoside kinase activation step (Figure 12.9). Administration of the NMP itself is ineffective due to the presence

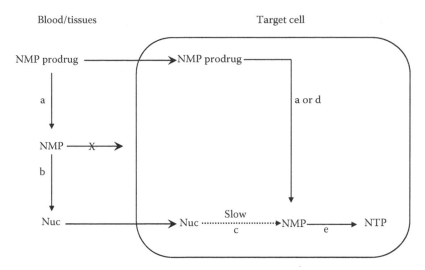

FIGURE 12.9 Nucleoside kinase bypass. Pathways and enzymes catalyzing nucleoside monophosphate (NMP) prodrug cleavage and conversion to corresponding nucleoside (Nuc) and nucleoside triphosphate (NTP): a, esterase or esterase and phosphoramidase; b, phosphatase; c, phosphodiesterase (cleaves monoacid); d, CYP3A; e, nucleoside kinase.

of phosphatases that rapidly dephosphorylate the NMP to the nucleoside. Consequently, numerous phosphate prodrug strategies were explored that both avoid NMP dephosphorylation as well as aid cellular uptake. Most of these strategies led to significant antiviral activity in HBV-infected cells, including cells that lack the nucleoside kinase.[56] In contrast, *in vivo* activity proved difficult to demonstrate presumably because most of the prodrug strategies cleaved through the action of esterases, which are not only catalytically efficient but also expressed in most tissues. Consequently, these prodrugs failed to deliver the NMP to the target cell due to extensive hydrolysis of the prodrug in the intestine and blood to the monophosphate followed by rapid conversion to the nucleoside. Another limitation posed by prodrug strategies relying on esterases stems from the presence of esterases in most tissues and therefore the ability of prodrug present in the circulation to distribute into nontarget tissues, undergo esterase-catalyzed hydrolysis to the NMP, and thereby bypass the nucleoside kinase, produce NTP, and result in NTP-related toxicity.

In contrast, HepDirect prodrugs of nucleoside monophosphates are stable in blood and extrahepatic tissues and thereby ensure greater hepatic exposure to the prodrug. Secondly, use of the HepDirect prodrug strategy targets NTP production to hepatocytes, the cells infected with the hepatitis B virus (HBV) or hepatitis C virus (HCV), and not to nonhepatic tissues. Targeting is expected to prevent or at least minimize NTP-related toxicities in extra-hepatic tissues, especially in tissues with rapidly multiplying cells, such as the bone marrow. Furthermore, liver targeting is expected to be particularly high for nucleosides that require nucleoside kinase bypass, since the nucleoside is the metabolite that is most often released into the circulation by the liver following prodrug conversion. This will preserve liver targeting since the released nucleoside is not converted to the corresponding NMP in extra-hepatic tissues.

HepDirect prodrugs of numerous NMP analogues containing base and/or sugar modifications have been synthesized and have been shown to undergo nucleoside kinase bypass in hepatocytes and *in vivo*. For example, relative to the anti-HBV nucleoside lamivudine, the HepDirect prodrug of lamivudine monophosphate resulted in 34-fold higher NTP levels in rat hepatocytes and a 320-fold higher liver NTP-to-plasma nucleoside ratio following intra-peritoneal (i.p.) administration.[57] Similarly, higher NTP levels were achieved in rat hepatocytes and in the livers of rats administered a HepDirect prodrug of the monophosphate of the anti-HCV nucleoside 2'-C-methyladenosine relative to the parent nucleoside.[58] A HepDirect prodrug of 2'-C-methylcytidine was reported to undergo efficient conversion to the NTP *in vitro* and to result in a marked reduction in viral load (3.6–4.8 $\log_{10}$) in HCV-infected chimpanzees after IV dosing at 4 mg/kg.[59]

HepDirect prodrugs have also been used to target certain nucleoside oncolytics[60] to the primary liver tumors, which retain CYP3A4 activity at near the same levels as found in the normal liver. Similar to nucleoside antivirals, these nucleoside analogs require conversion to the NTP for biological activity, which in this case entails inhibition of cell proliferation and cytotoxicity. MB07133, a HepDirect prodrug of cytarabine 5′-monophosphate, has entered into clinical trials. Results from preclinical studies and the phase 1/2 clinical trial on MB07133 are summarized in Section 12.5.2.1.

12.3.4   MB07811: HepDirect Prodrug of a Thyroid Receptor Agonist

HepDirect prodrugs have also been used to enhance the liver targeting of a novel class of phosphonate-containing thyroid hormone receptor (TR) agonists.[61] TR agonists have been intensely studied for over 40 years based on their ability to lower both low density lipoprotein-cholesterol (LDL-C) and triglycerides (TG). The development of these agents, however, has been hampered by the inability to find compounds that exhibit the desired lipid lowering activity without adverse effects on cardiac function and/or the hypothalamus–pituitary–thyroid (HPT) axis. Since lipid lowering occurs by the modulation of TR-sensitive gene expression in the liver and the side effects occur by the modulation of genes in extra-hepatic tissues, efforts have been on-going to identify TR agonists with high liver specificity.[62]

MB07811 is a HepDirect prodrug of a phosphonate-containing TR agonist, designated as MB07344 (Figure 12.10), that has been extensively evaluated in preclinical models[63–65] and in two human clinical trials. Liver targeting is evident from the measurement of drug levels in the liver relative to 25 other tissues over a 24 h period. Moreover, functional liver targeting was demonstrated by monitoring the expression of TR sensitive genes in the liver and five extra-hepatic tissues following the administration of MB07811, T3 (3,5,3′-triiodo-L-thyronine), and the nonliver targeted TR agonist KB-141 (3,5-dichloro-4-(4-hydroxy-3-isopropylphenoxy)phenylacetic acid (Figure 12.11).

Liver targeting appears to arise from multiple mechanisms (Figure 12.12). First, MB07811, like other HepDirect prodrugs, is activated predominantly by CYP3A4 in the liver. Second, after

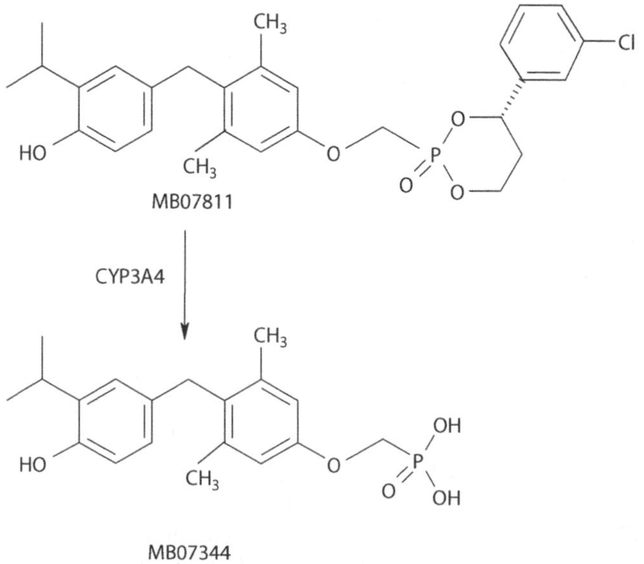

FIGURE 12.10   Conversion of the HepDirect prodrug MB07811 to MB07344.

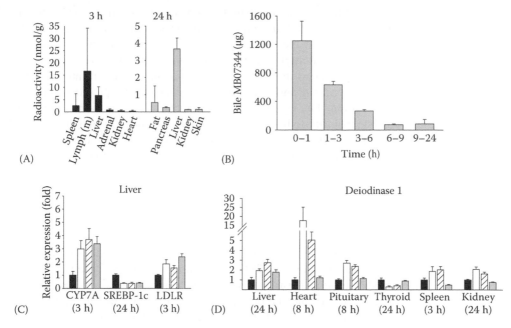

FIGURE 12.11 Tissue Targeting of MB07811, a HepDirect prodrug of the thyroid receptor agonist, MB07344, in rats. (A) Approximate mean tissue concentration (total radioactivity) 3 and 24 h after an oral dose of [^{14}C]-MB07811 (5 mg/kg) to male SD rats. (B) Mean MB07344 levels in bile samples collected over the indicated periods from bile duct-cannulated male SD rats treated with MB07344 (10 mg/kg, i.v.). (C–D) Relative expression of mRNA in tissues of male SD rats treated with vehicle (black bar), T3 (white bar), KB-141 (white hatched bar) or MB07811 (gray bar) at 10× the ED$_{50}$ dose for cholesterol lowering in the cholesterol fed rat.

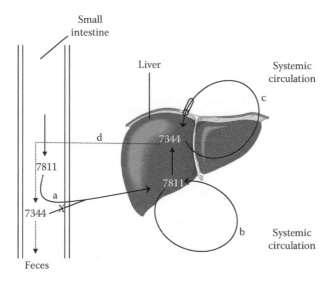

FIGURE 12.12 Uptake, metabolism and distribution of MB07811 (abbreviated 7811 in the figure) and the TR agonist MB07344 (abbreviated 7344 in the figure). MB07811 administered orally is absorbed via the portal vein (path a) and distributed to the liver. In the liver MB07811 is either metabolized to MB07344 via CYP3A or eliminated into the systemic circulation where it is stable and eventually returns to the liver (path b). MB07344 is either eliminated into the systemic circulation where it eventually returns to the liver via an organic anion transporter (path c). MB07344 is eliminated from the liver via the bile (path d) and not reabsorbed.

oral administration, MB07811 undergoes extensive first pass metabolism, which results in reduced prodrug exposure to extra-hepatic tissues[63] and increased prodrug activation in the liver. Third, a portion of the MB07344 produced in the hepatocytes is excreted into the bile and not likely reabsorbed from the intestine given the high negative charge (oral bioavailability is <2%). Also, the remainder of the MB07344 produced in hepatocytes is apparently excreted into the systemic circulation. Importantly, both the prodrug and circulating phosphonic acid appear to result in insignificant extra-hepatic TR activation. The lack of prodrug-mediated TR activation is related to its poor affinity for the TR and its inability to be converted to MB07344 in extra-hepatic tissues. The reduced activity from circulating MB07344 is attributed in part to the inability of phosphonic acids to cross cell membranes by passive diffusion at physiologic pH. Liver targeting has also been speculated to arise from differences in the tissue uptake of MB07344. Thyroid hormone agonists enter tissues predominantly via monocarboxylate transporters or MCTs (e.g., MCT-8),[66] a transporter that appears to recognize carboxylic acids but not phosphonic acids. In contrast, uptake by the liver of TR agonists can occur via MCT-8 as well as the more promiscuous organic anion transporters.[61]

These properties resulted in significant liver targeting and an improved therapeutic index (Figure 12.13). An extensive evaluation of MB07811 in six animal species and a variety of animal models of hyperlipidemia showed that MB07811 resulted in marked reductions in LDL-C and TG levels. Moreover, studies showed that the doses required for lipid lowering had a minimal impact on cardiac function. More recently, MB07811 was evaluated in a 14-day phase 1b trial

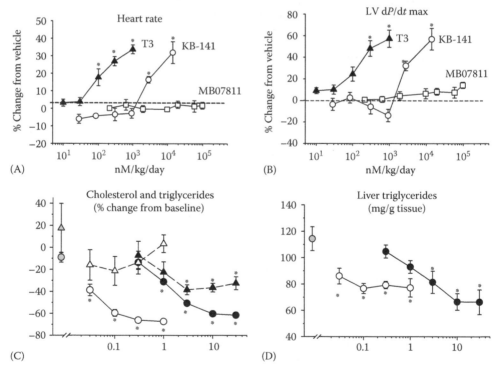

FIGURE 12.13 Therapeutic benefits of liver targeting. (A–B) Effects on Sprague Dawley (SD) rat cardiac function and thyroid hormone axis (THA). Dose–response of T3 (▲, 6.5–650 µg/kg/day), KB-141 (○, 0.01–5 mg/kg/day), and MB07811 (□, 0.1–50 mg/kg/day) on (A) heart rate; and (B) left ventricular (LV) dP/dt in SD rats (n = 3–6/dose) treated for 7 days. (C–D) Dose-response curves in diet induced obese (DIO) mice (n = 8/group) treated for 14 days with KB-141 (open symbols) and MB07811 (closed symbols). Vehicle is denoted by grey-filled symbols ±SEM. Percent change from baseline for (C) total plasma cholesterol (circles) and triglycerides (triangles); (D) effects of KB-141 and MB07811 on liver triglycerides.

in subjects with elevated LDL-C and was shown to significantly reduce both LDL-C and TG without affecting the heart rate, heart rhythm, or blood pressure (Metabasis Therapeutics press release, 2008).

12.3.5 SUMMARY

HepDirect prodrugs of drugs from several different drug classes have been extensively studied in preclinical studies and human clinical trials. These studies have provided an insight into the potential benefits of HepDirect prodrugs as well as the potential limitations of HepDirect prodrugs and their use in targeting certain drugs to the liver or in treating certain diseases (Table 12.1).

TABLE 12.1
Strengths and Weaknesses of HepDirect Prodrugs

	Strength	Weakness
Stability		
Aqueous	Stable at neutral pH. Long shelf life in contrast to standard phosph(on)ate prodrugs	
Plasma	High plasma stability enables prodrug delivery to the liver	
Intestine	HepDirect prodrugs have not shown significant drug levels in the GI nor GI toxicity	CYP3A4 is expressed in small intestine which could result in significant prodrug conversion especially with poorly absorbed prodrugs
Liver	Liver activation enhances liver specificity	Liver specificity restricts application of HepDirect prodrugs to drug targets in the liver and liver associated diseases
Therapeutic index		
Efficacy	Improved due to increased drug levels resulting from increased drug delivery	
Safety	Improved via liver targeting and avoidance of prodrug activation in nontarget tissues	
Pharmacokinetics		
Oral bioavailability	Good oral bioavailability demonstrated across species (rat, dog, monkey, human)	
Half-life	Long $t1/2$ relative to standard prodrugs enables higher liver prodrug exposure	
Conversion rate		Slow conversion could limit drug levels due to elimination of intact prodrug
Drug variability	Acceptable variability observed in humans with drugs absorbed rapidly from GI	Hepatic disease and/or prolonged GI exposure likely to show high variability
DDI potential	No CYP inhibition or CYP induction observed nor effects on CYP3A4-metabolized drug PK	Prodrug conversion affected by potent CYP3A4 inhibitors and inducers
Safety		
Toxicology	No by-product-related toxicity observed in animal toxicology studies	Potential toxicology risk at higher doses if production depletes glutathione stores
Genetic toxicology	No evidence in standard in vitro or in vivo tests	By-product is from class associated with genetic toxicology potential
Carcinogenicity	2 year carcinogenicity study on pradefovir found a NOAEL dose and tumors at higher doses attributed to anti-viral drug (PMEA)	

Significant liver targeting has been shown for HepDirect prodrugs of drugs that are eliminated by the bile (e.g., pradefovir), undergo extensive hepatic metabolism to an inactive metabolite (e.g., MB07133), or are unable to distribute into extra-hepatic tissues (e.g., MB07811). Targeting has been demonstrated in rodents by measuring tissue drug levels or by gaining indirect evidence of drug distribution by monitoring signature gene expression across tissues (e.g., MB07811). Indirect evidence of liver targeting has also been observed in humans based on differences in efficacy and drug levels between a HepDirect prodrug (pradefovir) and a nonliver targeted prodrug (adefovir dipivoxil). The benefits of liver targeting have been shown in animal pharmacology and toxicology studies as well as in humans. The benefits include enhanced efficacy through increased drug levels (e.g., MB07133 and HepDirect prodrugs of anti-HCV nucleosides), improved safety (e.g., MB07811, pradefovir), and/or increased therapeutic index.

HepDirect prodrugs are activated by CYP3A4 and after activation produce an aryl vinyl ketone. Both properties represent potential concerns that need to be evaluated on a case-by-case basis to ensure that neither will impede successful drug development. The HepDirect prodrugs that are in clinical development provide evidence that the development risks associated with these properties can be evaluated in preclinical models and in human clinical trials and that thus far have not limited the advancement of pradefovir, MB07133, or MB07811.

Prodrug activation by CYP3A4 leads to concerns regarding intra- and inter-patient drug variability and the drug–drug interaction potential. To date, the drug variability has been in the acceptable range presumably because both pradefovir and MB07811 are rapidly absorbed and therefore undergo limited activation by intestinal CYPs, which exhibit high inter-patient variability due in part to CYP3A5 polymorphisms. Drug–drug interactions are expected with HepDirect prodrugs since CYP3A4 inhibitors and inducers will affect HepDirect prodrug conversion. The impact of these interactions on the development of HepDirect prodrugs will depend on the potential safety risk of the interaction as well as the frequency in which these drugs are used by the target patient population. In contrast, no drug interactions are expected to be induced by HepDirect prodrugs at least based on the results to date that show that the HepDirect prodrugs advanced into development are neither CYP inhibitors nor inducers, and therefore are unlikely to affect the levels of drugs that undergo CYP metabolism.

The potential liability associated with the HepDirect prodrug by-product has been evaluated extensively in acute and chronic animal toxicology studies and in genotoxicology studies. The absence of toxicology is attributed to the presence of glutathione, which exists at high levels in the liver (>100× the amount of by-product produced) and effectively forms a conjugate with the by-product. The presence of glutathione prevents the covalent modification of proteins in standard covalent binding studies. As a consequence, no by-product toxicity has been identified for HepDirect prodrugs. Long-term studies with pradefovir in rats and monkeys showed no signs of toxicity other than that observed with adefovir dipivoxil. Similarly, results from the standard battery of *in vitro* and *in vivo* genotoxicology studies have not shown signs of by-product-related toxicity.

12.4 TISSUE TARGETED PRODRUGS

Prodrug strategies for organ-selective drug targeting are designed to exploit specific proteins that are enriched in the target organ and can be used in the uptake and/or activation of prodrugs or in the elimination of the active drug produced after prodrug cleavage. In addition, some organs exhibit unique anatomical features that can be exploited to enhance overall targeting.

12.4.1 LIVER

Drugs often achieve high liver concentrations as a result of the enormous capacity of the liver to take up drugs from the blood. This characteristic feature of the liver is derived from its high blood flow (25% of cardiac output), the large surface area that results from its fenestrated endothelium, and the presence of numerous transporters on the cell surface used to actively transport drugs unable to traverse the cell membrane by passive diffusion. Consequently, many drugs preferentially distribute to the liver and exhibit high liver-to-plasma ratios. Despite this natural organ selectivity, extra-hepatic toxicities can still be dose-limiting. For example, the thyroid receptor agonist GC-1,[67] which exhibits a 30-fold improvement in liver to cardiac tissue distribution relative to T3,[62] still exhibits extra-hepatic effects. These include increased oxygen consumption, decreased body fat, reduced TSH and T4 levels (consistent with direct effects on the HPT axis), and increased pancreatic cell proliferation in rats.[68] Accordingly, prodrug strategies that target the liver can be used to further enhance liver specificity and improve the therapeutic index.

Relative to other organs, the liver contains a large number of enzymes capable of metabolizing prodrugs. Some of the enzymes are relatively hepato-specific, e.g., CYP3A4, and as discussed in Section 12.3, can be used to gain liver specificity. Most of the enzymes expressed in the liver, however, are also expressed in extra-hepatic tissues (e.g., carboxyesterases). These enzymes are only useful for liver targeting if the prodrug distributes selectively to the liver. This can be achieved if the prodrug requires transporters for cellular uptake and is designed to be an efficient substrate for transporters primarily expressed by the liver.

Several families of transporters have been identified and characterized (Figure 12.14).[69] The most well studied is the sodium-dependent bile acid transporter family, now known as the Na+-taurocholate cotransporting polypeptide (NCTP in humans) family. This transporter is expressed on the basolateral surface of hepatocytes, where it functions as the transporter for conjugated bile acids and sulfated steroids. Other transporter families that are expressed on hepatocytes and are important for uptake include the sodium-independent bile acid transporters, known as the organic anion transporting polypeptides (OATPs in humans); the organic cation transporters (OCTs); and the organic anion transporters (OATs in humans).

Transporters are also used in the efflux of charged compounds from the hepatocytes. Efflux into the sinusoid uses transporters that are bi-directional (e.g., OATs, OATPs, and OCTs); whereas efflux into the bile uses transporters that belong to the ABC transporter superfamily and are expressed on the bile canalicular membrane. Included in this superfamily of transporters are the multidrug resistance proteins (MDR; e.g., MDR1 or P-glycoprotein) and the multidrug resistance-associated proteins (MRP; e.g., MRP2).[69]

Efforts to exploit liver-specific transporters have largely focused on bile acid conjugates that are orally absorbed and transported into the liver using sodium-dependent bile acid transporters expressed on the brush border membrane of ileal enterocytes and the sinusoidal membrane of hepatocytes,

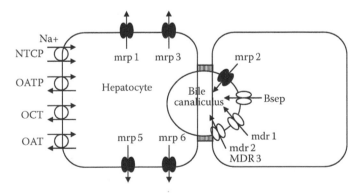

FIGURE 12.14 Liver transporters expressed on the basolateral and canalicular membranes participating in the uptake for drugs from the sinusoid and elimination into the systemic circulation or bile. The transporters include Na+-taurocholate cotransporting polypeptide (NTCP), organic anion-transporting polypeptide (OATP), organic cation transporter (OCT), organic anion transporter (OAT), multidrug resistance prodrugs (MDR), multidrug resistance-associated proteins (MRP) and bile salt export protein (BSEP). (Adapted and reprinted from Kullak-Ublick, G.A., *J. Hepatol.*, 31, 563, 1999. With permission.)

respectively.[70] These efforts illustrate the challenges faced in finding prodrugs that effectively deliver drugs to hepatocytes using cell surface transporters. First, the moiety linking the drug and bile acid must be relatively stable in the blood to ensure adequate delivery of the prodrug to the liver. Second, the moiety linking the drug and bile acid must cleave inside the hepatocyte faster than the prodrug is exported into the bile via bile acid transporters present on the bile canalicular membrane. High intra-hepatic drug levels, therefore, require a balancing of the rates of conjugate uptake and elimination by hepatocytes along with the rates of intra- and extra-hepatocyte conjugate cleavage.

Two of the most promising prodrugs exploiting liver transporters are shown in Figure 12.15. CGH 509H (Figure 12.15A) is a bile acid conjugate of the natural thyroid hormone L-T3.[71] Relative to L-T3, CGH 509H exhibited a 100-fold weaker binding affinity for the thyroid hormone receptor, but was only sixfold weaker in its cholesterol lowering activity *in vivo*. The authors suggested that the enhanced *in vivo* potency was due to the local production of L-T3 following the intra-hepatocyte cleavage of the amide bond. The high liver targeting achieved by the conjugate resulted in a 50- to 64-fold improvement in the therapeutic index for cardiac side effects and thyroid hormone suppression.

Another prodrug using this concept comprises coupling HMG CoA reductase inhibitors with bile acids using an aminoethyl spacer between the carboxylate of the statin mevinolin and the 7α-hydroxy of the bile acid[72] (Figure 12.15B). The prodrug was shown to interact with the hepatocyte and ileocyte bile acid uptake systems. Cholesterol biosynthesis was inhibited by the prodrug in HepG2 cells as well as *in vivo* 1 h following intravenous administration.[73] The bile acid-based prodrug showed small increases in drug levels in the liver and up to 10-fold lower levels in non-hepatic tissues. No data was reported demonstrating cleavage of the amide bond. Interestingly, the prodrug inhibited cholesterol synthesis in the liver but not in the small intestine, whereas mevinolin inhibited both liver and intestinal cholesterol synthesis. These results

> Relative to other organs, the liver contains a large number of enzymes capable of metabolizing prodrugs. Some of the enzymes are relatively hepato-specific, e.g., CYP3A4. Most of the enzymes expressed in the liver, however, are also expressed in extra-hepatic tissues, e.g., carboxyesterases. These enzymes are only useful for liver targeting if the prodrug distributes selectively to the liver. This can be achieved if the prodrug requires transporters for cellular uptake and is designed to be an efficient substrate for transporters primarily expressed by the liver.

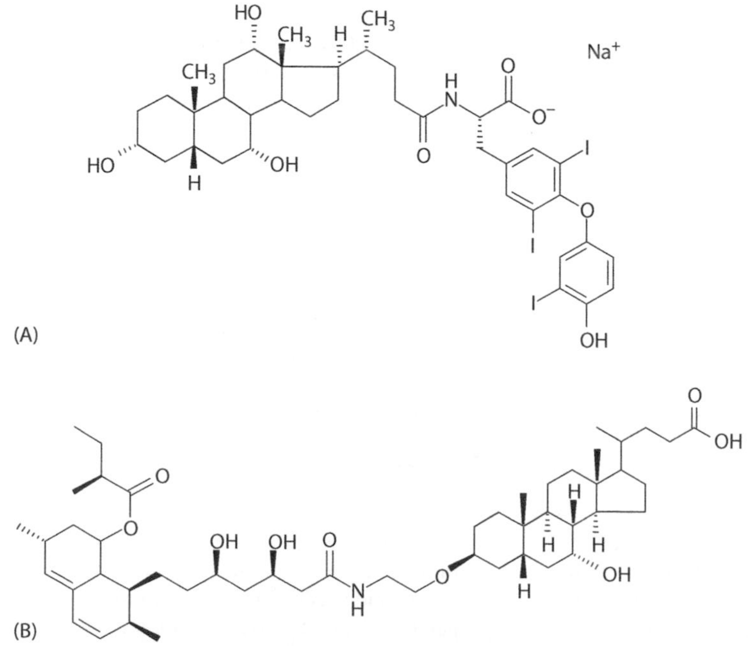

FIGURE 12.15   Structures of prodrugs targeting bile acid transporters.

provide some evidence for liver targeting assuming that the inhibition of cholesterol synthesis by the prodrug depends on prodrug cleavage.

12.4.2   CNS

In contrast to the liver, the brain is typically associated with the lowest drug levels and therefore represents the most difficult organ in which to deliver drugs. Limited drug distribution is a result of the ability of the endothelial cells within the brain capillaries to form tight junctions, called the blood–brain barrier, which restricts the passage of drugs into the brain. This cellular barrier further limits drug penetration by exhibiting limited pinocytic activity, transporter systems favoring efflux rather than drug influx, and high levels of drug metabolizing enzymes. Enhanced drug levels in the brain can be achieved by increasing drug lipophilicity through the removal and/or masking of polar groups that serve as hydrogen bond donors and acceptors. This is often accomplished by using lipophilic prodrugs, which increase drug distribution throughout the body, including the brain. Given these characteristics, it is not surprising that site-specific delivery of drugs to the brain is very challenging, especially since enzymes expressed in the CNS and used for prodrug conversion (e.g., xanthine oxidase, monoamine oxidase, and adenosine deaminase)[74] are expressed in other organs.

One strategy proven capable of the site-specific delivery of drugs to the brain is based on a redox chemical delivery system using dihydropyridine prodrugs[75] (Figure 12.16). Targeting arises following the distribution of the lipophilic prodrug throughout the body, including the brain, and its oxidation to the corresponding membrane-impermeable pyrimidine salt. The oxidation is catalyzed

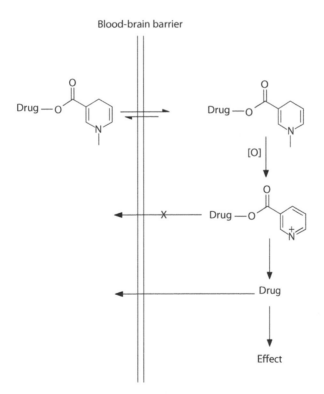

FIGURE 12.16   Chemical delivery system. Prodrugs containing a dihydropyridine distribute into tissues including the brain. In the brain, oxidation results in a hydrophilic pyridinium prodrug that is "trapped" in the CNS due to its inability to cross the blood–brain barrier. Esterase-catalyzed cleavage of the prodrug results in local drug delivery.

by oxidoreductases, analogous to those used in respiration and responsible for the oxidation of nicotinamide adenine dinucleotide (NADH) and its phosphorylated form (NADPH). The pyrimidine salt is eliminated in peripheral tissues; whereas in the CNS, the positively charged intermediate is effectively trapped and unable to diffuse out of the CNS due to the blood–brain barrier. The subsequent hydrolysis of the ester by carboxyesterases results in the brain-specific production of the drug.

Dihydropyridine prodrugs have been used to enhance the brain delivery of a large variety of pharmaceutical agents, including neurotransmitters, steroids, anticancer and antiviral drugs, antibiotics, anticonvulsants, and antidementia drugs.[76] Much of the initial efforts were focused on using dihydropyridine prodrugs for the delivery of neurochemicals such as dopamine and γ-aminobutyric acid (GABA) for the treatment of Parkinson's disease and epilepsy, respectively. *In vitro,* these prodrugs were transformed to the corresponding pyridinium salt, which was subsequently hydrolyzed to the active drug. *In vivo,* the corresponding pyridinium salts accumulated in the rat brain to relatively high levels. Evidence for the cleavage of the pyridinium salt was based on pharmacologic endpoints— with the dopamine prodrugs resulting in the suppression of serum prolactin and the GABA prodrugs in increased anxiolytic activity and protection from maximal electroconvulsive shock. Detectable levels of the parent drug in the brain were demonstrated using other dihydropyridine prodrugs (e.g., estradiol and zidovudine [AZT]), including a prodrug of the anti-cancer drug chlorambucil, which showed sustained levels of the active drug in the brain and drug levels that fell quickly in the blood.

12.4.3 KIDNEY

The kidney, like the liver, is an organ associated with high drug metabolism and clearance. Efforts to target the kidney using a prodrug strategy were first reported by Wilk et al.[77] who showed that a γ-glutamyl conjugate of 3,4-dihydroxyphenyl-L-alanine (L-DOPA) was metabolized by γ-glutamyl transpeptidase, followed by L-amino acid decarboxylase to produce dopamine (Figure 12.17A). Both enzymes are expressed at relatively high levels on the brush border of the proximal tubules, which putatively led to significantly higher dopamine levels in the kidney relative to levels in the blood, heart, liver, lung, muscle, and spleen 20 min after prodrug administration to rats. The result of the kidney-selective targeting of dopamine was a selective increase in renal vasodilation and, therefore, an increase in renal blood flow without a cardiovascular effect.

Application of the same prodrug strategy to the antibiotic sulfamethoxazole led to the preferential accumulation of sulfamethoxazole in the kidney.[78] Nevertheless, high drug levels were also observed in other tissues suggesting that low levels of γ-glutamyl transpeptidase might have been

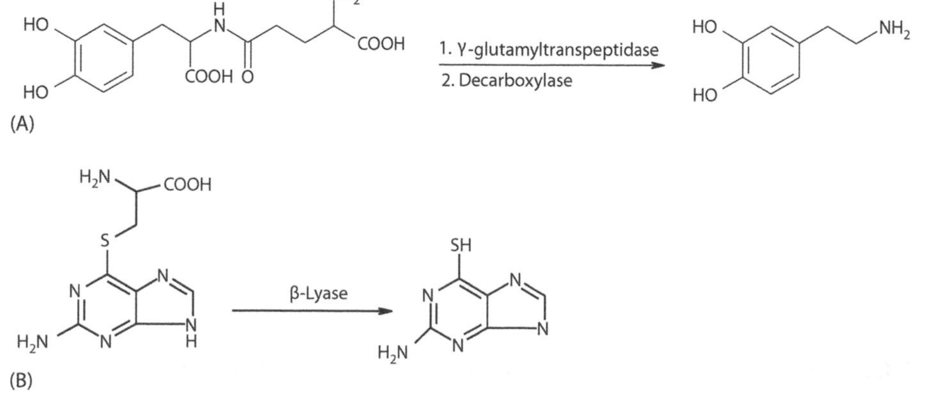

(A)

(B)

FIGURE 12.17   Prodrugs targeting drugs to the kidney. (A) Conversion of γ-glutamyl conjugate of L-DOPA to dopamine. (B) 6-thioguanine prodrug.

sufficient to diminish kidney specificity. To enhance kidney specificity, a prodrug that required both γ-glutamyl transpeptidase and *N*-acylamino acid deacylase was designed and shown to provide greater kidney specificity.

An alternative strategy has been explored that uses prodrugs activated by β-lyase, an enzyme present predominantly in the liver and the kidney (Figure 12.17B). Using this strategy, prodrugs of 6-mercaptopurine and 6-thioguanine were evaluated as potential agents for the treatment of renal carcinoma.[79] Prodrug levels were higher in the kidney than in the liver, which was attributed to the selective uptake of the prodrug by a kidney organic anion transporter. Renal levels of the active drug were also significantly higher than that found in the liver and in excess of the levels needed to inhibit cell proliferation by human renal carcinoma cell lines.

12.4.4 OTHER

Prodrugs have also been evaluated as a strategy for the selective delivery of drugs to other organs with limited success. Much of the difficulties have centered on finding prodrugs with suitable properties, i.e., prodrugs that either distribute specifically to the target organ and/or breakdown by an organ-specific enzyme.

Efforts to treat colonic diseases such as ulcerative colitis, colorectal cancer, and Crohn's disease have focused on strategies that would deliver anti-inflammatory agents, such as nonsteroidal anti-inflammatory drugs (NSAIDs) and steroids to the colon with minimal absorption in both the small and large intestine.[80] Colon specificity is achieved by using prodrugs sensitive to enzymes present in intestinal microflora. These include hydrolytic reactions catalyzed by β-glucuronidase, β-xylosidase, α-L-arabinosidase, and β-galactosidase. In addition, a variety of other bacterial specific enzymes exist including nitroreductase, azoreductase, deaminase, and urea dehydroxylase. For example, balsalzide is a colon-specific prodrug that uses a bacterial azoreductase to cleave an azo bond linkage to produce 5-aminosalicylic acid and an analogue of sulfasalazine (Figure 12.18).

Prodrugs have also been developed that target the bone as a possible treatment for bone diseases, including inflammatory diseases, conditions that result in bone loss, and cancers that have metastasized to the bone.[81] Bone targeting relies on the use of prodrugs containing bisphosphonates, which selectively distribute to the bone. Evidence for prodrug cleavage, however, is less clear although there is circumstantial evidence in the case of 17β-estradiol prodrugs that may suggest slow ester cleavage (Figure 12.19).

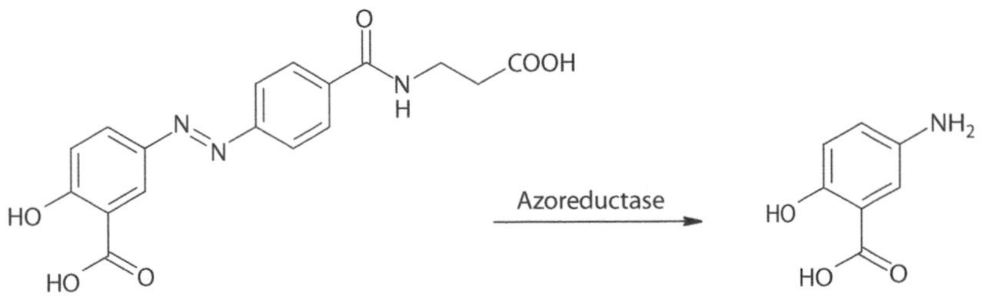

FIGURE 12.18 Colon-targeted prodrug of 5-aminosalicylic acid.

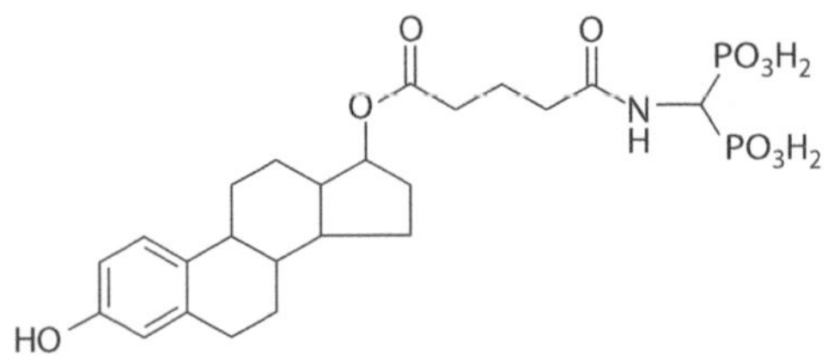

FIGURE 12.19 Bone targeted prodrug of estradiol.

12.5 TUMOR-TARGETED PRODRUGS

Prodrugs capable of targeting oncolytic agents to tumors with high specificity remain of high interest given the strong medical need for effective anti-cancer agents. Despite the advancement of numerous new cancer therapies, cytotoxic chemotherapy agents remain the drug class most likely to result in significant tumor reduction and a cure. The effectiveness of cytotoxic oncolytics, however, is severely hampered by acute and chronic toxicity. Accordingly, efforts have been focused on the identification of prodrug strategies that deliver cytotoxic oncolytics to tumors with a greater therapeutic index. The challenge is to identify prodrugs capable of exploiting differences between tumor and nontumor tissue, which comprise primarily differences in the local microenvironment and in enzyme expression.

12.5.1 HYPOXIA-ACTIVATED PRODRUGS

Solid tumors are usually less well oxygenated than normal tissues due to the combination of increased metabolic demand arising from uncontrolled tumor growth coupled with an imperfect neovascular system. This hypoxic microenvironment is reported to render the tumor resistant to both radiation and chemotherapy. Consequently, efforts were initiated over 25 years ago to identify hypoxia-activated prodrugs that could enable tumor-specific drug delivery. The most advanced prodrug, tirapazamine, is currently in phase 3 clinical trials for a variety of cancers.[82] Tirapazamine and related 1,2,4-benzotriazine-1,4-dioxides result in DNA strand cleavage following a one-electron reduction by a reductase (Figure 12.20).[83] Tumor specificity is achieved because the reductases (e.g., cytochrome P450 and P450 reductase) that activate the prodrug to a DNA-damaging transient intermediate under the hypoxic condition of solid tumors catalyze the deactivation of this intermediate[84] under normoxic conditions. Tirapazamine exhibits a 100-fold specificity for hypoxic cells in culture. Unfortunately, its *in vivo* potency appears to be limited by poor tumor penetration. Second generation prodrugs, banoxantrone[85] and PR-104, are[86] now in clinical evaluation based on their improved tumor distribution (Figure 12.21).

An alternative prodrug strategy investigated by Borch et al. led to a series of hypoxia-activated phosphoramidate mustards with high hypoxia selectivity and good *in vivo* efficacy.[87,88] This strategy uses a 2-nitroimidazole-5-yl methyl moiety as a hypoxia sensitive trigger that, following reduction by P450 reductase to the hydroxylamine, undergoes rapid 1,6-elimination to the

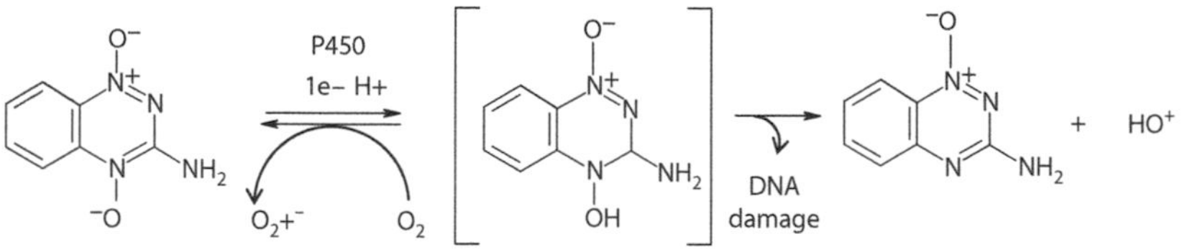

FIGURE 12.20 Metabolism of tirapazamine.

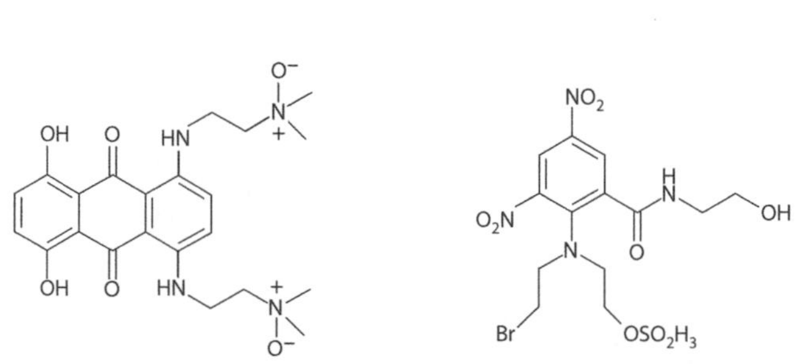

FIGURE 12.21 Structures of banoxantrone (AQ4N) and PR-104A.

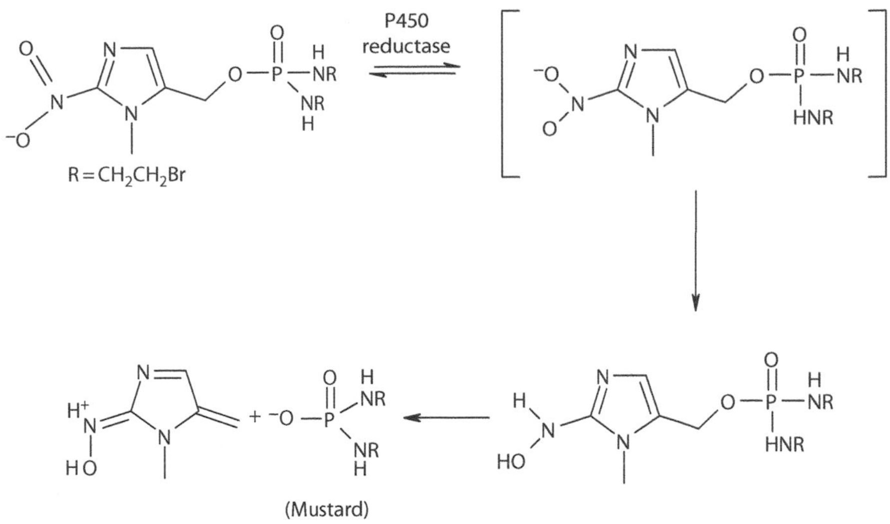

FIGURE 12.22 Hypoxia-activated prodrug of a phosphoramidate mustard.

activated mustard (Figure 12.22). The lead prodrug exhibits a 400-fold enhanced cytotoxicity toward cultured H460 cells tested under hypoxic conditions relative to aerobic conditions and marked anti-tumor activity in a pancreatic cancer orthotopic xenograft model.

12.5.2 Prodrugs of Oncolytic Nucleoside Monophosphates

Oncolytic nucleosides are generally ineffective against solid tumors because of their inefficient conversion to the anti-tumor metabolites, i.e., the corresponding nucleoside triphosphate (NTP). Much of the limitations in this conversion are attributed to nucleoside uptake via nucleoside transporters and intracellular conversion of the nucleoside to the monophosphate by a nucleoside kinase. As described in Section 12.3.3, prodrugs of the monophosphate represent a possible solution that could circumvent both limitations. To achieve a suitable therapeutic index, however, the prodrugs need to undergo tumor-selective activation since producing NTP in normal dividing cells could result in dose-limiting side effects. Two strategies are described in this section as potential solutions, namely the use of HepDirect prodrugs for the treatment of hepatocellular carcinoma (HCC)[60] and the use of hypoxia-activated prodrugs for the treatment of various solid tumors.

12.5.2.1 MB07133: HepDirect Prodrug of Cytarabine 5′-Monophosphate

Cytarabine (araC) is a well-known oncolytic nucleoside that has been in clinical use for several decades to treat acute myelocytic leukemia. In leukemic cells, araC is converted to araC triphosphate (araCTP) via the araC monophosphate (araCMP) intermediate. AraCTP inhibits cell proliferation through the inhibition of DNA polymerases as well as through chain termination following incorporation into the growing DNA strand. AraCTP is also produced in bone marrow cells resulting in concomitant bone marrow toxicity. In contrast, araCTP is not produced in most other tissues, including the liver and solid tumors due, in part, to the low levels of the kinase that phosphorylates araC to araCMP, namely deoxycytidine kinase (dCK).[89]

Unlike araC, the HepDirect prodrug of araCMP, MB07133, targets araCTP production to the liver and greatly reduces araCTP levels in bone marrow where CYP3A is not expressed. High levels of araCTP are produced in the liver because the prodrug enters hepatocytes independent of nucleoside transporters and then undergoes CYP3A-mediated cleavage to araCMP. The delivery of araCMP effectively bypasses the step limiting araCTP production from araC and avoids metabolism

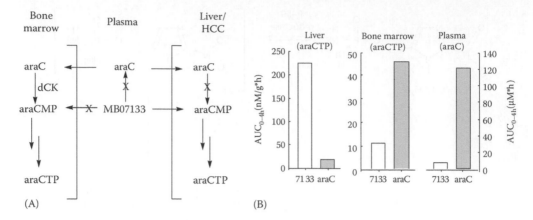

FIGURE 12.23   MB07133 is a liver-targeted prodrug of araCMP. (A) Pathways describing araC and MB07133 uptake and metabolism in liver (and HCC tumors) as well as bone marrow. (B) Mean liver and bone marrow araCTP area-under-the curve (AUC) 0–4h determined from samples collected from normal mice treated with 100-mg/kg araC-equivalent doses of MB07133 or araC administered i.p.

by cytidine deaminase, which is an enzyme expressed at high levels in the liver and responsible for the rapid deamination of araC to the inactive metabolite araU.

Studies in rodents comparing araC and MB07133 showed that MB07133 resulted in high araCTP levels in the liver and undetectable levels in the bone marrow; whereas araC produced high levels of araCTP in the bone marrow and undetectable levels in the liver[28] (Figure 12.23). The net effect of the HepDirect prodrug was an increase of at least 45-fold in the liver/bone marrow ratio for araCTP exposure. High levels of araCTP in the liver are not hepatotoxic, based on preclinical animal studies, presumably because the liver is a relatively quiescent organ. In contrast, primary liver tumors, which are reported to retain high levels of CYP3A4,[90] are expected to be sensitive to araCTP.

Liver targeting led to an improvement in safety as demonstrated by the decreased bone marrow suppression and death in mice treated with MB07133 relative to araC (30-fold shift in the dose–response). The finding of bone marrow suppression at high MB07133 doses correlated with plasma araC, which is derived from araCMP produced in the liver that undergoes intrahepatic dephosphorylation. A portion of the araC produced inside the hepatocytes is deaminated and effluxed into the circulation as araU. The rest is presumably effluxed as araC, which at high doses of MB07133 reaches levels that are toxic to the bone marrow.

12.5.2.2 Phosphoramidate Prodrugs

An alternative prodrug strategy for minimizing NTP production in dividing normal tissue is to use prodrugs of monophosphate nucleosides that are activated in hypoxic environments. Phosphoramidate-based prodrugs of nucleoside monophosphates (Figure 12.24), including the monophosphates of 5-fluoro-2′-deoxyuridine,[91] cytarabine,[92] and gemcitabine,[93] inhibit the growth of wild-type, nucleoside transport-deficient and nucleoside kinase-deficient cells. While these studies demonstrated an enhanced inhibitory activity in cells, previous efforts to use phosphoramidates as prodrugs of nucleoside antivirals have shown less promising results *in vivo*. This could be due to premature cleavage of the prodrug and the limited ability of the intermediate metabolites to be taken up by the target tissue.[94]

12.5.3 Prodrugs Activated by Enzymes Overexpressed in Tumors

Another strategy for targeting prodrugs to tumor cells entails the exploitation of enzymes that are expressed in tumor cells to a higher level than normal cells. Using this strategy, the potential

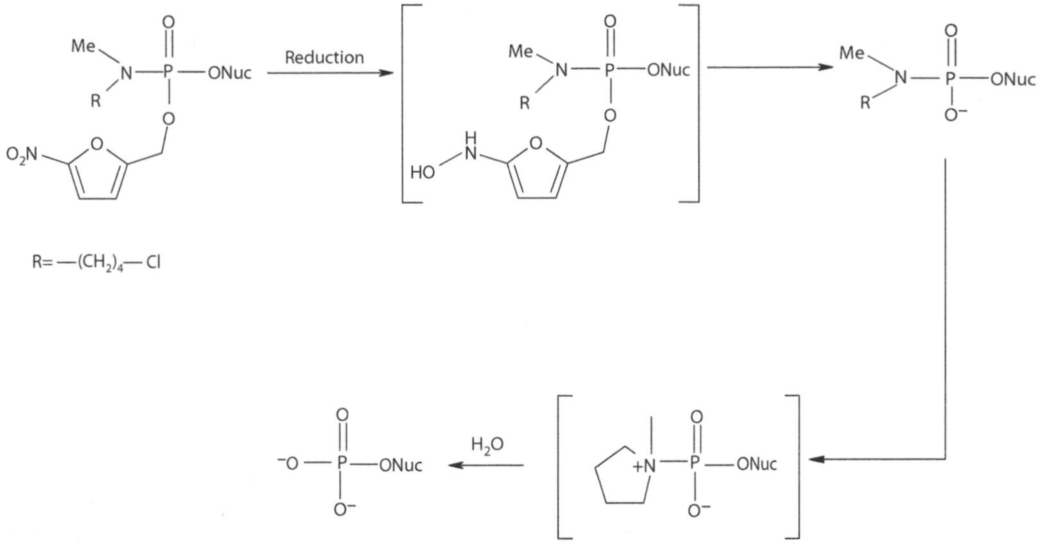

FIGURE 12.24 Mechanism of prodrug activation of phosphoramidate-based prodrugs of nucleoside monophosphates.

improvement in the therapeutic index is dependent on the fold difference in enzyme expression as well as other factors (e.g., hypoxia).[95] In this section, several prodrug strategies are summarized that target enzymes overexpressed in human tumors.

Glutathione-*S*-transferase (GST) is an attractive enzyme suitable for targeting prodrugs to human tumors. GST is not only elevated in tumors but is also associated with drug resistance and poor prognosis. GST catalyzes the addition of glutathione to various alkylating agents and, therefore, plays an important role in the detoxification of cytotoxic chemotherapeutics. Prodrugs cleaved by a reaction involving GST have shown promising activity in preclinical models. For example, TER286 is a cytotoxin that incorporates a glutathione moiety, wherein the sulfur atom exists as a sulfone. Prodrug cleavage occurs through the action of class pi GST (P1-1), which catalyzes a β-elimination reaction. This releases a nitrogen mustard that results in DNA alkylation and cytotoxicity.[96,97]

Another prodrug targeting GST is JS-K, which in contrast to TER286, catalyzes the addition of glutathione. The resulting conjugate undergoes an intramolecular rearrangement to produce an intermediate that generates nitric oxide (NO; Figure 12.25). The local production of NO avoids systemic vasodilation while eliciting NO-mediated anti-cancer activity. JS-K inhibited tumor growth in human xenograft mouse models.[98]

Another prodrug activating enzyme expressed in tumors is DT diaphorase (DTD). It catalyzes a two electron quinine reduction that protects cells from damage caused by the formation of semiquinone radicals and reactive oxygen species. DTD is overexpressed in some cancers and

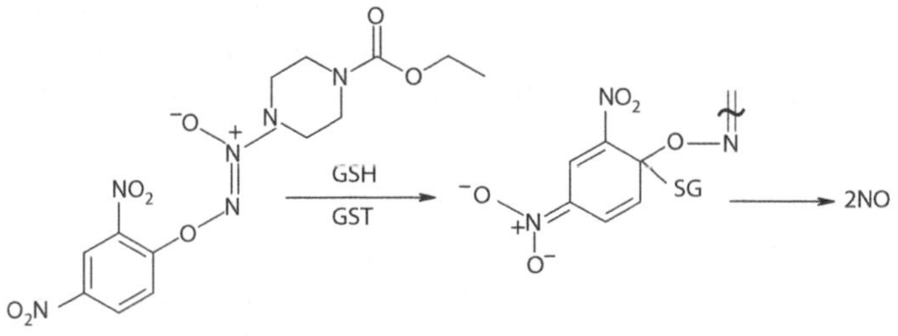

FIGURE 12.25 JS-K is a prodrug that is activated in tumors by GST to produce NO in a site-specific manner.

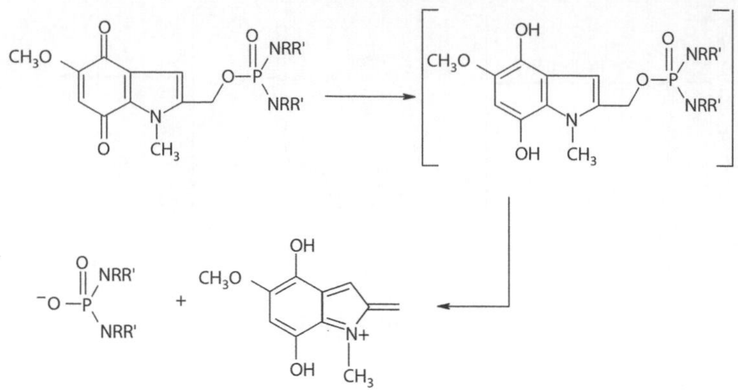

FIGURE 12.26 Mechanism for the bioreductive prodrug activation of 2-substituted indolequinone phosphoramidate by DT diaphorase.

appears to be the enzyme responsible for the bioreduction of the anti-cancer drug mitomycin C. Phosphoramidate prodrugs activated by DTD are toxic to human colon cancer cell lines[99] (Figure 12.26). Their toxicity is correlated with DTD activity.

Endoproteases represent another class of enzymes that are potential targets for tumor-selective prodrugs.[100] For example, a prostate specific antigen (PSA) is a serine protease with chymotrypsin-like activity that cleaves seminal fluid proteins within the prostate. A portion of the PSA in the prostate is secreted into the systemic circulation, where it is rapidly inactivated through complexation with α_1-antichymotrypsin. Efforts to use PSA for the local production of cytotoxic agents led to peptide conjugates of doxorubicin[101] and vinblastine[102] that undergo cleavage by PSA. These prodrugs exhibit high specificity for PSA-secreting cell lines relative to those that do not secrete PSA and were effective in xenograph models of prostate cancer.

Other proteases are expressed at high levels in tumors as a part of processes closely associated with tumor progression such as angiogenesis, invasion, and metastasis. For example, the protease legumain is present in tumors but not in tissues in which the tumor originated.[103] Legumain is present in endosomes and is involved in protein degradation. It is also present extracellularly, where it is available to activate prodrugs in the microenvironment of the tumor. Since legumain is the only mammalian protease specific for asparagines in the P1 position, prodrugs of doxorubicin containing a legumain-sensitive peptide arrested tumor growth and extended survival without the characteristic toxicities of doxorubicin (i.e., cardiac toxicity and myelosuppression).

GST is an attractive enzyme for targeting prodrugs to human tumors. GST is not only elevated in tumors but is also associated with drug resistance and poor prognosis. GST catalyzes the addition of glutathione to various alkylating agents and, therefore, plays an important role in the detoxification of cytotoxic chemotherapeutics. Prodrugs cleaved by a reaction involving GST have shown promising activity in preclinical models.

Thymidine phosphorylase (TP) is another enzyme known to be expressed at higher levels in tumor tissue relative to normal tissue. The prodrug 5′-deoxy-5-fluorouridine (DFUR) is converted by TP to the anti-tumor drug 5-FU. DFUR is used clinically to treat colorectal, gastric, and breast cancer with evidence in breast cancer that tumor effects correlate with TP activity.[104]

12.5.3.1 Capecitabine

One limitation in DFUR therapy is its gastrointestinal toxicity, which arises from high TP activity in the small intestine. Capecitabine is a prodrug of DFUR that avoids these dose-limiting side effects by undergoing a 3-step activation sequence using enzymes located in the liver and tumor tissue (Figure 12.27).[105,106]

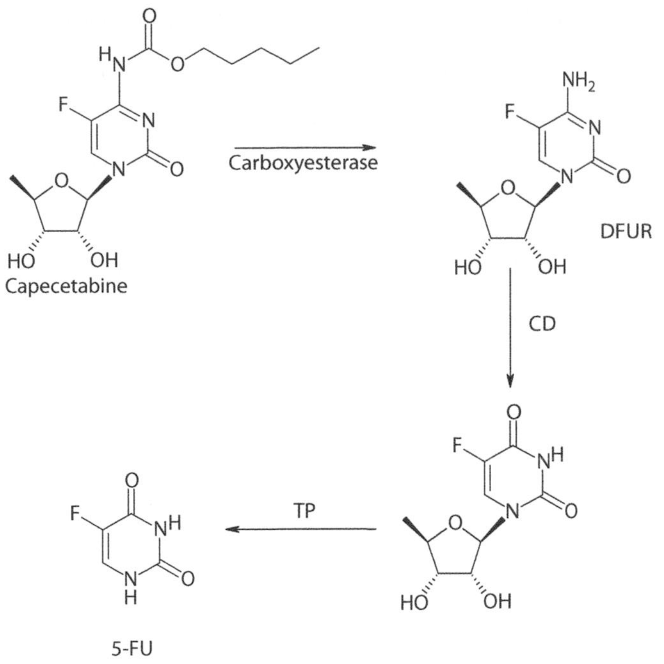

FIGURE 12.27 Capecitabine activation mechanism that results in delivery of 5-FU to tumors.

The first step entails cleavage of the carbamate, which is primarily catalyzed by carboxyesterases present in the liver. The second step generates DFUR via a deamination catalyzed by cytidine deaminase, which is expressed in both the liver and tumors. The final step is catalyzed by TP, which is overexpressed in tumors and thereby ensures high tumor specificity. Accordingly, capecitabine exhibits high tumor specificity and correspondingly an improved therapeutic index.

12.6 CONCLUDING REMARKS

The challenge in developing prodrug strategies for site-selective drug delivery largely stems from the lack of enzymes that both catalyze reactions useful for prodrug cleavage and are expressed in a tissue-specific manner. In some cases, this limitation can be overcome by targeting nontissue specific enzymes such as esterases using a prodrug that distributes selectively into the target tissue via a tissue-specific receptor or transporter. Prodrug strategies that deliver drugs to the liver, brain, kidney, and colon have been identified and shown in many cases to improve the drug safety profile and/or therapeutic effect. Prodrug strategies have also been discovered that gain tumor specificity through exploiting either the unique microenvironment of the tumor or enzymes that are overexpressed in the tumor relative to normal tissues.

REFERENCES

1. Albert A. Chemical aspects of selective toxicity. *Nature* 1958 (Aug 16);**182**(4633):421–422.
2. Ettmayer P, Amidon GL, Clement B, Testa B. Lessons learned from marketed and investigational prodrugs. *J Med Chem* 2004 (May 6);**47**(10):2393–2404.
3. Stella VJ. Prodrugs as therapeutics. *Expert Opin Ther Patents* 2004;**14**(3):277–280.
4. Hecker SJ, Erion MD. Prodrugs of phosphates and phosphonates. *J Med Chem* 2008 (Apr 24);**51**(8):2328–2345.
5. Rautio J, Kumpulainen H, Heimbach T, Oliyai R, Oh D, Jarvinen T, Savolainen J. Prodrugs: Design and clinical applications. *Nat Rev Drug Discov* 2008 (Mar);**7**(3):255–270.

6. Stella VJ, Himmelstein KJ. Prodrugs and site-specific drug delivery. *J Med Chem* 1980 (Dec);**23**(12):1275–1282.
7. Tomlinson E. Site-specific drugs and delivery systems: Rationale, potential and limitations. In: Timmerman H, ed. *Trends in Drug Research*. Elsevier, Amsterdam, the Netherlands; 1990. pp. 287–302.
8. Langer R. Drug delivery and targeting. *Nature* 1998 (Apr 30);**392**(6679 Suppl):5–10.
9. Arap W, Pasqualini R, Ruoslahti E. Cancer treatment by targeted drug delivery to tumor vasculature in a mouse model. *Science* 1998 (Jan 16);**279**(5349):377–380.
10. Ruoslahti E. Drug targeting to specific vascular sites. *Drug Discov Today* 2002 (Nov 15); **7**(22):1138–1143.
11. Meijer DK, Molema G. Targeting of drugs to the liver. *Semin Liver Dis* 1995 (Aug);**15**(3):202–256.
12. Iyer AK, Khaled G, Fang J, Maeda H. Exploiting the enhanced permeability and retention effect for tumor targeting. *Drug Discov Today* 2006 (Sep);**11**(17–18):812–818.
13. Liederer BM, Borchardt RT. Enzymes involved in the bioconversion of ester-based prodrugs. *J Pharm Sci* 2006 (Jun);**95**(6):1177–1195.
14. Olbe L, Carlsson E, Lindberg P. A proton-pump inhibitor expedition: The case histories of omeprazole and esomeprazole. *Nat Rev Drug Discov* 2003 (Feb);**2**(2):132–139.
15. Niculescu-Duvaz I, Spooner R, Marais R, Springer CJ. Gene-directed enzyme prodrug therapy. *Bioconjug Chem* 1998 (Jan–Feb);**9**(1):4–22.
16. Huttunen KM, Mahonen N, Raunio H, Rautio J. Cytochrome P450-activated prodrugs: Targeted drug delivery. *Curr Med Chem* 2008;**15**(23):2346–2365.
17. de Waziers I, Cugnenc PH, Yang CS, Leroux JP, Beaune PH. Cytochrome P 450 isoenzymes, epoxide hydrolase and glutathione transferases in rat and human hepatic and extrahepatic tissues. *J Pharmacol Exp Ther* 1990 (Apr);**253**(1):387–394.
18. Erion MD. Prodrugs for liver-targeted drug delivery in prodrugs: Challenges and rewards, part I. In: Stella VJ, Borchardt RT, Hageman DL, Oliyai R, Maag H, and Tilley J, eds. *Prodrugs: Challenges and Rewards*. Springer, New York; 2006. pp. 529–560.
19. Dechant KL, Brogden RN, Pilkington T, Faulds D. Ifosfamide/mesna. A review of its antineoplastic activity, pharmacokinetic properties and therapeutic efficacy in cancer. *Drugs* 1991 (Sep);**42**(3):428–467.
20. Altaner C. Prodrug cancer gene therapy. *Cancer Lett* 2008 (Nov 8);**270**(2):191–201.
21. Xu G, McLeod HL. Strategies for enzyme/prodrug cancer therapy. *Clin Cancer Res* 2001 (Nov);**7**(11):3314–3324.
22. Kievit E, Bershad E, Ng E, Sethna P, Dev I, Lawrence TS, Rehemtulla A. Superiority of yeast over bacterial cytosine deaminase for enzyme/prodrug gene therapy in colon cancer xenografts. *Cancer Res* 1999 (Apr 1);**59**(7):1417–1421.
23. Zhang Y, Parker WB, Sorscher EJ, Ealick SE. PNP anticancer gene therapy. *Curr Top Med Chem* 2005;**5**(13):1259–1274.
24. Oldfield EH, Ram Z, Culver KW, Blaese RM, DeVroom HL, Anderson WF. Gene therapy for the treatment of brain tumors using intra-tumoral transduction with the thymidine kinase gene and intravenous ganciclovir. *Hum Gene Ther* 1993 (Feb);**4**(1):39–69.
25. Chen L, Waxman DJ. Cytochrome P450 gene-directed enzyme prodrug therapy (GDEPT) for cancer. *Curr Pharm Des* 2002;**8**(15):1405–1416.
26. Jounaidi Y, Chen CS, Veal GJ, Waxman DJ. Enhanced antitumor activity of P450 prodrug-based gene therapy using the low Km cyclophosphamide 4-hydroxylase P450 2B11. *Mol Cancer Ther* 2006 (Mar);**5**(3):541–555.
27. Erion MD, Reddy KR, Boyer SH, Matelich MC, Gomez-Galeno J, Lemus RH, Ugarkar BG, Colby TJ, Schanzer J, Van Poelje PD. Design, synthesis, and characterization of a series of cytochrome P(450) 3A-activated prodrugs (HepDirect prodrugs) useful for targeting phosph(on)ate-based drugs to the liver. *J Am Chem Soc* 2004 (Apr 28);**126**(16):5154–5163.
28. Erion MD, van Poelje PD, Mackenna DA, Colby TJ, Montag AC, Fujitaki JM, Linemeyer DL, Bullough DA. Liver-targeted drug delivery using HepDirect prodrugs. *J Pharmacol Exp Ther* 2005 (Feb);**312**(2):554–560.
29. Mitchell JR, Jollow DJ, Potter WZ, Gillette JR, Brodie BB. Acetaminophen-induced hepatic necrosis. IV. Protective role of glutathione. *J Pharmacol Exp Ther* 1973 (Oct);**187**(1):211–217.
30. Ingelman-Sundberg M. Human drug metabolising cytochrome P450 enzymes: Properties and polymorphisms. *Naunyn Schmiedebergs Arch Pharmacol* 2004 (Jan);**369**(1):89–104.
31. Lin CC, Yeh LT, Vitarella D, Hong Z, Erion MD. Remofovir mesylate: A prodrug of PMEA with improved liver-targeting and safety in rats and monkeys. *Antivir Chem Chemother* 2004 (Nov);**15**(6):307–317.

32. Cummins CL, Jacobsen W, Christians U, Benet LZ. CYP3A4-transfected Caco-2 cells as a tool for understanding biochemical absorption barriers: Studies with sirolimus and midazolam. *J Pharmacol Exp Ther* 2004 (Jan);**308**(1):143–155.

33. Zhang CY, Baffy G, Perret P, Krauss S, Peroni O, Grujic D, Hagen T, Vidal-Puig AJ, Boss O, Kim YB, Zheng XX, Wheeler MB, Shulman GI, Chan CB, Lowell BB. Uncoupling protein-2 negatively regulates insulin secretion and is a major link between obesity, beta cell dysfunction, and type 2 diabetes. *Cell* 2001;**105**(6):745–755.

34. Lamba JK, Lin YS, Thummel K, Daly A, Watkins PB, Strom S, Zhang J, Schuetz EG. Common allelic variants of cytochrome P4503A4 and their prevalence in different populations. *Pharmacogenetics* 2002 (Mar);**12**(2):121–132.

35. Shimada T, Yamazaki H, Mimura M, Inui Y, Guengerich FP. Interindividual variations in human liver cytochrome P-450 enzymes involved in the oxidation of drugs, carcinogens and toxic chemicals: Studies with liver microsomes of 30 Japanese and 30 Caucasians. *J Pharmacol Exp Ther* 1994 (Jul);**270**(1):414–423.

36. Lin JH, Lu AY. Interindividual variability in inhibition and induction of cytochrome P450 enzymes. *Annu Rev Pharmacol Toxicol* 2001;**41**:535–567.

37. Salva P, Costa J. Clinical pharmacokinetics and pharmacodynamics of zolpidem. Therapeutic implications. *Clin Pharmacokinet* 1995 (Sep);**29**(3):142–153.

38. Fakhoury M, Litalien C, Medard Y, Cave H, Ezzahir N, Peuchmaur M, Jacqz-Aigrain E. Localization and mRNA expression of CYP3A and P-glycoprotein in human duodenum as a function of age. *Drug Metab Dispos* 2005 (Nov);**33**(11):1603–1607.

39. Lin CC, Xu C, Zhu N, Lourenco D, Yeh LT. Single-dose pharmacokinetics and metabolism of [14C]remofovir in rats and cynomolgus monkeys. *Antimicrob Agents Chemother* 2005 (Mar);**49**(3):925–930.

40. Gibbs MA, Hosea NA. Factors affecting the clinical development of cytochrome p450 3A substrates. *Clin Pharmacokinet* 2003;**42**(11):969–984.

41. Lin CC, Fang C, Benetton S, Xu GF, Yeh LT. Metabolic activation of pradefovir by CYP3A4 and its potential as an inhibitor or inducer. *Antimicrob Agents Chemother* 2006 (Sep);**50**(9):2926–2931.

42. Neudecker T, Eder E, Deininger C, Hoffman C, Henschler D. Mutagenicity of methylvinyl ketone in *Salmonella typhimurium* TA100—indication for epoxidation as an activation mechanism. *Mutat Res* 1989 (Oct);**227**(2):131–134.

43. Dinkova-Kostova AT, Massiah MA, Bozak RE, Hicks RJ, Talalay P. Potency of Michael reaction acceptors as inducers of enzymes that protect against carcinogenesis depends on their reactivity with sulfhydryl groups. *Proc Natl Acad Sci USA* 2001 (Mar 13);**98**(6):3404–3409.

44. MacCoss M, Baillie TA. Organic chemistry in drug discovery. *Science* 2004 (Mar 19);**303**(5665):1810–1813.

45. Hales BF, Ludeman SM, Boyd VL. Embryotoxicity of phenyl ketone analogs of cyclophosphamide. *Teratology* 1989 (Jan);**39**(1):31–37.

46. Reddy KR, Matelich MC, Ugarkar BG, Gomez-Galeno JE, DaRe J, Ollis K, Sun Z, Craigo W, Colby TJ, Fujitaki JM, Boyer SH, van Poelje PD, Erion MD. Pradefovir: A prodrug that targets adefovir to the liver for the treatment of hepatitis B. *J Med Chem* 2008 (Feb 14);**51**(3):666–676.

47. Dando T, Plosker G. Adefovir dipivoxil: A review of its use in chronic hepatitis B. *Drugs* 2003;**63**(20):2215–2234.

48. Marcellin P, Chang TT, Lim SG, Tong MJ, Sievert W, Shiffman ML, Jeffers L, Goodman Z, Wulfsohn MS, Xiong S, Fry J, Brosgart CL. Adefovir dipivoxil for the treatment of hepatitis B e antigen-positive chronic hepatitis B. *N Engl J Med* 2003 (Feb 27);**348**(9):808–816.

49. van Montfoort JE, Hagenbuch B, Groothuis GM, Koepsell H, Meier PJ, Meijer DK. Drug uptake systems in liver and kidney. *Curr Drug Metab* 2003 (Jun);**4**(3):185–211.

50. de Vrueh RL, Rump ET, van De Bilt E, van Veghel R, Balzarini J, Biessen EA, van Berkel TJ, Bijsterbosch MK. Carrier-mediated delivery of 9-(2-phosphonylmethoxyethyl)adenine to parenchymal liver cells: A novel therapeutic approach for hepatitis B. *Antimicrob Agents Chemother* 2000 (Mar);**44**(3):477–483.

51. Dallas S, Schlichter L, Bendayan R. Multidrug resistance protein (MRP) 4- and MRP 5-mediated efflux of 9-(2-phosphonylmethoxyethyl)adenine by microglia. *J Pharmacol Exp Ther* 2004 (Jun);**309**(3):1221–1229.

52. Lim S, Lee K, Chuang W-L, Hwang S, Cho M, Lai M-Y, Chao Y-C, Chang T-T, Xu Y, Sullivan-Bolyai J. Safety, tolerability, antiviral activity, and pharmacokinetics of pradefovir mesylate in patients with chronic hepatitis B virus infection: 24-week interim analysis of a phase II study. AASLD; 2005. p. Abs LB07.

53. Erion MD, Dang Q, Reddy MR, Kasibhatla SR, Huang J, Lipscomb WN, van Poelje PD. Structure-guided design of AMP mimics that inhibit fructose-1,6-bisphosphatase with high affinity and specificity. *J Am Chem Soc* 2007 (Dec 19);**129**(50):15480–15490.

54. Gumina G, Chong Y, Choo H, Song GY, Chu CK. L-nucleosides: Antiviral activity and molecular mechanism. *Curr Top Med Chem* 2002;**2**(10):1065–1086.

55. Yamanaka G, Wilson T, Innaimo S, Bisacchi GS, Egli P, Rinehart JK, Zahler R, Colonno RJ. Metabolic studies on BMS-200475, a new antiviral compound active against hepatitis B virus. *Antimicrob Agents Chemother* 1999;**43**(1):190–193.

56. Schultz C. Prodrugs of biologically active phosphate esters. *Bioorg Med Chem* 2003 (Mar) 20;**11**(6):885–898.

57. Reddy KR, Colby TJ, Fujitaki JM, van Poelje PD, Erion MD. Liver targeting of hepatitis-B antiviral lamivudine using the HepDirect prodrug technology. *Nucleosides Nucleotides Nucleic Acids* 2005;**24**(5–7):375–381.

58. Hecker SJ, Reddy KR, van Poelje PD, Sun Z, Huang W, Varkhedkar V, Reddy MV, Fujitaki JM, Olsen DB, Koeplinger KA, Boyer SH, Linemeyer DL, MacCoss M, Erion MD. Liver-targeted prodrugs of 2′-C-methyladenosine for therapy of hepatitis C virus infection. *J Med Chem* 2007 (Aug 9); **50**(16):3891–3896.

59. Carroll S, Koeplinger K, Vavrek M, Handt L, MacCoss M, Hecker SJ, Olsen DB. Administration of a HepDirect™ Prodrug of 2′-C-methylcytidine to hepatitis C virus infected Chimpanzees. *22nd International Conference on Antiviral Research*. Elsevier, Miami Beach, FL; 2009. p. A22.

60. Mackenna DA, Montag A, Boyer SH, Linemeyer DL, Erion MD. Delivery of high levels of anti-proliferative nucleoside triphosphates to CYP3A-expressing cells as a potential treatment for hepatocellular carcinoma. *Cancer Chemother Pharmacol* 2009 (Mar 13);**64**(5):981–991.

61. Erion MD, Cable EE, Ito BR, Jiang H, Fujitaki JM, Finn PD, Zhang BH, Hou J, Boyer SH, van Poelje PD, Linemeyer DL. Targeting thyroid hormone receptor-beta agonists to the liver reduces cholesterol and triglycerides and improves the therapeutic index. *Proc Natl Acad Sci USA* 2007 (Sep 25);**104**(39):15490–15495.

62. Trost SU, Swanson E, Gloss B, Wang-Iverson DB, Zhang H, Volodarsky T, Grover GJ, Baxter JD, Chiellini G, Scanlan TS, Dillmann WH. The thyroid hormone receptor-beta-selective agonist GC-1 differentially affects plasma lipids and cardiac activity. *Endocrinology* 2000 (Sep);**141**(9):3057–3064.

63. Fujitaki JM, Cable EE, Ito BR, Zhang BH, Hou J, Yang C, Bullough DA, Ferrero JL, van Poelje PD, Linemeyer DL, Erion MD. Preclinical pharmacokinetics of a HepDirect prodrug of a novel phosphonate-containing thyroid hormone receptor agonist. *Drug Metab Dispos* 2008 (Aug 14);**36**:2393–2403.

64. Boyer SH, Jiang H, Jacintho JD, Reddy MV, Li H, Li W, Godwin JL, Schulz WG, Cable EE, Hou J, Wu R, Fujitaki JM, Hecker SJ, Erion MD. Synthesis and biological evaluation of a series of liver-selective phosphonic acid thyroid hormone receptor agonists and their prodrugs. *J Med Chem* 2008 (Nov 1); **51**:7075–7093.

65. Ito BR, Zhang BH, Cable EE, Song X, Fujitaki JM, MacKenna DA, Wilker CE, Chi B, van Poelje PD, Linemeyer DL, Erion MD. Thyroid hormone beta receptor activation has additive cholesterol lowering activity in combination with atorvastatin in rabbits, dogs and monkeys. *Br J Pharmacol* 2009 (Feb);**156**(3):454–465.

66. Friesema EC, Kuiper GG, Jansen J, Visser TJ, Kester MH. Thyroid hormone transport by the human monocarboxylate transporter 8 and its rate-limiting role in intracellular metabolism. *Mol Endocrinol* 2006 (Aug 3);**20**(11):2761–2772.

67. Baxter JD, Webb P, Grover G, Scanlan TS. Selective activation of thyroid hormone signaling pathways by GC-1: A new approach to controlling cholesterol and body weight. *Trends Endocrinol Metab* 2004 (May–Jun);**15**(4):154–157.

68. Columbano A, Pibiri M, Deidda M, Cossu C, Scanlan TS, Chiellini G, Muntoni S, Ledda-Columbano GM. The thyroid hormone receptor-beta agonist GC-1 induces cell proliferation in rat liver and pancreas. *Endocrinology* 2006 (Jul);**147**(7):3211–3218.

69. Kullak-Ublick GA, Beuers U, Paumgartner G. Hepatobiliary transport. *J Hepatol* 2000;**32** (1 Suppl):3–18.

70. Kramer W, Wess G, Schubert G, Bickel M, Girbig F, Gutjahr U, Kowalewski S, Baringhaus KH, Enhsen A, Glombik H et al. Liver-specific drug targeting by coupling to bile acids. *J Biol Chem* 1992 (Sep 15); **267**(26):18598–18604.

71. Stephan ZF, Yurachek EC, Sharif R, Wasvary JM, Steele RE, Howes C. Reduction of cardiovascular and thyroxine-suppressing activities of L-T3 by liver targeting with cholic acid. *Biochem Pharmacol* 1992 (May 8);**43**(9):1969–1974.

72. Petzinger E, Nickau L, Horz JA, Schulz S, Wess G, Enhsen A, Falk E, Baringhaus KH, Glombik H, Hoffmann A et al. Hepatobiliary transport of hepatic 3-hydroxy-3-methylglutaryl coenzyme A reductase inhibitors conjugated with bile acids. *Hepatology* 1995 (Dec);**22**(6):1801–1811.

73. Kramer W, Wess G, Enhsen A, Bock K, Falk E, Hoffmann A, Neckermann G, Gantz D, Schulz S, Nickau L et al. Bile acid derived HMG-CoA reductase inhibitors. *Biochim Biophys Acta* 1994 (Nov 29);**1227**(3):137–154.

74. Pavan B, Dalpiaz A, Ciliberti N, Biondi C, Manfredini S, Vertuani S. Progress in drug delivery to the central nervous system by the prodrug approach. *Molecules* 2008;**13**(5):1035–1065.

75. Bodor N, Farag HH, Brewster ME, III. Site-specific, sustained release of drugs to the brain. *Science* 1981 (Dec 18);**214**(4527):1370–1372.

76. Prokai L, Prokai-Tatrai K, Bodor N. Targeting drugs to the brain by redox chemical delivery systems. *Med Res Rev* 2000 (Sep);**20**(5):367–416.

77. Wilk S, Mizoguchi H, Orlowski M. gamma-Glutamyl dopa: A kidney-specific dopamine precursor. *J Pharmacol Exp Ther* 1978 (Jul);**206**(1):227–232.

78. Orlowski M, Mizoguchi H, Wilk S. *N*-acyl-gamma-glutamyl derivatives of sulfamethoxazole as models of kidney-selective prodrugs. *J Pharmacol Exp Ther* 1980 (Jan);**212**(1):167–172.

79. Elfarra AA, Duescher RJ, Hwang IY, Sicuri AR, Nelson JA. Targeting 6-thioguanine to the kidney with *S*-(guanin-6-yl)-L-cysteine. *J Pharmacol Exp Ther* 1995 (Sep);**274**(3):1298–1304.

80. Kinget R, Kalala W, Vervoort L, van den Mooter G. Colonic drug targeting. *J Drug Target* 1998; **6**(2):129–149.

81. Uludag H. Bisphosphonates as a foundation of drug delivery to bone. *Curr Pharm Des* 2002; **8**(21):1929–1944.

82. Brown JM, Wang LH. Tirapazamine: Laboratory data relevant to clinical activity. *Anticancer Drug Des* 1998 (Sep);**13**(6):529–539.

83. Hwang JT, Greenberg MM, Fuchs T, Gates KS. Reaction of the hypoxia-selective antitumor agent tirapazamine with a C1'-radical in single-stranded and double-stranded DNA: The drug and its metabolites can serve as surrogates for molecular oxygen in radical-mediated DNA damage reactions. *Biochemistry* 1999 (Oct 26);**38**(43):14248–14255.

84. Patterson AV, Saunders MP, Chinje EC, Patterson LH, Stratford IJ. Enzymology of tirapazamine metabolism: A review. *Anticancer Drug Des* 1998 (Sep);**13**(6):541–573.

85. Lalani AS, Alters SE, Wong A, Albertella MR, Cleland JL, Henner WD. Selective tumor targeting by the hypoxia-activated prodrug AQ4N blocks tumor growth and metastasis in preclinical models of pancreatic cancer. *Clin Cancer Res* 2007 (Apr 1);**13**(7):2216–2225.

86. Patterson AV, Ferry DM, Edmunds SJ, Gu Y, Singleton RS, Patel K, Pullen SM, Hicks KO, Syddall SP, Atwell GJ, Yang S, Denny WA, Wilson WR. Mechanism of action and preclinical antitumor activity of the novel hypoxia-activated DNA cross-linking agent PR-104. *Clin Cancer Res* 2007 (Jul 1);**13**(13):3922–3932.

87. Borch RF, Liu J, Schmidt JP, Marakovits JT, Joswig C, Gipp JJ, Mulcahy RT. Synthesis and evaluation of nitroheterocyclic phosphoramidates as hypoxia-selective alkylating agents. *J Med Chem* 2000 (Jun 1); **43**(11):2258–2265.

88. Duan JX, Jiao H, Kaizerman J, Stanton T, Evans JW, Lan L, Lorente G, Banica M, Jung D, Wang J, Ma H, Li X, Yang Z, Hoffman RM, Ammons WS, Hart CP, Matteucci M. Potent and highly selective hypoxia-activated achiral phosphoramidate mustards as anticancer drugs. *J Med Chem* 2008 (Apr 24); **51**(8):2412–2420.

89. Arner ES, Eriksson S. Mammalian deoxyribonucleoside kinases. *Pharmacol Ther* 1995;**67**(2):155–186.

90. Zhang YJ, Chen S, Tsai WJ, Ahsan H, Lunn RM, Wang LY, Chen CJ, Santella RM. Expression of cytochrome P450 IA 1/2 and 3A4 in liver tissues of hepatocellular carcinoma cases and controls from Taiwan and their relationship to hepatitis B virus and aflatoxin B1- and 4-aminobiphenyl-DNA adducts. *Biomarkers* 2000;**5**(4):295–306.

91. Tobias SC, Borch RF. Synthesis and biological studies of novel nucleoside phosphoramidate prodrugs. *J Med Chem* 2001 (Dec 6);**44**(25):4475–4480.

92. Tobias SC, Borch RF. Synthesis and biological evaluation of a cytarabine phosphoramidate prodrug. *Mol Pharm* 2004 (Mar–Apr);**1**(2):112–116.

93. Wu W, Sigmond J, Peters GJ, Borch RF. Synthesis and biological activity of a gemcitabine phosphoramidate prodrug. *J Med Chem* 2007 (Jul 26);**50**(15):3743–3746.

94. McGuigan C, Harris SA, Daluge SM, Gudmundsson KS, McLean EW, Burnette TC, Marr H, Hazen R, Condreay LD, Johnson L, De Clercq E, Balzarini J. Application of phosphoramidate pronucleotide technology to abacavir leads to a significant enhancement of antiviral potency. *J Med Chem* 2005 (May 19);**48**(10):3504–3515.

95. Rooseboom M, Commandeur JN, Vermeulen NP. Enzyme-catalyzed activation of anticancer prodrugs. *Pharmacol Rev* 2004 (Mar);**56**(1):53–102.

96. Satyam A, Hocker MD, Kane-Maguire KA, Morgan AS, Villar HO, Lyttle MH. Design, synthesis, and evaluation of latent alkylating agents activated by glutathione *S*-transferase. *J Med Chem* 1996 (Apr 12); **39**(8):1736–1747.

97. Morgan AS, Sanderson PE, Borch RF, Tew KD, Niitsu Y, Takayama T, Von Hoff DD, Izbicka E, Mangold G, Paul C, Broberg U, Mannervik B, Henner WD, Kauvar LM. Tumor efficacy and bone marrow-sparing properties of TER286, a cytotoxin activated by glutathione *S*-transferase. *Cancer Res* 1998 (Jun 15);**58**(12):2568–2575.

98. Shami PJ, Saavedra JE, Wang LY, Bonifant CL, Diwan BA, Singh SV, Gu Y, Fox SD, Buzard GS, Citro ML, Waterhouse DJ, Davies KM, Ji X, Keefer LK. JS-K, a glutathione/glutathione *S*-transferase-activated nitric oxide donor of the diazeniumdiolate class with potent antineoplastic activity. *Mol Cancer Ther* 2003 (Apr);**2**(4):409–417.

99. Hernick M, Flader C, Borch RF. Design, synthesis, and biological evaluation of indolequinone phosphoramidate prodrugs targeted to DT-diaphorase. *J Med Chem* 2002 (Aug 1);**45**(16):3540–3548.

100. Atkinson JM, Siller CS, Gill JH. Tumour endoproteases: The cutting edge of cancer drug delivery? *Br J Pharmacol* 2008 (Apr);**153**(7):1344–1352.

101. Garsky VM, Lumma PK, Feng DM, Wai J, Ramjit HG, Sardana MK, Oliff A, Jones RE, DeFeo-Jones D, Freidinger RM. The synthesis of a prodrug of doxorubicin designed to provide reduced systemic toxicity and greater target efficacy. *J Med Chem* 2001 (Nov 22);**44**(24):4216–4224.

102. Brady SF, Pawluczyk JM, Lumma PK, Feng DM, Wai JM, Jones R, DeFeo-Jones D, Wong BK, Miller-Stein C, Lin JH, Oliff A, Freidinger RM, Garsky VM. Design and synthesis of a pro-drug of vinblastine targeted at treatment of prostate cancer with enhanced efficacy and reduced systemic toxicity. *J Med Chem* 2002 (Oct 10);**45**(21):4706–4715.

103. Wu W, Luo Y, Sun C, Liu Y, Kuo P, Varga J, Xiang R, Reisfeld R, Janda KD, Edgington TS, Liu C. Targeting cell-impermeable prodrug activation to tumor microenvironment eradicates multiple drug-resistant neoplasms. *Cancer Res* 2006 (Jan 15);**66**(2):970–980.

104. Hata Y, Takahashi H, Sasaki F, Ogita M, Uchino J, Yoshimoto M, Akasaka Y, Nakanishi Y, Sawada Y. Intratumoral pyrimidine nucleoside phosphorylase (PyNPase) activity predicts a selective effect of adjuvant 5′-deoxy-5fluorouridine (5′DFUR) on breast cancer. *Breast Cancer* 2000 (Jan);**7**(1):37–41.

105. Miwa M, Ura M, Nishida M, Sawada N, Ishikawa T, Mori K, Shimma N, Umeda I, Ishitsuka H. Design of a novel oral fluoropyrimidine carbamate, capecitabine, which generates 5-fluorouracil selectively in tumours by enzymes concentrated in human liver and cancer tissue. *Eur J Cancer* 1998 (Jul);**34**(8):1274–1281.

106. Ishikawa T, Utoh M, Sawada N, Nishida M, Fukase Y, Sekiguchi F, Ishitsuka H. Tumor selective delivery of 5-fluorouracil by capecitabine, a new oral fluoropyrimidine carbamate, in human cancer xenografts. *Biochem Pharmacol* 1998 (Apr 1);**55**(7):1091–1097.

107. Kullak-Ublick GA. Regulation of organic anion and drug transporters of the sinusoidal membrane. *J Hepatol* 1999;**31**:563–573.

13 Enzyme-Activated Prodrug Strategies for Targeted Drug Action

Jarkko Rautio, Krista Laine, Lanyan Fang, Bing Han, Kristiina Huttunen, and Duxin Sun

CONTENTS

13.1 WHAT ARE PRODRUGS?

Prodrugs are bioreversible derivatives of drug molecules that undergo an enzymatic and/or chemical transformation *in vivo* to release the active parent drug, which can then produce its desired pharmacological effect.[1–3] In most cases, prodrugs are simple chemical derivatives that are one or two chemical or enzymatic steps away from the parent drug. In some cases, a prodrug may consist of two pharmacologically active drugs that are coupled together in a single molecule, so that each drug acts as a promoiety for the other. Such derivatives are called co-drugs.[4] Prodrugs have also been called reversible or bioreversible derivatives, latentiated drugs, or biolabile drug-carrier conjugates, but the term "prodrug" is now standard. Some prodrugs lack an obvious carrier or promoiety, but result from a molecular modification of the active drug itself. This modification, which can be, for example, oxidation or reduction, generates a new active compound. These prodrugs are referred to as bioprecursor prodrugs. Finally, soft drugs also find applications in tissue targeting. In contrast to prodrugs, soft drugs are active drugs but are designed to transform to an inactive form *in vivo* after achieving their therapeutic effect.[5] The prodrug concept is illustrated in Figure 13.1.

The development of prodrugs is now well established as a strategy to improve the physicochemical, biopharmaceutical, or pharmacokinetic properties of pharmacologically potent compounds, and thereby increases the developability and usefulness of a potential drug. This is unquestioned

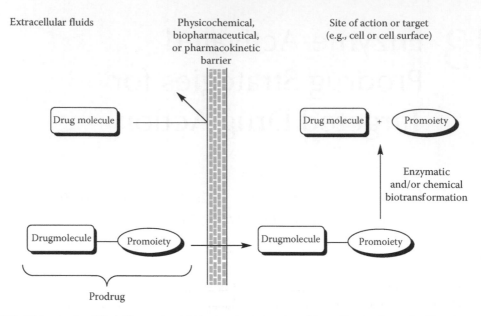

FIGURE 13.1 A simplified illustration of the prodrug concept. (From Rautio, J. et al., *Nat. Rev. Drug Discov.*, 7, 255, 2008.)

since currently by estimate 5%–7% of drugs approved worldwide can be classified as prodrugs, and approximately 15% of all new drugs approved in 2001 and 2002 were prodrugs.[6,7] Over the years, prodrugs have provided possibilities for overcoming various barriers to drug formulation and delivery, of which the most common include the following:

1. Poor aqueous solubility
   - Prevents the development of aqueous-based formulations (e.g., solutions, drops, infusions)
   - Leads to dissolution rate-limited and variable oral bioavailability
2. Poor lipid solubility
   - Results in low membrane permeation across various barriers including the gastrointestinal mucosa, the blood–brain barrier, cornea, skin, etc.
   - Limits the development of lipid-based formulations
3. Short duration of action (due to rapid elimination from the body or high first-pass metabolism)
   - Necessitates frequent administration of drug that often leads to poor patient compliance
4. Lack of site specificity (e.g., poor brain, tumor, or colon/kidney/liver targeting)
   - May lead to undesirable systemic effects
5. Economic barriers
   - The development of a prodrug of an existing drug with improved properties may represent a life-cycle management opportunity

13.2 WHY PRODRUGS FOR DRUG TARGETING?

Although the concept of targeted or site-specific drug delivery has been evolving for at least 100 years from Nobelist Paul Ehrlich's "magic bullet," which is an active agent delivered only at the desired site in the body, the challenge of making drugs with very selective treatment has not been completely resolved and is one of the ultimate goals in drug delivery. Rationally designed drug targeting is, therefore, one of the most attractive and actively pursued objectives of the prodrug approach. When the prodrug patent literature over the years 1993–2003 was analyzed, as many as

14.9% of the patents claimed targeting.[7] Since drug targeting is particularly attractive for highly toxic drugs and for drugs having a narrow therapeutic window, it is not surprising that the majority of patents mentioning drug targeting were directed toward cancer treatment. Several of these patents were for antibody-directed enzyme prodrug therapy (ADEPT), gene-directed enzyme prodrug therapy (GDEPT), and their variants.

In prodrug design, drug targeting can, in general, be achieved by *site-directed drug delivery* or *site-selective drug bioactivation*. With site-directed drug delivery, the bioreversible prodrug is selectively or primarily transported, as an intact prodrug, to the site of drug action. This can be achieved after localized drug delivery where the prodrug is applied directly to the target organ, as in the case of dermal and ocular drug delivery. Site-directed drug delivery after systemic administration constitutes a much more challenging task due to various complex and unpredictable barriers in the body, but has demonstrated some success, for example, in brain drug delivery.[8,9] With site-selective bioactivation, the prodrug can be widely distributed all over the body, but undergoes bioactivation and exerts activity by forming active drug selectively at the desired site. For site-selective prodrug activation, differences in various physiological conditions such as hypoxia and pH as well as enzymes that are preferably unique for the tissue, or present at a higher concentration compared with other tissues, can all be exploited. However, the ubiquitous distribution of most endogenous enzymes responsible for the bioactivation of prodrugs diminishes the possibilities for selective activation, and consequently, targeting. Therefore, the prodrug approaches that rely on bioactivation by exogenous enzymes selectively delivered via monoclonal antibodies (ADEPT) or generated from genes encoding an exogenous enzyme (GDEPT) have received considerable attention over the last decade especially in cancer therapy. In many prodrug applications, site-directed drug delivery and site-specific bioactivation have naturally been combined in order to achieve successful targeted drug delivery.

The use of prodrugs in targeted drug delivery has been reviewed in the literature. Stella and Himmelstein focused on defining, targeting, and resolving the pharmacokinetic characteristics of both the parent drug and the prodrug necessary for achieving targeted drug delivery.[10,11] Kearney reviewed simple pharmacokinetic models for targeting by prodrugs.[12] Moreover, his paper summarized the prodrug approaches developed so far to target various tissues and the use of the ADEPT. Han and Amidon gave a few examples of prodrugs designed to be activated by tissue-specific enzymes.[13] Much more attention was paid to prodrugs designed to target nutrient (e.g., glucose, amino acid, and peptide) transporters capable of facilitating the membrane transport of their substrates. Ettmayer et al. reviewed both marketed and investigational prodrugs and categorized tissue-selective drug delivery by prodrugs into four approaches. Of these, the approach of targeting tissue- or cell-specific enzymes is the one that gained the most attention.[14] Recently, Rajewski and McIntosh reviewed and improved the pharmacokinetic models developed by Stella and Himmelstein.[15] The authors described theoretical and computational models for drug targeting using the prodrug approach. While only a few reviews focused on targeting via so-called one-step prodrug approaches

(see below), there are a number of reviews that highlight two-step prodrug approaches, namely, ADEPT[16,17] and GDEPT.[18,19] The reader is directed to these reviews for an in-depth discussion on relevant topics.

Section 13.2.1 of this book discusses examples of when the prodrug approach has been utilized to achieve the targeted drug delivery by site-selective enzyme activation. These approaches fall into two main categories: one-step approaches, which include prodrugs that are designed for direct activation either by tissue-selective enzymes or pH conditions; and two-step approaches, in which the enzyme that is supposed to activate the prodrug is administered in the second step of the therapy and is targeted to the target tissue (typically tumor) for the

---

Simplified categorization of prodrug approaches to improve drug targeting

Site-directed drug delivery

Prodrug is selectively or primarily transported to the site of drug action:

- Localized drug delivery (e.g., dermal and ocular drug delivery)
- Prodrug improves drug delivery to specific tissue (e.g., improved CNS drug delivery)

Site-selective bioactivation

- Bioactivation takes place predominantly at the desired site of drug action

first step. The following discussion of one-step approaches describes examples in which some degree of success has been achieved by using prodrugs. These examples are categorized by the physiologic sites, e.g., liver, kidney, colon, and tumor tissue, that have been targeted. Of the two-step approaches, this chapter focuses mainly on ADEPT.

Finally, for successful drug targeting using prodrugs, the following properties of the prodrug as well as the active drug should be taken into consideration[10,11]:

1. The prodrug must be readily transported to the target site and uptake must be reasonably fast.
2. The prodrug must be selectively converted to the active drug at the target site relative to its conversion at other sites in the body.
3. The active drug, once selectively generated at the target site, must be somewhat retained by the tissue.

13.2.1 ONE-STEP PRODRUG APPROACHES FOR TARGETED DRUG DELIVERY

13.2.1.1 Targeting the Liver

The liver is the first organ to gain nutrients, drugs, and toxins after their absorption from the stomach and intestine. It plays a primary role in the synthesis and/or metabolism of biomolecules and xenobiotics.[20,21] The major cells of the liver are hepatocytes, which are the main metabolic site of action. Molecules are taken up into the hepatocytes through passive diffusion, transporters, or receptor-mediated endocytosis. The metabolism in the hepatocytes usually leads to the detoxification of xenobiotics. In phase I biotransformation reactions, the functional groups of xenobiotics are unveiled by oxidation, reduction, or hydrolysis reactions. In phase II metabolism reactions, the formed metabolite or xenobiotic itself is conjugated with hydrophilic endogenous substrates, like glucuronic acid, glutathione, sulphates, or amino acids. The more formed hydrophilic metabolites are then eliminated via the bile or kidneys from the body.[22]

Various acute and chronic liver diseases (e.g., several viral infections, a single overdose of particular drugs, toxins, or alcohol), as well as several metabolic disorders (e.g., diabetes and hyperlipidemia) can affect the normal functions of the liver. The liver may become, if untreated, cirrhotic and eventually kill the patient due to liver failure or liver cancer.[20,21] Since the liver is the major drug uptake and metabolism organ in the body, it possesses various cell surface carriers, transport proteins, and metabolizing enzymes. These may be used as targets for the liver-specific drug delivery to improve the efficacy and safety of drug molecules. Although many drugs used in the treatment of liver diseases do reach the liver in sufficient amounts, they may cause unwanted extrahepatic adverse effects.

Targeting the liver by prodrugs

- Targeting either specific cell surface carriers and transporters, or by specific enzymes inside the hepatocytes capable of prodrug bioactivation.
- HepDirect® prodrugs utilize cytochrome P450 enzymes, especially CYP3A4, to activate cyclic phosph(on)-ate prodrugs.
- A few HepDirect prodrugs are advanced into the clinical trials.

13.2.1.1.1 Targeting Liver-Specific Receptors

The most widely studied liver-specific drug delivery strategy is based on antibodies and macromolecules that are conjugated with an acid-labile covalent bond to the drug molecules. These prodrugs bind to the liver-specific receptors and are delivered by receptor-mediated endocytosis into the hepatocytes, where the parent drug molecules are liberated. The asialoglycoprotein (ASGP) receptor, located on the hepatocyte membrane, can recognize galactose or N-acetylgalactosamine residues of desialylated glycoproteins, and therefore, can be exploited for liver-specific drug delivery.[23–26] However, despite the extended studies and wide variety of macromolecules that have been explored with several (e.g., anti-viral) drugs to target the ASGP receptor, no such liver-specific prodrug has proceeded into clinical trials to date. Poor oral bioavailability, immunogenicity, chemical instability, and manufacturing difficulties have largely limited the use of these pharmaceutical carriers.

Furthermore, the reduced expression of the ASGP receptor in the liver diseases, the low internalization rate of the ASGP receptor, and the limited intrahepatic conversion of the prodrug to the active drug molecule may limit the use of this liver-specific drug delivery approach in the future.[27]

13.2.1.1.2 Targeting Liver-Specific Transporters

An alternative strategy for the liver-specific uptake of drugs relies on transporter proteins expressed on the surface of the liver cells. The prodrugs recognized by transporters are delivered into the hepatocytes and biotransformed to the active drug molecules by nonspecific enzymes. For example, sodium-taurocholate cotransporting polypeptide (NTCP) is a transport protein localized on the sinusoidal surface of the hepatocytes. NTCPs reabsorb produced bile acids, especially taurocholate, from the portal circulation into the hepatocytes.[28] Although a structurally related transporter, apical sodium-dependent bile acid transporter (ASBT), exists in the intestine, the NTCP may serve as a potential target for the liver-specific drug delivery.[29–32] Few studies have been reported to target the NTCPs by bile acid prodrugs. These include the cytostatic drug chlorambucil[33] and the 3-hydroxy-3-methylglutaryl coenzyme A (HMG CoA) reductase inhibitors lovastatin and HR 780.[34,35] However, this strategy has special limitations, such as the potential drug–drug interactions between the bile acid containing prodrugs and the drugs that use the NCTPs, and the decreased expression of the bile acid transporters and the subsequent reduced liver uptake of the bile acid prodrugs, in liver diseases.

13.2.1.1.3 Targeting Liver-Specific Enzymes

The most promising strategy involves targeting the liver-specific enzymes that biotransform the prodrugs to the active drug molecules in the hepatocytes. Liver-targeted prodrugs that are converted by cytochrome P450 (CYP) enzymes have been successfully developed during the last decades. CYP enzymes are a large class of heme-containing microsomal proteins that catalyze more than 40 different types of oxidation and reduction reactions of a great number of endogenous and exogenous substrates.[36] The liver is the predominant site for CYP-mediated reactions, although CYP enzymes are also expressed to a lesser extent in the intestine, kidney, brain, lung, testis, skin, and spleen. Within cells, CYP enzymes are mainly located in the endoplasmic reticulum.[37] More than 270 different CYP gene families are known today, with 18 of them identified in mammals.[38] CYPs can be classified into two functional groups: the ones that nonspecifically mediate the reactions of exogenous substrates, like drugs or chemicals (CYP forms in families 1, 2, and 3) and the ones with specific roles in the metabolism of endogenous substrates, such as steroid hormones and fatty acids (CYP forms in families 4, 5, 7, 8, 11, 17, 19, 21, 24, 27, 51).[36,38–40] Xenobiotic metabolizing CYPs have a wide substrate specificity, e.g., substrates can range in size from Mw 28 (ethylene) to Mw 1201 (cyclosporine A); whereas the CYP enzymes that metabolize endogenous compounds have a very strict substrate specificity.[38,41,42] The general features that characterize the usually lipophilic substrates of different CYP enzymes are listed in Table 13.1.[43] Since CYP enzymes convert drug substances into inactive metabolites, they can similarly be utilized to convert prodrugs into active drugs. However, when targeting CYP enzymes, special attention should be paid to potential species-related and patient-related specificities, genetic polymorphisms, and drug–drug interactions during development phases.[14]

There are several challenges in designing CYP-activated prodrugs because the crystal structures of most of the CYP enzymes are yet to be determined. Presently, drug design strategies are based on the knowledge of the substrate structure and the enzyme's mechanism of action.[39] The desired CYP-mediated activation of the prodrug depends to a great extent on the properties of the parent molecule and the structure of the prodrug promoiety. Finding a suitable and functioning prodrug structure does not guarantee success in developing a new CYP-activated prodrug. Despite these limitations, several liver-specific CYP-activated prodrugs have been successfully developed and some of them have advanced to clinical trials. One recent development to improve the local activation of CYP-activated prodrugs is the use of specific enzyme antibodies (ADEPT) or enzyme encoding genes (GDEPT).

The knowledge of CYP-catalyzed bioconversion mechanisms of anticancer prodrugs cyclophosphamide (CPA), ifosfamide (IFA), and trofosfamide led to the development of cyclic phosphate and

TABLE 13.1

Characteristics of Some of the Human Xenobiotic Metabolizing CYP Enzyme Substrates

CYP Form	Characteristics
1A2	Planar, neutral, or basic molecules
2A6	Relatively small, neutral molecules, usually with one aromatic ring
2B6	Angular, medium-sized, neutral, or basic molecules with 1–2 hydrogen bond donors/acceptors
2C8	Relatively large, acidic or neutral, elongated molecules
2C9	Medium-sized, acidic molecules with 1–2 hydrogen bond acceptors
2C19	Medium-sized, basic molecules with 2–3 hydrogen bond acceptors
2D6	Medium-sized, basic molecules with protonatable nitrogen 5–7 Å from the site of metabolism
2E1	Structurally diverse, small, neutral molecules
3A4	Structurally diverse, large molecules

Source: Lewis, D.F. and Dickins, M., *Drug Discov. Today*, 7, 918, 2002.

phosphonate prodrugs, which all show effective CYP-catalyzed oxidative cleavage reactions to their corresponding parent drugs as well as high liver-specific drug delivery.[27,44–49] The prodrugs, called HepDirect prodrugs (Metabasis Therapeutics, San Diego, California), are substituted cyclic 1,3-propanyl esters of phosphates and phosphonates that undergo CYP-catalyzed oxidation predominantly in the liver. Originally, HepDirect prodrugs were designed and applied to nucleosides, which are widely used for the treatment of viral infections and leukemia. In order to inhibit viral replication and cell proliferation, the nucleosides need to be bioconverted to nucleoside triphosphates (NTPs). The poor intracellular bioconversion of nucleosides to nucleoside monophosphates (NMPs) can be enhanced by cyclic phosphate prodrugs. The C4 aryl substituent in the ring renders prodrugs sensitive to the hydroxylation of the C4 methine, the benzylic carbon atom adjacent to a phosph(on)ate oxygen, which is catalyzed specifically by CYP3A4 (Figure 13.2). Hydroxylation results in an irreversible ring opening and the formation of a transient intermediate, which is a negatively charged form. A subsequent β-elimination reaction releases the phosphate or phosphonate, and an aryl vinyl ketone as a byproduct. The anionic intermediate and product after prodrug cleavage have poor diffusion across cell membranes. They are, therefore, retained in the hepatocytes, which augments the liver specificity. The highly electrophilic aryl vinyl ketone, which, along with other vinyl ketones, is associated with significant toxicity, is rapidly detoxified by intracellular glutathione as long as the glutathione levels remain at 20% of normal liver levels (0.5–1 mM). Structure–activity relationship (SAR) studies have shown that the C4 aryl group is essential for efficient prodrug cleavage, most likely due to the increased susceptibility of benzylic hydrogens to CYP-catalyzed oxidation.[44] The cleavage rates were clearly dependent on the relative configuration between C4 and phosphorus but less dependent on the absolute configuration at C4 or the NMP. Furthermore, different electron withdrawing aryl substituents, such as chlorine in the *meta*-position of the C4 aryl ring or pyridine, enhanced the cleavage of aryl vinyl ketone.

The particular limitations of this prodrug approach may be the potential bioactivation of the prodrug in the intestine, since the CYP3A4 is also expressed in the intestinal epithelia, as well as possible changes in the CYP3A4 levels in the diseased liver. However, studies in rats and monkeys have shown that the nonhepatic metabolism of the HepDirect prodrug pradefovir is only marginal and is accompanied by elevated levels of adefovir and its metabolites in the liver.[27]

Three aryl substituted cyclic phosphonate prodrugs have advanced to clinical trials. These are pradefovir (MB06866, remofovir), MB07133, and MB07811 (Figure 13.3), which are prodrugs of adefovir (PMEA), cytarabine (araC), and a thyroid receptor agonist, MB07344, respectively.[27,44–47,49] Pradefovir was developed to improve the therapeutic potential of the hepatitis B virus (HBV) prodrug,

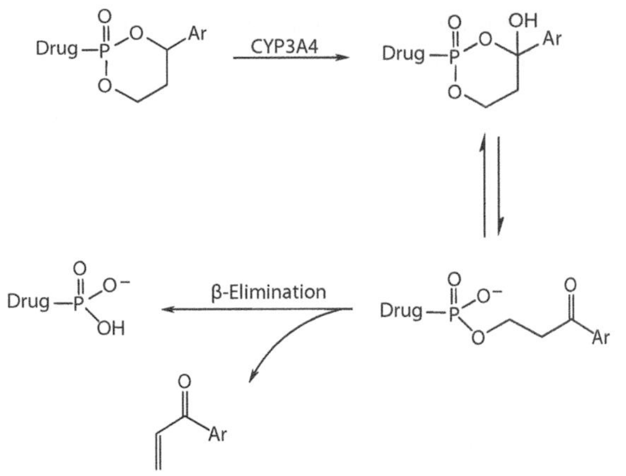

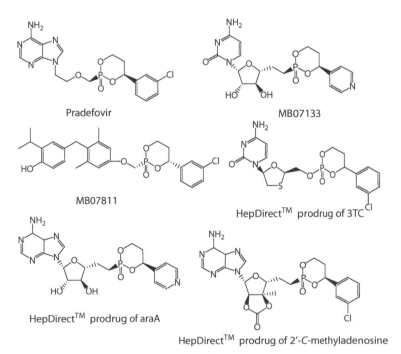

FIGURE 13.2 Conversion of HepDirect prodrugs to the corresponding phosphates or phosphonates and aryl vinyl ketone after a CYP3A4-catalyzed hepatic oxidation and consequent ring-opening and β-elimination. (From Erion, M.D. et al., *J. Am. Chem. Soc.*, 126, 5154, 2004.)

adefovir dipivoxil (Hepsera, Gilead Sciences, Foster City, California).[50] Adefovir dipivoxil is a bispivaloyloxymethyl (POM) prodrug of PMEA and is cleaved nonspecifically by esterases in the body. The phase III clinical studies have revealed that the exposure of PMEA to the kidneys and the subsequent kidney toxicity limits the use of adefovir dipivoxil. In contrast, the HepDirect prodrug pradefovir has a higher liver/kidney and liver/intestine targeting ratio relative to adefovir dipivoxil in rats and monkeys. In patients with hepatitis B, pradefovir has demonstrated good efficacy combined with the low systemic adefovir levels. Currently, pradefovir is undergoing phase II clinical trials for the treatment of hepatitis B infection (see Refs. [51,52] for reviews).[51,52] The cyclic 1-aryl-1,3-propanyl phosphonate prodrug, MB07133, of the anti-leukemic agent araC is also currently undergoing clinical evaluation.

FIGURE 13.3 Structures of HepDirect prodrugs in clinical trials, pradefovir, MB07133, and MB07811, and the investigational HepDirect prodrugs of 3TC, araA and 2′-*C*-methyladenosine.

AraC is converted to cytarabine triphosphate (araCTP) via cytarabine monophosphate (araCMP) mainly in the leukemic cells, but to a lesser extent also in the bone marrow cells, which results in bone marrow toxicity. On the contrary, the HepDirect prodrug MB07133 is bioactivated to araCTP in the hepatocytes, effluxed into the circulation, and transported directly into the leukemic cells. Studies in rodents have shown that with MB07133, the araCTP levels are much higher in the liver and are unsubstantial in the bone morrow, since there is no CYP3A4 activity in the bone marrow.

The HepDirect prodrug approach has also been applied to the antihyperlipidemic drug MB07344, the antiviral agents lamivudine (3CT) and vidarabine (araA), and the antiviral compound 2′-C-methyladenosine together with the 2′,3′-carbonate prodrug promoiety (Figure 13.3).[44,46,48,53]

13.2.1.2 Targeting Tumor Tissue

Cancer is characterized as a group of diseases with an uncontrolled proliferative growth and spread of abnormal tumor cells. Despite the fact that the first cancer chemotherapy agents were discovered over 60 years ago, it is still an increasing health problem and one of the leading causes of death worldwide.[54]

Numerous anti-tumor drugs have been developed that are available for the treatment of cancer. However, the anticancer drugs are often highly active and their clinical utility is limited due to systemic toxicity. The current chemotherapeutic agents cannot selectively differentiate their DNA replication and cell division interrupting actions between neoplastic and normal cells. Therefore, the unwanted damage of proliferating healthy cells, such as those in bone marrow, becomes one of their major problems.[55] Many antitumor drugs also possess a narrow therapeutic index, indicating that there is only a minor difference between the dose needed for therapeutic response and the dose causing potentially life-threatening adverse effects.[56] In addition, the tumors often develop resistance against anticancer drugs because of the up-regulation of multidrug resistance efflux pumps, increased glutathione S-transferase (GST) expression, and enhanced DNA-repair.[57]

One feasible strategy for overcoming the adverse effects and achieving more tumor-selective cancer treatment is the development of less toxic prodrug derivatives of anti-tumor agents that can be activated by a specific, tumor-selective enzyme in the tumor tissue. Ideally, the potential target enzyme for tumor-activated prodrug design should possess the following characteristics:[58]

- The tumor-targeted prodrug activating enzyme or enzyme family should be well characterized and have a known role in tumor phenotype, development, or progression.
- The expression of the prodrug activating enzyme should be significantly elevated in the tumor tissue compared with normal tissue, and it should have activity in the tumor environment.
- The activity of the enzyme should be minimal or lacking from nontumoral sites, including patient serum.
- The appropriate target-enzyme should possess a high catalytic activity for the investigational tumor-targeted prodrug derivative and the ability to selectively and rapidly activate the prodrug at the tumor tissue.

Targeting the tumor by prodrugs

Tumors over-express a number of enzymes, which can be exploited for tumor targeting by the following:

- Being rapidly activated by a target enzyme, which has no or only minimal expression in nontumoral tissues
- Not be activated at sites distant from the tumor
- Be less toxic than the parent anti-tumor drug
- Retain in tumor-tissue for a time-period that is sufficient to induce tumor cell death

---

Several classes of prodrug candidates have been developed to be activated in the tumor tissue by exploiting either the unique tumor-specific enzymes or the significant over-expression of a specific enzyme between the tumor and the healthy cells. Numerous endogenous target enzymes have been utilized for the local activation of these anti-tumor prodrugs (Table 13.2). The potential tumor-associated enzymes with examples of anticancer prodrugs utilizing the catalytic action of these enzymes are briefly outlined in the following sections.

TABLE 13.2
Endogenous Tumor-Associated Enzymes That Can Be Utilized in Local Activation of Anti-Tumor Prodrugs

Enzyme	Main Function	Main Expression	References
Oxidoreductases			
Amino acid oxidase	Oxidative deamination of amino acids	Kidney, liver	Rooseboom et al. [213]
Cytochrome P450 reductase[a]	One-electron reduction of cytochrome P450s	Variety of tissues; may be elevated in liver cancer tissue	Guise et al. [73]
DT-diaphorase[a]	Two-electron reduction of several substrates, *incl.*, quinones	Variety of tissues; strongly elevated in tumor tissue	Joseph et al. [214]
Cytochrome P450[a]	Catalyses several types of oxidation reactions	Variety of tissues; different levels in tumors	Chen et al. [215]
Tyrosinase	Oxidation of L-tyrosine to dopaquinone	Melanocytes and melanoma cells	Pawelek et al. [91]; Jordan et al. [93,94]
Transferases			
Thymidine phosphorylase	Phosphorolysis of thymidine to thymine and deoxyribose-1-phosphate	Variety of tissues; markedly elevated in tumors, particularly in hypoxic areas of solid tumors	Ackland and Peters [104]
Glutathione-*S*-transferase	Conjugation of GSH to electrophiles	Virtually in all tissues; P1-1 over-expressed in tumors	Mahajan and Atkins [95]; Tew [216]
Lyases			
Cysteine conjugate β-lyase	β-Elimination of various cysteine *S*-conjugates	Liver, kidney; increased in renal carcinoma	Nelson et al. [217]
Proteases			
Cathepsin B	Protein turnover within lysosomes	Lysosomes; high levels in tumors	Roshy et al. [218]
Prostate-specific antigen	Peptide bond cleavage in proteins	Selectively expressed in prostate cancer; active only in prostate cancer tissue	Lilja [219]
Plasmin	Peptide bond cleavage in fibrin network, Cleavage of extracellular matrix and basement membrane molecules	Blood circulation (inactive); bound in tumor cell surface (active)	Ellis et al. [220]; Irigoyen et al. [221]
uPa[b]	Cleavage of plasminogen to active plasmin	Various tissues, elevated in malignant tumors	Andreasen [222]; Wang [223]
Matrix metalloproteinases	Cleavage of extracellular matrix proteins	Minimally expressed in normal physiological conditions; elevated in malignant tumors	Skrzydlewska et al. [224]

[a] Utilized predominantly in development of *bioreductive prodrugs* that are activated by enzyme under hypoxic conditions.

[b] Urokinase plasminogen activator.

13.2.1.2.1 Hypoxia-Associated Reductive Enzymes

Many solid tumors are characterized with abnormal vasculature, which leads to hypoxia and reduced nutrient delivery to the tissue. The low oxygen content increases the tumor resistance to drug or radiation therapy and favors tumor progression.[59,60] This hypoxic state of solid tumors can be, however, turned to therapeutic advantage by designing cytotoxic prodrugs that are converted to the active drug in a hypoxic environment of tumor tissue, thus leaving the healthy well vascularized tissues unaffected. In designing the hypoxia-selective cytotoxic prodrugs, functionalities, such as quinones, *N*-oxides, and aromatic nitro groups that are readily reduced by endogenous reductive enzymes are usually incorporated in the active anti-tumor drug. Even though the bioreductive enzymes are often expressed in a variety of tissues, the hypoxia-specific activation of anti-tumor drugs can still be obtained since the reduction intermediate is rapidly re-oxidized back to the inactive prodrug in the oxygen-rich healthy tissues. In hypoxic solid tumors, this oxidation is significantly slower and results in higher concentrations of the active anticancer agent. Examples of reductive enzymes that have been successfully exploited in the bioreversible activation of anti-tumor prodrugs include cytochrome P450 reductase and cytochrome P450s (Table 13.2).

13.2.1.2.1.1   Cytochrome P450 Reductase   Cytochrome P450 reductase is the only flavoprotein that donates electrons to all microsomal cytochrome P450 enzymes for oxidation of their substrates. This one-electron reductase is located in endoplasmic reticulum. It is capable of reducing aldehydes to the corresponding alcohols and quinones to semiquinone free radicals, which are readily and automatically oxidized back to the parent quinone and superoxide anion in the presence of oxygen. These reductive reactions may occur directly or via CYP450s. Cytochrome P450 reductase is widely present in human tissues, but some variation in its levels between tumor versus normal tissue has been reported.[61–63]

Mitomycin C is a naturally occurring, potential bioreductive alkylating agent that was not originally designed as a prodrug. After clinical use for almost a decade, it was observed that the hypoxic tumor environment facilitated its activation.[64] Mitomycin C itself cannot attack DNA, but the reduction of quinone functionality triggers the formation of semiquinone radical anion, which covalently binds with DNA (Figure 13.4). In the presence of oxygen, the free semiquinone radical is oxidized back to inactive mitomycin C, thereby giving some selectivity toward hypoxic tissues.[65] Cytochrome P450 reductase has been reported as the predominant enzyme involved in the biore-duction of mitomycin C; although other bioreductive enzymes, such as DT-diaphorase, also seem to play an important role in the activation of mitomycin C.[62,64,66]

Another natural alkylating anticancer agent, porfiromycin (Figure 13.5), also requires biore-ductive activation prior to its cytotoxic action toward tumor cells. Porfiromycin is a methylated

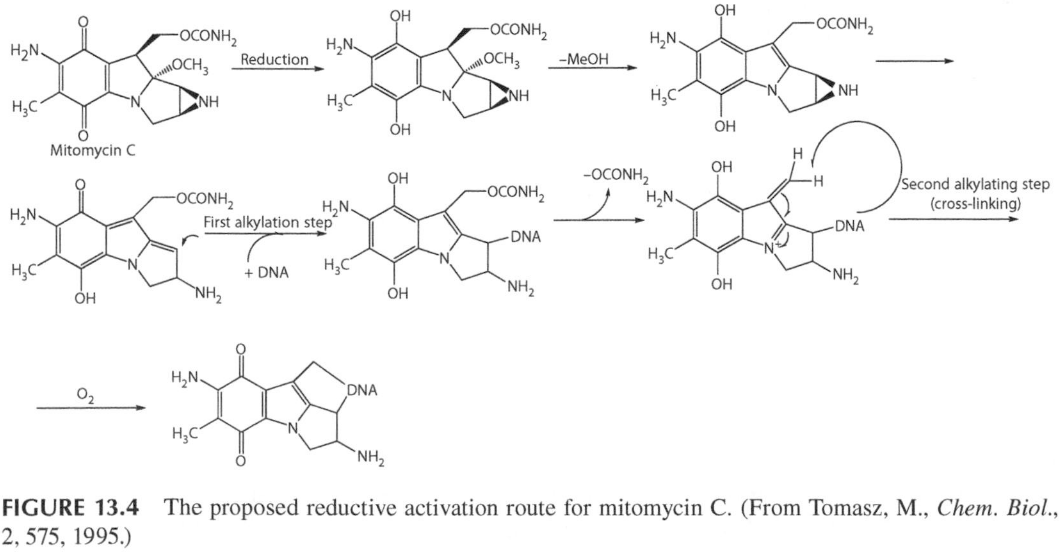

FIGURE 13.4   The proposed reductive activation route for mitomycin C. (From Tomasz, M., *Chem. Biol.*, 2, 575, 1995.)

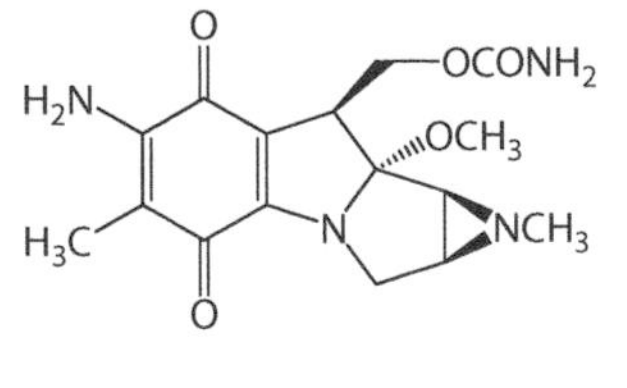

FIGURE 13.5 Chemical structure of mitomycin C-analogue porfiromycin.

derivative of mitomycin C that shows an enhanced toxicity toward hypoxic cells; but is less toxic to cells under aerobic conditions, indicating greater hypoxia selectivity. The increased selectivity of porfiromycin has been related to its preferential activation by cytochrome P450 reductase, in which DT-diaphorase plays a less important role.[67]

The bioreductive reaction catalyzed by cytochrome P450 reductase is also involved in the activation of tirapazamine (SR-4233), a heteroaromatic N-oxide, which is an extensively studied anticancer prodrug.[68,69] In the hypoxic environment, one-electron reduction of tirapazamine yields a highly reactive, cytotoxic free radical intermediate that can attack tumor DNA (Figure 13.6), prior to its reduction to a nontoxic metabolite.[70] In the presence of oxygen, the unstable, free radical intermediate can be rapidly oxidized back to the inactive parent prodrug with the concomitant generation of moderately cytotoxic superoxide radicals and other reactive oxygen species that mediate the anticancer effects of tirapazamine under aerobic conditions.[70,71]

The first hypoxia-activated nitrogen mustard alkylating agent, PR-104, is currently undergoing phase II clinical studies for small cell lung cancer (http://clinicaltrials.gov/ct2/show/NCT00544674, sponsored by Proacta Inc.). The activation of this novel dinitrobenzamide mustard is preceded by systemic cleavage of the water-soluble phosphate ester by phosphatases to yield the corresponding more lipophilic alcohol metabolite, PR-104A, which acts as a hypoxia-activated anti-tumor prodrug.[72] In the hypoxic regions of the tumor, the 5-nitro group of PR-104A is reduced selectively by cytochrome P450 reductase to the corresponding hydroxylamine (PR-104H), which exerts cytotoxic effects through the formation of DNA interstrand cross-links. Subsequently, PR-104H is reduced to its 5-amine metabolite (PR-104M) (Figure 13.7).[72,73] Albeit the cytochrome P450 reductase has the predominant role in the bioreductive activation of PR-104A, other intratumoral flavoenzymes may also contribute to its activation pathway.[72]

13.2.1.2.1.2 DT-Diaphorase   DT-Diaphorase (NAD(P)H:Quinone oxidoreductase) is a cytosolic two-electron transfer flavoprotein that catalyses the reduction of quinones to corresponding hydroquinones. This enzyme is present in virtually all mammalian tissues. Interestingly, its levels are

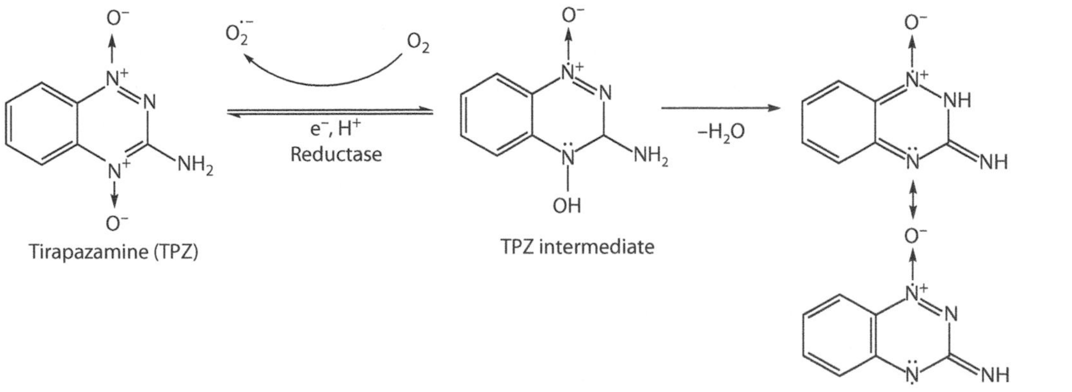

FIGURE 13.6 Suggested enzymatic activation mechanism for tirapazamine. Under aerobic conditions, TPZ radical is back-oxidized to inactive tirapazamine. (From Elwell, J.H. et al., *Biochem. Pharmacol.*, 54, 249, 1997.)

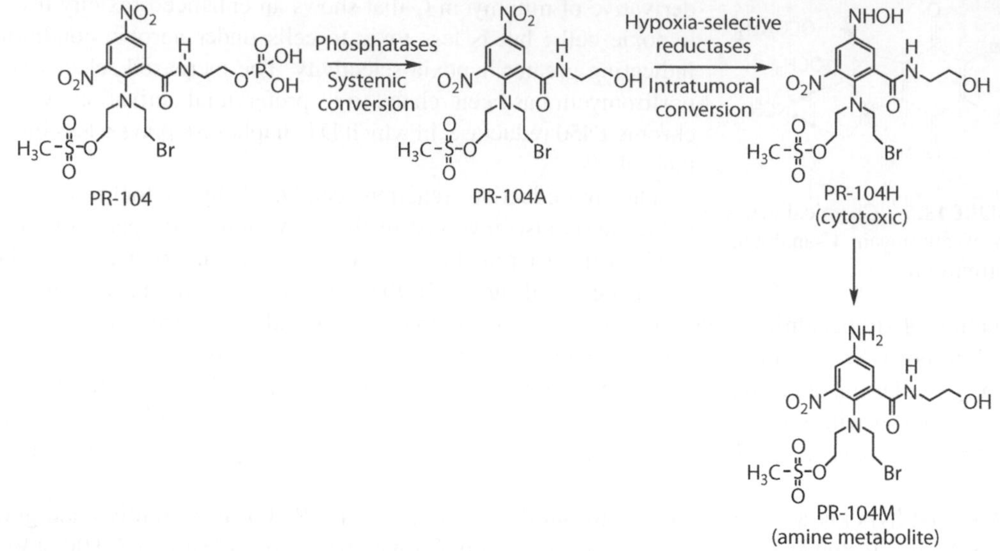

FIGURE 13.7 Two-step enzymatic cleavage of PR-104 to form an active cytotoxic drug PR-104H, and, subsequently, its metabolite, PR-104M. (From Guise, C.P. et al., *Biochem. Pharmacol.*, 74, 810, 2007.)

significantly elevated in certain cancer tissues, including breast, colon, liver, bladder, stomach, central nervous system (CNS), and lung tumors, as well as in melanomas. In human tissues, the majority of DT-diaphorase activity is accounted for by the enzyme NADPH:quinone oxidoreductase-1 (NQO1).[66,74,75]

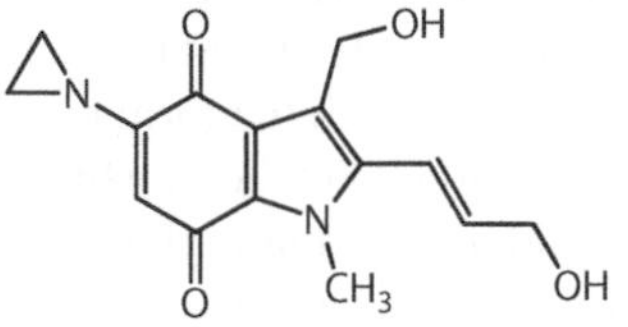

Research in the area of quinone-containing alkylating agents, such as mitomycin C and porfiromycin, led to the synthesis of novel indoloquinone compounds, including apaziquone (EO-9) (Figure 13.8).[76] Apaziquone is a bioreductive anticancer prodrug that generates a highly oxygen-sensitive drug radical and other

FIGURE 13.8 Chemical structure of alkylating antitumor prodrug apaziquone (EO-9).

reactive oxygen species after activation by intracellular reductases.[77–79] The mechanism of activation of apaziquone is not yet completely clear. Apaziquone is a good substrate for DT-diaphorase (NQO1), which is assumed to be the main enzyme involved in its activation under aerobic conditions.[78] However, cytochrome P450 reductase may also contribute to the antitumor activity of apaziquone in hypoxic cells.[79] Earlier, apaziquone failed to demonstrate clinical efficacy in phase II studies after intravenous administration.[80] Recently, its intravesical formulation has entered phase III clinical trials for noninvasive bladder cancer (EOquin®) (http://www.spectrumpharm.com/eoquin.html, Spectrum Pharmaceuticals, Inc.).

CB1954 is an anticancer prodrug that requires the reduction of its 2- or 4-nitro group prior to cytotoxic action (Figure 13.9). Additionally, both nitro groups of CB1954 can be metabolized to the corresponding hydroxylamine derivatives, which can further transform to amines by two-electron reduction. The most cytotoxic metabolite of CB1954 is the 5-(aziridin-1-yl)-4-hydroxyamino-2-nitrobenzamide, which can react with acetyl coenzyme A to produce a highly reactive nitrenium intermediate.[81] Other metabolites may also contribute to the cytotoxic DNA cross-linking action of CB1954.[82] The bioactivation of CB 1954 occurs by the reductive DT-diaphorase enzyme NQO2, whose activity is related to the expression of NQO1.[83] Other reductive enzymes such as rat NQO1, nitric oxide synthases (NOS), and nitroreductase also metabolize CB1954.[84–86]

Other anticancer drugs that are activated through bioreductive reaction by DT-diaphorase include diaziquone and streptonigrin (Figure 13.10). The enzymatic two-electron reduction of diaziquone

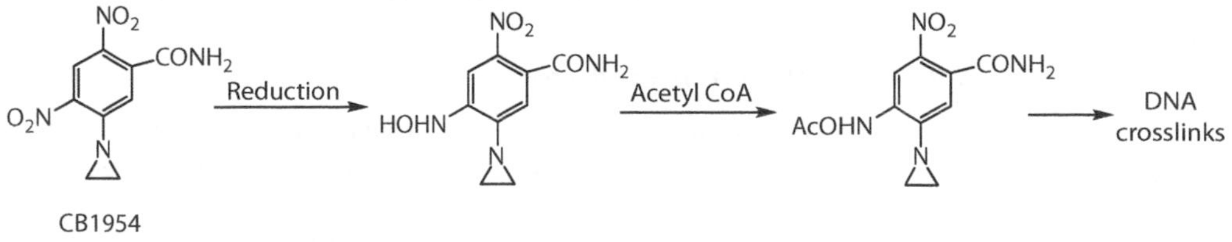

FIGURE 13.9 Activation of CB1954 to a cytotoxic intermediate by enzyme-catalyzed reduction of the 4-nitro group. (From Helsby, N.A. et al., *Br. J. Cancer*, 90, 1084, 2004.)

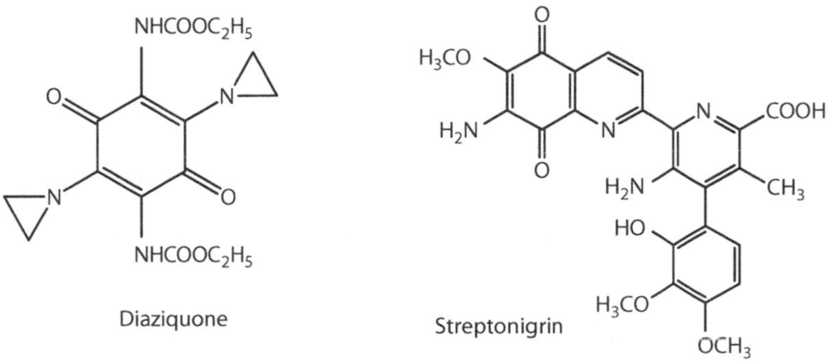

FIGURE 13.10 Chemical structures of DT-diaphorase-activated anticancer drugs, diaziquone and streptonigrin.

yields the corresponding hydroquinone, which can auto-oxidize in the presence of molecular oxygen to cytotoxic semiquinone radical and reactive oxygen species.[57]

13.2.1.2.1.3 Cytochrome P450s Cytochrome P450s (CYP450s) are a diverse superfamily of heme-containing enzymes that catalyze several types of reactions including the hydroxylation of alkanes to alcohols, the conversion of alkenes to epoxides, arenes to phenols, sulfides to sulfoxides or sulfones, and the oxidative split of C–N, C–O, C–C, or C–S bonds.[39] The CYP450 enzyme system is present in all mammalian tissues, with the highest levels observed in the liver. Members of CYP families 1, 2, and 3 have been identified in both healthy and cancerous extrahepatic tissues. Additionally, a tumor-selective expression of CYP1B1 and CYP2W1 has been reported.[87,88] The CYP enzymes can metabolize thousands of endogenous as well as exogenous compounds, and they are the major enzyme system involved in drug metabolism (see characteristic features of main CYP enzyme substrates in Table 13.1 and prodrugs explored for cancer treatment in Table 13.3).

Although CYP450s activate several anticancer prodrugs, most of them were originally not designed as prodrugs (Table 13.3). AQ4N (banoxantrone) (Figure 13.11) is a novel *N*-oxide prodrug of the active topoisomerase II inhibitor, AQ4. The activation of AQ4N is not targeted to a specific CYP isoenzyme, but local CYP expression is required for its activation. AQN4 is reduced to its active basic amine, AQ4, in the hypoxic tumor environment by CYP3A4, CYP1A, and CYP1B1.[89] A recent phase I study indicated a tumor-targeted and hypoxia-selective action of AQN4 in patients with advanced solid tumors.[90] AQ4N is currently under clinical development by Novacea Inc.

13.2.1.2.2 Other Tumor-Specific Enzymes

13.2.1.2.2.1 Tyrosinase Tyrosinase is an extracellular phenol oxidase that participates in the biosynthesis of melanin and other pigments. Tyrosinase catalyses the oxidation of *o*-phenols, such as L-tyrosine, to the corresponding *o*-quinones. This enzyme is naturally present in melanocytes and melanoma cells. Tyrosinase genes upregulate in malignancy, resulting in increased tyrosinase levels in cancerous cells.[91,92] The unique localization of tyrosinase makes it an interesting target

TABLE 13.3

Examples of CYP-Activated Anti-Tumor Prodrugs

Anticancer Prodrug	Active Cytotoxic Drug	CYP Isoforms Involved in Activation
4-Ipomeanol	Unidentified (highly reactive electrophile)	**CYP1A2**, CYP3A3, CYP3A4, CYP2F1, CYP4B1
Tegafur (ftorafur)	5-FU	**CYP1A2**, **CYP2A6**, CYP2C8, CYP2E1, CYP3A5
Dacarbazine	5-(3-Hydroxymethyl-3-methyltriazen-1-yl)-imidazole-4-carboxamide (MHHTIC)	CYP1A1, **CYP1A2**, CYP2E1
Cyclophosphamide	Phosphoramide mustard	CYP2B6, CYP2C, CYP3A4
Trofosfamide	Trofosfamide mustard	CYP2B6, **CYP3A4**
Ifosfamide	Isophophamide mustard	CYP2A6, CYP2B6, **CYP3A4**, CYP3A5, CYP2C9/18/19
AQ4N	AQ4	CYP1A1, CYP2B6, **CYP3A4**
Thiotepa	N,N',N''-Triethylenephosphoramide (TEPA)	CYP3B6, CYP3A

Source: Adapted from Rooseboom, M. et al., *Pharmacol. Rev.*, 56, 53, 2004; Purnapatre et al., 2008.

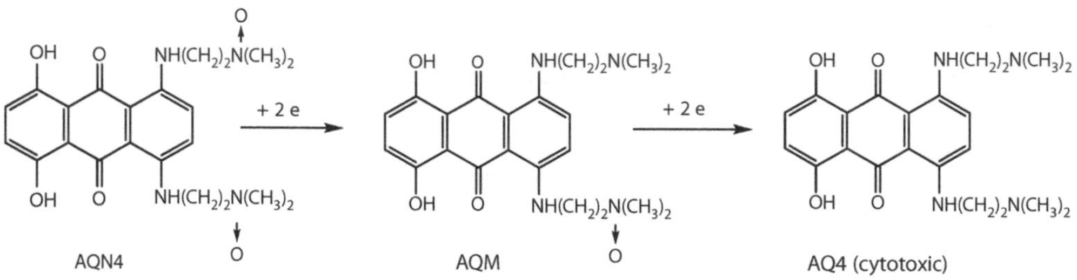

FIGURE 13.11 CYP450-catalyzed reduction of AQN4 to active anti-tumor drug, AQ4, through a formation of mono-*N*-oxide intermediate (AQM). (From Patterson, L.H. and McKeown, S.R., *Br. J. Cancer*, 83, 1589, 2000.)

enzyme for the activation of antimelanoma prodrugs. This targeting approach is known as melano-cyte-directed enzyme prodrug therapy (MDEPT).[93]

Jordan et al. developed several tyrosinase activated prodrugs of known cytotoxic agents, phenyl mustard, bisethyl amine mustard, and daunomycin.[93,94] A tyrosinase substrate was incorporated into the active anticancer drug by the carbamate linkage. Of the all prodrug candidates investigated, [2′-(4″-hydroxyphenyl)ethyl] carbamic acid (**1**, Figure 13.12) and [2′-(3″,4″-dihydroxyphenyl)-ethyl] carbamic acid (**2**, Figure 13.12) esters of phenyl mustard, as well as urea-linked bis-(2-chloroethylamino)-4-hydroxyphenylaminomethanone (**3**, Figure 13.12) were the most efficient substrates for mushroom tyrosinase oxidation. Additionally, prodrugs **1** and **2** were able to release the active phenyl mustard drug in mushroom tyrosinase assay; however, the detection of active bisethyl amine mustard was not possible for compound **3** due to its instability in aqueous media.

13.2.1.2.2.2 Glutathione S-Transferase The GST are a family of dimeric phase II detoxification enzymes that catalyze the conjugation of glutathione to electrophiles in a wide range of xenobiotics, resulting in the formation of corresponding glutathione conjugates. GST are cytosolic enzymes present in all species and virtually in all tissues. Glutathione *S*-transferase pi (GST P1-1) is the predominant form in cancer cells, and its over-expression has frequently been reported in a variety of rat and human tumors, including carcinomas of the colon, esophagus, lung, kidney, ovary,

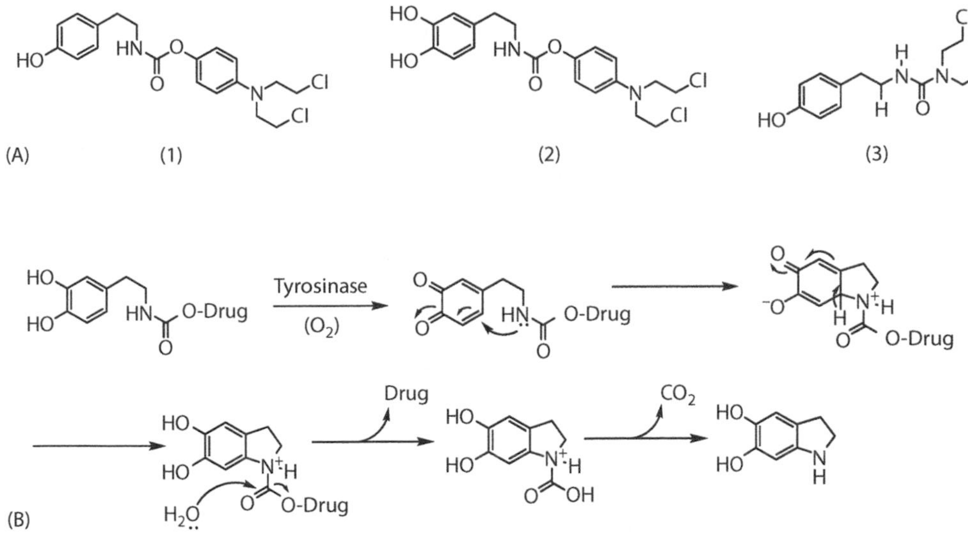

FIGURE 13.12 (A) Chemical structures of tyrosinase-activated anticancer prodrugs 1, 2, and 3. (B) The proposed mechanism for enzymatic drug release from prodrug 2. (From Jordan, A.M. et al., *Bioorg. Med. Chem.*, 9, 1549, 2001.)

pancreas, and stomach.[57,95] Furthermore, many tumors develop drug resistance by over-expressing GST enzymes. Drug resistance to alkylating agents, such as melphalan, clorambusil, and cyclophosphamide is associated with elevated levels of GST P1-1.[96]

A novel glutathione analog prodrug, canfosfamide (TLK286, formerly also TER286), exploits the tumor tissue over-expression of GST P1–1 in its cleavage to cytotoxic DNA alkylating phosphoroamidate mustard and vinyl sulfate derivative (Figure 13.13).[97,98] Cytotoxicity of canfosfamide correlates with GST P1-1 expression, i.e., the cells that have increased levels of GST P1-1 are more sensitive to the therapeutic effects of the prodrug.[99] Furthermore, the down-regulation of GST

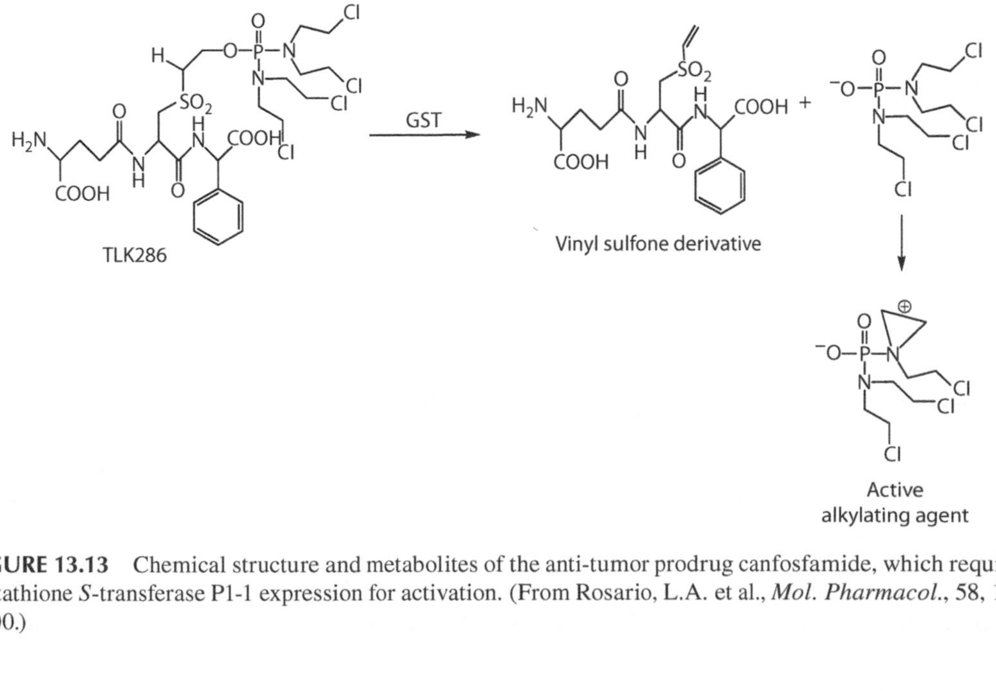

FIGURE 13.13 Chemical structure and metabolites of the anti-tumor prodrug canfosfamide, which requires glutathione *S*-transferase P1-1 expression for activation. (From Rosario, L.A. et al., *Mol. Pharmacol.*, 58, 167, 2000.)

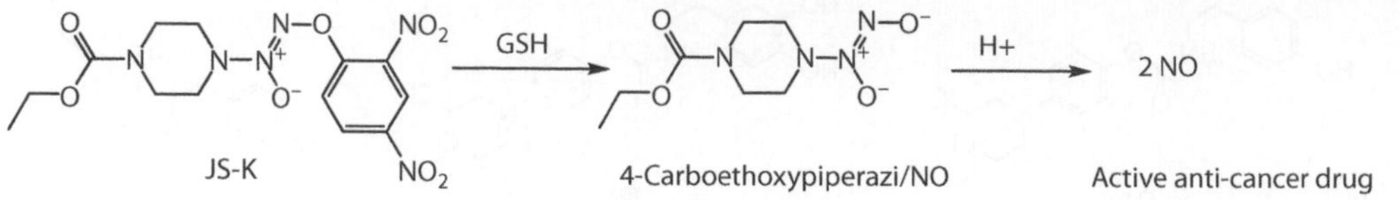

FIGURE 13.14 Glutathione *S*-transferase-dependent mechanism of nitric oxide (NO) release from antitumor prodrug JS-K. (From Chakrapani, H. et al., *Bioorg. Med. Chem. Lett.*, 18, 950, 2008.)

P1-1 by long-term chronic exposure to canfosfamide may also increase the therapeutic efficacy of other anti-tumor agents, to which the tumors may have developed GST-mediated drug resistance.[100] Canfosfamide showed clinical benefit in advanced non-small cell lung cancer and in platinium-resistant ovarian cancer.[100]

Another interesting example of GST-activated prodrugs is an O^2-aryl diazeniumdiolate compound, JS-K (Figure 13.14). JS-K is cleaved by GST in GST over-expressing cells to selectively release nitric oxide (NO), which can inhibit tumor growth.[101,102] The activation of JS-K occurs via a two-step reaction. First, the glutathione or another strong nucleophilic biomolecule is arylated with JS-K by GST to form 4-carboethoxypiperazi/NO, which subsequently releases NO spontaneously at physiological pH.[101] JS-K was shown to be effective against human leukemia, hepatoma, and prostate cancer *in vivo*.[101,103]

13.2.1.2.2.3 Thymidine Phosphorylase

Thymidine phosphorylase is a pentosyltransferase, which catalyses the reversible reaction of thymidine and phosphate to yield thymine and deoxyribose-1-phosphate. This enzyme also participates in the phosphorolytic cleavage of uridine and its derivatives. Thymidine phosphorylase is present in a wide variety of human tissues, and its levels are almost always increased in malignant tumor cells. A significant expression of thymidine phosphorylase was found in several tumors, including those of the colon, stomach, breast, cervix, bladder, and skin. Thymidine phosphorylase appears to be a poor prognostic factor in most tumors.[104]

Doxifluridine (5′-DFUR; Figure 13.15) is an orally administered anticancer prodrug that was developed to improve the tumor selectivity of an active antimetabolite drug, 5-fluorouracil (5-FU). The conversion of 5′-DFUR to active 5-FU occurs by thymidine phosphorylase, which is present in at least 10% of the elevated levels in many types of tumors compared with healthy normal tissue.[105] However, since thymidine phosphorylase also exists in intestinal tissue, the conversion of 5′-DFUR to 5-FU in the gastrointestinal tract caused dose-related diarrhea in clinical trials. This unwanted gastrointestinal toxicity limits its oral administration.[106,107]

A novel innovative fluoropyrimidine prodrug, capecitabine (Figure 13.15), was rationally developed to be more effective and to overcome the unwanted gastrointestinal adverse effects of 5′-DFUR. Capecitabine is activated to 5-FU through three reaction steps, which all are enzymatic. After rapid absorption from the gastrointestinal tract, capecitabine is first hydrolyzed to 5′-deoxy-5-fluorocytidine (5′-DFCR) in the liver by hepatic carboxylesterase. Subsequently, 5′-DFCR is converted into 5′-DFUR by cytidine deaminase either in the liver or in the tumor tissue. Finally, the release of cytotoxic 5-FU occurs selectively through thymidine phosphorylase at the tumor site.[105] Cabecitabine showed thymidine phosphorylase-dependent anti-tumor activity. It is currently approved for the treatment of metastatic colorectal cancer and breast cancer in over 70 countries worldwide.

13.2.1.2.3 Tumor-Associated Proteases

During metastases, the tumor cells escape from the primary tumors through the extracellular matrix, migrate and invade surrounding tissues; enter the vasculature, circulate, and reach secondary sites; extravasate, and establish metastatic loci.[108] Proteases are protein digesting enzymes that are capable of remodeling the extracellular matrix of encapsulated tumors, and thus play an important role in tumor invasion and metastasis.[109] Numerous tumor-associated proteases, such as

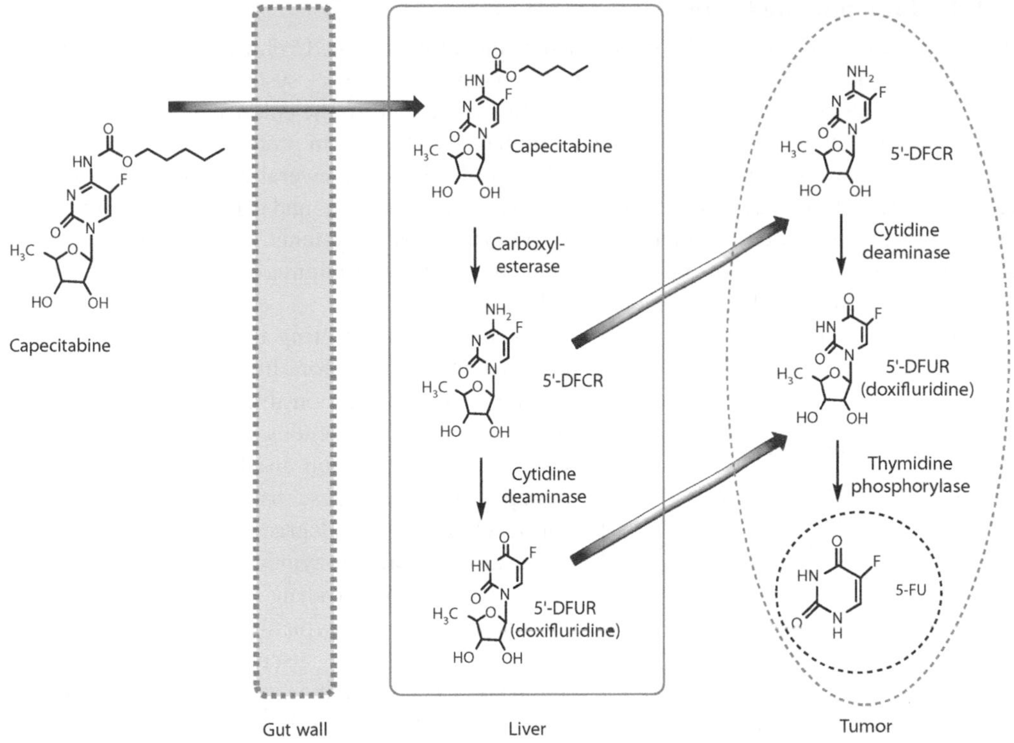

FIGURE 13.15 Three-step enzymatic activation of oral anticancer prodrug capecitabine to cytotoxic 5-FU.

cathepsins,[110] matrix metalloproteinases,[111] urokinase-type plasminogen activator (uPA),[112] plasmin,[113] prostate-specific antigen (PSA),[114] and other peptidases[115] have been exploited to design tumor-selective anticancer peptide prodrugs. Due to their elevated activity in the extracellular tumor environment and their ability to selectively cleave short peptide sequences, serine proteases, such as PSA, and matrix metalloproteinases, such as MMP-2 and MMP-9, comprise the most common target enzymes for tumor-activated macromolecular prodrug design (Figure 13.16).[58] The first results about the clinical evaluation of the PSA-activated doxorubicin peptide-conjugate prodrug L-377202 were published recently.[116] L-377202 was better tolerated than doxorubicin alone and was able to release its active metabolites leucine-doxorubicin and doxorubicinin in patients. However, additional studies are needed to confirm that L-377202 is active against prostate cancer and whether its active metabolites are targeted in tumor cells as compared with healthy cells.[116] An increased understanding of tumor-associated proteases will facilitate the discovery of novel target enzymes, protease substrates, and optimal substrate sequence requirements for individual proteases, which all are crucial for the development of entirely new tumor-associated protease-activated prodrugs.[58]

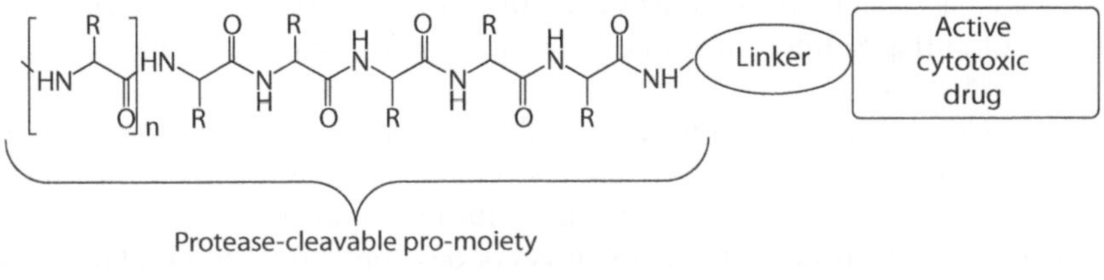

FIGURE 13.16 Schematic structure of tumor-associated protease-activated anticancer prodrugs. (Modified from Atkinson, J.M. et al., *Br. J. Pharmacol.*, 153, 1344, 2008.)

13.2.1.3 Targeting the Colon

There are a number of colonic disorders such as ulcerative colitis, Crohn's disease, and colorectal cancer that can be treated more efficiently by colon-specific delivery systems. Targeting drugs such as anti-inflammatory agents, antibiotics, and anticancer agents to the colon also have the advantage of fewer side-effects and improved patient compliance. Also, it can protect drugs from absorption and degradation in the upper gastrointestinal tract. To this end, several colon-targeting strategies have been explored, such as time-dependent formulations, pressure- and pH-sensitive polymers, and enzyme-activated drug delivery methods (e.g., prodrugs, coated systems, and hydrogel networks), in which the release of drug from systems is triggered by time, pressure, or pH change and specific enzymes present in the colon, respectively.[117,118]

The enzyme-activated drug delivery methods in colon targeting take advantage of certain enzymes present mainly in the colon. Colonic bacterial microflora produces various reductive enzymes that are responsible for the metabolism of endogenous and exogenous compounds that are not susceptible to digestion in the small intestine. For example, disaccharides, trisaccharides, and muco-polysaccharides are degraded to small saccharides by sugar-degrading enzymes produced by the colonic microflora.[119] The prodrug approaches for targeted colonic delivery are typically designed to contain a hydrophilic promoiety susceptible to cleavage by the bacterial enzymes such as azoreductase, glycosidases, and glucuronidases. Following oral administration, the absorption of the hydrophilic prodrug is decreased in the stomach and the small intestine; but within the colon, the more lipophilic parent drug gets liberated for site-specific absorption.[120] In the following sections, we describe some prodrugs of anti-inflammatory agents and steroids that are useful for the treatment of inflammatory bowel diseases (IBD).

> **Targeting the colon by prodrugs**
>
> - The aim is to protect drugs from absorption and degradation in the upper gastrointestinal tract but have them released site-specifically in the proximal colon.
> - Prodrugs typically contain a hydrophilic promoiety susceptible to cleavage by bacterial enzymes, such as azoreductase, glycosidases, and glucuronidases. The absorption of the hydrophilic prodrug is decreased in the stomach and the small intestine, but within the colon the more lipophilic parent drug is liberated and becomes available for site-specific absorption.
> - The best known colon-targeting prodrugs are azo-bond derivatives of 5-aminosalicylic acid (5-ASA).

13.2.1.3.1 Azo-Bond Prodrugs

The best known prodrugs that target the colon are azo-bond derivatives of 5-ASA—an anti-inflammatory drug used primarily for the treatment of IBD. These prodrugs are formed by attaching a hydrophilic promoiety to 5-ASA. They have very limited absorption from the upper gastrointestinal tract due to their polar nature, but are converted to their lipophilic constituent entities by azoreductases in the colon, produced by anaerobic colonic bacteria.[117]

One of the first prodrugs with site-specific activation in the colon, sulfasalazine, consists of 5-ASA bound to sulfapyridine by azo-linkage (Figure 13.17). After oral administration, only a small amount of the prodrug (3%–12%) is absorbed from the small intestine, and most of the dose reaches the colon.[121,122] In the colon, sulfasalazine is converted to 5-ASA and sulfapyridine by azoreductases associated with the bacterial microflora. However, this prodrug causes side-effects most likely due to the formation of sulfapyridine. Therefore, other less toxic carrier molecules (i.e., promoieties) were developed for 5-ASA.

In balsalazine (Colazal®), 4-amino benzoyl-β-alanine was used as the promoiety and *p*-aminohippurate (4-amino benzoyl glycine) was used in ipsalazine.[123] Balsalazine was therapeutically more effective than sulfasalazine in clinical trials with fewer side effects.[124] However, in spite of promising pharmacokinetic results, ipsalazine was not developed further. Olsalazine (Dipentum®) is a dimer of two 5-ASA molecules linked by an azo-bond. Olzalazine has very limited absorption

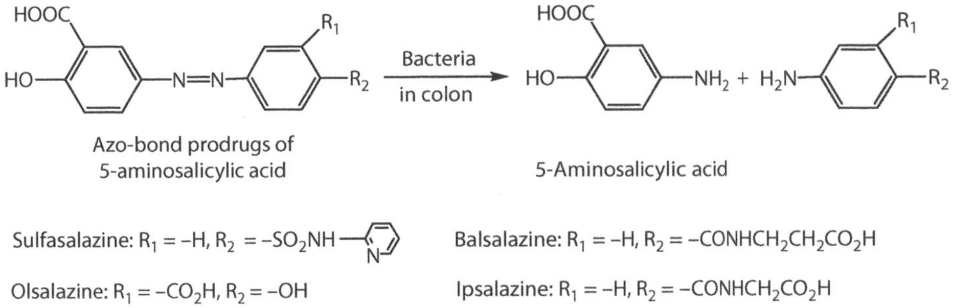

Sulfasalazine: R_1 = –H, R_2 = –SO$_2$NH—⟨N⟩   Balsalazine: R_1 = –H, R_2 = –CONHCH$_2$CH$_2$CO$_2$H

Olsalazine: R_1 = –CO$_2$H, R_2 = –OH   Ipsalazine: R_1 = –H, R_2 = –CONHCH$_2$CO$_2$H

FIGURE 13.17 Azo-bond prodrugs of 5-aminosalisylic acid (5-ASA).

from the small intestine, but releases two 5-ASA molecules per each olsalazine molecule by reduction in the colon.[125]

With the aim of reducing the absorption of prodrugs from the upper part of the intestine, various polymeric prodrugs with less cleavable, sterically hindered azo-bonds were considered for colon-targeted drug delivery. As the high molecular weight polymeric carrier is poorly absorbed, drugs linked to a polymeric backbone traverse the small intestine to the colon, where they are susceptible to absorption after azo-bond cleavage. Although these polymeric prodrugs can be delivered successfully to the colon intact, they tend to release the parent, active drug slowly, often resulting in poor therapeutic effect. Moreover, a very large amount of polymeric prodrug is needed for effective oral administration, reducing patient compliance. Several drug-polymer conjugates have been tested in preclinical species, with varying degrees of success. The water-soluble N-(2-hydroxypropyl) methacrylamide copolymer (HPMA polymer) conjugates are among the most studied. Readers are directed to the following references for further information.[117,126]

13.2.1.3.2 Glucuronide and Glycoside Prodrugs

Glucuronide formation is a major route for the metabolism of a variety of drugs to water-soluble conjugates. Moreover, several drugs can be conjugated with different sugar moieties resulting in the formation of glycosides. The reductive enzymes that are produced by colonic bacteria include, for example, β-glucuronidase and glycosidase, which can also degrade a variety of drugs. Both glucuronides and glycosides are hydrophilic conjugates and are generally poorly absorbed from the small intestine. Nevertheless, they are capable of undergoing degradation in the colon. Thus, glucuronide and glycoside prodrugs have been explored for their colon-targeting potential.[126]

Dexamethasone and prednisolone-21-β-D-glucosides and naloxone-, nalmefene-, budesonide-, and dexamethasone-β-D-glucuronides were evaluated for their colon-targeting potential.[127–130] *In vivo* studies in rats revealed that nearly 60% of the orally administered 21-β-D-glucosidic prodrug of dexamethasone reached the colon in the form of the free drug. In the case of prednisolone-β-D-glucoside, 15% of the dose reached the colon. When unmodified steroids were administered orally, they were absorbed from the small intestine, and less than 1% of the dose reached the colon. Moreover, *in vivo* studies in guinea pigs demonstrated that a lower dose of dexamethasone, as its glucoside prodrug, was needed to reduce the total number of ulcers, compared with the treatment with dexamethasone itself. Similarly, β-D-glucuronide prodrugs showed improved colon delivery compared with their parent drugs. Only 0.2%–0.5% of the dose of the narcotic antagonists, naloxone and nalmefene, administered in rats as glucuronide prodrugs was systemically absorbed. Moreover, the glucuronide prodrugs resulted in the delay of the onset of diarrhea caused by the parent drugs. Both are indirect evidences of colon targeting.[128] Also budesonide- and dexamethasone-β-D-glucuronides (Figure 13.18) showed colon targeting both in healthy and colitic rats—the delivery of dexamethasone from its prodrug was somewhat more effective compared with budesonide from its prodrug.[131] None of these prodrugs have, however, advanced to the clinic.

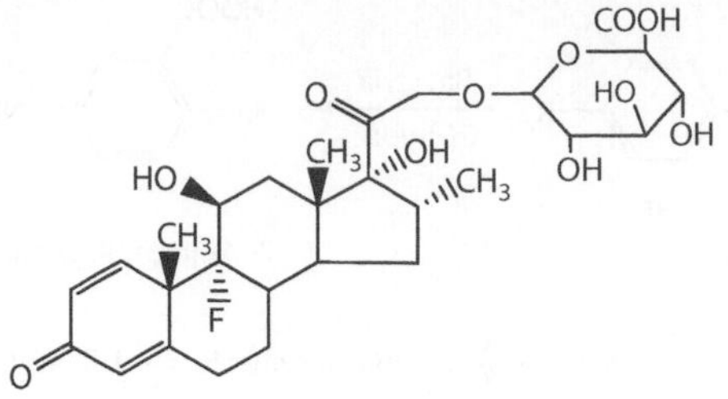

FIGURE 13.18 Dexamethasone-β-D-glucuronide.

13.2.1.3.3 Other Prodrugs

Other commonly explored colon-targeting promoieties in prodrug design are polysaccharides, such as cyclodextrins, and various amino acids. While cyclodextrins (cyclic oligosaccharides consisting of six to eight glucose units attached through α-1,4 glucosidic bonds) are typically used to form water-soluble inclusion complexes with drug molecules, they can also serve as hydrophilic carriers in colon-targeting prodrugs after a drug is covalently bound to one of the primary hydroxyl groups of the cyclodextrin molecule through a bioreversible bond.[126] This prodrug approach was utilized with the nonsteroidal anti-inflammatory drugs (NSAIDs) flurbiprofen, naproxen, and sulindac. These drugs were conjugated to the hydroxyl groups of both α-cyclodextrin (consists of six glucose units) and β-cyclodextrin (consists of seven glucose units).[132] Both flurbiprofen-cyclodextrin prodrugs were chemically stabile in the pH environment of the gastrointestinal tract, but were hydrolyzed to free flurbiprofen by the colonic enzymes. Furthermore, the β-cyclodextrin prodrug decreased the extent and severity of colonic damage in rats.

Similarly, various polar amino acids, such as aspartic acid and glutamic acid, have shown promising results as colon-targeting promoieties with minimal absorption and degradation in the upper gastrointestinal tract.[132,133] Common to both cyclodextrins and amino acids is their polar nature resulting in only negligible absorption in the passage through the stomach and small intestine and their ability to ferry their conjugate drugs to the colon.

13.2.1.4 Renal-Specific Prodrugs

While the liver is the most important metabolizing organ in the body, the kidneys are the major excretion ones.[134,135] The functional unit of the kidney is a nephron, in which four different process occur that contribute to renal clearance. These processes are (1) glomerular filtration (in the glomerulus), (2) active secretion (mainly in the proximal tubule), (3) passive reabsorption (mainly in the distal tubule), and (4) renal metabolism. Several diseases, such as nephritis, inherited polycystic kidney disease (PCKD), pyelonephritis, renovascular disease, diabetes mellitus, and obstructive nephropathy, can cause chronic kidney failure, which almost always progresses to a condition called end-stage renal failure (ESRF) and the kidneys stop working almost completely. Today, the only treatments for ESRF are dialysis or a kidney transplantation. Currently, several renal-specific prodrugs are at the preclinical stages of investigation.

Although all drugs are eventually excreted by the kidneys, many of them are inactivated before they reach the kidneys, and the drugs that reach the kidneys in active form may cause unwanted extrarenal adverse effects. Therefore, renal-specific prodrugs for targeting the kidneys may be useful in overcoming these limitations. The mesangial cells of the glomerulus and the proximal tubular cells are the primary choice of targets for renal-specific drug delivery, since they play a pivotal role in many kidney diseases.[136] To date, only a limited number of studies have focused on the drug delivery to the mesangial cells with a modest degree of selectivity, while more extensive research has been performed on targeting drugs to the proximal tubular cells. The proximal tubular cells are the most active cells in the kidneys, since they actively transport various endogenous and exogenous compounds from the blood into the urine and vice versa.[136] Furthermore, the proximal tubular cells are involved in phase I and II metabolism (i.e., the reactivation of substrates and the degradation of proteins and oligopeptides by lysosomal proteases).

13.2.1.4.1 Alkylylglucoside Prodrugs

The alkylylglucoside vector has been shown to be a kidney-specific drug delivery carrier for peptides.[137–139] The alkylylglucosides deliver therapeutic agents from the blood via the basolateral membrane of the proximal tubular cells. This renal targeting vector should have a hydrophobic group linked to the sugar moiety by a β-glycoside bond.[140] The therapeutic agents should be of moderate size and neutral charge.[137] However, more studies are needed to fully evaluate the potential of this renal-specific drug targeting method.

13.2.1.4.2 Amino Acid Prodrugs

Certain amino acid prodrugs can be delivered selectively into the proximal tubular cell where they are activated by specific enzymes, like γ-glutamyl transpeptidase at the brush border or the basolateral side of the proximal tubular cells or β-lyase, N-acetyl transferase, and L-amino acid decarboxylase on the cytosolic side of the proximal tubular cells. γ-Glutamyl-L-dopa (gludopa) (Figure 13.19) is a double prodrug that is activated specifically in the proximal tubular cells by γ-glutamyl transpeptidase and subsequently by L-amino acid decarboxylase. It may be used as a renal vasodilator,[141–143] although the oral bioavailability of gludopa may be unsubstantial.[144] Similarly, N-acyl-γ-glutamyl derivatives of sulfamethoxazole (Figure 13.19) and the vasodilative drug CGP 18137 (2-hydrazine-5-n-butyl pyridine) are selectively activated in the proximal tubular cells by the sequential action of the kidney-specific acylase and γ-glutamyl transpeptidase.[145–147] However, not every N-acyl-γ-glutamyl prodrug is transported into the proximal tubular cells, e.g., N-acyl-γ-glutamyl-4′-aminowarfarin (AGAW) is not renally selective. This may be due to the lack of carrier-mediated transport and high plasma protein binding.[148,149] In addition, the chemotherapeutic prodrugs S-(guanine-6-yl)-L-cysteine (Figure 13.19) and selenocysteine Se-conjugates have been studied as a kidney-selective prodrugs of 6-mercaptopurine[150–153] and selenol compounds,[154–156] respectively. These prodrugs are activated by renal cysteine conjugate β-lyases. Furthermore, low molecular weight proteins (LMWP) have been evaluated as renal specific drug carriers.[136,157] However, being drug carriers, not actual prodrugs, LMWPs are not discussed further in this chapter.

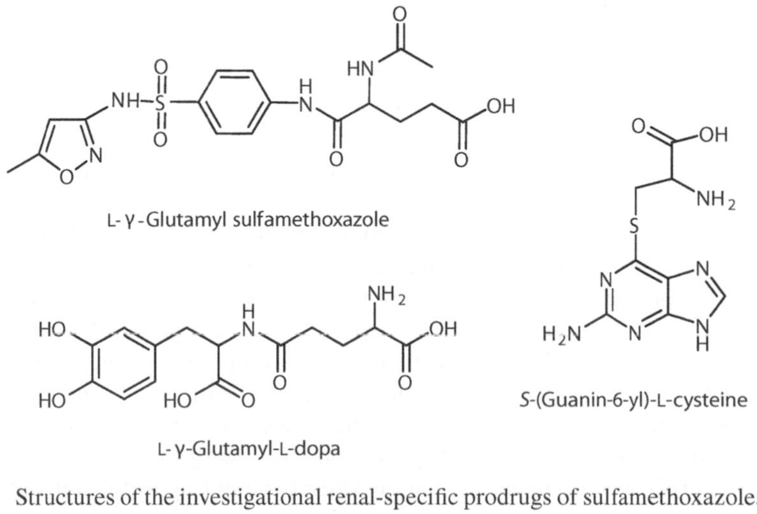

L-γ-Glutamyl sulfamethoxazole

L-γ-Glutamyl-L-dopa

S-(Guanin-6-yl)-L-cysteine

FIGURE 13.19 Structures of the investigational renal-specific prodrugs of sulfamethoxazole, dopamine, and 6-mercaptopurine.

13.2.2 TWO-STEP APPROACHES FOR TARGETED DRUG DELIVERY: ADEPT

ADEPT was proposed by Dr. Bagshawe over two decades ago.[158,159] ADEPT is a two-step process. In the first step, a drug-activating enzyme is targeted to the tumors by a tumor-targeting antibody (via an antibody-enzyme conjugate [AbE]); in the second step, a nontoxic prodrug is administered systemically. This prodrug then gets converted to the active drug by the localized enzyme, resulting in high tumor concentration. However, the prodrug remains inactive in normal tissues (without drug-activating enzyme), thus resulting in lower nonspecific toxicity.

ADEPT provides many advantages:[160]

- Amplification. Each localized AbE molecule converts a larger number of nontoxic prodrugs to potent active drugs and increases the tumor active drug concentration.
- Bystander effect. The locally activated drug molecules with high lipophilicity can diffuse into the cancer cells regardless of the heterogeneous antigen expression. The bystander effect addresses the issues of the poor tumor penetration of AbE.
- AbE does not need to be internalized into each cancer cell for prodrug activation.

13.2.2.1 Requirements for the Success of ADEPT

ADEPT is a rather complex therapeutic regimen, considering the following facts:[161]

- At least two components or steps are required, i.e., the delivery of AbE specifically to the desired tumor site followed by the activation of nontoxic prodrug in the target site by the pre-delivered enzyme. Increasing therapeutic steps always makes the whole therapy harder to control and to predict the outcome. This necessitates a thorough understanding of the therapy itself and the optimal design.
- High expression levels of antigens in tumors, but low levels in normal tissues are required for AbE tumor targeting.
- A sufficient amount of AbE might not be able to penetrate into the target tissues.
- Elimination of the biological molecules (AbE) might be nonlinear.
- The prodrug needs to be enzyme-specifically activated in the tumors with minimal nonspecific activation. A large difference of cytotoxicity and other properties between the prodrug and activated drug is desired, such as low permeability to the cell membrane, which is preferred for the prodrug, while high permeability is preferred for the activated drug.[162]
- Since hypoxia induces drug resistance, it is ideal to select a drug that is active under hypoxia for prodrug design.

Careful consideration of the following factors will increase the success rate of the ADEPT approach. First, the antibodies that target the extracellular antigen may be preferred, since they will likely overcome the limitation due to the poor penetration of the antibody-enzyme complex. For example, HuCC49ΔCH2 is an anti-TAG-72 antibody that is localized at the extracellular matrix (not the cell membrane). The large amount of antigen in the extracellular space will trap a large amount of the AbE.[163] The tumor antigen on the cell membrane could have a maximal binding capacity, while the extracellular antigen is less likely to have this binding limitation. In addition, it is easier for the conjugate to be exposed to the antigen in the extracellular space, than on the tumor cell surface. Because of the large molecular size of the conjugate, the conjugate may have a low diffusion rate of penetration into the tumor tissue for binding to the antigen on the tumor cell surface. Thus, it is expected that more conjugate can be trapped when the rich antigen is present in the extracellular space, compared with the cellular surface. This will also overcome the problem of internalization of AbE after binding to the antigen for lysosomal degradation.

Second, the minimization of immunological response is critical for the clinical use of ADEPT. Most murine antibodies are known to cause human anti-mouse antibody (HAMA) response, which may change the pharmacokinetics of the AbE and limit the repeat dosing of AbEs. In order to eradicate the tumor cells, multiple dosing or repeated cycles of ADEPT might be desired. Thus, the most desired conjugate should cause no immune response. For instance, the humanized anti-TAG-72 antibody (HuCC49ΔCH2) for tumor detection has shown no detectable immunological response in human clinical trials, thus making it a good candidate for ADEPT.

Third, the selection of drug candidates for prodrug design may also affect the efficacy of ADEPT. Ideally, the drug should be active under hypoxic conditions. Thus, the Hsp90 inhibitor (geldanamycin [GA]) may be advantageous for prodrug design. GA has higher anticancer activity under hypoxia. GA targets multiple oncogenic proteins via Hsp 90. These oncogenic proteins, such as hypoxia-inducible factor 1α (HIF-1α), vascular endothelial growth factor (VEGF), and AKT, are over-expressed under hypoxic conditions. Thus, GA is very effective under hypoxia.

In addition, the permeability difference between active drug and prodrug should be optimized. For ADEPT to succeed, active drug should have higher lipophilicity than the prodrug.[164] If the prodrug is very lipophilic, it will leak back from the tissues and tumors to blood circulation rapidly; leading to its lack of retention in the tumor and lower prodrug conversion. On the other hand, a lipophilic-active drug would better penetrate the tumor.

As shown in Figure 13.20, the anti-TAG-72 (tumor-associated glycoprotein-72) antibody (HuCC49ΔCH2) has been utilized *in vitro* to deliver a drug-activating enzyme for GA prodrug activation in ADEPT.[165,166] HuCC49ΔCH2-β-galactosidase conjugates were highly specific and enzymatically active. The conjugates activated the GA prodrug and reduced the median inhibition concentration (IC50) of the prodrug to 1 μM from 25 μM against LS174T, colorectal cancer cells with high levels of TAG-72 expression. A key advantage of using the anti-TAG-72 antibody and GA prodrug is the TAG-72 antigen expression primarily in tumors, with almost no expression in normal tissues. This provides the selectivity and specificity of the AbE to the tumor cells. This step is very critical for the success of ADEPT since the undesired binding of conjugate to normal cells may cause the systemic activation of prodrug and general toxicity.

13.2.2.2 Component Selection Criteria of ADEPT

ADEPT is meant to restrict the action of the active cytotoxic drug to tumor sites; thus increasing its efficacy within tumors and reducing the toxicity to normal tissues. In this complex strategy, three important components, i.e., antibody, enzyme, and prodrug, need to be carefully chosen. The following describes some general criteria for their selection.

13.2.2.1.1 Antibody

The principle of ADEPT is to deliver enzymes to tumor sites via the reaction between a tumor-associated antigen and an antibody-enzyme conjugate. Ideally, the antibody should recognize a tumor-specific antigen and bind to it tightly. Consequently, the antibody is restrained at tumor sites after it is cleared from the blood and normal tissue. Thus, antibodies are utilized to deliver a high concentration of enzymes to tumor sites. However, there is a wide variation in the degree of antibody localization among individual subjects, which depends on the specificity and accessibility of

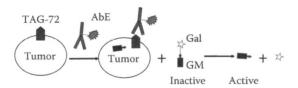

FIGURE 13.20 Scheme of ADEPT using HuCC49ΔCH2-β-galactosidase conjugates and GM prodrugs for colorectal cancer treatment.

the antigen. For instance, colorectal adenocarcinomas are composed of glandular structures separated from fibrovascular stroma by a basal lamina, which may represent a significant barrier to extravasated antibody. In addition to TAG-72, basement membrane-associated carcinoembryonic antigen (CEA) epitopes may be more accessible to antibodies than those which are cytoplasmic or lumenal. For example, the tumor localization of two monoclonal antibodies (A5B7 and EA77) recognizing nonoverlapping CEA epitopes were different, which may be due to the accessibility of epitopes on tumor cells.[167] The antigen specificity of the antibodies facilitates efficient enzyme loading and the amplification of the target-specific activity. For example, monoclonal antibody A33 recognizes a cell-surface antigen that is expressed on ~95% of colon cancers. In clinical trials, radiolabelled A33 localized specifically to colon cancer cells, where it was retained for several weeks, while it cleared within days from a normal colon.[168] In another clinical trial, specific antigen binding and enzyme activity were utilized to increase the toxicity of 5-fluorocytosine to A33 antigen positive tumor cells by 300-fold.[169]

13.2.2.1.2   Enzyme

Theoretically, the selected enzyme should minimize nonspecific prodrug activation in normal tissues. So, the enzymes in ADEPT should not be present in normal tissue. For example, the enzyme could be a bacterial enzyme without mammalian homolog, such as carboxypeptidase G2,[170] cytosine deaminase,[171] and beta-lactamase.[172–174] Other bacterial enzymes with mammalian homolog or mammalian enzymes with low expression in normal tissues can also be used, such as beta-glucuronidase[175,176] and alpha-galactosidase.[177]

Bacterial enzymes have several properties that make them very suitable for ADEPT. They tend to be stable, have high catalytic activity, and are generally easier to manufacture in large quantities than mammalian enzymes. Importantly, they have a unique specificity of substrates, which allows the design of prodrugs that are not activated by human enzymes.

The AbE should be nonimmunogenic. To meet the specific requirement that the prodrug not be activated by enzymes endogenous to humans, bacterial enzymes have typically been employed in ADEPT studies. The administration of a foreign protein typically elicits a vigorous antibody response that limits the repeated administration of the protein. Thus, immunogenicity has been a concern in the clinical studies of ADEPT.[178] In order to suppress antibody responses against the AbE, the immunosuppressive agent cyclosporine has been used in early clinical studies of the ADEPT approach.[179] Immunosuppression in cancer, however, is not desirable and offers only limited mitigation of an immune response against the conjugate. Thus, the immunogenicity of the enzyme component of ADEPT remains a major problem seriously limiting the use of this approach.

In addition, the enzyme needs to activate the prodrug with high selectivity and turnover at physiological conditions. A single enzyme molecule typically has the potential to cleave many prodrug molecules. For example, the benzoic acid mustard substrates of carboxypeptidase G2 can cleave up to 800 mol/mol of enzyme per second,[180] thus providing an amplification effect and high levels of drug localized at the tumor. This may be an important advantage in the clinic, in view of the typically low localization of immunoconjugates in humans.

13.2.2.1.3   Prodrug

Prodrugs are derivatives of drug that are activated in the body to release or generate the active drug. Potential advantages of ADEPT are the delivery of prodrug and the production of high concentrations of extremely potent drug at tumor sites, such as nitrogen mustards and palytoxin, which are too toxic to be readily used in conventional chemotherapy. Prodrug forms of both clinically used anticancer agents and novel cytotoxic compounds have been developed to take advantage of a variety of enzymes with widely different substrate specificities. Hence, it is important that the drug generated from the prodrug should produce a linear dose-related cell kill, while the prodrug remains inactive in normal tissue. A wide spectrum of clinically established anticancer agents can be considered for designing prodrugs, such as benzoic acid mustard, doxorubicin,[170,181] methotrexate,[182–184] camptothecin, 5-fluorouracil,[175,176] nitrogen mustards, paclitaxel,[172–174] and camptothecin.[185]

Another concern with regard to chemotherapy is the drug resistance to many cytotoxic agents. Therefore, avoiding the drug resistance is an important criterion for prodrug development. Drug resistance may be mediated by the P-glycoprotein pump, thus developing multi-drug resistance through the exclusion of the drug from the cell.[186] This mechanism does not appear to operate with alkylating agents.[187] Besides efflux by the P-glycoprotein pump, drug resistance may develop through repairing DNA damage, such as that caused by alkylating agents.[188,189] So, overcoming drug resistance caused by efflux and DNA repair is preferred for increasing drug effects.

Another important consideration for prodrug development is coupled with the enzyme selectivity. The prodrug should be enzyme-specifically activated in tumors, with minimal nonspecific activation. The prodrug should be designed so that it is only catalytically converted to the active drug by the enzyme-antibody conjugate localized at the tumor site and not by endogenous enzymes. This issue is coupled with the selectivity of the enzyme. Also, the active drug's tumor distribution and pharmacokinetic properties should also be considered. Active drug, generated by cleaving an inactivating component from the prodrug, could diffuse to neighboring cells in the tumor so that cells that do not express the target antigen would be killed through the so-called bystander effect.[187] It may also leak out of tumors and be carried to normal tissues via the blood stream, causing systemic toxicity. Thus, the drug generated in tumor sites should have a short half-life.

For example, A5CP, which consists of a F(ab)2 fragment of a mouse monoclonal antibody conjugated to CEA (A5B7), was linked to the bacterial enzyme carboxypeptidase (CPG2) as the antibody-enzyme targeting agent. This was used in combination with a benzoic acid mustard prodrug, CMDA, which is activated by cleavage of its glutamate moiety. These trials showed tumor response.[190] However, toxicity was thought to have resulted from the long half-life of the activated drug, which diffused back into the circulation to cause myelosuppression.[179,191] A new prodrug, bis-iodo phenol mustard (ZD2767P), was designed whose activated form is highly potent and has a short half-life. It cleared rapidly from circulation and the activated drug was not measurable in the blood. The drug-related toxicities were milder.[192]

In addition, the locally active drug molecules should be highly lipophilic in order to diffuse into the cancer cells. For example, nitrogen mustard drugs are relatively lipophilic and can readily diffuse through cell membranes, making them appropriate for prodrug candidates.

It is challenging to meet all the selection criteria of antibody-enzyme conjugation and prodrug design. Many ADEPT attempts met some, but not all, of these criteria. The selection of components has to take into consideration all the factors involved to give an overall benefit. Some of these issues are elaborated in detail in the following important ADEPT studies.

13.2.2.3 Case Studies

Numerous prodrug/drug systems have been developed for activation by a variety of enzymes. Although many have shown potential in preclinical studies, clinical development is restricted to a few phase I studies. No ADEPT products have yet been marketed.

Notwithstanding the complexity, ADEPT has been widely tested by many research groups. Among these studies, researchers from London (UK) using CEA as the target antigen have made the greatest progress in clinical trials. Some improvements of ADEPT that were successfully executed in their clinical studies are covered in this section.

In the early clinical trials from 1997 to 2000, limited colorectal cancer patients were enrolled in the study.[179,190] Colorectal cancer is a common epithelial tumor. Response to conventional treatment is limited due to drug resistance and lack of selectivity. ADEPT is preferred to overcome these problems by selective generation of a high concentration of drug in the tumor. The tumor was associated with a high level of the target antigen, CEA. It is an oncofetal antigen, expressing abundantly at tumor sites. It is expressed in normal tissue, but is limited to the luminal surface of the gut—where it is inaccessible to systemically administered AbE. The A5B7 F(ab')2 antibody (against CEA) was conjugated to carboxypeptidase G2 (CPG2). CPG2, a bacterial enzyme, was expected to be immunogenic, but otherwise had the required characteristic of a high rate of turnover of substrate molecules. It cleaves the terminal glutamates of molecules, such as natural and synthetic folates.[193] To accelerate the clearance of AbE from blood circulation, a clearing antibody SB43-gal (against the active site of CPG2) was administered. Consequently, with the help of a clearing antibody, a high tumor:plasma ratio (exceeding 10,000:1) was obtained for AbE around 50h post administration, ideal for selective prodrug activation in the tumor site. Benzoic acid mustard-glutamate, which can be converted to the alkylating agent, was the selected prodrug. Although there was evidence of tumor response by the active drug, dose-limiting myelosuppression was observed for the majority of the patients. This myelosuppression was attributed to the presence of active drug in the plasma, since prodrug itself did not cause toxicity in a previous study. It was suggested that active drug in the circulation was the result of "leak back" from the tumor, given that no active enzyme was found in the plasma.

In 2002, a new phase I clinical trial using a new prodrug and galactosylated AbE was undertaken.[192] The galactosylated AbE was expected to be cleared faster from circulation, without the help of a second clearing antibody. The elegantly designed prodrug was converted to highly potent active drug with a short half-life. This was expected to prevent the "leak back" of active drug to circulation. The result of this clinical trial was rather unexpected. Inadequate tumor localization of AbE (the median tumor:normal tissue ratios are less than 1) was observed. Therefore, selective prodrug conversion in the tumor tissue was not observed for almost all the patients. The study concluded that each component (or step) of ADEPT must be strictly monitored in order to achieve the optimal therapeutic outcome. AbE with more efficient tumor localization and less immunogenicity was suggested, if a second clearing antibody were not to be used.

Another important study was published by Sharma et al. in 2005.[194] In this study, a recombinant genetic fusion protein, composed of a single-chain Fv antibody and an enzyme, was expressed in *Pichia pastoris*. This resulted in a glycosylated protein with branched mannose. The mannosylated fusion protein's clearance from the circulation was accelerated (rapid clearance from plasma within 6h) via mannose receptors, without inducing toxicity. This was confirmed in two morphologically different human colon carcinoma xenografts (LS174T and SW1222). Also, the high AbE tumor to plasma ratios of 1400:1 and 339:1 were observed for the LS174T and SW1222 models, respectively. In 2006, the clinical trial result was published.[195] In this phase I study, MFECP1, a recombinant antibody-enzyme fusion protein of an anti-CEA single-chain Fv antibody and the bacterial enzyme carboxypeptidase G2 followed by a bis-iodo phenol mustard prodrug, was administered. The study involved 80-fold dose escalation from the starting dose of prodrug to evaluate the therapeutic benefit. AbE was cleared rapidly via the liver in normal tissue and was less immunogenic than other conjugates of carboxypeptidase G2. Its tumor localization was sufficient and prodrug conversion was effective. This study is the first clinical report of ADEPT with the recombinant antibody-enzyme fusion protein MFECP1. However, these trials of ADEPT, based on the bacterial enzyme carboxypeptidase G2, were limited in the number of treatment cycles by the antibodies formed by patients against the nonhuman proteins. Thus, immunogenicity was a key obstacle to further development in this case. The use of human derived enzymes may reduce the risk of eliciting an immune response.

Some reports suggested that engineered human-derived enzymes could be nonimmunogenic.[196] For example, a stabilized variant of human prolyl endopeptidase has been engineered for use in ADEPT.[197] Human-derived enzymes need to be designed carefully to avoid the risk of prodrug conversion in normal tissue. In addition, the use of enzymes with human homolog brings the risk of triggering an autoimmune response. Furthermore, human enzymes will only be suitable with appropriate prodrugs if their kinetics are comparable with bacterial enzymes. It remains to be proven if human enzymes can be used in ADEPT.

An alternative to the use of human enzymes is the use of low immunogenic bacterial enzymes, such as beta-lactamase. Beta-lactamase is the most widely used enzyme in ADEPT for the broad specificity of substrates linked to the lactam ring of cephalosporins. The Genencor group has constructed a beta-lactamase mutant that is associated with reduced immunogenicity in human patients and retains functional properties suitable for application in ADEPT.[198] Beta-lactamase from *Enterobacter cloacae* was the parent enzyme, which activated prodrugs of chemotherapeutic agents. To reduce its immunogenic potential, several CD4+ T-cell epitopes from beta-lactamase sequence were modified, while sufficient protein stability and enzyme activity were preserved. Besides reduced immunogenicity, beta-lactamase is a monomeric protein and showed sufficiently fast plasma clearance when studied *in vivo*.[199,200] The evaluation of a conjugate between antibody fragments and beta-lactamase variant is in progress.

Although ADEPT has great potential, improvements in design and the use of optimal conditions is necessary. The other two enzymatic-prodrug strategies, GDEPT and VDEPT, have practical advantages and clinical limitations as well. A comparison of these three major enzyme-prodrug approaches is listed in Table 13.2.[161]

13.2.2.4   The Application of Modeling and Simulation in ADEPT

Due to the complexity of ADEPT, it would be ideal to use predictive models to estimate the therapeutic outcome before large-scale, lengthy, and costly preclinical and clinical studies are undertaken. Pharmacokinetic (PK) and pharmacodynamic (PD) studies have been shown to guide and expedite drug development.[202] The urgency of PK/PD modeling is clearly demonstrated in U.S. Food and Drug Administration (FDA) guidance.[203] It is without question that using mathematical modeling and fragmenting the complex system into elementary components will help understand the complex ADEPT and optimize the therapeutic regimen. Some researchers have used mathematical modeling to provide insights and guides for ADEPT.[204–206] However, these studies assumed a simple compartment model for AbE, prodrug, and the active drug. Although informative, compartmental models are very limited in describing the pharmacokinetic properties of biological molecules.

Physiology-based pharmacokinetic (PBPK) modeling has been proposed to predict the pharmacokinetics of antibodies itself.[207–210] The PBPK approach is more physiologically relevant and allows for the integration of all anatomical compartments together, as they are in the biological system. This will enable the accurate prediction of the system change with each compartment variation. In our previously published study, PBPK modeling and simulation were applied to predict the outcome of ADEPT.[211] PBPK modeling would be able to incorporate special features of ADEPT components, such as convection, which is more likely to contribute to the AbE distribution process; the neonatal Fc Receptor (FcRn), which is important for antibody recycling and elimination; and the tumor size, which might change significantly during the course of ADEPT.

As mentioned above, a PBPK approach was used to understand the complexity of ADEPT and to guide AbE selection, AbE dose regimen (dose and dosing interval before prodrug administration), prodrug design, and prodrug dose in our previous study.[211] The objectives were the following: (A) To build three levels of PBPK model for AbE, prodrug, and active drug and to provide a quantitative basis to carry out ADEPT *in vivo*. (B) To identify the sensitive factors or parameters controlling the ADEPT process, including antigen expression in tumor tissues, antibody affinity to antigen, clearance and depletion of AbE, and prodrug and active drug permeability. (C) Dosing regimen optimization for AbE and prodrug administration to achieve maximum active drug concentration in tumors and minimum active drug in blood and normal tissues.

PBPK simulation models for AbE, prodrug, and active drug were successfully constructed and applied for dose regimen selection.[211] All the pharmacokinetics for these molecules were interconnected through prodrug activation to active drug by the pretargeted AbE. This PBPK model is advantageous compared with the compartmental model in the following aspects:

- This PBPK model is more physiologically relevant. It integrates all the tissues/organs into the system as they are in the biological body. Thus, they reflect the real biological system much better than the compartmental model. For example, the previous compartmental model does not consider the flow collection back from normal organs into the circulation, while this is captured in the current PBPK model.[205] Indeed, this phenomenon is confirmed by the clinical studies. The "leak back" of active drug from regular organs or tumors to the circulation was the main reason for the observed toxicity.[190] The PBPK model helps understand the "leak back" issue better.

- The PBPK model captures and predicts individual organs/tissue concentration–time response based on each organ's characteristics. For example, the skin and muscle are unique compared with other organs. It would be difficult for a compartmental model to incorporate these unique features. Thus, the PBPK model is much more flexible in this aspect.

It is also important to note that further refinement of the current PBPK model is necessary. For example, active drug trapping in the tissues is not considered. It is likely that the active drug may be trapped in the tumor cells. For example, the active metabolite of 17-AG was trapped in the tumor more than the parent compound, 17-AAG, itself.[212] Therefore, it is reasonable to expect that the active drug would behave similarly, since the active drug may bind to its target inside the tumor cells. Consequently, the active drug tumor/plasma area under the curve (AUC) ratio might be even higher.

13.2.3 Future Prospects

Targeting prodrugs to tissue-selective enzymes is a promising strategy for precise and efficient site-selective drug delivery and improved therapeutic efficacy. However, to be successful, the designing and development of targeted prodrugs require considerable knowledge of enzymes and their molecular and functional characteristics as well as pharmacokinetic characteristics of the parent drug and corresponding prodrug. This chapter divides enzyme-activated prodrug strategies into two main categories. Of one-step approaches, where prodrugs are designed for direct activation by tissue-selective enzymes, two successful examples are especially worth highlighting. HepDirect prodrugs (Metabasis Therapeutics) undergo a CYP-catalyzed oxidation predominantly in the liver where carefully selected parent drugs are released and retained to demonstrate good efficacy combined with the low systemic levels of parent drugs. The HepDirect approach has already been applied to several drugs of which three have advanced to clinical trials. Capecitabine, on the other hand, is the oral tumor-activated prodrug of 5-FU that is sequentially converted to 5′-DFCR by hepatic carboxylesterase in the liver, to 5′-DFUR by cytidine deaminase either in liver or tumor tissues, and eventually to cytotoxic 5-FU by thymidine phosphorylase preferentially expressed at the tumor site. These examples demonstrate that an enzyme-activated prodrug strategy can be useful for targeting drugs. Table 13.4 summarizes some of the merits and demerits of one-step prodrug targeting strategies discussed in this chapter.

The main drawback of the enzyme-activated prodrug strategy is the ubiquitous distribution of most endogenous enzymes responsible for the bioactivation of prodrugs, which diminishes the possibilities for selective activation, and consequently, targeting. Hence, targeting by prodrugs can be further improved by delivering prodrug-activating enzymes to target cells, especially to tumor cells, by using antibodies (ADEPT) and genes (GDEPT). Some ADEPT systems have progressed to clinical phase I studies, and one GDEPT has reached phase III clinical studies (Cerebro®, Ark Therapeutics, London, United Kingdom) and is likely to become the first gene-based product for the treatment of patients with glioma. Due to the large molecular size, AbEs cannot easily penetrate into tumor cells, while most enzymes need cofactors, which are present only inside the cells, for enzymatic activity. So, it is expected that the future ADEPT will use small molecules as targeting agents. Comparison of ADEPT, GDEPT, and VDEPT is summarized in Table 13.5.

TABLE 13.4

Summary of One-Step Prodrug Approaches for Targeted Drug Action

Target Tissue	Specific Enzyme(s) for Prodrug Activation	Successful Example(s)	Limitations
Liver	Cytochrome P450s, particularly CYP3A4	HepDirect prodrugs	Cytochrome P450s are expressed also in gut wall; possible changes in cytochrome P450s' levels in diseased liver and due to genetic polymorphism; probability of drug–drug interactions due to likely inhibition or induction of P450s
Tumor	Several hypoxia-specific and tumor-associated enzymes	Cabecitabine	Narrow therapeutic index of active cytotoxic drugs; full tumor selectivity and delivery of therapeutical concentrations of an active drug at the tumor site may be difficult to achieve
Colon	Reductive enzymes produced by colonic microflora	Azo-bond prodrugs	Absorption of prodrug in the upper gastrointestinal tract
Kidney	—	Still in preclinical studies	No kidney-specific enzymes for prodrug activation characterized yet

TABLE 13.5

Comparison of ADEPT, GDEPT, and VDEPT

Principle	GDEPT	Physical delivery of a gene encoding drug-activating enzyme
	VDEPT	Viral vector to deliver a gene encoding drug-activating enzyme
	ADEPT	Monoclonal antibody linked to a drug-activating enzyme to target deliver drug-activating enzyme to tumors
Advantages	GDEPT	Directly delivered inside tumor cells, thus the enzyme is accessible to all the cofactors required for enzymatic activity
	VDEPT	Similar to GDEPT, gene-encoding enzyme can be specifically delivered to the target tissue and drive the expression within cells
	ADEPT	Highly selective and low mutagenesis risk; bystander effect: the locally activated drug molecules with high lipophilicity can diffuse into the cancer cells regardless of the heterogeneous antigen expression
Limitations	GDEPT	Insertional mutagenesis, anti-DNA antibody formation, local infection, and tumor nodule ulceration; difficulties with the selective delivery and expression of genes
	VDEPT	Mutagenesis risk of the host's genome; retroviral vectors only target dividing cells, thus the majority of the tumor would not be sensitive to killing mediated by retroviral VDEPT
	ADEPT	Immunogenicity; due to large AbE molecular size, enzymes might need to gain access inside cells to interact with cofactors, required for enzymatic activity; cost and difficulties with development and purification of antibodies
Reference	GDEPT	Pandha et al.[201]
	VDEPT	FDA and Varner[203,204]
	ADEPT	Mayer et al. and Bagshawe[195,196]

Finally, when one wants to consider an enzyme-activated prodrug strategy for drug targeting, irrespective of the prodrug strategy that is being utilized, there are key issues that are important to keep in mind. The prodrug should be readily transported to the target site and uptake should be reasonably fast compared with distribution to other tissues. The prodrug should also be stable against ubiquitous enzymes present in the body but be exclusively converted to the active drug at the site of drug action. Additionally, the active drug, once selectively generated at the target site, should be retained by the tissue, and by-products formed during prodrug conversion should ideally be safe and rapidly excreted from the body. Although appearing complicated, more successful enzyme-activated prodrug strategies can be expected to originate as the future research will unravel the location and function of specific enzymes that are available for therapeutic intervention such as prodrug targeting.

REFERENCES

1. Stella, V., Hageman, M., Oliyai, R., Tilley, J., and Maag, H. (Eds.) *Prodrugs: Challenges and Rewards* (AAPS Press/Springer, New York, 2007).
2. Rautio, J. et al. Prodrugs: Design and clinical applications. *Nat Rev Drug Discov* 7, 255–270 (2008).
3. Stella, V. J., Charman, W. N., and Naringrekar, V. H. Prodrugs. Do they have advantages in clinical practice? *Drugs* 29, 455–473 (1985).
4. Leppanen, J. et al. Design and synthesis of a novel L-dopa-entacapone codrug. *J Med Chem* 45, 1379–1382 (2002).
5. Bodor, N. and Buchwald, P. Soft drug design: General principles and recent applications. *Med Res Rev* 20, 58–101 (2000).
6. Stella, V. In *Optimizing the "Drug-Like" Properties of Leads in Drug Discovery* (Borchardt, R., Hageman, M., Stevens, J., Kerns, E., and Thakker, D., Eds.), pp. 221–242 (Springer, New York, 2006).
7. Stella, V. J. Prodrugs as therapeutics. *Expert Opin Ther Pat* 14, 277–280 (2004).
8. Bodor, N. and Buchwald, P. Recent advances in the brain targeting of neuropharmaceuticals by chemical delivery systems. *Adv Drug Deliv Rev* 36, 229–254 (1999).
9. Bodor, N. and Buchwald, P. Barriers to remember: Brain-targeting chemical delivery systems and Alzheimer's disease. *Drug Discov Today* 7, 766–774 (2002).
10. Stella, V. J. and Himmelstein, K. J. In *Directed Drug Delivery* (Borchardt, R. T., Repta, A. J. and Stella, V. J., Eds.), pp. 247–267 (Humana Press, Clifton, NJ, 1985).
11. Stella, V. J. and Himmelstein, K. J. In *Design of Prodrugs* (Bundgaard, H., Ed.), pp. 177–198 (Elsevier Science Publishers BV, Amsterdam, the Netherlands, 1985).
12. Kearney, A. S. Prodrugs and targeted drug delivery. *Adv Drug Deliv Rev* 19, 225 (1996).
13. Han, H. K. and Amidon, G. L. Targeted prodrug design to optimize drug delivery. *AAPS Pharm Sci* 2, E6 (2000).
14. Ettmayer, P., Amidon, G. L., Clement, B., and Testa, B. Lessons learned from marketed and investigational prodrugs. *J Med Chem* 47, 2393–2404 (2004).
15. Rajewski, R. A. and McIntosh, M. P. In *Prodrugs: Challenges and Rewards*. Part 1 (Stella, V. J. et al., Eds.), pp. 429–445 (AAPS Press/Springer, New York, 2007).
16. Bagshawe, K. D., Sharma, S. K., and Begent, R. H. Antibody-directed enzyme prodrug therapy (ADEPT) for cancer. *Expert Opin Biol Ther* 4, 1777–1789 (2004).
17. Sharma, S. K., Bagshawe, K. D., and Begent, R. H. Advances in antibody-directed enzyme prodrug therapy. *Curr Opin Investig Drugs* 6, 611–615 (2005).
18. Dachs, G. U., Tupper, J., and Tozer, G. M. From bench to bedside for gene-directed enzyme prodrug therapy of cancer. *Anticancer Drugs* 16, 349–359 (2005).
19. Niculescu-Duvaz, I., Spooner, R., Marais, R., and Springer, C. J. Gene-directed enzyme prodrug therapy. *Bioconjug Chem* 9, 4–22 (1998).
20. Boyer, T. D., Wright, W. L., and Manns, M. P. (Eds.) *Zakim and Boyer's Hepatology: A Textbook of Liver Diseases* (Elsevier, Inc., Philadelphia, PA, 2006).
21. Worman, H. J. *The Liver Disorders and Hepatic Sourcebook* (McGraw-Hill, Inc., New York, 2006).
22. Kwon, Y. *Handbook of Essential Pharmacokinetics, Pharmacodynamics and Drug Metabolism for Industrial Scientists* (Kluwer Academic Publishers, Hingham, MA, 2001).
23. Meijer, D. K. and Molema, G. Targeting of drugs to the liver. *Semin Liver Dis* 15, 202–256 (1995).

24. Wu, J., Nantz, M. H., and Zern, M. A. Targeting hepatocytes for drug and gene delivery: Emerging novel approaches and applications. *Front Biosci* 7, d717–d725 (2002).

25. Stockert, R. J. The asialoglycoprotein receptor: Relationships between structure, function, and expression. *Physiol Rev* 75, 591–609 (1995).

26. Fiume, L. et al. Liver targeting of antiviral nucleoside analogues through the asialoglycoprotein receptor. *J Viral Hepat* 4, 363–370 (1997).

27. Erion, M. D. *Prodrugs for Liver-targeted Drug Delivery* (Stella, V. J. et al., Eds.) (AAPS Press, Arlington, VA/Springer Science, New York, 2007).

28. St-Pierre, M. V., Kullak-Ublick, G. A., Hagenbuch, B., and Meier, P. J. Transport of bile acids in hepatic and non-hepatic tissues. *J Exp Biol* 204, 1673–1686 (2001).

29. Sievanen, E. Exploitation of bile acid transport systems in prodrug design. *Molecules* 12, 1859–1889 (2007).

30. Kramer, W. et al. Liver-specific drug targeting by coupling to bile acids. *J Biol Chem* 267, 18598–18604 (1992).

31. Kramer, W. et al. Intestinal absorption of peptides by coupling to bile acids. *J Biol Chem* 269, 10621–10627 (1994a).

32. Balakrishnan, A. and Polli, J. E. Apical sodium dependent bile acid transporter (ASBT, SLC10A2): A potential prodrug target. *Mol Pharm* 3, 223–230 (2006).

33. Kullak-Ublick, G. A. et al. Chlorambucil-taurocholate is transported by bile acid carriers expressed in human hepatocellular carcinomas. *Gastroenterology* 113, 1295–1305 (1997).

34. Kramer, W. et al. Bile acid derived HMG-CoA reductase inhibitors. *Biochim Biophys Acta* 1227, 137–154 (1994b).

35. Petzinger, E. et al. Hepatobiliary transport of hepatic 3-hydroxy-3-methylglutaryl coenzyme A reductase inhibitors conjugated with bile acids. *Hepatology* 22, 1801–1811 (1995).

36. Guengerich, F. P. Common and uncommon cytochrome P450 reactions related to metabolism and chemical toxicity. *Chem Res Toxicol* 14, 611–650 (2001).

37. Park, B. K., Pirmohamed, M., and Kitteringham, N. R. The role of cytochrome P450 enzymes in hepatic and extrahepatic human drug toxicity. *Pharmacol Ther* 68, 385–424 (1995).

38. Nebert, D. W. and Russell, D. W. Clinical importance of the cytochromes P450. *Lancet* 360, 1155–1162 (2002).

39. Bruno, R. D. and Njar, V. C. Targeting cytochrome P450 enzymes: A new approach in anti-cancer drug development. *Bioorg Med Chem* 15, 5047–5060 (2007).

40. Lewis, D. F., Watson, E., and Lake, B. G. Evolution of the cytochrome P450 superfamily: Sequence alignments and pharmacogenetics. *Mutat Res* 410, 245–270 (1998).

41. Isin, E. M. and Guengerich, F. P. Complex reactions catalyzed by cytochrome P450 enzymes. *Biochim Biophys Acta* 1770, 314–329 (2007).

42. Smith, D. A., Ackland, M. J., and Jones, B. C. Properties of cytochrome P450 isoenzymes and their substrates. Part 1: Active site characteristics. *Drug Discov Today* 2, 406–414 (1997).

43. Lewis, D. F. and Dickins, M. Substrate SARs in human P450s. *Drug Discov Today* 7, 918–925 (2002).

44. Erion, M. D. et al. Design, synthesis, and characterization of a series of cytochrome P(450) 3A-activated prodrugs (HepDirect prodrugs) useful for targeting phosph(on)ate-based drugs to the liver. *J Am Chem Soc* 126, 5154–5163 (2004).

45. Erion, M. D. et al. Liver-targeted drug delivery using HepDirect prodrugs. *J Pharmacol Exp Ther* 312, 554–560 (2005).

46. Erion, M. D. et al. Targeting thyroid hormone receptor-beta agonists to the liver reduces cholesterol and triglycerides and improves the therapeutic index. *Proc Natl Acad Sci USA* 104, 15490–15495 (2007).

47. Boyer, S. H. et al. Synthesis and characterization of a novel liver-targeted prodrug of cytosine-1-beta-D-arabinofuranoside monophosphate for the treatment of hepatocellular carcinoma. *J Med Chem* 49, 7711–7720 (2006).

48. Hecker, S. J. et al. Liver-targeted prodrugs of 2′-C-methyladenosine for therapy of hepatitis C virus infection. *J Med Chem* 50, 3891–3896 (2007).

49. Reddy, K. R. et al. Pradefovir: A prodrug that targets adefovir to the liver for the treatment of hepatitis B. *J Med Chem* 51, 666–676 (2008).

50. Dando, T. and Plosker, G. Adefovir dipivoxil: A review of its use in chronic hepatitis B. *Drugs* 63, 2215–2234 (2003).

51. Erion, M. D., Bullough, D. A., Lin, C. C., and Hong, Z. HepDirect prodrugs for targeting nucleotide-based antiviral drugs to the liver. *Curr Opin Investig Drugs* 7, 109–117 (2006).

52. Tillmann, H. L. Pradefovir, a liver-targeted prodrug of adefovir against HBV infection. *Curr Opin Investig Drugs* 8, 682–690 (2007).

53. Reddy, K. R., Colby, T. J., Fujitaki, J. M., van Poelje, P. D., and Erion, M. D. Liver targeting of hepatitis-B antiviral lamivudine using the HepDirect prodrug technology. *Nucleosides Nucleotides Nucleic Acids* 24, 375–381 (2005).

54. Varmus, H. The new era in cancer research. *Science* 312, 1162–1165 (2006).

55. Denny, W. A. Tumor-activated prodrugs—A new approach to cancer therapy. *Cancer Invest* 22, 604–619 (2004).

56. Huang, P. S. and Oliff, A. Drug-targeting strategies in cancer therapy. *Curr Opin Genet Dev* 11, 104–110 (2001).

57. Rooseboom, M., Commandeur, J. N., and Vermeulen, N. P. Enzyme-catalyzed activation of anticancer prodrugs. *Pharmacol Rev* 56, 53–102 (2004).

58. Atkinson, J. M., Siller, C. S., and Gill, J. H. Tumour endoproteases: The cutting edge of cancer drug delivery? *Br J Pharmacol* 153, 1344–1352 (2008).

59. Brown, J. M. The hypoxic cell: A target for selective cancer therapy—Eighteenth Bruce F. Cain Memorial Award lecture. *Cancer Res* 59, 5863–5870 (1999).

60. Brahimi-Horn, M. C., Chiche, J., and Pouyssegur, J. Hypoxia and cancer. *J Mol Med* 85, 1301–1307 (2007).

61. Hall, P. M., Stupans, I., Burgess, W., Birkett, D. J., and McManus, M. E. Immunohistochemical localization of NADPH-cytochrome P450 reductase in human tissues. *Carcinogenesis* 10, 521–530 (1989).

62. Fitzsimmons, S. A. et al. Reductase enzyme expression across the National Cancer Institute Tumor cell line panel: Correlation with sensitivity to mitomycin C and EO9. *J Natl Cancer Inst* 88, 259–269 (1996).

63. Yu, L. J. et al. P450 enzyme expression patterns in the NCI human tumor cell line panel. *Drug Metab Dispos* 29, 304–312 (2001).

64. McKeown, S. R., Cowen, R. L., and Williams, K. J. Bioreductive drugs: From concept to clinic. *Clin Oncol (R Coll Radiol)* 19, 427–442 (2007).

65. Tomasz, M. Mitomycin C: Small, fast and deadly (but very selective). *Chem Biol* 2, 575–579 (1995).

66. Spanswick, V. J., Cummings, J., and Smyth, J. F. Current issues in the enzymology of mitomycin C metabolic activation. *Gen Pharmacol* 31, 539–544 (1998).

67. Begleiter, A. Clinical applications of quinone-containing alkylating agents. *Front Biosci* 5, E153–E171 (2000).

68. Patterson, A. V. et al. Importance of P450 reductase activity in determining sensitivity of breast tumour cells to the bioreductive drug, tirapazamine (SR 4233). *Br J Cancer* 72, 1144–1150 (1995).

69. Saunders, M. P., Patterson, A. V., Chinje, E. C., Harris, A. L., and Stratford, I. J. NADPH:cytochrome c (P450) reductase activates tirapazamine (SR4233) to restore hypoxic and oxic cytotoxicity in an aerobic resistant derivative of the A549 lung cancer cell line. *Br J Cancer* 82, 651–656 (2000).

70. Lloyd, R. V., Duling, D. R., Rumyantseva, G. V., Mason, R. P., and Bridson, P. K. Microsomal reduction of 3-amino-1,2,4-benzotriazine 1,4-dioxide to a free radical. *Mol Pharmacol* 40, 440–445 (1991).

71. Elwell, J. H., Siim, B. G., Evans, J. W., and Brown, J. M. Adaptation of human tumor cells to tirapazamine under aerobic conditions: Implications of increased antioxidant enzyme activity to mechanism of aerobic cytotoxicity. *Biochem Pharmacol* 54, 249–257 (1997).

72. Patterson, A. V. et al. Mechanism of action and preclinical antitumor activity of the novel hypoxia-activated DNA cross-linking agent PR-104. *Clin Cancer Res* 13, 3922–3932 (2007).

73. Guise, C. P. et al. Identification of human reductases that activate the dinitrobenzamide mustard prodrug PR-104A: A role for NADPH:cytochrome P450 oxidoreductase under hypoxia. *Biochem Pharmacol* 74, 810–820 (2007).

74. Belinsky, M. and Jaiswal, A. K. NAD(P)H:quinone oxidoreductase1 (DT-diaphorase) expression in normal and tumor tissues. *Cancer Metastasis Rev* 12, 103–117 (1993).

75. Jaiswal, A. K. Regulation of genes encoding NAD(P)H:quinone oxidoreductases. *Free Radic Biol Med* 29, 254–262 (2000).

76. Speckamp, W. N. and Oostveen, E. A. (United States Patent 5079257, 1992).

77. Hendriks, H. R. et al. EO9: A novel bioreductive alkylating indoloquinone with preferential solid tumour activity and lack of bone marrow toxicity in preclinical models. *Eur J Cancer* 29A, 897–906 (1993).

78. Bailey, S. M. et al. Reduction of the indoloquinone anticancer drug EO9 by purified DT-diaphorase: A detailed kinetic study and analysis of metabolites. *Biochem Pharmacol* 56, 613–621 (1998).

79. Bailey, S. M. et al. Involvement of NADPH: Cytochrome P450 reductase in the activation of indoloquinone EO9 to free radical and DNA damaging species. *Biochem Pharmacol* 62, 461–468 (2001).

80. Dirix, L. Y. et al. EO9 phase II study in advanced breast, gastric, pancreatic and colorectal carcinoma by the EORTC Early Clinical Studies Group. *Eur J Cancer* 32A, 2019–2022 (1996).
81. Knox, R. J., Friedlos, F., Marchbank, T., and Roberts, J. J. Bioactivation of CB 1954: Reaction of the active 4-hydroxylamino derivative with thioesters to form the ultimate DNA-DNA interstrand crosslinking species. *Biochem Pharmacol* 42, 1691–1697 (1991).
82. Helsby, N. A., Ferry, D. M., Patterson, A. V., Pullen, S. M., and Wilson, W. R. 2-Amino metabolites are key mediators of CB 1954 and SN 23862 bystander effects in nitroreductase GDEPT. *Br J Cancer* 90, 1084–1092 (2004).
83. Knox, R. J. et al. Bioactivation of 5-(aziridin-1-yl)-2,4-dinitrobenzamide (CB 1954) by human NAD(P) H quinone oxidoreductase 2: A novel co-substrate-mediated antitumor prodrug therapy. *Cancer Res* 60, 4179–4786 (2000).
84. Knox, R. J. et al. The nitroreductase enzyme in Walker cells that activates 5-(aziridin-1-yl)-2,4-dinitrobenzamide (CB 1954) to 5-(aziridin-1-yl)-4-hydroxylamino-2-nitrobenzamide is a form of NAD(P)H dehydrogenase (quinone) (EC 1.6.99.2). *Biochem Pharmacol* 37, 4671–4677 (1988).
85. Anlezark, G. M. et al. The bioactivation of 5-(aziridin-1-yl)-2,4-dinitrobenzamide (CB1954)–I. Purification and properties of a nitroreductase enzyme from *Escherichia coli*—A potential enzyme for antibody-directed enzyme prodrug therapy (ADEPT). *Biochem Pharmacol* 44, 2289–2295 (1992).
86. Chandor, A. et al. Metabolic activation of the antitumor drug 5-(Aziridin-1-yl)-2,4-dinitrobenzamide (CB1954) by NO synthases. *Chem Res Toxicol* 21, 836–843 (2008).
87. McFadyen, M. C. and Murray, G. I. Cytochrome P450 1B1: A novel anticancer therapeutic target. *Future Oncol* 1, 259–263 (2005).
88. Karlgren, M. et al. Tumor-specific expression of the novel cytochrome P450 enzyme, CYP2W1. *Biochem Biophys Res Commun* 341, 451–458 (2006).
89. Patterson, L. H. and McKeown, S. R. AQ4N: A new approach to hypoxia-activated cancer chemotherapy. *Br J Cancer* 83, 1589–1593 (2000).
90. Albertella, M. R. et al. Hypoxia-selective targeting by the bioreductive prodrug AQ4N in patients with solid tumors: Results of a phase I study. *Clin Cancer Res* 14, 1096–1104 (2008).
91. Pawelek, J., Korner, A., Bergstrom, A., and Bologna, J. New regulators of melanin biosynthesis and the autodestruction of melanoma cells. *Nature* 286, 617–619 (1980).
92. Riley, P. A. Melanogenesis and melanoma. *Pigment Cell Res* 16, 548–552 (2003).
93. Jordan, A. M., Khan, T. H., Osborn, H. M., Photiou, A., and Riley, P. A. Melanocyte-directed enzyme prodrug therapy (MDEPT): Development of a targeted treatment for malignant melanoma. *Bioorg Med Chem* 7, 1775–1780 (1999).
94. Jordan, A. M. et al. Melanocyte-Directed enzyme prodrug therapy (MDEPT): Development of second generation prodrugs for targeted treatment of malignant melanoma. *Bioorg Med Chem* 9, 1549–1558 (2001).
95. Mahajan, S. and Atkins, W. M. The chemistry and biology of inhibitors and pro-drugs targeted to glutathione *S*-transferases. *Cell Mol Life Sci* 62, 1221–1233 (2005).
96. Aliya, S., Reddanna, P., and Thyagaraju, K. Does glutathione *S*-transferase Pi (GST-Pi) a marker protein for cancer? *Mol Cell Biochem* 253, 319–327 (2003).
97. Lyttle, M. H. et al. Glutathione-*S*-transferase activates novel alkylating agents. *J Med Chem* 37, 1501–1507 (1994).
98. Satyam, A. et al. Design, synthesis, and evaluation of latent alkylating agents activated by glutathione *S*-transferase. *J Med Chem* 39, 1736–1747 (1996).
99. Rosario, L. A., O'Brien, M. L., Henderson, C. J., Wolf, C. R., and Tew, K. D. Cellular response to a glutathione *S*-transferase P1-1 activated prodrug. *Mol Pharmacol* 58, 167–174 (2000).
100. Townsend, D. M. and Tew, K. D. The role of glutathione-*S*-transferase in anti-cancer drug resistance. *Oncogene* 22, 7369–7375 (2003).
101. Shami, P. J. et al. JS-K, a glutathione/glutathione *S*-transferase-activated nitric oxide donor of the diazeniumdiolate class with potent antineoplastic activity. *Mol Cancer Ther* 2, 409–417 (2003).
102. Chakrapani, H. et al. Synthesis and in vitro anti-leukemic activity of structural analogues of JS-K, an anti-cancer lead compound. *Bioorg Med Chem Lett* 18, 950–953 (2008).
103. Shami, P. J. et al. Antitumor activity of JS-K [O2-(2,4-dinitrophenyl) 1-[(4-ethoxycarbonyl)piperazin-1-yl]diazen-1-ium-1,2-diolate] and related O2-aryl diazeniumdiolates in vitro and in vivo. *J Med Chem* 49, 4356–4366 (2006).
104. Ackland, S. P. and Peters, G. J. Thymidine phosphorylase: Its role in sensitivity and resistance to anticancer drugs. *Drug Resist Updat* 2, 205–214 (1999).

105. Miwa, M. et al. Design of a novel oral fluoropyrimidine carbamate, capecitabine, which generates 5-fluorouracil selectively in tumours by enzymes concentrated in human liver and cancer tissue. *Eur J Cancer* 34, 1274–1281 (1998).

106. Budman, D. R. Capecitabine. *Invest New Drugs* 18, 355–363 (2000).

107. Ebi, H. et al. Pharmacokinetic and pharmacodynamic comparison of fluoropyrimidine derivatives, capecitabine and 5'-deoxy-5-fluorouridine (5'-DFUR). *Cancer Chemother Pharmacol* 56, 205–211 (2005).

108. Deryugina, E. I. and Quigley, J. P. Matrix metalloproteinases and tumor metastasis. *Cancer Metastasis Rev* 25, 9–34 (2006).

109. Takahashi, H. et al. Antiproteases in preventing the invasive potential of pancreatic cancer cells. *Jop* 8, 501–508 (2007).

110. Dubowchik, G. M., Mosure, K., Knipe, J. O., and Firestone, R. A. Cathepsin B-sensitive dipeptide prodrugs. 2. Models of anticancer drugs paclitaxel (Taxol), mitomycin C and doxorubicin. *Bioorg Med Chem Lett* 8, 3347–3352 (1998).

111. Bellacchio, E. and Paggi, M. G. Protease-mediated arsenic prodrug strategy in cancer and infectious diseases: A hypothesis for targeted activation. *J Cell Physiol* 214, 681–686 (2008).

112. Chung, D. E. and Kratz, F. Development of a novel albumin-binding prodrug that is cleaved by urokinase-type-plasminogen activator (uPA). *Bioorg Med Chem Lett* 16, 5157–5163 (2006).

113. Devy, L. et al. Plasmin-activated doxorubicin prodrugs containing a spacer reduce tumor growth and angiogenesis without systemic toxicity. *Faseb J* 18, 565–567 (2004).

114. Graeser, R. et al. Synthesis and biological evaluation of an albumin-binding prodrug of doxorubicin that is cleaved by prostate-specific antigen (PSA) in a PSA-positive orthotopic prostate carcinoma model (LNCaP). *Int J Cancer* 122, 1145–1154 (2008).

115. Janssen, S. et al. Pharmacokinetics, biodistribution, and antitumor efficacy of a human glandular kallikrein 2 (hK2)-activated thapsigargin prodrug. *Prostate* 66, 358–368 (2006).

116. DiPaola, R. S. et al. Characterization of a novel prostate-specific antigen-activated peptide-doxorubicin conjugate in patients with prostate cancer. *J Clin Oncol* 20, 1874–1879 (2002).

117. Roldo, M. et al. Azo compounds in colon-specific drug delivery. *Expert Opin Drug Deliv* 4, 547–560 (2007).

118. Friend, D. R. New oral delivery systems for treatment of inflammatory bowel disease. *Adv Drug Deliv Rev* 57, 247–265 (2005).

119. Rubinstein, A. Microbially controlled drug delivery to the colon. *Biopharm Drug Dispos* 11, 465–475 (1990).

120. Hirayama, F. and Uekama, K. In *Prodrugs: Challenges and Rewards. Part 1* (Stella, V. J. et al., Eds.), pp. 683–699 (Springer/AAPS Press, New York/Arlington, 2007).

121. Azad Khan, A. K., Piris, J., and Truelove, S. C. An experiment to determine the active therapeutic moiety of sulphasalazine. *Lancet* 2, 892–895 (1977).

122. Azadkhan, A. K., Truelove, S. C., and Aronson, J. K. The disposition and metabolism of sulphasalazine (salicylazosulphapyridine) in man. *Br J Clin Pharmacol* 13, 523–528 (1982).

123. Jain, A., Gupta, Y., and Jain, S. K. Azo chemistry and its potential for colonic delivery. *Crit Rev Ther Drug Carrier Syst* 23, 349–400 (2006).

124. Qureshi, A. I. and Cohen, R. D. Mesalamine delivery systems: Do they really make much difference? *Adv Drug Deliv Rev* 57, 281–302 (2005).

125. Wadworth, A. N. and Fitton, A. Olsalazine. A review of its pharmacodynamic and pharmacokinetic properties, and therapeutic potential in inflammatory bowel disease. *Drugs* 41, 647–664 (1991).

126. Chourasia, M. K. and Jain, S. K. Pharmaceutical approaches to colon targeted drug delivery systems. *J Pharm Pharm Sci* 6, 33–66 (2003).

127. Friend, D. R. and Chang, G. W. A colon-specific drug-delivery system based on drug glycosides and the glycosidases of colonic bacteria. *J Med Chem* 27, 261–266 (1984).

128. Simpkins, J. W., Smulkowski, M., Dixon, R., and Tuttle, R. Evidence for the delivery of narcotic antagonists to the colon as their glucuronide conjugates. *J Pharmacol Exp Ther* 244, 195–205 (1988).

129. Cui, N., Friend, D. R., and Fedorak, R. N. A budesonide prodrug accelerates treatment of colitis in rats. *Gut* 35, 1439–1446 (1994).

130. McLeod, A. D., Fedorak, R. N., Friend, D. R., Tozer, T. N., and Cui, N. A glucocorticoid prodrug facilitates normal mucosal function in rat colitis without adrenal suppression. *Gastroenterology* 106, 405–413 (1994).

131. Nolen, H. W., 3rd, Fedorak, R. N., and Friend, D. R. Steady-state pharmacokinetics of corticosteroid delivery from glucuronide prodrugs in normal and colitic rats. *Biopharm Drug Dispos* 18, 681–695 (1997).

132. El-Kamel, A. H., Abdel-Aziz, A. A., Fatani, A. J., and El-Subbagh, H. I. Oral colon targeted delivery systems for treatment of inflammatory bowel diseases: Synthesis, in vitro and in vivo assessment. *Int J Pharm* 358, 248–255 (2008).

133. Jung, Y. J., Lee, J. S., and Kim, Y. M. Colon-specific prodrugs of 5-aminosalicylic acid: Synthesis and in vitro/in vivo properties of acidic amino acid derivatives of 5-aminosalicylic acid. *J Pharm Sci* 90, 1767–1775 (2001).

134. *Brenner & Rector's The Kidney* (Benner, B. M., Ed.) (Elsevier, Inc., Philadelphia, PA, 2004).

135. Stein, A. and Wild, J. *Kidney Failure Explained* (Class Publishing, London, U.K., 2002).

136. Haas, M., Moolenaar, F., Meijer, D. K., and de Zeeuw, D. Specific drug delivery to the kidney. *Cardiovasc Drugs Ther* 16, 489–496 (2002).

137. Shirota, K., Kato, Y., Suzuki, K., and Sugiyama, Y. Characterization of novel kidney-specific delivery system using an alkylglucoside vector. *J Pharmacol Exp Ther* 299, 459–467 (2001).

138. Suzuki, K., Susaki, H., Okuno, S., and Sugiyama, Y. Renal drug targeting using a vector "alkylglycoside." *J Pharmacol Exp Ther* 288, 57–64 (1999).

139. Suzuki, K. et al. Specific renal delivery of sugar-modified low-molecular-weight peptides. *J Pharmacol Exp Ther* 288, 888–897 (1999).

140. Suzuki, K. et al. Structural requirements for alkylglycoside-type renal targeting vector. *Pharm Res* 16, 1026–1034 (1999).

141. Wilk, S., Mizoguchi, H., and Orlowski, M. gamma-Glutamyl dopa: A kidney-specific dopamine precursor. *J Pharmacol Exp Ther* 206, 227–232 (1978).

142. Barthelmebs, M., Caillette, A., Ehrhardt, J. D., Velly, J., and Imbs, J. L. Metabolism and vascular effects of gamma-L-glutamyl-L-dopa on the isolated rat kidney. *Kidney Int* 37, 1414–1422 (1990).

143. Drieman, J. C. et al. Regional haemodynamic effects of dopamine and its prodrugs L-dopa and gludopa in the rat and in the glycerol-treated rat as a model for acute renal failure. *Br J Pharmacol* 111, 1117–1122 (1994).

144. Lee, M. R. Five years' experience with gamma-L-glutamyl-L-dopa: A relatively renally specific dopaminergic prodrug in man. *J Auton Pharmacol* 10(Suppl 1), s103–s108 (1990).

145. Orlowski, M., Mizoguchi, H., and Wilk, S. *N*-acyl-gamma-glutamyl derivatives of sulfamethoxazole as models of kidney-selective prodrugs. *J Pharmacol Exp Ther* 212, 167–172 (1980).

146. Drieman, J. C., Thijssen, H. H., and Struyker-Boudier, H. A. Renal selective *N*-acetyl-gamma-glutamyl prodrugs. II. Carrier-mediated transport and intracellular conversion as determinants in the renal selectivity of *N*-acetyl-gamma-glutamyl sulfamethoxazole. *J Pharmacol Exp Ther* 252, 1255–1260 (1990a).

147. Drieman, J. C., Thijssen, H. H., Zeegers, H. H., Smits, J. F., and Struyker Boudier, H. A. Renal selective *N*-acetyl-gamma-glutamyl prodrugs: A study on the mechanism of activation of the renal vasodilator prodrug CGP 22979. *Br J Pharmacol* 99, 15–20 (1990b).

148. Drieman, J. C. and Thijssen, H. H. Renal selective *N*-acetyl-L-gamma-glutamyl prodrugs. III. *N*-acetyl-L-gamma-glutamyl-4′-aminowarfarin is not targeted to the kidney but is selectively excreted into the bile. *J Pharmacol Exp Ther* 259, 766–771 (1991).

149. Drieman, J. C., Thijssen, H. H., and Struyker-Boudier, H. A. Renal selective *N*-acetyl-L-gamma-glutamyl prodrugs: Studies on the selectivity of some model prodrugs. *Br J Pharmacol* 108, 204–208 (1993).

150. Hwang, I. Y. and Elfarra, A. A. Cysteine *S*-conjugates may act as kidney-selective prodrugs: Formation of 6-mercaptopurine by the renal metabolism of *S*-(6-purinyl)-L-cysteine. *J Pharmacol Exp Ther* 251, 448–454 (1989).

151. Hwang, I. Y. and Elfarra, A. A. Kidney-selective prodrugs of 6-mercaptopurine: Biochemical basis of the kidney selectivity of *S*-(6-purinyl)-L-cysteine and metabolism of new analogs in rats. *J Pharmacol Exp Ther* 258, 171–177 (1991).

152. Elfarra, A. A. and Hwang, I. Y. Targeting of 6-mercaptopurine to the kidneys. Metabolism and kidney-selectivity of *S*-(6-purinyl)-L-cysteine analogs in rats. *Drug Metab Dispos* 21, 841–845 (1993).

153. Elfarra, A. A., Duescher, R. J., Hwang, I. Y., Sicuri, A. R., and Nelson, J. A. Targeting 6-thioguanine to the kidney with *S*-(guanin-6-yl)-L-cysteine. *J Pharmacol Exp Ther* 274, 1298–1304 (1995).

154. Andreadou, I., Menge, W. M., Commandeur, J. N., Worthington, E. A., and Vermeulen, N. P. Synthesis of novel Se-substituted selenocysteine derivatives as potential kidney selective prodrugs of biologically active selenol compounds: Evaluation of kinetics of beta-elimination reactions in rat renal cytosol. *J Med Chem* 39, 2040–2046 (1996).

155. Commandeur, J. N. et al. Bioactivation of selenocysteine Se-conjugates by a highly purified rat renal cysteine conjugate beta-lyase/glutamine transaminase K. *J Pharmacol Exp Ther* 294, 753–761 (2000).

156. Rooseboom, M., Vermeulen, N. P., Andreadou, I., and Commandeur, J. N. Evaluation of the kinetics of beta-elimination reactions of selenocysteine Se-conjugates in human renal cytosol: Possible implications for the use as kidney selective prodrugs. *J Pharmacol Exp Ther* 294, 762–769 (2000).

157. Franssen, E. J. et al. Low molecular weight proteins as carriers for renal drug targeting. Preparation of drug-protein conjugates and drug-spacer derivatives and their catabolism in renal cortex homogenates and lysosomal lysates. *J Med Chem* 35, 1246–1259 (1992).

158. Bagshawe, K. D. Antibody directed enzymes revive anti-cancer prodrugs concept. *Br J Cancer* 56, 531–532 (1987).

159. Bagshawe, K. D. et al. A cytotoxic agent can be generated selectively at cancer sites. *Br J Cancer* 58, 700–703 (1988).

160. Bagshawe, K. D., Sharma, S. K., Burke, P. J., Melton, R. G., and Knox, R. J. Developments with targeted enzymes in cancer therapy. *Curr Opin Immunol* 11, 579–583 (1999).

161. Xu, G. and McLeod, H. L. Strategies for enzyme/prodrug cancer therapy. *Clin Cancer Res* 7, 3314–3324 (2001).

162. Syrigos, K. N. and Epenetos, A. A. Antibody directed enzyme prodrug therapy (ADEPT): A review of the experimental and clinical considerations. *Anticancer Res* 19, 605–613 (1999).

163. Knox, R. J. and Melton, R. G. *Enzyme-Prodrug Strategies for Cancer Therapy* (Kluwer Academic/Plenum Publishers, New York, 1999).

164. Tietze, L. F. et al. Proof of principle in the selective treatment of cancer by antibody-directed enzyme prodrug therapy: The development of a highly potent prodrug. *Angew Chem Int Ed Engl* 41, 759–761 (2002).

165. Fang, L. et al. Enzyme specific activation of benzoquinone ansamycin prodrugs using HuCC49DeltaCH2-beta-galactosidase conjugates. *J Med Chem* 49, 6290–6297 (2006).

166. Cheng, H. et al. Synthesis and enzyme-specific activation of carbohydrate-geldanamycin conjugates with potent anticancer activity. *J Med Chem* 48, 645–652 (2005).

167. Boxer, G. M., Abassi, A. M., Pedley, R. B., and Begent, R. H. Localisation of monoclonal antibodies reacting with different epitopes on carcinoembryonic antigen (CEA)—Implications for targeted therapy. *Br J Cancer* 69, 307–314 (1994).

168. Welt, S. et al. Phase I/II study of iodine 125-labeled monoclonal antibody A33 in patients with advanced colon cancer. *J Clin Oncol* 14, 1787–1797 (1996).

169. Deckert, P. M. et al. A33scFv-cytosine deaminase: A recombinant protein construct for antibody-directed enzyme-prodrug therapy. *Br J Cancer* 88, 937–939 (2003).

170. Blakey, D. C. et al. Antitumor effects of an antibody-carboxypeptidase G2 conjugate in combination with a benzoic acid mustard prodrug. *Cell Biophys* 22, 1–8 (1993).

171. Wallace, P. M. et al. Intratumoral generation of 5-fluorouracil mediated by an antibody-cytosine deaminase conjugate in combination with 5-fluorocytosine. *Cancer Res* 54, 2719–2723 (1994).

172. Kerr, D. E. et al. Regressions and cures of melanoma xenografts following treatment with monoclonal antibody beta-lactamase conjugates in combination with anticancer prodrugs. *Cancer Res* 55, 3558–3563 (1995).

173. Svensson, H. P. et al. In vitro and in vivo activities of a doxorubicin prodrug in combination with monoclonal antibody beta-lactamase conjugates. *Cancer Res* 55, 2357–2365 (1995).

174. Rodrigues, M. L. et al. Synthesis and beta-lactamase-mediated activation of a cephalosporin-taxol prodrug. *Chem Biol* 2, 223–227 (1995).

175. Florent, J. C. et al. Prodrugs of anthracyclines for use in antibody-directed enzyme prodrug therapy. *J Med Chem* 41, 3572–3581 (1998).

176. Leu, Y. L., Roffler, S. R., and Chern, J. W. Design and synthesis of water-soluble glucuronide derivatives of camptothecin for cancer prodrug monotherapy and antibody-directed enzyme prodrug therapy (ADEPT). *J Med Chem* 42, 3623–3628 (1999).

177. Gesson, J. P. et al. Prodrugs of anthracyclines for chemotherapy via enzyme-monoclonal antibody conjugates. *Anticancer Drug Des* 9, 409–423 (1994).

178. Senter, P. D. Activation of prodrugs by antibody-enzyme conjugates: A new approach to cancer therapy. *Faseb J* 4, 188–193 (1990).

179. Martin, J. et al. Antibody-directed enzyme prodrug therapy: Pharmacokinetics and plasma levels of prodrug and drug in a phase I clinical trial. *Cancer Chemother Pharmacol* 40, 189–201 (1997).

180. Springer, C. J. et al. Ablation of human choriocarcinoma xenografts in nude mice by antibody-directed enzyme prodrug therapy (ADEPT) with three novel compounds. *Eur J Cancer* 27, 1361–1366 (1991).

181. Niculescu-Duvaz, I., Friedlos, F., Niculescu-Duvaz, D., Davies, L., and Springer, C. J. Prodrugs for antibody- and gene-directed enzyme prodrug therapies (ADEPT and GDEPT). *Anticancer Drug Des* 14, 517–538 (1999).

182. Smith, G. K. et al. Toward antibody-directed enzyme prodrug therapy with the T268G mutant of human carboxypeptidase A1 and novel in vivo stable prodrugs of methotrexate. *J Biol Chem* 272, 15804–15816 (1997).

183. Smal, M. A. et al. Activation and cytotoxicity of 2-alpha-aminoacyl prodrugs of methotrexate. *Biochem Pharmacol* 49, 567–574 (1995).

184. Deckert, P. M. et al. Specific tumour localisation of a huA33 antibody—Carboxypeptidase A conjugate and activation of methotrexate-phenylalanine. *Int J Oncol* 24, 1289–1295 (2004).

185. Pessah, N. et al. Bioactivation of carbamate-based 20(S)-camptothecin prodrugs. *Bioorg Med Chem* 12, 1859–1866 (2004).

186. Sparreboom, A., and Nooter, K. Does P-glycoprotein play a role in anticancer drug pharmacokinetics? *Drug Resist Updat* 3, 357–363 (2000).

187. Bagshawe, K. D. Antibody-directed enzyme prodrug therapy (ADEPT) for cancer. *Expert Rev Anticancer Ther* 6, 1421–1431 (2006).

188. Webley, S. D. et al. Measurement of the critical DNA lesions produced by antibody-directed enzyme prodrug therapy (ADEPT) in vitro, in vivo and in clinical material. *Br J Cancer* 84, 1671–1676 (2001).

189. Zheng, H., Wang, X., Legerski, R. J., Glazer, P. M., and Li, L. Repair of DNA interstrand cross-links: Interactions between homology-dependent and homology-independent pathways. *DNA Repair (Amst)* 5, 566–574 (2006).

190. Napier, M. P. et al. Antibody-directed enzyme prodrug therapy: Efficacy and mechanism of action in colorectal carcinoma. *Clin Cancer Res* 6, 765–772 (2000).

191. Springer, C. J., Poon, G. K., Sharma, S. K., and Bagshawe, K. D. Identification of prodrug, active drug, and metabolites in an ADEPT clinical study. *Cell Biophys* 22, 9–26 (1993).

192. Francis, R. J. et al. A phase I trial of antibody directed enzyme prodrug therapy (ADEPT) in patients with advanced colorectal carcinoma or other CEA producing tumours. *Br J Cancer* 87, 600–607 (2002).

193. Sherwood, R. F., Melton, R. G., Alwan, S. M., and Hughes, P. Purification and properties of carboxypeptidase G2 from Pseudomonas sp. strain RS-16. Use of a novel triazine dye affinity method. *Eur J Biochem* 148, 447–453 (1985).

194. Sharma, S. K. et al. Sustained tumor regression of human colorectal cancer xenografts using a multifunctional mannosylated fusion protein in antibody-directed enzyme prodrug therapy. *Clin Cancer Res* 11, 814–825 (2005).

195. Mayer, A. et al. A phase I study of single administration of antibody-directed enzyme prodrug therapy with the recombinant anti-carcinoembryonic antigen antibody-enzyme fusion protein MFECP1 and a bis-iodo phenol mustard prodrug. *Clin Cancer Res* 12, 6509–6516 (2006).

196. Bagshawe, K. D. The First Bagshawe lecture. Towards generating cytotoxic agents at cancer sites. *Br J Cancer* 60, 275–281 (1989).

197. Heinis, C., Alessi, P., and Neri, D. Engineering a thermostable human prolyl endopeptidase for antibody-directed enzyme prodrug therapy. *Biochemistry* 43, 6293–6303 (2004).

198. Harding, F. A. et al. A beta-lactamase with reduced immunogenicity for the targeted delivery of chemotherapeutics using antibody-directed enzyme prodrug therapy. *Mol Cancer Ther* 4, 1791–1800 (2005).

199. Siemers, N. O. et al. Construction, expression, and activities of L49-sFv-beta-lactamase, a single-chain antibody fusion protein for anticancer prodrug activation. *Bioconjug Chem* 8, 510–519 (1997).

200. Cortez-Retamozo, V. et al. Efficient cancer therapy with a nanobody-based conjugate. *Cancer Res* 64, 2853–2857 (2004).

201. Pandha, H. S. et al. Genetic prodrug activation therapy for breast cancer: A phase I clinical trial of erbB-2-directed suicide gene expression. *J Clin Oncol* 17, 2180–2189 (1999).

202. Galluppi, G. R. et al. Integration of pharmacokinetic and pharmacodynamic studies in the discovery, development, and review of protein therapeutic agents: A conference report. *Clin Pharmacol Ther* 69, 387–399 (2001).

203. FDA. http://www.fda.gov/cber/gdlns/popharm.htm (1999).

204. Varner, J. D. Systems biology and the mathematical modelling of antibody-directed enzyme prodrug therapy (ADEPT). *Syst Biol* (Stevenage) 152, 291–302 (2005).

205. Yuan, F., Baxter, L. T., and Jain, R. K. Pharmacokinetic analysis of two-step approaches using bifunctional and enzyme-conjugated antibodies. *Cancer Res* 51, 3119–3130 (1991).

206. Baxter, L. T. and Jain, R. K. Pharmacokinetic analysis of the microscopic distribution of enzyme-conjugated antibodies and prodrugs: Comparison with experimental data. *Br J Cancer* 73, 447–456 (1996).

207. Ferl, G. Z., Wu, A. M., and DiStefano, J. J., 3rd. A predictive model of therapeutic monoclonal antibody dynamics and regulation by the neonatal Fc receptor (FcRn). *Ann Biomed Eng* 33, 1640–1652 (2005).

208. Friedrich, S. W. et al. Antibody-directed effector cell therapy of tumors: Analysis and optimization using a physiologically based pharmacokinetic model. *Neoplasia* 4, 449–463 (2002).

209. Baxter, L. T., Zhu, H., Mackensen, D. G., and Jain, R. K. Physiologically based pharmacokinetic model for specific and nonspecific monoclonal antibodies and fragments in normal tissues and human tumor xenografts in nude mice. *Cancer Res* 54, 1517–1528 (1994).

210. Baxter, L. T., Zhu, H., Mackensen, D. G., Butler, W. F., and Jain, R. K. Biodistribution of monoclonal antibodies: Scale-up from mouse to human using a physiologically based pharmacokinetic model. *Cancer Res* 55, 4611–4622 (1995).

211. Fang, L. and Sun, D. Predictive physiologically based pharmacokinetic model for antibody-directed enzyme prodrug therapy. *Drug Metab Dispos* 36, 1153–1165 (2008).

212. Xu, L., Eiseman, J. L., Egorin, M. J., and D'Argenio, D. Z. Physiologically-based pharmacokinetics and molecular pharmacodynamics of 17-(allylamino)-17-demethoxygeldanamycin and its active metabolite in tumor-bearing mice. *J Pharmacokinet Pharmacodyn* 30, 185–219 (2003).

213. Rooseboom, M., Vermeulen, N. P., van Hemert, N., and Commandeur, J. N. Bioactivation of chemopreventive selenocysteine Se-conjugates and related amino acids by amino acid oxidases novel route of metabolism of selenoamino acids. *Chem Res Toxicol* 14, 996–1005 (2001).

214. Joseph, P., Xie, T., Xu, Y., and Jaiswal, A. K. NAD(P)H: Quinone oxidoreductase1 (DT-diaphorase): Expression, regulation, and role in cancer. *Oncol Res* 6, 525–532 (1994).

215. Chen, C. S., Jounaidi, Y., and Waxman, D. J. Enantioselective metabolism and cytotoxicity of R-ifosfamide and S-ifosfamide by tumor cell-expressed cytochromes P450. *Drug Metab Dispos* 33, 1261–1267 (2005).

216. Tew, K. D. TLK-286: A novel glutathione S-transferase-activated prodrug. *Expert Opin Investig Drugs* 14, 1047–1054 (2005).

217. Nelson, J. A., Pan, B. F., Swanson, D. A., and Elfarra, A. A. Cysteine conjugate beta-lyase activity in human renal carcinomas. *Cancer Biochem Biophys* 14, 257–263 (1995).

218. Roshy, S., Sloane, B. F., and Moin, K. Pericellular cathepsin B and malignant progression. *Cancer Metastasis Rev* 22, 271–286 (2003).

219. Lilja, H. Structure, function, and regulation of the enzyme activity of prostate-specific antigen. *World J Urol* 11, 188–191 (1993).

220. Ellis, V., Behrendt, N., and Dano, K. Plasminogen activation by receptor-bound urokinase. A kinetic study with both cell-associated and isolated receptor. *J Biol Chem* 266, 12752–12758 (1991).

221. Irigoyen, J. P., Munoz-Canoves, P., Montero, L., Koziczak, M., and Nagamine, Y. The plasminogen activator system: Biology and regulation. *Cell Mol Life Sci* 56, 104–132 (1999).

222. Andreasen, P. A., Kjoller, L., Christensen, L., and Duffy, M. J. The urokinase-type plasminogen activator system in cancer metastasis: A review. *Int J Cancer* 72, 1–22 (1997).

223. Wang, Y. The role and regulation of urokinase-type plasminogen activator receptor gene expression in cancer invasion and metastasis. *Med Res Rev* 21, 146–170 (2001).

224. Skrzydlewska, E., Sulkowska, M., Koda, M., and Sulkowski, S. Proteolytic-antiproteolytic balance and its regulation in carcinogenesis. *World J Gastroenterol* 11, 1251–1266 (2005).

Part V

Organ- or Tissue-Specific Drug Delivery

14 Targeting Colon and Kidney: Pathophysiological Determinants of Design Strategy

Ajit S. Narang and Ram I. Mahato

CONTENTS

14.1 INTRODUCTION

Targeted drug delivery to an organ or tissue is intended to bring the drug to its primary site of action. Thus, it can help improve the efficacy of the drug or prevent its undesired toxicities in other tissues or organs. In addition, sometimes targeted strategies are intended to avoid drug exposure to a specific organ or tissue. This can help avoid specific drug-related toxicities, increase systemic exposure, and achieve higher concentration at the target site. Most targeted drug delivery systems involve the use of macromolecular or particulate carriers, with the aim of modifying the pharmacokinetics and cellular distribution of the drug. In addition to achieving higher drug concentrations and/or prolonged exposure within the target cells, strategies can be designed to target organelles or specific compartments within the target cells. The overall goal of all drug-targeting strategies is the improvement of the efficacy and/or safety profile of a drug substance.

The most significant advantages of targeted drug delivery are realized in the advanced disease states. A majority of targeted drug delivery research has focussed on cytotoxic anticancer drugs. Drug targeting to tumor tissues and the tumor vasculature have been extensively studied. Among the organs, drug delivery to the brain, lungs, liver, kidney, and colon have been widely investigated.[1–8] The selection of target tissues is governed by the pharmacological need of the disease state and the drug substance, while the selection of the targeted drug delivery strategy is governed by the pathophysiology of the target tissue. For example, the leaky vasculature of the tumor tissue has been utilized for passive drug targeting as it allows for the tissue-selective extravasation of particulate systems.[9]

Several drug-targeting approaches have successfully transitioned from the proof-of-concept to the clinical application and have become a state of the art. Examples of targeted drug delivery platforms that have become well accepted in the clinical practice include the enteric coating of oral solid dosage forms to overcome chemical instability or adverse effects of the drug in the gastric environment, pulmonary drug delivery by dry powder inhalation, the use of ocular inserts for drug delivery to the eye, and transdermal and implantable drug delivery systems for systemic absorption of low molecular weight drugs such as steroid hormones. In addition, several drug delivery strategies being explored are at different preclinical and clinical stages of advancement.

A majority of targeted drug delivery research has focused on cytotoxic anticancer drugs. Drug targeting to tumor tissues and the tumor vasculature have been extensively studied. Among the organs, drug delivery to the brain, lungs, liver, kidney, and colon have been widely investigated.

In this chapter, we discuss colon and kidney targeting as examples of strategies at relatively different stages of development, with the former being more established than the latter. We highlight the role that disease mechanism and tissue physiology play in the identification of target organ or tissue and the drug-targeting strategy.

14.2   COLON-SPECIFIC DRUG DELIVERY

Traditionally, colonic drug delivery is focused on the treatment of local conditions such as ulcerative colitis, colorectal cancer, irritable bowl syndrome, amebiasis, and Crohn's disease. However, the systemic delivery of potent compounds such as proteins, peptides, and oligonucleotides that are unstable in the harsh conditions of the upper gastrointestinal (GI) tract have been gaining importance. The colon is rich in lymphoid tissues, thus offering opportunities for the oral delivery of vaccines targeted for release and absorption in the lower GI tract. Also, colon delivery can be exploited to improve the bioavailability of drugs that are extensively metabolized by cytochrome P450 enzymes in the upper GI tract, since the activity of these metabolizing enzymes is relatively lower in the colonic mucosa.[10,11] Colon-specific drug delivery may also help overcome the GI side effects of drugs. For example, the conversion of flurbiprofen to a glycine prodrug, hydrolysable by colonic microfloral enzymes (amidases), reduced its ulcerogenic activity in rats.[12] Targeted drug delivery to the colon has been extensively studied.[13–22]

Colon-specific drug delivery is challenged by its distal location in the GI tract. Even localized delivery through the rectum, however, only reaches a small part of the colon and is not a patient-friendly mode of administration. Therefore, oral delivery has been explored, utilizing physiological differences in the colonic microenvironment and physiology. The aspects of colon physiology that have been exploited to develop drug-targeting strategies include the presence of unique colonic microflora, high pH, the relatively predictable transition time in the small intestine, and high intra-luminal pressure inside the colon. In addition, osmotically controlled drug delivery systems, oxidation-potential-controlled drug delivery systems, and bioadhesive polymers have been used for colonic drug delivery.

The aspects of colon physiology that have been exploited to develop drug-targeting strategies include the presence of unique colonic microflora, high pH, the relatively predictable transition time in the small intestine, and high intra-luminal pressure inside the colon. In addition, osmotically and oxidation potential controlled drug delivery systems, and bioadhesive polymers have been used for colonic drug delivery.

14.2.1   Utilization of the Unique Colonic Microflora

Human colonic microflora consists predominantly of bacteria, which also make up to 60% of the dry mass of feces. The metabolic activities of this microflora result in the salvage of absorbable nutrients from the diet by fermenting unused energy substrates, trophic effects on the epithelium, and protection of the colonized host against invasion by alien microbes.[23] Colonic bacteria is mostly gram negative and anaerobic, except cecum, which can have high amounts of aerobic bacteria. Bacteria in the proximal part of the colon are primarily involved in fermenting carbohydrates, while the latter part breaks down proteins and amino acids.

The unique metabolic ability of these microbes has been exploited to develop polymerics and prodrugs that are degraded by the unique enzymatic activities of colonic microflora. In particular, the azo reductase and glycosidase activities of the microflora help degrade the azo bound and glycosidic linkages. The prodrug strategy for colonic drug delivery utilizes drug conjugation with a promoiety through an azo bond, which is degraded by the colonic bacteria. Examples of such prodrugs include sulfasalazine, balsalazide, ipsalazide, olsalazide, and salicylazosulfapyridine for the treatment of inflammatory bowl disease. As shown in Figure 14.1, all of these prodrugs contain an azo bond, which is reductively cleaved by the colonic anaerobic bacteria to release the anti-inflammatory compound 5-amino salicylic acid (5-ASA). Sulfasalazine was first introduced for the treatment of rheumatoid arthritis and inflammatory bowel disease. In the colon, it degrades into 5-ASA and sulfapyridine, which is responsible for most of the side effects of sulfasalazine. This problem was overcome by the use of other promoieties, such as 4-amino benzoyl glycine in ipsalazine and 4-aminobenzoyl-β-alanine in balsalazide, or azo bond conjugation of sulfasalazine with itself to

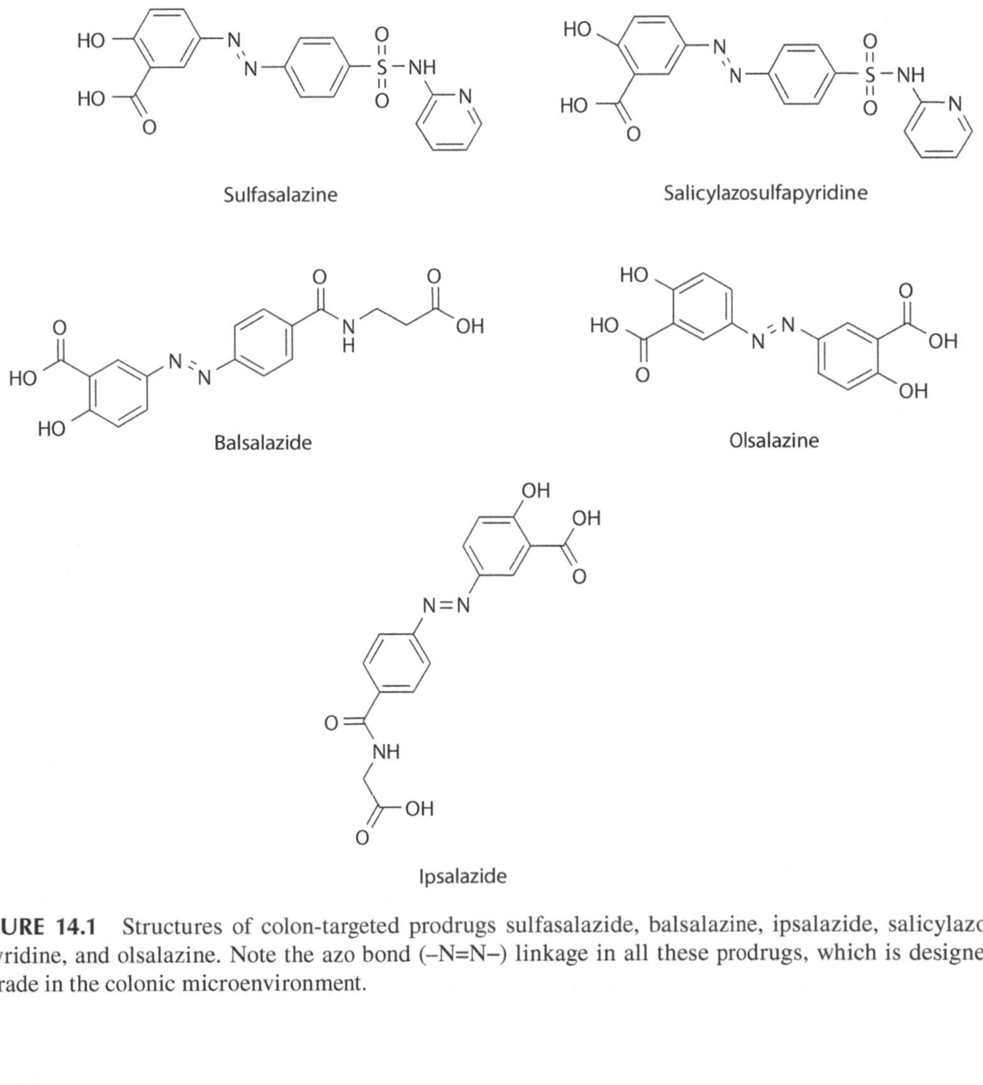

FIGURE 14.1 Structures of colon-targeted prodrugs sulfasalazide, balsalazine, ipsalazide, salicylazosulfapyridine, and olsalazine. Note the azo bond (–N=N–) linkage in all these prodrugs, which is designed to degrade in the colonic microenvironment.

form olsalazine. In addition, the drug has been covalently conjugated to a polymeric backbone of polysulfonamidoethylene by azo bond (Figure 14.1).[24]

Polymers that degrade specifically in the colon have been used for drug targeting by surface coating to form a barrier to drug release or as matrix systems embedding the drug substance. For example, azo-linked acrylate copolymers and poly(ester–ether) copolymers have been used for the delivery of proteins, peptide drugs, and small molecular weight compounds such as ibuprofen, sulfasalazine, and betamethasone.[25–28] For embedding the drug in polymer matrices, natural polysaccharides have been used in the oral solid dosage forms to protect the drug during GI transit and release in the colon upon polymer degradation by the microflora. They offer advantages such as the presence of derivatizable functional groups and a range of molecular size, in addition to their low toxicity. The hydrogel (hydrophilic and swelling) properties of these polymers, however, can lead to the dosage form swelling and disintegration in the presence of water before reaching the colon. Therefore, these dosage forms require protection from the aqueous environment during upper GI transit. This is usually accomplished by the use of protective surface coating or chemical crosslinking with linkers that are degraded in the colon. Polymers that are stable in the upper GI tract and degraded by colonic microflora include azo-crosslinked synthetic polymers and plant polysaccharides, such as amylose, pectin, inulin, and guar gum.[29–37]

A disadvantage of polymeric coating or embedding approaches for colonic drug delivery is their dependence on the bacterial microflora in the large intestine. Although the microflora is fairly constant in a healthy population, it can be affected by the dietary fermentation precursors, type of diet consumed, and coadministration of antibiotics. In addition, the natural polymers are often not available in pure form, which can lead to the physicochemical incompatibility with the drug substance and/or inconsistency of product performance.

14.2.2 pH-Dependent Dosage Forms

pH-sensitive polymers have been widely used for the enteric coating of dosage forms to facilitate pH-dependent drug release. As the pH level increases progressively from the stomach (pH 1–2) to the small intestine (pH 6–7) and the distal ileum (pH 7–8), dosage forms can be coated with polymers that dissolve only above specific pH ranges. For colon targeting, the polymeric coating should be able to withstand the acidic pH level of the stomach and the higher pH level of the proximal small intestine, but dissolve in the neutral to slightly basic pH level of the terminal ileum. However, most of the commonly used enteric coating polymeric systems have a pH threshold of 6.0 or lower for dissolution. These include the methacrylic acid/methyl methacrylate copolymers, (Eudragits® L100, L-30D, L100-55), polyvinylacetate phthalate (PVAP), hydroxypropyl methylcellulose phthalate (HPMCP), cellulose acetate phthalate (CAP), and cellulose acetate trimelliate (CAT). Only Eudragit S100 and FS 30D have a higher pH threshold of 6.8 and 7.0, respectively.[17]

Eudragit S100 coating is used, for example, in the mesalamine (Asacol®, Procter & Gamble) delayed-release tablets for topical anti-inflammatory action in the colon. Eudragit L100 and S100 are copolymers of methacrylic acid and methyl methacrylate with a ratio of carboxyl to ester groups of 1:1 or 1:2, respectively. The carboxylate groups form salts, leading to polymer dissolution at a basic pH level. Drug release from these acrylate polymers also depends upon the plasticizer, the nature of the salt in the dissolution medium, and the permeability of the film. Colon-targeted dosage forms utilizing methacrylate resins for coating or matrix formation have been reported for several molecules such as bisacodyl, indomethacin, 5-fluorouracil, and budesonide.[38–41]

The use of a pH trigger for drug delivery to the colon, however, has the disadvantage of a lack of consistency in the dissolution of the polymer at the desired site due to inter- and intra-individual pH variation, among other factors. For example, Ashford et al. observed significant variability in the disintegration time and location of Eudragit S coated tablets in human volunteers.[42] Also, based on the GI motility, polymer dissolution can complete toward the end of the ileum or deep in the colon. In addition, factors such as the presence of short chain fatty acids, residues of bile acids in the luminal contents, and the locally formed fermentation products can reduce the local pH level, thus influencing the drug release mechanism.[17]

14.2.3 TIME-DEPENDENT DRUG RELEASE

Human small intestinal transit time for pharmaceutical dosage forms was measured using gamma scintigraphy and was found to be about 3–4 h.[43] While the transit time does vary with the amount of food and the type of dosage form, it is less variable than the gastric-emptying time.[44] Timed release dosage forms to target the colon are, thus, typically formulated to prevent drug release in the acidic gastric environment and to prevent the release of drug until 3–4 h after leaving the acidic gastric environment.

An example of such timed release dosage form is the Pulsincap® device. In this device, the drug formulation is sealed in an impermeable capsule body with a hydrogel polymer plug. The hard gelatin capsule body may be made insoluble by exposure to formaldehyde vapor, which crosslinks gelatin. The plug expands in the aqueous GI tract fluid and exits the body, thus releasing the drug after a time delay determined by the rate of expansion and the length of the plug.[45,46]

Another approach utilized a three layer coated dosage form with an inner coating of an acid soluble polymer, Eudragit E, followed by a water soluble coat and the outer enteric coating of Eudragit L. An organic acid (succinic acid) was used as a part of the formulation. Upon oral administration, the dosage form is protected in the acidic gastric environment by the enteric coating. In intestinal conditions, water ingress into the formulation lowers the pH level inside the dosage form by the dissolution of the organic acid. This, in turn, causes the inner, acid-labile coat to dissolve, thus releasing the drug. The drug release rate and lag time is controlled by the coating thickness of the acid soluble layer and the amount of organic acid in the formulation. Using this approach, Fukui et al. prepared timed-release press-coated tablets with the core tablets containing diltiazem hydrochloride (DIL) and the outer, water soluble, layer containing phenylpropanolamine hydrochloride (PPA) as a marker for gastric-emptying time.[47] Upon administration to beagle dogs, the gastric-emptying time and lag time after gastric emptying were evaluated by determining the times at which PPA and DIL first appeared in the plasma, which were about 4 and 7 h, respectively. The 3 h lag time between the time of appearance of these drugs in the plasma correlated well with the expected intestinal transit time.

An inherent limitation of the time-dependent drug release systems is the inter- and intra-individual variability in gastric emptying, and small intestinal and colonic transit time. This can result in variations in the site of drug release in the small intestine or within the colon, which can impact drug absorption since absorption by the transcellular route diminishes in the distal colon.[48]

14.2.4 OSMOTICALLY CONTROLLED DRUG DELIVERY SYSTEMS

Osmotic drug delivery systems, such as the OROS-CT® system of Alza Corporation, are based on the incorporation of an osmotic agent, such as a salt, in the dosage form. The dosage form is encapsulated in a semipermeable membrane with an orifice for drug release. Upon ingestion, osmotic pressure gradient forces the ingress of water, which leads to the formation of flowable gel in the drug compartment and generates pressure to force the drug gel out of the orifice at a controlled rate.[17] The amount of the osmotic agent, rate of water permeation, and size of the laser-drilled orifice primarily determine the drug release rate. The release rate can be extended for 4–24 h in the colon and each osmotic unit is designed for a 3–4 h post-gastric delay for drug release.

A modification of the osmotic pump suitable for colonic drug delivery involves a microbially triggered release mechanism. Liu et al. exploited the gelation of chitosan under acidic conditions and its degradation in the colon to use it as an osmotic agent and as a pore-forming agent in the impermeable cellulose acetate membrane.[49] The authors designed a dosage form containing citric acid and chitosan in the drug containing core, which had a coating of cellulose acetate and chitosan, followed by an enteric coat of methacrylic acid/methyl methacrylate copolymer, Eudragit L100. As shown in Figure 14.2A, upon reaching the small intestine, the enteric coat dissolves followed by water permeation into the core, which leads to the formation of a flowable gel through the dissolution of citric acid and the swelling of chitosan. However, chitosan in the cellulose acetate membrane is completely dissolved only in the colonic microenvironment, thus preventing significant drug release until the dosage form reaches the colon. As shown in Figure 14.2B, using budesonide as a model drug, the authors showed drug release inhibition at gastric and intestinal pH levels and controlled release in the simulated colonic fluid (SCF), which was a function of the amounts of chitosan, citric acid, and the coating thickness. On similar lines, Kumar et al. designed a metronidazole delivery system using guar gum as a pore-forming agent and showed *in vitro* drug release characteristics that demonstrated its potential for colon targeting.[20]

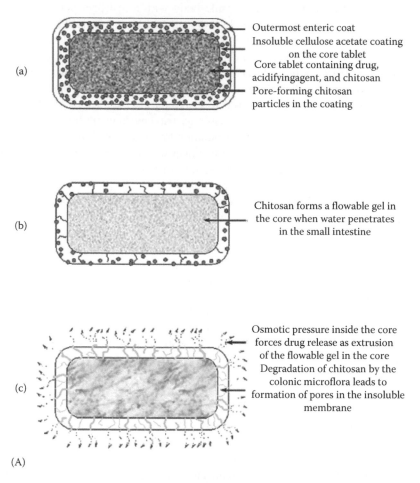

FIGURE 14.2 An osmotic pump colonic drug delivery system that utilizes gelation of chitosan under acidic conditions and its degradation in the colon by the local microflora. (A) Core tablets contain both the drug and chitosan. Cores are coated with a semipermeable membrane of cellulose acetate and chitosan, followed by the outermost enteric coating of Eudragit L 100. The dosage form stays intact in the stomach environment (a). Dissolution of the enteric coat in the small intestine is followed by water penetration into the core and formation of a flowable gel (b). When the dosage form arrives in the colon, the colonic microflora degrade chitosan particles in the coating leading to pore formation in the coat (c). This allows the flowable gel in the core of the tablet to extrude out from the semipermeable cellulose acetate coating in the colon.

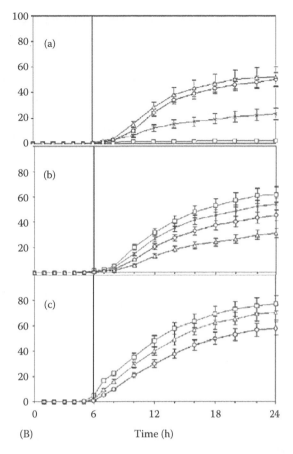

(B)   Time (h)

FIGURE 14.2 (continued) (B) *In vitro* drug release from this formulation was inhibited in the simulated gastric and intestinal fluids, which represent the first 6 h of dissolution profile in Figure 14.3B. The dosage form was exposed to the simulated colonic fluid (SCF) from 6 h to 24 h. In SCF, drug release was a function of chitosan/citric acid ratio (a; where weight ratio of chitosan/citric acid is represented by —□—, 1:1; —✶—, 1:1.6; —◇—, 1:2; and —△—, 1:2.6), amount of chitosan in the core (b; where the amount of chitosan is represented by —□—, 55 mg; —✶—, 60 mg; —◇—, 50 mg; and —△—, 40 mg), and the thickness of the cellulose acetate coating (c; where % weight gain of the coating is represented by —□—, 10%; —△—, 12%; —◇—, 14%). (Modified from Liu, H. et al., *Int. J. Pharm.*, 332, 115, 2007.)

14.2.5 COMBINATION AND OTHER STRATEGIES FOR COLON TARGETING

Physiological differences between the colon and the small intestine, such as intra-luminal pressure and the level of hydration, can also be utilized to design a colon targeted drug delivery system. For example, Takada and colleagues[50] utilized the higher intra-luminal pressure in the colon and its low hydration state as a trigger mechanism for drug release. To utilize this as a trigger for drug release, the authors prepared liquid-filled hard gelatin capsules coated with an insoluble ethyl cellulose film. The drug was dissolved in a water soluble or insoluble semisolid base, such as polyethylene glycol 1000 (PEG 1000), which liquifies at body temperature. After oral administration of the capsule, it behaves as a flexible membrane balloon with encapsulated drug, thus maintaining integrity during small intestinal transit. Upon reaching the colon, the reabsorption of water leads to an increased viscosity of the contents of the ethyl cellulose balloon, leading to its fragility and disintegration under higher pressure. The authors identified the thickness of the water-insoluble ethyl cellulose membrane as the key factor that controls drug release. Using this system, they demonstrated targeted delivery to the human colon using caffeine as a model drug[51,52] and glycyrrhizin in dogs.[53]

In addition to targeted drug release in the colon, the dosage form may incorporate a bioadhesive polymer to prolong the duration of time the dosage form stays in the colon. The polymers that can be used for this purpose include polycarbophils, polyurethanes, and poly(ethylene oxide—proplylene oxide) copolymers. Utilizing this strategy, Kakoulides et al. synthesized azo cross-linked bioadhesive acrylic polymers. The cross-linking prevents hydration and swelling in the upper intestinal tract.[54] Upon degradation of azo bonds in the large intestine, hydrogel swelling and bioadhesion was expected to lead to drug release and prolonged residence in the colonic environment.[55,56]

Similarly, Gao et al. synthesized a conjugate of bioadhesive polymer N-(2-hydroxypropyl) methacrylamide (HPMA) and the drug 9-aminocamptothecin (9-AC) via a spacer containing a combination of an aromatic azo bond and a 4-aminobenzylcarbamate group.[57] The spacer was designed to release the drug by azo bond cleavage in the colonic microenvironment. In subsequent studies, the authors observed colon targeting in mouse[58] and rat[59] models for the treatment of colon cancer. After oral administration of equal doses of the polymer conjugate or free 9-AC to mice, the colon-specific release of 9-AC produced high local concentrations with the mean peak concentration of 9-AC in cecal contents, feces, cecal tissue, and colon tissue being 3.2, 3.5, 2.2, and 1.6-fold higher, respectively. Therefore, the authors anticipated higher antitumor efficacy of the polymer conjugate due to prolonged colon tumor exposure to higher and more localized drug concentrations.

Combination strategies for colon-specific drug delivery commonly utilize a combination of pH and colonic microflora-based strategies. For example, Kaur and Kim prepared prednisolone beads with multiple coating layers for colonic delivery of the anti-inflammatory compound.[60] The authors coated prednisolone on nonpareil beads followed by a hydrophobic coat of Eudragit RL/RS; followed by a layer containing chitosan, succinic acid, and Eudragit RL/RS; followed by an outermost enteric coat layer (Figure 14.3). *In vitro* experiments showed an absence of drug release in simulated gastric and intestinal fluids, followed by drug release in the pathological colonic fluid with rate dependence on the presence of succinic acid in the formulation and the enzyme β-glucosidase. The authors proposed a combination mechanism of drug release that involved pH-triggered enteric dissolution of the outermost layer, followed by chitosan and Eudragit swelling in the presence of succinic acid, and biodegradation of chitosan by the colonic bacteria. Organic acid interacts with the amine groups in Eudragit and chitosan polymers, leading to increased permeability of the coating and facilitated drug release at the colonic site. Upon oral administration of this formulation to male Sprague-Dawley rats, a significant delay in the time to maximum plasma drug concentration (T_{max}) was obtained compared with both unmodified powder and enteric-coated tablet formulations, thus indicating colonic targeting (Figure 14.3).

14.3 DRUG DELIVERY TO THE KIDNEY

Renal targeting is valuable to avoid extrarenal side effects of drugs used in the treatment of kidney diseases or to optimize the intra-renal distribution of a drug candidate, thus increasing its therapeutic index. Although renal drug delivery is not the most studied area in drug targeting, it highlights the challenges and opportunities inherent in developing a targeted drug delivery system. The drugs used for the treatment of kidney diseases, among others, are anti-inflammatory and anti-fibrotic compounds. Specific drug delivery to the kidney may also be helpful during shock, renal transplantation, ureteral obstruction, diabetes, renal carcinoma, and other diseases such as Fanconi

> Renal targeting is valuable to avoid extrarenal side effects of drugs used in the treatment of kidney diseases or to optimize the intrarenal distribution of a drug candidate, thus increasing its therapeutic index. Three cellular drug targets have been identified within the kidney—proximal tubular cells, mesangial cells, and fibroblasts.

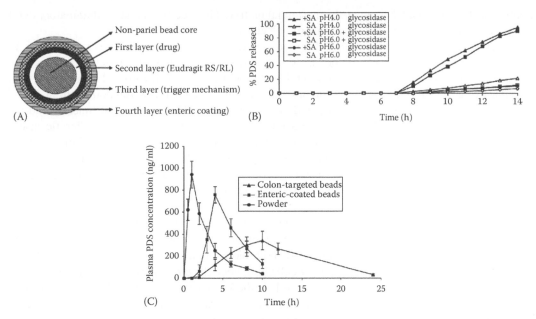

FIGURE 14.3 Combination strategy for colonic drug targeting using an oral solid dosage form. (A) Design of the targeted drug delivery system. Predniosolone (PDS, drug) was coated on nonpariel beads (first layer), followed by a hydrophobic coat of Eudragit RS/RL polymers (second layer), which was followed by a layer of Eudragit RS/RL polymers in combiation with chitosan and succinic acid (third layer), and the outermost enteric coating layer of Eudragit L 100 (fourth layer). (B) *In vitro* drug release from the system as a function of pH, succinic acid (SA) content in the formulation, and β-glucosidase content in the dissolution medium. The formulation dissolution was carried out in the gastric fluid for the first 2 h, followed by the small intestinal fluid for next 5 h, and the pathological colonic fluid for the last 7 h. (C) Plasma drug concentration after oral administration of powder, enteric-coated, or colon-targeted drug delivery sytsems in rats. (Modified from Kaur, K. and Kim, K., *Int. J. Pharm.*, 366, 140, 2009.)

and Bartter's syndrome.[61] Also, renal targeting can be helpful for drugs that would otherwise be rapidly metabolized and inactivated before reaching the kidney and to overcome or minimize the effects of pathological conditions, such as proteinuria, on drug distribution to the target site.

14.3.1 CELLULAR DRUG TARGETS

Three cellular drug targets have been identified within the kidney—proximal tubular cells, mesangial cells, and fibroblasts.[61] Nephron, the functional unit of the kidney, consists of a renal corpuscle and a renal tubule. The renal corpuscle is responsible for the filtration of blood. It consists of the glomerulus and the Bowman's capsule. The renal tubule consists of proximal and distal convoluted tubules interconnected by the loop of Henle. After blood filtration through the glomerulus, the proximal convoluted tubule is responsible for pH regulation and reabsorption of salts and organic solutes from the filtrate. The luminal surface of the proximal tubular cells has a brush border epithelium, with densely packed microvilli, which help increase the luminal surface area.

Mesangium, or the mesangial tissue, constitutes the inner layer of the glomerulus within the basement membrane of the renal corpuscle. It surrounds the glomerular arteries and arterioles both within (intraglomerular) and outside (extraglomerular) the glomerulus. The glomerular epithelium is fenestrated and there is no basement membrane between the glomerular capillaries and the mesangial cells. Hence, mesangial cells are separated from the capillary lumen by only a layer of endothelial cells. Mesangial cells are phagocytic in nature and secrete an amorphous, basement membrane-like material, known as the mesangial matrix. These cells generate inflammatory cytokines and are involved in the uptake of macromolecules.

Fibroblasts synthesize the extracellular matrix (ECM) and collagen. Excessive production and accumulation of the ECM leads to fibrosis. Renal fibrosis is the underlying process that leads to the progression of chronic kidney disease to end-stage renal disease. It involves changes in the renal vasculature, glomerulosclerosis, and tubulointerstitial fibrosis. Of these, tubulointerstitial fibrosis is considered to be the most consistent predictor of an irreversible loss of renal function and progression to end-stage renal disease.[62] The accumulation of ECM components in fibrotic disease is attributed to the activation of resident interstitial fibroblasts. Therefore, targeted drug delivery to renal fibroblasts has been attempted. For example, Kushibiki et al. used cationized gelatin to complex an enhanced green fluorescent protein (EGFP) expressing plasmid, which was injected into the left kidney of mice through the ureter. The authors observed significant EGFP expression in the fibroblasts residing in the renal interstitial cortex.[63] Similarly, Xia et al. reported the delivery of small interfering RNA (siRNA) targeted against heat shock protein 47 (HSP47) using cationized gelatin microspheres to the mice kidneys with tubulointerstitial fibrosis. The authors observed that the cationized gelatin microspheres enhanced and prolonged the antifibrotic effect of the siRNA.[64]

Of these cell types, the proximal tubular cells have been the target for most drug delivery strategies. They are metabolically the most active cells in the kidney and are involved with the transport[65] and metabolism[66] of several organic and inorganic substrates. Consequently, they have specific transporter receptors on their luminal and basolateral membranes for substrate exchange between the blood and the urine. These transport and metabolic functions of the proximal tubular epithelial cells are utilized for drug targeting.

14.3.2 Particulate Systems

The lack of basement membrane in the glomerular capillaries causes the mesangial cells to come in closer contact with the bloodstream, being separated from the capillary lumen by only a layer of endothelial cells. The mesangial cells, therefore, can be targeted using particulate carrier systems that may not filter through the glomeruli. Tuffin et al. used OX7 coupled immunoliposomes to target renal mesangial cells.[67] The authors coupled OX7 monoclonal antibody F(ab')$_2$ fragments, directed against the mesangial cell expressing Thy1.1 antigen, on the surface of doxorubicin-loaded immunoliposomes. The authors observed specific targeting to rat mesangial cells *in vitro* and *in vivo* upon intravenous administration (Figure 14.4). The administration of doxorubicin encapsulated immunoliposomes resulted in significant glomerular damage, with low damage to other parts of the kidney and other organs. The targeted localization was not observed with free drug or liposomes, and immunoliposome localization was blocked by the coadministration of free antibody fragments.

In a later study, the authors attempted to correlate the biodistribution of these immunoliposomes with the tissue distribution of the antigen.[68] The Thy1.1 antigen showed a high expression in rat glomeruli, brain cortex and striatum, and thymus; and moderate expression in the collecting ducts of the kidney, lung, and spleen. The biodistribution of immunoliposomes did not correlate well with the tissue distribution of Thy1.1 antigen, with the highest levels seen in the spleen, followed by the lungs, liver, and kidney. Within the kidney, specific localized delivery to the mesangial cells was observed, which was sensitive to competition with the unbound OX7 monoclonal antibody fragments. The authors concluded that the absence of endothelial barriers and high target antigen density are important factors governing tissue localization of immunoliposomes.

An application of drug targeting to glomerular endothelial cells to reduce the systemic side effects of drug therapy was reported by Asgeirsdottir et al., who used immunoliposomes to target glomerular endothelial cells in mice.[69] Glomerulonephritis, a spectrum of inflammatory diseases specifically affecting renal glomeruli, is characterized by the activation of proinflammatory pathways, resulting in glomerular injury and proteinuria. These disorders are frequently treated with glucocorticoids, such as dexamethasone, in combination with cytotoxic agents, such as

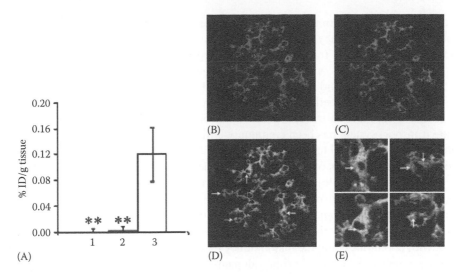

FIGURE 14.4 Tissue distribution and immunohistochemical localization of OX7 labeled immunoliposomes. (A) Shows that higher percentage of injected dose (% ID) of immunoliposomes (labeled 3) was observed in the kidney as compared to unlabeled liposomes (1) and immunoliposomes administered with 10-fold excess of free antibody fragments as competitive targeting inhibitor (2). (B) through (D) show the sub-renal distribution of immunoliposomes. Immunostaining for the mesangium in kidney sections (B) corresponds to the green signal for fluorescein isothiocyante (FITC) (C), which is evident in the superimposed (D) and (E). (Modified from Tuffin, G. et al., *J. Am. Soc. Nephrol.*, 16, 3295, 2005.)

cyclophosphamide, as anti-inflammatory and immunosuppressive agents. These drugs, however, present serious extrarenal side effects including an increase in blood glucose levels with dexamethasone.[70,71] Asgeirsdottir et al. coupled monoclonal rat anti-mouse E-selectin antibody, MES-1, to the surface of liposomes. The selection of this antibody was designed to target glomerular endothelial cells in glomerulonephritis, wherein endothelial cell expression of inflammation-related cell adhesion molecules, such as E-selectin and VCAM-1, is upregulated. The authors obtained the site-specific delivery of the immunoliposome-encapsulated anti-inflammatory agent dexamethasone and observed a reduction in glomerular proinflammatory gene expression with no effect on blood glucose levels.

In addition to liposomes, nanoparticles have been utilized for drug targeting to the mesangial cells. For example, Manil et al. used isobutylcyanoacrylate nanoparticles for targeting the antibiotic actinomycin D to rat mesangial cells.[72] Compared with the free drug, the uptake of drug-loaded nanoparticles in the whole kidneys was over twofold at both 30 min and 120 min after intravenous injection. Similar or higher uptake ratios were obtained for isolated rat glomeruli, but not for tubules. The glomerular uptake of nanoparticles was even higher in rats with experimental glomerulonephritis. Mesangial cell targeting was indicated by *in vitro* experiments, which demonstrated a fivefold higher uptake by mesangial cells than the epithelial cells. In a separate study, Guzman et al. also obtained about a twofold higher *in vitro* uptake of drug-loaded nanoparticles in rat mesangial cells using polycaprolactone as the polymeric carrier and digitoxin as the drug candidate.[73]

14.3.3 PRODRUG APPROACH

Prodrugs are drug conjugates designed to modify the physicochemical and/or biopharmaceutical properties of the drug candidate. Their derivatization is bioreversible and is designed to improve drug properties with respect to solubility, stability, permeability, presystemic metabolism, and targeting.[74] Prodrugs retain the advantages of low molecular weight compounds such as low immunogenicity and feasibility of oral administration. Renal specificity of prodrugs would depend on the renal-specific metabolism and/or the uptake of the promoiety. For this purpose, amino acid prodrugs, which can be activated by kidney specific enzymes, have been evaluated for renal targeting.

Amino acid prodrugs have the advantage of biodegradability in addition to receptor-mediated uptake, which can help in both oral absorption and organ- or tissue-specific targeting. For example, valine prodrugs of acyclovir and ganciclovir showed 3–5 times higher bioavailability than the parent compounds.[75,76] The enhanced oral absorption of amino acid prodrugs is attributed to the carrier-mediated intestinal uptake via transporters.[77–80] For organ- and tissue-specific drug targeting, the L-glutamate transport system has been commonly utilized.[81]

The prodrug design for renal targeting is aimed at utilizing kidney-specific enzymes. The proximal tubular cells contain high levels of metabolizing enzymes in the cytosol (such as L-amino acid decarboxylase, β-lyase, and N-acetyl transferase) and at the brush border (such as γ-glutamyl transpeptidase). Examples of renal-targeted prodrugs include the γ-glutamyl prodrugs of L-dopa and sulfamethoxazole.

Gludopa (γ-L-glutamyl-L-dopa) is a kidney-specific dopamine prodrug. Cummings et al. reported its pharmacokinetic and tissue distribution in rats.[82] Gludopa was metabolized primarily in the liver and kidney, with dopamine being the major kidney metabolite. The pharmacokinetics of gludopa in healthy human volunteers indicated urinary dopamine excretion in parallel with urinary levodopa excretion, supporting the view that levodopa was the precursor of urinary dopamine.[83] Based on these results, Boateng et al. indicated that gludopa may be useful in conditions where the renal effects of dopamine are indicated. However, Lee noted the limitations in clinical practice posed by its low oral bioavailability in humans.[84]

The kidney-specific delivery of parent compounds after the intravenous administration of γ-L-glutamyl (G) and N-acetyl-γ-L-glutamyl (AG) prodrugs of p-nitroaniline, sulfamethoxazole, and sulphamethizole was investigated by Murakami et al. in rats.[85] The authors observed a higher plasma stability with AG over G prodrugs for all compounds. The concentration of parent compounds was higher in the kidney than the pulmonary and hepatic tissue for all compounds, with markedly increased kidney distribution of AG prodrugs of p-nitroaniline and sulfamethoxazole. The activation of AG prodrugs requires the action of two enzymes—deacylation by N-acylamino acid deacylase and hydrolysis by γ-glutamyl transpeptidase, whereas G prodrugs can be activated by the action of γ-glutamyl transpeptidase alone. When the biodistribution of G prodrugs of sulfamethoxazole was studied in mice, relatively high concentrations of sulfamethoxazole were found in nonrenal tissues as well an indication of the rapid kinetics of the enzymatic cleavage of G prodrugs even in tissues with low γ-glutamyl transpeptidase activity.[86] However, kidney-selective accumulation was obtained after the administration of AG prodrugs. Drieman et al. hypothesized that the renal selectivity of AG prodrugs of sulfamethoxazole was due to a carrier-mediated transport followed by the intracellular conversion of the prodrug to the active compound.[87,88]

> Amino acid prodrugs, which can be activated by kidney-specific enzymes, have been evaluated for renal targeting. The proximal tubular cells contain high levels of metabolizing enzymes in the cytosol (such as L-amino acid decarboxylase, β-lyase, and N-acetyl transferase) and at the brush border (such as γ-glutamyl transpeptidase). For example, gludopa (γ-L-glutamyl-L-dopa) is a kidney-specific dopamine prodrug.

The effective utilization of the prodrug strategy requires the intensive investigation of the role of variables such as the linker groups and the promoiety modifications.[89,90] This results in inherent complexity in prodrug design and utilization for organ- or tissue-targeted drug delivery.

14.3.4 BIOCONJUGATION APPROACHES

The bioconjugation of a drug to a carrier that is significantly larger than the molecular size of the drug allows the biopharmaceutical properties of carriers to dominate the absorption and biodistribution of the conjugate. In the case of renal drug targeting to the proximal tubular cells, the conjugates would need to be filtered through the glomerular capillaries and reabsorbed by the tubular cells. Particles with a hydrodynamic diameter below 5–7 µm are rapidly filtered through the glomerulus.[91]

For this purpose, the carriers that naturally accumulate in the proximal tubular cells can be used as drug carriers. These include the low (less than about 30 kDa) molecular weight proteins (LMWPs), such as lysozyme, aprotinin, and cytochrome *C*. They are readily filtered through the glomerulus but selectively reabsorbed by the proximal tubular cells (Figure 14.5).[92] Thus, LMWP-drug conjugates that are stable in the plasma but cleaved within the proximal tubular cells after endosomal/lysosomal uptake can be used as effective vehicles for drug targeting. Drugs may be conjugated to LMWPs directly using the lysine amino groups or through the use of a spacer.[93] The relatively large size of the LMWPs allows the pharmacokinetic properties of the LMWPs to override those of the

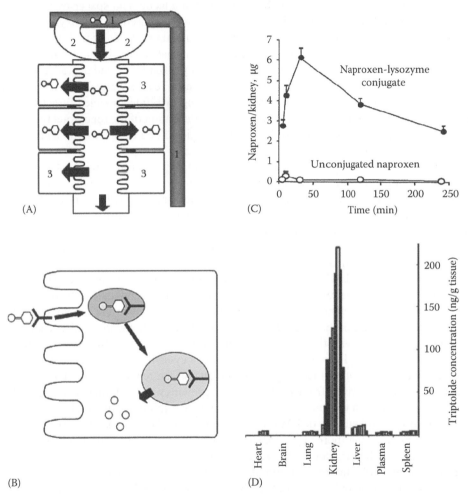

FIGURE 14.5 Proximal tubular cell targeting pathway and the biodistribution advantage of low molecular weight protein (LMWP) conjugation of small molecule drugs, using lysozyme-drug conjugate as an example. (A) The conjugate (o-O) in the bloodstream (1) is filtered through glomeruli (2) and actively endocytosed by the proximal tubular cells (3) through the megalin receptor (>−) on its luminal brush border endothelium. (B) The conjugate (o-O) is entrapped within the endosome (⊙o>), which converts to a lysosome with the lowering of pH and degradation of the protein, thus releasing the drug. (C) Renal accumulation of naproxen after intravenous injection of naproxen (open symbols) or naproxen-lysozyme (closed symbols) conjugate in rats. (D) Biodistribution of triptolide as a function of time (0.08, 0.25, 0.5, 1, 1.5, 2, 4, 8, and 12 h, from right to left in each organ) after intravenous injection of triptolide-lysozyme conjugate in rats. (Modified from Dolman, M.E. et al., *Int. J. Pharm.*, 364, 249, 2008; Haas, M. et al., *Kidney Int.*, 52, 1693, 1997; and Zhang, Z. et al., *Biomaterials*, 30, 1372, 2009.)

drug candidate in the LMWP-drug conjugates. This approach, however, is limited by the requirement of parenteral administration and the potential immunogenicity of the conjugates.

The internalization of proteins in the proximal convoluted tubule epithelium cells is mediated via the multiligand megalin and cubilin receptors.[94] These cells have very high endocytic activity. After endocytosis, the protein is degraded in the lysosomes, wherein the attached drug may be released (Figure 14.5B). Lysozymes have been used as renal carriers for the nonsteroidal anti-inflammatory drug (NSAID) naproxen,[95,96] the acetylcholinesterase (ACE) inhibitor compound captoril,[97–99] and the nephroprotective compound triptolide.[100]

Naproxen is a carboxylic acid group bearing compound that could be conjugated to the amine group in lysozymes directly by an amide bond or through a lactic acid spacer by an ester bond.[98] The biodistribution and degradation of these conjugates was compared with lysozyme and naproxen by themselves in rats. Drug conjugation did not affect the renal uptake or degradation of lysozymes in the rat kidney.[95] The pharmacokinetic profile of the conjugates was similar to that of lysozyme, but markedly different from the drug. The drug was rapidly taken up by and degraded in the kidney with no detectable levels in the plasma (Figure 14.5C). Similar results were obtained when captopril was conjugated with lysozyme through a spacer utilizing disulfide linkage. Targeting this ACE inhibitor to the kidney was hypothesized to prevent the attenuation of the renoprotective (antiproteinuric) efficacy of captopril under high sodium concentrations. The drug was efficiently targeted to the kidney with rapid release of the drug.[99]

Triptolide is an immunosuppressive and anti-inflammatory natural compound with low water solubility and significant toxicity. Renal targeting of the triptolide–lysozyme conjugate linked through succinyl residue was investigated in rats.[100] The authors obtained a significantly higher targeting efficiency of the drug conjugate to the kidney with a reversal of disease progression in a renal ischemia-reperfusion injury rat model, lower hepatotoxicity, and no effect on immune and genital systems, compared with the free drug (Figure 14.5D). These results demonstrated the potential therapeutic benefits of renal drug targeting.

In addition to the use of LMWPs as drug-targeting ligands, their receptor-mediated uptake can also be utilized to mitigate the renal toxicity of drugs. For example, endocytosis by proximal tubular cells is responsible for the renal accumulation and toxicity of aminoglycoside antibiotics, such as gentamicin, which is a substrate of the megalin receptors. Watanabe et al. found that the coadministration of cytochrome C competes with the receptor-mediated renal uptake of gentamicin, thus reducing its renal accumulation in rats.[101] However, the required dose of cytochrome C was quite high; the authors tested the relative efficacy of peptide fragments in reducing the renal accumulation of gentamicin. Three peptide fragments derived from actin-regulating proteins were identified that reduced the renal accumulation of gentamicin without affecting its plasma concentration–time profile.[101]

In addition to the exploitation of LMWPs for modulating the pharmacokinetics and biodistribution of drugs by utilizing their physiological disposition to modify drug biodistribution, drugs and enzymes can also be targeted to the renal proximal tubular epithelial cells by their surface modification. For example, Inoue et al. modified the enzyme superoxide dismutase (SOD), which disproportionates the superoxide free radical into oxygen and hydrogen peroxide, thus reducing free radical and oxidative stress in the cells.[102] Intravenously administered Cu, Zn-SOD was rapidly removed from the circulation with a half-life of about 5 min and appeared intact in the urine, thus indicating that it is filtered through the glomerulus. The authors conjugated hexamethylene diamine (AH) to SOD. The conjugate (AH-SOD) was rapidly filtered through the glomeruli but bound apical plasma membranes of proximal tubular cells followed by localized action in these cells. The authors observed more than 80% of the radioactivity derived from AH-SOD localized in the kidney at 30 min after injection, most of which was localized in the proximal tubular cells (Figure 14.6). *In vitro* kinetic studies revealed that the specific binding of AH-SOD to the apical surface of the tubular cells was attributable to AH.[102]

Polymeric carriers have also been described for renal drug targeting. These include the anionized derivatives of polyvinyl pyrrolidone (PVP),[103,104] low molecular weight N-(hydroxypropyl)

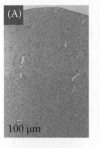

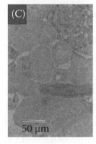
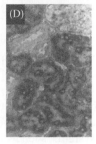

Distribution of radioactivity derived from SOD samples

Tissues	AH-SOD (%)	SOD (%)
Kidney	160,795 ± 34,560 (80.4)	13,371 ± 390 (9.2)
Urine	5,816 ± 2,345 (2.9)	145,875 ± 28,436 (72.9)
Brain	252 ± 92 (0.13)	132 ± 23 (0.07)
Heart	488 ± 123 (0.24)	122 ± 24 (0.03)
Lung	980 ± 357 (0.49)	163 ± 32 (0.03)
Liver	1,428 ± 640 (0.62)	235 ± 34 (0.12)
Spleen	744 ± 178 (0.37)	127 ± 27 (0.05)

(E)

FIGURE 14.6 Localization of hexamethylene diamine (AH) conjugate of superoxide dismutase (SOD) in rat kidney after intravenous administration, compared to SOD alone. (A) through (D) show immunohistochemical straining for human SOD at 30 minutes post-injection of either saline (A and C) or AH-SOD (B and D) at different magnifications. (E) Shows the accumulation of radioactivity predominantly in the kidney after AH-SOD was administered, compared to that of SOD alone. (Modified from Inoue, M. et al., *Arch. Biochem. Biophys.*, 368, 354, 1999.)

methylacrylamide (HPMA),[105] and low molecular weight chitosan.[106] The use of synthetic polymers requires surface modification and derivatizing groups for optimum renal accumulation. For example, PVP by itself does not accumulate in the tubular epithelial cells, but upon copolymerization with maleic acid, it is selectively distributed into the kidneys upon intravenous injection in mice.[104] When anionized derivatives of PVP were prepared, the plasma clearance of these derivatives decreased with the increasing size of anionic groups. Also, even though the clearance of carboxylated PVP and sulfonated PVP from the blood was similar, renal accumulation of carboxylated PVP was severalfold higher than that of sulfonated PVP.[104]

> LMWPs can be used as drug-targeting ligands. The receptor-mediated uptake of LMWPs can also be utilized to mitigate renal toxicity of drugs. For example, endocytosis by proximal tubular cells is responsible for the renal accumulation and toxicity of aminoglycoside antibiotics, such as gentamicin, which is a substrate of the megalin receptors. Coadministration of cytochrome *C* reduced the renal accumulation of gentamicin in rats.

In summary, these studies demonstrate not only the potential for renal targeting of drugs where it may be beneficial but also the potential to prevent accumulation in the kidney for drugs that have renal toxicity.

14.4 CONCLUDING REMARKS

Organ- and tissue-specific targeted drug delivery approaches are based on the unique elements of organ physiology and take into account any disease-state-induced pathological changes. These concepts were exemplified in this chapter using the relatively well established and nascent disciplines of colon- and kidney-specific drug targeting.

Colon- and kidney-specific drug delivery have been used for both local and systemic benefits. The targeted drug delivery for the treatment of diseases that have localized pathology can help increase local drug concentration and reduce systemic exposure, resulting in increased efficacy and decreased systemic toxicity. Site-specific drug delivery for local therapy is exemplified by the targeting of anti-inflammatory agents to the large intestine for the treatment of ulcerative colitis. In addition, due to the presence of lymphoid tissue and relatively mild conditions in the lumen, colonic delivery has been explored for the oral delivery of vaccines and the absorption of proteins and peptides from the GI tract. Colon targeting has also been explored to help reduce the serious upper GI side effects of drugs such as flurbiprofen.[12]

Drug targeting to the kidney has been used both for local drug action and for minimizing the renal or extrarenal side effects of drugs. Targeted renal delivery for local action is exemplified by the delivery of anti-inflammatory and antifibrotic compounds for glomerulonephritis and renal fibrosis. In addition, the kidney-specific delivery of dexamethasone minimized its extrarenal side effects.[69] The modulation of the renal effects of drugs can be done without drug modification or incoporation in a delivery system. For example, the renal specificity of coadministered LMWPs was used to minimize the renal toxicity of the aminoglycoside antibiotic gentamicin.[101]

Organ physiology is the key determinant of organ- or tissue-specific drug delivery strategy. Thus, colon targeting utilizes the presence of unique colonic microflora for the colon-specific degradation of polymeric carriers, coating agents, and prodrugs. In addition, the higher pH of the large intestine and intestinal transit time have been used for the design of dosage forms that release drug in the colon. In the kidney, drug targeting within the renal tissue is based on the anatomical location of cellular targets and their physiological function. The lack of an endothelial barrier to mesangial cells in the glomeruli allows them to be targeted by particulate systems, such as immunoliposomes, that may not be filtered through the glomeruli. In contrast, targeting proximal tubular cells requires glomerular filtration for anatomical access and utilizes their physiological function in the reabsorption of essential nutrients for targeted drug uptake.

In addition, specific case-studies and examples discussed in this chapter highlight that the potential value of targeted drug delivery depends on the unique elements of the clinical profile of the drug candidate. For example, targeted drug delivery can increase local drug concentration and enhance therapeutic efficacy depending on the mechanism and location of drug action. These are exemplified by the delivery of anti-inflammatory compounds to the colon and the renal mesangial cells. In addition, targeting approaches can also be used to overcome organ- or tissue-specific drug toxicities. Thus, the coadministration of LMWPs reduced the renal toxicity of gentamicin.[101] Also, liposomal encapsulation reduced the cardiotoxicity of doxorubicin due to reduced liposomal permeation through the relatively tight endothelial barriers in the cardiac tissue.[107] Therefore, optimal benefits and the value of targeted drug delivery can only be realized through a holistic consideration of the drug characteristics and clinical need in combination with organ physiology and tissue pathology.

REFERENCES

1. Molema, G and Meijer, KF, *Drug Targeting: Organ Specific Strategies* (Wiley-VCH Verlag GmbH, Weinheim, Germany, 2001).
2. Faraji, AH and Wipf, P. Nanoparticles in cellular drug delivery. *Bioorg. Med. Chem.* 2009; **17**(8): 2950–2962.
3. Raju, J, Srinivas, A, and Bairi, A. Drug targeting: Approaches to colonic drug delivery. *J. Chem. Pharm. Sci.* 2008; **1**(2): 52–55.
4. Gershkovich, P, Wasan, KM, and Barta, CA. A review of the application of lipid-based systems in systemic, dermal/transdermal, and ocular drug delivery. *Crit. Rev. Ther. Drug Carrier Syst.* 2008; **25**(6): 545–584.
5. Mayer, CR, Geis, NA, Katus, HA et al. Ultrasound targeted microbubble destruction for drug and gene delivery. *Expert Opin. Drug Deliv.* 2008; **5**(10): 1121–1138.
6. Temming, K, Fretz, MM, and Kok, RJ. Organ- and cell-type specific delivery of kinase: A novel approach in the development of targeted drugs. *Curr. Mol. Pharmacol.* 2008; **1**(1): 1–12.
7. Lim, CS. Organelle-specific targeting in drug delivery and design. *Adv. Drug Deliv. Rev.* 2007; **59**(8): 697.
8. Braun, K, Pipkorn, R, and Waldeck, W. Development and characterization of drug delivery systems for targeting mammalian cells and tissues: A review. *Curr. Med. Chem.* 2005; **12**(16): 1841–1858.

9. Di Paolo, A. Liposomal anticancer therapy: Pharmacokinetic and clinical aspects. *J. Chemother.* 2004; **16**(Suppl 4): 90–93.

10. Zhang, Q-Y, Dunbar, D, Ostrowska, A et al. Characterization of human small intestinal cytochromes P-450. *Drug Metab. Dispos.* 1999; **27**(7): 804–809.

11. Peters, WH, Kock, L, Nagengast, FM et al. Biotransformation enzymes in human intestine: Critical low levels in the colon? *Gut* 1991; **32**(4): 408–412.

12. Philip, AK, Dubey, RK, and Pathak, K. Optimizing delivery of flurbiprofen to the colon using a targeted prodrug approach. *J. Pharm. Pharmacol.* 2008; **60**(5): 607–613.

13. Singh, BN. Modified-release solid formulations for colonic delivery. *Recent Pat. Drug Deliv. Formul.* 2007; **1**: 53–63.

14. Gazzaniga, A, Maroni, A, Sangalli, ME et al. Time-controlled oral delivery systems for colon targeting. *Expert Opin. Drug Deliv.* 2006; **3**(5): 583–597.

15. Hovgaard, L and Brondsted, H. Current applications of polysaccharides in colon targeting. *Crit. Rev. Ther. Drug Carrier Syst.* 1996; **13**(3–4): 185–223.

16. Ashford, M and Fell, JT. Targeting drugs to the colon: delivery systems for oral administration. *J. Drug Target.* 1994; **2**(3): 241–257.

17. Chourasia, MK and Jain, SK. Pharmaceutical approaches to colon targeted drug delivery systems. *J. Pharm. Pharm. Sci.* 2003; **6**(1): 33–66.

18. Chourasia, MK and Jain, SK. Polysaccharides for colon targeted drug delivery. *Drug Deliv.* 2004; **11**(2): 129–148.

19. Kosaraju, SL. Colon targeted delivery systems: Review of polysaccharides for encapsulation and delivery. *Crit. Rev. Food Sci. Nutr.* 2005; **45**(4): 251–258.

20. Kumar, P and Mishra, B. Colon targeted drug delivery systems—An overview. *Curr. Drug Deliv.* 2008; **5**(3): 186–198.

21. Haupt, S and Rubinstein, A. The colon as a possible target for orally administered peptide and protein drugs. *Crit. Rev. Ther. Drug Carrier Sys.* 2002; **19**(6): 499–551.

22. Jain, SK and Jain, A. Target-specific drug release to the colon. *Expert Opin. Drug Deliv.* 2008; **5**(5): 483–498.

23. Guarner, F and Malagelada, JR. Gut flora in health and disease. *Lancet* 2003; **361** (9356): 512–519.

24. Brown, JP, McGarraugh, GV, Parkinson, TM et al. A polymeric drug for treatment of inflammatory bowel disease. *J. Med. Chem.* 1983; **26**(9): 1300–1307.

25. Kalala, W, Kinget, R, Van den Mooter, G et al. Colonic drug-targeting: In vitro release of ibuprofen from capsules coated with poly(ether–ester) azopolymers. *Int. J. Pharm.* 1996; **139**(1,2): 187–195.

26. Van den Mooter, G, Samyn, C, and Kinget, R. In vivo evaluation of a colon-specific drug delivery system: An absorption study of theophylline from capsules coated with azo polymers in rats. *Pharm. Res.* 1995; **12**(2): 244–247.

27. Saffran, M, Kumar, GS, Neckers, DC et al. Biodegradable azopolymer coating for oral delivery of peptide drugs. *Biochem. Soc. Trans.* 1990; **18**(5): 752–754.

28. Van den Mooter, G, Samyn, C, and Kinget, R. Azo polymers for colon-specific drug delivery. *Int. J. Pharm.* 1992; **87**(1–3): 37–46.

29. Vaidya, A, Jain, A, Khare, P et al. Metronidazole loaded pectin microspheres for colon targeting. *J. Pharm. Sci.* 2009; **98**(11): 4229–4236.

30. Hodges, LA, Connolly, SM, Band, J et al. Scintigraphic evaluation of colon targeting pectin-HPMC tablets in healthy volunteers. *Int. J Pharm.* 2009; **370**(1–2): 144–150.

31. Freire, C, Podczeck, F, Veiga, F et al. Starch-based coatings for colon-specific delivery. Part II: Physicochemical properties and in vitro drug release from high amylose maize starch films. *Eur. J. Pharm. Biopharm.* 2009; **72**(3): 587–594.

32. Calinescu, C and Mateescu, MA. Carboxymethyl high amylose starch: Chitosan self-stabilized matrix for probiotic colon delivery. *Eur. J. Pharm. Biopharm.* 2008; **70**(2): 582–589.

33. Wilson, PJ and Basit, AW. Exploiting gastrointestinal bacteria to target drugs to the colon: An in vitro study using amylose coated tablets. *Int. J. Pharm.* 2005; **300**(1–2): 89–94.

34. Pitarresi, G, Tripodo, G, Calabrese, R et al. Hydrogels for potential colon drug release by thiol-ene conjugate addition of a new inulin derivative. *Macromol. Biosci.* 2008; **8**(10): 891–902.

35. Maris, B, Verheyden, L, Van Reeth, K et al. Synthesis and characterisation of inulin-azo hydrogels designed for colon targeting. *Int. J. Pharm.* 2001; **213**(1–2): 143–152.

36. Ji, CM, Xu, HN, and Wu, W. Guar gum as potential film coating material for colon-specific delivery of fluorouracil. *J. Biomater. Appl.* 2009; **23**(4): 311–329.

37. Ji, C, Xu, H, and Wu, W. In vitro evaluation and pharmacokinetics in dogs of guar gum and Eudragit FS30D-coated colon-targeted pellets of indomethacin. *J. Drug Target.* 2007; **15**(2): 123–131.

38. Kelm, GR, Kondo, K, and Nakajima, A. Bisacodyl dosage form with multiple enteric polymer coatings for colonic delivery. Patent No. 5843479 (1998).

39. Makhlof, A, Tozuka, Y, and Takeuchi, H. pH-Sensitive nanospheres for colon-specific drug delivery in experimentally induced colitis rat model. *Eur. J. Pharm. Biopharm.* 2009; **72**(1): 1–8.

40. Asghar, LF, Chure, CB, and Chandran, S. Colon specific delivery of indomethacin: effect of incorporating pH sensitive polymers in xanthan gum matrix bases. *AAPS Pharm. Sci. Tech.* 2009; **10**(2): 418–429.

41. Zambito, Y, Baggiani, A, Carelli, V et al. Matrices for site-specific controlled-delivery of 5-fluorouracil to descending colon. *J. Control. Release* 2005; **102**(3): 669–677.

42. Ashford, M, Fell, JT, Attwood, D et al. An in vivo investigation into the suitability of pH dependent polymers for colonic targeting. *Int. J. Pharm.* 1993; **95**(1–3): 193–199.

43. Wilson, CG and Washington, N. Assessment of disintegration and dissolution of dosage forms in vivo using gamma scintigraphy. *Drug Dev. Ind. Pharm.* 1988; **14**(2–3): 211–281.

44. Davis, SS, Hardy, JG, and Fara, JW. Transit of pharmaceutical dosage forms through the small intestine. *Gut* 1986; **27**(8): 886–892.

45. Stevens, HNE. Pulsincap and hydrophilic sandwich (HS) capsules: Innovative time-delayed oral drug delivery technologies. *Drugs Pharm. Sci.* 2003; **126**(Modified-Release Drug Delivery Technology): 257–262.

46. Stevens, HNE, Wilson, CG, Welling, PG et al. Evaluation of pulsincap to provide regional delivery of dofetilide to the human GI tract. *Int. J. Pharm.* 2002; **236**(1–2): 27–34.

47. Fukui, E, Miyamura, N, Uemura, K et al. Preparation of enteric coated timed-release press-coated tablets and evaluation of their function by in vitro and in vivo tests for colon targeting. *Int. J. Pharm.* 2000; **204**(1–2): 7–15.

48. Hebden, JM, Wilson, CG, Spiller, RC et al. Regional differences in quinine absorption from the undisturbed human colon assessed using a timed release delivery system. *Pharm. Res.* 1999; **16**(7): 1087–1092.

49. Liu, H, Yang, X-G, Nie, S-F et al. Chitosan-based controlled porosity osmotic pump for colon-specific delivery system: Screening of formulation variables and in vitro investigation. *Int. J. Pharm.* 2007; **332**(1–2): 115–124.

50. Hu, Z, Kimura, G, Mawatari, S et al. New preparation method of intestinal pressure-controlled colon delivery capsules by coating machine and evaluation in beagle dogs. *J. Control. Release* 1998; **56**(1–3): 293–302.

51. Hu, Z, Mawatari, S, Shimokawa, T et al. Colon delivery efficiencies of intestinal pressure-controlled colon delivery capsules prepared by a coating machine in human subjects. *J. Pharm. Pharmacol.* 2000; **52**(10): 1187–1193.

52. Muraoka, M, Hu, Z, Shimokawa, T et al. Evaluation of intestinal pressure-controlled colon delivery capsule containing caffeine as a model drug in human volunteers. *J. Control. Release* 1998; **52**(1–2): 119–129.

53. Shibata, N, Ohno, T, Shimokawa, T et al. Application of pressure-controlled colon delivery capsule to oral administration of glycyrrhizin in dogs. *J. Pharm. Pharmacol.* 2001; **53**(4): 441–447.

54. Mahkam, M and Doostie, L. The relation between swelling properties and cross-linking of hydrogels designed for colon-specific drug delivery. *Drug Deliv.* 2005; **12**(6): 343–347.

55. Kakoulides, EP, Smart, JD, and Tsibouklis, J. Azocross-linked poly(acrylic acid) for colonic delivery and adhesion specificity: Synthesis and characterisation. *J. Control. Release* 1998; **52**(3): 291–300.

56. Kakoulides, EP, Smart, JD, and Tsibouklis, J. Azocrosslinked poly(acrylic acid) for colonic delivery and adhesion specificity: In vitro degradation and preliminary ex vivo bioadhesion studies. *J. Control. Release* 1998; **54**(1): 95–109.

57. Gao, SQ, Lu, ZR, Petri, B et al. Colon-specific 9-aminocamptothecin-HPMA copolymer conjugates containing a 1,6-elimination spacer. *J. Control. Release* 2006; **110**(2): 323–331.

58. Gao, SQ, Lu, ZR, Kopeckova, P et al. Biodistribution and pharmacokinetics of colon-specific HPMA copolymer—9-aminocamptothecin conjugate in mice. *J. Control. Release* 2007; **117**(2): 179–185.

59. Gao, SQ, Sun, Y, Kopeckova, P et al. Pharmacokinetic modeling of absorption behavior of 9-aminocamptothecin (9-AC) released from colon-specific HPMA copolymer-9-AC conjugate in rats. *Pharm. Res.* 2008; **25**(1): 218–226.

60. Kaur, K and Kim, K. Studies of chitosan/organic acid/Eudragit RS/RL-coated system for colonic delivery. *Int. J. Pharm.* 2009; **366**: 140–148.

61. Haas, M, Moolenaar, F, Meijer, DK et al. Specific drug delivery to the kidney. *Cardiovasc. Drugs Ther.* 2002; **16**(6): 489–496.

62. Nangaku, M. Mechanisms of tubulointerstitial injury in the kidney: Final common pathways to end-stage renal failure. *Intern. Med.* 2004; **43**(1): 9–17.
63. Kushibiki, T, Nagata-Nakajima, N, Sugai, M et al. Targeting of plasmid DNA to renal interstitial fibroblasts by cationized gelatin. *Biol. Pharm. Bull.* 2005; **28**(10): 2007–2010.
64. Xia, Z, Abe, K, Furusu, A et al. Suppression of renal tubulointerstitial fibrosis by small interfering RNA targeting heat shock protein 47. *Am. J. Nephrol.* 2008; **28**(1): 34–46.
65. Christensen, EI, Birn, H, Verroust, P et al. Membrane receptors for endocytosis in the renal proximal tubule. *Int. Rev. Cytol.* 1998; **180**: 237–284.
66. Pacifici, GM, Viani, A, Franchi, M et al. Profile of drug-metabolizing enzymes in the cortex and medulla of the human kidney. *Pharmacol.* 1989; **39**(5): 299–308.
67. Tuffin, G, Waelti, E, Huwyler, J et al. Immunoliposome targeting to mesangial cells: A promising strategy for specific drug delivery to the kidney. *J. Am. Soc. Nephrol.* 2005; **16**(11): 3295–3305.
68. Tuffin, G, Huwyler, J, Waelti, E et al. Drug targeting using OX7-immunoliposomes: correlation between Thy1.1 antigen expression and tissue distribution in the rat. *J. Drug Target.* 2008; **16**(2): 156–166.
69. Asgeirsdottir, SA, Kamps, JA, Bakker, HI et al. Site-specific inhibition of glomerulonephritis progression by targeted delivery of dexamethasone to glomerular endothelium. *Mol. Pharm.* 2007; **72**(1): 121–131.
70. Chadban, SJ and Atkins, RC. Glomerulonephritis. *Lancet* 2005; **365**(9473): 1797–1806.
71. Tam, FW. Current pharmacotherapy for the treatment of crescentic glomerulonephritis. *Expert Opin. Investig. Drugs* 2006; **15**(11): 1353–1369.
72. Manil, L, Davin, JC, Duchenne, C et al. Uptake of nanoparticles by rat glomerular mesangial cells in vivo and in vitro. *Pharm. Res.* 1994; **11**(8): 1160–1165.
73. Guzman, M, Aberturas, MR, Rodriguez-Puyol, M et al. Effect of nanoparticles on digitoxin uptake and pharmacologic activity in rat glomerular mesangial cell cultures. *Drug Deliv.* 2000; **7**(4): 215–222.
74. Stella, VJ. Prodrugs as therapeutics. *Expert Opin. Ther. Pat.* 2004; **14**(3): 277–280.
75. Jung, D and Dorr, A. Single-dose pharmacokinetics of valganciclovir in HIV- and CMV-seropositive subjects. *J. Clin. Pharm.* 1999; **39**(8): 800–804.
76. Weller, S, Blum, MR, Doucette, M et al. Pharmacokinetics of the acyclovir pro-drug valaciclovir after escalating single- and multiple-dose administration to normal volunteers. *Clin. Pharm. Ther.* 1993; **54**(6): 595–605.
77. Amidon, GL and Walgreen, CR, Jr. 5′-Amino acid esters of antiviral nucleosides, acyclovir, and AZT are absorbed by the intestinal PEPT1 peptide transporter, *Pharm. Res.* 1999; **16**(2): 175.
78. Borner, V, Fei, YJ, Hartrodt, B et al. Transport of amino acid aryl amides by the intestinal H+/peptide cotransport system, PEPT1. *Eur. J Biochem./FEBS* 1998; **255**(3): 698–702.
79. Han, H, de Vrueh, RL, Rhie, JK et al. 5′-Amino acid esters of antiviral nucleosides, acyclovir, and AZT are absorbed by the intestinal PEPT1 peptide transporter. *Pharm. Res.* 1998; **15**(8): 1154–1159.
80. Umapathy, NS, Ganapathy, V, and Ganapathy, ME. Transport of amino acid esters and the amino-acid-based prodrug valganciclovir by the amino acid transporter ATB(0,+). *Pharm. Res.* 2004; **21**(7): 1303–1310.
81. Sakaeda, T, Siahaan, TJ, Audus, KL et al. Enhancement of transport of D-melphalan analogue by conjugation with L-glutamate across bovine brain microvessel endothelial cell monolayers. *J. Drug Target.* 2000; **8**(3): 195–204.
82. Cummings, J, Matheson, LM, Maurice, L et al. Pharmacokinetics, bioavailability, metabolism, tissue distribution and urinary excretion of gamma-L-glutamyl-L-dopa in the rat. *J. Pharm. Pharmacol.* 1990; **42**(4): 242–246.
83. Boateng, YA, Barber, HE, MacDonald, TM et al. Disposition of gamma-glutamyl levodopa (gludopa) after intravenous bolus injection in healthy volunteers. *Br. J. Clin. Pharmacol.* 1991; **31**(4): 419–422.
84. Lee, MR. Five years' experience with gamma-L-glutamyl-L-dopa: a relatively renally specific dopaminergic prodrug in man. *J. Auton. Pharmacol.* 1990; **10**(Suppl 1): s103–108.
85. Murakami, T, Kohno, K, Yumoto, R et al. *N*-acetyl-L-gamma-glutamyl derivatives of *p*-nitroaniline, sulphamethoxazole and sulphamethizole for kidney-specific drug delivery in rats. *J. Pharm. Pharmacol.* 1998; **50**(5): 459–465.
86. Orlowski, M, Mizoguchi, H, and Wilk, S. *N*-acyl-gamma-glutamyl derivatives of sulfamethoxazole as models of kidney-selective prodrugs. *J. Pharmacol. Exp. Ther.* 1980; **212**(1): 167–172.
87. Drieman, JC, Thijssen, HH, and Struyker-Boudier, HA. Renal selective *N*-acetyl-gamma-glutamyl prodrugs. II. Carrier-mediated transport and intracellular conversion as determinants in the renal selectivity of *N*-acetyl-gamma-glutamyl sulfamethoxazole. *J. Pharmacol. Exp. Ther.* 1990; **252**(3): 1255–1260.

88. Drieman, JC, Thijssen, HH, Zeegers, HH et al. Renal selective *N*-acetyl-gamma-glutamyl prodrugs: A study on the mechanism of activation of the renal vasodilator prodrug CGP 22979. *Br. J. Pharmacol.* 1990; **99**(1): 15–20.

89. Hashida, M, Akamatsu, K, Nishikawa, M et al. Design of polymeric prodrugs of prostaglandin E(1) having galactose residue for hepatocyte targeting. *J. Control. Release* 1999; **62**(1–2): 253–262.

90. Akamatsu, K, Yamasaki, Y, Nishikawa, M et al. Synthesis and pharmacological activity of a novel water-soluble hepatocyte-specific polymeric prodrug of prostaglandin E(1) using lactosylated poly(L-glutamic hydrazide) as a carrier. *Biochem. Pharmacol.* 2001; **62**(11): 1531–1536.

91. Choi, HS, Liu, W, Misra, P et al. Renal clearance of quantum dots. *Nat. Biotechnol.* 2007; **25**(10): 1165–1170.

92. Haas, M, de Zeeuw, D, van Zanten, A et al. Quantification of renal low-molecular-weight protein handling in the intact rat. *Kidney Int.* 1993; **43**(4): 949–954.

93. Franssen, EJ, Koiter, J, Kuipers, CA et al. Low molecular weight proteins as carriers for renal drug targeting. Preparation of drug–protein conjugates and drug-spacer derivatives and their catabolism in renal cortex homogenates and lysosomal lysates. *J. Med. Chem.* 1992; **35**(7): 1246–1259.

94. Christensen, EI and Verroust, PJ. Megalin and cubilin, role in proximal tubule function and during development. *Pediat. Nephrol.* 2002; **17**(12): 993–999.

95. Haas, M, Kluppel, ACA, Wartna, ES et al. Drug-targeting to the kidney: Renal delivery and degradation of a naproxen–lysozyme conjugate in vivo. *Kidney Int.* 1997; **52**(6): 1693–1699.

96. Franssen, EJF, Moolenaar, F, de Zeeuw, D et al. Low-molecular-weight proteins as carriers for renal drug targeting: Naproxen coupled to lysozyme via the spacer L-lactic acid. *Pharm. Res.* 1993; **10**(7): 963–969.

97. Windt, WAKM, Prakash, J, Kok, RJ et al. Renal targeting of captopril using captopril–lysozyme conjugate enhances its antiproteinuric effect in adriamycin-induced nephrosis. *JRAAS* 2004; **5**(4): 197–202.

98. Prakash, J, van Loenen-Weemaes, AM, Haas, M et al. Renal-selective delivery and angiotensin-converting enzyme inhibition by subcutaneously administered captopril-lysozyme. *Drug Metab. Dispos.* 2005; **33**(5): 683–688.

99. Kok, RJ, Grijpstra, F, Walthuis, RB et al. Specific delivery of captopril to the kidney with the prodrug captopril–lysozyme. *J. Pharm. Exp. Ther.* 1999; **288**(1): 281–285.

100. Zhang, Z, Zheng, Q, Han, J et al. The targeting of 14-succinate triptolide–lysozyme conjugate to proximal renal tubular epithelial cells. *Biomaterials* 2009; **30**(7): 1372–1381.

101. Watanabe, A, Nagai, J, Adachi, Y et al. Targeted prevention of renal accumulation and toxicity of gentamicin by aminoglycoside binding receptor antagonists. *J. Control. Release* 2004; **95**(3): 423–433.

102. Inoue, M, Nishikawa, M, Sato, E et al. Synthesis of superoxide dismutase derivative that specifically accumulates in renal proximal tubule cells. *Archiv. Biochem. Biophys.* 1999; **368**(2): 354–360.

103. Kamada, H, Tsutsumi, Y, Sato-Kamada, K et al. Synthesis of a poly(vinylpyrrolidone-*co*-dimethyl maleic anhydride) co-polymer and its application for renal drug targeting. *Nat. Biotechnol.* 2003; **21**(4): 399–404.

104. Kodaira, H, Tsutsumi, Y, Yoshioka, Y et al. The targeting of anionized polyvinylpyrrolidone to the renal system. *Biomaterials* 2004; **25**(18): 4309–4315.

105. Kissel, M, Peschke, P, Subr, V et al. Detection and cellular localisation of the synthetic soluble macromolecular drug carrier pHPMA. *Eur. J. Nucl. Med. Mol. Imaging* 2002; **29**(8): 1055–1062.

106. Yuan, ZX, Sun, X, Gong, T et al. Randomly 50% *N*-acetylated low molecular weight chitosan as a novel renal targeting carrier. *J. Drug Target.* 2007; **15**(4): 269–278.

107. Wigler, N, O'Brien, M, and Rosso, R. Reduced cardiac toxicity and comparable efficacy in a phase III trial of pegylated liposomal doxorubicin (Caelyx®/Doxil®) vs. doxorubicin for first-line treatment of metastatic breast cancer. In *Conference Proceeding, American Society of Clinical Oncology,* 2002, Orlando, FL.

108. Dolman, ME, Fretz, MM, Segers, GJ et al. Renal targeting of kinase inhibitors. *Int. J. Pharm.* 2008; **364**(2): 249–257.

15 Principles and Practice of Pulmonary Drug Delivery

Vivek Gupta, Chandan Thomas, and Fakhrul Ahsan

CONTENTS

15.1 INTRODUCTION

The lungs have been extensively used for medicinal and recreational purposes for hundreds or even thousands of years. Pulmonary drug delivery refers to a noninvasive route of administration for delivering drugs to the body via the lungs for local and systemic effects by inhalation. The human lungs have the capacity to actively exchange various materials between the external environment and the interior of the body. This ability of the lungs makes them a very convenient and safe route for administration of a number of drugs that are considered unsuitable for administration via other routes, such as oral and parenteral routes.

Although some consider inhalation therapy as a new drug delivery approach, it has been in practice since ancient times. The use of leaves from the *Atropa belladonna* plant for the treatment of throat and chest diseases was described in Ayurvedic medicine more than 4000 years ago. Belladonna leaves containing atropine used to be smoked for the treatment of various diseases. During the industrial revolution, "asthma cigarettes" containing stramonium from *Datura stramonium* were introduced for the first time.[1,2] In the late 1820s, first generation nebulizers were developed for the inhalation of droplets instead of vapors. Despite a lot of research in the field of inhaled drugs over the first half of the nineteenth century, the second half of the century evidenced the development of highly effective inhaled asthma medications with portable delivery devices. Considering this fact, it can be argued that inhaled drugs have been in practice for more than 50 years now. About 25–30 inhalation products for the treatment of various lung diseases are now commercially available.[3–5]

Although currently there is no inhaled formulation in the market for the treatment of systemic diseases, an ever-increasing number of inhalable drugs for treating systemic diseases are in the pipeline. Recent advances in drug delivery systems have made it possible to formulate and deliver almost any drug via the lungs.[6] According to recent reports, at least 5–10 pharmaceutical industries have been conducting extensive research in the area of inhalable drug delivery. A report published by the Kalorama Foundation suggests that the market for pulmonary drug delivery systems reached

25.5 billion in 2006—an annual increase of about 12% since 2002. As per a report published by the Kalorama Foundation, the market for pulmonary drug delivery is expected to grow to 34 billion by 2010 with a 10% increase in annual growth.[7]

Pulmonary drug delivery can be utilized for the delivery of a variety of molecules into the body. This may include drugs for the treatment of various lung and systemic diseases. The major class of molecules being investigated includes systemically active peptides and proteins, such as insulin, interferons, growth hormone–releasing peptides, and, more recently, hepatitis-B vaccine.[8–10] The pulmonary drug delivery approach has also been used for many small molecules that act locally in the lungs.[1,11] Moreover, over the past few years, many research groups have explored the possibility of targeting drugs to various regions of the lungs to maximize therapeutic efficacy at the affected region while eliminating the exposure of drugs to other parts of the lungs and body. The drug targeting approach has been utilized mainly for the treatment of various lung diseases such as non-small-cell lung cancer, cystic fibrosis, and pulmonary arterial hypertension (PAH).[12–14]

Drug delivery via the pulmonary route offers various advantages over other routes of administration. The most important advantage is the possibility of needle-free treatment. Another major advantage is the ease of administration without the help of health professionals. This eliminates the risks associated with the use of needles and catheters. Furthermore, the lungs provide an enormous absorptive surface area ($100 m^2$) and a thin, highly permeable mucous membrane. These features of the lungs make them highly permeable to macromolecules in comparison with any other ports of entry to the body. Drugs delivered via the pulmonary route bypass metabolism and degradation by the enzymes in the gut and liver, thus delivering the drugs to the body very efficiently without generating toxic metabolites. This may result in a similar therapeutic effect at a fraction of the dose administered by other noninvasive routes. Pulmonary delivery provides a quicker absorption of drugs than that achieved by other noninvasive routes, resulting in a rapid clinical response and improved bioavailability. For example, inhaled insulin provides a faster and more physiological response when compared with subcutaneously injected insulin. Macromolecular drugs with very low absorption rates are extensively absorbed from the lungs and may have prolonged residence time. Moreover, pulmonary delivery being independent of complications associated with food intake and variability due to metabolic degradation gives reproducible absorption profiles. However, there are several disadvantages with pulmonary drug delivery systems that include limited absorption due to the physical barrier of the mucus layer, interactions of many drugs with the mucus, reduced retention time due to lungs' clearance mechanisms, and the inaccessibility of lung surfaces for targeted delivery.[1,6,11]

To understand the delivery and absorption of drugs via the pulmonary route, and the physiological factors influencing it, one must be familiar with the details of the anatomy and physiology of the lungs or of the respiratory system in a broader sense.

15.2 ANATOMY AND PHYSIOLOGY OF RESPIRATORY SYSTEM

The human respiratory system can be divided broadly into (1) conducting airways carrying air to the alveoli—the gas exchange region of the lungs and (2) the respiratory region comprising of the chest structures responsible for air movement in and out of the lungs—the respiratory pump.

15.2.1 ANATOMY OF THE AIRWAYS

Conducting airways are made up of different structures including the nasal cavity, nasopharynx, oropharynx, trachea, bronchi, and bronchioles, i.e., the first 16 generations of the tracheobronchial tree, as described by Weibel.[15] Conducting airways are incapable of gaseous exchanges with venous blood and, thus, create the anatomical dead space.

Different regions of the respiratory system differ in blood supply. Anatomical structures of the lung in the conducting zone, i.e., bronchi and bronchioles, derive their nutrition from systemic blood supply. The structures in the respiratory zone receive nutrition from the pulmonary circulation.

15.2.1.1 Nose

In the respiratory system, the nose functions to warm, humidify, and filter the air entering the human body. In addition, it also acts as a very efficient barrier against invading pathogens and large particles. The entire nasal cavity is lined with pseudostratified squamous epithelium covered with a thin layer of mucus. The cilia of the epithelium move at 1000 times/min, leading to a surface mucus movement of 3–25 mm/min. The transport in the nasal cavity is unidirectional.[16]

15.2.1.2 Pharyngeal Region

After passing through the nose, inhaled air enters the pharynx. The pharynx is a funnel-shaped tube that starts at the nasal passages and extends up to the cricoid cartilage lying just above the trachea. The pharynx is composed of skeletal muscles lined with a mucus membrane and is a major site of impaction. The lower portion of the pharynx gives rise to the larynx. Inhaled air passes through the larynx before reaching the trachea and finally reaches the lungs. The larynx also has a major role to play in influencing breathing patterns and delivery of drugs to the lungs.

15.2.1.3 Trachea

Weibel's tracheobronchial tree starts with the trachea considering it as generation "0." The trachea may be represented as a cylindrical tube, lined with ciliated epithelium, 10–12 cm long, with a mean diameter of about 1.7–1.8 cm. There are 16–20 C-shaped cartilage rings present in the tracheal wall providing rigidity to the trachea. As discussed earlier, the trachea may be considered as a trunk of the pulmonary tree, which divides to give rise to the main bronchi at the level of fifth thoracic vertebra. At the point of bifurcation, an internal cartilaginous ridge lined with mucus membrane, carina, is present. The right bronchus is wider and shorter than the left one, and thus is more likely to provide a passage to any inhaled foreign body. Moving forward, the main bronchi divide to form smaller bronchi, which, in turn, lead to the individual lobes of the lungs—3 on the right side and 2 on the left side. The division continues even inside the lobes to form the bronchioles, the terminal bronchioles, respiratory bronchioles, alveolar ducts, and finally alveolar sacs. As described in the classical model of the airways, each airway divides to form two smaller daughter airways. Thus, with each generation, the number of airways doubles in Weibel's tracheobronchial tree. There are 24 such generations, which start from the trachea as the 0th generation and end at the alveolar sac, the 23rd generation.[15]

The major changes that occur as we progress from 0th to 23rd generation include (1) a decrease in the airway diameter—the tracheal diameter is 1.8 cm, while the alveolar diameter is 0.04 cm and (2) a tremendous increase in the airways' surface area. The total surface area is about 140 m^2 at the level of the alveolus, the primary site for the gaseous exchange between the alveolar space and blood in the alveolar capillaries in the respiratory region. There is a relatively small change in the surface area of the airways for over 19 generations up to the terminal bronchioles, facilitating the rapid flow of inspired air to the terminal bronchioles. On the contrary, the surface area increases tremendously, 180 cm^2–100 m^2, in later 4 generations, thus decreasing the velocity of the inspired air even lesser than the diffusing oxygen molecules. Thus, diffusion may be regarded as the major player in determining gaseous movements.[17]

As discussed earlier, the airways can be categorized on the basis of their functions: (1) the conducting zone not participating in the gas exchange, up to the terminal bronchioles and (2) the respiratory zone involved with gas exchange, up to the alveolar sacs. Another important change that occurs is the disappearance of cartilage from the bronchial wall after the 11th generation. Thus, based on the cartilage, different regions of the airways may be classified into three categories: (1) incomplete rings in the trachea; (2) irregularly shaped, plated in the bronchi; and (3) absent from bronchioles.

Different regions of the respiratory system differ in the blood supply as well. In the conducting zone, bronchi and bronchioles derive their nutrition from the systemic blood supply, while the structures in the respiratory zone receive nutrition from the pulmonary circulation.

15.2.1.4 Alveolus

The alveolus is a hollow cavity and is considered to be the primary site for gas exchange between the lungs and blood circulation. Human lungs contain about 300–500 million alveoli, with a total surface area of 75–90 m^2.[18] The alveoli primarily derive from respiratory bronchioles with increasing generations of Weibel's tracheobronchial tree. Alveolar ducts arise from respiratory bronchioles that give rise to alveolar sacs, which in turn give rise to alveoli. Adult alveoli have an average diameter of 0.2–0.3 mm and are wrapped with a fine network of capillaries. Some alveolar walls demonstrate the presence of "pores of Kohn," which help in collateral ventilation. Two adjacent alveoli are separated by an alveolar wall with two layers of alveolar epithelium (AE). The interstitial space between the alveolar and capillary epithelial cells is known as the "air–blood carrier." The thickness of this interstitial space is asymmetric, <0.4 μm on the active side and ~1–2 μm on the service side. Such variations are important to maintain the lung's geometry. The presence of tight intracellular connections prevents the penetration of inhaled particles through intercellular pathways. However, this may change in certain disease states, which can consequently lead to an increase in permeability.[15]

15.2.2 HISTOLOGY OF THE AIRWAYS

15.2.2.1 Cells of Airway Epithelium

As shown in Figure 15.1, the airway epithelium is a sheet of cells lining the luminal surface of the airways and is composed of a variety of cell types. It also serves as a barrier to prevent inhaled substances access to the internal environment of the body. In the major airways, the epithelium is pseudostratified and columnar.[17] Four major types of cells make up the epithelium: (1) *ciliated cells*, which are present up to the terminal bronchioles. The cilia on this cell surface beat synchronously, thus facilitating movement of the mucus layer. (2) *Goblet cells* (6000–7000 cells/mm^3) in the human trachea secrete mucus, which covers the luminal surface of the epithelium. The beating of the cilia

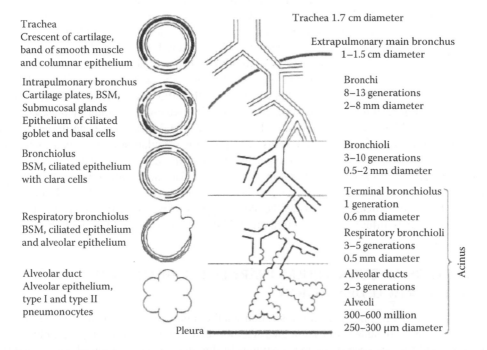

FIGURE 15.1 Number and dimensions of the airways in the adult lung and the structure of the airway wall. (Reproduced from Stocks, J. and Hislop, AA, Structure and function of the respiratory system: Developmental aspects and their relevance to aerosol therapy, in *Drug Delivery to the Lung*, Marcel Dekker, New York, 2002, pp. 47–104. With permission from Informa Healthcare.)

causes the movement of mucus up the pulmonary tree, known as the mucociliary escalator. This is a defense function of the body against large inhaled particles trapped in the mucus. There are no goblet cells in distal airways. Mucus secretion is enhanced by coughing, and may be an indication of cystic fibrosis or chronic bronchitis. (3) *Basal cells* are the primary stem cells giving rise to ciliated and mucus cells. (4) *Clara cells*, the primary cells of small airways, are found up to terminal bronchioles. These are involved in fluid absorption and may produce bronchiolar surfactant.[17]

15.2.2.2   Cells of Alveoli

The luminal epithelium of the alveolus is made up of (1) *alveolar type I cells, pneumonocytes*, the primary sites of gas exchange with blood and (2) *alveolar type II cells*. Type II cells are cuboidal in shape and possess microvilli. These are responsible for epithelial renewal and secretion of surfactant, a phospholipid, which reduces alveolar surface tension.[19,20]

15.2.2.3   Smooth Muscle Cells

Smooth muscles are found in the trachea and extrapulmonary bronchi in the gap between cartilage plates and in the intrapulmonary bronchi circling the lumen internal to the cartilage. It is separated from the epithelium by lamina propria. The contraction and relaxation of smooth muscles controlled by neurotransmitters, hormones, and inflammatory mediators directly affects the airflow in the airways.

15.2.2.4   Alveolar Macrophages

Alveolar macrophages are the migrating defensive cells of the respiratory system. These mononuclear cells are present in the interstitium and alveoli's luminal surface. They clear foreign substances and microorganisms in the alveoli by phagocytosis and enzymatic degradation.[21]

15.2.3   Blood Supply to the Respiratory System

The blood supply to the respiratory system can be divided into two categories: (1) systemic circulation, which supplies blood to the conducting airways and (2) pulmonary circulation, which supplies blood to the respiratory airways. Pulmonary circulation carries deoxygenated blood from the right ventricle to the lungs and carries back oxygenated blood to the left atrium. The main pulmonary artery emerges from the right ventricles, rapidly divides to form smaller arteries, and finally pulmonary capillaries forming the network pass from one alveolus to the other. At a given time, about 75% of the capillary bed is filled with blood. This varies due to the influence of gravity, which is the basis of the vertical gradient of the ventilation/perfusion ratio.[22,23] Alveolar inflation increases the capillaries' resistance to blood flow by decreasing their cross-sectional area. These capillaries drain into venules, which finally make pulmonary veins. The systemic circulation carries oxygenated blood from the left ventricle and returns it in deoxygenated form to the right atrium. The blood pressure in the pulmonary artery is about 1/6th of that in systemic circulation. For this reason, the pulmonary arterial wall is thinner than the systemic arterial wall with fewer smooth muscles.[17] Several investigators have shown the differences between the blood supply to the conducting and respiratory zones by using various dyes infused into the circulation. This distinction should be kept in mind while dealing with the aerosol absorption from conducting or respiratory airways.[24]

15.3   FACTORS AFFECTING PULMONARY DRUG ABSORPTION AND PARTICLE DEPOSITION

The absorption of drugs following administration via the pulmonary route is influenced by a number of factors, which include (1) physiological factors such as airway geometry, humidity, pattern of breathing, and the presence of various enzymes in the lungs; (2) pathophysiological conditions; (3) mucociliary clearance; and (4) the physicochemical properties of the drug. Furthermore, the physical characteristics of the inhaled particles and their site of deposition in the lungs also play important roles in the absorption of drugs following pulmonary administration.

15.3.1 PHYSIOLOGICAL FACTORS

15.3.1.1 Air–Blood Barrier

As mentioned earlier, the lung is the only organ in the body that receives entire cardiac output. Drug absorption through the lungs is regulated by the permeability of a thin alveolar–vascular barrier present between the alveoli and the fine mesh of pulmonary capillaries. There are several mechanisms by which drug molecules pass through various barriers—the epithelium, basement membrane, lung surfactant, and surface lining fluid—before reaching the blood circulation. These include absorptive transcytosis, paracellular transport, or transport through the large pores created by cell injury/apoptosis.

15.3.1.2 Airway Geometry

Due to continuous branching, airways become narrow with increasing generations of Weibel's tracheobronchial tree and, thus, influence the flow of air through the airways. The smaller the airway radius, the greater the velocity of incoming air, the greater the bend angle of bifurcations, and the greater the probability of particle deposition in any specific area.

15.3.1.3 Breathing Pattern

The breathing rate and pattern can significantly influence the rate and extent of drug absorption from the respiratory route. During deep and slow respiration, inhaled substances are deposited in the peripheral airway region; while with shallow and fast breathing, substances get deposited in the central and/or respiratory zone. Also, an increased respiratory rate with low tidal volume results in more drug wastage in dead space, thus, decreased drug absorption and residence time in the lungs. An optimum peak inspiratory flow (>30 L/min) is necessary for successful inhaled therapy. At the same time, the ratio of inspiratory to total respiratory cycle, the duty cycle, determines the adequate deposition.

> An optimum peak inspiratory flow (>30 L/min) is necessary for successful inhaled therapy. At the same time, the ratio of inspiratory to total respiratory cycle, the duty cycle, determines the adequate deposition.

15.3.1.4 Humidity

The lungs have a high relative humidity reaching up to $44\,\mu g/cm^3$ in the alveolar lumen. These high levels of humidity can significantly affect the particle size of generally hygroscopic drug particles, and consequently their deposition patterns in the lungs. Depending on the water content and tonicity, hygroscopic aerosolized droplets may increase in size. This may affect the amount of drug deposited and more importantly, change the distribution pattern. A reduced deposition of particles of $1\,\mu m$ in size ranging from peripheral to larger, i.e., central airways has been observed.[25]

15.3.1.5 Presence of Enzymes

The drug metabolizing activity of the lung may affect the concentration and efficacy of the inhaled drugs. For many xenobiotics, the lungs act as the primary site for metabolism/degradation. There are >40 cell types present in the lungs, all with different metabolic capacities depending on the enzymes present. The lungs have almost all the metabolizing enzymes present in the liver and GI tract, though at a much lower concentration, 5–20 times less than that in the liver. The major enzymes present in the lungs include phase I-metabolizing (CYP450) enzymes, monoamine oxidases, aldehyde dehydrogenases, esterases, NADPH-CYP450 reductase, and proteases such as endopeptidases and cathepsin H. The monooxygenases metabolize fatty acids, steroids, and lipophilic molecules; while proteases are responsible for the inactivation of various inhaled proteins and peptide molecules. Enzymes in the lungs are broadly distributed in the lung tissues. Phase I-metabolizing enzymes are present ubiquitously in the lower respiratory tract with a high concentration in the epithelial and Clara cells. Proteases are mainly localized in alveolar macrophages and inflammatory cells.[26,27] It has been reported that the coadministration of protein drugs and protease inhibitors such as bacitracin improves the pulmonary absorption of many drugs by reducing the extent of protein degradation.[28]

15.3.2 Pathophysiological Conditions of the Respiratory System

A variety of lung diseases can affect drug absorption and particle deposition in the lungs, mainly because of airway narrowing, bronchoconstriction, and the presence of inflammation. The accumulation of unwanted materials in the airway lumen results in airway obstruction. Generally, airway obstruction occurs because of factors such as mucus accumulation due to mucus gland hypertrophy, an increase in smooth muscle tone, mucosal edema, and an increase in inflammatory and epithelial cells. In emphysema, airway narrowing occurs due to the loss of supporting elastic tissue elements in the airways. Airway obstruction leads to a reduction in the surface area of the lungs, diversion of inspired air to unobstructed regions leading to uneven and decreased absorption of drug in the tissue, increased airflow resistance, and elevated residual volume resulting in increased deposition of drug in the central airways.[29,30] Forced expired volume at 1 s (FEV_1) is the most common parameter to assess the degree of airway obstruction, which decreases in the case of increased obstruction. Bronchial constriction in chronic obstructive pulmonary disease (COPD) (low FEV_1) enhances the central airway deposition of radioaerosol particles. Laube and coinvestigators showed that in COPD, the distribution of a radiolabeled aerosol was extremely uneven and the clearance from the central airways was inversely related to FEV_1.[31]

15.3.3 Lung Clearance Mechanisms

15.3.3.1 Mucociliary Clearance

Mucociliary clearance is an important function of the respiratory system. It is utilized to clear unwanted debris, secretions, or particles from the system. Upon pulmonary drug delivery, larger drug particles are deposited in the conducting airways. These are mostly cleared by mucociliary clearance. In conducting airways, the epithelium is ciliated and covered with a double-layer mucus film secreted by goblet cells. The beating of the epithelial cilia (1000–1200 beats/min) causes the upward movement of mucus. Particles trapped in the upper gel layer of mucus are transported toward the pharynx and then to the GI tract.[32] The normal mucociliary transport rate in humans is about 5.5 mm/min in the trachea and about 2.4 mm/min in bronchi.[33] For normal mucociliary clearance, the epithelial ciliary structures should be normal and intact. Also, the depth, rheology, and chemical composition of the fluid should be optimal. In various lung diseases, such as asthma, cystic fibrosis, and bronchitis, mucociliary clearance is adversely affected due to impaired ciliary function and the presence of thick mucus in the airways.[34,35] In these conditions, the unwanted secretions are cleared by coughing. The mucociliary clearance mechanism plays an important role in the pulmonary delivery of drug particles by clearing a significant amount of particles that have settled in the conducting airways. Thus, for efficient absorption, facilitating deep lung deposition of aerosolized formulations is advised.[36]

15.3.3.2 Pulmonary Endocytosis

Pulmonary endocytosis is an important clearance mechanism for microorganisms and insoluble drug particles deposited in the alveolar region of the respiratory system. This is carried out by alveolar macrophages by several mechanisms that include (1) transport of the particles toward the mucociliary escalator, (2) enzymatic degradation, and (3) particle translocation to the lymphatic system. A combination of mucociliary transport and lymphatic clearance may also be involved. The transport to mucociliary and lymphatic systems is insignificant compared with total alveolar clearance. Enzymatic phagocytosis is considered to be the major player in pulmonary endocytosis. Macrophages phagocytose insoluble particles deposited in the alveolar region within a few minutes to an hour. The contribution of pulmonary endocytosis to overall clearance is based upon particle size, shape, solubility, particle burden to the airways, and the chemical nature of the aerosol.[37]

15.3.4 Physicochemical Properties of the Drugs

Absorption of the drugs following administration via the pulmonary route is influenced not only by physiological factors and clearance mechanisms in the lungs but also by physicochemical properties of drug molecules including molecular weight, partition coefficient, aqueous solubility, pH, and osmolarity. The effect of molecular weight on the absorption of drugs has been studied in detail. These studies consider that lung epithelia act as a sieve allowing only molecules up to a certain size to pass through. Taylor and colleagues demonstrated that 60 kDa urea is cleared 7 times faster than 180 kDa glucose molecules. Also, low molecular weight compounds dissolve and, thus, diffuse more readily than large ones.[38] This represents a good correlation between the molecular weight and the time to maximum concentration in the blood (T_{max}) of the compound being investigated. Brown and Schanker demonstrated that compounds with molecular weights <1000 are absorbed at a faster rate ($t_{1/2} = 90$ min) compared with larger molecules (with an absorption half-life ($t_{1/2}$) of 3–27 h).[39]

Lipophilicity and particle size are often considered as the major determinants of pulmonary absorption rates. Some studies suggest that alveolar wall permeability increases with an increase in the lipophilicity of the compound. Lipophilic compounds are absorbed more rapidly than hydrophilic ones. Many groups have reported the existence of a sigmoidal relationship between permeability coefficients and partition coefficients of the drugs administered via the pulmonary route. Another study by Schanker and colleagues has shown that the relationship between the absorption and lipophilicity of the molecules is species dependent. In mice, lipid insoluble drugs are absorbed 5 times faster than in rats, whereas lipophilic drugs were absorbed at comparable rates in all the species.[40]

At the same time, another important factor affecting drug absorption is the aqueous solubility of the drug. This could be because the pulmonary epithelium is kept moist by mucus secretion and is also well supplied with blood vessels.

15.3.5 Morphological Properties of the Particles

One of the most critical factors in pulmonary delivery is the particle size of the formulations. As the majority of pulmonary formulations are composed of different-sized particles, there is a direct relationship between drug absorption and distribution within the lungs to the mass median aerodynamic diameter (MMAD) of the particles. MMAD is a complex parameter, which does not reflect the real particle dimension. MMAD can be described as the equivalent diameter of a sphere flying as the real particle. MMAD reflects particle properties such as size, density, and shape. The optimal particle size for reproducible drug delivery to the lung is in the range between 1 and 5 µm.[41] Particles that are smaller than 1 µm have short transit times in the lung and may be deposited in the alveoli. This is ideal for the treatment of cystic fibrosis, where the particles must reach the bronchioles since the disease usually extends to the bronchi.[42] Particles larger than 5 µm may be deposited in the airway and later cleared out by the mucociliary clearance mechanism of the respiratory tract. Some delivery devices may not be able to force those particles out of the device. Particle size and, at the same time, the rate of nebulization can significantly influence the deposition pattern. These can affect the therapeutic efficacy and systemic absorption of the pulmonary formulations. However, the influence of particle shape on drug deposition is not well studied. Drug formulations with sustained release particles provide selective delivery to the lung periphery.[43] However, particle shape may have little or no influence on the respirable fraction of the drug.[44]

15.4 DEVICES FOR PULMONARY DRUG DELIVERY

Both, the types of drug delivery system and delivery device can affect drug absorption via the pulmonary route. The choice of delivery systems depends on the physiochemical properties of the drug, its desired site of action, and, more importantly, patient compliance and elegance. Based on the device used, the required particle size, deposition patterns, and MMAD may vary. These may eventually affect drug absorption and therapeutic efficacy. The delivery device and the formulation must be able to generate a respirable dose, with a particle size of 1–5.0 μm. Other patient and formulation factors that should be considered for the rational design of pulmonary drug delivery systems include the physicochemical properties of drug substances (such as the ionization constant [pK_a] and lipophilicity [log P]), drug stability, interaction with containers, ability of aerosolization, patient population, therapeutic goals, and regulatory issues.

The most widely used pulmonary delivery systems are nebulizers, metered dose inhalers (MDIs), and dry powder inhalers (DPIs). Particle size is also influenced by the particle generation device. Particle size, for example, is inversely related to the gas flow rate in jet nebulizers. In ultrasonic nebulizers, the particle size is a function of the capillary waves produced on the surface of the liquid.[45,46] Nebulizers can also vary in their mass output. Several studies showed that there is large variability in particle size and mass output. For example, Matthys et al. (1985) showed that mass output varies from 47% to 81% depending on the brand and type of nebulizers.[47] The compressor flow of nebulizers and the viscosity of the inhalation solution can also affect the deposition of drug administered and drug absorption via the pulmonary route.

Similarly, dry-powder inhalers may affect drug deposition in the lungs. In powder-based formulations, lactose is used as a bulking and deagglomerating agent. During inhalation, the inspired air aerosolizes the blend of lactose and drug and separates the drug crystals from the lactose. Drug deposition from a dry-powder inhaler may vary depending on the type of inhaler, drug formulation, and inspiratory flow rate.[48] A comparative study between the ISF® inhaler and Rotahaler® using a radiolabeled sodium cromoglycate/lactose blend showed that the drug deposition from ISF was 16.4%, while with Rotahaler, the deposition was 6.2%.[49] Zanen and Laube pointed out that efficient delivery from the DPI depends on the inspiratory flow rate generated by the patient. An increase or decrease in the flow may affect the drug deposition by increasing or decreasing MMAD and mass output[48]. Various types of delivery devices that are currently available are described in the following section. Table 15.1 summarizes the advantages and disadvantages of commonly used inhaler devices.

> In powder-based formulations, lactose is used as a bulking and deagglomerating agent. During inhalation, the inspired air aerosolizes the blend of lactose and drug, and separates the drug crystals from the lactose. Drug deposition from a dry-powder inhaler may vary depending on the type of inhaler, drug formulation, and inspiratory flow rate.

15.4.1 Pressurized Metered Dose Inhalers

A pressurized metered dose inhaler (pMDI) can be regarded as a compact droplet dispenser, which can be used for dispensing multiple doses—typically 200 actuations—of the medication. The key components of the pMDI include a reservoir, a metering valve, an actuator, and a spray nozzle. The spray nozzle controls the spray angle, size distribution of droplets, and atomization process. The structure of a typical pMDI is depicted in Figure 15.2a. The formulations to be delivered through the pMDI have a therapeutic agent and a propellant, with one or more surfactants and lubricants. Chlorofluorocarbons (CFCs) were typically used as propellants in pMDIs. The use of CFCs has been discontinued because of their adverse effects on the ozone layer. As a result, hydrofluoroalkane (HFA)-based propellants are becoming popular as a replacement. The transition from CFCs to HFA resulted in a modification of the formulation and structural elements in pMDIs. Several studies suggest that CFC-pMDIs deliver 80%–90% of the dose into the oropharyngeal region, thus resulting in about 10%–20% of the dose entering the central lung zones. On the contrary, HFA-pMDIs deliver 60%–70% of the dose into the central lung zones. The delivery can be increased with the use of spacers with pMDIs, which results in a smaller particle size of the aerosol spray. Figure 15.3 demonstrates a simulated droplet transport and deposition patterns for HFA-pMDIs with and without a spacer.[50]

TABLE 15.1
Summary of Three Types of Commonly Used Inhaler Devices

Type	Advantages	Disadvantages	Appropriate Users
Nebulizer	Easy to use; effective use requires only simple, tidal breathing	Device preparation required; more time-consuming for treatment	Can be used at any age and for any disease severity or acuity
	High dose and dose modification possible	Contamination possible, i.e., equipment maintenance and cleaning required	
	Can deliver combination therapies if compatible (jet nebulizer)	Jet nebulizers lack portability and ultrasonic nebulizers may be expensive	
		Does not aerosolize suspensions well; not all medication is available in solution form	
pMDI	Small and portable; can be used very quickly	The technique and coordination of breathing and actuation required for efficient use; potential for abuse	Preferred device for asthma and COPD therapy
	No drug preparation required; treatment time is short	No dose counter to determine remaining drug amount	Children under 4 years old use chambers with face masks
	No contamination of content	High pharyngeal deposition without spacer or holding chamber	
	Dose–dose reproducibility high; some can be used with breath-actuated mouthpiece	Upper limit of unit dose content; not all medications available	
DPI	The newest type of aerosol delivery device with many different forms (single-dose, multi-dose, etc.)	Moderate to high inspiratory flow required	Not applicable for very young children and patients with low levels of lung functions; generally recommended for patients ≥5 years old who have adequate inspiratory flow and lung volume
	Breath-actuated and easier to use than pMDIs	Can result in high pharyngeal deposition	
	No propellant, small, portable, and quick to use	Not all medications available	
	Short treatment time		
	Spacers not required and dose counters incorporated in most newer designs		

Source: Reproduced from Kleinstreuer, C. et al., *Annu. Rev. Biomed. Eng.*, 10, 195, 2008. With permission from Annual Reviews.

15.4.2 NEBULIZED DRUG DELIVERY SYSTEMS

In nebulized drug delivery systems, the aqueous solution or micronized suspension of a drug is aerosolized. Most of the nebulizer solutions are water based, but may contain some cosolvents such as glycerine, propylene glycol, and ethanol. Like other liquid pharmaceutical formulations, nebulizer solution may also contain antioxidants, preservatives, buffers, and chelating agents. In addition, a tonicity adjustor, such as sodium chloride, is added to make the drug solution isotonic. For optimal

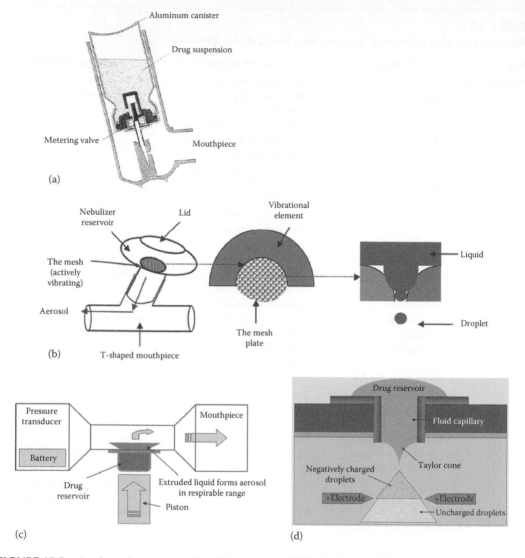

FIGURE 15.2 A schematic representation of (a) a typical pMDI; (b) Aeroneb® Pro, an active vibrating mesh nebulizer; (c) AERx® pulmonary dosing system; and (d) electrohydrodynamic aerosol generation mechanism in the Mystic® EHD. (Reproduced from Watts, A.B. et al., *Drug. Dev. Ind. Pharm.*, 34, 913, 2008. With permission from Taylor and Francis.)

performance of the nebulizers, the interfacial and surface tension of the nebulizer solution is optimized to avoid irritation and mucosal thinning and flow. Solutions for nebulizers are aseptically filled in unit dose glass or plastic containers. The aerosolization of a nebulizer solution is carried out by either a high velocity airstream or ultrasonic energy. For this reason, nebulizers are often called air jet or ultrasonic nebulizers. Various types of nebulizers are briefly described in Table 15.2.

15.4.2.1   Air-Jet Nebulizers

The air-jet nebulizer operates by passing compressed air over the open end of a narrow capillary tube immersed in a liquid reservoir. The liquid is drawn from the reservoir by a region of negative pressure above the capillary tube and is dispersed into aerosol by the high shearing action of the airflow. Larger droplets return to the reservoir because of impaction with baffles, while the smaller ones pass out with the air stream and are inhaled by the patient through a mouth piece or face mask.

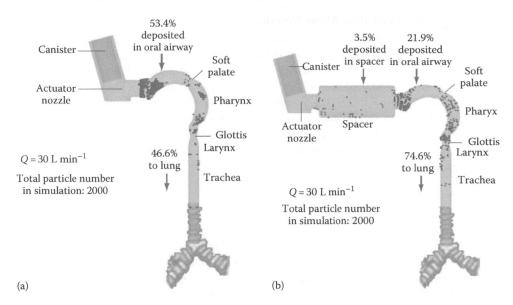

FIGURE 15.3 Simulation results of HFA-propelled pMDI droplet transport and deposition (a) without and (b) with spacer, illustrating the impact of a simple spacer in terms of enhanced droplet percentage reaching the tracheobronchial tree. Q = airflow rate. (Reproduced from Kleinstreuer, C. et al., *Annu. Rev. Biomed. Eng.*, 10, 195, 2008. With permission from Annual Reviews.)

TABLE 15.2
Different Types of Nebulizers Available in the Market under Development

Type	Example	Manufacturer	Advantages
Air-jet nebulizers	Pari LC® Star	Pari GmbH	Breath actuated nebulizers
	AeroEclipse II® BAN	Trudell Medical International	Only droplets in respirable range pass with air stream
	Halolite®	Philips Respironics	Recently developed jet nebulizers operated by a compressor
	Circulaire®	Lifelink Monitoring	Computerized aerosol delivery system
			Reduces aerosol waste emission
			Increases the accuracy and total dose delivered
Ultrasonic/vibrating mesh nebulizers	Omron Micro*Air*®	Omron	More particles are generated in the respirable fraction range with low velocity
	Aeroneb® Pro	Aerogen	
Smart nebulizers	I-neb® AAD®	Philips Respironics	High accuracy in drug delivery
			Determines the duration of aerosol production needed to target beginning of a breath
	eFlow®	Pari Pharma	Precision dosing through patient feedback option
			Formulation/dose specific settings
			Well suited for easily degraded formulations

Few of the major disadvantages of air-jet nebulizers are that they are expensive, bulky, and cumbersome to use. Furthermore, they are considered to be inefficient drug delivery systems since only 5%–20% of the nominal dose placed in the nebulizer reaches the lung. Moreover, because of the requirement for compressed air from an air or oxygen cylinder in the nebulization systems, the use of air-jet nebulizers is limited to hospitals.

15.4.2.2   Ultrasonic/Vibrating Mesh Nebulizers

Ultrasonic nebulizers utilize oscillating piezoelectric crystals and direct high frequency ultrasonic waves (1–3 MHz) through a reservoir of drug solution. These high frequency waves produce a dense aerosol plume in the respirable range, which is inhaled by the patient. Ultrasonic nebulizers are portable and expensive compared with air-jet nebulizers. An example of a vibrating mesh nebulizer is the Aeroneb® Pro (Figure 15.2b). Briefly, vibrating mesh nebulizers work with micropump technology. In vibrating mesh nebulizers, the vibrating piezoelectric crystals have been replaced with a laser-bored mesh plate, the oscillation of which pumps liquid through numerous tapered holes producing primary aerosol droplets in the respirable range (1–5 μm). Vibrating mesh nebulizers produce a high respirable fraction and low velocity aerosols.

15.4.2.2.1   Newly Developed Nebulizers

Recently developed air-jet and ultrasonic nebulizers have addressed some of the inconvenience associated with traditional nebulizers. A detailed discussion of new nebulizer technology is beyond the scope of this chapter. Interested readers are directed to two recent chapters on this topic.[51,52]

Halolite® and Circulaire®, for example, are two recently developed air-jet nebulizers. Halolite is a portable jet nebulizer operated by a compressor. It has a computerized aerosol delivery system that can monitor patient breathing parameters, such as inhalation flow, breathing frequency, and inspiratory time, to deliver a precise dose to each patient. This device maximizes the lung deposition by delivering aerosols during the initial inspiratory phase of the inhalation cycle. One of the most convenient features of Halolite is that it can record the date, time, and dose received. The system is fully automatic and requires no individual adjustment. The Circulaire nebulizer significantly reduces aerosol waste emission to the environment. Aerosol generated during patient exhalation is stored in a flexible reservoir until the next inhalation. These nebulizers increase the accuracy and total aerosol dose delivered to the patient compared with traditional nebulizers. Newly developed ultrasonic nebulizers include Omron® and Aeroneb nebulizers. Both are portable devices and do not require a compressor to operate.

15.4.2.3   Smart Nebulizers

The ever-developing range of pulmonary formulations demand better control over the dose delivered from the nebulizer, thus delivering the drug efficiently, while adapting to changes in the patient's physiological factors such as breathing patterns. This control can be achieved by combining smart devices with the benefits of vibrating mesh technology.

15.4.2.3.1   I-neb® Adaptive Aerosol Delivery (AAD®) System

I-neb has been designed for high accuracy and low variability in pulmonary drug delivery. This system determines the duration of aerosol production based on the breathing pattern of the patient by monitoring the peak flow of patient's first three inhalations. Sufficient time is allowed for the nebulized droplets to reach the deep lung. It also takes into account the change in breathing pattern with the progression of treatment. By optimizing operating parameters, it enables the development of inhalation devices specific to formulations.[53]

15.4.2.3.2   eFlow®

The eFlow aerosolization technique has been developed for easily degraded formulations, and produces high respirable fraction aerosols. It requires only 2–3 min to complete its operations. It works based on the principle of vibrating mesh technology as discussed earlier (TouchSpray®). However, the delivery efficiency is lower than in I-Neb due to wastage of drug during continuous aerosol generation.

15.4.3   DRY POWDER INHALERS

DPIs are devices used for the delivery of active pharmaceutical ingredients in powdered form. Like nebulizers, dry powder inhalation drug delivery systems have two components: the device and the formulation. As the name implies, the formulation component of this delivery system is powder suitable for administration to the respiratory tract.

Powder properties including particle morphology, interparticle forces, particle size distribution, hygroscopicity, density, and flowability affect drug absorption. To obtain maximum absorption, the drug should have adequate solubility in the respiratory mucus. Other formulation factors that affect drug deposition include crystal habit, surface texture, and porosity. Finer particles may adhere to the surface of the device due to electrostatic attraction. Lactose is frequently used to increase the particle size in inhalable formulations. Good aerosolization or dispersibility of powder formulation also depends on their compressibility and dustability. These affect the deposition and absorption from pulmonary drug delivery systems.

Some examples of devices for dry powder inhalation include Turbuhaler®, Diskus®, Diskhaler®, Novolizer®, and Aerolizer®. Drug deposition can be significantly affected by the delivery devices.[54]

15.4.4 METERED DOSE LIQUID INHALERS

As pMDIs have been shown to be inefficient in terms of delivered dose and deposition, a new class of MDIs have emerged that work on the principle of aerosol generation by mechanical and electro-mechanical forces called metered dose liquid inhalers (MDLIs). MDLIs are propellant free inhalers, which provide greater flexibility during formulation development. Some of the commercially available MDLIs are exemplified below.

15.4.4.1 AERx®

The AERx system was developed by Aradigm (Hayward, California). It delivers a unit dose through small laser drilled holes via extrusion of a solution containing the required concentration of a drug. It uses a microprocessor controlled device (Figure 15.2c)[55,56] that allows flexibility in terms of aerosol droplet size, flow rate, and aerosol production rate. Farr et al. showed that inhalation by AERx resulted in the deposition of 6.9% of the dose in the oropharynx compared with 42% in the case of pMDIs.[57]

15.4.4.2 Mystic®

Mystic generates aerosol through electrohydrodynamic disruption. In this system, the aerosol is generated by passing the liquid through a capillary, thus forming a conical shape due to the electrical field. The liquid at the crest aerosolizes into electrically excited droplets, thus forming a respirable mist.[58] The aerosol droplets get neutralized subsequently (Figure 15.2d). The main advantages of this instrument are (1) a short actuation cycle of ~2 s, (2) the generation of monodispersed aerosols, and (3) the deposition of a very high fraction of drug to deep lungs.[59,60]

15.5 ENHANCING DRUG ABSORPTION VIA THE PULMONARY ROUTE

Although the lung is a very attractive route for the administration of drugs due to its large surface area, thin air–blood barrier, and low enzyme activity, there are still major obstacles in the widespread acceptance of pulmonary drug delivery. One of these obstacles is the lungs' relative impermeability to most drugs. Small molecules may pass through and get absorbed through the epithelium, but this remains a challenge for large molecular weight drugs. Numerous absorption enhancers have been studied to promote absorption of large molecular weight drugs via the lungs.

The mechanisms by which these agents work are not clear. One of the proposed mechanisms is the irreversible damage to the alveolar epithelial cell layer, thus making the lungs more susceptible to the entry of exogenous substances during inhalation.[61] This is, in fact, a major concern with regard to the safety of absorption enhancers in pulmonary drug delivery. Recent studies suggest that some agents are relatively nontoxic at high doses. Also, reversible damage with the short-term use of absorption enhancers has been demonstrated.[62] Absorption enhancers that have been used in pulmonary drug delivery include (1) protease inhibitors, (2) surface active agents, (3) cyclodextrins, and (4) liposomes.

TABLE 15.3
Effect of Protease Inhibitors on the Pulmonary Absorption of Insulin Microcrystals

	Concentration	D%	%MBGC[a]	T%MBGC[b] (h)	Time[c] (h)
Insulin 5 U/kg	—	42.68±1.62	52.46±7.29	4	0.6–24
+Soybean-trypsin	1	51.49±5.27*	28.25±2.05***	7	3–17
inhibitor (mg/mL)	5	55.78±0.71*	30.59±9.47**	5	3–24
	10	48.86±3.24	42.66±5.78*	7	4–24
+Aprotinin (mg/mL)	1	56.90±3.42***	44.06±4.10*	7	0.6–24
	5	51.77±1.98**	48.07±5.36	5	1.3–24
	10	52.57±8.78	35.84±4.46	1.3	0.6–24

Source: Reproduced from Park, S.H. et al., *Int. J. Pharm.*, 339, 205, 2007. With permission from Elsevier.
Note: Each value represents the mean±SD ($n=3$–6).
[a] %MBGC, the percent of minimum blood glucose concentration.
[b] T%MBGC, the time required to attain %MBGC.
[c] Time: the time during which less than 70% of blood glucose is held.
Statistical significance: $^*P < 0.05$, $^{**}P < 0.01$ and $P < 0.001$.

15.5.1 Protease Inhibitors

Protease inhibitors have been reported to work by reducing the proteolytic activity of enzymes responsible for the degradation of macromolecules such as insulin and calcitonin. Komada et al. showed that nafamostat mesilate, a trypsin and plasmin inhibitor, when coadministered with insulin doubled the relative bioavailability of insulin following intratracheal administration (data not shown).[63] Recently, Park et al. showed the effect of various protease inhibitors (aprotinin, bacitracin, and soybean-trypsin inhibitor) on pulmonary absorption of insulin microcrystals in male Sprague-Dawley rats. As can be seen in Table 15.3, the pharmacodynamic properties of insulin improved in the presence of aprotinin and soybean-trypsin inhibitor. The decrease in blood glucose level (*D%*) and the percent of minimum blood glucose concentration (%MBGC) reached 48.9%–56.9% and 28.3%–48.1%, respectively in the presence of the soybean-trypsin inhibitor and aprotinin, in comparison with 42.7% and 52.5% in the absence of the soybean-trypsin inhibitor and aprotinin.[64]

15.5.2 Surface Active Agents

Surface active agents increase the transcellular transport via fluidization of the cell membrane, thus making it more permeable. They also modulate the tight junctions for enhanced movements of the large sized molecules. Surface active agents that have been used in pulmonary drug delivery include (1) bile salts and acids such as sodium salts of cholic acid and chenodeoxycholic acid, (2) fatty acids, and (3) nonionic surfactants such as octyl-β-D-maltoside. Johansson et al. showed the effects of different concentrations of sodium taurocholate (NaTC) when coadministered with insulin via the pulmonary route. As evident from the data shown in Figure 15.4, the absolute bioavailability (%) of insulin increased by up to ninefold when coadministered with 30 mM NaTC (23.2±4.4% as compared with 2.6±0.3% for pure insulin).[65]

15.5.3 Cyclodextrins

Cyclodextrins, cyclic oligomers of glucose, form inclusion complexes with drug molecules that fit into their lipophilic cavities. They may promote pulmonary absorption by disrupting the alveolar epithelial membrane. For example, Kobayashi et al. showed the effects of different absorption enhancers on the pulmonary absorption of salmon calcitonin following both dry powder and solution administration. As can be seen in Table 15.4, administration of the calcitonin complex

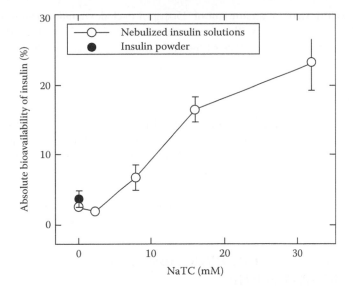

FIGURE 15.4 Effect of NaTC on the absolute bioavailability of nebulized insulin. Solutions containing insulin and different concentrations of NaTC were given as nebulized solutions (open circles) or powder (closed circle) to anesthetized, intubated beagle dogs. Data represent mean±SD, $n=4$. (Reproduced from Johansson, F. et al., *J. Pharm. Sci.*, 17, 63, 2002. With permission from Elsevier.)

TABLE 15.4

Effect of Absorption Enhancers on the Pulmonary Absorption of Salmon Calcitonin from Dry Powder and Solution in Rats

Enhancer	Amount of Enhancer (μg/Dose)	Dry Powder		Solution	
		AUC (%)[a]	ACR (%)[b]	AUC (%)[a]	ACR (%)[b]
None		29±5[c]	34±7	25±6	30±9
Oleic acid	25	43±7[*]	58±10[c]	29±9	34±8
	250	80±12[d]	120±25[c,d]	40±11	52±16
Dimethyl-β- cyclodextrin	25	35±9[c,d]	39±12	29±8	31±10
	250	60±18[c]	70±20[c]	60±12[c]	76±15[c]
Lecithin	25	41±12	46±10	27±9	30±11
	250	53±13[c,d]	67±16[c,d]	38±9	42±10
Taurocholic acid	25	32±8	36±10	27±5	31±8
	250	54±10[c,d]	61±13[c,d]	34±10	45±9
Octyl-β-D- glucoside	25	30±6	34±9	26±8	30±10
	250	47±9[c]	57±14[c]	34±12	45±14
Citric acid	25	41±14	49±13	27±9	30±8
	250	63±12[c,d]	66±14[c,d]	38±7	42±11

Source: Reproduced from Kobayashi, S. et al., *Pharm. Res.*, 13, 80, 1996. With permission from Elsevier.

Note: Dose of salmon calcitonin: 1 μg/kg. Values shown are means±SE ($n=4 < 6$).

[a] Area under the curve.

[b] Area of calcium reduction as a percentage of the value measured after intramuscular injection of salmon calcitonin at 1 μg/kg.

[c] Between control group (without enhancer) and group given enhancer.

[d] Between group given dry powder and group given solution.

[*] Statistically significant difference ($P < 0.05$).

with dimethyl-β-cyclodextrin (at an amount of 250 μg of cyclodextrin/dose) significantly increased the absorption of calcitonin in rats (the area under the curve [AUC] increased from 29 ± 5% to 60 ± 18%, when measured as a percentage of the AUC measured after the subcutaneous injection of calcitonin).[66]

15.5.4 LIPOSOMES

Besides being sustained release carriers of various drugs, liposomes act as absorption enhancers by promoting the surfactant recycling process in alveolar cells, thus increasing drug uptake into the systemic circulation. Li and Mitra suggest that the liposomes' ability to promote pulmonary absorption depends on the concentration, charge, and acyl chain length of phospholipid present in liposomes.[67]

In addition to the above listed agents, many other agents such as EDTA, polyethylene glycol (PEG), and lanthanide ions have shown efficacy as permeation enhancers.[68,69]

15.6 MODELS FOR STUDYING DRUG ABSORPTION VIA PULMONARY ROUTE

The respiratory system represents a very complex organ system in terms of anatomy and function. To understand the mechanisms involved in the pulmonary absorption and clearance of inhaled molecules, several models have been developed for preclinical investigations on pulmonary drug delivery systems.[70] These models fall into three major categories: (1) *in vivo* models, (2) *in vitro* cell culture models, and (3) *in situ* models.

15.6.1 *IN VIVO* MODELS

In vivo models provide a real time assessment of the deposition and absorption of drug molecules and formulations following pulmonary administration. Schanker et al. did pioneering work in the late 1970s and 1980s in establishing *in vivo* models for the determination of drug absorption and disposition in the lungs.[71–73] Small animals, such as rats and guinea pigs, were used for *in vivo* studies because of their ease of handling and low drug dose requirement. In pulmonary delivery, a number of variables such as tracheal access, delivery site, anesthesia, and animal posture can influence the kinetics of drug deposition and absorption.

The intratracheal administration of molecules of interest was first proposed by Enna and Schanker.[74] This method involves surgically exposing the trachea and inserting an endotracheal tube until just before the tracheal bifurcation. The drug is instilled through the tube using a microsyringe. The initial studies used destructive tissue sampling, such as removal of a lung at each timepoint, to determine the drug disappearance profiles. This method was adapted to collect blood samples from the same animal at multiple timepoints by catheterizing a vein. This allowed for the pharmacokinetic analysis of plasma and serum data, and comparison of pulmonary drug absorption with intravenous (IV) drug profiles. Ahsan's group and others established the technique of blood collection by milking the tail vein, thus making it possible to reuse animals after a 7 day wash-out period.[10,75–78]

Since Schanker's seminal work, several other more sophisticated approaches have been developed for lung dosing in small rodents. This includes the use of the PennCentury® Liquid Microsprayer® (Philadelphia, Pennsylvania). Upon visualization of the trachea with a small animal laryngoscope, the PennCentury microsprayer is inserted into the trachea through the mouth. It atomizes a plume of liquid droplets with a mass median diameter of ~16–22 μm.[79] Recently, a handheld dry powder insufflator was introduced by PennCentury, thus making possible the administration of liquid and powder formulations via the pulmonary route.[80,81] Also, several studies have used positive pressure ventilation along with endotracheal administration to maximize deep lung deposition.[82–84]

Large animals, such as rabbits, dogs, sheep, and monkeys, have also been extensively used to study pulmonary drug absorption. Large animals offer advantages of multiple sampling and pharmacokinetic analyses due to large blood volume. In a widely used model, aerosols are administered to rabbits or other large animals via nasotracheal or orotracheal intubation with or without ventilation.[85–87] A recent tool for the assessment of drug absorption and deposition following pulmonary administration is the use of imaging technology. A number of studies have been performed to visualize the fate of radiolabeled drugs and particles after intratracheal administration. Gamma scintigraphy and positron emission tomography (PET) are the most commonly used techniques. These techniques can also be used to determine the regional distribution of formulations in the lungs. Real time *in vivo* fluorescent imaging is another new technique used to study the distribution of fluorescent-labeled drugs in whole animal bodies.[88,89]

> In pulmonary delivery, a number of variables such as tracheal access, delivery site, anesthesia, and animal posture can influence the kinetics of drug deposition and absorption.

15.6.2 *In Vitro* Cell Culture Models

Compared with *in vivo* methods, *in vitro* models offer reproducibility, simplicity, and better control of data acquisition along with reduced operation cost. Models of lung epithelial cell monolayers help predict *in vivo* absorption by determining the transepithelial transport kinetics (P_{app}) prior to performing actual *in vivo* work. Primary cell culture models of lung epithelia involve the isolation of fresh epithelial cells from lung cells. As >97% of the lung epithelial area is represented by AE, the most common barrier for systemic absorption, they represent the most widely used primary culture cells. AE type I (AEI) cell cultivation has not yet been possible. AE type II (AEII) cells have been extensively used. AEII cells were first isolated by Dobbs[90] and Cheek et al.[91] When cultured, AEII cells acquire biochemical and morphological characteristics similar to AEI, and then they are referred to as ATI-like cells.

AE cell monolayers have been used to study the transport mechanisms and permeability of peptide and protein drugs across the lung epithelium. Several continuous cell lines of human lung epithelium have been developed and tested for transepithelial transport kinetics for prediction of *in vivo* drug absorption. For example, Calu-3, derived from human bronchial carcinoma; 16HBE14o-, a transformed epithelial cell line; and CFBE41o-, a transformed cystic fibrotic tracheobronchial cell line, are extensively used for transport, absorption, and safety studies. To adequately mimic the epithelial barrier properties and be suitable for transport studies, cell culture monolayers should form a tight polarized monolayer with a high transepithelial electrical resistance value (TEER) of >2 K$\Omega \cdot$cm^2 and a low P_{app} value for mannitol, ~0.2 cm/s. As cell culture models are used to predict P_{app} values to predict drug absorption from lungs, cell monolayer models forming leaky tight junctions are not suitable for determining the diffusive transport kinetics of different molecules. Calu-3 and 16HBE14o- cell lines have significantly higher TEER values and, hence, show excellent *in vitro-in vivo* correlation.

15.6.3 *Ex Vivo* Lung Tissue Model

Isolated perfused lung (IPL) is one of the most popular *ex vivo* models that is used to study the mechanisms of drug transport and disposition in lungs.[92–95] In IPL, lungs are housed in an artificial thoracic chamber after isolation from the body and are perfused with a physiological buffer by cannulating the pulmonary artery and veins. The trachea is also cannulated to maintain the respiration of the lungs under positive pressure ventilation, and to administer the drug of interest (Figure 15.5). This model eliminates the complications associated with the whole body system, while maintaining the architecture and functionality of the tissue. It also allows for the regulation of lung volume, ventilation rates, and respiratory patterns. IPL has been used for drug uptake, metabolism, and disposition studies. In addition, it has also been used for pharmacokinetic modeling for the systemic

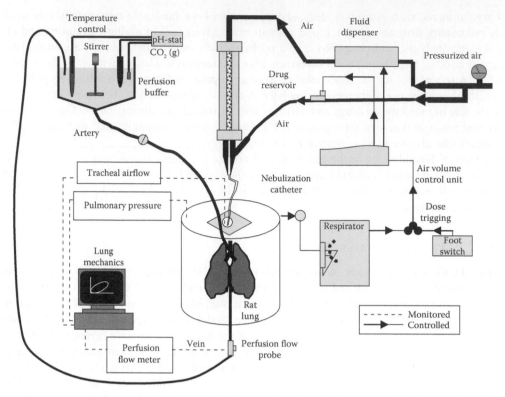

FIGURE 15.5   Schematic diagram representing isolated perfused rat lung (IPRL) system. Isolated lungs are housed in an artificial thoracic chamber, and are perfused with physiological buffer via pulmonary artery and veins through a cannula. Trachea is cannulated to maintain respiration of lungs under positive pressure ventilation, and to administer drugs of interest.

delineation of the lung's disposition processes. One of the main concerns with IPL is the viability of tissues over a period of time. Up to 4 h of viability has been reported with the handling and perfusion of the tissue.[96]

15.7   LARGE POROUS MICROPARTICLES FOR PULMONARY DELIVERY OF THERAPEUTIC AGENTS

Drug delivery to the lungs by means of inhalable particulate carriers has been a topic of interest for many years now. Aerosolized microparticles can be effective therapeutic carriers for the treatment of various respiratory diseases, such as lung inflammation and cystic fibrosis, and for providing the continuous release of medications via the lungs to the systemic circulation.[82,97] However, for effective delivery of therapeutic agents into the lungs, microparticles need to be deposited into the deep lung regions. For deep lung deposition, the particles should have a mass median geometric diameter in the range of 1–5 μm. As discussed before, this size range is important to avoid excessive deposition in the oropharyngeal cavity and on the surface of inhaler devices for dry powder.[98] At the same time, the existing size limitations make the microparticulate drug delivery systems, not falling in the specific size range, more susceptible to the lungs' clearance mechanisms. As discussed above, the human lungs are efficient in the removal of inhaled particles by various mechanisms, including mucociliary clearance in the upper airways and phagocytosis by alveolar macrophages in the deep lung regions. These clearance mechanisms cause a reduction in the residence time of the drug in the lungs and, thus, play a vital role in determining the release of the entrapped therapeutic agents into the circulation.

Large porous microparticulate delivery systems provide a means to escape the lungs' natural clearance mechanisms. These may, thus, provide sustained release of the drugs from the delivery systems. Pioneering work in the field of large porous particle technology has been conducted by David A. Edwards of Harvard University and Robert Langer at the Massachusetts Institute of Technology.[99,100] Some of their work has been discussed in detail in the next paragraph. Porous microspheres have hollow spaces and channels to release the drug in a controlled fashion.

Based on the pore diameter, microspheres can be macro- (3 μm), meso- (1–3 μm), or nanoporous (200–500 nm), as shown in Figure 15.6.[101] Porous microspheres of larger diameters have shown promise in the long-acting formulations for pulmonary delivery. The presence of pores and channels gives these microspheres a low density. Furthermore, porous particles of larger size can overcome both formulation and physiological barriers to facilitate the efficient deposition of the encapsulated drugs in the respiratory tract. As discussed earlier, in conventional inhaled formulations, the mass mean geometric diameter of inhaled particles should be 1–5 μm. Outside this size range, particles are either exhaled or deposited in the upper respiratory tract. In other words, particles within this size range are considered respirable. In a seminal paper, Edwards et al. proposed that particles with mass densities <0.4 g/cm^3 and a geometric diameter >5 μm could be used to facilitate the respirability and enhance the residence time of drugs in the lungs.[100] This assumption was based on the observation that the deposition of particles in the respiratory tract is a function of the aerodynamic diameter of the particles—a size-dependent parameter that depends on the settling velocity of the particles in the respiratory tract, rather than the actual geometric diameter of the particles:[99]

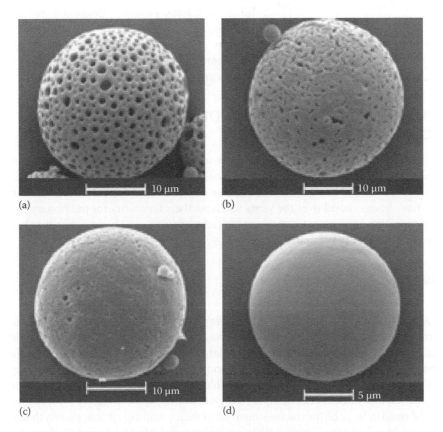

(a)   (b)   (c)   (d)

FIGURE 15.6 SEM images of (a) macroporous, (b) mesoporous, (c) nanoporous, and (d) nonporous microspheres. (Reproduced from Kim, H.K. et al., *J. Control Release*, 112, 167, 2006. With permission from Elsevier.)

$$d_a = \sqrt{\frac{\rho}{\rho_a}}\, d$$

where

d_a is the aerodynamic diameter
d is the particle's geometric diameter
ρ is the mass density of the particle
ρ_a is the reference density ($1\,g/cm^3$)

Furthermore, it was hypothesized that particles larger than $5\,\mu m$ can circumvent the lungs' clearance mechanism, reside in the lungs for a longer period of time, and produce a sustained release effect. Large porous microspheres are too big to be phagocytosed by alveolar macrophages. Also, since large porous particles would be lighter than corresponding conventional particles, their aerodynamic diameter will be within the respirable range despite them having a geometric diameter that is larger than those of particles used in conventional inhaled formulations. Consequently, microparticles containing the drug will reside longer in the lungs and will release the drug for a longer period of time. In addition, large porous particles tend to have a lower tendency to aggregate and form larger particles. Although large porous particle technology has generated tremendous interest in long-acting pulmonary formulations, this technology has thus far been used for only a limited number of biopharmaceuticals and conventional therapeutic agents, including insulin, testosterone, estradiol, deslorelin, tobramycin, and para-aminosalicylic acid.[100,102–105] Recent studies by Ungaro et al. exemplifying the use of large porous microparticle technology for the pulmonary delivery of insulin are discussed later in this chapter.[106,107]

> Large porous microparticulate delivery systems provide a means for escaping the lungs' natural clearance mechanisms. These may, thus, provide a sustained release of the drug from the delivery systems. Based on the pore diameter, microspheres can be macro-($3\,\mu m$), meso-($1–3\,\mu m$), or nano-porous ($200–500\,nm$).

15.8 PULMONARY DELIVERY OF PEPTIDE AND LARGE MOLECULAR WEIGHT DRUGS

Recent progress in biotechnology has resulted in a thrust in the search for noninvasive delivery routes for peptides, proteins, and other large molecular weight drugs. Pulmonary and nasal delivery are generally considered to be the lead noninvasive alternatives to injectable formulations. A number of drugs have been studied over the years to assess their feasibility for pulmonary delivery. The following section summarizes various drugs, delivery systems, and approaches that have recently been explored in the area of pulmonary delivery.

15.8.1 INSULIN

Beta cells of the islets of Langerhans in the pancreas produce insulin. It is made up of two peptide chains, having 21 and 30 amino acid residues, respectively. These chains are held together by disulfide linkages between cysteine residues. The molecular weight of insulin is about 6000. It was first successfully used for the treatment of diabetes mellitus in 1922. Today, insulin is widely used in the treatment of both insulin-dependent and non-insulin-dependent diabetes mellitus.[108,109] It has been about nine decades since noninjectable insulin administration was first proposed in 1922, when Woodyatt[110] studied the nasal delivery of insulin. Approximately 3 years after the commercial use of insulin in 1922 for the treatment of diabetes mellitus, it was shown that aerosolized insulin reduces blood glucose levels following pulmonary administration.[111] Ever since then, a variety of agents and drug delivery systems have been developed and studied for the delivery of inhaled insulin.

For inhaled insulin to be a viable therapy for diabetes, the delivery of insulin to the distal lung is required. This is because insulin may diffuse more readily across this region with a large surface and a thin alveolar membrane.[112–114] However, the main problem of pulmonary insulin is its low bioavailability after inhalational delivery.[100,115,116] A significant amount of research has been carried out over the past decade to overcome the obstacles of inhalable insulin.

Exubera® (Pfizer Labs, New York) was recently marketed as the first insulin and first biotechnology-based medication for the treatment of a systemic disorder that can be administered without needles as a dry powder aerosol. The Exubera system is a dry powder aerosol with a particle size of <5 μm made from short-acting human insulin. It can be instilled into the deep lung regions for the efficient and reproducible delivery of insulin. This dry powder formulation is packaged in single-dose blisters and the dose administered is controlled by the number of blister packs inhaled by the patient. A pneumatic mechanism is involved in the puncture of the blister, which is responsible for the consistency in the delivery of the drug. Though initially it generated interest among clinicians and patients, it failed to gain widespread acceptance. In comparison with the patients receiving Exubera, subcutaneous insulin showed a clear advantage when long-term pulmonary safety studies were conducted recently in type 2 diabetic patients. Clinically nonmeaningful treatment group differences in the change in FEV_1 were found during the first 3 months of treatment with Exubera as compared with subcutaneous insulin.[117] In October 2007, this product was taken off the market.[118] In general, it may be said that with an increasing number of setbacks, the patient compliance as far the convenience the route offers for chronic usage makes it a very promising area to continue dwelling in; hence despite this setback, pulmonary insulin delivery is still an intensive area of research and a number of other systems that are in various stages of developments are summarized below.

The AERx® Insulin Diabetes Management System (iDMS) has been developed by Aradigm Corporation (Hayward, California) in collaboration with Novo Nordisk (Copenhagen, Denmark). In this system, a microprocessor-controlled piston extrudes liquid insulin under pressure through laser-drilled perforations that yield aerosolized droplets of 2–3 μm. The system then uses a green light as an indicator to guide the patient to breathe at an optimal speed and depth for deep lung delivery, which is accomplished by means of a system called "Breath Check." A 400 mL chaser volume of fresh air follows the patient's breath to deliver aerosolized insulin to the deep lungs.[119] The phase III long-term safety and efficacy of the AERx system are being evaluated.[119,120] Recently, Aradigm Corporation reported that inhalation of insulin using the AERx iDMS does not seem to be associated with lung cancer.[121]

Large porous particles have also been studied as carriers for pulmonary delivery of insulin. Alkermes (Cambridge, Massachusetts), in collaboration with Eli Lilly (Indianapolis, Indiana), developed porous particles 5–30 μm in diameter for the deep lung deposition of insulin.[119] However, in March 2008, Eli Lilly and Company decided not to move forward with inhaled insulin. The company released a statement that the decision was not due to safety concerns but was more due to the increasing regulatory requirements that have been laid out recently. Technosphere® (Bergenfield, New Jersey) insulin uses a small organic molecule, 3,6-bis[N-fumaryl-N-(n-butyl) amino]-2,5-diketopiperazine, that self-assembles in an acidic environment into microspheres of ~2 μm. This delivery approach uses a MedTone® inhaler device for pulmonary delivery of the insulin formulation. Clinical studies have demonstrated the efficacy of this formulation and delivery system.[122] For instance, a very rapid uptake of systemic insulin was accompanied by a fast onset and a short duration of action in healthy volunteers and in patients with type 2 diabetes. Commercially available inhalers showed a relative bioavailability of ~26% for the first 3 h and 16% for the entire study period of 6 h, while the Technosphere insulin formulation using the MedTone inhaler device showed a relative bioavailability of around 50% at 3 h and 30% over the 6 h period.[122] In a separate study, Technosphere insulin formulation showed improved postprandial sugar control compared with subcutaneously administered regular insulin.[119,123]

Very recently, PROMAXX® inhaled insulin (Baxter, Norwood, Massachusetts) has been shown to be safe and efficacious after pulmonary administration.[124] This technology is based on the temperature-controlled precipitation of an aqueous insulin solution in the presence of PEG. This formulation, called recombinant human insulin inhalation powder (RHIIP), was administered to 30 healthy male volunteers in a clinical trial using a Cyclohaler® DPI. The ability of the formulations to reduce blood glucose levels was compared with subcutaneous regular insulin (SCIns). RHIIP inhalation was well received by the patients with no signs of cough or shortness of breath. It also showed a faster onset of action than the subcutaneously administered regular insulin. The RHIIP formulation took around 73 ± 2.4 min to reach 10% of the total area under the glucose curve, as compared with 94.9 ± 3.2 min for SCIns ($P < 0.0001$). The relative bioavailability was around 12%.

In addition to the above described clinical studies, preclinical studies on inhalable insulin have used absorption enhancers to address low bioavailability.[68,125–128] In this chapter, we will exemplify our work using some of these agents and novel delivery approaches.

15.8.1.1 Alkylmaltosides

Chemically, alkylglycosides are alkyl derivatives of disaccharides, such as maltose or sucrose, or monosaccharides, such as glucose. Hussain et al. showed that the pulmonary absorption of insulin increases when insulin is formulated with tetradecylmaltoside (TDM). Insulin administered with saline at a dose of 1.25 U/kg failed to lower the initial plasma glucose level, but the plasma glucose concentration was significantly decreased when insulin was formulated with 0.06% TDM in Sprague-Dawley rats. An increase in the concentration of TDM from 0.06% to 0.25% further decreased the plasma glucose level. A proportional increase in the plasma insulin levels was observed (Figure 15.7). The total exposure (measured as the area under the plasma concentration–time curve extrapolated to infinite time, $AUC_{0-\infty}$) of the plasma insulin-time curve as well as the plasma glucose-time profile against the TDM concentrations showed a dose-dependent effect of TDM on insulin absorption. When TDM concentration was increased from 0.25% to 0.5%, no further increase in AUC was observed. The pharmacokinetic parameters of insulin also showed a substantial increase in maximum plasma level (C_{max}) with the increasing concentrations of TDM. The time to reach the maximum concentration (T_{max}) for insulin formulations containing TDM was reduced from 10 min in the absence of TDM to 5 min. The relative bioavailability of insulin was 0.34 without and 0.84 with the 0.25% TDM, showing an increase in the bioavailability.[62]

The rate of absorption of monomeric insulin was found to be 2–3 times faster than hexameric insulin after the subcutaneous route of delivery. Furthermore, the blood glucose levels produced

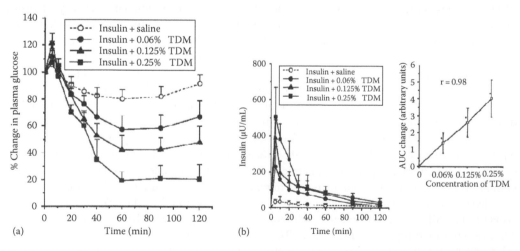

FIGURE 15.7 Changes in plasma glucose (a) and plasma insulin (b) after intratracheal administration of insulin in saline or in the presence of increasing concentrations of TDM. Inset shows changes in $AUC_{0-\infty}$ for plasma insulin–time curve with increasing concentrations of TDM. Data represent mean $\pm$ SD, $n = 3$–5. (Reproduced from Hussain, A. et al., *Pharm. Res.*, 20, 1551, 2003. With permission from Springer.)

by monomeric insulin administered just before a meal were found to be comparable with that produced by hexameric insulin administered 30 min prior to food intake in a study in the early 1990s.[129] Monomeric and hexameric insulin administered via the pulmonary route were compared in the presence or absence of TDM.[130] Regular hexameric insulin showed an increase in pulmonary absorption with an increasing dose and a corresponding decrease in plasma glucose levels. Similarly, all doses of regular insulin showed a significant increase in systemic exposure compared with the control group without TDM. The pharmacokinetics and pharmacodynamics of monomeric insulin were similar to that of hexameric insulin. These data were in contrast to those obtained after subcutaneous administration, wherein monomeric insulin was absorbed much faster than that of hexameric insulin.

In another set of studies, Hussain et al.[131] showed that dry powder formulations of inhaled insulin were better absorbed compared with the solution form of insulin. Both insulin solution and dry powder formulations showed a gradual increase in the plasma insulin curve, and corresponding reduction in plasma glucose levels, with increasing doses of insulin. However, when the absorption profiles of insulin solution and dry powder were compared, the increase in insulin absorption from dry powder was significantly higher. Interestingly, there was not much difference between the absorption profiles when the dose of insulin was 1.5 U. This anomaly was attributed to the saturability of insulin absorption from the lungs after dry powder administration (Figures 15.8 and 15.9).

Similarly, when the lyophilized formulation containing insulin (0.375 U), 4.6 mmol of C-8 maltoside, and lactose was administered pulmonarily, the increase in insulin absorption was significantly

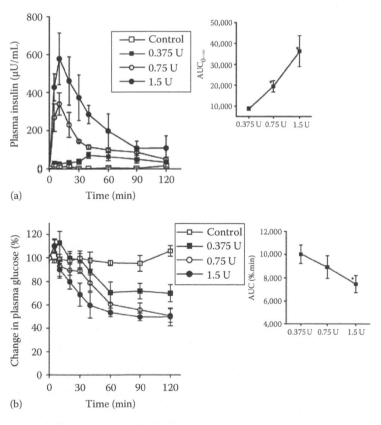

FIGURE 15.8 Changes in (a) plasma insulin and (b) plasma glucose after pulmonary administration of increasing doses of insulin solution. Figure insets show area under the curve (AUC) changes with increasing doses of insulin. Data represent mean ± SD, $n = 4$. (Reproduced from Hussain, A. et al., *Pharm. Res.*, 23, 138, 2006. With permission from Springer.)

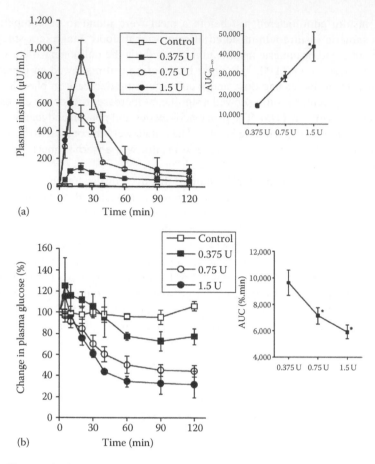

FIGURE 15.9 Changes in (a) plasma insulin and (b) plasma glucose after pulmonary administration of increasing doses of insulin powder. Figure insets show AUC changes with increasing doses of insulin. Data represent mean ± SD, $n = 4$. (Reproduced from Hussain, A. et al., *Pharm. Res.*, 23, 138, 2006. With permission from Springer.)

higher than the corresponding solution. The increased plasma insulin levels correlated with the reduction in plasma glucose levels. The authors suggested that lyophilization of the insulin formulations led to particles with lighter density, due to the presence of pores, which made particles travel a longer distance and deposit in the alveolar region. Also, the dry powder formulations were administered by insufflators that use a relatively large amount of air to force the dry powder through the delivery device for inhalation into rats. This forceful delivery may have caused a deeper lung deposition of the powder, thereby producing increased drug absorption compared with the solution. They also tested the safety of the formulations in the rat model using bronchoalveolar lavage (BAL) studies by studying different alkylglycosides (C-8 to C-14 maltosides). The effect of the formulations on different enzyme markers such as lactate dehydrogenase (LDH), alkaline phosphatase (ALP), and *N*-acetyl glucosaminidase (NAG) was evaluated. These enzyme markers have been frequently used as a tool for the re-evaluation of lung injury after pulmonary administration. Of the enzymes studied, LDH, ALP, and NAG are known to provide important insights as to the cell injury produced by exogenous substances. LDH is a well-known injury marker released upon cell damage. ALP, a membrane bound enzyme, has been regarded as an indicator of alveolar type II cell proliferation in response to type I cell damage.[132,133] Shorter chain length alkylmaltosides (C-8) caused the least increase in enzyme levels compared with saline control. Hence, these formulations were considered a safe delivery option for the pulmonary administration of insulin.

15.8.1.2 Cell-Penetrating Peptides for Pulmonary Absorption

Patel et al.[134] used cell-penetrating peptides to increase the pulmonary absorption of insulin. A heterobifunctional cross linker was used to conjugate insulin to the cationic cell penetrating peptides Tat, oligoarginine (r9), or oligolysine (k9) via a disulfide bridge to a D-isoform cysteine, to make insulin conjugates INS-cTat, INS-cr9, and INS-ck9, respectively. When compared with the native insulin, these conjugates showed higher insulin transport across the cultured rat AE in the order INS-cr9 > INS-cTat > INS-ck9. The transport across the AE for the INS-cr9 was both temperature- and time-dependent. When the INS-cr9 conjugate was administered by the pulmonary route in diabetic rats, it showed a steady decrease in the blood glucose levels, which was much more sustained compared with native insulin. The authors concluded that oligoarginine could be used as a potential means to increase the alveolar absorption of insulin.

15.8.1.3 Cyclodextrins

We have previously studied the use of cyclodextrins in increasing the pulmonary absorption of insulin. Dimethyl-β-cyclodextrins were less effective than alkylmaltosides in increasing pulmonary insulin absorption. The relative bioavailability of alkylmaltosides was 0.34–0.84, compared with dimethyl β cyclodextrin of 0.19–0.84, at different concentrations of the absorption enhancer employed.[62] Ungaro et al. used large porous particles (LPP) of poly (lactic-*co*-glycolic acid) (PLGA)-cyclodextrin for the dry powder inhalable formulation of insulin.[106,107] Hydroxypropyl-β-cyclodextrin (HPβCD) was used to enhance aerodynamic properties of large porous particles. The authors developed large porous particles of different loading capacities of insulin and HPβCD. When HPβCD was combined with insulin, it led to particles with surface pores. The concentration of HPβCD in the microspheres played a role in the release and aerodynamic properties of the large porous particles. The authors concluded that HPβCD containing large porous particles show flow properties and dimensions suitable for aerosolization and deposition in deep lung regions following inhalation as a dry powder.

In vitro aerosolization properties and release features of large porous particles were further tested in simulated lung fluids.[107] In these studies, insulin-loaded large porous particles made of PLGA were prepared with good yield using HPβCD as porosigen. The particles prepared with HPβCD were a mean diameter of ~26.2 μm and had widespread external and internal pores as shown in Figure 15.10. The experimental mass mean aerodynamic diameter ($MMAD_{exp}$) was in the range of 4.01–7.00 μm and the fine particle fraction (FPF) was between 26.9%–89.6% at different airflow rates. The fine-particle fraction is usually defined as the amount of powder with an aerodynamic size <4.7 mm (particles deposited at stage 3 and lower) divided by the initial total powder loaded in the DPI used in the studies being performed. Confocal microscopy studies were performed after the administration of labeled PLGA-HPβCD-insulin particles to rat lungs using DPI. These studies

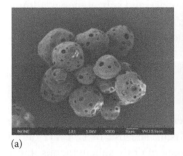
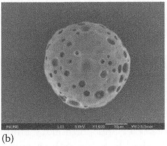
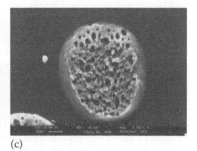

(a)   (b)   (c)

FIGURE 15.10   SEM micrographs of PLGA/HPβCD/insulin large porous particles (LPP): (a) overall picture (×900 magnification); (b) detail (×1600 magnification); (c) particle cross-section. Field is representative of the formulation. (Reproduced from Ungaro, F. et al., *J. Control Release*, 135, 25, 2009. With permission from Elsevier.)

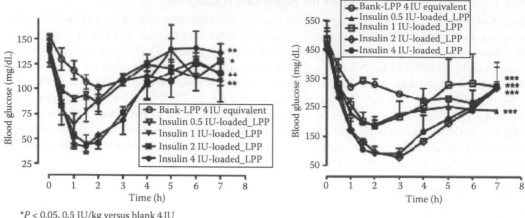

(a) **P < 0.005 1 IU/kg, 2 IU/kg and 4 IU/kg versus blank 4 IU   (b) ***P < 0.0001 all doses versus blank

FIGURE 15.11 Fasting blood glucose level in normoglycemic ($n = 15$) (panel a) and streptozotocin-induced diabetic ($n = 16$) (panel b) rats after intra-tracheal administration of different doses (0.5, 2, and 4 IU/kg) of PLGA/HPβCD/insulin LPP. Unloaded PLGA/HPβCD LPP equivalent to 4 IU/kg, were used as control. Data are reported as mean ± SEM (3–4 animals each group) expressed as mg/dL of glucose and analyzed by two way analysis of variance (ANOVA) followed by Bonferroni's as posttest. The values of $P < 0.05$ were taken as significant. (Reproduced from Ungaro, F. et al., *J. Control Release*, 135, 25, 2009. With permission from Elsevier.)

showed that particles reached the alveoli and remained for a longer time after delivery as is evident from the prolonged control over blood glucose.

When bovine insulin solutions were administered at different doses (0.5, 2, and 4 IU/kg), they did not result in a significant change of blood glucose levels in normoglycemic or hyperglycemic rats. Only a mild reduction in glycemia was seen when 4 IU/kg of bovine insulin were spray-instilled into normoglycemic rats. However, PLGA-HP-βCD-insulin large porous particles produced a significant reduction in blood glucose levels in a dose- and time-dependent fashion compared with the control groups. In normoglycemic conditions, a 0.5 IU/kg dose caused a significant reduction in fasting blood glucose. In the hyperglycemic rats, all the administered doses showed a very significant reduction in fasting blood glucose when compared with the control group. For all doses tested, normoglycemic rats showed a maximum reduction in blood sugar levels 1 h after pulmonary administration of PLGA-HPβCD-insulin particles. In streptozotocin-induced diabetic rats, a maximal reduction in blood glucose was observed after 3 h and a reduced level of sugar was maintained for about 5 h (Figure 15.11a and b). The relative pharmacodynamic availability (PA%) of the inhaled insulin was determined by taking into account the AUC after pulmonary and subcutaneous administration. The PA% of the solution and PLGA-HPβCD-insulin large porous particles were ~10.2 and 94.0 respectively in normoglycemic rats, whereas was determined to be ~44.3 and 152.0 in streptozotocin induced diabetic rats.

15.8.2 LOW MOLECULAR WEIGHT HEPARINS

Low molecular weight heparins (LMWHs) are negatively charged oligosaccharides used in the treatment of deep vein thrombosis (DVT) and pulmonary embolism. The use of LMWH on an outpatient basis, however, has been limited because of the requirement of daily subcutaneous injections. Attempts have been made to deliver LMWH via noninvasive routes, including the nasal and pulmonary routes.[78,135,136] However, the presence of carboxylic acid and sulfate groups in the glycosaminoglycan units of the LMWH renders the molecule highly anionic and an unlikely candidate for absorption via the mucosa, including the nasal and pulmonary routes.

We used cationic dendrimers as carriers for delivery of LMWHs.[77] Dendrimers are tree-like macromolecules showing tremendous potential in drug and gene delivery. Each dendrimer molecule has three distinct features: (1) a central core, consisting of either a single atom or a group of atoms attached to at least two chemical functional groups; (2) branches of repeating units that flow from the core, as is in a tree. These are repeated in a radial concentric fashion, each layer being called a generation; and (3) the outer surfaces of the tree have many functional groups determining dendrimers' chemical and physical properties. These unique structural features make dendrimers ideal drug delivery vehicles as many drugs and macromolecules are encapsulated in the central core or bound to the surface of the dendrimer by ionic or covalent interactions. We hypothesized that negatively charged LMWHs can form a complex with positively charged dendrimers to facilitate LMWH absorption across biological membranes. Generations 2 (G2), 2.5 (G2.5), and 3 (G3) polyamidoamine (PAMAM) dendrimers were used in these studies. G2 and G3 are full-generation (with terminal amine functional groups) dendrimers, whereas G2.5 is a half-generation (with terminal anionic carboxylic acid groups) dendrimer. *In vitro* studies assessed the differences in the interaction and/or complexation between LMWHs and dendrimers of different generations. Fourier transform infrared (FTIR) spectroscopy and the azure A assay were used to evaluate the interactions between dendrimers and enoxaparin, a commercially available LMWH. The azure A assay is a colorimetric assay involving the binding of a positively charged phenothiazine dye with the negatively charged sulfate groups in a heparin molecule. This method has previously been used to study the interaction between neutrophil elastase and heparin.[137,138] The results of both the FTIR analysis and azure assay demonstrated that an electrostatic interaction occurs between the LMWH and dendrimer. Similar interactions also occur between DNA and dendrimers.[139]

The ability of PAMAM dendrimers to enhance the pulmonary absorption of negatively charged LMWHs was evaluated in a rodent model. A LMWH formulated with only saline failed to show an increase in the plasma anti-factor Xa level, which is required for an antithrombotic effect in rats. A plasma anti-factor Xa level of 0.2 U/mL or higher is considered to produce a therapeutic effect in rodent models. A LMWH was formulated with different concentrations of G2 PAMAM dendrimers (0.25%, 0.5%, 1%, and 2%, respectively) with 0.25% and 0.5% showing no appreciable increase, and at the same time 1.0% and 2.0% PAMAM dendrimers showed a significant increase in plasma anti-factor Xa levels. In the case of G3 dendrimers, plasma anti-factor Xa levels were above therapeutic levels only when the concentration of the dendrimer was 0.5%. Interestingly, at 0.25%, 1%, and 2% levels, the anti-factor Xa levels were sub-therapeutic. The half-generation (G2.5) dendrimer failed to show an increase in anti-factor Xa levels at any of the concentrations employed in the study. The relative bioavailability of a 1% G2 or 0.5% G3 dendrimer-based formulation was twofold higher than the saline control. However, other formulations used in the studies failed to show a statistically significant change in the relative bioavailability.

We hypothesized that the higher pulmonary absorption with the G2 and G3 dendrimers was due to the positive surface charge of the dendrimers, which formed a complex with the negatively charged LMWH. The complexation led to either a reduction in the net negative charge of the LMWH or made the complex electrostatically neutral. The reduction in negative surface charge aids in the absorption of the negatively charged LMWH to a greater extent. The efficacy of PAMAM dendrimers and LMWH formulations in the treatment of DVT was studied in a rat jugular vein thrombosis model using two formulations that showed the highest bioavailability (1% G2 PAMAM dendrimer plus LMWH and 0.5% G3 PAMAM dendrimer plus LMWH). The thrombus weight was used as an indicator of antithrombotic effect. The efficacy of the formulations was compared against a saline control and plain LMWH administered by both the pulmonary and subcutaneous routes. A significant reduction in thrombus weight was observed when the LMWH plus 1% G2 or 0.5% G3 dendrimer was administered via the pulmonary route. When LMWH plus saline was administered by the subcutaneous route, thrombus weights reduced significantly compared with the pulmonary formulations of LMWH plus dendrimer. The *in vivo* data suggest that the dendrimer-based LMWH formulation was effective in preventing DVT in a rodent model. The safety of the optimized formulations was tested by analyzing the effect of the formulations on levels of different injury markers (LDH, ALP, and wet lung weight) in BAL fluid and on the mucociliary transport rate in a frog palate model. The frog palate model is a method used to determine the mucociliary clearance against inhaled particulate matter. Frog palates possess a pseudostratified epithelium with mucus secreting cells and numerous ciliated cells closely resembling the epithelium of human conductive airways. In this model, a mustard seed or a marker particle is put on the isolated frog palate and its movement from one point to the other is monitored. This study is done by spraying the palate with either the physiological ringer's solution, or the formulations being studied.

In 2004, Qi et al. reported the use of particulate carriers for pulmonary delivery of unfractionated heparin and LMWHs. This group reported that the bioavailability of LMWH, when formulated into particles, increases 10–20 times as compared with other noninvasive routes of administration. The particles for pulmonary delivery of LMWHs were prepared by two different methods—spray drying or by mechanical grinding followed by mechanical sieving. Particles prepared by both the methods possessed identical properties. Only certain particles such as the ones containing 60% dipalmitoyl phosphatidylcholine were prepared by spray drying, and the ones containing only heparin or LMWHs were prepared by mechanical sieving. The pulmonary delivery of LMWH particles resulted in therapeutic blood levels of the anti-coagulant, and the dose–response curve was linear. In addition, pulmonary delivery of LMWHs resulted in the rapid absorption of the drug, thus achieving the C_{max} before subcutaneous administration.[140]

We also investigated the efficacy of PEG conjugated (PEGylated) dendrimeric nanocarriers for the pulmonary delivery of LMWHs.[76] PEGylation has been shown to prolong the circulation time of the formulation in the body by retarding clearance by the reticuloendothelial system (RES).[141] In this study, G3 PAMAM dendrimers were PEGylated with methoxy PEG 2000 (mPEG 2000). The conjugation between PEG and G3 PAMAM dendrimers was confirmed by FTIR, nuclear magnetic resonance (NMR) spectra, and thin layer chromatography (TLC). The LMWH was loaded onto the mPEG-PAMAM dendrimers by mixing aliquots of mPEG-dendrimer solution and LMWH. PEG-dendrimers increased the pulmonary absorption of LMWH significantly in adult male Sprague-Dawley rats. The relative bioavailability of the formulation was 60.6% as compared with subcutaneous LMWH. Also, the half-life of the PEGylated dendrimeric formulation of LMWHs was 11.9 h (2.4 times higher than LMWH's half-life in saline controlled formulations; Figure 15.12).

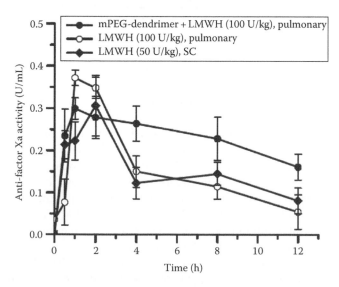

FIGURE 15.12 Changes in anti-factor Xa activity after pulmonary or subcutaneous administration of LMWH formulated in saline or with PEGylated dendrimers. Data represent mean ± SD, $n = 3$–5. (Reproduced from Bai, S. and Ahsan, F., *Pharm. Res.*, 26, 539, 2009. With permission from Springer.)

In addition, when these formulations were tested in the rodent model of DVT, PEGylated dendrimers showed a decrease in thrombus weight comparable with the subcutaneous injections.

We have also shown the increased pulmonary absorption of the drug from poly-L-arginine (PLA)/LMWH complexes.[142] PLA is a cationic polyamino acid, which has the unique ability of increasing the permeability of cell membranes, thus enhancing the absorption of drug molecules. The low toxicity and biodegradability of PLA make it an ideal candidate as an absorption enhancer and drug carrier. The effect of LMWH complexation with PLA on its absorption was studied after pulmonary administration. The *in vitro* characterization of the PLA/LMWH complex was done by particle size, zeta potential, and the amount of drug complexed with PLA using the azure A assay. Immortalized Calu-3 lung epithelium cell lines were used for performing cell membrane transport studies for PLA. Transport studies were performed by studying and measuring mannitol transport and determining changes in TEER in the presence of various enoxaparin-PLA complexes across the cell monolayer in collagen-coated polycarbonate transwells®. 14C-mannitol transport was determined by a Beckman LS-6500 liquid scintillation counter, thus calculating the apparent permeability coefficient and flux across the cell monolayer (cpm/s). Changes in TEER were determined using an EVOM® epithelial voltohmmeter (World Precision Instruments, Sarasota, Florida). *In vivo* absorption studies performed in rats demonstrated that complexation of LMWH with 93 kDa PLA (0.0125% or 0.0625%) increased the pharmacological activity of the formulation by twofold, as compared with LMWH + saline formulation (Figure 15.13). The PLA formulations were safe

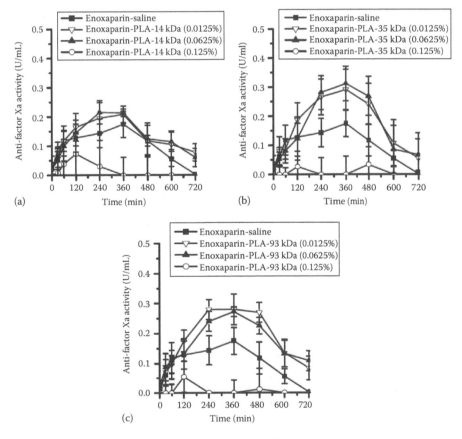

FIGURE 15.13 Changes in plasma anti-factor Xa activity after pulmonary administration of enoxaparin (50 U/kg) in the absence or presence of PLA-14 kDa (a), PLA-35 kDa (b) or PLA-93 kDa (c). Data represent mean ± SD, *n* = 5–6. (Reproduced from Rawat, A. et al., *Pharm. Res.*, 25, 936, 2008. With permission from Springer.)

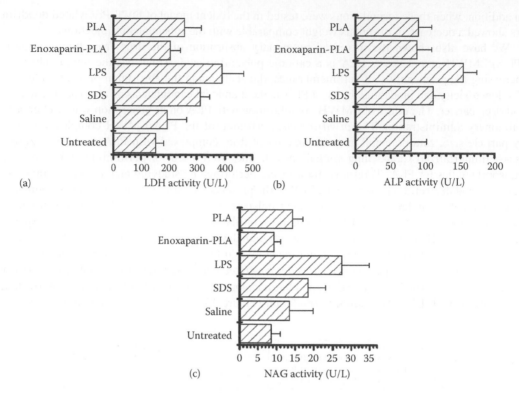

FIGURE 15.14 Enzyme activities of (a) LDH, (b) ALP, and (c) NAG following BAL fluid analysis at 24 h after pulmonary administration of enoxaparin-0.125% PLA-93 kDa complexes. Data represent mean ± SD, $n = 5-6$. (Reproduced from Rawat, A. et al., *Pharm. Res.*, 25, 936, 2008. With permission from Springer.)

for pulmonary administration based on BAL studies. BAL studies are performed to investigate the biochemical and cellular changes in the lungs due to administration of various formulations and different excipients. For collection of BAL fluid, adult male rats were sacrificed; the lungs were isolated and lavaged with sterile saline, so as to collect the inflammatory cells. The cells were centrifuged and the supernatant was collected and assayed for the presence of various injury markers (LDH, ALP, and NAG). The results of these experiments, as shown in Figure 15.14, indicate that enoxaparin-PLA 93 kDa complex does not induce any cellular damage in the lungs, when compared with liposaccharide (LPS) and sodium dodecyl sulfate (SDS).

Recently, Rawat et al. developed large porous PLGA microparticulate formulations for pulmonary delivery of LMWH.[143] In this study, PLGA microparticles entrapped LMWH in the core. At the same time, various core modifying agents were used to change microparticles' morphology, release characteristics, and *in vivo* performance. Modifying the core of the microparticles with positively charged absorption enhancers (polyethyleneimine [PEI] and stearylamine [SA]) increased the entrapment efficiency of the microparticles. PEI increased the entrapment efficiency from $16.22 \pm 1.32\%$ to $54.82 \pm 2.79\%$. PEI also made the particles bulky and porous, thus ensuring deep lung deposition. *In vivo* absorption studies in rats showed an increase in the relative bioavailability by 2.5- to 3.0-fold as compared with the plain LMWH administered via the pulmonary route. At the same time, biological $t_{1/2}$ increased to 20.13 ± 1.68 h (PEI microparticles) and 25.28 ± 2.81 h (SA microparticles) as compared with 4.35 ± 0.33 h for subcutaneous administration and 4.28 ± 0.31 h for pulmonary administration of plain LMWH (Figure 15.15 and Table 15.5). At the same time, cytotoxicity studies performed using the lung epithelial cell line, Calu-3, showed no or negligible toxic effects of PEI, SA, or PLGA.

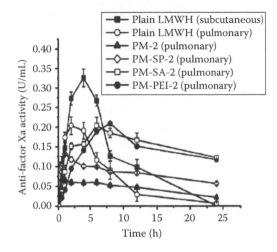

FIGURE 15.15   Changes in plasma anti-factor Xa activity after pulmonary administration of LMWH (50 U/kg) in plain and core-modified PLGA microspheres (*n* = 5–6). (Reproduced from Rawat, A. et al., *J. Control Release*, 128, 224, 2008. With permission from Elsevier.)

TABLE 15.5
Pharmacokinetic Parameters of LMWH-Loaded PLGA Microspheric Formulations

			Pharmacokinetic Parameters				
Formulations	C_{max} **(U/mL)**	T_{max} **(h)**	AUC_{0-24} **(U h/mL)**	$AUMC_{0-24}$	$T_{1/2}$ **(h)**	**MRT(h)**	$F_{relative}$ **(%)**
Plain LMWH subcutaneous	0.33 ± 0.03	4.4 ± 0.31	3.98 ± 0.22	36.6 ± 1.72	4.35 ± 0.33	7.79 ± 0.60	—
Plain LMWH pulmonary	0.20 ± 0.01	2.2 ± 0.44	1.58 ± 0.12	9.63 ± 0.77	4.28 ± 0.31	6.63 ± 0.47	39.7 ± 3.0
PM-2	0.07 ± 0.04	0.8 ± 0.4	1.05 ± 0.11	10.57 ± 2.04	12.13 ± 0.93	18.43 ± 1.42	26.38 ± 2.8
PM-SP-2	0.13 ± 0.03	1.7 ± 0.3	1.98 ± 0.29	21.22 ± 1.86	23.75 ± 2.97	34.33 ± 4.29	49.74 ± 7.31
PM-SA-2	0.20 ± 0.04	6.9 ± 0.89	3.64 ± 0.36	43.14 ± 3.7	25.28 ± 2.81	39.09 ± 4.34	91.45 ± 9.01
PM-PEI-2	0.21 ± 0.03	7.6 ± 0.70	3.37 ± 0.40	40.8 ± 2.38	20.13 ± 1.68	32.39 ± 2.70	84.67 ± 0.11

Source: Reproduced from Rawat, A. et al., *J. Control Release*, 128, 224, 2008. With permission from Elsevier.
Note: Data represent mean ± SEM (*n* = 5–6).

15.9   PULMONARY DELIVERY OF NONPEPTIDE SMALL MOLECULAR WEIGHT DRUGS

We present some case studies of the small molecular weight, nonpeptide drugs that have been studied for delivery via the pulmonary route.

15.9.1   Iloprost

Iloprost is a synthetic analogue of prostacyclin (PGI$_2$), which is used for the treatment of PAH, a rare but debilitating disorder of pulmonary circulation. PAH results from an imbalance among the neurochemical mediators responsible for maintaining the vascular tone in pulmonary circulation. These mediators include prostacyclin and nitric oxide, which serve as vasodilators, while endothelin-1 and cytokines serve as vasoconstrictors. The pathophysiology of PAH includes the elevated mean pulmonary arterial pressure (MPAP) of >25 mm of Hg at rest or >30 mm of Hg after exercise. These abnormalities and elevated MPAP result in pulmonary vascular remodeling, endothelial cell proliferation, and increased pulmonary vascular resistance (PVR).[144] Prostacyclin is one of the major and most potent vasodilators for both the pulmonary and systemic circulations. The synthesis of prostacyclin is severely diminished in PAH patients.[145,146] For this reason, prostacyclin analogues have been extensively investigated for PAH treatment.

Iloprost is a potent vasodilator for systemic and pulmonary arterial vascular beds. It is one of three PGI_2 analogues currently approved by the FDA for PAH treatment. Epoprostenol and treprostinil are the other two currently available prostacyclin analogues. One of the major problems associated with PGI_2 analogues is their instability at physiological conditions and short biological half-lives. The half-life of iloprost is ~20–30 min. The short half-life requires them to be delivered via continuous IV or subcutaneous infusion.[147] In 2006, the FDA approved the first inhalable formulation of iloprost (Ventavis®) for PAH treatment. Besides providing an increased availability of the drug in circulation, inhalable formulations may also provide selectivity of the hemodynamic effects to the pulmonary vasculature thus eliminating systemic side effects.[148] The efficacy of inhaled iloprost in PAH treatment, and in various pathological conditions associated with PAH, has been studied in various animal models. These animal models include monocrotaline (MCT) and hypoxia-induced rodent models of PAH.

Schermuly et al. demonstrated the efficacy of inhaled iloprost to reverse vascular remodeling in a chronic monocrotaline-induced rodent model of PAH. Iloprost, when administered in the nebulized form for 15 min, 12 times a day, at a dose of 6 μg/kg/day to MCT-induced PAH rats caused a reduction in right ventricular systolic pressure, an increase in cardiac output, and a decrease in the PVR index. Also, inhaled iloprost significantly decreased the degree of muscularization. The percentage of fully vascularized vessels and median wall thickness was decreased significantly in inhaled iloprost-treated rats (21.8 ± 2.8% compared with 32.0 ± 5.0% for MCT-treated rats). The authors also demonstrated that inhaled iloprost decreased the expression of matrix metalloproteinases (MMP), especially MMP-2 in MCT-treated rats.[149]

In another study, Schermuly et al. compared the pharmacokinetics and vasodilatory effects of inhaled iloprost with an infused formulation of iloprost in an isolated rabbit lung model. PAH (MPAP ≈ 32 mm) was induced by infusing U46619, a thromboxane A2 agonist, over the period of experiment. Administration of 75 ng iloprost by nebulization over a period of 10 min resulted in a significant decrease in pulmonary arterial pressure (PAP). The anti-hypertensive effect was maintained for 50 min and then leveled off at the end of the 210 min experiment. On the other end, when iloprost was administered as an IV infusion at a dose of 200 ng bolus + 33 ng/h infusion, the PAP decreased by a mean of 9.5 mm of Hg, but the effects started to diminish within 40–60 min of the experiment and completely disappeared after 210 min (data not shown).[150]

In a clinical study performed by Olschewski et al., the efficacy of inhaled iloprost in reversing the symptoms of PAH was investigated. Iloprost was administered to patients at a total inhaled dose of 5.0 μg, 6 to 9 times a day. The effects were compared with patients receiving placebo. As shown in Figure 15.16, there was a significant improvement in the distance walked (mean of 36.4 m) in 6 min, when compared with placebo. As is evident from Table 15.6, the hemodynamics such as PAP, cardiac output, PVR, and many other determinants also improved significantly when compared with the placebo group.[151]

In 2006, the FDA approved the first inhalable formulation of iloprost (Ventavis®) for PAH treatment. Besides providing an increased availability of the drug in circulation, inhalable formulations may also provide selectivity of the hemodynamic effects to the pulmonary vasculature thus eliminating systemic side effects.

As is evident from the studies discussed above, iloprost has to be inhaled 6 to 9 times a day to maintain the drug levels within the therapeutic range. To overcome the problem of multiple dosing, there is an urgent need to develop a controlled release formulation of iloprost. Recently, Kleeman et al. reported the preparation and optimization of iloprost containing liposomes for pulmonary delivery. Further investigations are required to

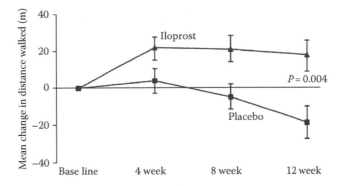

FIGURE 15.16 Effect of inhaled iloprost and placebo on the mean (±SE) change from base line in the distance walked in 6 min, according to an intention-to-treat analysis. *P* value was obtained with Wilcoxon's test for two independent samples. (Reproduced from Olschewski, H. et al., *N. Engl. J. Med.*, 347, 322, 2002. With permission from Massachusetts Medical Society.)

TABLE 15.6
Mean ± SD Changes from Baseline in Hemodynamic Values during 12 Weeks of Therapy with Inhaled Iloprost or Placebo

Variable	Placebo Group	Iloprost Group[a]	
		Before Inhalation	**After Inhalation**
		Mean ± SD	
Pulmonary-artery pressure (mm Hg)	−0.2 ± 6.9	−0.1 ± 7.3	−4.6 ± 9.3[*]
Cardiac output (L/min)	−0.19 ± 0.81[**]	+0.05 ± 0.86	+0.55 ± 1.1[*]
PVR (dyn · s · cm^{-5})	+96 ± 322[**]	−9 ± 275[***]	−239 ± 279[*]
SAP (mm Hg)	−0.2 ± 12.4	−1.7 ± 12.8	−4.3 ± 13.6[****]
Right arterial pressure (mm Hg)	+1.4 ± 4.8[**]	+0.5 ± 4.6	−0.8 ± 4.6
Pulmonary-artery wedge pressure (mm Hg)	+0.7 ± 3.6	+1.1 ± 4.7[**]	+1.8 ± 5.3[****]
Arterial oxygen saturation (%)	−1.6 ± 4.4[**]	−0.4 ± 3.7	−14 ± 3.7[**]
Mixed venous oxygen saturation (%)	−3.2 ± 6.7[*]	−1.1 ± 7.6	+1.8 ± 8.3
Heart rate (beats/min)	−1.2 ± 9.5	−1.8 ± 12.4	−2.25 ± 12.6

Source: Reproduced from Olschewski, H. et al., *N. Engl. J. Med.*, 347, 322, 2002. With permission from Massachusetts Medical Society.

Note: For the iloprost group, both preinhalation and postinhalation values after 12 weeks are compared with the baseline values at study entry.

[*] P < 0.001 for the difference from baseline values.

[**] P < 0.05 for the difference from baseline values.

[***] P < 0.01 for die comparison with the placebo group.

[****] P < 0.01 for the difference from baseline values.

---

evaluate the pharmacokinetics and efficacy of iloprost liposomes in the treatment of pulmonary hypertension.[152]

15.9.2 Treprostinil

As discussed earlier, treprostinil is one of the stable tricyclic benzidene prostacyclin (PGI$_2$) analogues currently approved by the FDA for the treatment of PAH. As a PGI$_2$ analogue, treprostinil has antiplatelet and vasodilatory effects both in pulmonary and systemic circulation. It causes vascular smooth muscle relaxation by binding to a membrane-associated G-protein-coupled receptor. It activates adenylate cyclase, resulting in the formation of cyclic adenosine monophosphate (cAMP). Despite being structurally similar to iloprost and PGI_2, treprostinil has a comparatively longer biological half-life of 2–4 h following subcutaneous injection, which can be attributed to its improved chemical stability at room temperature.[153,154] The FDA approved treprostinil for the treatment of PAH as a subcutaneous infusion (Remodulin®). A subcutaneous infusion of treprostinil is preferred over an IV infusion of epoprostenol as the former is less cumbersome and does not require a surgically implanted central catheter. Though the terminal half-life of treprostinil is comparatively longer than epoprostenol or iloprost, it still needs to be administered as a continuous subcutaneous infusion. This leads to the same complications associated with epoprostenol, such as infection at the site of infusion and discomfort due to needle-based delivery. These complications have led to the development of an inhaled formulation of treprostinil, which has recently entered clinical trials.

The efficacy of the inhaled treprostinil formulation for treating PAH symptoms has been studied by several independent investigators both in animals and human subjects. Sandifer et al. compared the efficacy of aerosolized and intravenously administered treprostinil on pulmonary circulation in a PAH-induced sheep model. PAH was induced by infusing a prostaglandin H_2 (PGH_2) analogue, U-44069, at a rate of 1000 ng/kg/min for 180 min. As shown in Figure 15.17a and b, aerosolized treprostinil was more effective as a pulmonary vasodilator even at a dose of 250 ng/kg/min. At the highest dose used in the experiment (1000 ng/kg/min), treprostinil decreased both PAP and PVR to the baseline level, even with the continuous infusion of the vasoconstricting agent. Pulmonary delivery also resulted in more localized delivery of treprostinil into the alveolar regions. As is evident from Figure 15.17c, aerosolized treprostinil had little or no effects on the systemic hemodynamics even at a dose of 1000 ng/kg/min, while treprostinil administered via IV infusion showed a marked increase in cardiac output and heart rate. In addition, when aerosolized, the duration of action of treprostinil was much greater than infused epoprostenol or treprostinil.[155]

In another clinical trial, Voswinckel et al. showed that treprostinil, when inhaled, demonstrates sustained pulmonary vasodilatory effects with excellent tolerability at relatively low doses when compared with inhaled iloprost. As seen in Figure 15.18, inhalation of both iloprost and treprostinil decreased the MPAP and PVR, but no significant differences were observed between the AUCs of PVR for iloprost and that for treprostinil (12.6 ± 7.0% vs. 13.3 ± 3.2%). As discussed earlier, treprostinil did not show any significant changes in cardiac output and systemic arterial pressure (SAP) (Figure 15.18). In addition, the maximum effects of iloprost and treprostinil on PVR were comparable. The maximal effect of treprostinil was observed 18 ± 2 min after inhalation, while for iloprost it took 8 ± 1 min for the maximal effect to occur. Importantly, the effect of the former lasted for ~60–180 min.[156]

Voswinckel et al. reported the efficacy of treprostinil after delivery by a MDI at a dose of 30, 45, and 60 μg at one time. Various efficacy parameters were recorded for 180 min. The authors demonstrated that the AUC of PVR and PAP decreased significantly with all the three doses of treprostinil delivered by MDI, whereas changes in systemic hemodynamics—SAP, cardiac output, heart rate—were minimal or unaltered (Table 15.7).[157]

15.9.3 AMPHOTERICIN B

Amphotericin B is a polyene antifungal drug used for the treatment of systemic fungal infections in immunocompromised patients. It acts by associating with ergosterol, a chemical in the fungal membrane, thus causing fungal cell death by inducing K^+ leakage. The use of amphotericin B has been limited due to dose-dependent toxicity and organ damage associated with IV administration. Lipid-based formulations of amphotericin B have been used to subside the side-effects. An alternative approach is the development of aerosolized inhalable formulations of amphotericin B.[158–160]

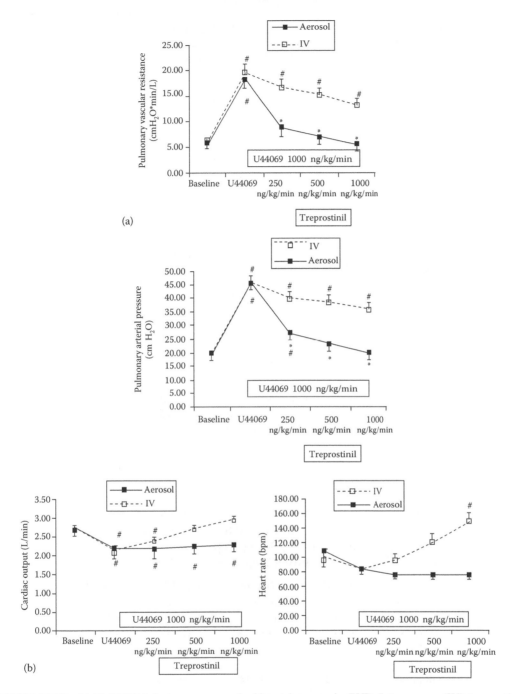

FIGURE 15.17 (a) U-44069 infusion causes a significant increase in PVR. Intravenous (IV) treprostinil caused a dose-dependent decrease in PVR that remained significantly elevated above baseline ($P < 0.05$). Aerosol treprostinil caused a dose-dependent decrease in PVR that was significantly lower compared with intravenous delivery ($P < 0.05$). (b) U-44069 caused a significant increase in MPAP. Intravenous treprostinil caused a dose dependent decrease in PAP that remained significantly elevated above baseline ($P < 0.05$). Aerosol delivery caused a dose-dependent decrease in PAP that was significantly lower compared with intravenous delivery ($P < 0.05$). Values are means ± SEM; $n = 6$ animals. (c) U-44069 caused a decline in cardiac output ($P < 0.05$) and heart rate (not significant). (Reproduced from Sandifer, B.L. et al., *J. Appl. Physiol.*, 99, 2363, 2005. With permission from The American Physiological Society.)

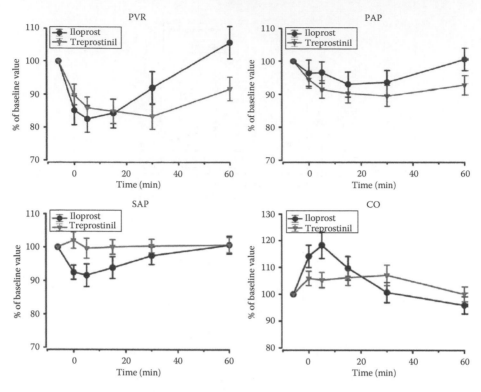

FIGURE 15.18 Hemodynamic response to inhalation of treprostinil versus iloprost. Data from 44 patients who inhaled both drugs in randomized order, shown as percent of baseline values (mean±95% confidence interval). (Reproduced from Voswinckel, R. et al., *J. Am. Coll. Cardiol.*, 48, 1672, 2006. With permission from Elsevier.)

TABLE 15.7
Maximal Changes of Hemodynamic Parameters in Percent from Baseline Values Following Metered Dose Inhaler Delivery of Placebo ($n = 4$), 30 mg Treprostinil ($n = 12$), 45 mg Treprostinil ($n = 9$), or 60 mg Treprostinil ($n = 20$)

	Placebo	30 µg TRE	45 µg TRE	60 µg TRE
PAP (min)	−0.6±3.0	−16.6±3.2	−22.4±6.8	−20.5±2.4
PVR (min	+1.4±1.9	−15.6±4.4	−28.6±8.9	−22.5±3.7
CO (max)	−0.3±1.1	+8.8±3.8	+8.6±5.6	+3.8±2.0
SVR (min)	+4.3±4.3	−2.3±4.2	−8.0±3.9	−8.7±2.1
SAP (min)	+2.7±1.7	−2.7±1.9	−3.9±1.5	−6.4±2.9
HR (max)	+5.0±2.1	+6.1±2.9	−0.9±2.4	+1.1±0.9

Source: Reproduced from Voswinckel, R. et al., *Pulm. Pharmacol. Ther.*, 22, 50, 2009. With permission from Elsevier.

Notes: PAP, pulmonary artery pressure; PVR, pulmonary vascular resistance; SVR, systemic vascular resistance; CO, cardiac output; SAP, systemic arterial pressure; HR, heart rate. Highest (max) or lowest (min) values observed during the observation period are shown. Data are given mean±SEM.

Ruijgrok et al. demonstrated the *in vivo* deposition of amphotericin B as desoxycholate (Fungizone®) and as liposomal (AmBisome®) formulations in rats following aerosol delivery. The concentration of amphotericin B was similar in both lobes of the lung in rats treated with Fungizone or AmBisome (data not shown).[161] Borro et al. investigated the efficacy of Abelcet® (Amphotericin B lipid complex, ABLC) in the prophylaxis of invasive fungal infections following lung transplantation. A total of 50 mg of ABLC administered once every 2 days for 2 weeks and then once per week for 13 weeks resulted in the achievement of an efficient prophylaxis in 98.3% of the patients.[162]

15.9.4 AMIKACIN

Amikacin is an aminoglycoside antibiotic used for the treatment of bacterial infections. Amikacin acts by binding with the 30S ribosomal subunit, leading to the misreading of mRNA, leaving the bacteria unable to synthesize vital proteins. Amikacin is prescribed for a variety of lung and respiratory tract infections including cystic fibrosis, nontuberculosis mycobacterial (NTM) infection, and ventilator associated pneumonia (VAP).

Aerosolized antibiotic delivery has many advantages over oral or IV delivery in treating lung infections. These include high lung drug concentrations and low systemic absorption and toxicity. Recently, a liposomal formulation of amikacin (Arikace®) has entered phase II clinical trials for the treatment of cystic fibrosis. Several groups investigated the efficacy of amikacin, both as plain drug and as controlled release formulations, for the treatment of a variety of lung infections.[163,164] Goldstein et al. investigated the efficiency of nebulized amikacin in the treatment of *E. coli* pneumonia in ventilated pigs. They compared the lung tissue concentrations of amikacin after IV (15 mg/kg) and aerosolized (45 mg/kg) administration. Figure 15.19a shows the concentration of amikacin in various lung regions measured 1 h after drug administration and performed 48 h after inoculation with *E. coli*. As can be seen in Figure 15.19b, lung tissue concentrations of amikacin were almost 3- to 30-fold higher than that achieved after IV infusion. Although lung segments with severe bronchopneumonia showed less accumulation of drug than regions with mild bronchopneumonia, nebulization always resulted in better lung deposition of amikacin than intravenously administered amikacin.[165]

Dhillon et al. demonstrated the efficacy of the liposomal formulation of amikacin in treating pulmonary tuberculosis in a murine model. They demonstrated that liposomal amikacin, when administered intravenously at a dose of 160, 80, and 40 mg/kg, is 2.4–5.0 times more active than free amikacin in treating the infection.[166] Recently, Li et al. reported the preparation of aerosolized liposomal formulations of amikacin (Arikace) for the treatment of gram negative infections. Arikace has now entered phase II clinical trials for the treatment of cystic fibrosis.[167]

15.10 INHALABLE siRNA AS THERAPEUTIC AGENT

Gene therapy based on small interfering RNA (siRNA)-induced RNA interference (RNAi) has been widely used to explore and develop new treatment options for diseases involving the dysregulation of protein synthesis. RNAi was first introduced by Andrew Fire and Craig Mello (Noble Prize recipients in 2006). RNAi is involved in the cellular defense against viral invasion and is referred to as a unique form of posttranscriptional gene silencing.[168–170] The siRNA molecules can be custom synthesized and introduced into a cell to promote gene silencing.[171] Briefly, RNAi starts when cells encounter ectopic double-stranded DNA, which is cleaved into siRNAs (19–25 bases). The siRNAs are incorporated into RISC (an RNA-induced silencing complex). Binding of the siRNA results in the site-specific cleavage of mRNA, thus silencing the message. This, in turn, results in a prominent reduction in the levels of corresponding proteins. RNAi offers several advantages over small drug molecules and antisense oligonucleotides, such as robust and specific inhibition, diminished risk of toxic effects, expansion of potential targets, and design of drugs in silico.

RNAi-induced gene silencing has been investigated for the treatment of a variety of lung diseases including lung cancer, cystic fibrosis, respiratory syncytial virus (RSV) infection, and severe acute

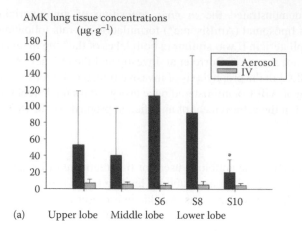

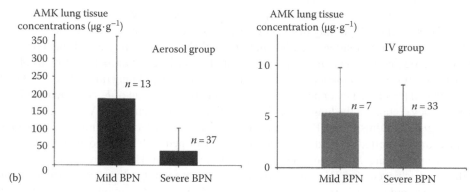

FIGURE 15.19 (a) Lung tissue concentrations of amikacin (AMK) measured 1 h after second administration performed 48 h after the bacterial inoculation (aerosol group in black bars, $n = 10$, and intravenous [IV] group kinetics in gray bars, $n = 8$) in different lung segments. In the lower lobe, specimens were sampled from dependent (segment 8), nondependent (segment 6), and posterocaudal (segment 10) lung regions. Significantly higher lung tissue concentrations were found in lung specimens obtained in animals of the aerosol group. In the aerosol group, AMK lung tissue concentrations were significantly lower in S10 region than in the other segments ($P < 0.001$). Data are expressed as mean ± SD. (b) AMK lung tissue concentrations according to the histological grade of bronchopneumonia (BPN) characterizing lung segments in the aerosol (left panel) and intravenous (IV) groups (right panel); n indicates the number of lung segments belonging to each histological category in each group. In the aerosol group, AMK lung tissue concentrations were greater in lung segments with mild BPN than in lung segments with severe BPN (*$P < 0.05$). (Reproduced from Goldstein, I. et al., *Am. J. Respir. Crit. Care Med.*, 166, 1375, 2002. With permission from American Thoracic Society.)

respiratory syndrome (SARS). The siRNA-mediated treatment approach to these diseases requires an efficient delivery system to target the siRNAs at the site of action. Major barriers to the efficient delivery of siRNA to lung cells include the branched anatomy of the lungs, mucociliary clearance, presence of airway cell membrane, and lung surfactants. Moreover, siRNA is rapidly inactivated by RNAses and macrophages. The aerosol delivery of siRNA has many advantages including local targeting, instant access, and a high level of deposition in the lungs. Moreover, siRNA is water soluble and effective at low concentrations, thus making it an ideal candidate for aerosol delivery. After lung deposition, the siRNA complex should have a particle diameter of less than 200 nm to avoid phagocytosis.[172]

Various viral and nonviral carriers have been studied to develop an efficient siRNA delivery system to lung cells. The viral vectors include retroviral and adenoviral vectors,[173,174] which induce gene silencing and RNAi in a range of animal tissues. Despite being effective carriers, viral vectors suffer from limitations of complications associated with the body's immune response to viruses. The nonviral vectors include lipid- and polymer-based carriers. siRNA, being negatively charged, forms a complex with positively charged lipid- and polymer-based delivery systems to enhance its uptake by the cells and prevent degradation.[175]

A number of cationic lipid-based systems are available as transfection reagents for siRNA. Many of those transfection reagents are liposome-based systems that include Dharmafect 1®, TranIT-TKO®, Lipofectamine®, and sIMPORTER®. Bitko et al. reported that the intranasal administration of the siRNA complex with cationic lipid TranIT-TKO resulted in an almost 1.5 times increase in transfection efficiency when compared with naked siRNA in the treatment of respiratory syncytial virus (RSV) and parainfluenza virus (PIV) infections (Figure 15.20).[176] In addition, liposomes can be modified with ligands, such as folate, to achieve targeted siRNA delivery to specific cell types.[177] However, cationic lipidic systems show poor transfection efficiency and cytotoxicity. Various polymers have also been investigated for siRNA delivery. PEI, a cationic polymer, has been used for DNA delivery *in vivo*, but the toxicity and nonbiodegradability of PEI makes it an unlikely carrier

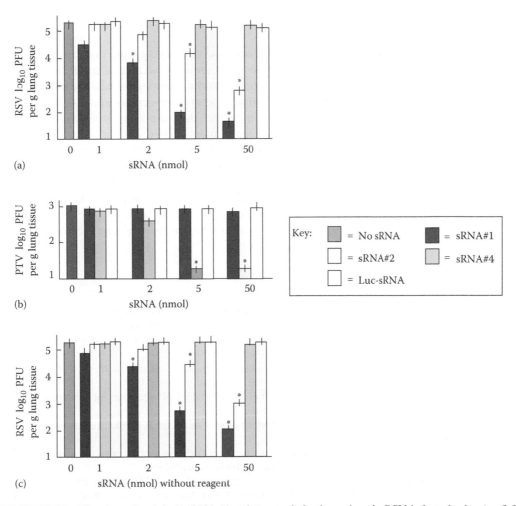

FIGURE 15.20 Titration of antiviral siRNA (a) pulmonary infectious virus in RSV-infected mice ($n=8$ for each data point); (b) pulmonary infectious virus in PIV-infected mice ($n=8$ for each data point); (c) as in b, except that naked siRNA was administered without any transfection reagent. Asterisks indicate significant inhibition ($P < 0.05$). (Reproduced from Bitko, V. et al., *Nat. Med.*, 11, 50, 2005. With permission from Nature Publishing Group.)

for gene delivery. A copolymer of PEI and PEG has been synthesized by Ahn et al. but this copolymer showed unsatisfactory transfection efficiency.[178]

Recently, many research groups have used branched polyesters—with hydrophilic positively charged amine groups attached to hydrophilic backbone—as carriers for the delivery of siRNA. These polyesteramine copolymers have high transfection efficiency but less toxic effects compared with nonbiodegradable polycations. Nguyen et al. demonstrated the efficacy of polyesters as nanocarriers for the pulmonary delivery of siRNA. They showed that anti-luciferase siRNA, when encapsulated in diethylaminopropylamine (DEAPA)-(68)-PVA-PLGA nanoparticles, demonstrates a rapid release of siRNA within 4 h. Following nebulization, these nanoparticles showed knock down efficiency against luciferase comparable with non-nebulized samples.[179] In another study, Xu et al. demonstrated that the aerosol delivery of Akt1 (a protein kinase B, an important regulator of cell survival and cell proliferation) siRNA complexed with poly(ester amine) in a mice model of lung cancer suppresses lung tumorigenesis by regulating proteins important for Akt1-related signals and cell cycle regulation, without affecting the protein expression of Akt1 in other organs.[180]

15.11 CONCLUDING REMARKS

There has been a tremendous increase in pulmonary drug delivery systems over the past decade. Drug delivery via the lungs for systemic effect has been an intensive area of research, which has paved the way for the development of the first inhaled insulin. Although inhaled insulin has been withdrawn from the market, it has demonstrated clinical proof of concept for systemic drug therapy using pulmonary delivery. In addition to the systemic effect, there are many drug delivery opportunities for localized pulmonary disorders including lung cancer, acute respiratory distress syndrome, and PAH. More studies should be directed toward studying the transport mechanism of particulate drug delivery systems across the lungs to the systemic circulation. Gene delivery for the treatment of cystic fibrosis and asthma are two important avenues that need to be explored further. Furthermore, there is little information on the safety of nanoparticle-based carriers for pulmonary drug delivery systems. Considering the short viability of lungs when used *ex vivo*, the development of an alternative to the isolated lung perfusion model would speed up the studies involving the disposition and metabolism of drugs after pulmonary administration.

REFERENCES

1. Gonda I. The ascent of pulmonary drug delivery. *J Pharm Sci* 2000; **89**:940–945.
2. Grossman J. The evolution of inhaler technology. *J Asthma* 1994; **31**:55–64.
3. Siekmeier R, Scheuch G. Systemic treatment by inhalation of macromolecules—Principles, problems, and examples. *J Physiol Pharmacol* 2008; **59**(Suppl 6):53–79.
4. Sobande PO, Kercsmar CM. Inhaled corticosteroids in asthma management. *Respir Care* 2008; **53**:625–633; discussion 633–624.
5. Steiropoulos P, Trakada G, Bouros D. Current pharmacological treatment of pulmonary arterial hypertension. *Curr Clin Pharmacol* 2008; **3**:11–19.
6. Patton JS, Fishburn CS, Weers JG. The lungs as a portal of entry for systemic drug delivery. *Proc Am Thorac Soc* 2004; **1**:338–344.
7. Kalorama Research Foundation 2007. Total pulmonary drug delivery market expected to top $34 billion by 2010. http://www.kaloramainformation.com/about/release.asp?id=891.
8. Gonda I. Systemic delivery of drugs to humans via inhalation. *J Aerosol Med* 2006; **19**:47–53.
9. Moses RG, Bartley P, Lunt H, O'Brien RC, Donnelly T, Gall MA, Vesterager A, Wollmer P, Roberts A. Safety and efficacy of inhaled insulin (AERx iDMS) compared with subcutaneous insulin therapy in patients with type 1 diabetes: 1-year data from a randomized, parallel group trial. *Diabet Med* 2009; **26**:260–267.
10. Thomas C, Rawat A, Bai S, Ahsan F. Feasibility study of inhaled hepatitis B vaccine formulated with tetradecylmaltoside. *J Pharm Sci* 2008; **97**:1213–1223.

11. Yu J, Chien YW. Pulmonary drug delivery: Physiologic and mechanistic aspects. *Crit Rev Ther Drug Carrier Syst* 1997; **14**:395–453.
12. Gettinger S. Targeted therapy in advanced non-small-cell lung cancer. *Semin Respir Crit Care Med* 2008; **29**:291–301.
13. Haj RM, Cinco JE, Mazer CD. Treatment of pulmonary hypertension with selective pulmonary vasodilators. *Curr Opin Anaesthesiol* 2006; **19**:88–95.
14. Ramalingam S, Belani CP. Recent advances in targeted therapy for non-small cell lung cancer. *Expert Opin Ther Targets* 2007; **11**:245–257.
15. Weibel ER. Morphological basis of alveolar-capillary gas exchange. *Physiol Rev* 1973; **53**:419–495.
16. Stocks J, Hislop AA. Structure and function of the respiratory system: Developmental aspects and their relevance to aerosol therapy. *Drug Delivery to the Lung* 2002; Marcel Dekker, New York: pp. 47–104.
17. Hickey AJ, Thompson DC. Physiology of the airways. *Pharmaceutical Inhalational Aerosol Technology* 1992; Marcel Dekker, New York: pp. 1–28.
18. Weibel ER. How to make an alveolus. *Eur Respir J* 2008; **31**:483–485.
19. Crapo JD, Young SL, Fram EK, Pinkerton KE, Barry BE, Crapo RO. Morphometric characteristics of cells in the alveolar region of mammalian lungs. *Am Rev Respir Dis* 1983; **128**:S42–S46.
20. Gail DB, Lenfant CJ. Cells of the lung: Biology and clinical implications. *Am Rev Respir Dis* 1983; **127**:366–387.
21. Crapo JD, Barry BE, Gehr P, Bachofen M, Weibel ER. Cell number and cell characteristics of the normal human lung. *Am Rev Respir Dis* 1982; **126**:332–337.
22. Glazier JB, Hughes JM, Maloney JE, West JB. Vertical gradient of alveolar size in lungs of dogs frozen intact. *J Appl Physiol* 1967; **23**:694–705.
23. Davies P, Jones RC, Schloo BL, Reid LM. Endothelium of the pulmonary vasculature in health and disease. *Pulmonary Endothelium in Health and Disease* 1987; Marcel Dekker, New York: pp. 375–446.
24. Munoz NM, Chang SW, Murphy TM, Stimler-Gerard NP, Blake J, Mack M, Irvin C, Voelkel NF, Leff AR. Distribution of bronchoconstrictor responses in isolated-perfused rat lung. *J Appl Physiol* 1989; **66**:202–209.
25. Rosenthal FS. The distribution of inhaled particles in aerosol measurements of pulmonary airspace size. *J Aerosol Med* 2000; **13**:315–324.
26. De Marzo N, Di Blasi P, Boschetto P, Mapp CE, Sartore S, Picotti G, Fabbri LM. Airway smooth muscle biochemistry and asthma. *Eur Respir J Suppl* 1989; **6**:473s–476s.
27. Philpot RM, Smith BR. Role of cytochrome P-450 and related enzymes in the pulmonary metabolism of xenobiotics. *Environ Health Perspect* 1984; **55**:359–367.
28. Shen Z, Zhang Q, Wei S, Nagai T. Proteolytic enzymes as a limitation for pulmonary absorption of insulin: In vitro and in vivo investigations. *Int J Pharm* 1999; **192**:115–121.
29. Labiris NR, Dolovich MB. Pulmonary drug delivery. Part I: Physiological factors affecting therapeutic effectiveness of aerosolized medications. *Br J Clin Pharmacol* 2003; **56**:588–599.
30. Dolovich MB, Sanchis J, Rossman C, Newhouse MT. Aerosol penetrance: A sensitive index of peripheral airways obstruction. *J Appl Physiol* 1976; **40**:468–471.
31. Laube BL, Swift DL, Wagner HN Jr., Norman PS, Adams III, GK. The effect of bronchial obstruction on central airway deposition of a saline aerosol in patients with asthma. *Am Rev Respir Dis* 1986; **133**:740–743.
32. Lippmann M, Schlesinger RB. Interspecies comparisons of particle deposition and mucociliary clearance in tracheobronchial airways. *J Toxicol Environ Health* 1984; **13**:441–469.
33. Foster WM, Langenback E, Bergofsky EH. Measurement of tracheal and bronchial mucus velocities in man: Relation to lung clearance. *J Appl Physiol* 1980; **48**:965–971.
34. Messina MS, O'Riordan TG, Smaldone GC. Changes in mucociliary clearance during acute exacerbations of asthma. *Am Rev Respir Dis* 1991; **143**:993–997.
35. Svartengren K, Ericsson CH, Svartengren M, Mossberg B, Philipson K, Camner P. Deposition and clearance in large and small airways in chronic bronchitis. *Exp Lung Res* 1996; **22**:555–576.
36. Suarez S, Hickey AJ. Drug properties affecting aerosol behavior. *Respir Care* 2000; **45**:652–666.
37. Green GM, Jakab GJ, Low RB, Davis GS. Defense mechanisms of the respiratory membrane. *Am Rev Respir Dis* 1977; **115**:479–514.
38. Taylor AE, Guyton AC, Bishop VS. Permeability of the alveolar membrane to solutes. *Circ Res* 1965; **16**:353–362.
39. Brown RA Jr., Schanker LS. Absorption of aerosolized drugs from the rat lung. *Drug Metab Dispos* 1983; **11**:355–360.

40. Schanker LS, Mitchell EW, Brown RA Jr. Species comparison of drug absorption from the lung after aerosol inhalation or intratracheal injection. *Drug Metab Dispos* 1986; **14**:79–88.

41. Touw DJ, Brimicombe RW, Hodson ME, Heijerman HG, Bakker W. Inhalation of antibiotics in cystic fibrosis. *Eur Respir J* 1995; **8**:1594–1604.

42. Kuhn RJ. Formulation of aerosolized therapeutics. *Chest* 2001; **120**:94S–98S.

43. Gonda I. The use of aerosol medication in respiratory disease. *Aust Fam Physician* 1992; **21**:575–576.

44. Ferron GA, Kreyling WG, Haider B. Inhalation of salt aerosol particles—II. growth and deposition in the human respiratory tract. *J Aerosol Sci* 1988; **19**:611–631.

45. Goddard RF, Mercer TT, O'Neill PX, Flores RL, Sanchez R. Output characteristics and clinical efficacy of ultrasonic nebulizers. *J Asthma Res* 1968; **5**:355–368.

46. Newman SP, Pellow PG, Clarke SW. Droplet size distributions of nebulised aerosols for inhalation therapy. *Clin Phys Physiol Meas* 1986; **7**:139–146.

47. Matthys H, Kohler D. Pulmonary deposition of aerosols by different mechanical devices. *Respiration* 1985; **48**:269–276.

48. Zanen P, Laube BL. Targeting the lungs with therapeutic aerosols. *Drug Delivery to the Lung* 2002; Marcel Dekker, New York: pp. 211–268.

49. Vidgren M, Käkäinen A, Karjalainen P, Paronen P, Nuutinen J. Effect of powder inhaler design on drug disposition in the respiratory tract. *Int J Pharm* 1998; **42**:211–216.

50. Kleinstreuer C, Zhang Z, Donohue JF. Targeted drug-aerosol delivery in the human respiratory system. *Annu Rev Biomed Eng* 2008; **10**:195–220.

51. Smaldone GC, Lesouef PN. Nebulization: The device and clinical considerations. *Drug Delivery to the Lung* 2002; Marcel Dekker, New York: pp. 269–302.

52. Dennis JH, Nerbrink O. New nebulizer technology. *Drug Delivery to the Lung* 2002; Marcel Dekker, New York: pp. 303–336.

53. McGuire S. The I-neb adaptive aerosol delivery (AAD) system—A holistic approach to inhaled drug delivery including regulatory approval. *Drug Deliv Rep (Spring/Summer)* 2006:68–71.

54. Son YJ, McConville JT. Advancements in dry powder delivery to the lung. *Drug Dev Ind Pharm* 2008; **34**:948–959.

55. Schuster J, Rubsamen R, Lloyd P, Lloyd J. The AERX aerosol delivery system. *Pharm Res* 1997; **14**:354–357.

56. Watts AB, McConville JT, Williams III, RO. Current therapies and technological advances in aqueous aerosol drug delivery. *Drug Dev Ind Pharm* 2008; **34**:913–922.

57. Farr SJ, Warren SJ, Lloyd P, Okikawa JK, Schuster JA, Rowe AM, Rubsamen RM, Taylor G. Comparison of in vitro and in vivo efficiencies of a novel unit-dose liquid aerosol generator and a pressurized metered dose inhaler. *Int J Pharm* 2000; **198**:63–70.

58. Cloupeau M, Prunet-Foch B. Electrostatic spraying of liquids in cone-jet mode. *J Electrostatics* 1989; **22**:135–159.

59. Zimlich WC, Ding JY, Busick DR, Moutvic RR, Placke ME, Hirst PH. The development of a novel electrohydrodynamic pulmonary drug delivery device. *Respir Drug Deliv* 2000; **7**:241–246.

60. Williams L. Novel pulmonary delivery technology [electronic version]. *Pharmamag* 2007:4–5.

61. Hussain A, Arnold JJ, Khan MA, Ahsan F. Absorption enhancers in pulmonary protein delivery. *J Control Release* 2004; **94**:15–24.

62. Hussain A, Yang T, Zaghloul AA, Ahsan F. Pulmonary absorption of insulin mediated by tetradecyl-beta-maltoside and dimethyl-beta-cyclodextrin. *Pharm Res* 2003; **20**:1551–1557.

63. Komada F, Okumura K, Hori R. Fate of porcine and human insulin at the subcutaneous injection site. II. In vitro degradation of insulins in the subcutaneous tissue of the rat. *J Pharmacobiodyn* 1985; **8**:33–40.

64. Park SH, Kwon JH, Lim SH, Park HW, Kim CW. Characterization of human insulin microcrystals and their absorption enhancement by protease inhibitors in rat lungs. *Int J Pharm* 2007; **339**:205–212.

65. Johansson F, Hjertberg E, Eirefelt S, Tronde A, Hultkvist Bengtsson U. Mechanisms for absorption enhancement of inhaled insulin by sodium taurocholate. *Eur J Pharm Sci* 2002; **17**:63–71.

66. Kobayashi S, Kondo S, Juni K. Pulmonary delivery of salmon calcitonin dry powders containing absorption enhancers in rats. *Pharm Res* 1996; **13**:80–83.

67. Li Y, Mitra AK. Effects of phospholipid chain length, concentration, charge, and vesicle size on pulmonary insulin absorption. *Pharm Res* 1996; **13**:76–79.

68. Shen ZC, Cheng Y, Zhang Q, Wei SL, Li RC, Wang K. Lanthanides enhance pulmonary absorption of insulin. *Biol Trace Elem Res* 2000; **75**:215–225.

69. Suzuka T, Furuya A, Kamada A, Nishihata T. Effect of phenothiazines, disodium ethylenediaminetetraacetic acid and diethyl maleate on in vitro rat colonic transport of cefmetazole and inulin. *J Pharmacobiodyn* 1987; **10**:63–71.

70. Sakagami M. In vivo, in vitro and ex vivo models to assess pulmonary absorption and disposition of inhaled therapeutics for systemic delivery. *Adv Drug Deliv Rev* 2006; **58**:1030–1060.

71. Burton JA, Schanker LS. Absorption of sulphonamides and antitubercular drugs from the rat lung. *Xenobiotica* 1974; **4**:291–296.

72. Enna SJ, Schanker LS. Absorption of drugs from the rat lung. *Am J Physiol* 1972; **223**:1227–1231.

73. Schanker LS. Drug absorption from the lung. *Biochem Pharmacol* 1978; **27**:381–385.

74. Enna SJ, Schanker LS. Absorption of saccharides and urea from the rat lung. *Am J Physiol* 1972; **222**:409–414.

75. Ahsan F, Arnold JJ, Meezan E, Pillion DJ. Mutual inhibition of the insulin absorption-enhancing properties of dodecylmaltoside and dimethyl-beta-cyclodextrin following nasal administration. *Pharm Res* 2001; **18**:608–614.

76. Bai S, Ahsan F. Synthesis and evaluation of pegylated dendrimeric nanocarrier for pulmonary delivery of low molecular weight heparin. *Pharm Res* 2009; **26**:539–548.

77. Bai S, Thomas C, Ahsan F. Dendrimers as a carrier for pulmonary delivery of enoxaparin, a low-molecular weight heparin. *J Pharm Sci* 2007; **96**:2090–2106.

78. Yang T, Mustafa F, Bai S, Ahsan F. Pulmonary delivery of low molecular weight heparins. *Pharm Res* 2004; **21**:2009–2016.

79. Suarez S, Garcia-Contreras L, Sarubbi D, Flanders E, O'Toole D, Smart J, Hickey AJ. Facilitation of pulmonary insulin absorption by H-MAP: Pharmacokinetics and pharmacodynamics in rats. *Pharm Res* 2001; **18**:1677–1684.

80. Codrons V, Vanderbist F, Ucakar B, Preat V, Vanbever R. Impact of formulation and methods of pulmonary delivery on absorption of parathyroid hormone (1–34) from rat lungs. *J Pharm Sci* 2004; **93**:1241–1252.

81. Suarez S, O'Hara P, Kazantseva M, Newcomer CE, Hopfer R, McMurray DN, Hickey AJ. Airways delivery of rifampicin microparticles for the treatment of tuberculosis. *J Antimicrob Chemother* 2001; **48**:431–434.

82. Niven RW. Delivery of biotherapeutics by inhalation aerosol. *Crit Rev Ther Drug Carrier Syst* 1995; **12**:151–231.

83. Oberdorster G, Cox C, Gelein R. Intratracheal instillation versus intratracheal-inhalation of tracer particles for measuring lung clearance function. *Exp Lung Res* 1997; **23**:17–34.

84. Sakagami M, Sakon K, Kinoshita W, Makino Y. Enhanced pulmonary absorption following aerosol administration of mucoadhesive powder microspheres. *J Control Release* 2001; **77**:117–129.

85. Bitonti AJ, Dumont JA, Low SC, Peters RT, Kropp KE, Palombella VJ, Stattel JM, Lu Y, Tan CA, Song JJ, Garcia AM, Simister NE, Spiekermann GM, Lencer WI, Blumberg RS. Pulmonary delivery of an erythropoietin Fc fusion protein in non-human primates through an immunoglobulin transport pathway. *Proc Natl Acad Sci USA* 2004; **101**:9763–9768.

86. Byron PR, Clark AR. Drug absorption from inhalation aerosols administered by positive-pressure ventilation. I: Administration of a characterized, solid disodium fluorescein aerosol under a controlled respiratory regime to the beagle dog. *J Pharm Sci* 1985; **74**:934–938.

87. Colthorpe P, Farr SJ, Taylor G, Smith IJ, Wyatt D. The pharmacokinetics of pulmonary-delivered insulin: A comparison of intratracheal and aerosol administration to the rabbit. *Pharm Res* 1992; **9**:764–768.

88. Perkins AC, Frier M. Radionuclide imaging in drug development. *Curr Pharm Des* 2004; **10**:2907–2921.

89. Richard JC, Zhou Z, Chen DL, Mintun MA, Piwnica-Worms D, Factor P, Ponde DE, Schuster DP. Quantitation of pulmonary transgene expression with PET imaging. *J Nucl Med* 2004; **45**:644–654.

90. Dobbs LG. Isolation and culture of alveolar type II cells. *Am J Physiol* 1990; **258**:L134–147.

91. Cheek JM, Evans MJ, Crandall ED. Type I cell-like morphology in tight alveolar epithelial monolayers. *Exp Cell Res* 1989; **184**:375–387.

92. Byron PR, Roberts NS, Clark AR. An isolated perfused rat lung preparation for the study of aerosolized drug deposition and absorption. *J Pharm Sci* 1986; **75**:168–171.

93. Niven RW, Rypacek F, Byron PR. Solute absorption from the airways of the isolated rat lung. III. Absorption of several peptidase-resistant, synthetic polypeptides: Poly-(2-hydroxyethyl)-aspartamides. *Pharm Res* 1990; **7**:990–994.

94. Pang Y, Sakagami M, Byron PR. The pharmacokinetics of pulmonary insulin in the in vitro isolated perfused rat lung: Implications of metabolism and regional deposition. *Eur J Pharm Sci* 2005; **25**:369–378.

95. Tronde A, Norden B, Jeppsson AB, Brunmark P, Nilsson E, Lennernas H, Bengtsson UH. Drug absorption from the isolated perfused rat lung—Correlations with drug physicochemical properties and epithelial permeability. *J Drug Target* 2003; **11**:61–74.

96. Orton TC, Anderson MW, Pickett RD, Eling TE, Fouts JR. Xenobiotic accumulation and metabolism by isolated perfused rabbit lungs. *J Pharmacol Exp Ther* 1973; **186**:482–497.

97. Einarsson O, Geba GP, Zhou Z, Landry ML, Panettieri RA Jr., Tristram D, Welliver R, Metinko A, Elias JA. Interleukin-11 in respiratory inflammation. *Ann NY Acad Sci* 1995; **762**:89–100; discussion 100–101.

98. Adjei A, Garren J. Pulmonary delivery of peptide drugs: Effect of particle size on bioavailability of leuprolide acetate in healthy male volunteers. *Pharm Res* 1990; **7**:565–569.

99. Edwards DA, Ben-Jebria A, Langer R. Recent advances in pulmonary drug delivery using large, porous inhaled particles. *J Appl Physiol* 1998; **85**:379–385.

100. Edwards DA, Hanes J, Caponetti G, Hrkach J, Ben-Jebria A, Eskew ML, Mintzes J, Deaver D, Lotan N, Langer R. Large porous particles for pulmonary drug delivery. *Science* 1997; **276**:1868–1871.

101. Kim HK, Chung HJ, Park TG. Biodegradable polymeric microspheres with "open/closed" pores for sustained release of human growth hormone. *J Control Release* 2006; **112**:167–174.

102. Koushik K, Dhanda DS, Cheruvu NP, Kompella UB. Pulmonary delivery of deslorelin: Large-porous PLGA particles and HPbetaCD complexes. *Pharm Res* 2004; **21**:1119–1126.

103. Newhouse MT, Hirst PH, Duddu SP, Walter YH, Tarara TE, Clark AR, Weers JG. Inhalation of a dry powder tobramycin PulmoSphere formulation in healthy volunteers. *Chest* 2003; **124**:360–366.

104. Tsapis N, Bennett D, O'Driscoll K, Shea K, Lipp MM, Fu K, Clarke RW, Deaver D, Yamins D, Wright J, Peloquin CA, Weitz DA, Edwards DA. Direct lung delivery of para-aminosalicylic acid by aerosol particles. *Tuberculosis (Edinb)* 2003; **83**:379–385.

105. Wang J, Ben-Jebria A, Edwards DA. Inhalation of estradiol for sustained systemic delivery. *J Aerosol Med* 1999; **12**:27–36.

106. Ungaro F, De Rosa G, Miro A, Quaglia F, La Rotonda MI. Cyclodextrins in the production of large porous particles: Development of dry powders for the sustained release of insulin to the lungs. *Eur J Pharm Sci* 2006; **28**:423–432.

107. Ungaro F, d'Emmanuele di Villa Bianca R, Giovino C, Miro A, Sorrentino R, Quaglia F, La Rotonda MI. Insulin-loaded PLGA/cyclodextrin large porous particles with improved aerosolization properties: In vivo deposition and hypoglycaemic activity after delivery to rat lungs. *J Control Release* 2009; **135**(1):25–34.

108. Bliss M. The history of insulin. *Diabetes Care* 1993; **16**(Suppl 3):4–7.

109. Triplitt CL, Reasner CA, Isley W (Eds.) *Pharmacotherapy: A Pathophysiological Approach.* 6th edn. 2005; McGraw-Hill Comp., New York.

110. Woodyatt RT. The clinical use of insulin. *J Metab Res* 1922; **2**:793–801.

111. Gänsslen M. Über inhalation von insulin. *Klin Wochensubcutaneoushr* 1925; **4**:71.

112. Farr SJ, McElduff A, Mather LE, Okikawa J, Ward ME, Gonda I, Licko V, Rubsamen RM. Pulmonary insulin administration using the AERx system: Physiological and physicochemical factors influencing insulin effectiveness in healthy fasting subjects. *Diabetes Technol Ther* 2000; **2**:185–197.

113. Forbes B, Wilson CG, Gumbleton M. Temporal dependence of ectopeptidase expression in alveolar epithelial cell culture: Implications for study of peptide absorption. *Int J Pharm* 1999; **180**:225–234.

114. Morimoto K, Yamahara H, Lee VH, Kim KJ. Transport of thyrotropin-releasing hormone across rat alveolar epithelial cell monolayers. *Life Sci* 1994; **54**:2083–2092.

115. Katz IM, Schroeter JD, Martonen TB. Factors affecting the deposition of aerosolized insulin. *Diabetes Technol Ther* 2001; **3**:387–397.

116. Klonoff DC. Inhaled insulin. *Diabetes Technol Ther* 1999; **1**:307–313.

117. Rosenstock J, Cefalu WT, Hollander PA, Belanger A, Eliaschewitz FG, Gross JL, Klioze SS, St Aubin LB, Foyt H, Ogawa M, Duggan WT. Two-year pulmonary safety and efficacy of inhaled human insulin (Exubera) in adult patients with type 2 diabetes. *Diabetes Care* 2008; **31**:1723–1728.

118. Siekmeier R, Scheuch G. Inhaled insulin—does it become reality? *J Physiol Pharmacol* 2008; **59**(Suppl 6):81–113.

119. Mastrandrea LD, Quattrin T. Clinical evaluation of inhaled insulin. *Adv Drug Deliv Rev* 2006; **58**:1061–1075.

120. Anonymous. Pulmonary medicine: Novo Nordisk, Aradigm start phase II studies of AERx insulin delivery system. *Diabetes Week* 2002:16.

121. Inhalation of insulin using the AERx insulin Diabetes Management System (iDMS) does not appear to be associated with lung cancer. *Reactions Weekly* May 10, 2008; **1201**:3.

122. Pfutzner A, Mann AE, Steiner SS. Technosphere/Insulin—A new approach for effective delivery of human insulin via the pulmonary route. *Diabetes Technol Ther* 2002; **4**:589–594.
123. Boss AH, Cheatham WW, Rave K, Heise T. Markedly reduced postprandial glucose excusrsions through inhaled Technosphere/Insulin in comparison to SC injected regular insulin in subjects with type 2 diabetes. *EASD Preview, Summer Street Research Partners* 2005:9 of 12.
124. Heise T, Brugger A, Cook C, Eckers U, Hutchcraft A, Nosek L, Rave K, Troeger J, Valaitis P, White S, Heinemann L. PROMAXX(R) inhaled insulin: Safe and efficacious administration with a commercially available dry powder inhaler. *Diabetes Obes Metab* 2009; **11**(5):455–459.
125. Hoffman A, Ziv E. Pharmacokinetic considerations of new insulin formulations and routes of administration. *Clin Pharmacokinet* 1997; **33**:285–301.
126. Morimoto K, Fukushi N, Chono S, Seki T, Tabata Y. Spermined dextran, a cationized polymer, as absorption enhancer for pulmonary application of peptide drugs. *Pharmazie* 2008; **63**:180–184.
127. Seki T, Fukushi N, Chono S, Morimoto K. Effects of sperminated polymers on the pulmonary absorption of insulin. *J Control Release* 2008; **125**:246–251.
128. Yamamoto A, Umemori S, Muranishi S. Absorption enhancement of intrapulmonary administered insulin by various absorption enhancers and protease inhibitors in rats. *J Pharm Pharmacol* 1994; **46**:14–18.
129. Brange J, Owens DR, Kang S, Volund A. Monomeric insulins and their experimental and clinical implications. *Diabetes Care* 1990; **13**:923–954.
130. Hussain A, Ahsan F. State of insulin self-association does not affect its absorption from the pulmonary route. *Eur J Pharm Sci* 2005; **25**:289–298.
131. Hussain A, Majumder QH, Ahsan F. Inhaled insulin is better absorbed when administered as a dry powder compared to solution in the presence or absence of alkylglycosides. *Pharm Res* 2006; **23**:138–147.
132. DeNicola DB, Rebar AH, Henderson RF. Early damage indicators in the lung. V. Biochemical and cytological response to NO2 inhalation. *Toxicol Appl Pharmacol* 1981; **60**:301–312.
133. Henderson RF, Benson JM, Hahn FF, Hobbs CH, Jones RK, Mauderly JL, McClellan RO, Pickrell JA. New approaches for the evaluation of pulmonary toxicity: Bronchoalveolar lavage fluid analysis. *Fundam Appl Toxicol* 1985; **5**:451–458.
134. Patel LN, Wang J, Kim KJ, Borok Z, Crandall ED, Shen WC. Conjugation with cationic cell-penetrating peptide increases pulmonary absorption of insulin. *Mol Pharm* 2009; **6**(2):492–503.
135. Mustafa F, Yang T, Khan MA, Ahsan F. Chain length-dependent effects of alkylmaltosides on nasal absorption of enoxaparin. *J Pharm Sci* 2004; **93**:675–683.
136. Yang T, Mustafa F, Ahsan F. Alkanoylsucroses in nasal delivery of low molecular weight heparins: In-vivo absorption and reversibility studies in rats. *J Pharm Pharmacol* 2004; **56**:53–60.
137. Cadene M, Boudier C, de Marcillac GD, Bieth JG. Influence of low molecular mass heparin on the kinetics of neutrophil elastase inhibition by mucus proteinase inhibitor. *J Biol Chem* 1995; **270**:13204–13209.
138. Gundry SR, Klein MD, Drongowski RA, Kirsh MM. Clinical evaluation of a new rapid heparin assay using the dye azure A. *Am J Surg* 1984; **148**:191–194.
139. Braun CS, Vetro JA, Tomalia DA, Koe GS, Koe JG, Middaugh CR. Structure/function relationships of polyamidoamine/DNA dendrimers as gene delivery vehicles. *J Pharm Sci* 2005; **94**:423–436.
140. Qi Y, Zhao G, Liu D, Shriver Z, Sundaram M, Sengupta S, Venkataraman G, Langer R, Sasisekharan R. Delivery of therapeutic levels of heparin and low-molecular-weight heparin through a pulmonary route. *Proc Natl Acad Sci USA* 2004; **101**:9867–9872.
141. Moghimi SM, Hunter AC, Murray JC. Long-circulating and target-specific nanoparticles: Theory to practice. *Pharmacol Rev* 2001; **53**:283–318.
142. Rawat A, Yang T, Hussain A, Ahsan F. Complexation of a poly-L-arginine with low molecular weight heparin enhances pulmonary absorption of the drug. *Pharm Res* 2008; **25**:936–948.
143. Rawat A, Majumder QH, Ahsan F. Inhalable large porous microspheres of low molecular weight heparin: In vitro and in vivo evaluation. *J Control Release* 2008; **128**:224–232.
144. Martin KB, Klinger JR, Rounds SI. Pulmonary arterial hypertension: New insights and new hope. *Respirology* 2006; **11**:6–17.
145. Berger M, Haimowitz A, Van Tosh A, Berdoff RL, Goldberg E. Quantitative assessment of pulmonary hypertension in patients with tricuspid regurgitation using continuous wave Doppler ultrasound. *J Am Coll Cardiol* 1985; **6**:359–365.
146. Tuder RM, Cool CD, Geraci MW, Wang J, Abman SH, Wright L, Badesch D, Voelkel NF. Prostacyclin synthase expression is decreased in lungs from patients with severe pulmonary hypertension. *Am J Respir Crit Care Med* 1999; **159**:1925–1932.
147. Gomberg-Maitland M, Preston IR. Prostacyclin therapy for pulmonary arterial hypertension: New directions. *Semin Respir Crit Care Med* 2005; **26**:394–401.

148. Diot P, Magro P, Vecellio L, Smaldone GC. Advances in our understanding of aerosolized iloprost for pulmonary hypertension. *J Aerosol Med* 2006; **19**:406–407.

149. Schermuly RT, Yilmaz H, Ghofrani HA, Woyda K, Pullamsetti S, Schulz A, Gessler T, Dumitrascu R, Weissmann N, Grimminger F, Seeger W. Inhaled iloprost reverses vascular remodeling in chronic experimental pulmonary hypertension. *Am J Respir Crit Care Med* 2005; **172**:358–363.

150. Schermuly RT, Schulz A, Ghofrani HA, Breitenbach CS, Weissmann N, Hildebrand M, Kurz J, Grimminger F, Seeger W. Comparison of pharmacokinetics and vasodilatory effect of nebulized and infused iloprost in experimental pulmonary hypertension: Rapid tolerance development. *J Aerosol Med* 2006; **19**:353–363.

151. Olschewski H, Simonneau G, Galie N, Higenbottam T, Naeije R, Rubin LJ, Nikkho S, Speich R, Hoeper MM, Behr J, Winkler J, Sitbon O, Popov W, Ghofrani HA, Manes A, Kiely DG, Ewert R, Meyer A, Corris PA, Delcroix M, Gomez-Sanchez M, Siedentop H, Seeger W. Inhaled iloprost for severe pulmonary hypertension. *N Engl J Med* 2002; **347**:322–329.

152. Kleemann E, Schmehl T, Gessler T, Bakowsky U, Kissel T, Seeger W. Iloprost-containing liposomes for aerosol application in pulmonary arterial hypertension: Formulation aspects and stability. *Pharm Res* 2007; **24**:277–287.

153. Skoro-Sajer N, Lang I. The role of treprostinil in the management of pulmonary hypertension. *Am J Cardiovasc Drugs* 2008; **8**:213–217.

154. Skoro-Sajer N, Lang I, Naeije R. Treprostinil for pulmonary hypertension. *Vasc Health Risk Manag* 2008; **4**:507–513.

155. Sandifer BL, Brigham KL, Lawrence EC, Mottola D, Cuppels C, Parker RE. Potent effects of aerosol compared with intravenous treprostinil on the pulmonary circulation. *J Appl Physiol* 2005; **99**:2363–2368.

156. Voswinckel R, Enke B, Reichenberger F, Kohstall M, Kreckel A, Krick S, Gall H, Gessler T, Schmehl T, Ghofrani HA, Schermuly RT, Grimminger F, Rubin LJ, Seeger W, Olschewski H. Favorable effects of inhaled treprostinil in severe pulmonary hypertension: Results from randomized controlled pilot studies. *J Am Coll Cardiol* 2006; **48**:1672–1681.

157. Voswinckel R, Reichenberger F, Gall H, Schmehl T, Gessler T, Schermuly RT, Grimminger F, Rubin LJ, Seeger W, Ghofrani HA, Olschewski H. Metered dose inhaler delivery of treprostinil for the treatment of pulmonary hypertension. *Pulm Pharmacol Ther* 2009; **22**:50–56.

158. Drew R. Potential role of aerosolized amphotericin B formulations in the prevention and adjunctive treatment of invasive fungal infections. *Int J Antimicrob Agents* 2006; **27**(Suppl 1):36–44.

159. Gavalda J, Martin MT, Lopez P, Gomis X, Ramirez JL, Rodriguez D, Len O, Puigfel Y, Ruiz I, Pahissa A. Efficacy of nebulized liposomal amphotericin B in treatment of experimental pulmonary aspergillosis. *Antimicrob Agents Chemother* 2005; **49**:3028–3030.

160. Slobbe L, Boersma E, Rijnders BJ. Tolerability of prophylactic aerosolized liposomal amphotericin-B and impact on pulmonary function: Data from a randomized placebo-controlled trial. *Pulm Pharmacol Ther* 2008; **21**:855–859.

161. Ruijgrok EJ, Vulto AG, Van Etten EW. Aerosol delivery of amphotericin B desoxycholate (Fungizone) and liposomal amphotericin B (AmBisome): Aerosol characteristics and in-vivo amphotericin B deposition in rats. *J Pharm Pharmacol* 2000; **52**:619–627.

162. Borro JM, Sole A, de la Torre M, Pastor A, Fernandez R, Saura A, Delgado M, Monte E, Gonzalez D. Efficiency and safety of inhaled amphotericin B lipid complex (abelcet) in the prophylaxis of invasive fungal infections following lung transplantation. *Transplant Proc* 2008; **40**:3090–3093.

163. Donald PR, Sirgel FA, Venter A, Smit E, Parkin DP, Van de Wal BW, Mitchison DA. The early bactericidal activity of a low-clearance liposomal amikacin in pulmonary tuberculosis. *J Antimicrob Chemother* 2001; **48**:877–880.

164. Mohr AM, Sifri ZC, Horng HS, Sadek R, Savetamal A, Hauser CJ, Livingston DH. Use of aerosolized aminoglycosides in the treatment of Gram-negative ventilator-associated pneumonia. *Surg Infect (Larchmt)* 2007; **8**:349–357.

165. Goldstein I, Wallet F, Nicolas-Robin A, Ferrari F, Marquette CH, Rouby JJ. Lung deposition and efficiency of nebulized amikacin during *Escherichia coli* pneumonia in ventilated piglets. *Am J Respir Crit Care Med* 2002; **166**:1375–1381.

166. Dhillon J, Fielding R, Adler-Moore J, Goodall RL, Mitchison D. The activity of low-clearance liposomal amikacin in experimental murine tuberculosis. *J Antimicrob Chemother* 2001; **48**:869–876.

167. Li Z, Zhang Y, Wurtz W, Lee JK, Malinin VS, Durwas-Krishnan S, Meers P, Perkins WR. Characterization of nebulized liposomal amikacin (Arikace) as a function of droplet size. *J Aerosol Med Pulm Drug Deliv* 2008; **21**:245–254.

168. DeVincenzo JP. RNA interference strategies as therapy for respiratory viral infections. *Pediatr Infect Dis J* 2008; **27**:S118–S122.
169. Durcan N, Murphy C, Cryan SA. Inhalable siRNA: Potential as a therapeutic agent in the lungs. *Mol Pharm* 2008; **5**:559–566.
170. Novina CD, Sharp PA. The RNAi revolution. *Nature* 2004; **430**:161–164.
171. Aigner A. Gene silencing through RNA interference (RNAi) in vivo: Strategies based on the direct application of siRNAs. *J Biotechnol* 2006; **124**:12–25.
172. Chono S, Tanino T, Seki T, Morimoto K. Influence of particle size on drug delivery to rat alveolar macrophages following pulmonary administration of ciprofloxacin incorporated into liposomes. *J Drug Target* 2006; **14**:557–566.
173. Narvaiza I, Aparicio O, Vera M, Razquin N, Bortolanza S, Prieto J, Fortes P. Effect of adenovirus-mediated RNA interference on endogenous microRNAs in a mouse model of multidrug resistance protein 2 gene silencing. *J Virol* 2006; **80**:12236–12247.
174. Zentilin L, Giacca M. In vivo transfer and expression of genes coding for short interfering RNAs. *Curr Pharm Biotechnol* 2004; **5**:341–347.
175. Demeneix B, Behr JP. Polyethylenimine (PEI). *Adv Genet* 2005; **53**:217–230.
176. Bitko V, Musiyenko A, Shulyayeva O, Barik S. Inhibition of respiratory viruses by nasally administered siRNA. *Nat Med* 2005; **11**:50–55.
177. Felgner PL, Ringold GM. Cationic liposome-mediated transfection. *Nature* 1989; **337**:387–388.
178. Ahn CH, Chae SY, Bae YH, Kim SW. Biodegradable poly(ethylenimine) for plasmid DNA delivery. *J Control Release* 2002; **80**:273–282.
179. Nguyen J, Steele TW, Merkel O, Reul R, Kissel T. Fast degrading polyesters as siRNA nano-carriers for pulmonary gene therapy. *J Control Release* 2008; **132**:243–251.
180. Xu CX, Jere D, Jin H, Chang SH, Chung YS, Shin JY, Kim JE, Park SJ, Lee YH, Chae CH, Lee KH, Beck GR Jr., Cho CS, Cho MH. Poly(ester amine)-mediated, aerosol-delivered Akt1 small interfering RNA suppresses lung tumorigenesis. *Am J Respir Crit Care Med* 2008; **178**:60–73.

16 Recent Advances in Ocular Drug Delivery: Role of Transporters, Receptors, and Nanocarriers

*Gyan P. Mishra, Ripal Gaudana,
Viral M. Tamboli, and Ashim K. Mitra*

CONTENTS

16.1 INTRODUCTION

The treatment of ocular disorders is challenging due to the anatomical and physiological constraints. Drug elimination via precorneal tear clearance, blinking, and nasolacrimal drainage restricts the entry of the drug molecule to the anterior segment of the eye. In addition, the presence of efflux pumps, such as P-glycoprotein (P-gp), multidrug resistance–associated proteins, and breast cancer–resistant proteins (BCRPs), also limit the ocular bioavailability of drugs, such as antibiotics, steroids, and antitumor agents. Drug delivery to the posterior segment of the eye is challenged by barriers such as the inner and outer blood–retinal barriers (BRBs) and efflux pumps.

Recent developments in ocular drug delivery have attempted to overcome these barriers. Transporter- and receptor-targeted drug delivery is one such exciting area of investigation. Drug transport to the anterior or posterior segment requires an understanding of these barriers and mechanisms that may be exploited to overcome them through the transporter- and receptor-targeted delivery approaches. Several transporters (both efflux and influx) and receptors have been identified on various ocular tissues, such as the cornea, retina, iris–ciliary body (ICB), and conjunctiva. These transporters and receptors possess different substrate specificity and capacity. Targeting drugs to these influx carriers can overcome significant hurdles imposed by epithelial tight junctions and efflux pumps and can increase selectivity. In recent years, prodrug design based on targeting transporters or receptors has been applied for optimizing ocular drug delivery.

In addition, nanocarriers have been evaluated for their ability to overcome various barriers to ocular drug delivery. Nanoparticles, microparticles, and vesicular systems can target and sustain drug release at the desired ocular sites. Ocular implants and hydrogel-based delivery systems have been evaluated for sustained drug release. Such delivery systems may be advantageous in diseases states that require constant drug levels at the target site for a long duration, such as age-related macular degeneration (AMD), proliferative vitreoretinopathy (PVR), and diabetic macular edema. Recently, noninvasive delivery systems, such as iontophoresis, have demonstrated the potential to deliver drugs to both anterior and posterior ocular segments.

In this chapter, we summarize the molecular presence and functional activity of transporters (both efflux and influx) and receptors in various ocular tissues. We also discuss the transporter-targeted prodrug approach and its potential in ocular drug delivery, among other ocular drug delivery techniques.

16.2 ANATOMY AND PHYSIOLOGY OF THE EYE

The eye is divided into two chambers commonly known as the anterior chamber and the posterior chamber (Figure 16.1). The anterior chamber is mainly comprised of the cornea, conjunctiva, iris, ciliary body, and lens. The posterior chamber includes the sclera, choroid, vitreous humor, and retina.

16.2.1 ANTERIOR CHAMBER

16.2.1.1 Cornea

The cornea is the outermost transparent membrane of the eye. It is avascular in nature and receives nourishment from the aqueous humor and capillaries originating in the limbal area. The human cornea is about 0.5 mm thick and composed of five layers: the corneal epithelium, Bowman's membrane, stroma, Descemet's membrane, and endothelium (in this sequence from the outermost layer to the innermost layer). The epithelial layer consists of five to six layers of columnar cells. The outermost layer is composed of nonkeratinized squamous cells with tight junctions between the adjacent cells. The innermost layer is columnar in shape and commonly known as the germinal layer. Bowman's membrane is mainly formed from collagen fibrils. The stroma, also known as substantia propria, is composed primarily of collagen fibrils. Descemet's membrane is a thick basal lamina between the stroma and the endothelium. The endothelium is composed of a single layer of squamous cells.[1]

16.2.1.2 Iris

The iris is composed of pigmented epithelial cells and the constrictor iridial sphincter muscles (circular muscle of the iris). These muscles are innervated by cholinergic nerves that, upon contraction, cause miosis (the constriction of the pupil). The iris also contains the dilator muscles, oriented radially, which mediate mydriasis (the dilation of the pupil) upon sympathetic stimulation.[2]

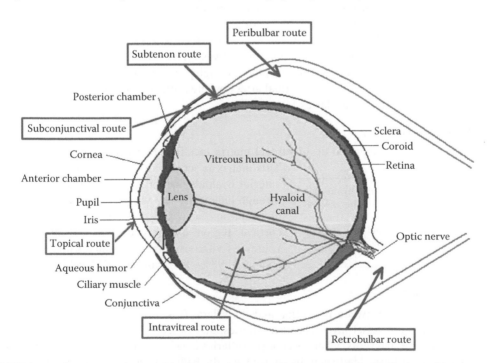

FIGURE 16.1 Structure and schematic representation of various routes of drug delivery to the eye.

16.2.1.3 Ciliary Body

The ciliary body is formed from ciliary muscles and ciliary processes. The ciliary muscle is a smooth muscle comprised of fibrous bundles that are vascularized with folding that extends into the posterior chamber. Its non-pigmented epithelial cells form the blood–aqueous barrier (BAB), which restricts the movement of proteins and colloids into the aqueous humor.[2]

16.2.1.4 Conjunctiva

The conjunctiva consists of a clear mucous membrane consisting of four parts: the palpebral, fornical, bulbar, and an underlying basement membrane. The membrane covers the inner part of the eyelid as well as the visible part of the sclera (the white part of the eye). It is composed of nonkeratinized stratified columnar epithelial cells.[2] It helps to lubricate the eye by producing mucus and some tears.

16.2.1.5 Aqueous Humor

The aqueous humor is the nutritive and protective fluid between the lens and the cornea. It is composed of 99% water, proteins, glucose, ascorbates, amino acids, and ions such as bicarbonate, chloride, sodium, potassium, calcium, and phosphate. It is secreted from the ciliary body ($2–3\,\mu L/min$) and circulates from the posterior to the anterior chambers before most of it is drained through the trabecular meshwork, then to the canal of Schlemm. A minor route of aqueous outflow is through the uveoscleral pathway. The impaired outflow of aqueous humor causes elevated intraocular pressure, which leads to the permanent damage of the optic nerve and consequential visual field loss that can progress to blindness.[3]

16.2.2 POSTERIOR CHAMBER

16.2.2.1 Retina

The retina is a light sensitive tissue comprised of two major layers: the retinal pigmented epithelium (RPE) and the neural retina. The RPE is the outermost layer, which is directly in contact with the rods and cones (the light sensing neural cells). These photoreceptors are linked to bipolar cells and ganglionic cells. The optic nerve is directly in contact with the ganglionic cells, which are coupled through the amacrine cells. The primary function of the RPE is to provide nutrients to the retina from the choroid. The RPE forms a tight junction between the choroid and the retina. These cells also aid in the removal of shredded photoreceptors through phagocytosis. The innermost retina primarily receives a blood supply from the retinal artery, whereas the outermost retina receives oxygen and nutrients from the choriocapillaries.[4]

16.2.2.2 Vitreous Humor

The vitreous humor is comprised of a hydrogel matrix localized between the retina and the lens. This matrix is separated from the anterior chamber by anterior hyaloids membrane and is linked to the retina through ligaments. The vitreous is primarily composed of hyaluronic acid and collagen fibrils. However, the cortical region contains dispersed hyalocytes. The volume of vitreous humor is around 4 mL with a water content of 98%–99.7% and the pH level is around 7.5.[5]

> The vitreous is primarily composed of hyaluronic acid and collagen fibrils. However, the cortical region contains dispersed hyalocytes. The volume of vitreous humor is around 4 mL with a water content of 98%–99.7% and the pH level is around 7.5.

16.2.2.3 Choroid

The choroid is situated between the retina and the sclera. It is a highly vascularized tissue that can be divided into the vessel layer, choriocapillaries, and Bruch's membrane. The vessel layer is comprised of arteries and veins, whereas choriocapillaries consist of a dense network of capillaries. Bruch's membrane is located between the choroid and the RPE. It is composed of basal lamellae of the RPE and the endothelial cells of the choroid.[4,6]

16.2.2.4 Sclera

The sclera is an external layer above the choroid, which primarily protects the inner organs of the eye. It is about 0.5–1 mm thick and is mainly composed of collagen bundles with some dispersed melanocytes and elastic fibers.[7]

16.3 BARRIERS TO OCULAR DRUG DELIVERY

The barriers to ocular drug delivery exist at both the molecular and tissue level, as classified in Figure 16.2.

16.3.1 PRECORNEAL TEAR CLEARANCE

Precorneal tear clearance is a major rate limiting factor in the ocular drug absorption of topically administered drugs because the instilled drug is eliminated from the corneal surface by lacrimal fluid drainage. An applied dose can also be eliminated by systemic absorption through the conjunctival sac and/or the nasolacrimal duct.[8] All these factors limit the ocular bioavailability of topically administered drugs to less than 5%.[9]

16.3.2 CORNEAL AND CONJUNCTIVAL BARRIERS

The corneal epithelial cells limit the permeation of hydrophilic drug molecules across the cornea due to the presence of tight junctions and the lipid-rich epithelial membrane. Tight junctions act as a seal around the epithelium, which restricts the entry of polar drug molecules into the cornea. These tight junctions are formed around the epithelial cell membranes, which are bound by cell adhesion proteins such as occludin, zonula occludens-1 (ZO-1), and ZO-2.[10] The tight junctions hinder the paracellular transport of polar drugs across the cornea, whereas lipophilic drugs can permeate through the lipid bilayer by passive diffusion.

Permeation enhancers, such as L-arginine, can improve the permeability of polar molecules, e.g., fluorescein isothiocyanate FITC-dextran, across the cornea by modulating tight junctions.[11] Ionization can also decrease the transcellular permeability, whereas molecular size does not have any significant effect on corneal permeability. Therefore, the pH of topical ocular formulations is an important factor in optimizing the ocular bioavailability of ionizable compounds.[12]

The stroma, which lies beneath the corneal epithelium, constitutes a major barrier to lipophilic drug absorption. This layer is composed of 90% water. Therefore, lipophilic drugs cannot readily partition into the stroma. Thus, it may act as a depot for hydrophobic drug molecules.[13]

The Bowman's and Descemet's membranes do not provide any significant resistance to drug permeation, whereas a single layer of endothelial cells presents a weak lipophilic barrier for drug

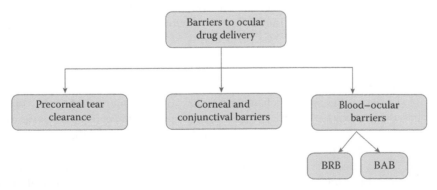

FIGURE 16.2 Classification of major barriers to ocular drug delivery. BRB, blood–retinal barrier; BAB, blood–ocular barrier.

molecules. The conjunctival epithelium leaks more and has approximately 20 times more area, 2 times larger pore size, 16 times higher pore density, and 230 times more paracellular space relative to the cornea. As a result, it allows easy permeation of the hydrophilic macromolecules and serves as a potential route for the delivery of macromolecules.[14] The apical conjunctival epithelial cells are attached by desmosomes, which connect the intracellular spaces and thus restrict the movement of proteins and peptides.[15]

The conjuctival permeability of peptides and proteins such as insulin (molecular weight 5800) and p-aminoclonidine (molecular weight 245.7) is higher than the corneal permeability.[16] Studies by Hamalainen et al. showed that the permeability of polyethylene glycols (PEGs) across the cornea was 15–20 times less than the sclera or conjunctiva. However, permeability across the sclera is about half of the conjunctival permeability, but it is 10 times more than the cornea.[17]

16.3.3 BLOOD–OCULAR BARRIERS

16.3.3.1 Blood–Retinal Barrier

The BRB is similar in function to the blood–brain barrier (BBB) and has similar capillary endothelial cell permeability to mannitol and sucrose.[18] However, interendothelial junctions of BRB are slightly different than BBB. The retinal capillary endothelium constitutes the inner blood–retinal barrier (i-BRB). The endothelial cells are sealed with zonulae occludens that acts as a barrier to hydrophilic molecules, such as trypan blue and fluorescein.[18] The BRB also acts as a barrier to small protein tracers (such as microperoxidase with a molecular weight of 1.9 kDa and a hydrodynamic radius of 2 nm) and large protein tracers (such as horseradish peroxidase with a molecular weight of ~40 kDa with a hydrodynamic radius of 5 nm).[19]

The i-BRB restricts bidirectional drug transport from both luminal and abluminal sides.[20] It primarily prevents the entry of drug molecules into the posterior segment. This barrier is formed by the RPE and the retinal endothelium. The RPE forms the outer BRB between the choroid and the neural retina. It regulates the transport of molecules from the choriocapillaries into the retina. Blood flow through the choroid and the BRB allows only a limited percentage of orally administered drug molecules to reach the retina. The apical junctional complex of the RPE is formed of tight junctions and adherent junctions. The tight junctions are formed with actin filaments, which encircle each cell at the apical end to form junctional complexes. Studies with trypan blue and fluorescein showed the localization of these dyes at the RPE, which confirmed the presence of tight junctions. A few studies also correlated an increase in the tight junction-associated protein ZO-1 content with decreased permeability across the RPE.[21]

The development of these barrier properties was studied with chick RPE, where the barrier starts developing from the embryonic state at day 7 and becomes fully functional within day 15–19.[22] The permeability across the RPE depends upon the pore radius. It was characterized by permeation studies of various solutes with different shapes, charges, molecular weight, and lipophilicity. Studies by Vargus et al. suggested that compounds with large molecular radii (such as insulin, 14 Å, and sucrose, 5.3 Å) cannot permeate into the vitreous humor, whereas smaller molecules (such as glycerol, 3 Å) permeate very slowly.[23] The permeability of various molecules of different sizes and polarity is summarized in Tables 16.1 and 16.2.[24,25]

16.3.3.2 Blood–Aqueous Barrier

The BAB, also known as the anterior chamber barrier, primarily prevents the entry of exogenous compounds into the aqueous humor. It is formed from the endothelial cells of the uvea, which is the middle vascular layer of the eye, and is comprised of three parts: the iris, ciliary body, and choroid. It restricts the movement of drug molecules from the plasma into the anterior chamber.[26,27]

The BAB is not as effective as the BRB due to the leaky nature of non-pigmented epithelium. After intravenous administration, higher concentrations of test substances, particularly proteins, urea, inorganic salts (sodium, potassium, chloride), and antibiotics, are found in the anterior part of the vitreous humor.[26,27]

TABLE 16.1
The Permeability of Various Molecular Weight Fluorescent Probes across Rabbit RPE-Choroid

Probe	Molecular Weight (Da)	Molecular Radius (nm)	Diffusion Direction[a]	Permeability Coefficient ($\times 10^{-7}$ cm/s)
Carboxyfluorescein	376	0.5	Inward	9.56 ± 3.87
			Outward	23.3 ± 10.6
FITC-dextran 4 kDa	4,400	1.3	Inward	2.36 ± 1.56
FITC-dextran 10 kDa	9,300	2.2	Inward	2.14 ± 1.02
			Outward	2.04 ± 1.03
FITC-dextran 20 kDa	21,200	3.2	Inward	1.34 ± 1.80
FITC-dextran 40 kDa	38,200	4.5	Inward	0.46 ± 0.29
FITC-dextran 80 kDa	77,000	6.4	Inward	0.27 ± 0.32

Source: Modified from Pitkanen, L. et al., *Invest. Ophthalmol. Vis. Sci.*, 46, 641, 2005.

[a] Inward is the choroid-to-retina direction; outward is the retina-to-choroid direction.

TABLE 16.2
The Permeability of Molecules with Different Lipophilicity across Rabbit RPE-Choroid

Solute	Molecular Weight	log p	Diffusion Direction[a]	Permeability Coefficient ($\times 10^{-6}$ cm/s)
Atenolol	266	0.16	Inward	2.21 ± 0.50
			Outward	2.00 ± 0.47
Nadolol	309	0.93	Inward	2.24 ± 0.54
			Outward	2.03 ± 0.46
Pindolol	248	1.75	Inward	5.62 ± 1.87
			Outward	3.48 ± 1.69
Metoprolol	267	1.88	Inward	18.8 ± 4.34
			Outward	10.6 ± 3.19
Timolol	316	1.91	Inward	14.5 ± 3.48
			Outward	8.41 ± 2.67
Betaxolol	307	3.44	Inward	16.7 ± 4.48
			Outward	10.3 ± 3.65

Sources: Modified from Pitkanen, L. et al., *Invest. Ophthalmol. Vis. Sci.*, 46, 641, 2005; Hughes, P.M. et al., *Adv. Drug Deliv. Rev.*, 57, 2010, 2005.

[a] Inward is the choroid-to-retina direction; outward is the retina-to-choroid direction.

16.4 SIGNIFICANCE OF ADMINISTRATION ROUTES FOR TARGETED OCULAR DRUG DELIVERY

The selection of the appropriate route for drug administration plays a critical role in the targeted drug delivery to the eye. Both local and systemic routes are used for ocular drug delivery. Local routes include topical, intravitreal (IVT), and periocular administration as mentioned in Figure 16.1. The barriers for drug delivery through various routes and strategies to overcome these barriers are summarized in Table 16.3 and Figures 16.3 and 16.4.

TABLE 16.3
Overview of Various Routes of Ocular Drug Delivery

Routes of Drug Administrations	Target Area	Advantages	Disadvantages	Major Barriers	Strategies to Overcome These Barriers
Topical route	Anterior segment diseases	Ease of administration	Low ocular bioavailability	Precorneal tear clearance, conjunctival absorption, drug metabolism by the ICB, elimination through the canal of Schlemn	Gel systems, prodrugs, viscosity and penetration enhancers
IVT route	Posterior segment diseases	Circumvents BRB	Repeated injections required that cause retinal detachment	Toxicity and patient noncompliance	Prodrugs, micro and nanoparticles, liposomes
Periocular routes Examples: retrobulbar, peribulbar, subtenon, sub-conjunctival	Both anterior and posterior segment diseases	Lower risk of injury, least invasive route, provide large surface area, easy accessibility, high permeability across sclera	Ocular hemorrhage, artery occlusion and globe perforation	Loss of drug by choriocapillaries and through conjunctival and lymph circulation	Implants, in situ-gelling systems, micro/ nanoparticles

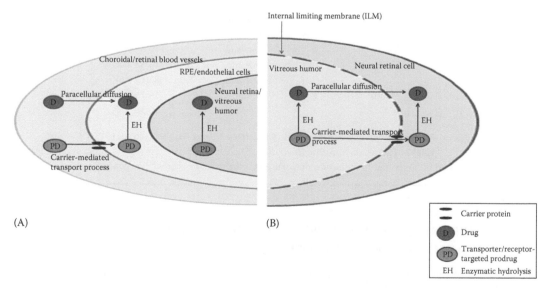

FIGURE 16.3   Schematic representation of retinal drug levels following: (A) IVT administration of drug and transporter targeted prodrug; (B) systemic administration of a drug and a transporter-targeted prodrug.

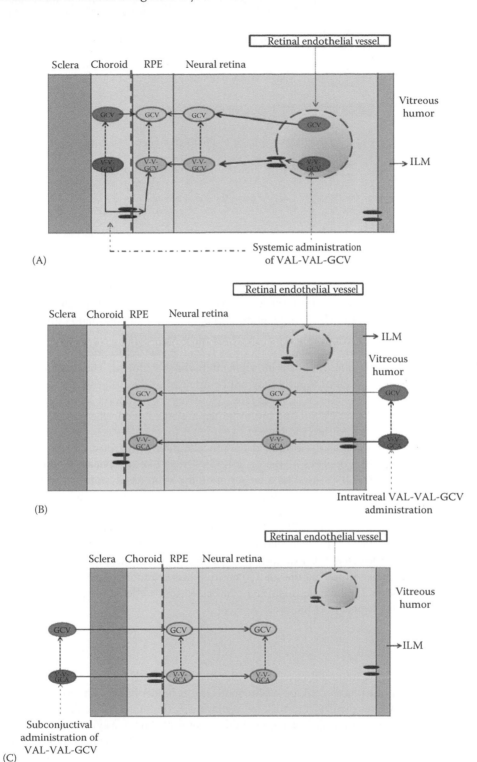

FIGURE 16.4 Schematic representation of transporter-targeted drug delivery by various routes to enhance drug delivery to the posterior segment. (A) Systemic administration, (B) IVT administration, and (C) *trans-scleral/subconjunctival administration.*

(*continued*)

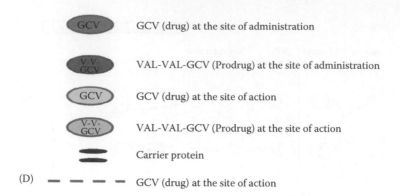

FIGURE 16.4 (continued)

16.4.1 Topical Route

The topical route is commonly utilized for the treatment of anterior segment diseases. Various constraints such as precorneal tear clearance and conjunctival absorption limit the ocular bioavailability (to even less than 1%). Also, drug metabolism by the ICB and elimination through the canal of Schlemm (a scleral-venous sinus that collects aqueous humor from the anterior chamber and delivers it to the bloodstream) results in further loss from the anterior segment.

The application of this route for posterior segment diseases is limited. Therapeutic drug concentrations in the posterior segment usually may not be attained as the drug would need to permeate through the cornea, aqueous humor, and the lens.[9] However, some reports suggest that therapeutic levels of some drugs, like verapamil and brominidine, are attainable in the posterior segment following topical instillation into the rabbit eye.[28]

Earlier, it was believed that the overall drug concentration in the posterior segment depends upon the physiochemical properties of the drug itself. Drugs like nepafenac, a nonsteroidal anti-inflammatory drug (NSAID), is used as a prescription eye drop (0.1% solution) to treat pain and inflammation associated with cataract surgery. Nepafenac reaches the posterior segment on topical application and inhibits choroidal and retinal neovascularization by lowering the production of vascular endothelial growth factors (VEGFs).[29] Other studies have indicated that even macromolecules like insulin can reach therapeutic concentrations in the retina.[30] Some of these topically applied drugs cause systemic toxicity. For example, phenylephrine causes tachycardia and hypertension, whereas timolol can cause bradycardia and congestive heart failure.[30] Thus, even though topical drug delivery has some limitations, this route can be used for targeted drug delivery to both the anterior and posterior segments of the eye.[31]

16.4.2 Systemic Route

The systemic route is not frequently used for ocular drug delivery. However, the systemic administration of acetazolamide is preferred for severe glaucoma as higher intraocular pressure reduces the absorption of drug from topically administered eye drops.[32] Treatments of ocular conditions utilizing systemic administration has also been used for the treatment of human cytomegalovirus (HCMV) retinitis. However, the drug concentration achieved at the targeted ocular tissues is only 1%–2% of the plasma concentration.[33] Following systemic administration, drug penetration from the blood into the ocular fluid is less in the vitreous humor compared with the aqueous humor. This is due to the presence of the blood–ocular barrier (BOB). Studies by Macha and Mitra have shown

> The systemic route is not frequently used for ocular drug delivery. However, systemic administration of acetazolamide is preferred for severe glaucoma as higher intraocular pressure reduces the absorption of drug from topically administered eye drops.

that only 1%–2% of the plasma concentration can be detected in the vitreous humor.[33] Therefore, the maintenance of the minimum therapeutic concentration in the eye may require frequent systemic drug administration, which may cause adverse effects in other tissues. Therefore, systemic administration may not be considered a desired route for the treatment of ocular pathologies.[33]

16.4.3 INTRAVITREAL ADMINISTRATION

IVT injection is mainly utilized for the treatment of posterior segment diseases such as diabetic retinopathy using drugs such as bevacizumab (Avastin®), triamcinolone (Kanalog®), and pegaptanib sodium (Macugen®). Also, viral infections like HCMV retinitis and endophthalmitis have been treated by IVT administration of antivirals like ganciclovir (GCV), cidofovir, and foscarnet.[34] This route circumvents the BRB. Thus, it is more efficient than both topical and systemic routes.

IVT administration is limited by patient noncompliance due to repeated administration, which may cause retinal detachment followed by vision loss.[35] Various strategies have been developed to reduce the frequency of administration by prolonging drug residence time in the vitreous humor by using prodrugs, microparticles, nanoparticles, and liposomes.[36] Reports from our laboratory have indicated that the administration of the GCV monoester prodrug provides sustained GCV levels for a prolonged period in the vitreous humor as compared with the parent drug.[37] However, the toxicity and noncompliance associated with this route restrict the applicability in the treatment of ocular pathologies.

16.4.4 PERIOCULAR ADMINISTRATION

Periocular administration is one of the least invasive routes of drug administration for the back of the eye. This route provides direct access to the sclera. Transscleral delivery can provide drug concentration both in the anterior and posterior segments. This route can be further classified into the retrobulbar, peribulbar, subtenon, and subconjunctival depending upon the site of injection.

16.4.4.1 Retrobulbar Injection

The retrobulbar injection is given directly into retrobulbar space. It is generally utilized for drug delivery into the macular region (highly pigmented yellow spot near the center of the retina, rich in ganglion cells and responsible for central vision). Hyndiuk et al. showed that steroids get localized near the macular region after retrobulbar injection.[38] Generally, a special type of 23-gauge needle with a 10° bend is utilized for this injection. The major disadvantage of this technique is damage to the blood vessels.

16.4.4.2 Peribulbar Injection

This route possesses the advantage of a lower risk of injury to the ocular structure in comparison with the retrobulbar injection. The injection can be performed by a 26-gauge needle.[39] Based on the site of administration, it can be classified into circumocular, periocular, periconal, and apical.[40] This route is generally useful for the administration of analgesics, but it may cause complications like ocular hemorrhage, artery occlusion, and globe perforation.

16.4.4.3 Subtenon Injection

The subtenon route is mostly used for drug delivery to the posterior segment. It involves drug administration into the tenon space, which is formed by the void between the tenon's capsule and the sclera. The major limitation of this route is rapid clearance by choriocapillaries and drug diffusion across the sclera.[41]

16.4.4.4 Subconjunctival Injection

It is one of the least invasive routes among all periocular routes for drug administration. The subconjunctival space can accommodate up to 500 µL of drug solution and an injection can be made through a 30-gauge needle.[42] This route can be utilized for the treatment of both anterior and posterior segment diseases. It provides a large surface area, easy accessibility, and high permeability across the sclera. This mode of administration can be utilized for sustained drug delivery in various chronic diseases, like glaucoma and AMD. A higher dexamethasone concentration could be achieved in the retina following a subconjunctival injection relative to a peribulbar injection or oral administration.[43] Ambati et al. reported that large hydrophilic molecules, such as proteins and peptides, can be successfully delivered through this route.[44] Similarly, Kim et al. reported a higher concentration of Gadolinium (III)-diethyltriaminepentaacetic acid Gd-DTPA in the ICB following subconjunctival injection as compared with other parts of the eye. This route can also be utilized for the administration of intraocular pressure lowering drugs, such as mitomycin-C and 5-fluorouracil, to treat glaucoma. The main limitation of this route is the loss of drug, mainly through conjunctival blood and lymph circulation.[45]

16.5 ROLE OF EFFLUX AND INFLUX TRANSPORTERS IN OCULAR DRUG DELIVERY

Efflux and influx transporters can be avoided or utilized, respectively, for targeted drug delivery to ocular fluids and tissues. Efflux transporters mainly limit ocular bioavailability, whereas influx transporters can act as carriers and, thereby, improve drug bioavailability in both the anterior and the posterior segment of the eye.

16.5.1 EFFLUX PUMPS AS A BARRIER

Efflux pumps are an ATP-binding cassette (ABC) family of transporters and are responsible for the extrusion of drugs out of cells and tissues. These transporters can act as a barrier for drug absorption into both anterior and posterior segments.

16.5.1.1 Efflux Pumps as Barriers to the Anterior Segment

Efflux pumps like P-gps, multiple drug resistance proteins (MRPs), and breast cancer resistance proteins (BCRPs) play a crucial role in lowering the ocular bioavailability of many therapeutic agents. These efflux pumps are expressed on the rabbit and human corneal epithelial cells.

16.5.1.1.1 P-glycoprotein

P-gp, an ABC-type transporter, was discovered in 1970.[46] It was initially found in cancerous tissue.[47] Its constitutive expression on the corneal epithelium limits ocular bioavailability of drugs such as antibiotics (e.g., erythromycin and ciprofloxacin) and steroids (e.g., prednisolone and dexamethasone). The mechanism of drug extrusion by P-gp is not well understood. However, it has been suggested that P-gp has common drug binding sites, whereas the binding of unrelated structures is explained by the substrate-induced fit by residues from transmembrane domains (4–6 and 9–12).[48,49] P-gp can act as a flipase and transfer drug substrate from the inner lipid bilayer to the outer layer,[50,51] or the efflux might originate from the intracellular region.[52] An understanding of the exact mechanism is further complicated by the presence of two or more binding sites. Therefore, a new model or structure activity relationship needs to be developed to elucidate the exact extrusion mechanism.[53] Erythromycin, a macrolide antibiotic indicated for various ocular infections, is a known substrate of both P-gp and MRP. These efflux transporters can be inhibited by steroids, such as prednisolone, which can be coadministered to control ocular inflammation.[54]

> P-gp is an ABC-type transporter. Its constitutive expression on the corneal epithelium limits the ocular bioavailability of drugs such as antibiotics (e.g., erythromycin and ciprofloxacin) and steroids (e.g., prednisolone and dexamethasone).

16.5.1.1.2 Multiple Drug Resistance Protein Family

The MRP family is composed of nine ABC-type transporters (MRPs 1–9), which differ in their substrate selectivity.[55] It is an ATP-dependent efflux pump. Previously the family was commonly known as the canalicular multispecific organ anion transporter, as it mainly effluxes lipophilic anions into the bile. These transporters are overexpressed in various neoplasms, such as colorectal, breast, and ovarian cancers. They show significantly different substrate specificity relative to P-gp.

Karla et al. have described the molecular expression and functional activity of MRP-1, -2 and -5 on rabbit pigmented corneal epithelial cells.[56] Macrolides (e.g., erythromycin), quinolones (e.g., ciprofloxacin and grepafloxacin), and steroids (e.g., prednisolone), which are widely used in ocular therapeutics, are known substrates of MRP. The ocular bioavailability of these agents could be enhanced by the coadministration of the second substrate, where the efflux of one substrate was reduced by the coadministration of another.

16.5.1.1.3 Breast Cancer–Resistant Protein

The BCRP is known as the half transporter that is composed of one nucleotide binding domain (NBD) followed by one membrane spanning domain (MSD) whereas P-gp and MRP have two repeated halves. It may function as either a homodimer or heterodimer with an ABC transporter.[57] It effluxes structurally diverse compounds, such as mitoxantrone, anthracyclines, topotecan, doxorubicin, and daunorubicin. The BCRP is commonly expressed on the apical membrane of the small intestine and the colon.[38,39]

Recently, Karla et al. reported the presence of this transporter on human corneal epithelial cells and demonstrated its functional activity.

The presence of this efflux pump confers drug resistance by the extrusion of drug molecules into the precorneal fluid, thereby lowering ocular bioavailability. The substrate specificity of this efflux pump overlaps with other efflux pumps.[58]

16.5.1.2 Efflux Pumps as Barriers to the Posterior Segment

Efflux pumps limit the transport of drugs to the retina. These pumps, particularly P-gp, MRP, and BCRP, are expressed on the RPE. Kenedy and Magnini found the molecular expression of P-gp on the RPE, whereas the functional activity of this pump was reported by Duvvuri et al., who showed that the ocular bioavailability and vitreal half-life of quinidine were higher in the presence of verapamil. Steuer et al. reported the molecular expression of both P-gp and MRP in porcine RPE. The permeability of rhodamine 123 and verapamil in the retina to choroid direction was 2.6- and 3.6-fold higher, respectively, which suggests the presence of P-gp on the choroidal side of the BRB.[60] Another report suggested the presence of MRP4 and MRP5 on the human RPE cell line (ARPE-19).[61,62] The BCRP was also found on the luminal side of the mouse RPE.

Steroids, such as dexamethasone and triamcinolone, indicated in the treatment of macular edema, are known substrates of the BCRP. Therefore, the ocular bioavailability of these drugs to the retina may be significantly limited by efflux pumps.

16.5.2 Influx Transporters and Receptors in Ocular Drug Delivery

Drug delivery facilitated through transporters and receptors involves targeting various nutrient transporters, e.g., amino acids, monocarboxylic acid, vitamins, bile acid, peptides, nucleoside, nucleobase, organic cation, and organic anion transporters. These transporters are targeted through a carrier-based approach involving the conjugation of a drug molecule or nanocarrier to an endogenous substrate, which is recognized by the particular transporter or receptor. These transporters/receptors assist in the translocation of prodrugs or nanocarriers across the cell membrane through the carrier-mediated process. Thus, transporter-based drug delivery could be an effective strategy for targeting drugs to both anterior and posterior segments.

16.5.2.1 Transporters and Receptors Expressed on Anterior Segment

16.5.2.1.1 Transporters on Cornea

The corneal epithelium is a major barrier for drug delivery by the topical route. The transporters and receptors expressed on the cornea have been utilized for targeted drug delivery. The transporters include the solute carrier type (SLC-1, SLC-6, SLC-14A, SLC-15, SLC-16, SLC-28, SLC-29, and SLCO) and the glucose transporters. A brief overview of these transporters follows:

- SLC-1 includes five glutamate transporters and two neutral amino acid transporters, namely, ASCT 1 and 2 (the transport system for alanine, serine, and cysteine). ASCT-1 was found on the corneal epithelium and on the apical side of the pigmented rabbit corneal epithelial cells.[63]
- SLC-6 is also known as a neurotransmitter transporter, which regulates the transport of norepinephrine, serotonin, dopamine, and gamma amino butyric acid (GABA). Studies on a transfected human corneal epithelial (tHCEC) cell line demonstrated that the taurine transporter is also expressed on the corneal epithelium.[64,65]
- SLC-6 isoform A14 is commonly known as ATB0+ and is mainly responsible for the transport of neutral and cationic amino acids.[66]
- Amino acid transporters can be classified as anionic, cationic, and neutral amino acid transporters. These transport proteins are also classified as sodium-dependent and sodium-independent on the basis of their functionality.
- SLC-7 includes large amino acid transporters (LATs). These proteins are sodium-independent and translocate large neutral amino acids and related compounds like melphlan and L-DOPA (3,4-dihydroxy-L-phenylalanine). Two isoforms of these transporters, LAT1 and LAT2, have been identified, which differ in terms of substrate specificity and affinity.[67–70] LAT1 is expressed on the human cornea. Corneal transporters offer a promising strategy to increase the ocular bioavailability of poorly permeable compounds. LATs mainly transport amino acids like L-arginine (Michaelis constant $K_M = 106 \pm 72\,\mu$M) and have been used to transport prodrugs like valacyclovir and valganciclovir.
- SLC-15 transporters are important in drug delivery, due to their broad substrate specificity and high capacity. The family mainly includes oligopeptide transporters (PEPT1, PEPT2) and phosphate transporters (PHT 1, PHT 2). Mitra et al. reported the presence of an oligopeptide transporter (PEPT1) on the rabbit cornea. This transporter recognizes peptide prodrugs and enhances their transport across rabbit cornea.[71–73] It mainly transports oligopeptides and the presence of this transporter was confirmed on the corneal epithelium through permeability studies of peptide prodrugs of acyclovir (ACV), cephalexin, and a known substrate, glycine–sarcosine.
- SLC-16 is a monocarboxylate transporter (MCT), which is responsible for the transport of lactate and pyruvate across the plasma membrane.[74] These transporters facilitate the translocation of drugs like salicylic acid and simvastatin.[75] It also assists in the removal of glycolytic products from the corneal epithelial surface to the aqueous humor, which helps maintain pH balance.[76] Chidlow et al. confirmed the presence of MCT 1, MCT 2, MCT 3, and MCT 4 on the surface of the cornea.[77]
- SLC-28 and 29 are also known as nucleoside transporters that are either Na$^+$-dependent or Na$^+$-independent. SLC-28 acts against the concentration gradient and is Na$^+$-dependent, whereas SLC-29 is expressed on most tissues and is a Na$^+$-independent transporter.[78] Rabbit cornea mainly expresses SLC-28 isoform A3, which primarily carries both purine and pyrimidine analogues.[79]
- SLCO transporters are organic anion transporters that regulate anionic amphipathic compounds. Their substrates include bile salts, steroids, hormones, and thyroids. Expression of these transporters was found on the basal cells of the rat corneal epithelium.[80]

- Glucose transporters: Bildin et al. have identified the glucose transporter (GLUT-1) in the bovine corneal epithelium.[81] Diabetic rats express higher amounts of these transporters due to higher glucose requirements for cell growth and differentiation.[82] These transporters have high affinity, but have limited applications in terms of drug delivery due to their low substrate specificity.[83–86]

16.5.2.1.2 Receptors on the Cornea

Various receptors expressed on the cornea, such as, growth factor, bardykinin, insulin, and folate receptors, could be utilized for targeted drug delivery.

- Growth factor receptors: these factors are responsible for corneal wound healing and the maintenance of epithelial thickness. Common growth factors include epidermal growth factor (EGF), hepatocyte growth factor (HGF), and kertinocyte growth factor (KGF). Growth factors assist in cell proliferation and stratification during wound healing. The enhanced expression of growth factors has been shown during corneal epithelial injury. HGF and KGF play a dominant role in corneal wound healing, whereas EGF mainly helps regulate homeostasis in corneal epithelium.[87,88] Growth factors, e.g., the nerve growth factor, have been indicated in the treatment of diseases of the retina and optic nerve. These factors are administered through the topical route in the form of an ointment. Receptor-based drug delivery utilizing growth factors may improve the therapeutic outcome for both anterior and posterior segment diseases.
- Bradykinin receptor: bradykinin, also known as an inflammatory mediator, exerts its effect by interacting with the bradykinin receptors B1 and B2. These inflammatory mediators are generated from the precursor kininogen, primarily by proteolysis. Wiernas et al. have confirmed the expression of the bradykinin receptor on human primary corneal epithelial cells.[89]
- Insulin receptor: ocular tissues, particularly conjuctiva and cornea, express insulin receptors, like insulin-like growth factor receptor 1 (IGFR-1). IGFR-1 may be responsible for regulating the metabolic and mitogenic activity on the ocular surface.[90] This is further supported by the fact that the topical insulin therapy promotes corneal healing.[91] Thus, drug delivery through the insulin receptor could be a potential strategy for enhancing ocular therapy.
- Miscellaneous receptors: various other receptors are also expressed on the cornea, such as vascular endothelial growth factor-C (VEGF-C), tumor necrosis factor (TNF) receptors TNF-R-I and TNF-R-II, hyaluronan receptors, and retinol receptors.[92]

16.5.2.1.3 Transporters on the Conjunctiva

- Acid-base transporters regulate cytoplasmic pH through ion-channel activity.[93] The two common transporters found on the rabbit conjuctival epithelium are the Na^+-K^+-Cl^- cotransporter and the Na^+-K^+-ATPase transporter. Chloride-based transporters (e.g., Cl^-/HCO_3^- transporter) are also expressed on the conjuctival epithelium. It is involved in the regulation of Cl^- ion and the maintenance of electrophysiological balance.[94] Kompella et al. and Shi and Candia have established the molecular presence of these transporters on rabbit conjuctival epithelial cells.[95,96]
- Glucose transporters are responsible for providing D-glucose to the conjunctival tissue to meet the energy requirement. Gherzi et al. reported the presence of the glucose transporter GLUT 1 on the conjuctival epithelium. It regulates the re-absorption of D-glucose and maintains fluid balance.[97] This transporter also helps in Na^+ influx into the conjuctival epithelium for maintaining solute absorption.[98]
- Other transporters for nucleosides, arginine, monocarboxylates, and dipeptides are also expressed on the conjuctival epithelium.[99]

16.5.2.1.4   Transporters and Receptors on Iris–Ciliary Body

The role of transporters expressed on the ICB has not been explored much in drug delivery. Glucose (GLUT1 and GLUT4) and nucleoside transporters are present in the ICB.[100,101] Vessey et al. identified the muscarinic receptor in chick ocular tissue.[102] Schmitt et al. confirmed the expression of the adrenergic receptor subtype-2 in rabbit on ICB.[103] Mukhopadhyay et al. studied the expression of prostaglandin receptors (EP1 and FP) in human ocular tissues.[104] However, all of the EP receptor subtypes are not yet characterized. Other receptors expressed on the ICB include androgen, oestrogen, and serotonin autoreceptors; and mineralocorticoid, melatonin, and glucocorticoid receptors.

16.5.2.1.5   Transporters and Receptors on the Lens

The lens expresses transporters such as amino acid (L-alanine, L-serine, and L-cysteine), vitamin C, glutathione, and glucose (GLUT1 and GLUT3) transporters.[105] These transporters are required for the supply of nutrients from aqueous humor to meet the metabolic energy needs of the lens. Collison et al. observed the muscarinic receptor on the lens epithelium. The utility of these transporters and receptors in drug delivery has not been explored much but their presence may allow for designing targeted drug delivery systems.

16.5.2.2   Transporters on the Posterior Segment

The RPE expresses transporters and receptors for the transport of nutrients and waste products. These transporters help in maintaining the ion and fluid balance of the retina. The various transporters expressed are amino acid, oligopeptide, monocarboxylate, folate, organic cation, nucleoside, and organic anion transporters.[106]

- Amino acid transporters are expressed in the RPE and retinal capillary endothelial cells. These proteins regulate the transport of amino acids, like glutamine.
- SLC-1 regulates the transport and removal of glutamine. There are five glutamate transporters excitatory amino acid transporters (EAAT 1 to EAAT 5). Several studies show the functional evidence of glutamate transporters in RPE cells.[107,108]
- SLC-6 regulates the transport of neurotransmitters, like taurines. This protein is localized throughout the RPE and regulates the transport process based on the concentration gradient of taurine.[109] The RPE also expresses transporters for the neurotransmitter GABA. Three major types of GABA transporters are expressed on rat RPE, viz., γ-aminobutyric acid transporters (GAT 1, GAT 2, and GAT 3).[110]
- SLC-7 is commonly known as a LAT. Nakauchi et al. reported the expression on LAT 1 and LAT 2 on the RPE cells.[111]
- SLC-15 is responsible for the transport of oligopeptides in the retina. Ochletre et al. confirmed the expression of these transporters on human and bovine retina.[113] Atluri et al. have shown its functional presence by the systemic administration of Gly-Sar, which is actively transported across the BRB and BAB.[114]
- SLC 16 is a MCT, which regulates the level of lactate, a glycolysis product, in the retina. Two major MCTs found in RPE are MCT-1 and MCT-3.[115,116] MCT-1 is located on the apical side, whereas MCT-3 is located on the basolateral side. Weak expression of MCT-2 and MCT-4 on the retina has also been suggested. This transporter could be successfully utilized for drug delivery since it transports monocarboxylates from the blood to the retina.
- The SLC-19 protein regulates the transport of folate to the RPE through the reduced folate transporter expressed on the apical side of RPE.[117,118] Bridges et al. studied the transport of folate from the basolateral side to the apical side of the ARPE-19 cells.[119] Such transporters may be utilized for drug delivery through a prodrug approach.
- SLC-22A is also known as an organic cation transporter and mainly translocates endogenous substances like epinephrine, guanidine, histidine; and agents like antineoplastics, antihistamines, and vitamins.

- Organic cation transporter 3 is mainly localized in the RPE. It is a high-capacity transporter and regulates the passage of various cationic drugs.[120]
- SLC-28 and 29 are known as nucleoside transporters that are pH-, Na$^+$-, and energy-dependent. Various types of ENT 1, ENT 2, CNT 1, and CNT 2 are also expressed on RPE.[121]

16.6 PRODRUGS: A TRANSPORTER-TARGETED TOOL FOR DRUG DELIVERY

Prodrugs are an inactive derivative of parent drugs which, upon chemical or enzymatic hydrolysis, generate the parent compound. Traditionally, prodrugs have been used for improving physiochemical properties, such as solubility or lipophilicity, of the parent drug. However, prodrugs can also be designed to target nutrient transporters or receptors expressed on cell membranes. In this approach, the pro-moiety, which is an amino acid, peptide, or vitamin, is conjugated to the parent molecule. The prodrug is recognized by the transporters or the receptors expressed on the cell surface, which translocate the prodrug into the cell. This is followed by the enzymatic cleavage into the parent drug molecule inside the cell. This approach had a very significant impact on the delivery of many therapeutic molecules such as ACV, GCV, and quinidine.

> The prodrug is recognized by the transporters or the receptors expressed on the cell surface, which translocate the prodrug into the cell. This is followed by the enzymatic cleavage into the parent drug molecule inside the cell. This approach had a significant impact on the delivery of many therapeutic molecules such as ACV, GCV, and quinidine.

16.6.1 ACYCLOVIR

The targeted prodrug strategy was employed for ACV, (9-(2-hydroxyethoxymethyl) guanine), a potent antiviral agent indicated for herpes simplex virus (HSV) type-I infections. It exerts therapeutic activity after transformation into ACV-triphosphate. ACV is highly efficacious in the treatment of HSV infection, but its ophthalmic application was less effective due to poor corneal permeability.

We synthesized a series of lipophilic acyl ester prodrugs of ACV. These prodrugs showed higher corneal permeability, but ophthalmic solutions of these prodrugs could not be formulated at high concentrations due to low aqueous solubility.[122]

An ACV prodrug was developed by attaching L-valine to the parent moiety (Figure 16.5), which resulted in higher permeability across the rabbit cornea.[71] This prodrug was recognized by PEPT1 and PEPT2, resulting in higher bioavailability than the parent drug. The carrier-mediated transport of L-valine ACV was confirmed by the competitive inhibition of the various substrates of peptide transporters.[71] The dipeptide prodrug of ACV, Val–Val–ACV, has shown significant stability in buffer pH5.4 as compared with the amino acid (Val–ACV). The cytotoxicity of the prodrugs was significantly reduced compared with the marketed formulation triflurothymidine (TFT). The solubility of prodrugs was also found to be dramatically increased compared with free drug. The dipeptide prodrugs, such as Val–Val–ACV and Gly–Val–ACV, have higher affinity for peptide transporters. Amino acid prodrugs have shown greater efficacy against HSV-1 and HSV-2 as mentioned in Table 16.4.[83,123]

To target peptide transporters present on the BAB following oral administration, we synthesized the stereoisomeric dipeptide ester prodrugs of ACV. Four prodrugs (LD ACV, DL ACV, DD ACV, and LL ACV) have shown different affinities toward the PEPT transporter and permeability across Caco-2 cell monolayers. The half-lives of these prodrugs are summarized in Table 16.5. The order of permeability across Caco-2 was LD ACV > LL ACV > DD ACV > DL ACV.[122]

The pharmacokinetics, metabolism, and corneal uptake of these stereoisomeric dipeptide prodrugs were compared with L ACV and ACV in rats. We have also evaluated uptake by corneal cells following the administration of LD ACV and L ACV by the oral route. Following IV administration, L ACV was metabolized to a higher extent than LD ACV and DL ACV. Following oral

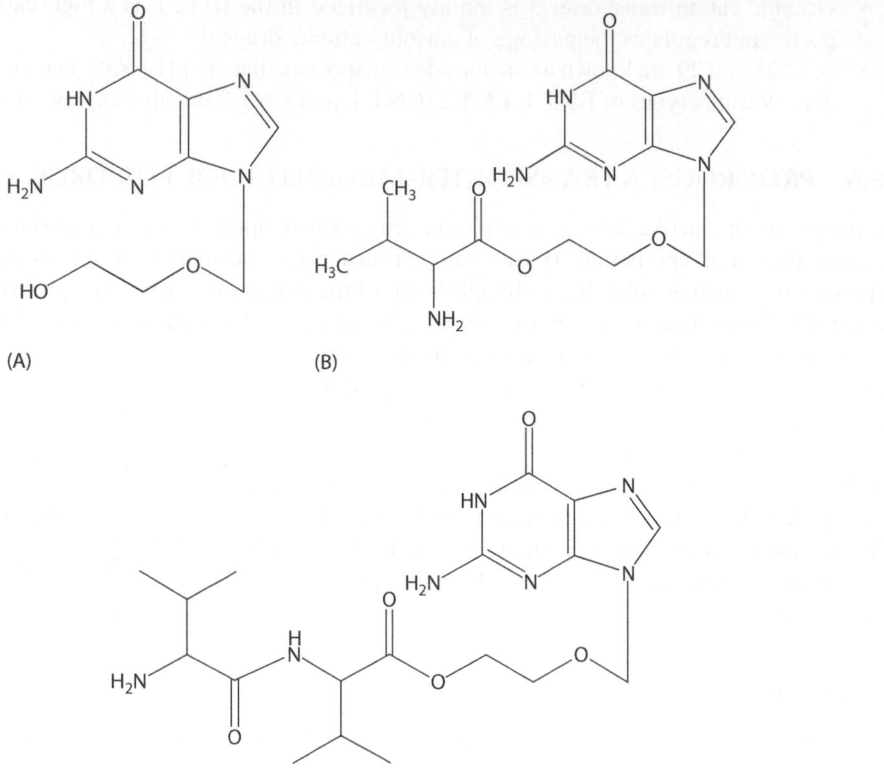

FIGURE 16.5　Chemical structures: (A) acyclovir, (B) valine–acyclovir, and (C) valine–valine–acyclovir.

TABLE 16.4
***In Vitro* Antiviral Activity of ACV and Its Prodrugs against HSV-1 and HSV-2**

Drug	HSV-1 (μM) CPE Inhibition	HSV-2 (μM) CPE Inhibition
ACV	$EC_{50}=7.11$	$EC_{50}=6.64$
Val-ACV	$EC_{50}=9.1$	$EC_{50}=7.77$
(VACV)	$CC_{50}>277$	$CC_{50}>277$
	$SI>30.3$	$SI>35.7$
Tyr-ACV	$EC_{50}=6.17$	$EC_{50}=7.77$
(YACV)	$CC_{50}>199$	$CC_{50}>199$
	$SI>32.2$	$SI>25.6$

Source:　Modified from Anand, B.S. et al., *Curr. Eye Res.*, 29, 153, 2004.

Note:　ACV: acyclovir; VACV: valecyclovir; YACV: L-tyrosine-ACV; HSV, herpes simplex virus; EC_{50}, the concentration required to inhibit virus cytopathogenicity by 50%; CC_{50}, the concentration required to inhibit cell proliferation by 50%; SI (selectivity index)$=CC_{50}/EC_{50}$.

TABLE 16.5
Half-Life of Various Stereo Isomeric Prodrugs in Caco-2, Rat Intestine, and Liver Homogenate

Prodrug	Caco-2	Rat Intestine	Rat Liver
LL ACV	7.52 ± 0.40 h	<0.08 h	<0.08 h
LD ACV	52.80 ± 8.42 h	1.01 ± 0.07 h	0.49 ± 0.02 h
DL ACV	a	6.27 ± 0.25 h	2.82 ± 0.18 h
DD ACV	a	a	a

Source: Modified from Talluri, R.S. et al., *Int. J. Pharm.*, 361, 118, 2008.

Note: h, hours; ACV, acyclovir, LL ACV, L-valine–L-valine ACV; LD ACV, L-valine–D-valine ACV; DL ACV, D-valine–L-valine ACV; DD ACV, D-valine–D-valine ACV.

a No appreciable degradation of the prodrug was found at the end of 1 week.

administration, ACV, L ACV, and LD ACV showed an exposure area under the curve (AUC) of 178 ± 34, 1077 ± 236, and 1141 ± 73, respectively. Almost fourfold higher values of the maximum concentration (C_{max}) and AUC of the intact prodrug were observed in the blood stream for LD ACV as compared with L ACV.[122]

Following the oral administration of these stereoisomeric prodrugs, a twofold higher amount of ACV was observed at its target site, the cornea, as compared with L ACV. Talluri et al. targeted the peptide transporters present on the BAB following oral administration of these stereoisomeric prodrugs of ACV. Apparently, due to the higher stability of the prodrug against its metabolic enzyme, the prodrug remains intact in the blood over a longer period of time, thus being recognized by peptide transporters on the cornea.[122] This targeting strategy to peptide transporters would also allow for the design of higher efficacy drugs for the treatment of diseases like genital and cutaneous herpes. This strategy can be potentially useful to other similar drugs, such as GCV.

16.6.2 QUINIDINE

The prodrug strategy can also be used to bypass efflux pumps, such as P-gp and MRP. Most of the topically applied drugs are substrates of P-gp. Therefore, the prodrug modification of these drugs has potential utility in ocular drug delivery.

Quinidine, a model P-gp substrate, was converted into its amino acid and peptide prodrugs, such as Val–quinidine (VQ) and Val–Val–quinidine (VVQ). Katragadda et al. reported that Val–quinidine and Val–Val–quinidine inhibited [^{3}H] Gly-Sar uptake at pH 5.0, which suggests the interaction of these prodrugs with peptide transporters. Furthermore, the inhibition of the corneal transport of VQ and VVQ in the presence of Gly-Sar suggests the interaction of these prodrugs with peptide transporters. Interestingly, the corneal permeability of VQ and VVQ prodrugs was 1.5 and 3 times higher than the parent drug, respectively. This could be attributed to their potential interaction with a peptide transporter present on the cornea. Peptide transporters have broad substrate specificity and a rapid turnover rate. This is a novel approach for bypassing an efflux pump by targeting the nutrient influx transporter present on the corneal surface.

The same strategy could be applied to antibiotics and steroids that are substrates of these efflux transporters, such as erythromycin, ofloxacin, dexamethasone, and prednisolone. A prodrug approach to these molecules can result in a dramatic increase in the bioavailability of these molecules.[124]

16.6.3 GANCICLOVIR

The prodrug strategy can also be applicable for the treatment of posterior segment diseases. The RPE expresses various nutrient transporters for peptides and vitamins. GCV is a 2′-deoxyguanosine analog with high activity against HCMV retinitis infection. RPE targeting by systemic delivery of GCV is challenging due to the presence of the BRB. Higher systemic doses can cause serious side effects, like neutropenia and thrombocytopenia. An IVT or subconjunctival injection may deliver GCV directly to the retina; its short IVT half-life necessitates frequent administration. Therefore, prodrug modification of GCV by attaching a peptide was developed to improve its IVT half-life and to provide the targeting capability to peptide transporters expressed on the basolateral side of RPE.[125]

We have shown that peptide prodrugs of GCV (particularly Gly–Val–GCV and Val–Val–GCV) are substrates for retinal peptide transporters. These dipeptide monoester prodrugs of GCV have higher permeability (almost two times higher than the parent drug GCV) across the sclera and retina, potentially due to their interaction with peptide transporters present on the retina.[126] This targeting strategy could be very valuable in the treatment of back of the eye diseases, such as CMV retinitis. Gly–Val–GCV provides a better IVT pharmacokinetic profile than the parent GCV, due to a slower elimination rate. This prodrug can be encapsulated into PLGA poly(lactic-*co*-glycolic acid) microspheres to provide a sustained release.[127]

16.7 NOVEL OCULAR DRUG DELIVERY SYSTEMS

Nanocarriers offer advantages such as lower degradation by enzymes, control over release parameters, and the enhancement of drug efficacy.[128] In addition, various formulation strategies can be used to deliver drugs to various ocular tissues, such as microemulsion, nanosuspension, nanoparticles, vesicular drug delivery (liposomes and niosomes), dendrimers, implants, and hydrogels.

The ubiquitous presence of efflux pumps on ocular tissues is a major barrier to ocular drug delivery. Colloidal delivery systems, such as microemulsions, liposomes, and niosomes, may contain polyoxyethylene-based nonionic surfactants. Anticancer drugs (e.g., doxorubicin and daunorubicin), steroids (e.g., hydrocortisone and dexamethasone), and beta-blockers (e.g., timolol and acebutolol) are substrates of this transporter.

The use of surfactants and polymers in the eye has been clinically accepted. The surfactants increase drug permeability by various mechanisms, such as the inhibition of efflux pumps like P-gp.[129] The exact mechanism of inhibition by surfactant is not known. A recent review summarized the relative efflux inhibition effectiveness of polyoxyethylated nonionic surfactants.[129] The authors cited the effectiveness to inhibit P-gp in the descending order, D-alpha-tocopheryl PEG 1000 succinate (Vitamin E-TPGS) > Cremophor® EL > Polysorbate 80 > Pluronic® F85 > Tyloxapol® > PEG 300.

Some polymers also inhibit P-gp-mediated efflux, such as poloxamers, poly-(ethyleneoxide)/poly-(propyleneoxide) block copolymers, and amphiphilic diblock copolymers methoxypolyethylene glycol-block-polycaprolactone. The mechanism of inhibition for efflux pumps is not yet clear, but has been hypothesized as their capability to inhibit ATPase.[130] The use of these excipients in formulations, such as various colloidal carriers or hydrogels, might result in better bioavailability due to the inhibition of efflux pumps. In this section, we will describe some of the key formulations that are widely used.

16.7.1 MICRO AND NANOCARRIERS FOR DRUG DELIVERY

Microemulsions are clear, isotropic mixtures of oil and water stabilized by a surfactant and a cosurfactant. They can provide higher thermodynamic stability, small droplet size, and clear appearance when compared with normal emulsion. Compared with emulsions, they have different characteristics because they do not exhibit physical instability such as agglomeration or separation of the dispersed phase.[131]

Microemulsion-based delivery systems can significantly enhance the solubility of drugs, such as indomethacin and chloramphenicol. This system can also provide higher stability, e.g., for timolol, sirolimus, and chloramphenicol.[132,133]

Nanosuspensions are submicron colloidal systems stabilized by surfactants. They have been used to deliver poorly water-soluble drug, such as flurbiprofen, methylprednisolone acetate, and glucocorticoids (e.g., hydrocortisone, prednisolone, and dexamethasone).[134–136] Nanosuspensions also impart stability to the drugs, such as cloricromene (AD6).[137] The excipients used in the formulation of this dosage form can also inhibit efflux pumps.

Nanoparticles are defined as particles with a diameter of less than 1 μm, comprising of various biodegradable or nonbiodegradable polymers, lipids, phospholipids, or metals. Nanoparticles have been used to control drug release and also to target a particular site. Various studies have also examined the efficiency of nanocarriers in bypassing efflux pumps such as P-gp and MRP.[138] Various formulation parameters affect their *in vivo* performance. For example, their particle size determines the potential distribution in the various tissues. Recently, Kompella et al. have carried out a study to understand the effect of nanoparticle size on their ocular distribution following periocular administration.[139] They have selected 20 and 200 nm nanoparticles. After periocular administration, they observed very little accumulation of 20 nm particles into the retinal tissue. They hypothesized that because of blood and lymphatic circulation, distribution inside the intraocular tissues was limited. The blood and lymphatic circulation will take up the nanoparticles immediately resulting in very minor distribution into intraocular tissues. At the same time, particles with 200 nm of size would be retained in the periocular space. So, for drug delivery perspective, it is important to consider the fate of different sizes of particles following periocular administration.

Table 16.6 summarizes the recent developments in the field of nanoparticle (NP)-based ocular delivery. The distribution and disposition of NPs also depend on various factors such as the size and presence of circulations (blood and lymph) following periocular administration.[139]

Recently, researches have hypothesized making a microsphere-based formulation encapsulating the nanocomplex of antisense TGF-β2 phosphorothioate oligonucleotides with polyethylenimine. They also prepared controlled microspheres using just TGF-β2 phosphorothioate oligonucleotides. A double emulsion method was used for microsphere preparation and PLGA was chosen as the polymer material for microsphere preparation. Investigators have observed that presence of polyethylenimine has significantly affected the release profile due to the formation of pores on the surface. The release from the microsphere was very high due to the presence of the pores. The same investigators performed *in vivo* studies in the rabbit model following subconjunctival administration. In the case of microsphere formulation containing nanocomplexes, they observed higher intracellular penetration of TGF-β2 phosphorothioate oligonucleotides in conjunctival cells. Due to the higher penetration of nanocomplexes, they observed enhanced bleb survival in a rabbit experimental model of filtering surgery.[140]

In a different approach, Kompella et al. evaluated the uptake of unmodified and surface-modified nanoparticles in various corneal layers. Surface-modified nanoparticles were prepared by attaching deslorelin (a luteinizing hormone-releasing hormone [LHRH] agonist) and transferrin. The higher uptake of the surface-modified nanoparticles was attributed to receptor-mediated endocytosis relative to the unmodified nanoparticles. It was hypothesized that these nanoparticles would be endocytosed at a higher extent relative to unmodified nanoparticles, due to the presence of surface modifying agents. They compared the uptake of these nanoparticles in a bovine eye by separating different layers of the cornea, such as the epithelium, stroma, and endothelium. The corneal epithelium was identified as the main barrier. At the end of 60 min of the uptake experiment of modified and unmodified nanoparticles in the cornea, deslorelin- and transferrin-modified nanoparticles had a higher uptake in the corneal epithelium. The uptake was almost 3- and 4.5-fold higher at 5 min and 4.5- and 3.8-fold higher at 60 min, for deslorelin- and transferin-conjugated nanoparticles, respectively. The uptake of these nanoparticles in excised cornea and conjunctiva was higher than

TABLE 16.6
Nanoparticulate-Based Drug Delivery System for Therapeutic Molecules

Drug Molecule	Characteristic of the Formulation	Reference
Tobramycin	Topical drug delivery retained for longer duration on the corneal surface and on the conjunctival sac compared with solution	[157]
GCV and ODN	Both oppositely charged molecules can be entrapped in albumin	[158]
Dexamethasone acetate	PLGA NPs administered by the IVT route caused higher drug levels to treat CMV	[159]
Gatifloxacin	Mucoadhesive chitosan–sodium alginate provided sustained release up to 24 h	[160]
Macugen	*In vitro* release study has shown a release of macugen (2 μg/day) up to 20 days across the sclera	[161]
Charged fluorescent nanoparticles	The positive charge on NP demonstrated better penetration abilities into inner ocular tissues compared with the negative charge NP	[162]
CK30-PEG compacted DNA NP	Higher transfection efficiency and longer duration of expression than other nonviral vectors without any toxicity	[163]
Cornea-specific promoters of keratin 12 and keratocan genes	Nonionic (PEO–PPO–PEO) polymeric micelles resulted in corneal epithelium and stroma-specific gene expression	[164]
Cu, Zn superoxide dismutase (SOD1) gene	Nonviral vector for ocular delivery	[165]
DNA nanoparticles	Nonviral gene transfer to ocular tissues like retina was obtained	[166]
Liposome–chitosan nanoparticle complexes (LCS-NP)	No alteration was macroscopically observed in *in vivo* after ocular surface exposure to LCS-NP	[167]
Surface-modified lipid nanocontainers	A homolipid templated with a heterolipid was used as a surface modifier	[168]
Brimonidine	NPs were prepared using polycarboxylic (polyacrylic and polyitaconic) acid to get sustained release	[169]
Np containing either Rh-6G (Rh) or Nile red (Nr)	NP localization was studied followed by intravitreous injection in intraocular tissues	[170]
Acyclovir	Optimization of formulation parameters of PLA NPs and effect of PEG coating on ocular drug bioavailability was studied	[171]

Note: GCV, ganciclovir; ODN, oligonucleotide; PLA, polylactide acid; PEG, polyethelene glycol; NPs, nanoparticles; PEO–PPO–PEO, poly(ethylene oxide)–poly(propylene oxide)–poly(ethylene oxide); PLGA, poly(lactic-*co*-glycolic acid; CMV, cytomegalovirus.

the unmodified nanoparticles. This could be related to the expression of the LHRH and transferin receptors observed in the corneal epithelium as well as the conjunctiva.[141]

A recent review has extensively covered the perspectives of particulate delivery systems (micro and nanoparticles) in ophthalmology.[142]

16.7.2 VESICULAR DRUG DELIVERY SYSTEMS

Liposomes are lipid vesicles containing an aqueous core. Vesicular drug delivery systems, like liposomes and niosomes, have been widely exploited in ophthalmic drug delivery. Niosomes are similar to liposomes except only nonionic surfactants are used in their preparations. These systems offer advantages such as protection against degradation by enzymes, higher capability to cross cell membranes, sustained release, and targeting intracellular components by avoiding efflux. Recently, some researchers have prepared a liposomal formulation of Avastin, which was given by IVT injection into the rabbit eye.[143] They prepared the formulation using the dehydration-rehydration method.

TABLE 16.7
Vesicular Delivery of Drug Molecules

Drug Molecule	Characteristic of Formulation	Reference
GCV	Permeability of liposomal formulation of GCV was higher than GCV solution in a rabbit model	[172]
Vasoactive intestinal peptide	High concentration of VIP following IVT injection of liposomal formulation than solution alone	[173]
Ciprofloxacin	Liposomal formulation lowered tear-driven dilution in the conjunctival sac	[174]
Acetazolamide	Liposomal formulation for delivery via topical route	[175]
gB1s and DTK peptides	Studied in the treatment of HSV-1 keratitis	[176]
Tropicamide and ACV	Positively charged formulation has shown higher absorption across the cornea	[177]
ODNs	PEGylated liposome-containing ODNs, results into inhibition of VEGF	[178]
Cyclopentolate	Niosomal formulation released the drug independent of pH resulting in higher ocular bioavailability	[179]
Timolol maleate	Less systemic drainage and large residence time in the cul-de-sac was observed due to size and shape	[180]

Note: GCV, ganciclovir; ACV, acyclovir; ODN, oligonuceotides; HSV 1, herpes simplex virus I; VEGF, vascular endothelial growth factor; VIP, vasoactive intestinal peptide; PEG, polyethylene glycol; DTK PEPTIDE, *Drosophila* tachykininrelated peptides.

An ELISA was used to study the release pattern, which revealed sustained release for more than 40 days. At 28 and 42 days, the liposomal formulation provided two and five times higher drug levels compared with the free solution. This study explains the significant advantage of liposomal formulation compared with free drug solution. Controlled release obtained by the vesicular system can also limit the systemic exposure of drug resulting in higher therapeutic benefit. Recently, one such study was done with ciprofloxacin liposomal formulation.[144] This formulation has shown a sustained release after administration into the eye for 24 h. Due to sustained release, systemic exposure was less, which can result in significantly fewer side effects in other parts of the body. Table 16.7 summarizes the recent developments in the field of vesicular drug systems.

16.7.3 INTRAOCULAR IMPLANTS

Implants have been developed for the drug molecules indicated for both anterior and posterior segment diseases. Implants for the posterior segment have been used in the treatment of PVR, CMV retinitis, and endophthalmitis. Both biodegradable and nonbiodegradable implants have been used using a wide variety of polymers, such as polylactic acid (PLA), polyglycolic acid (PGA), polylactic-*co*-glycolic acid (PLGA), polyglycolide-*co*-lactide-*co*-caprolactone copolymer (PGLC), poly-caprolactone (PCL), polyanhydrides, and polyorthoesters (POE).

For example, PLGA implants have been used for the sustained delivery of dexamethasone (Surodex®) after phacotrabeculectomy.[145] This implant contains 60 µm of dexamethasone in a pellet made up of the PLGA polymer, which will slowly release the drug. This is usually implanted in the patients before cataract surgery so that after surgery topical administration of the steroid can be avoided. Another intracameral (i.e., administered within the eye) implant containing cyclosporine in PLGA was developed to prevent corneal graft rejection or postoperative inflammation in rats.[146] In a novel attempt to treat PVR, an implant containing a combination 5-fluorouridine, triamcilone acetonide, and recombinant tissue plasminogen activator was developed utilizing PLGA as the copolymer matrix.[147] In a similar approach, *cis*-4-hydroxyproline was delivered by a combination of different grades of polymers, like PLGA 65/35 and PLGA 50/50.[148] Different grades of PLGA are available depending upon the composition of the copolymer (lactide or glycolide), e.g., PLGA 50/50 has equal lactide and glycolide content. Heparin was also delivered by encapsulating in PLGA for posterior capsular opacification (PCO) in rabbits.[149] An episcleral implant made up of ethylene vinyl acetate (EVA) was used to deliver betamethasone for the treatment of retinal inflammation.[150] Betamethasone was shown to release in a sustained manner from the implant. A zero order release profile was achieved from this implant and drug concentration in the retina choroid tissue was higher than in the vitreous humor. Histology and electroretinography studies revealed no significant toxicity of the implant. Similarly, Polyvinyl alcohol (PVA) was used to deliver triamcinolone acetonide and fluocinolone acetate for the treatment of choroidal neovascularisation (CNV) and uveitis, respectively.[151,152] PGLC was used to control the release of various hydrophilic and hydrophobic molecules, such as FK506 and cyclosporine A for the treatment of corneal allograft rejection and uveitis, respectively.[153,154]

16.7.4 HYDROGEL SYSTEMS

These are three-dimensional, hydrophilic, polymeric networks capable of absorbing a large amount of water. Gelation in the hydrogel can be achieved through optimizing parameters such as ion concentration, temperature, and pH. Recently, a theromosensitive gel was designed to deliver drug to the posterior segment diseases. Investigators have cross-linked poly(*N*-isopropylacrylamide) (PNIPAAm) using poly(ethylene glycol) diacrylate (PEG-DA). They intented to deliver protein using this hydrogel. The release of bovine serum albumin, bevacizumab, and ranibiumab was shown to depend upon the degree of cross-linker density. They have shown a sustained release of the protein up to 3 weeks from this gel. *In vitro* cell proliferation was also carried out, which has shown no loss in the bioactivity of the protein. Another group has developed a quaternized chitosan-based pH and temperature sensitive gel. They observed that at a lower pH level, it remains in solution form while at neutral or alkaline pH, it converts into a gel-like structure. These authors have hypothesized using this transparent gel for ocular applications as well.

In our laboratory, we have developed a PLGA–PEG–PLGA copolymer-based thermosensitive gel-based formulation of GCV. A microsphere-based formulation of GCV was suspended into this gel. Following single IVT administration, an effective drug level was maintained for up to 14 days in the vitreous humor.[155]

Pefloxacin mesylate, indomethacin, ciprofloxacin hydrochloride, and timolol maleate were delivered in a hydrogel formulation using Gelrite® (gellan gum).[92] The gelation was achieved by changing ionic strength. Ofloxacin and puerarin were delivered using Carbopol® 940 and hydroxypropyl methylcellulose. This was pH-triggered gelation, which led to controlled drug release. Temperature-triggered gelation for molecules like timolol maleate and pilocarpine were also developed.[92]

16.7.5 IONTOPHORESIS

Iontophoresis is a noninvasive method that has been used to deliver the ionized form of the drug across a particular tissue using small electrical current. This current enhances the permeation of the drug. Table 16.8 summarizes the recent developments in iontophoretic drug delivery to both anterior and posterior segments of the eye. Apart from small molecules, this technique also allows delivery of macromolecules such as antisense oligonucleotides and plasmids. Important drug delivery parameters include the properties of drug, selection of site of administration, and voltage applied. The safety and efficacy of iontophoresis in ocular tissue has been proven in several studies. OcuPhor® and Visulex® are recently developed iontophoretic methods for drug delivery into ocular tissues.[156] The inventors of the OcuPhor® technology have delivered radiolabeled [¹⁴C] diclofenac

TABLE 16.8
Recent Development of Iontophoresis-Based Delivery of Therapeutic Agents

Route	Name of the Molecule	Characteristic/Used in the Treatment of	Reference
TC	Ciprofloxacin hydrochloride	A sustained release of the drug was obtained that caused drug concentration high enough to treat intraocular infections	[181]
TS	GFP plasmid	Good transfection was obtained in retinal cells, which could be useful for the treatment of retinal degenerations	[182]
TS	Methylprednisolone	This has potential to treat posterior segment inflammatory diseases	[183]
TS	Carboplastin	This could be useful to treat intraocular retinoblastoma	[184]
TS-TC	Dexamethasone phosphate	Higher concentration of drug was observed following iontophoresis	[185]
TS	Methotrexate	Ocular inflammatory diseases and intraocular lymphoma	[186]
TC	Gentamicin	Pseudomonas keratitis in rabbit eyes	[187]
TP	ODNs	This therapy was targeted for survival of photoreceptors	[188]
TC	AS-ODNs	This AS-ODN was targeted to treat angiogenesis in cornea	[189]
TS	Amicacin	Therapeutically significant amount of drug was observed	[190]
TS-TC	6-FAM labeled ODNs	High concentration of gene was observed in both anterior and posterior segment tissues	[191]
TC	Anti-NOSII ODN	This therapy was successfully tested in the treatment of endotoxin-induced uveitis	[192]
TS	DNA, DNA–RNA hybrids, and dyes	51 bp oligonucleotides to a 3 kb plasmid were successfully delivered via this strategy	[193]

Note: TC, transcorneal; TS, transscleral; TP, transpalpebral; AS-ODN, antisense oligonucleotides; GFP, green fluorescence protein; anti-NOSII ODN, anti-nitric oxide synthase II oligonucleotides; 6-FAM, fluorescence dye; DNA, deoxyribonucleic acid; RNA, ribonucleic acid.

into rabbit eyes using 4 mA current for 20 min. They placed an electrode under the lower eyelid. They found a significantly higher concentration of diclofenac inside the retina-choroid tissue compared with the control (more than 16 times) without any ocular side effects. They claimed that this technology can also be used to deliver other drugs noninvasively for the treatment of wet AMD and PVR.

16.8 CONCLUDING REMARKS

Ocular drug delivery has always been a major challenge to drug delivery scientists. Anatomical and physiological understanding of the barriers is crucial in optimizing drug delivery to the eye. The presence of the BAB and BRB has posed a significant barrier. Posterior segment ocular diseases such as wet AMD, DR, and PVR require constant administration of the drugs. The ubiquitous presence of efflux pumps has made ocular delivery even more challenging. The role of various nutrient transporters and receptors in delivering the drug to targeted ocular tissues has gained significant attention. Targeting nutrient transporters can assist in overcoming the efflux transporter, thereby increasing ocular bioavailability. In this regard, the anatomical localization, functions, and substrate specificities of the transporters play a crucial role in optimizing ocular delivery systems. For example, transporters on the cornea and retina can be targeted following periocular administration. This strategy can overcome the traditional problems associated with other delivery routes, such as topical and IVT administration. Recent developments in the field of nanocarriers that can provide targeted and sustained drug release are also exciting. New strategies can be designed to exploit the potential of nanocarriers and the various excipients used in formulation that can evade efflux pumps. Other delivery systems, such as implants and hydrogel-based delivery systems hold promise for noninvasive, controlled, and targeted therapy. This strategy has particular importance because it can be very critical for the patients suffering from posterior segment diseases. The pharmaceutical industry has adapted a multidisciplinary approach to deal with the gigantic problems related to drug development and delivery. In the near future, the development of sustained released, noninvasive, and patient-friendly formulations will gain momentum. The development of new biomaterial, polymers, and transporter-targeted formulations will also receive much of attention. The current momentum in the field of ocular drug delivery holds great promise for the development of targeted, noninvasive, and controlled release formulation for the treatment of vision-threatening ocular diseases.

REFERENCES

1. Klyce SD, Beuerman RW. Structure and function of the cornea. In: Kaufman HE, Barron, BA, Mcdonald MB, Waltman, SR (Eds.), *The Cornea*. Churchil Livingstone, New York, 1988; p. 3.
2. Stjernschantz J, Astin M. Anatomy and physiology of the eye. Physiological aspects of ocular drug therapy. In: P. Edman (Ed.), *Biopharmaceutics of Ocular Drug Delivery*. CRC Press, Boca Raton, FL, 1993; pp. 1–26.
3. Hazin R, Hendrick AM, Kahook MY. Primary open-angle glaucoma: Diagnostic approaches and management. *J Natl Med Assoc* 2009; **101**: 46–50.
4. Sharma RJ, Ehinger BEJ. Development and structure of retina. In: Kaufman PL, Alam A, Moses RA (Eds.), *Physiology of the Eye*. C. V. Mosby, St. Louis, MO, 2003; pp. 319–347.
5. Andersen HL, Sander B. The vitreous. In: Kaufman PL, Alam A, Moses RA (Eds.), *Physiology of the Eye*. C. V. Mosby, St. Louis, MO, 2003; pp. 293–318.
6. Cour M. The retinal pigmented epithelium. In: Kaufman PL, Alam A, Moses RA (Eds.), *Physiology of the Eye*. C. V. Mosby, St. Louis, MO, 2003; pp. 348–357.
7. Edelhauser HF, Ubels JL. Cornea and sclera. In: Kaufman PL, Alam A, Moses RA (Eds.), *Physiology of the Eye*. C. V. Mosby, St. Louis, MO, 2003; pp. 47–116.
8. Urtti A, Salminen L, Periviita L. Ocular distribution of topically applied adrenaline in albino and pigmented rabbits. *Acta Ophthalmol (Copenh)* 1984; **62**: 753–762.
9. Urtti A, Salminen L. Minimizing systemic absorption of topically administered ophthalmic drugs. *Surv Ophthalmol* 1993; **37**: 435–456.
10. Yi X, Wang Y, Yu FS. Corneal epithelial tight junctions and their response to lipopolysaccharide challenge. *Invest Ophthalmol Vis Sci* 2000; **41**: 4093–4100.
11. Nemoto E, Takahashi H, Kobayashi D et al. Effects of poly-L-arginine on the permeation of hydrophilic compounds through surface ocular tissues. *Biol Pharm Bull* 2006; **29**: 155–160.
12. Brechue WF, Maren TH. pH and drug ionization affects ocular pressure lowering of topical carbonic anhydrase inhibitors. *Invest Ophthalmol Vis Sci* 1993; **34**: 2581–2587.
13. Prausnitz MR, Noonan JS. Permeability of cornea, sclera, and conjunctiva: A literature analysis for drug delivery to the eye. *J Pharm Sci* 1998; **87**: 1479–1488.
14. Watsky MA, Jablonski MM, Edelhauser HF. Comparison of conjunctival and corneal surface areas in rabbit and human. *Curr Eye Res* 1988; **7**: 483–486.
15. Pfister RR. The normal surface of conjunctiva epithelium. A scanning electron microscopic study. *Invest Ophthalmol* 1975; **14**: 267–279.
16. Chien DS, Sasaki H, Bundgaard H et al. Role of enzymatic lability in the corneal and conjunctival penetration of timolol ester prodrugs in the pigmented rabbit. *Pharm Res* 1991; **8**: 728–733.
17. Hamalainen KM, Kananen K, Auriola S et al. Characterization of paracellular and aqueous penetration routes in cornea, conjunctiva, and sclera. *Invest Ophthalmol Vis Sci* 1997; **38**: 627–634.
18. Cunha-Vaz J. The blood–ocular barriers. *Surv Ophthalmol* 1979; **23**: 279–296.
19. Smith RS, Rudt LA. Ocular vascular and epithelial barriers to microperoxidase. *Invest Ophthalmol* 1975; **14**: 556–560.
20. Peyman GA, Bok D. Peroxidase diffusion in the normal and laser-coagulated primate retina. *Invest Ophthalmol* 1972; **11**: 35–45.
21. Stevenson BR, Anderson JM, Goodenough DA et al. Tight junction structure and ZO-1 content are identical in two strains of Madin-Darby canine kidney cells which differ in transepithelial resistance. *J Cell Biol* 1988; **107**: 2401–2408.

22. Ban Y, Rizzolo LJ. A culture model of development reveals multiple properties of RPE tight junctions. *Mol Vis* 1997; **3**: 18.
23. Cunha-Vaz JG. The blood-retinal barriers. *DOC Ophthalmol* 1976; **2**: 287–327.
24. Pitkanen L, Ranta VP, Moilanen H et al. Permeability of retinal pigment epithelium: Effects of permeant molecular weight and lipophilicity. *Invest Ophthalmol Vis Sci* 2005; **46**: 641–646.
25. Hughes PM, Olejnik O, Chang-Lin JE et al. Topical and systemic drug delivery to the posterior segments. *Adv Drug Deliv Rev* 2005; **57**: 2010–2032.
26. Cunha-Vaz JG. The blood–retinal barriers system. Basic concepts and clinical evaluation. *Exp Eye Res* 2004; **78**: 715–721.
27. Davson H, Duke-Elder WS, Maurice DM et al. The penetration of some electrolytes and non-electrolytes into the aqueous humour and vitreous body of the cat. *J Physiol* 1949; **108**: 203–217.
28. Kent AR, King L, Bartholomew LR. Vitreous concentration of topically applied brimonidine–purite 0.15%. *J Ocul Pharmacol Ther* 2006; **22**: 242–246.
29. Lindstrom R, Kim T. Ocular permeation and inhibition of retinal inflammation: An examination of data and expert opinion on the clinical utility of nepafenac. *Curr Med Res Opin* 2006; **22**: 397–404.
30. Koevary SB. Pharmacokinetics of topical ocular drug delivery: Potential uses for the treatment of diseases of the posterior segment and beyond. *Curr Drug Metab* 2003; **4**: 213–222.
31. Rait JL. Systemic effects of topical ophthalmic beta-adrenoceptor antagonists. *Aust N Z J Ophthalmol* 1999; **27**: 57–64.
32. Rosenberg LF, Krupin T, Tang LQ et al. Combination of systemic acetazolamide and topical dorzolamide in reducing intraocular pressure and aqueous humor formation. *Ophthalmology* 1998; **105**: 88–92; discussion-3.
33. Macha S, Mitra AK. Ocular pharmacokinetics in rabbits using a novel dual probe microdialysis technique. *Exp Eye Res* 2001; **72**: 289–299.
34. Cheng L, Hostetler KY, Lee J et al. Characterization of a novel intraocular drug-delivery system using crystalline lipid antiviral prodrugs of ganciclovir and cyclic cidofovir. *Invest Ophthalmol Vis Sci* 2004; **45**: 4138–4144.
35. Baum J, Peyman GA, Barza M. Intravitreal administration of antibiotic in the treatment of bacterial endophthalmitis. III. Consensus. *Surv Ophthalmol* 1982; **26**: 204–206.
36. Lopez-Cortes LF, Pastor-Ramos MT, Ruiz-Valderas R et al. Intravitreal pharmacokinetics and retinal concentrations of ganciclovir and foscarnet after intravitreal administration in rabbits. *Invest Ophthalmol Vis Sci* 2001; **42**: 1024–1028.
37. Macha S, Mitra AK. Ocular disposition of ganciclovir and its monoester prodrugs following intravitreal administration using microdialysis. *Drug Metab Dispos* 2002; **30**: 670–675.
38. Hyndiuk RA, Reagan MG. Radioactive depot-corticosteroid penetration into monkey ocular tissue. I. Retrobulbar and systemic administration. *Arch Ophthalmol* 1968; **80**: 499–503.
39. Ebner R, Devoto MH, Weil D et al. Treatment of thyroid associated ophthalmopathy with periocular injections of triamcinolone. *Br J Ophthalmol* 2004; **88**: 1380–1386.
40. van den Berg AA. An audit of peribulbar blockade using 15 mm, 25 mm and 37.5 mm needles, and sub-Tenon's injection. *Anaesthesia* 2004; **59**: 775–780.
41. Canavan KS, Dark A, Garrioch MA. Sub-Tenon's administration of local anaesthetic: A review of the technique. *Br J Anaesth* 2003; **90**: 787–793.
42. Kim TW, Lindsey JD, Aihara M et al. Intraocular distribution of 70-kDa dextran after subconjunctival injection in mice. *Invest Ophthalmol Vis Sci* 2002; **43**: 1809–1816.
43. Weijtens O, Schoemaker RC, Lentjes EG et al. Dexamethasone concentration in the subretinal fluid after a subconjunctival injection, a peribulbar injection, or an oral dose. *Ophthalmology* 2000; **107**: 1932–1938.
44. Ambati J, Gragoudas ES, Miller JW et al. Transscleral delivery of bioactive protein to the choroid and retina. *Invest Ophthalmol Vis Sci* 2000; **41**: 1186–1191.
45. Kim H, Robinson MR, Lizak MJ et al. Controlled drug release from an ocular implant: An evaluation using dynamic three-dimensional magnetic resonance imaging. *Invest Ophthalmol Vis Sci* 2004; **45**: 2722–2731.
46. Juliano RL, Ling V. A surface glycoprotein modulating drug permeability in Chinese hamster ovary cell mutants. *Biochim Biophys Acta* 1976; **455**: 152–162.
47. Thiebaut F, Tsuruo T, Hamada H et al. Cellular localization of the multidrug-resistance gene product P-glycoprotein in normal human tissues. *Proc Natl Acad Sci USA* 1987; **84**: 7735–7738.
48. Loo TW, Clarke DM. Location of the rhodamine-binding site in the human multidrug resistance P-glycoprotein. *J Biol Chem* 2002; **277**: 44332–44438.

49. Loo TW, Clarke DM. Vanadate trapping of nucleotide at the ATP-binding sites of human multidrug resistance P-glycoprotein exposes different residues to the drug-binding site. *Proc Natl Acad Sci USA* 2002; **99**: 3511–3516.

50. Higgins CF, Gottesman MM. Is the multidrug transporter a flippase? *Trends Biochem Sci* 1992; **17**: 18–21.

51. Eytan GD, Kuchel PW. Mechanism of action of P-glycoprotein in relation to passive membrane permeation. *Int Rev Cytol* 1999; **190**: 175–250.

52. Sharom FJ. The P-glycoprotein efflux pump: how does it transport drugs? *J Membr Biol* 1997; **160**: 161–175.

53. Didziapetris R, Japertas P, Avdeef A et al. Classification analysis of P-glycoprotein substrate specificity. *J Drug Target* 2003; **11**: 391–406.

54. Hariharan S, Gunda S, Mishra GP et al. Enhanced corneal absorption of erythromycin by modulating P-glycoprotein and MRP mediated efflux with corticosteroids. *Pharm Res* 2009; **26**: 1270–1282.

55. Dolfini E, Dasdia T, Arancia G et al. Characterization of a clonal human colon adenocarcinoma line intrinsically resistant to doxorubicin. *Br J Cancer* 1997; **76**: 67–76.

56. Karla PK, Quinn TL, Herndon BL et al. Expression of multidrug resistance associated protein 5 (MRP5) on cornea and its role in drug efflux. *J Ocul Pharmacol Ther* 2009; **25**: 121–132.

57. Mao Q, Unadkat JD. Role of the breast cancer resistance protein (ABCG2) in drug transport. *AAPS J* 2005; **7**: E118–E133.

58. Litman T, Brangi M, Hudson E et al. The multidrug-resistant phenotype associated with overexpression of the new ABC half-transporter, MXR (ABCG2). *J Cell Sci* 2000; **113**(Pt 11): 2011–2021.

59. Rocchi E, Khodjakov A, Volk EL et al. The product of the ABC half-transporter gene ABCG2 (BCRP/MXR/ABCP) is expressed in the plasma membrane. *Biochem Biophys Res Commun* 2000; **271**: 42–46.

60. Steuer H, Jaworski A, Elger B et al. Functional characterization and comparison of the outer blood–retina barrier and the blood–brain barrier. *Invest Ophthalmol Vis Sci* 2005; **46**: 1047–1053.

61. Aukunuru JV, Sunkara G, Bandi N et al. Expression of multidrug resistance-associated protein (MRP) in human retinal pigment epithelial cells and its interaction with BAPSG, a novel aldose reductase inhibitor. *Pharm Res* 2001; **18**: 565–572.

62. Kelly SL, Lamb DC, Jackson CJ et al. The biodiversity of microbial cytochromes P450. *Adv Microb Physiol* 2003; **47**: 131–186.

63. Kanai Y, Hediger MA. The glutamate and neutral amino acid transporter family: Physiological and pharmacological implications. *Eur J Pharmacol* 2003; **479**: 237–247.

64. Chen NH, Reith ME, Quick MW. Synaptic uptake and beyond: The sodium- and chloride-dependent neurotransmitter transporter family SLC6. *Pflugers Arch* 2004; **447**: 519–531.

65. Shioda R, Reinach PS, Hisatsune T et al. Osmosensitive taurine transporter expression and activity in human corneal epithelial cells. *Invest Ophthalmol Vis Sci* 2002; **43**: 2916–2922.

66. Jain-Vakkalagadda B, Pal D, Gunda S et al. Identification of a Na^+-dependent cationic and neutral amino acid transporter, B(0,+), in human and rabbit cornea. *Mol Pharm* 2004; **1**: 338–346.

67. Kanai Y, Segawa H, Miyamoto K et al. Expression cloning and characterization of a transporter for large neutral amino acids activated by the heavy chain of 4F2 antigen (CD98). *J Biol Chem* 1998; **273**: 23629–23632.

68. Kanai Y, Endou H. Functional properties of multispecific amino acid transporters and their implications to transporter-mediated toxicity. *J Toxicol Sci* 2003; **28**: 1–17.

69. Verrey F. System L: Heteromeric exchangers of large, neutral amino acids involved in directional transport. *Pflugers Arch* 2003; **445**: 529–533.

70. Wagner CA, Lang F, Broer S. Function and structure of heterodimeric amino acid transporters. *Am J Physiol Cell Physiol* 2001; **281**: C1077–C1093.

71. Anand BS, Mitra AK. Mechanism of corneal permeation of L-valyl ester of acyclovir: Targeting the oligopeptide transporter on the rabbit cornea. *Pharm Res* 2002; **19**: 1194–1202.

72. Anand B, Nashed Y, Mitra A. Novel dipeptide prodrugs of acyclovir for ocular herpes infections: Bioreversion, antiviral activity and transport across rabbit cornea. *Curr Eye Res* 2003; **26**: 151–163.

73. Majumdar S, Nashed YE, Patel K et al. Dipeptide monoester ganciclovir prodrugs for treating HSV-1-induced corneal epithelial and stromal keratitis: In vitro and in vivo evaluations. *J Ocul Pharmacol Ther* 2005; **21**: 463–474.

74. Halestrap AP, Meredith D. The SLC16 gene family-from monocarboxylate transporters (MCTs) to aromatic amino acid transporters and beyond. *Pflugers Arch* 2004; **447**: 619–628.

75. Enerson BE, Drewes LR. Molecular features, regulation, and function of monocarboxylate transporters: Implications for drug delivery. *J Pharm Sci* 2003; **92**: 1531–1544.

76. Bonanno JA. Lactate-proton cotransport in rabbit corneal epithelium. *Curr Eye Res* 1990; **9**: 707–712.
77. Chidlow G, Wood JP, Graham M et al. Expression of monocarboxylate transporters in rat ocular tissues. *Am J Physiol Cell Physiol* 2005; **288**: C416–C428.
78. Kong W, Engel K, Wang J. Mammalian nucleoside transporters. *Curr Drug Metab* 2004; **5**: 63–84.
79. Majumdar S, Gunda S, Mitra A. Functional expression of a sodium dependent nucleoside transporter on rabbit cornea: Role in corneal permeation of acyclovir and idoxuridine. *Curr Eye Res* 2003; **26**: 175–183.
80. Mikkaichi T, Suzuki T, Tanemoto M et al. The organic anion transporter (OATP) family. *Drug Metab Pharmacokinet* 2004; **19**: 171–179.
81. Bildin VN, Iserovich P, Fischbarg J et al. Differential expression of Na:K:2Cl cotransporter, glucose transporter 1, and aquaporin 1 in freshly isolated and cultured bovine corneal tissues. *Exp Biol Med (Maywood)* 2001; **226**: 919–926.
82. Takahashi H, Kaminski AE, Zieske JD. Glucose transporter 1 expression is enhanced during corneal epithelial wound repair. *Exp Eye Res* 1996; **63**: 649–659.
83. Wright EM. The intestinal Na+/glucose cotransporter. *Annu Rev Physiol* 1993; **55**: 575–589.
84. Thorens B. Facilitated glucose transporters in epithelial cells. *Annu Rev Physiol* 1993; **55**: 591–608.
85. Silverman M. Structure and function of hexose transporters. *Annu Rev Biochem* 1991; **60**: 757–794.
86. Shepherd PR, Kahn BB. Glucose transporters and insulin action—implications for insulin resistance and diabetes mellitus. *N Engl J Med* 1999; **341**: 248–257.
87. Wilson SE, Liang Q, Kim WJ. Lacrimal gland HGF, KGF, and EGF mRNA levels increase after corneal epithelial wounding. *Invest Ophthalmol Vis Sci* 1999; **40**: 2185–2190.
88. Wilson SE, Chen L, Mohan RR et al. Expression of HGF, KGF, EGF and receptor messenger RNAs following corneal epithelial wounding. *Exp Eye Res* 1999; **68**: 377–397.
89. Wiernas TK, Davis TL, Griffin BW et al. Effects of bradykinin on signal transduction, cell proliferation, and cytokine, prostaglandin E2 and collagenase-1 release from human corneal epithelial cells. *Br J Pharmacol* 1998; **123**: 1127–1137.
90. Rocha EM, Cunha DA, Carneiro EM et al. Identification of insulin in the tear film and insulin receptor and IGF-1 receptor on the human ocular surface. *Invest Ophthalmol Vis Sci* 2002; **43**: 963–967.
91. Rocha EM, Cunha DA, Carneiro EM et al. Insulin, insulin receptor and insulin-like growth factor-I receptor on the human ocular surface. *Adv Exp Med Biol* 2002; **506**: 607–610.
92. Gaudana R, Jwala J, Boddu SH et al. Recent perspectives in ocular drug delivery. *Pharm Res* 2008; **5**: 1197–1216.
93. Watsky MA. Characterization of voltage-gated, whole-cell ionic currents from conjunctival epithelial cells. *Invest Ophthalmol Vis Sci* 1998; **39**: 351–357.
94. Turner HC, Alvarez LJ, Candia OA. Identification and localization of acid-base transporters in the conjunctival epithelium. *Exp Eye Res* 2001; **72**: 519–531.
95. Kompella UB, Kim KJ, Lee VH. Active chloride transport in the pigmented rabbit conjunctiva. *Curr Eye Res* 1993; **12**: 1041–1048.
96. Shi XP, Candia OA. Active sodium and chloride transport across the isolated rabbit conjunctiva. *Curr Eye Res* 1995; **14**: 927–935.
97. Gherzi R, Melioli G, De Luca M et al. High expression levels of the "erythroid/brain" type glucose transporter (GLUT1) in the basal cells of human eye conjunctiva and oral mucosa reconstituted in culture. *Exp Cell Res* 1991; **195**: 230–236.
98. Xiao-ping S, Candia OA. Contribution of Na(+)-glucose cotransport to the short-circuit current in the pigmented rabbit conjunctiva. *Curr Eye Res* 1996; **15**: iii–iv.
99. Hosoya K, Lee VH, Kim KJ. Roles of the conjunctiva in ocular drug delivery: A review of conjunctival transport mechanisms and their regulation. *Eur J Pharm Biopharm* 2005; **60**: 227–240.
100. Harik SI, Kalaria RN, Andersson L et al. Immunocytochemical localization of the erythroid glucose transporter: Abundance in tissues with barrier functions. *J Neurosci* 1990; **10**: 3862–3872.
101. Williams EF, Chu TC, Socci RR et al. Comparison of nucleoside transport binding sites in rabbit iris–ciliary body and cultured rabbit nonpigmented ciliary epithelial cells. *J Ocul Pharmacol Ther* 1996; **12**: 461–469.
102. Vessey KA, Cottriall CL, McBrien NA. Muscarinic receptor protein expression in the ocular tissues of the chick during normal and myopic eye development. *Brain Res Dev Brain Res* 2002; **135**: 79–86.
103. Schmitt CJ, Gross DM, Share NN. Beta-adrenergic receptor subtypes in iris–ciliary body of rabbits. *Graefes Arch Clin Exp Ophthalmol* 1984; **221**: 167–170.
104. Mukhopadhyay P, Bian L, Yin H et al. Localization of EP(1) and FP receptors in human ocular tissues by in situ hybridization. *Invest Ophthalmol Vis Sci* 2001; **42**: 424–428.
105. Collison DJ, Coleman RA, James RS et al. Characterization of muscarinic receptors in human lens cells by pharmacologic and molecular techniques. *Invest Ophthalmol Vis Sci* 2000; **41**: 2633–2641.

106. Basu SK, Haworth IS, Bolger MB et al. Proton-driven dipeptide uptake in primary cultured rabbit conjunctival epithelial cells. *Invest Ophthalmol Vis Sci* 1998; **39**: 2365–2373.

107. Miyamoto Y, Del Monte MA. Na(+)-dependent glutamate transporter in human retinal pigment epithelial cells. *Invest Ophthalmol Vis Sci* 1994; **35**: 3589–3598.

108. Kanai Y, Hediger MA. The glutamate/neutral amino acid transporter family SLC1: Molecular, physiological and pharmacological aspects. *Pflugers Arch* 2004; **447**: 469–479.

109. Hosoya K, Tomi M. Advances in the cell biology of transport via the inner blood–retinal barrier: Establishment of cell lines and transport functions. *Biol Pharm Bull* 2005; **28**: 1–8.

110. Honda S, Yamamoto M, Saito N. Immunocytochemical localization of three subtypes of GABA transporter in rat retina. *Brain Res Mol Brain Res* 1995; **33**: 319–325.

111. Nakauchi T, Ando A, Ueda-Yamada M et al. Prevention of ornithine cytotoxicity by nonpolar side chain amino acids in retinal pigment epithelial cells. *Invest Ophthalmol Vis Sci* 2003; **44**: 5023–5028.

112. Tomi M, Mori M, Tachikawa M et al. L-type amino acid transporter 1-mediated L-leucine transport at the inner blood–retinal barrier. *Invest Ophthalmol Vis Sci* 2005; **46**: 2522–2530.

113. Ocheltree SM, Keep RF, Shen H et al. Preliminary investigation into the expression of proton-coupled oligopeptide transporters in neural retina and retinal pigment epithelium (RPE): Lack of functional activity in RPE plasma membranes. *Pharm Res* 2003; **20**: 1364–1372.

114. Atluri H, Anand BS, Patel J et al. Mechanism of a model dipeptide transport across blood–ocular barriers following systemic administration. *Exp Eye Res* 2004; **78**: 815–822.

115. Philp NJ, Yoon H, Grollman EF. Monocarboxylate transporter MCT1 is located in the apical membrane and MCT3 in the basal membrane of rat RPE. *Am J Physiol* 1998; **274**: R1824–R1828.

116. Philp NJ, Wang D, Yoon H et al. Polarized expression of monocarboxylate transporters in human retinal pigment epithelium and ARPE-19 cells. *Invest Ophthalmol Vis Sci* 2003; **44**: 1716–1721.

117. Chancy CD, Kekuda R, Huang W et al. Expression and differential polarization of the reduced-folate transporter-1 and the folate receptor alpha in mammalian retinal pigment epithelium. *J Biol Chem* 2000; **275**: 20676–20684.

118. Huang W, Prasad PD, Kekuda R et al. Characterization of N5-methyltetrahydrofolate uptake in cultured human retinal pigment epithelial cells. *Invest Ophthalmol Vis Sci* 1997; **38**: 1578–1587.

119. Bridges CC, El-Sherbeny A, Ola MS et al. Transcellular transfer of folate across the retinal pigment epithelium. *Curr Eye Res* 2002; **24**: 129–138.

120. Rajan PD, Kekuda R, Chancy CD et al. Expression of the extraneuronal monoamine transporter in RPE and neural retina. *Curr Eye Res* 2000; **20**: 195–204.

121. Nagase K, Tomi M, Tachikawa M et al. Functional and molecular characterization of adenosine transport at the rat inner blood–retinal barrier. *Biochim Biophys Acta* 2006; **1758**: 13–19.

122. Talluri RS, Samanta SK, Gaudana R et al. Synthesis, metabolism and cellular permeability of enzymatically stable dipeptide prodrugs of acyclovir. *Int J Pharm* 2008; **361**: 118–124.

123. Anand BS, Katragadda S, Nashed YE et al. Amino acid prodrugs of acyclovir as possible antiviral agents against ocular HSV-1 infections: Interactions with the neutral and cationic amino acid transporter on the corneal epithelium. *Curr Eye Res* 2004; **29**: 153–166.

124. Katragadda S, Talluri RS, Mitra AK. Modulation of P-glycoprotein-mediated efflux by prodrug derivatization: An approach involving peptide transporter-mediated influx across rabbit cornea. *J Ocul Pharmacol Ther* 2006; **22**: 110–120.

125. Patel K, Trivedi S, Luo S et al. Synthesis, physicochemical properties and antiviral activities of ester prodrugs of ganciclovir. *Int J Pharm* 2005; **305**: 75–89.

126. Kansara V, Hao Y, Mitra AK. Dipeptide monoester ganciclovir prodrugs for transscleral drug delivery: Targeting the oligopeptide transporter on rabbit retina. *J Ocul Pharmacol Ther* 2007; **23**: 321–334.

127. Janoria KG, Mitra AK. Effect of lactide/glycolide ratio on the in vitro release of ganciclovir and its lipophilic prodrug (GCV-monobutyrate) from PLGA microspheres. *Int J Pharm* 2007; **338**: 133–141.

128. Lee VH, Robinson JR. Topical ocular drug delivery: Recent developments and future challenges. *J Ocul Pharmacol* 1986; **2**: 67–108.

129. Werle M. Natural and synthetic polymers as inhibitors of drug efflux pumps. *Pharm Res* 2008; **25**: 500–511.

130. Huang J, Si L, Jiang L et al. Effect of pluronic F68 block copolymer on P-glycoprotein transport and CYP3A4 metabolism. *Int J Pharm* 2008; **356**: 351–353.

131. Narang AS, Delmarre D, Gao D. Stable drug encapsulation in micelles and microemulsions. *Int J Pharm* 2007; **345**: 9–25.

132. Ansari MJ, Kohli K, Dixit N. Microemulsions as potential drug delivery systems: A review. *PDA J Pharm Sci Technol* 2008; **62**: 66–79.

133. Vandamme TF. Microemulsions as ocular drug delivery systems: Recent developments and future challenges. *Prog Retin Eye Res* 2002; **21**: 15–34.

134. Pignatello R, Bucolo C, Spedalieri G et al. Flurbiprofen-loaded acrylate polymer nanosuspensions for ophthalmic application. *Biomaterials* 2002; **23**: 3247–3255.

135. Adibkia K, Omidi Y, Siahi MR et al. Inhibition of endotoxin-induced uveitis by methylprednisolone acetate nanosuspension in rabbits. *J Ocul Pharmacol Ther* 2007; **23**: 421–432.

136. Kassem MA, Abdel Rahman AA, Ghorab MM et al. Nanosuspension as an ophthalmic delivery system for certain glucocorticoid drugs. *Int J Pharm* 2007; **340**: 126–133.

137. Pignatello R, Ricupero N, Bucolo C et al. Preparation and characterization of eudragit retard nanosuspensions for the ocular delivery of cloricromene. *AAPS PharmSciTech* 2006; **7**: E27.

138. Esmaeili F, Ghahremani MH, Ostad SN et al. Folate-receptor-targeted delivery of docetaxel nanoparticles prepared by PLGA-PEG-folate conjugate. *J Drug Target* 2008; **16**: 415–423.

139. Amrite AC, Edelhauser HF, Singh SR et al. Effect of circulation on the disposition and ocular tissue distribution of 20 nm nanoparticles after periocular administration. *Mol Vis* 2008; **14**: 150–160.

140. Gomes dos Santos AL, Bochot A, Doyle A et al. Sustained release of nanosized complexes of polyethylenimine and anti-TGF-beta 2 oligonucleotide improves the outcome of glaucoma surgery. *J Control Release* 2006; **112**: 369–381.

141. Kompella UB, Sundaram S, Raghava S et al. Luteinizing hormone-releasing hormone agonist and transferrin functionalizations enhance nanoparticle delivery in a novel bovine ex vivo eye model. *Mol Vis* 2006; **12**: 1185–1198.

142. Moshfeghi AA, Peyman GA. Micro- and nanoparticulates. *Adv Drug Deliv Rev* 2005; **57**: 2047–2052.

143. Abrishami M, Ganavati SZ, Soroush D et al. Preparation, characterization, and in vivo evaluation of nanoliposomes-encapsulated bevacizumab (avastin) for intravitreal administration. *Retina* 2009; **29**: 699–703.

144. Mehanna MM, Elmaradny HA, Samaha MW. Ciprofloxacin liposomes as vesicular reservoirs for ocular delivery: Formulation, optimization, and in vitro characterization. *Drug Dev Ind Pharm* 2009; **35**: 583–593.

145. Seah SK, Husain R, Gazzard G et al. Use of surodex in phacotrabeculectomy surgery. *Am J Ophthalmol* 2005; **139**: 927–928.

146. Xie L, Shi W, Wang Z et al. Prolongation of corneal allograft survival using cyclosporine in a polylactide-*co*-glycolide polymer. *Cornea* 2001; **20**: 748–752.

147. Zhou T, Lewis H, Foster RE et al. Development of a multiple-drug delivery implant for intraocular management of proliferative vitreoretinopathy. *J Control Release* 1998; **55**: 281–295.

148. Yasukawa T, Kimura H, Tabata Y et al. Sustained release of *cis*-hydroxyproline in the treatment of experimental proliferative vitreoretinopathy in rabbits. *Graefes Arch Clin Exp Ophthalmol* 2002; **240**: 672–678.

149. Xie L, Sun J, Yao Z. Heparin drug delivery system for prevention of posterior capsular opacification in rabbit eyes. *Graefes Arch Clin Exp Ophthalmol* 2003; **241**: 309–313.

150. Kato A, Kimura H, Okabe K et al. Feasibility of drug delivery to the posterior pole of the rabbit eye with an episcleral implant. *Invest Ophthalmol Vis Sci* 2004; **45**: 238–244.

151. Ciulla TA, Criswell MH, Danis RP et al. Choroidal neovascular membrane inhibition in a laser treated rat model with intraocular sustained release triamcinolone acetonide microimplants. *Br J Ophthalmol* 2003; **87**: 1032–1037.

152. Jaffe GJ, Yang CH, Guo H et al. Safety and pharmacokinetics of an intraocular fluocinolone acetonide sustained delivery device. *Invest Ophthalmol Vis Sci* 2000; **41**: 3569–3575.

153. Shi W, Liu T, Xie L et al. FK506 in a biodegradable glycolide-*co*-clatide-*co*-caprolactone polymer for prolongation of corneal allograft survival. *Curr Eye Res* 2005; **30**: 969–976.

154. Dong X, Shi W, Yuan G et al. Intravitreal implantation of the biodegradable cyclosporin A drug delivery system for experimental chronic uveitis. *Graefes Arch Clin Exp Ophthalmol* 2006; **244**: 492–497.

155. Duvvuri S, Janoria KG, Pal D et al. Controlled delivery of ganciclovir to the retina with drug-loaded poly(D,L-lactide-*co*-glycolide) (PLGA) microspheres dispersed in PLGA-PEG-PLGA Gel: A novel intravitreal delivery system for the treatment of cytomegalovirus retinitis. *J Ocul Pharmacol Ther* 2007; **23**: 264–274.

156. Eljarrat-Binstock E, Domb AJ. Iontophoresis: A non-invasive ocular drug delivery. *J Control Release* 2006; **110**: 479–489.

157. Cavalli R, Gasco MR, Chetoni P et al. Solid lipid nanoparticles (SLN) as ocular delivery system for tobramycin. *Int J Pharm* 2002; **238**: 241–245.

158. Irache JM, Merodio M, Arnedo A et al. Albumin nanoparticles for the intravitreal delivery of anticytomegaloviral drugs. *Mini Rev Med Chem* 2005; **5**: 293–305.

159. Xu J, Wang Y, Li Y et al. Inhibitory efficacy of intravitreal dexamethasone acetate-loaded PLGA nanoparticles on choroidal neovascularization in a laser-induced rat model. *J Ocul Pharmacol Ther* 2007; **23**: 527–540.

160. Motwani SK, Chopra S, Talegaonkar S et al. Chitosan–sodium alginate nanoparticles as submicroscopic reservoirs for ocular delivery: Formulation, optimisation and in vitro characterisation. *Eur J Pharm Biopharm* 2008; **68**: 513–525.

161. Carrasquillo KG, Ricker JA, Rigas IK et al. Controlled delivery of the anti-VEGF aptamer EYE001 with poly(lactic-*co*-glycolic)acid microspheres. *Invest Ophthalmol Vis Sci* 2003; **44**: 290–299.

162. Eljarrat-Binstock E, Orucov F, Aldouby Y et al. Charged nanoparticles delivery to the eye using hydrogel iontophoresis. *J Control Release* 2008; **126**: 156–161.

163. Cai X, Conley S, Naash M. Nanoparticle applications in ocular gene therapy. *Vision Res* 2008; **48**: 319–324.

164. Tong YC, Chang SF, Liu CY et al. Eye drop delivery of nano-polymeric micelle formulated genes with cornea-specific promoters. *J Gene Med* 2007; **9**: 956–966.

165. Mo Y, Barnett ME, Takemoto D et al. Human serum albumin nanoparticles for efficient delivery of Cu, Zn superoxide dismutase gene. *Mol Vis* 2007; **13**: 746–757.

166. Farjo R, Skaggs J, Quiambao AB et al. Efficient non-viral ocular gene transfer with compacted DNA nanoparticles. *PLoS ONE* 2006; **1**: e38.

167. Diebold Y, Jarrin M, Saez V et al. Ocular drug delivery by liposome–chitosan nanoparticle complexes (LCS-NP). *Biomaterials* 2007; **28**: 1553–1564.

168. Attama AA, Muller-Goymann CC. Investigation of surface-modified solid lipid nanocontainers formulated with a heterolipid-templated homolipid. *Int J Pharm* 2007; **334**: 179–189.

169. De TK, Bergey EJ, Chung SJ et al. Polycarboxylic acid nanoparticles for ophthalmic drug delivery: An ex vivo evaluation with human cornea. *J Microencapsul* 2004; **21**: 841–855.

170. Bourges JL, Gautier SE, Delie F et al. Ocular drug delivery targeting the retina and retinal pigment epithelium using polylactide nanoparticles. *Invest Ophthalmol Vis Sci* 2003; **44**: 3562–3569.

171. Giannavola C, Bucolo C, Maltese A et al. Influence of preparation conditions on acyclovir-loaded poly-D,L-lactic acid nanospheres and effect of PEG coating on ocular drug bioavailability. *Pharm Res* 2003; **20**: 584–590.

172. Shen Y, Tu J. Preparation and ocular pharmacokinetics of ganciclovir liposomes. *AAPS J* 2007; **9**: E371–E377.

173. Lajavardi L, Bochot A, Camelo S et al. Downregulation of endotoxin-induced uveitis by intravitreal injection of vasoactive intestinal Peptide encapsulated in liposomes. *Invest Ophthalmol Vis Sci* 2007; **48**: 3230–3238.

174. Budai L, Hajdu M, Budai M et al. Gels and liposomes in optimized ocular drug delivery: Studies on ciprofloxacin formulations. *Int J Pharm* 2007; **343**: 34–40.

175. Hathout RM, Mansour S, Mortada ND et al. Liposomes as an ocular delivery system for acetazolamide: In vitro and in vivo studies. *AAPS PharmSciTech* 2007; **8**: 1.

176. Cortesi R, Argnani R, Esposito E et al. Cationic liposomes as potential carriers for ocular administration of peptides with anti-herpetic activity. *Int J Pharm* 2006; **317**: 90–100.

177. Nagarsenker MS, Londhe VY, Nadkarni GD. Preparation and evaluation of liposomal formulations of tropicamide for ocular delivery. *Int J Pharm* 1999; **190**: 63–71.

178. Bochot A, Mashhour B, Puisieux F et al. Comparison of the ocular distribution of a model oligonucleotide after topical instillation in rabbits of conventional and new dosage forms. *J Drug Target* 1998; **6**: 309–313.

179. Kaur IP, Garg A, Singla AK et al. Vesicular systems in ocular drug delivery: An overview. *Int J Pharm* 2004; **269**: 1–14.

180. Vyas SP, Mysore N, Jaitely V et al. Discoidal niosome based controlled ocular delivery of timolol maleate. *Pharmazie* 1998; **53**: 466–469.

181. Vaka SR, Sammeta SM, Day LB et al. Transcorneal iontophoresis for delivery of ciprofloxacin hydrochloride. *Curr Eye Res* 2008; **33**: 661–667.

182. Souied EH, Reid SN, Piri NI et al. Non-invasive gene transfer by iontophoresis for therapy of an inherited retinal degeneration. *Exp Eye Res* 2008; **87**: 168–175.

183. Eljarrat-Binstock E, Orucov F, Frucht-Pery J et al. Methylprednisolone delivery to the back of the eye using hydrogel iontophoresis. *J Ocul Pharmacol Ther* 2008; **24**: 344–350.

184. Eljarrat-Binstock E, Domb AJ, Orucov F et al. In vitro and in vivo evaluation of carboplatin delivery to the eye using hydrogel-iontophoresis. *Curr Eye Res* 2008; **33**: 269–275.

185. Raiskup-Wolf F, Eljarrat-Binstock E, Rehak M et al. Transcorneal and transscleral iontophoresis of the dexamethasone phosphate into the rabbit eye. *Cesk Slov Oftalmol* 2007; **63**: 360–368.
186. Eljarrat-Binstock E, Domb AJ, Orucov F et al. Methotrexate delivery to the eye using transscleral hydrogel iontophoresis. *Curr Eye Res* 2007; **32**: 639–646.
187. Frucht-Pery J, Raiskup F, Mechoulam H et al. Iontophoretic treatment of experimental pseudomonas keratitis in rabbit eyes using gentamicin-loaded hydrogels. *Cornea* 2006; **25**: 1182–1186.
188. Andrieu-Soler C, Doat M, Halhal M et al. Enhanced oligonucleotide delivery to mouse retinal cells using iontophoresis. *Mol Vis* 2006; **12**: 1098–1107.
189. Berdugo M, Valamanesh F, Andrieu C et al. Delivery of antisense oligonucleotide to the cornea by iontophoresis. *Antisense Nucleic Acid Drug Dev* 2003; **13**: 107–114.
190. Vollmer DL, Szlek MA, Kolb K et al. In vivo transscleral iontophoresis of amikacin to rabbit eyes. *J Ocul Pharmacol Ther* 2002; **18**: 549–558.
191. Asahara T, Shinomiya K, Naito T et al. Induction of gene into the rabbit eye by iontophoresis: Preliminary report. *Jpn J Ophthalmol* 2001; **45**: 31–39.
192. Voigt M, de Kozak Y, Halhal M et al. Down-regulation of NOSII gene expression by iontophoresis of anti-sense oligonucleotide in endotoxin-induced uveitis. *Biochem Biophys Res Commun* 2002; **295**: 336–341.
193. Davies JB, Ciavatta VT, Boatright JH et al. Delivery of several forms of DNA, DNA–RNA hybrids, and dyes across human sclera by electrical fields. *Mol Vis* 2003; **9**: 569–578.

Part VI

Polymer–Drug Conjugates and Micelles

17 Injectable Polymers for Regional Drug Delivery

*Rajendra P. Pawar, Niteen R. Shinde, Narsinha M. Andurkar,
Satish A. Dake, and Abraham J. Domb*

CONTENTS

17.1　INTRODUCTION

Advances in drug development and site-specific delivery have evolved in several phases. It began with the botanical phase of human civilization, via the synthetic chemistry era, and is presently in the biotechnology era. Researchers are continuously developing new and more powerful drugs. Increasing attention is being given to the delivery methods of these active substances. Drug delivery systems transport drugs in the biological system. The delivery system not only carries a single or multiple therapeutic agents, but also performs certain functions to increase the effectiveness of drug therapy.

The use of combinatorial chemistry and its advances in screening, functional genomics, and proteomics have increased the number of therapeutic moieties. Suitable strategies have to be adopted to deliver these potent molecules. The most conventional routes of administration are oral ingestion and intravenous (IV) and intramuscular (IM) injections. These routes are used to distribute drug molecules to all parts of the body, including targeted as well as nontargeted sites. The distribution of drugs to nontargeted sites may cause toxicity to healthy tissues; however, the drug is only required at specific sites in the body. In addition, conventionally delivered drugs get diluted in the blood and body fluids, resulting in an insufficient drug concentration at the diseased site. Therefore, localized drug delivery is most suitable for the delivery of pharmacologically active compounds. Using localized delivery, a lower dose of active compound may be administered. Hence, the chances of systemic adverse effects are reduced or completely eliminated; short half-life therapeutic agents, such as proteins and peptides, and other biologically unstable biomolecules like nucleic acids and oligonucleotides have been delivered locally with negligible loss in therapeutic activity.

A number of strategies have been explored to deliver drugs to a specific site or body compartment. Site-specific drug delivery using polymeric carriers is one of the simplest and most useful approaches. The polymers used for localized application play an important structural and functional role. A range of the polymers has been developed, with the focus on biodegradable polymers and copolymers for use in drug delivery systems.

Targeted delivery has been achieved by the use of biodegradable and biocompatible polymeric drug delivery systems. Higher demand for these polymers has led to tremendous advancement in polymer sciences. These include chemical modifications, synthesis of copolymers, and the development of new delivery systems. *In situ* drug delivery systems have been developed to address the need for prolonged and controlled drug administration. In polymeric implant systems, several biodegradable products including drugs are injected into the body through a syringe. After injection, these materials solidify to form a semisolid depot.[1] Various strategies have been explored to achieve this goal, including solvent removal,[2] *in situ* cross-linking,[3,4] and temperature-responsive polymeric systems.[5–7]

Fast growing R&D and continuous improvement in polymeric materials have played an important role in the advancement of this technology. In the last few years, the increasing number of publications and patents in this area show a considerable increase in the interest of this technology. Numerous drug delivery systems have been reported, including implants and injectable systems such as microspheres and *in situ* gelling systems. Drug delivery systems have been successfully administered in neurological disorders, vascular complications, bone infections, retinal diseases, and brain tumors.

17.2　IMPLANTS

Injectable solid implants are devices in which the drug is dispersed throughout a polymer matrix. They are designed to release the drug at a specific rate. A polymeric matrix controls the release rate of the drug from the implant. This dosage form is suitable over a prolonged period of time.

Long-acting implants have been developed with both biodegradable and nonbiodegradable polymers. Biodegradable implants are degraded and eliminated by the body after drug release.

Nonbiodegradable implants can be retrieved either during or after drug release. The main advantage of these systems is their small size, which has been utilized for easier administration and local delivery. Other advantages of these systems include the potential for high drug loading and the low risk of dose dumping.

In situ forming systems have been extensively used for the delivery of various therapeutic agents, including small molecules, proteins, peptides,[7] polysaccharides, and nucleic acid–based drugs. Numerous approaches have been utilized to prepare *in situ* setting systems. These include solvent removal for the depot formation by precipitation, *in situ* cross-linking by heating, irradiation or ionic interaction, and temperature-responsive polymeric systems.

On the basis of the solidification process, these injectable implant systems are categorized into six types: (1) thermoplastic pastes, (2) *in situ* cross-linked systems, (3) *in situ* precipitates, (4) thermally induced gelling systems, (5) *in situ* solidifying organogels, and (6) hydrophobic fatty acid–based injectable pastes. An ideal *in situ* forming drug delivery system should possess good syringe ability and form a (semi-)solid depot at the injection site.

17.2.1 Types of *In Situ* Depot Systems

In situ forming systems have been extensively used for the delivery of various therapeutic agents including small drug molecules, proteins, peptides,[7] polysaccharides, and nucleic acid–based drugs. These systems cover every segment of the pharmaceutical field. Numerous approaches have been utilized to prepare *in situ* setting systems. They include the solvent removal of the depot formation by precipitation, *in situ* cross-linking by heating, irradiation or ionic interaction, and temperature-responsive polymeric systems. On the basis of the solidification process, these injectable implant systems are categorized into six types as discussed below.

17.2.1.1 Thermoplastic Pastes

Thermoplastic pastes are polymeric systems that are injected into the body in melted form and turned to a semisolid at body temperature. Usually, they are low melting polymers (with a melting point ranging from 25°C to 65°C) with low intrinsic viscosity. Systems having an intrinsic viscosity below 0.05 dL/g do not show a delayed release profile, whereas viscosity above 0.08 dL/g creates problems in administration as they become too viscous to pass through a needle. Monomers such as D,L-lactide, glycolide, ε-caprolactone, trimethylene carbonate, dioxanone, and ortho esters have been used in thermoplastic pastes.[7] These monomers are biocompatible and, therefore, have been used in the development of new materials for drug delivery.

Thermoplastic biodegradable polymeric paste formulations have been prepared using a triblock system composed of poly(D,L-lactide)-block–poly(ethylene glycol)–block-poly(D,L-lactide) (PLA–PEG–PLA) and have been studied for paclitaxel delivery.[8] Upon subcutaneous (SC) injection, this system releases the drug over a period of 2 months by the diffusion and polymer erosion process. It has been shown to reduce the side effects of paclitaxel as compared with the system administration of Taxol®. However, its melting point is above 60°C. Administration at such a high temperature causes pain at the injection site, and increases the risk of necrosis and scar tissue formation.[1]

Polycaprolactone (PCL) and its blends with methoxypolyetylene glycol (MePEG) were used in surgical pastes, which showed a decrease in the melting point of PCL upon the addition of MePEG and facilitated administration at a lower temperature. Furthermore, MePEG acts as a plasticizer and reduces the tensile strength of PCL. MePEG diffused out of the polymer matrix and enhanced water uptake by PCL, without increasing the *in vitro* release of paclitaxel. A slightly modified polymer composition in thermoplastic paste was tested in human prostate LNCaP tumors, which were grown subcutaneously in castrated athymic mice and offered promising results.[9]

A class of highly flexible thermoplastic elastomers were synthesized from PEO/PLA/-poly(ether–ester–urethane) multiblock copolymers. Triblock copolymer PLA–PEO–PLA was synthesized by the ring-opening polymerization of L-lactide using hexamethylene diisocyanate (HDI), wherein urethane groups were generated along the polymeric backbone. Amorphous poly(ethylene oxide) (PEO) chains work as a molecular spring and the crystalline PLA blocks formed strong noncovalent cross-linking domains. The hard blocks formed strong domains and were utilized in cross-linking. The soft, conformationally flexible segments render with remarkable flexibility and extendibility. These highly flexible thermoplastic elastomers attained tensile strength as high as 30 MPa and elongation at break levels well above 1000%. Furthermore, the crystalline and hydrophobic PLA domains are enabled to retain strength (8–9 MPa), even in a hydrated state.[10]

Versatile poly(orthoester) (POE)s are also used as thermoplastic pastes. Their consistency and controlling ability depends upon the nature of diols used. The viscous semisolid materials are directly injected for localized drug action. This system is mainly used for ocular drug delivery, in the treatment of periodontal diseases, and for veterinary applications. The POE-based tetracycline delivery system was obtained by solubilizing a tetracycline base and poly(orthoester)-lactic acid POE95LA5 in an organic solvent followed by drying and compression molding. It resulted in a viscous formulation. These systems were designed to be placed or injected into the periodontal pocket to maintain therapeutic concentrations for 14 days (Figure 17.1).[11]

> Upon SC injection of thermoplastic polymeric paste formulations of paclitaxel prepared using PLA–PEG–PLA triblock polymer, the drug releases over a period of 2 months by diffusion and polymer erosion process. It has shown to reduce side effects of paclitaxel as compared to the systemic administration of Taxol®.

17.2.1.2 *In Situ* Cross-Linked Systems

The cross-linking processes between polymeric chains can be used for the *in situ* formation of solid polymer systems or gels. *In situ* cross-linking proceeds via a free radical mechanism, usually initiated by heat or photon absorption, or by ionic interactions between small cations and polymer anions.[1] Depending on the source of the cross-link, these systems are categorized into thermosets, photo-cross-linked gels, and ion-mediated gelation.

Thermosetting polymers are molded in a specific shape only on heating. A macromolecular network is formed through covalent cross-links. Limited information is available in this area because of the several limitations and adverse effects associated with this system.[1] Biodegradable copolymers of D,L-lactide or L-lactide with ε-caprolactone were used with a polyol initiator to form a thermosetting system for prosthetic implants and lower the release of drug from the delivery system. However, certain disadvantages were associated with this system including a burst release during

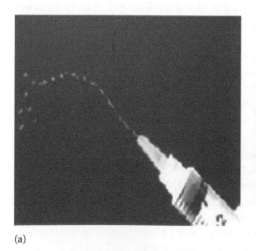
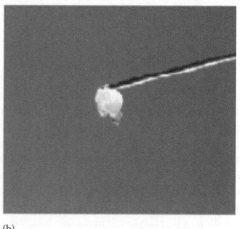

(a)   (b)

FIGURE 17.1 Typical appearance of a periodontal site after the administration of the delivery system POE/TB. (From Igor, G. and Bo, M., *Smart Polymer: Applications in Biotechnology and Biomedicines*, CRC Press, Boca Raton, FL, 2008.)

the first hour and the generation of free radicals causing tissue injury. Free radical producing agents may promote tumor growth. Furthermore, the heat released during curing may cause necrosis of the surrounding tissues.[1]

Photo-cross-linked gels are preferred over chemically initiated thermoset systems. In this approach, the photo-curing process is done through fiber optic cables immediately after the introduction of the polymer to a desired site via injection.[1] A novel supramolecular α-CD$_{[n17]}$s gelation is being threaded onto an oligo(L-lactide)–poly(ethylene glycol)–oligo(L-lactide) (LA–PEG–LA) amphiphilic copolymer finished with$_{[n18]}$ methacryloyl moieties.[12] They could be photopolymerized *in situ* by UV irradiation with a photo initiator to chemically cross-linked biodegradable hydrogels with the markedly improved mechanical strength. The experimental results reveal that the swelling ratio and the *in vitro* degradation of these supramolecular hydrogels are different from those without α-CDs.

Succinic acid and PEG-based polyester polyol macromers and their acrylates were synthesized.[4] The acrylate end groups polymerized on UV irradiation in the presence of a photo-initiator. Water equilibrium swell, mechanical strength, and *in vitro* degradation of the cross-linked matrices reflected a trend based on equilibrium swelling in water, which increased with the increasing PEG chain length. The addition of *N*-vinyl pyrrolidinone as a reactive diluent increased the tensile strength of these formulations. *In vitro* burst strength determinations suggested that they are quite useful as tissue sealants. Lastly, *in vitro* release studies with sulfamethoxazole suggest that they can also be used for the localized controlled delivery of antibiotics over a short period of time (3 days).

Ion-mediated gelation has been achieved through a naturally occurring polymer alginate, form gel in the presence of divalent calcium ions. Recently, sodium alginate-calcium chloride hydrogel was used to deliver combined therapeutic modalities, i.e., radiation (^{188}Re) and chemotherapy (cisplatin) in a tumor-bearing animal model.[3] A delay in tumor growth was observed in the ^{188}Re-hydrogel group as compared with the ^{188}Re control. The use of hydrogel prolonged survival more than two times that of untreated groups. Calcium performs a dual function in this system as it cross-links with sodium alginate and forms a complex with ^{188}Re, leading to gel formation and lowering the release of cisplatin coupled with the trapping of ^{188}Re at the site of injection. The problems associated with the use of calcium alginates in drug delivery devices are its potential immunogenicity and long *in vivo* degradation time.[13]

A new class of injectable and bioabsorbable supramolecular hydrogels derived from PEOs and α-cyclodextrin (α-CD) have been studied for controlled drug delivery.[14] PEO was fixed$_{[n20]}$ in the inner cavity of cyclodextrines to form necklace-like supramolecular structures. A chemical cross-linking reagent was not required in this complex formation. These hydrogels were thixotropic and reversible. On agitation, the viscosity of the hydrogel greatly diminished, which renders the hydrogel injectable even through a fine needle. On cooling at room temperature, the hydrogel regained its viscosity. Fluorescein isothiocyanate-labeled dextran (dextran-FITC) was entrapped in these hydrogels. The dextran-FITC release was prolonged to 5 days *in vitro*.

A drug-loaded nanoparticulate system forming a hydrogel in the presence of ions was reported.[15] The positively charged surface of nanoparticles was responsible for the ion-mediated gelation process, since they were formulated using a novel amine-modified branched polyester. These polymers consisted of a poly(vinyl alcohol) backbone modified with amines such as diethylaminopropylamine (DEAEA), dimethylaminopropylamine (DMAPA), and diethylaminoethylamine (DEAEA) using a *N,N'*-carbonyldiimidazole (CDI) linker. The hydrophilic backbones were grafted with poly(D,L-lactide-*co*-glycolide) (PLGA) side chains of 10–20 repeating units. A degradation time from several hours to months was achieved by altering the degree of amine-substitution, PLGA side-chain lengths, and/or the graft density.

17.2.1.3 *In Situ* Polymer Precipitation

An injectable drug delivery depot can be obtained by polymer precipitation from its solution. The solvent is removed by a change in temperature or pH.[1] In the solvent removal method, an injectable implant system consists of a hydrophobic biodegradable polymer dissolved in a physiologically compatible solvent. Upon injecting the polymeric implant, *in situ* precipitation of the polymer takes place by the diffusional loss of solvent into the aqueous environment. The problem associated with this system is the burst release, which occurs in the first few hours because of the lag time between the injection and the solid implant formation.

A PLGA/*N*-methyl-2-pyrrolidinine (NMP) depot system was designed and utilized for protein release. The protein release rate was directly related to the phase inversion kinetics and morphological characteristics of the membrane2. Additive increases the burst effect with maintaining the morphology constant. Uniform and more desirable protein release rates were achieved by controlling the aqueous miscibility of the depot. In depots, the concentration is reduced with the lowering of the solvent affinity of the polymer, resulting in interconnected polymer-lean phase structures. Mass transfer kinetics within the polymer rich phase controls the protein release.[16]

The effect of the pluronic® concentration and PEO block length on the phase inversion and *in vitro* protein release kinetics of injectable PDLA/pluronic® depots have been studied. An increased pluronic concentration and PEO block length resulted in a burst release, though the release profiles retained the typical burst-type shape. The burst effect is reduced because the hydrophilic PEO segments extend into the interconnected release pathway and reduce open pores through which the entrapped protein diffuses. A transition from an extended-release profile occurred by increasing the pluronic® concentration beyond a critical concentration. A polymer-lean[n26] phase with the pluronic® material forms a diffusion barrier within the entire interconnected release pathway, thus extending the protein release to minimize the burst.[17]

17.2.1.4 Thermally Induced Gelling Systems

Temperature is widely used to cause gelling of responsive polymer systems. The change in temperature is applicable both *in vitro* and *in vivo*. The polymer implants show thermo-reversible sol–gel transitions characterized by lower critical solution temperature (LCST).[18,19] These polymers are liquid at room temperature and form a gel at body temperature.

The thermosensitive polymer poly(*N*-isopropyl acryl amide) (poly-NIPAAM) exhibits a sharp LCST of 32°C.[19] Unfortunately, poly-NIPAAM is not suitable for biomedical applications because of its nonbiodegradable[1] nature and cytotoxicity. Triblock poly(ethylene oxide)–poly(propylene oxide)–poly(ethylene oxide) copolymers (PEO–PPO–PEO), commonly known as poloxamers or pluronics®, form gel at body temperature. The drawbacks of poloxamer gels include weak mechanical strength, rapid erosion, and nonbiodegradability.[20]

Low molecular weight, thermosensitive, biodegradable triblock copolymers (ABA and BAB) were developed by MacroMed, Inc. wherein, A represents the hydrophobic polyester blocks and B represents the hydrophilic PEG blocks (ReGel®). These water-soluble copolymers show reverse thermal gelation properties.[21] OncoGel®, an injectable controlled release formulation of paclitaxel, demonstrated efficacy in the treatment of esophageal and breast cancers[n30].

The release of several drugs, including paclitaxel and proteins (such as pGH, G-CSF, insulin, and rHbsAg[n31]), has been reported from the ReGel® formulation.[7] The gel provided a controlled release of paclitaxel over approximately 50 days. Direct intratumoral injection of ReGel®/paclitaxel (OncoGel®) resulted in the slow clearance of paclitaxel from the injection site, with minimal distribution into any organ. The OncoGel® treatment groups exhibited a dose response equal or superior to the systemic treatments. Hydrophobic paclitaxel and cyclosporine A showed significantly higher solubility (400- to >2000-fold) in ReGel®. Additionally, the chemical stability of these drugs in aqueous co-solvent solutions was substantially improved in the presence of ReGel®.

The triblock copolymer of poly(lactide-*co*-glycolide)–poly(ethylene glycol)–poly(lactide-*co*-glycolide) (PLGA–PEG–PLGA) is used as a drug delivery carrier for the continuous release of human insulin.[6] This formulation is used to achieve basal insulin levels over a week by a single insulin injection. This system is also used for the sustained delivery of glucagon like peptide-1 (GLP) for the treatment of type 2 diabetes mellitus.[5]

Phase sensitive and thermosensitive smart polymer-based delivery systems have been used for delivering testosterone.[22] Poly(lactide) (PLA) with a mixture of benzyl benzoate (BB) and benzyl alcohol (BA) solvents was used in phase sensitive polymeric delivery systems. The effects of the formulation on testosterone release were investigated in different solvent systems and at different drug loading levels. A series of low-molecular-weight PLGA–PEG–PLGA triblock copolymers with different lactide/glycolide (LA/GA, 2.0–3.5) ratios were studied to control the release of testosterone.

A poly(caprolactone-*b*-ethylene glycol-*b*-caprolactone) (PCL–PEG–PCL) triblock copolymer underwent a temperature-dependent sol–gel–sol transition. Both PEG–PCL–PEG and PCL–PEG–PCL polymers are used in biodegradable thermogelling systems. In this system, they are lyophilized in a powder form. It makes them easy to handle and to redissolve to a clear solution. They show a little syneresis[n34] through the gel phase.[23]

17.2.1.5 *In Situ* Solidifying Organogels

Organogels or oleaginous gels are made up of water-insoluble amphiphilic lipids, which swell in water and form various types of lyotropic liquid crystals. The structural properties of the lipid, temperature, nature of the incorporated drug, and the amount of water determines the nature of the liquid crystalline phase formed. Primarily, glycerol esters of fatty acids such as glycerol monooleate, glycerol monopalmitostearate, and glycerol monolinoleate have been used. These esters are wax at room temperature and form a cubic liquid crystal phase upon injection into an aqueous medium. The cubic phase consists of a three-dimensional lipid bilayer separated by water channels. The liquid crystalline structure is highly viscous and behaves like a gel.[1] Several drugs have been delivered using these gels. The glycerol monooleate system was used for the delivery of somatostatin subcutaneously in rabbits.

The water content of the organogel formed is approximately 35%. The organogel lowered the release of hydrophilic drugs. Formulations comprising of interferon-α in aluminum monostearate and peanut oil have been developed. The glycerol palmitostearate (Precirol®) system was employed to deliver the lipophilic drugs levonorgestrel and ethinyl estradiol. The *in vitro* release of levonorgestrel was slowed for 14 days, while *in vivo* studies of levonorgestrel in the organogel injected subcutaneously into rabbits demonstrated an estrus blockage for up to 40 days.[1]

Organogels are a promising injectable delivery system for lipophilic compounds. However, it has some disadvantages. The purity of the waxes and the stability of the oils are the major issues of concern. Oils need a stabilizer, antioxidant, and preservative to increase their shelf life and stability. Moreover, the difference between the melting point of waxes and oils makes this system susceptible to phase separation. Another drawback of this system is that it needs a higher temperature to mix the oil and the wax phase. Temperatures of up to 60°C for 30 min have been used.

> The organogel lowered the release of hydrophilic drugs when water content of the organogel formed was approximately 35%.

17.2.1.6 Hydrophobic Fatty Acid–Based Injectable Pastes

Recently, poly(sebacic-*co*-ricinoleic acid) fatty acid biodegradable polymers were reported.[24–26] These polymers are hydrophobic in nature and are obtained from natural fatty acids. They can be used to entrap both hydrophobic and hydrophilic drugs. Polymers P(SA:RA) having 70% and higher ricinoleic acid content resemble *in situ* forming organogels. The high content of water in organogel leads to a relatively faster release of hydrophilic drugs (6 h for somatostatin), while P(SA:RA) in 3:7 w/w ratio release of hydrophilic drugs (5FU, cisplatin) lasted for 5–7 days. Polymers P(SA:RA) are suitable for hydrophobic drugs.

A three-dimensional structure of this polymer explained the hydrogen bonding between the carboxylic end groups, which resulted in slow hydrolytic degradation. The same mechanism was also suggested for lecithin bridging by hydrogen bonds in the organogel, where lipid functional groups exhibit an affinity for solvents. This polymeric system is less sensitive with respect to the purity of the polymer or the solvents. Furthermore, drugs may be incorporated by trituration at room temperature without applying heat.[26]

17.3   BIODEGRADABLE POLYMERIC CARRIERS IN REGIONAL THERAPY

Developments in the field of polymer science have resulted in the development of a wide range of biodegradable polymers of natural and synthetic origin possessing specific properties beneficial to the desired applications. Natural biodegradable polymers like chitin, chitosan, alginate, gelatin, and hyaluronan and synthetic polymers, such as polyesters, PCL, POEs, polyanhydrides, etc., are customized for regional therapy. Synthetic polymers are preferred for regional therapy, since they are chemically pure and potentially have low immunogenicity. Also their physicochemical properties are predictable, reproducible, and easier to modify. They can be fabricated according to the need into wafers, flexible films, or linked beads and rods to fit diseased sites. However, the advantages of polymers' usefulness must be weighed against the risks. It is associated with drug release dumping or drug release failure. The toxicity of the polymer, its biodegradability, degradation products, and biocompatibility have to be evaluated. The following sections provide a brief overview of the biodegradable polymers used *in situ* to form a drug delivery system.[20]

17.3.1   Natural Polymers

The properties of natural polymers have been tailored to suit their application in site-specific drug delivery. Chitosan has been explored in drug delivery, tissue engineering, and gene delivery. Alginates have been used to form microparticles and nanoparticulates gels. Natural polymers have also been used in combination with each other with other synthetic polymers to achieve better control of drug delivery.

17.3.1.1   Chitosan

Chitosan is a polysaccharide derived from chitin by the deacetylation process. It is a copolymer of *N*-acetyl-glucosamine and *N*-glucosamine units randomly distributed throughout the polymeric chain (Table 17.1).[27] Biocompatibility, biodegradability, nonbioactivity, low toxicity, and low allergenicity make chitosan attractive for several biomedical applications,[28] including drug-delivery systems, tissue engineering,[29–31] and orthopedics.[32,33] Chitin and chitin–pluronic® F-108 microparticles were used to encapsulate paclitaxel for localized delivery in solid tumors.[34] Chitosan gel beads and microspheres were chemically cross-linked with glutaraldehyde and ethylene glycol diglycidyl ether

TABLE 17.1
List of Implantable Drug Delivery Products

Drug	Product Name	Manufacturing Company
Doxycycline	Atridox	CollaGenex
Leuprolide	Eligard	Sanofi
BCNU	Gliadel	MGI Pharmaceuticals, Inc.
Leuprolide	Luprogel	Medigene AG
Norgestrel	Norplant	Wyeth Ayerst
Buserelin	Profact Depot	Aventis
Histerlin	Vantas	Valera
Leuprolide	Viadur	ALZA
Goserelin	Zoladex	AstraZeneca

for stabilization. Recently, their polyelectrolyte complexes have been proposed for drug delivery systems. Cationic chitosan forms complexes with nontoxic multivalent anionic counterions such as polyphosphate[35] and sodium alginate.[36] Moreover, matrices of polyglycolide chitosan were found to have high strength and porosity.[33] An injectable thermogel has also been prepared by grafting PEG onto the chitosan backbone and has been explored for drug release *in vitro* using bovine serum albumin as a model protein.[37]

17.3.1.2 Hyaluronic Acid

Hyaluronic acid (HA) is a polysaccharide composed of alternating D-glucuronic acid and *N*-acetyl-D-glucosamine (Table 17.2). It is a linear, uniform, and unbranched molecule made up of the same multiple disaccharide units.[38] It is distributed throughout the extracellular matrix, connective tissues, and organs of all higher animals. HA is nonimmunogenic. Hence, it is used as an ideal biomaterial for tissue engineering and drug as well as gene delivery.

For example, HA was used as a substitute for a vitreous body in retinal-reattachment surgery.[39] A variety of hydrophobic and chemical cross-linking strategies have been reported to produce insoluble or gel-like HA materials. The stability and cytotoxicity of disulfide cross-linked thiolated HA films *in vitro* and the biocompatibility of these films *in vivo* have been reported.[40] In localized drug delivery, microspheres and thin films of hyaluronan benzyl esters have been found more suitable for drug and peptide delivery. The hydrophobic, mucoadhesive properties of HA facilitated intranasal, buccal, ocular, and vaginal delivery. High-viscosity gels of HA and the nonsteroidal anti-inflammatory drug (NSAID) naproxen sodium prevented postsurgical tendon adhesions.[41] Recently, regulatory approval in the United States, Canada, and Europe was granted for 3% w/w diclofenac in 2.5% w/w HA gel Solarazc® for the topical skin treatment of actinic keratoses.[42] Various glucocorticoid and HA formulations are currently available in the market for intra-articular drug injection to treat osteoarthritis.[43]

17.3.1.3 Alginates

Alginates are the linear unbranched polysaccharides having 1,4-linkage between ß-D-mannuronic acid and α-L-glucuronic acid residues.[44] Commercial alginates are extracted from brown algae (kelp) *Laminaria hyperborea*, *Ascophyllum nodosum*, and *Macrocystis pyrifera*. Multivalent calcium cations form gels with alginates upon forming a complex with carboxylic acid groups. This brings glucuronate chains together stoichiometrically in an egg-box-like conformation, leaving the mannuronate intact.[45]

Alginate beads prepared by the cross-linking of calcium ions with sodium alginate polymer were evaluated as biodegradable implants containing teicoplanin for the prevention or treatment of bone infections.[46] Also, 5-fluorouracil (5-FU) alginate beads were prepared by the gelation of alginate with calcium cations. In this system, polymer concentration and drug loading affected the release of 5-FU.[47] In addition, a novel hydrogel formulation of alginate was designed for the local delivery of antineoplastic agents methotrexate, doxorubicin, and mitoxantrone. It allowed the release of single or combined antineoplastic agents for localized delivery.[48]

17.3.1.4 Gelatin

Gelatin is a natural polymer derived from collagen.[49] Its high biodegradability and biocompatibility makes it suitable for use in pharmaceutical and medical applications. It is clinically safe and can preserve the bioactivity of the therapeutic agent. It possesses unique gelation property, which may be modified during the processing.

Numerous applications have been studied for gelatin-mediated drug delivery, including bone infection and repair and cancer chemotherapy. It provided the controlled release of cisplatin *in vivo* from a biodegradable hydrogel.[50] It was used for the trans-tissue delivery of ciplatin and adriamycin from a biodegradable hydrogel, resulting in improved antitumor effect.[50]

TABLE 17.2
Representative Structures of Natural Polymers

Polymer	Structure
Chitosan	
Hyaluronic acid	
Alginate	
Gelatin	
Poly(hydroxy-alkanoate)s	

Source: Igor, G. and Bo, M., *Smart Polymer: Applications in Biotechnology and Biomedicines*, CRC Press, Boca Raton, FL, 2008. With permission.

17.3.1.5 Poly(hydroxyalkanoate)s

Poly(hydroxyalkanoate)s (PHAs) are the thermoplastic polymers obtained from various bacteria that harbor them as intracellular reserve materials. The type of bacteria and their growth conditions determine the chemical composition and molecular weight of the PHAs. Isolated PHAs have interesting properties such as biodegradability and biocompatibility. Depending on the size of the R group and the composition of the polymer, they are rigid and brittle or flexible plastics with high strength and elasticity.

The applications of PHAs include implants, as scaffolds in tissue engineering, or as drug carriers. For example, a localized formulation of gentamicin PHA prevented implant-related Staphylococcus infections.[51] Various copolyesters of 3-hydroxybutyrate, 3-hydroxyvalerate, 3-hydroxybutyrate, and 4-hydroxybutyrate have also been used in biodegradable implantable rods for the local delivery of antibiotics in chronic osteomyelitis therapy.[52]

17.3.2 SYNTHETIC POLYMERS

The controlled and modifiable properties of synthetically prepared biodegradable polymers make them the preferred material for localized drug delivery. This class of polymers comprises a broad family of polyesters such as poly(glycolic acid) (PGA), poly(lactic acid) (PLA), their (PGA and PLA) copolymers, PCL, polyanhydrides, and POE (Table 17.3). Copolymers and other materials of desired and reproducible characteristics are often used in drug delivery systems and tissue engineering. The copolymers of polyesters with amides, imides, urethanes, anhydrides, and ethers have been prepared to improve physical properties and control the degradation rate.

17.3.2.1 Polyesters

Biodegradable polyesters constitute the family of synthetic condensation polymers investigated in the 1930s.[53,54] PGA is a linear aliphatic polyester. It is widely used in clinical applications, especially for sutures. PGA sutures have been available under the trade name Dexon® since the 1970s. However, a practical drawback of the use of Dexon® is that it loses mechanical strength within 2–4 weeks after implantation. PGA has been also used for the design of internal bone-fixation devices like bone pins. These pins are available commercially under the trade name Biofix®.

Lactic acid is a chiral molecule and forms four types of morphologically different polymers: D-PLA and L-PLA, racemic form DL-PLA, and *meso*-PLA. *meso*-PLA is obtained from DL-lactide, which is rarely used in practice. D-PL and L-PLA are semi-crystalline solids, whereas optically inactive DL-PLA is amorphous in nature. A complete range of lactic acid and glycolic acid copolymers has been investigated.

PLA was used to design an injectable scaffold from microcarriers and cross-linked chitosan hydrogels. This injectable scaffold is used in tissue engineering particularly in orthopedics regenerative medicine.[55] Microparticles of PLA were also used to design injectable drug-loaded biodegradable devices that form *in situ*. The slow release of solvent from these implants in an aqueous medium resulted in less porous microparticles that reduced the initial drug release.[56]

The first commercial PLGA suture was Vicryl® (Polyglactin 910) and was composed of 8% PL–LA and 92% PGA. It has been studied as a substrate for biodegradation and a controlled-release matrix system. A biodegradable drug delivery system was developed for naltrexone hydrochloride from an injectable *in situ* forming PLGA implant. The additives inversely affected the drug release rate and solvent removal from the formulation.[57] Biodegradable PLGA injectable implants with microencapsulated *N*-acetylcysteine (NAC) were used for site-specific controlled NAC. This system was used as a chemopreventive agent for persons with previously excised head and neck cancers.[58]

> The first commercial PLGA suture was Vicryl® (Polyglactin 910), composed of 8% PL-LA and 92% PGA. It has been studied as a biodegradable controlled-release matrix system. A biodegradable drug delivery system was developed for naltrexone hydrochloride from an injectable *in situ* forming PLGA implant. The additives inversely affected drug release rate and solvent removal from the formulation.

TABLE 17.3
Representative Structures of Synthetic Polymers

Polymer	Structure

PLA

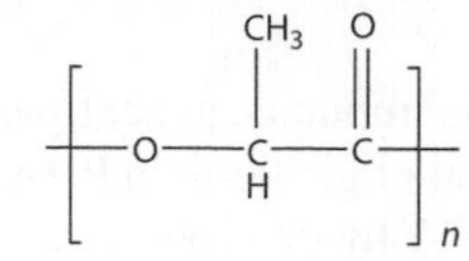

PGA

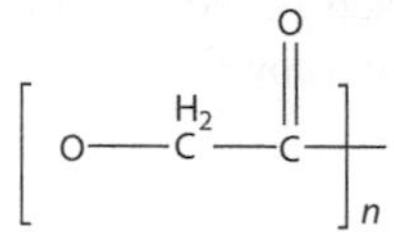

(PCPP-SA)

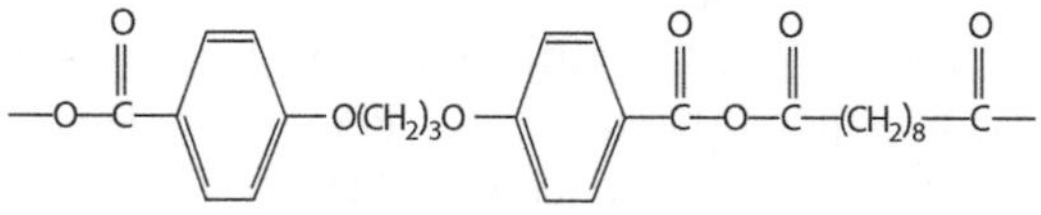

PCL

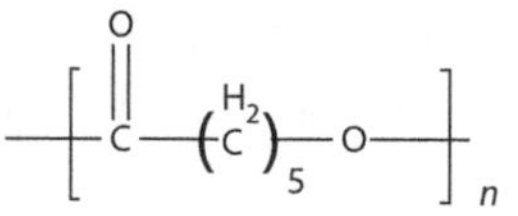

POE I

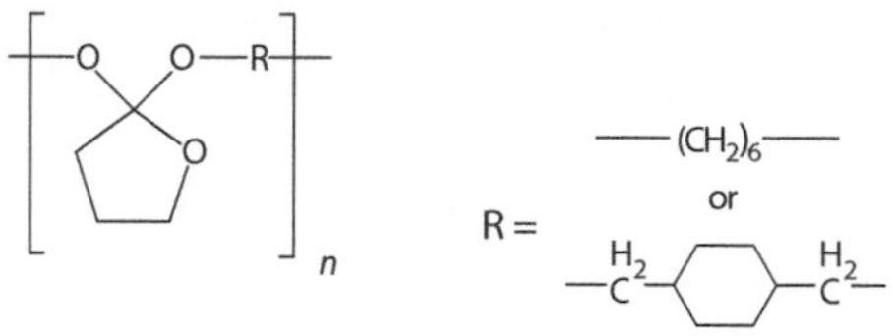

$$R = ---(CH_2)_6---$$
or

POE II

$$R = ---(CH_2)_8---$$
or

POE III

$$R = ---CH_3$$
$$R' = ---(CH_2)_4--- \text{ or } ---(CH_2)_6---$$

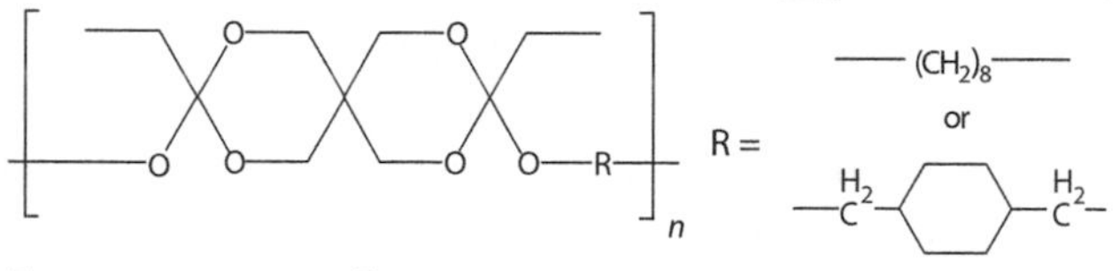

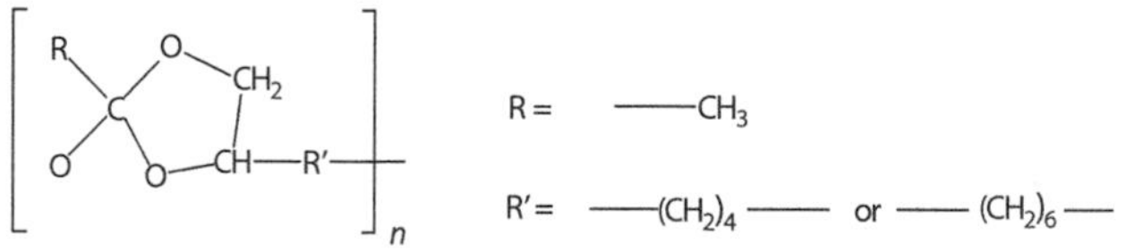

POE IV

$$R = ---H \text{ or } ---CH_3$$
$$R' = ---(CH_2)_{10}--- \text{ or } ---(CH_2)_{12}---$$

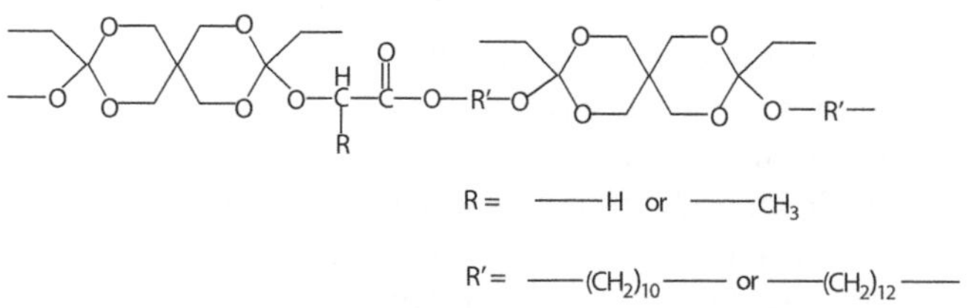

Source: Igor, G. and Bo, M., *Smart Polymer: Applications in Biotechnology and Biomedicines*, CRC Press, Boca Raton, FL, 2008. With permission.

17.3.2.2 Polyanhydrides

Polyanhydrides have been used for the sustained release of drugs. They are hydrolytically unstable and have nontoxic metabolites. The high hydrolytic reactivity of anhydride linkages controls the degradation rates of these bioerodible polymers. Gliadel®, an FDA-approved device of polyanhydride (P[CPP-SA 20:80]) is used for delivering carmustine (BCNU) in the adjuvant therapy of brain tumors (Figure 17.2). Polyanhydrides were also used for the local delivery of antibiotics in the treatment of osteomyelitis.[59,60] For example, Septaciñis® is a polyanhydride implant of erucic acid dimmer and sebacic acid copolymer in a 1:1 by weight ratio containing gentamicin sulfate, which is dispersed into a polyanhydride polymer matrix (Figure 17.3).[61]

17.3.2.3 Polycaprolactone

PCL has been widely used in drug delivery systems, since it degrades very slowly *in vivo*. It forms compatible blends with a wide range of other polymers. PCL was used in clinical trials for the 1 year implantable contraceptive device, Capronor®. Various PCL copolymers have been evaluated as delivery systems as microparticles,[62,63] polymeric paste,[64] nanoparticles,[65] and micelles.[66]

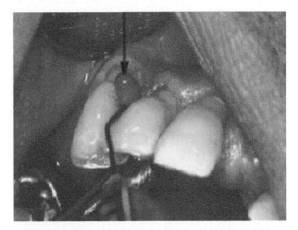

FIGURE 17.2   Molded Septacin™ beads with linkers. (From Igor, G. and Bo, M., *Smart Polymer: Applications in Biotechnology and Biomedicines*, CRC Press, Boca Raton, FL, 2008.)

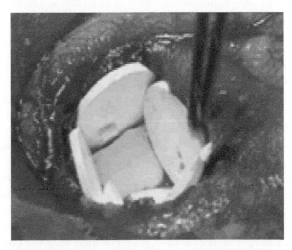

FIGURE 17.3   Gliadel wafers being inserted into the tumor cavity. (From Igor, G. and Bo, M., *Smart Polymer: Applications in Biotechnology and Biomedicines*, CRC Press, Boca Raton, FL, 2008.)

Recently, pH and temperature sensitive biodegradable poly(ε-caprolactone-*co*-lactide)-poly(ethylene glycol) (PCLA–PEG) block copolymers were synthesized with oligomeric sulfamethazine (OSM). The properties of this biodegradable block copolymer are an ideal injectable carrier for various protein-based drugs.[67]

17.3.2.4 Poly(ortho esters)

Poly(ortho esters) (POE) have been developed and used since the 1970s in controlled drug release systems. They were first designated as Chronomer®, later as Alzamer®, and have evolved through four families, viz., POE I, POE II, POE III, and POE IV.

Depending on the nature of the diols used, POEs can be obtained as (a) solid polymers, which can be fabricated into desired shapes such as wafers, strands, and microspheres or (b) directly injectable viscous semisolid materials of specific viscosity.[68] These materials are used in the treatment of postsurgical pain, osteoarthritis, and ophthalmic diseases and for the delivery of proteins and DNA. Ophthalmic applications of POE can be exemplified by the use of POE III for the delivery of antiproliferative agents like 5-FU and mitomycin C. POE III exhibits good subconjunctival biocompatibility and efficacy to prevent the failure of trabeculectomy by providing a sustained release of 5-FU.[69] A bioerodible delivery system, based on POE IV and tetracycline base (TB), has been designed for injection into the periodontal cavity. It is capable of maintaining therapeutic concentrations in the gingival crevicular fluid (GCF) for 10–14 days.[69] *In vivo* results suggest that the POE-based formulation was well tolerated without any pain during application and no irritation or discomfort was felt after treatment.

The local anesthetic agent, mepivacaine, was incorporated into a viscous, injectable POE IV and was used in nonclinical models to provide long-acting anesthesia for postsurgical pain management.

17.4 BIOCOMPATIBILITY AND BIODEGRADIBILITY OF SYNTHETIC POLYMERS

Different synthetic biodegradable polymers like poly(lactic acid), poly(glycolic acid), and their copolymers have been used in several clinical applications. The major applications. include drug delivery systems and orthopedic devices such as pins, rods, and screws.[70,71] Among these synthetic polymers, the polyesters have also been used in several applications because of easy degradation by hydrolysis. Furthermore, the development of several *in situ* polymerizable compositions has been used for drug delivery in the form of an injectable liquid or paste. The polymeric material used for localized drug delivery should satisfy certain requirements. These include biocompatibility and biodegradation to nontoxic products in the specific time.

Usually, the prepolymers are liquid or paste sterilized without any chemical change. This injected prepolymeric mixture bonds to the biological surface and cures to a solid. The curing of polymeric systems has been done with minimal heat generation and without any damage to cells or adjacent tissues. The cured polymers are degraded to biocompatible components that are easily absorbed or released from the body.[72]

Both *in vitro* and *in vivo* studies have been done to determine the biocompatibility of PLA and PGA. The degradation of PLA, PGA, and PLA/PGA copolymers was done because of the hydrolysis of their ester bonds (see Table 17.4). PLA degrades to lactic acid, which further enters to a tricarboxylic acid cycle and excreted as water and carbondioxide. No significant amounts of accumulated degradation products of PLA have been reported in any vital organ.[73] PGA hydrolysis has been made possible by esterase active enzymes.[74] PGA hydrolyzed to glycolic acid, which is also excreted through urine. The rate of degradation is determined from the configurational structure, copolymer ratio, crystallinity, molecular weight, morphology, stresses, amount of residual monomer, porosity, and site of implantation. These polymers are found to be sufficiently biocompatible.

TABLE 17.4
List of the Degradable Polymers and Their Degradation Products

Polymer	Approximate Degradation Time (Months)	Degradation Products	Reference
Poly(glycolic acid)	6–12	Glycolic acid	[72]
Poly(lactic acid)	>24	Lactic acid	[72]
Poly(caprolactone)	>24	Caproic acid	[72]
Poly(propylene fumarate)	Several months	Propylene glycol and fumaric acid	[72]

Recent studies show that PLA–PGA scaffolds may be used for systemic or localized drug delivery. Devices made up of the PLA–PGA copolymer are used in bone repairing also. They are more biocompatible, nontoxic, and noninflammatory.[75,76] Since PLA–PGA copolymers have been used successfully in clinical use as sutures, their use in fixation devices or replacement implants in musculoskeletal tissues may be considered safe. The biocompatibility concern of these materials shows that PLA and PGA produced toxic solutions because of acidic degradation.[77] Another concern is the release of small particles during degradation, which can trigger an inflammatory response.

Homopolymer material takes two to three years for degradation.[71] A total of 50,000 average molecular weight PCLs required about three years for complete degradation *in vitro*.[78] The rate of hydrolysis can be altered by copolymerization with other lactones, for example a copolymer of caprolactone and valerolactone degrades more readily.[79] Copolymers of Σ-caprolactone with DL-lactide have degraded more rapidly (e.g., a commercial suture MONOCRYL, Ethicon).[71] PCL is considered to be a nontoxic and tissue compatible material. Poly(propylene fumarate) (PPF) degrades in bulk degradation and its degradation time depends on the polymer structure and some other components. PPF on hydrolysis gave fumaric acid and propylene glycol. It does not exhibit a harmful and long-term inflammatory response when injected subcutaneously into rats. Initially, a mild inflammatory response was observed and a fibrous capsule formed around the implant in 12 weeks.[80]

Polyanhydrides are more biocompatible and are used clinically in drug delivery systems.[81] Polyanhydrides hydrolyzed through anhydride linkage and degrades to the simple diacid monomers. Poly(sebacic acid) degrades within 54 days in saline. Whereas, poly(1,6-bis(-*p*-arboxy phenoxy)hexane degrades very slowly—about 1 year. According to the need, combinations of different monomers result in polymers with specific degradation properties.[82] Minimal inflammatory responses to sebacic acid/1,3-bis(*p*-carboxyphenoxy) propane (SA/CPP) systems have been reported when implanted subcutaneously in rats up to 28 weeks.

> Homopolymer material takes two to three years time for degradation. 50,000 average molecular weight PCL required about three years for complete degradation *in vitro*. The rate of hydrolysis can be altered by copolymerization with other lactones. For example a copolymer of caprolactone and valerolactone degrades more readily. Copolymers of caprolactone and DL-lactide degrade more rapidly (e.g., a commercial suture MONOCRYL®).

17.5 REGIONAL DRUG THERAPY

Regional drug therapy has been widely employed for several diseases, particularly for the treatment of ailments localized in a specific organ or tissue. The work in this field has mainly focused on cancer chemotherapy due to the high toxicity and lack of specificity of anticancer agents. In addition, these delivery systems have been used for the treatment of brain disorders, bacterial infections, cardiovascular diseases, thrombosis, restenosis, osteomyelitis,[65] pain (as local anesthetics), local infections,[83] glaucoma, and retinal disorders,[84] which are difficult to treat by systemic therapy.[64]

17.5.1 CANCER

The modality of the administration of drugs is an important aspect in cancer chemotherapy. Systemic therapy can be useful in some cases, but is less effective in the treatment of solid malignant tumors of the brain or the liver. The delivery of therapeutic agents to solid tumors is impeded by their unique structural properties.[85] The unequal distribution of blood vessels results in uneven and slow blood flow within the tumors. Additionally, the absence of a functional lymphatic system results in high interstitial pressure, causing the retardation of the transport of high-molecular-weight drugs. Furthermore, the chemo-therapeutic and radio-therapeutic agents are usually nonselective. They are toxic to the healthy cells as well as to the tumor cells, leading to undesirable systemic side effects. If the dose is decreased to avoid the undesirable side effects, the efficacy of therapy also decreases. Whereas, increasing dose controls tumor growth but with high toxicity.[85]

Localized drug delivery systems are used to overcome this problem. Low dose localized delivery is found in the treatment of common solid tumors, such as breast, brain, and prostate cancer.[86] Adjuvant chemotherapy is usually used for the local treatment of breast, colon, and rectal cancers. The localized delivery of therapeutic agents accompanied by the implantation of drugs directly into the brain also helps to overcome inadequate penetration through the blood–brain barrier. In addition, these implants are placed at specific regions of the brain and avoid an undesirable distribution of the drug throughout the brain.[58]

The initial studies of brain drug delivery in the treatment of malignant glioma using a polyanhydride implant were performed with the chemotherapeutic alkylating agent 1,3-bis-(2-chloroethyl)-1-nitrosourea (BCNU, carmustine).[87] BCNU (3.8% w/w) loaded in small polymer wafers was tested in rats, rabbits, and monkeys for their safety and effectiveness before use in humans.[88] Gliadel®, the drug-loaded polymer wafers of carmustine in poly(bis[p-carboxy phenoxy] propane-sebacic acid) P(CPP-SA, 20:80), was approved as a polymeric implant for the treatment of brain tumors.[89] A polyanhydride-film-releasing cisplatin was also effective in inhibiting tumor growth. This could be used for human squamous cell carcinoma of the head and neck.[90]

A concept of carrier-based radiochemotherapy was proposed for treating advanced solid malignancies. For example, N-(2-hydroxypropyl) methylacrylamide (HPMA) copolymers were used with model drugs doxorubicin and gemcitabine in the targeted delivery system.[91]

Recently, a study reported an intratumoral injection of a polymeric paste loaded with paclitaxel in orthotopic prostate tumor rat models. This intervention prevented tumor metastases compared with the control group.

This study used the biodegradable polymer poly(sebacic acid-co-ricinoleic acid) ester/anhydride in a 2:8 w/w ratio. The compositions were mixed to smooth pastes, which were injectable at room temperature. Various concentrations of paclitaxel were loaded in the polymer. The formulations were injected in orthotopic prostate cancer rat models and the results were recorded after several days. The increasing concentration of paclitaxel slowed the drug release from the polymer and decreased the polymer's degradation rate. A 10% paclitaxel formulation was the most efficacious in heterotopic tumor models. This study provides a formulation of the biodegradable polymer loaded with paclitaxel to prevent the metastasis and prolong the lifespan of orthotopic prostate cancer rat models.[92]

17.5.2 BONE INFECTIONS

Osteomyelitis is a chronic bone inflammation caused by dead vascular bone and is difficult to diagnose and cure. The current treatment suggests surgical debridement (removal of dead mass) of the infected area, followed by high-dose systemic antibiotic therapy for 4–6 weeks. However, the systemic antibiotic therapy leads to insufficient antibiotic concentrations in the infected tissues.[93] This may be due to inadequate blood supply at the infected site in the bone, especially in diabetes patients. The use of local antibiotic delivery using a biodegradable polymer can obviate these problems.

Various polymers have been used as implantable carriers for the local delivery of antibiotics.[93,94] The nondegradable polymeric carrier poly(methylmethacrylate) was used clinically in Europe (Septopal®, E. Merck & Co., Darmstadt, Germany) for the delivery of gentamicin in bone. Later on, several biodegradable polymers like polylactide, poly(propylene fumarate), polyanhydride, and natural polymers such as collagen, gelatin, and inorganic phosphates have been used. Antibiotic gentamicin encapsulated in cross-linked biodegradable polyanhydride beads was implanted in the surgical treatment of osteomyelitis and soft-tissue infection. These beads degrade over a week and release gentamicin at high local concentrations required to kill most of the organisms associated with osteomyelitis. Copolyesters such as 3-hydroxybutyrate with 3-hydroxyvalerate and 4-hydroxybutyrate have also been used to build biodegradable implantable rods for the local delivery of antibiotics (Sulperazone® and Duocid®, respectively) in chronic osteomyelitis.[52] PLGA microspheres containing tobramycin were also used to treat osteomyelitis. The use of biodegradable microspheres of tobramycin in combination with parenteral treatment with cefazolin was the most successful treatment in a rabbit osteomyelitis model.[95] Teicoplanin microspheres and vancomycin beads of biodegradable polymer have also been used in the treatment of bone infections.[96,97] PLGA microspheres of ofloxacin were used in the treatment of bacterial biofilm infections associated with the bone.[98]

Injectable biodegradable poly(sebacic-*co*-ricinoleic-ester-anhydride)s, designated as p(SA:RA)s, were used in the treatment of solid tumors.[26] p(SA:RA) was also used for the treatment of osteomyelitis induced by *Staphylococcus aureus*. In this study, a poly(sebacic-*co*-ricinoleic-ester-anhydride) 2:8 w/w ratio was used. All the animals developed osteomyelitis within 3 weeks following inoculation. The involvement of the surrounding soft tissue in the inflammation process was noticed and confirmed by clinical evidence. After three weeks, a reduction of bony abscess formation at the infection site was confirmed by histopathology.[99] Degradation of poly(ricinoleic-*co*-sebacic-ester-anhydride)s in buffer solution was studied by following the composition of released degradation products into the medium and the degraded polymer.[100]

In a recent study, osteomyelitis of both tibiae was induced in 13 female Fischer rats by injecting a suspension containing approximately 105 CFU/mL *S. aureus* into the tibial medullar canal. Three weeks later, both tibiae were x-rayed, drilled down the medullar canal, washed with gentamicin solution (80 mg/2 mL), and then injected with 50 μL p(SA-RA) + gentamycin 20% w/v in the right tibia and 50 μL p(SA-RA) without gentamicin in the left tibia. After an additional 3 weeks, the rats were sacrificed and radiographs of the tibiae were taken. A histological evaluation revealed significant differences between the right and left tibiae in 10 rats. In the left tibia, moderate intramedullary abscess formation occurred. In most drug-treated (right) tibiae, the typical changes included the absence (or minimal grade only) of abscesses. The treated group developed significantly less intramedullary abscesses.[101]

A reduction in bacterial count was found in treated rats with a gentamicin-containing collagen sponge or PMMA-containing gentamicin. The therapy was more effective in combination with systemic cephazolin.[102] Researchers mostly evaluated the treatment results on the basis of bacterial count.[102–104]

17.5.3 VASCULAR DISORDERS

Vascular surgery generally faces the complications of intravascular thrombosis and delayed stenosis. In addition, restenosis of the coronary artery used in coronary angioplasty causes a localized injury to the vessel wall. It leads to the release of vasoactive thrombogenic and mitogenic factors causing renarrowing at the injured site. Mechanical devices have been designed to provide a larger lumen on completion of the procedure. These devices are designed to inhibit the neointimal proliferation and to reduce restenosis. Debulking processes like directional coronary atherectomy, rotational atherectomy, and laser angioplasty do not reduce restenosis. However, localized drug delivery through a coronary artery stent[105] reduces the post-coronary angioplasty restenosis rate to approximately 50%.

Pharmacological agents used to interfere with the local neointimal formation are classified as antiproliferative, anti-inflammatory immune modulating, antimigratory, antithrombotic, and prohealing agents.[106,107] Clinical studies show a greater reduction in restenosis with drug-eluting stents than with bare-metal stents. The first human experience with a sirolimus drug-eluting stent (Cypher®, Cordis Corp., Miami Beach, Florida), the Ravel trial, and the SIRIUS multicenter U.S. phase III trial, have demonstrated a substantial reduction in angiographic restenosis (>50% stenosis).[106,108,109]

Drug-eluting polymeric matrices were also used to inhibit injury-induced thrombosis and neointimal thickening. Heparin-releasing polymers were evaluated in rats after carotid artery balloon catheter injury. A thin and flexible biodegradable matrix of polyanhydrides and polyesters loaded with heparin has been evaluated *in vitro* and *in vivo*. Heparin was released for 1–3 weeks from these films at a constant concentration. The control showed a significant reduction in the internal diameter of the artery, while the treated rats showed minimal or no proliferation of smooth muscle cells.

Other agents, such as dexamethasone (anti-inflammatory agent), hirulog (thrombin inhibitor), and antisense oligonucleotides incorporated in a polymeric system also prevented smooth muscle cell proliferation after endothelial injury.[110]

17.5.4 Neurological Disorders

Polymeric microspheres have been used to deliver neuroactive agents at specific sites within the brain. Drug delivery is controlled and prolonged without any risk of infection. Small-sized microparticles are implanted precisely at the affected areas of the brain without damaging the surrounding tissue. This method is often applied in neuro-oncology and neurodegenerative diseases.[111]

A potential treatment for Alzheimer's disease was reported via the intracerebral delivery of cholinergic agent bethanecol.[112] In this study, polymeric microspheres with bethanecol were injected into the brain of memory deficit rats by bilateral fimbria-fomix lesions. A remarkable improvement was found within 10 days and lasted for the entire 40 days of testing. Injectable microspheres releasing dopamine were developed as an effective treatment for Parkinson's disease. Rats implanted with dopamine microspheres exhibited contralateral rotations with an amplitude comparable to a previously administered test dose of apomorphine for long durations. Control animals injected with placebo microspheres did not show any reliable rotational behavior. It confirmed that the direct delivery of the neurotransmitter to the brain through a biodegradable polymer restores functions for a prolonged period.[113]

A method for the localized delivery of therapeutic agents to the injured spinal cord utilized dispersing therapeutic agents to form a gel in a polymeric solution after injection into the subarachnoid space. The drug delivery system provided a safe and alternative method of delivering therapeutic agents intrathecally.[114]

17.5.5 Retinal Disorders

The systemic administration of drugs in retinal diseases is not preferred because of the blood–retinal barrier and systemic toxicity. In human cytomegalovirus (CMV) infection, vitritis, retinitis, and optic neuritis were cured by the inoculation of antiviral ganciclovir microspheres in rabbit eyes, without any adverse tissue reactions and minimal focal disruption of the retinal structure.[115] Similarly, intravitreal corticosteroid budesonide injection is administered to treat diabetic retinopathy since it prevents neovascularization and microvascular alterations, which are the common manifestations of ocular diseases.[116]

Drug-loaded microspheres were prepared for the controlled intravitreous release of retinoic acid. A sustained release of retinoic acid from PLGA microspheres was obtained *in vitro* for 40 days. A single injection of retinoic acid-loaded microspheres suspension in bismuth salicylate

(BS) efficiently reduced the retinal detachment after two months in a rabbit model of proliferative vitreoretinopathy.[117]

17.5.6 TUBERCULOSIS

Antitubercular drugs (ATD) like rifampicin, isoniazid, and pyrazinamide make tuberculosis (TB) curable. However, after a certain period of time, because of the clinical improvement, patients stop the intake of the ATDs leading to noncompliance, failure of therapy, and increased microbial drug resistance. Drug-resistant cases are increasing especially rapidly in cases of coexisting HIV and TB patients. Therefore, modified-release ATDs are valuable in reducing the doses and improving patient compliance.

Rifampicin and isoniazid were encapsulated in liposomes. These preparations are stable, non-toxic, and are administered by a single IV injection. In addition, SC delivery using polymeric PLG microparticle-based ATD delivery was investigated. PLG-based SC injection not only maintained the therapeutic drug level for 6–7 weeks, but also demonstrated significant chemotherapeutic efficacy in the murine rat TB model. The PLG nanoparticulate system has advantages in terms of low polymer amount, high drug loading, and desirable release profile.

In addition, alginate microsphere-based ATD release systems were effective drug carriers and showed complete bacterial clearance.[118]

17.5.7 LOCAL ANESTHESIA

Drug delivery systems that allow high doses of effective and nontoxic analgesic agents with a slow and constant release are useful in conditions that require local anesthesia.[119,120] These agents improve postoperative pain management, particularly the healing process after the surgery. Local anesthetic blocks the nerve conduction reversibly at the administered site and produces a temporary loss of sensation at a specific site in the body.

A biodegradable polyester-*co*-anhydride polymer of ricinoleic acid prolonged the effect of bupivacaine for 8–30 h. Hydrolysis sensitive anhydride bonds degraded rapidly and released the drug. Thus, new hydrophobic polymer carriers were developed. These new polymers, castor oil–based polyesters, reduced the polymer degradation rate and prolonged the drug release period.[3] Increasing the castor oil content of the polymer reduced the drug release rate. These polymers increased the overall viscosity of the system. The p(DLLA:CO) 3:7 system was too viscous, hence it was administered easily[n70] at room temperature *in vivo*. This castor oil–based formulation prolonged the sensory anesthesia to 48 h and motor block for 24 h.[121,122]

17.6 CONCLUDING REMARKS

Driving the therapeutically active molecules into the drug delivery pipeline has provided strong motivation to develop new polymeric materials. Available drug therapies for diseases localized at a specific organ or tissue provide opportunities for alternative means of drug administration through a polymeric device.

The idea of biodegradable polymers as carriers for regional therapy has gained the attention of researchers and clinicians. The utility of delivery systems and the use of different biodegradable polymer-based localized drug delivery devices have been recognized. Gliadel® is a polyanhydride wafer used to deliver BCNU for the treatment of brain tumors. Macromed has been developing an *in situ* gelling system derived from biodegradable poly(ether-esters) for treating various anticancer agents. This system is now in phase 2 clinical trials.

Polymeric drug delivery systems have great potential for regional therapy. Currently, most polymeric carriers are used for cancer chemotherapy and infectious diseases where high concentrations of therapeutic drugs are required. However, these polymeric devices can also be used in the treatment of other diseases. They also serve as long-acting drug delivery systems.

REFERENCES

1. Hatefi, A. and Amsden, B. 2002. Biodegradable injectable in-situ forming drug delivery systems. *J. Control. Release* 80:9–28.
2. Graham, P. D., Brodbeck, K. J., and McHugh, A. J. 1999. Phase inversion dynamics of PLGA solutions related to drug delivery. *J. Control. Release* 58:233–245.
3. Azhdarinia, A., Yang, D. J., Yu, D. F., Mendez, R., Oh, C., Kohanim, S., Bryant, J., and Kim, E. E. 2005. Regional radiochemotherapy using in situ hydrogel. *Pharm. Res.* 22:776–783.
4. Nivasu, V. M., Reddy, T. T., and Tammishetti, S. 2004. In situ polymerizable polyethyleneglycol containing polyesterpolyol acrylates for tissue sealant applications. *Biomaterials* 25:3283–3291.
5. Choi, S., Baudys, M., and Kim, S. W. 2004. Control of blood glucose by novel GLP-1 delivery using biodegradable triblock copolymer of PLGA-PEG-PLGA in type 2 diabetic rats. *Pharm. Res.* 21:827–831.
6. Choi, S. and Kim, S. W. 2003. Controlled release of insulin from injectable biodegradable triblock copolymer depot in ZDF rats. *Pharm. Res.* 20:2008–2010.
7. Zentner, G. M., Rathi, R., Shih, C., McRea, J. C., Seo, M., Oh, H., Rhee, B. G., Mestecky, J., Moldoveanu, Z., Morgan, M., and Weitman, S. 2001. Biodegradable block copolymers for delivery of proteins and water-insoluble drugs. *J. Control. Release* 72:203–215.
8. Jackson, J. K., Gleave, M. E., Yago, V., Beraldi, E., Hunter, W. L., and Burt, H. M. 2000. The suppression of human prostate tumor growth in mice by the intratumoral injection of a slow-release polymeric paste formulation of paclitaxel. *Cancer Res.* 60:4146–4151.
9. Igor, G. and Bo, M. 2008. Polymeric carriers for regional drug therapy, in *Smart Polymer: Applications in Biotechnology and Biomedicines*, CRC Press, Boca Raton, FL.
10. Cohn, D. and Hotovely-Salomon, A. 2005. Biodegradable multiblock PEO/PLA thermoplastic elastomers: Molecular design and properties. *Polymer*, 46:2068–2075.
11. Schwach-Abdellaoui, K., Monti, A., Barr, J., Heller, J., and Gurny, R. 2001. Optimization of a novel bioerodible device based on auto-catalyzed poly(ortho esters) for controlled delivery of tetracycline to periodontal pocket. *Biomaterials* 22:1659–1666.
12. Hongliang, W., Jiyu, H., Ling-gang, S., Kaiqiang, Z., and Zeng-guo, F. 2005. Gel formation and photopolymerization during supramolecular self-assemblies of α-CDs with LA–PEG–LA copolymer end-capped with methacryloyl groups. *Eur. Polym. J.* 41:948–957.
13. Balakrishnan, B. and Jayakrishnan, A. 2005. Self-cross-linking biopolymers as injectable in situ forming biodegradable scaffolds. *Biomaterials* 26:3941–3951.
14. Li, J. Ni, X., and Leong, K. W. 2003. Injectable drug-delivery systems based on supramolecular hydrogels formed by poly(ethylene oxide)s and α-cyclodextrin. *J Biomed. Mater. Res.* 65:196–202.
15. Oster, C. G., Wittmar, M., Unger, F., Barbu-Tudoran, L., Schaper, A. K., and Kissel, T. 2004. Design of amine-modified graft polyesters for effective gene delivery using DNA-loaded nanoparticles. *Pharm. Res.* 21:927–931.
16. Brodbeck, K. J., DesNoyer, J. R., and McHugh, A. J. 1999. Phase inversion dynamics of PLGA solutions related to drug delivery Part II. The role of solution thermodynamics and bath-side mass transfer. *J. Control. Release* 62:333–344.
17. DesNoyer, J. R. and McHugh, A. J. 2003. The effect of pluronic on the protein release kinetics of an injectable drug delivery system. *J. Control Release* 86:15–24.
18. Packhaeuser, C. B., Schnieders, J., Oster, C. G., and Kissel, T. 2004. In situ forming parenteral drug delivery systems: An overview. *Eur. J. Pharm. Biopharm.* 58:445–455.
19. Peppas, N. A., Bures, P., Leobandung, W., and Ichikawa, H. 2000. Hydrogels in pharmaceutical formulations. *Eur. J. Pharm. Biopharm.* 50:27–46.
20. Ruel-Gariépy, E. and Leroux, J. C. 2004. In situ-forming hydrogels—Review of temperature-sensitive systems. *Eur. J. Pharm. Biopharm.* 58:409–426.
21. Kwon, K. W., Park, M. J., Bae, Y. H., Kim, H. D., and Char, K. 2002. Gelation behavior of PEO–PLGA–PEO triblock copolymers in water. *Polymer* 43:3353–3358.
22. Chen, S. and Singh, J. 2005. Controlled delivery of testosterone from smart polymer solution based systems: In vitro evaluation. *Int. J. Pharm.* 295:183–190.
23. Bae, S. J., Suh, J. M., Sohn, Y. S., Bae, Y. H., Kim, S. W., and Jeong, B. 2005. Thermogelling poly(caprolactone-*b*-ethylene glycol-*b*-caprolactone) aqueous solutions, *Macromolecules*, 38(12): 5260–5265.
24. Krasko, M. Y., Shikanov, A., Ezra, A., and Domb, A. J. 2003. Poly(ester anhydride)s prepared by the insertion of ricinoleic acid into poly(sebacic acid) *J. Polym. Sci. Polym. Chem.* 41:1059–1069.

25. Shikanov, A., Domb, A. J., Shikanov, A., Vaisman, B., Krasko, M. Y., Nyska, A. and Domb, A. J. 2006. Poly(sebacic acid-*co*-ricinoleic acid) biodegradable injectable in situ gelling polymer. *Biomacromolecules* 7:288–296.

26. Shikanov, A., Vaisman, B., Krasko, M. Y., Nyska, A., and Domb, A. J. 2004. Pasty injectable biodegradable polymers derived from natural acids. *J Biomed. Mater. Res.* 69:47–54.

27. Khor, E. and Lim, L. Y. 2003. Implantable applications of chitin and chitosan, *Biomaterials* 24:2339.

28. Senel, S. and McClure, S. J. 2004. Potential applications of chitosan in veterinary medicine. *Adv. Drug. Deliv. Rev.* 56:1467.

29. Hsieh, C. Y. et al. Preparation of [gamma]-PGA/chitosan composite tissue engineering matrices. *Biomaterials* 26:5617.

30. Dhiman, H. K. Ray, A. R., and Panda, A. K. 2004. Characterization and evaluation of chitosan matrix for in vitro growth of MCF-7 breast cancer cell lines, *Biomaterials* 25:5147.

31. Dhiman, H. K., Ray, A. R., and Panda, A. K. 2005. Three-dimensional chitosan scaffoldbased MCF-7 cell culture for the determination of the cytotoxicity of tamoxifen. *Biomaterials* 26:979.

32. Hu, Q. et al. 2004. Preparation and characterization of biodegradable chitosan/hydroxyapatite nanocomposite rods via in situ hybridization: A potential material as internal fixation of bone fracture. *Biomaterials* 25:779.

33. Wang, Y. C. et al. 2003. Fabrication of a novel porous PGA-chitosan hybrid matrix for tissue engineering. *Biomaterials* 24:1047.

34. Nsereko, S. and Amiji, M. 2002. Localized delivery of paclitaxel in solid tumors from biodegradable chitin microparticle formulations. *Biomaterials* 23:2723.

35. Gan, Q. et al. 2005. Modulation of surface charge, particle size and morphological properties of chitosan-TPP nanoparticles intended for gene delivery. *Colloids Surf* 44:65

36. Anal, A. K. and Stevens, W. F. 2005. Chitosan-alginate multilayer beads for controlled release of ampicillin. *Int. J. Pharm.* 290:45.

37. Bhattarai, N. et al. 2005. PEG-grafted chitosan as an injectable thermosensitive hydrogel for sustained protein release. *J. Control. Release* 103:609.

38. Andre, P. 2004. Hyaluronic acid and its use as a "rejuvenation" agent in cosmetic dermatology. *Semin. Cutan. Med. Surg.* 23:218.

39. Reinmuller, J. 2003. Hyaluronic acid. *Aesth. Surg. J* 23:309.

40. Liu, Y., Zheng Shu, X., and Prestwich, G. D. 2005. Biocompatibility and stability of disulfide-crosslinked hyaluronan films. *Biomaterials* 26:4737.

41. Miller, J. A. et al. 1998. Efficacy of hyaluronic acid/nonsteroidal anti-inflammatory drug systems in preventing postsurgical tendon adhesions. *J. Biomed. Mater. Res.* Part A, 38:25.

42. Brown, M. and Jones, S. 2005. Hyaluronic acid: A unique topical vehicle for the localized delivery of drugs to the skin. *J. Eur. Acad. Dermatol. Venereol.* 19:305.

43. Gerwin, N., Hops, C., and Lucke, A. 2006. Intraarticular drug delivery in osteoarthritis. *Adv. Drug Deliv. Rev.* 58:226–242.

44. Gombotz, W. R. and Wee, S. 1998. Protein release from alginate matrices. *Adv. Drug Deliv. Rev.* 31:267.

45. Tu, J. et al. 2005. Alginate microparticles prepared by spray-coagulation method: Preparation, drug loading and release characterization. *Int. J. Pharm.* 303:171.

46. Yenice, I. et al. 2002. Biodegradable implantable teicoplanin beads for the treatment of bone infections. *Int. J. Pharm.*, 242:271.

47. Arica, B. et al. 2002. 5-Fluorouracil encapsulated alginate beads for the treatment of breast cancer. *Int. J. Pharm.* 242:267.

48. Bouhadir, K. H. Alsberg, E., and Mooney, D. J. 2001. Hydrogels for combination delivery of antineoplastic agents. *Biomaterials* 22:2625.

49. Lim, S. T. et al. 2002. In vivo evaluation of novel hyaluronan/chitosan microparticulate delivery systems for the nasal delivery of gentamicin in rabbits. *Int. J. Pharm.* 231:73.

50. Konishi, M. et al. 2005. In vivo anti-tumor effect of dual release of cisplatin and adriamycin from biodegradable gelatin hydrogel. *J. Control. Release* 103:7.

51. Rossi, S. Azghani, A. O., and Omri, A. J. 2004. Antimicrobial efficacy of a new antibiotic-loaded poly(hydroxybutyric-*co*-hydroxyvaleric acid) controlled release system. *Antimicrob. Chemother.* 54:1013.

52. Türesin, F., Gürsel, I., and Hasirci, V. J. 2001. Biodegradable polyhydroxyalkanoate implants for osteomyelitis therapy: In vitro antibiotic release. *Biomater. Sci.* 12:195.

53. Carothers, W. H. 1929. An introduction to the general theory of condensation polymers. *J. Am. Chem. Soc.* 51:2548.
54. Carothers, W. H. and Arvin, G. A. 1929. Polyesters. *J. Am. Chem. Soc.* 51:2560.
55. Hong, Y., Gong, Y., Gao, C., and Shen, J. 2007. Collagen-coated polylactide microcarriers/chitosan hydrogel composite: Injectable scaffold for cartilage regeneration. *J. Biomed. Mater. Res.* Part A, 85A:628–637.
56. Kranz, H. and Bodmeier, R. 2008. Structure formation and characterization of injectable drug loaded biodegradable devices: In situ implants versus in situ microparticles. *Eur. J. Pharmaceut. Sci.* 34:164–172.
57. Bakshi, R. Ebrahim, V. F., Mobedi, Jamshidi, H., and Khakpour, M. 2006. *Polym. Adv. Technol.* 17:354–359.
58. Desai, K. H., Mallery, S. R., and Schwendeman, S. P. 2008. Formulation and characterization of injectable poly(DL-lactide-co-glycolide) implants loaded with N-acetylcysteine, a MMP inhibitor. *Pharmaceut. Res.* 25(3):586–597.
59. Stephens, D. et al. 2000. Investigation of the in vitro release of gentamycin from a polyanhydride matrix. *J. Control. Release* 63:305.
60. Tian, Y. et al. 2002. The effect of storage temperatures on the in vitro properties of a polyanhydride implant containing gentamycin. *Drug Dev. Ind. Pharm*, 28:897.
61. Li, L. C., Deng, J., and Stephens, D. 2002. Polyanhydride implant for antibiotic delivery: From the bench to the clinic. *Adv. Drug Deliv. Rev*, 54:963.
62. Chen, D. R., Bei, J. Z., and Wang, S. G. 2000. Polycaprolactone microparticles and their biodegradation. *Polym. Degrad. Stab*. 67:455.
63. Benoit, M. A. Baras, B., and Gillard, J. 1999. Preparation and characterization of protein-loaded poly(o-caprolactone) microparticles for oral vaccine delivery. *Int. J. Pharm.*184:73.
64. Jackson, J. K. et al. 2004. The characterization of novel polymeric paste formulations for intratumoral delivery. *Int. J. Pharm*. 270:185.
65. Varela, M. C. et al. 2001. Cyclosporine-loaded polycaprolactone nanoparticles: Immunosuppression and nephrotoxicity in rats. *Eur. J. Pharm. Sci*. 12:471.
66. Allen, C. et al. 2000. Polycaprolactone-b-poly(ethylene oxide) copolymer micelles as a delivery vehicle for dihydrotestosterone. *J. Control. Release* 275.
67. Woo, S. S., Sung, W. K., and Doo, S. L. 2006. Sulfonamide-based pH- and temperature-sensitive biodegradable block copolymer hydrogels. *Biomacromolecules* 7:1935–1941.
68. Barr, J. et al. 2002. Postsurgical pain management with poly(ortho esters). *Adv. Drug Deliv. Rev*. 54:1041.
69. Einmahl, S. et al. 2001. Therapeutic applications of viscous and injectable poly(ortho esters). *Adv. Drug Deliv. Rev*. 53:45.
70. Behravesh, E., Yasko, A. W., Engle, P. S., and Mikos, A. G. 1999. Synthetic biodegradable polymers for orthopaedic applications. *Clin. Orthop*. 367S:118–185.
71. Middleton, J. C. and Tipton, A. J. 2000. Synthetic biodegradable polymers as orthopaedic devices. *Biomaterials* 21:2335–2346.
72. Gunatillake, P. A. and Adhikari, R. 2003. Biodegradable synthetic polymers for tissue engineering. *Eur. Cells Mater*. 5:1–16.
73. Vert, M., Christel, P., Chabot, F., Leray, J., Hastings, G. W., and Ducheyne, P. eds. 1984. *Macromolecular Biomaterials*. CRC Press, Boca Raton, FL, pp. 119–142.
74. William, D.F. and Mort, E. 1977. Enzyme-accelerated hydrolysis of polyglycolic acid. *J. Bioeng*. 1:231–238.
75. Nelson, J. F., Stanford, H. G., and Cutright, D. E. 1977. Evaluation and comparison of biodegradable substances as osteogenic agents. *Oral Surg*. 43:836–843.
76. Hollinger, J. O. 1983. Preliminary report on osteogenic potential of a biodegradable copolymer of polylactide (PLA) and polyglycolide (PGA). *J. Biomed. Mater. Res*. 17:71–82.
77. Tayler, M. S. Daniels, A. U. Andriano, K. P., and Heller, J. 1994. Six bioabsorbale polymers: In-vitro acute toxicity of accumulated degradation products. *J. Appl. Biomater*. 5:151–157.
78. Gabelnick, H. L. 1983. Long acting steroid contraception. In: Mishell, D. R. Jr., ed. *Advances in Human Fertility and Reproductive Endocrinology*, Raven Press, New York. Vol. 3:149–173.
79. Pitt, C. G., Marks, T. A., and Schindler, A. 1981. In: Willette. R.E. and Barnet, G. eds. *Narcotic Antagonists: Naltrexone Pharmacochemistry and Sustained-Release Preparations*, National Institute on Drug Abuse Research Monograph 28, National Institute on Drug Abuse, Bethesda, MD, pp. 232–253.
80. Peter, S. J. Miller, S. T. Zhu, G. Yasko, A. W., and Mikos, A. G. 1998. In vivo degradation of a poly(propylene fumarate)/ß-tricalcium phosphate injectable composite scaffold. *J. Biomed. Mater. Res*. 41:1–7.

81. Leong, K. W. Brott, B. C., and Langer, R. 1985. Bioerodible polyanhydrides as drug-carrier matrices. I: Characterization, degradation, and release characteristics. *J Biomed. Mater. Res.* 19:941–955.
82. Temenoff, J. S. and Mikos, A. G. 2000. Injectable biodegradable materials for orthopaedic tissue engineering. *Biomaterials* 21:2405–2412.
83. Park, E. S. Maniar, M., and Shah, J. C. 1998. Biodegradable polyanhydride devices of cefazolin sodium, bupivacaine, and taxol for local drug delivery: Preparation and kinetics and mechanism of in vitro release. *J. Control. Release.* 52:179.
84. Jampel, H. D. et al. 1993. Glaucoma filtration surgery in nonhuman primates using taxol and etoposide in polyanhydride carriers. *Invest. Opthalmol. Vis. Sci.* 34:3076.
85. Chilkoti, A. et al. 2002. Targeted drug delivery by thermally responsive polymers. *Adv. Drug Deliv. Rev.* 54:613.
86. Chabner, B. A. et al. 2001. *Goodman and Gilman's the Pharmacological Basis of Therapeutics*, 10th edn., McGraw Hill, New York, p. 1389.
87. Lesniak, M. S. and Brem, H. 2004. Targeted therapy for brain tumors. *Nature Rev. Drug Discov.* 3:499.
88. Byrd, K. E. and Hamilton-Byrd, E. L. 1992. Polymer chemotherapy of neurotransmitters and neuromodulators polymeric site-specific pharmacotherapy, 141.
89. Domb, A. J. et al. 1999. Preparation and characterisation of carmustine loaded polyanhydride wafers for treating brain tumors. *Pharm. Res.* 16:762.
90. Shikani, A., Eisele, D. W., and Domb, A. J. 1994. Polymer chemotherapy for squamous cell carcinoma of the head and neck. *Arch. Otolaryngol. Headneck Surg.* 120:1242.
91. Lammers, T., Subr, V., Peschke, P., Kuhnlein, R., Hennink, W. E., Ulbrich, K., Kiessling, F., Heilmann, M., and Debus, J., Huber, P. E., and Strom G. 2008. Image-guided and passively tumour-targeted polymeric nanomedicines for radiochemotherapy, *Br. J. Cancer*, 99:900–910.
92. Shikanov, S., Shikanov, A., Gofrit, O., Nyska, A., Corn, B., and Domb, A. J. 2008. Intratumoral delivery of paclitaxel for treatment of orthotopic prostate cancer. *J. Pharm. Sci.* 9999:1–11.
93. Rens, T. J. G. and Kayser, F. H. 1980. Local antibiotic treatment in osteomyelitis and soft-tissue infections. *Int. Congr. Ser.* 556.
94. Domb, A. J. and Amselem, S. 1994. Antibiotic delivery systems for the treatment of chronic bone infections polymeric site-specific. *Pharmacother.* 243.
95. Yeh, H. Y. and Huang, Y. Y. 2003. Injectable biodegradable polymeric implants for the prevention of postoperative infection: Implications for antibacterial resistance *Am. J. Drug Deliv.* 1:149.
96. Yenice, I. et al. 2003. In vitro/in vivo evaluation of the efficiency of teicoplanin loaded biodegradable microparticles formulated for implantation to infected bone defects. *J. Microencapsul.* 20:705.
97. Ueng, S.W. N. et al. 2002. In vivo study of hot compressing molded 50:50 poly (DL-lactide-*co*-glycolide) antibiotic beads in rabbits. *J. Orthop. Res.* 20:654.
98. Habib, M. et al. 1999. Preparation and characterization of ofloxacin microspheres for the eradication of bone associated bacterial biofilm. *J. Microencapsul.* 16:27.
99. Shikanov, A., Ezra, A., and Domb, A. J. 2005. Poly(sebacic acid-*co*-ricinoleic acid) biodegradable carrier for paclitaxel-effect of additives, *J. Control. Release* 105:52–67.
100. Krasko, M. Y. and Domb, A. J. 2005. Hydrolytic degradation of ricinoleic-sebacic-ester-anhydride copolymers. *Biomacromolecules* 6 (4):1877–1884.
101. Yaron, S. B., Jacob, G., Boaz, M., Guy, M., Abraham, J. D., Shyamal, P., Shmuel, T., Abraham, N., and Meir, N. 2008. Treatment of osteomyelitis in rats by injection of degradable polymer releasing gentamicin, *J. Control. Release* 131(2):121–127.
102. Krasko, M. Y., Golenser, J. N., A Nyska, M., Brin, Y. S., and Domb, A. J. 2007. Gentamicin extended release from an injectable polymeric implant, *J. Control. Release* 117(1):90–96.
103. Mendel, V., Simanowski, H. J., Scholz, H. C., and Heymann, H. 2005. Therapy with gentamicin-PMMA beads, gentamicin-collagen sponge, and cefazolin for experimental osteomyelitis due to *Staphylococcus aureus* in rats, *Arch. Orthop. Trauma Surg.* 125(6):363–368.
104. Kamel, A. H. and Baddour, M. M. 2007. Gatifloxacin biodegradable implant for treatment of experimental osteomyelitis: In vitro and in vivo evaluation, *Drug Deliv.* 14(6):349–356.
105. Sigwart, U. et al. 1987. Intravascular stents to prevent occlusion and restenosis after transluminal angioplasty. *N. Engl. J. Med.* 316:701.
106. Sousa, J. Costa, M., and Abizaid, A. 2001. Lack of neointimal proliferation after implantation of sirolimus-coated stents in human coronary arteries: A quantitative coronary angiography and three-dimensional intravascular ultrasound study. *Circulation* 103:192.
107. Sousa, J. E. Serruys, P. W. and Costa, M. A. 2003. New frontiers in cardiology: Drug eluting stents. *Circulation* 107:2274.

108. Morice, M. C., Serruys, P. W., and Sousa, J. E. 2002. A randomized comparison of a sirolimus-eluting stent with a standard stent for coronary revascularization. *N. Engl. J. Med.* 346:1173.
109. Moses, J. W., Leon, M. B., and Popma, J. J. 2003. Sirolimus-eluting stents versus standard stents in patients with stenosis in a native coronary artery. *N. Engl. J. Med.* 349:1315.
110. Orloff, L. A. et al. 1995. Prevention of venous thrombosis in microvascular surgery by transmural release of heparin from a polyanhydride polymer. *Surgery* 117:554.
111. Menei, P. et al. 1994. Drug targeting into the central nervous system by stereotactic implantation of biodegradable microspheres. *Neurosurg* 34:1058.
112. Howard, M. A. et al. 1989. Intracerebral drug delivery in rats with lesion-induced memory deficits. *J. Neurosurg* 71:105.
113. Mason, D. W. 1988. Biodegradable poly(D,L,-lactide-*co*-glycolide) microspheres for the controlled release of catecholamines to the CNS Proc. *Int. Symp. Control Rel. Bioact. Mater.* 15:270.
114. Hamann, M. C. J. et al. 2003. Novel intrathecal delivery system for treatment of spinal cord injury. *Exp. Neurol* 182:300.
115. Veloso, A. A. et al. 1997. Ganciclovir-loaded polymer microspheres in rabbit eyes inoculated with human cytomegalovirus. *Invest. Opthalmol. Vis. Sci.* 38:665.
116. Ciulla, T. A. et al. 2004. Corticosteroids in posterior segment disease: An update on new delivery systems and new indications *Curr. Opin. Ophthalmol.* 15:211.
117. Giordano, G. G., Refojo, M. F., and Arroyo, M. H. 1993. Sustained delivery of retinoic acid from microspheres of biodegradable polymer in PVR invest. *Ophthalmol. Vis. Sci.* 34:2743.
118. Khuller, G. K. and Pandey, R. 2003. Sustained release drug delivery systems in management of tuberculosis. *Indian J. Chest Dis. Allied Sci.* 45:229–230.
119. Grant, G. J., Piskoun, B., and Bansinath, M. 2003. Analgesic duration and kinetics of liposomal bupivacaine after subcutaneous injection in mice, *Clin. Exp. Pharmacol. Physiol.* 30:966–968.
120. Grant, G. J., Barenholz, B., Piskoun, B., Bansinath, M., Turndorf, H., and Bolotin, E. M. 2001. DRV liposomal bupivacaine: Preparation, characterization and in vivo evaluation in mice, *Pharma. Res.* 18:336–343.
121. Shikanov, A., Domb, A. J., and Weiniger, C. F. 2007. Long acting local anesthatic polymer formulation to prolong the effect of analgesia, *J. Control. Release* 117:97–103.
122. Sokolsky-Papkov. M., Golovanevski. L., Domb, A. J., and Weiniger. C. F. 2009. Prolonged local anesthetic action through slow release from poly(lactic acid co castor oil), *Pharm. Res.* 26(1):32–39.

18 Polymer–Drug Conjugates

Lucienne Juillerat-Jeanneret and Feride Cengelli

CONTENTS

18.1 INTRODUCTION

The treatment of human diseases such as cancer, inflammatory disorders, or degenerative disorders is challenging because these pathologies involve the dysregulation of endogenous and often essential cellular processes. Human diseases are generally heterogeneous entities; not all cells present with the same distorted phenotype and/or genotype. In addition, several different cell types are involved in diseased tissues: the diseased cells, the normal cell populations from which the disease evolved, vascular cells, fibroblasts, and immune cells. As a consequence, there is a need to protect the normal cells of the diseased tissue, as well as other tissues and organs from the toxicity of therapeutic agents. Most therapeutic drugs distribute to the whole body, which results in the general toxicity and poor acceptance of the treatment by patients. The targeted delivery of chemotherapeutics to defined cells, for example, either stromal or cancer cells in cancer lesions, defined inflammatory cells in immunological disorders, or macrophages in degeneration or atheromatosis, is one of the main challenges and is a very active field of research in the development of treatment strategies to enhance the efficacy and minimize the side effects of drugs. Disease-associated cells express molecules that are different or differently expressed than their normal counterparts. Therefore, one goal in the field of targeted therapies is to develop chemically derivatized drug vectors that are able to target defined cells via specific recognition mechanisms that are also able to overcome biological barriers. This general toxicity to the whole body of many chemotherapeutics results in important side effects and suboptimal drug concentrations at the desired site, and is a challenge facing the development of new modalities of treatment for human diseases. Therefore, in order to improve treatment, it is necessary to increase the selectivity of drugs for defined organs, tissues, or cells by devising therapeutic formulations selective for target cells in a tissue that are able to overcome the biological barriers that prevent drugs from efficiently reaching their targets. However, the achievement of such goals faces formidable challenges, which include the identification of biological targets, their evolution over time, disease progression, and the development of the biotechnologies to prepare these formulated drugs. Several strategies may be employed to achieve drug targeting in human diseases; the choice will depend on the disease and its tissue characteristics, the drug chemical and biological properties, and the rate and time-course of the drug application. The aims of this chapter are (1) to critically summarize the characteristics of human diseases that can be used to develop targeted drug delivery systems using polymeric devices, in particular polymer-functionalized drugs; (2) to review and discuss the advantages and drawbacks of some systems for selected human diseases; and (3) to define and discuss the chemical, biophysical, and biological characteristics of an optimized system.

18.2 PRINCIPLES AND BACKGROUND FOR DRUG DELIVERY USING POLYMERIC DRUG CONJUGATES

18.2.1 BIOLOGICAL ISSUES AND STRATEGIES FOR TARGETED DRUG DELIVERY

Long circulation times are efficient for treating circulatory disorders or for vascular imaging. Direct systemic injection is the most frequent route of administration of therapeutics, but drugs may also be applied orally or by inhalation. However, whatever the administration routes, drugs must be transported through blood vessels, then across the vascular wall into the surrounding tissues and the interstitial space. These processes are determined by (1) the characteristics of the drug, (2) the characteristics of the delivery system, or (3) the biological properties of the tissue. One strategy may rely on the *general characteristics of the diseased cells*, mainly the increased metabolism and active proliferation of cancer cells or the cellular activation of immune cells. However, cell selectivity is low, collateral side effects are important, and resistance of the diseased cells to chemotherapeutic agents is a major cause for treatment failure, which will not be discussed in detail in this chapter. Another strategy, *active molecular targeting*, relies on the expression of the disease-selective molecular markers using agonists and antagonists of selective recognition mechanisms expressed by diseased cells. For example, functional and morphological differences exist between the normal and diseased vasculature offering therapeutic opportunities and windows for the delivery of therapeutic agents. Thus, another strategy relies on the diseased tissue characteristics, mainly the leaky vessels associated with many human cancers and inflammatory disorders, the so-called *enhanced permeability and retention* (EPR) effect. These two latter possibilities will be discussed in more detail in this chapter, using drug-loaded delivery devices.

Therefore, following the vascular location, drugs can leave the blood stream either using passive mechanisms (passive targeting) or after being actively targeted to and transported across the vascular wall (active targeting). Passive targeting depends on vascular leakage and on passive diffusion via the EPR effect of polymeric vectors to achieve drug delivery. The escape of polymeric structures from the vasculature is restricted to the endothelial fenestration (between 150 and 300 nm) of leaky areas in inflammation, tumors, or splenic filtration. Active ligand-targeting using selective recognition mechanisms can be achieved with more recent devices, presently under clinical development and evaluation, and may follow passive diffusion. For these devices, the *engineering of the surface of polymeric structures* is a crucial determinant of their biological behavior, and many efforts are currently being undertaken to improve these modifications. A thorough understanding of the elaborate cell transport machinery as well as understanding and finding the targets to achieve selective delivery will be necessary to fulfill the expectancy of drug–polymer conjugates in the treatment of human diseases.

The challenges of these developments are to design the means of escaping the reticulo-endothelial system by developing stealth nanoparticles "invisible" to macrophages that are long-lasting in the blood compartment. For this effect, the surface modification (hydrophilic/hydrophobic) and size (<100 nm) of the colloidal carrier as well as controlled drug release from the carrier are essential factors for successful development. A previous breakthrough was the use of poly(ethylene glycol) (PEG) or polysaccharides to coat the nanoparticle surface, which avoids the unwanted adsorption of plasma proteins.

Most drugs are agonists or antagonists of molecules inappropriately produced by diseased cells. "Intelligent therapeutics" systems should respond to differences in the concentration of these molecules or the changes in external biological conditions. The delivery of therapeutic agents precisely where and when they are needed in the human body is becoming a reality due to progress in polymer technology, improvement in targeting and local residence time, and enhancement in the local concentration of the therapeutic agents where they are needed. The present research in this field aims at achieving these goals. Chemical bonding, ionic or hydrophobic adsorption, or embedding of drugs into nanoparticles have been devised to be sensitive to the modified properties of diseased tissues, including high proteolytic or glycolytic activity, high metabolism, low pH, and high oxidative environments, to ensure the selective release of the drug. These combined approaches would result not only in increased efficacy but also in decreased collateral side effects. However, targeting strategies and chemical synthesis routes need to be improved, and the mechanisms of interactions of these functionalized polymers with living materials need to be better understood.

Two main approaches can be attempted and will be briefly reviewed below: *passive targeting and active targeting* are illustrated by a few examples.

Passive targeting relies on the EPR effect of the vascular system of diseased tissue in chronic or acute human diseases, including degenerative, neoplasic, inflammatory disorders, or wounding. Fluid movement across leaky vessels by passive diffusion or convection depends on the hydrostatic and osmotic pressure differences between blood and the interstitial space. Small molecules mainly diffuse whereas large molecules are transported by convection/pressure differences. High molecular weight polymer–drug conjugates can take advantage of these features and act as a vehicle to selectively and specifically deliver therapeutic drugs. To take advantage of these defects, drugs have been linked to macromolecular structures, polymers, or nanostructures as vectors;[1–11] however, their penetration into diseased tissue is generally not far away from the nearest capillary. The heterogeneity of the blood flow in diseased tissue and the trapping of these high molecular weight conjugates by the reticulo-endothelial system, mainly of the spleen and the liver, are challenging issues to be solved. These processes are determined both by the characteristics of the drug–delivery system complex and by the biological properties of tissues. An additional problem in cancer therapy resides in the fact that tumors smaller than 2–3 mm in diameter receive nutrients, oxygen, etc. from the surrounding host tissue by diffusion and do not develop their own vasculature, thus they will not be reached by therapeutic agents using passive targeting. In more advanced disease, the passive diffusion of polymeric materials (20–150 nm) at sites of vascular leakage is possible. Drug release, in the vicinity of the cancer, by the carrier must follow extravasation and drug therapeutic dosages must be achieved. The release rates depend on both the drug and the chemical and biophysical properties of the polymeric materials and on the biological characteristics (pH, redox state, etc.) of the tissue where the drugs have to be released and active. Drug release from its carrier remains an issue, some polymeric materials do not allow drug release at levels and rates that are compatible with those necessary for treatment efficacy.

Active targeting involves the design of delivery systems selective for cells expressing specific molecules at their surface. To achieve active targeting and drug delivery to the right cells based on molecular recognition processes, including ligand-receptor and antibody-antigen, the high expression at the cell-surface of disease-specific molecules has to be known and used. Such molecules must be disease-specific and not expressed by other cells in normal human tissues. Drug–polymer conjugates, whose activation depends on the specific biological properties of diseased cells, can also achieve treatment selectivity. Among these approaches, peptidase- or acid-sensitive linkers have been evaluated. For example, adriamycin conjugated to PEG via a linker containing Ala-Val, Ala-Pro, Gly-Pro sequences, which can be cleaved by proteolytic enzymes, displayed tumor cell selectivity.[12] Liposomes that may be destabilized by enzymes, for example, phospholipases or proteases, which are highly expressed and secreted in many cancers, depending on the lipid composition and structure, pH changes, or high redox potential associated with the cancer environment can also be useful for this purpose. The effects of the surface modification have also been evaluated. For example, poly(lactic-*co*-glycolic acid) nanoparticles have been coated with vitamin E TPGS.[7,9] Polysaccharide-decorated nanoparticles have also been developed.[13]

Therefore, to achieve active drug targeted delivery using polymeric devices, it is necessary to develop and validate the necessary chemistry to modify the polymers with "addressing" molecules, provide devices still able to bind drugs to the polymers, and design such complex devices that allow the release of the drugs at the right place, concentration, and time from its vector by developing "intelligent linkers." In addition, the delivery systems of active therapeutic agents must overcome biological barriers, cellular resistance mechanisms to treatment, and biodegradation pathways.

> "Intelligent therapeutics" systems should respond to the changes in pathophysiological conditions. Delivery of therapeutic agents precisely where and when they are needed in the human body is becoming a reality due to the progress in polymer technology, which helps in improving targeting, local residence time, and enhancing the local concentration of the therapeutic agents.

18.2.2 Characteristics of Polymeric Drug Delivery Systems in Human Diseases

Most of the studies performed up to now with polymer–drug conjugates have addressed cancer therapy and inflammatory diseases. In this present description, we will focus mainly on the delivery of chemical drugs in cancer therapy for illustrative purposes, excluding gene therapeutic attempts since they are not in clinical use yet. The present treatments for cancer include approaches encompassing the total or partial surgical excision of tumor tissue, radiotherapy, and chemotherapy. In chemotherapy, anticancer drugs are generally administered intravenously leading to general systemic distribution. Because drugs used in chemotherapy are mostly nonselective for tumor or tumor-associated cells, important and deleterious side effects result from their use. These secondary effects in patients result in their loss of quality of life and necessitate the use of drugs to alleviate these side effects. Therefore, means to deliver drugs to specific areas of the body maximizing drug action exclusively in diseased cells, together with minimizing side effects, and consequently increasing treatment efficiency, are needed. Selective or targeted drug delivery systems, and in particular nanoparticles, have the potential to achieve the goal of drug-targeted delivery to a particular organ, cell, or a structure within a cell, for example, the nucleus, if targeting to the nucleus is a prerequisite for efficacy.

The efficiency of drug delivery depends strongly on the characteristics of the polymeric vector; these characteristics control the fate of a drug in the organism and the selectivity of drug delivery. The control of the release of a drug in a defined localization in an organism, organ, tissue, at the cell surface, or intracellularly and the kinetics of drug release must be defined, and the means to achieve these goals must be designed. The stability and cytotoxicity of the mechanisms of cell uptake and the biodegradation of the vectors are also important parameters. Therefore, the vector size, surface charge, coating hydrophilicity/hydrophobicity, and release characteristics of the drug from the polymeric vectors, which depends on the encapsulation efficiency and/or the linkers binding the drug to its polymeric carriers, as well as the device biocompatibility and biodegradability, are the main factors in determining efficient drug delivery. Passive (EPR effect) versus active (ligand-targeting, cationic lipids or polymer cytotoxicity, and poor circulating times) delivery is also a choice to consider for efficient delivery, and this choice must be dictated by the characteristics of the cancer to be treated, whether a marked angiogenesis is present or not. The expression at the surface of these polymeric vectors of cell-specific ligands, "the biological addresses", may further increase tissue selectivity using active targeting.

Various vectors are available to achieve drug delivery, such as liposomes, micro/nanospheres, nanoemulsions, and micro/nanocapsules. They can be used to deliver hydrophilic drugs, hydrophobic drugs, proteins, nucleic acids, vaccines, biological macromolecules, etc. Vectors, such as liposomes, protect drugs from degradation and biological metabolism, however, liposomes have shown a low encapsulation efficiency, poor storage stability, and rapid leakage of water-soluble drugs in the blood. As such, their ability to control the release of many drugs is not optimal. Particles made of colloidal suspensions and biodegradable polymers offer better stability than liposomes and allow controlled release. Finally, the efficiency of drug delivery may be increased using magnetic vectors, which can be targeted with an external magnetic field combined with the potential to record the drug delivery sites as contrast agents in magnetic resonance imaging (MRI) for diagnostics (see below for more details). The characteristics, composition, etc. of polymeric drug-conjugates in clinical use, clinical trials, or under development that are necessary to achieve the targeted delivery of anticancer agents to treat human cancers will be reviewed as a function of the particle physicochemical properties, the drug chemical properties, and the biological properties or the disease characteristics.

In summary, drug delivery using drug–polymer conjugates and strategies using physicochemical, biological, or chemical methods can improve the distribution of drugs and the outcome of chemotherapy. Physicochemical methods mainly rely on the surface properties of the vector to avoid unselective trapping in the liver and the spleen by the reticulo-endothelial system and the EPR effects of the disturbed vasculature of the diseased tissue. Chemical methods involve the use of modified forms of active drugs, for example prodrugs, by exploiting the differences in the pathophysiological conditions within the target tissues (e.g., pH, redox state, enzyme content) and normal tissues. The biological methods involve the display at the surface of the vector of ligands "the biological addresses" for specific molecules expressed at the surface of the target tissue.

18.2.3 Drug–Polymer Conjugate Nanoparticles

The era of polymer therapeutics started with the improved knowledge of polymer characteristics and the development of polymer chemistry (review[10,11]). Initially polymer–drugs, polymer–proteins, and in particular, PEGylated derivatives and HPMA (N-(hydroxypropyl-methacrylamide) copolymers had been used in the context of anticancer therapy,[5] and are the precursors of nanoparticulate systems. Then self-assembling block-copolymer systems were evaluated to deliver drugs to treat cancer. A pluronic block copolymer-doxorubicin was able to circumvent drug resistance,[14] and PEG-polyAsp–doxorubicin was shown to accumulate preferentially in tumors due to vascular leakage,[15] while increased size prevented back-diffusion and renal clearance when evaluated in clinical trials. These approaches opened the way to nanotechnology for drug delivery. Basically, three possibilities exist for the devices (Figure 18.1), with a lot of variants, and two possibilities exist for the drugs. The drugs are included in the core of the polymeric micro/nanoparticles, which represents the vast majority of the possibilities currently under clinical use or clinical evaluation for treating human diseases or the drugs are displayed at the surface of the particles, allowing for the core to play the role of reporter for tissue localization, such as SPIOs or QDs, which are currently mostly experimental devices.

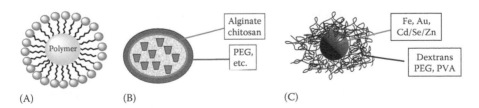

FIGURE 18.1 Nanoparticulate polymeric drug delivery devices. (A) Liposome (drugs are embedded in the polymer). (B) Nanocapsule (drugs are embedded in the core of the capsule). (C) Imaging agent (drugs are bound or adsorbed at the surface).

Drugs can be adsorbed onto or into the polymers or covalently linked to the polymer(s) mostly via linkers. The adsorption depends on the reciprocal characteristics of the drugs and the polymers, such as hydrophobicity/hydrophilicity, ionic bonds, hydrogen bonds, etc. The release of the drugs is mediated by either the degradation or dissolution of the polymers in the biological environment, diffusion of the drugs out of the polymers mediated by a concentration or ionic gradient, or changes in the external conditions of the devices in the biological environment, for example, an increase or decrease in pH, of ionic strength, of hydrophobicity, or hydrophilicity. Thus, these ways of releasing drugs are mainly *passive* means depending on the physicochemical characteristics of the device *and* the biological medium. A more *active* approach involves the design of environment-sensitive linker-drug bonds, again an increase or decrease in pH, but also redox-sensitive bonds or bonds susceptible to hydrolysis by defined enzymatic activities, resulting in the cleavage of the drug-linker bond and release of the free drug. Alternatively, the covalent binding of the drug-linker entity to the polymer(s) may be a stable one in biological systems, not allowing the release of the drugs in the cell environment, rather than a biologically labile one. The biologically stable systems may be preferred for therapeutic agents that must act at the cell surface and the biologically labile systems may be preferred for agents active inside the cells. Basically, three types of bonds have been mostly explored in this latter context: ester bonds and drug release by cellular esterases, amide bonds and drug release by proteolytic enzymes, or disulfide bonds and drug release form its carrier in an oxidative environment, such as is observed in tumors or inflammation.

Alternatively, thermo-responsive, pH-responsive, and biodegradable nanoparticles of poly(D,L-lactide)-graft-poly(N-isopropyl acrylamide-co-methacrylic acid) have been developed as a core-shell type nanoparticle with high drug-loading capacity. A hydrophilic outer shell and a hydrophobic inner core, with a phase transition above 37°C were prepared. Heating above the phase transition temperature or pH modification caused leakage of the drugs demonstrating the potential of these nanoparticles as drug carriers for intracellular delivery of anticancer drugs.[16] Monodisperse polymeric nanoparticles of polyacrylic/isopropylacrylamide were prepared by the seed-and-feed method displaying inverse thermogellation at 33°C. Therefore, drug–polymer mixtures that are liquids at room temperature become a gel at body temperature without chemical reaction, allowing for a sustained release of drugs.[17] Oxidation-sensitive polymeric nanoparticles of cross-linked polysulfides were also developed as oxidation-sensitive vehicles for hydrophilic or hydrophobic drugs able to release drugs in the more oxidative environment of cancer and inflammation.[18]

Creating a toolbox that allows for therapeutics to be hierarchically assembled into an ordered, spatially, and chemically defined architecture into micro/nanoparticles or displayed at the surface of particles is a major synthetic challenge.

> Creating a toolbox that allows for therapeutics to be hierarchically assembled by an ordered, spatially and chemically defined architecture into micro/nanoparticles or displayed at the surface of particles is a major synthetic challenge.

18.2.4 Nanoparticles for Human Therapy

As stated above, the treatment of many human diseases is limited by the inadequacy to deliver therapeutic agents in such a way that most drug molecules will selectively reach the desired targets, and with only marginal collateral damages. Therefore, in order to achieve such efficient treatments, two main goals must be achieved:

- Increase the targeting selectivity of drug–polymer conjugates for defined organs, tissues, or cells.
- Devise a therapeutic formulation able to overcome the biological barriers, such as the respiratory, digestive and cerebral cellular barriers, that prevent drugs from efficiently reaching their targets, the blood–brain barrier (BBB) being the most challenging for transporting therapeutics into the central nervous system (CNS) for the treatment of neurological, degenerative or neoplasic disorders.

However, the development of such systems faces formidable challenges, which include the identification of disease biomarkers as "biological addresses" and the development of the biotechnologies necessary to develop biomarker-targeted delivery of therapeutic agents, coupled with the possibility of avoiding biological barriers. Submicroscopic (nano)particles, smaller in one of their dimensions than 100 nm (subcellular size), may act as drug vehicles either as matrix systems in which the drug is dispersed or as reservoirs in which the drug is confined in a hydrophobic or hydrophilic core surrounded by a polymeric membrane.[10,11,19–21] The other possibilities involve the drugs being displayed at the surface of the nanoparticles.

Several possibilities exist for developing nanoparticles made of polymer–drug conjugates:

- Polymer–protein conjugates.
- Polyelectrolyte complexes formed by a polycation and an anion, such as an oligonucleotide or carboxyl carbohydrates such as the hyaluronic acid.
- Dendrimers—highly branched macromolecules containing symmetrically arranged branches arising from a multifunctional core, to which a precise number of terminal groups are added stepwise, covalently binding drugs.
- Drug nanosuspensions—insoluble nanocrystals of drugs, generally coated with a surfactant or a stabilizing agent for biocompatibility.
- Liposomes—closed vesicles forming by the hydration of synthetic or natural phospholipids above their transition temperature. Nanoliposomes are bilayer structures of less than 100 nm, surrounding the drug entrapped in the aqueous space. Drugs can also be contained in the lipid space between bilayers. Surface modification is possible, and nucleic acids are adsorbed on cationic liposomes by ion-pairing. Liposome nanoparticles are biodegradable and flexible, may be either liquid or solid lipids at body temperature and these structures have been the first to reach clinical use. Drugs encapsulated in liposomes under evaluation or in clinics include paclitaxel, lurtotecan, platinum derivatives, vincristine, and doxorubicin.
- Micelles—self-assembling amphipathic colloidal aggregates of hydrophilic (A) and hydrophobic (B) block copolymers (AB or ABA), in which hydrophobic or hydrophilic drugs are physically trapped or covalently bound. Polymeric micelles are biodegradable.
- Polymeric nanospheres—synthetic or natural polymer aggregates, such as (poly(lactide-co-glycolide), polyvinylpyrrolidone, poly(ε-caprolactone), in which the drug is either dissolved, entrapped, or encapsulated allowing the controlled drug to release from the polymer, or to covalently attach. Surface modification is possible by covalent binding or adsorption of drug, antibodies, nucleic acid, targeting agents, and the core may be used as imaging contrast agents, such as gadolinium or iron oxide nanosized contrast agents for MRI or quantum dots (QDs) for imaging by fluorescence.

Colloidal delivery systems such as the encapsulation of therapeutic agents in colloidal carriers, including liposomes, emulsion, solid lipid nanoparticles, polymeric particles, and polymeric micelles are being used clinically (for more extensive reviews, see[22–24]). Drugs covalently bound to the polymer may be active either when still coupled to the polymer, or may need to be released from the polymer to be active. Release of drugs from polymers may be devised to be selective using drug-polymer bonds sensitive to pH or redox changes or to a defined enzymatic activity. Alternatively, the polymer may be chosen to be biodegradable to release the drugs.

The stability and extracellular or cellular distribution of nanoparticles is dependent on their surface properties, chemical composition, morphology, and size. The main challenges for intravenously injected nanoparticles are the rapid opsonization and clearance by the reticulo-endothelial system of the liver and the spleen or excretion by the kidneys. Opsonization renders nanoparticles recognizable by the major defence systems of the body: the reticulo-endothelial system, mainly in the liver and spleen, and the mononuclear phagocyte system, depending on the surface properties of nanoparticles, their size (<200 or >200 nm), and surface characteristics. Nanoparticles with a largely hydrophobic surface are efficiently coated with plasma components, trapped in the liver, and rapidly removed from circulation, while smaller particles can stay in circulation. More hydrophilic nanoparticles can resist the coating process to a variable extent and are more slowly cleared from the bloodstream.[20] Therefore, clearance kinetics depends on the chemical and physical properties of the nanoparticles: surface changes and charge density, lipophilic/hydrophilic area ratio, and the presence of functional and chemically reactive groups. Consequently, in order to successfully achieve drug delivery, the physicochemical properties of nanovectors (size and surface) must be carefully controlled. The suppression of opsonization will increase the retention of nanoparticles in locations different from macrophages and will increase the circulation times. In addition, macrophages are heterogeneous in different tissues and within a tissue. The PEGylation (the coating of the surface by PEG) of nanoparticles has been the main approach up to now for solving the opsonization problems and short circulation times. PEG coating decreases liver, spleen, or kidney clearance. A large surface area is also an issue in the aggregation of nanoparticles in the biological environment, determining the effective clearance rates and mechanisms. However, the potential cytotoxicity of the carrier or of its degradation products and drug release from the nanocarrier at levels and rates that are compatible with those necessary for treatment efficacy remain issues to be solved.

PEG has been widely used to coat the surface of polyester or polyalkylcyanoacrylate particles, delaying phagocytosis by macrophages and making them compatible for passive targeting by increased vascular permeability associated with cancer.[8,25,26] Polysaccharide coating may be a valuable alternative to PEG for this purpose, having the additional advantages of providing targeting by themselves for saccharide cell surface receptors, being biocompatible and biodegradable,[13] and controlling the interactions with cells. The polysaccharides evaluated up to now include the following:

1. Dextran, pullulan, and glycolipid or sialic acid, for decreased macrophage uptake
2. Hyaluronic acid provides bioadhesive properties
3. Functionalized dextran allows vascular targeting
4. Galactose containing copolymer achieves liver targeting

The results depend on the relative polysaccharide and nanoparticle surface characteristics and chemical composition: hydrophobic, hydrophilic, and covalent photopolymerization. The methods of preparation include the following:

1. Adsorption on pre-formed nanoparticles
2. Incorporation during the nanoparticle preparation
3. Copolymerization
4. Using preformed copolymer where the polysaccharide backbone was grafted with preformed polyester chains, and a core-shell structure

Nanoparticles are interesting for medical application since they present a large surface for functionalization with drugs or addressing molecules when compared with larger particles made of the same materials, and when conveniently modified, may achieve targeted drug delivery and can pass, under certain conditions, epithelial and vascular barriers with their cargo. Thus, nanoparticles have the potential to provide opportunities to meet the therapeutic challenges of targeted drug delivery.

Therefore, nanocarriers using the following polymer-conjugates can be used not only for the (targeted) delivery of therapeutic drugs, but also as imaging agents:

- Polymeric micelles
- Liposomes
- Soluble polymer conjugate
- Dendrimers

- Polymeric vesicles
- Polymeric nanosphere, nanogel
- Gd-complexed polymer matrix
- QD
- Iron core nanoparticle

18.2.5 POLYMER DRUG CONJUGATE DELIVERY SYSTEMS

Lipid-based or polymer–drug conjugate nanoparticles can improve the pharmacological properties, pharmacokinetics, biodistribution, and sustained release of free drugs. But they also present new challenges and issues to solve (review[22]). Their potency depends on the drug loading—the fewer the carrier can carry, the more potent the drug must be. The stability of the drug-carrier, either the shelf life or stability in the biological environment, the solubility of the drug, the relative size of the carrier and of the cargo (for example, using nanosized carriers as vectors for proteins around the same size), the surface charge of the device, the carrier biocompatibility, and the potential cytotoxicity of the degradation products are all issues to consider when choosing a polymeric drug delivering system. On the other hand, the drug must resist the chemical procedures and coupling routes, and the system must support therapeutically efficient rates and efficacy of drug release in the tissue. For example, for schedule-dependent anticancer drug therapies, drugs must stay above the minimal efficacy levels for several hours or days; for schedule-independent anticancer drug therapies, a large burst is more important than a constant release. A hypersentivity reaction to the carrier-drug conjugates is also an issue to be taken into account for drug-delivering polymers to reach clinical use. In rare events and for some therapeutic agents, the drug linked to its carrier may have similar biological activity to the free drug; thus, the drug release for the carrier is not a relevant issue for therapeutic efficacy. However, in most cases, the pharmacological properties of the drug may be modified, either improved or in most cases decreased when considering the drug–polymer conjugate, either drug adsorbed or chemically linker to the carrier. For example, the cytotoxicity of liposomal vincristine is similar to that of the free drug, but its potency is augmented and liposomal topotecan is protected from biodegradation whereas the free drug is very unstable in the biological environment, or doxorubicin-linked N-2-hydroxypropyl methacrylamide copolymer displays a slow release but an increased maximal tolerated dose compared with the free drug.

The factors controlling the rate of drug release are not well understood, but depend on the assembly morphology, drug molecular weight, chemical composition, etc., and these factors have also been addressed. Biodegradable polymers are preferred for the controlled drug delivery systems, and are made of natural or synthetic polymers, which have the advantage over natural polymers of being tailored to obtain defined properties. They must match the mechanical properties and degradation rates that are needed for the application. Commonly used biodegradable polymers for biomedical applications include polyglycolic acid, L-, D-, DL-polylactic acid, polycaprolactone, poly(DL-lactide-co-glycolide), and poly(vinyl alcohol). These polymers have features such as controllable mechanical properties, controllable degradation rates, minimal toxicity, and immune responses.[1,2]

Targeted drug delivery nanoparticulate systems are the most recent development in the field of drug–polymer conjugates, currently only at an experimental stage. Drugs may be chemically conjugated to ligands for specific cellular receptors or to antibodies, or incorporated into carriers bearing ligands or antibodies for recognition by cell surface receptors expressed by target cells. For example, doxorubicin-nanoparticles targeting HerB2/neu for breast cancer are under development. The major obstacles include the definition of selective cell-specific targets and the physiological barriers the systems must cross for the tissue delivery of anticancer drugs, in particular the epithelial and BBBs. For example, approaches using nanoparticles that mimic LDL targeting the LDL receptors on brain endothelial cells[27] or a galactose-HPMA copolymer bearing a doxorubicin system for the asialoglycoprotein receptors in liver tumors that is under clinical trial[28] have been attempted. One major problem in these approaches is the identification of relevant targeting entities in human

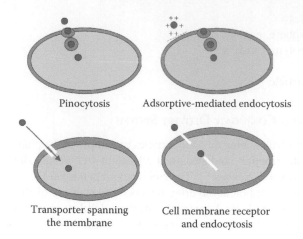

Pinocytosis   Adsorptive-mediated endocytosis

Transporter spanning   Cell membrane receptor
the membrane   and endocytosis

FIGURE 18.2   Mechanisms of uptake of nanoparticles by cells.

diseases, compared with normal cells of the whole body. A few of them have been identified and are evaluated in preliminary trials, for example, the folate receptors or the prostate-specific-antigen (PSA)-doxorubicin conjugates for PSA-positive prostate cancer.

For some therapeutic devices, drugs must reach their appropriate targets in the appropriate location within cells, which may be located in the cytosol, the nucleus, or in cell organelles such as the mitochondria, thus intracellular drug delivery must be achieved for maximal efficacy. For example, in cancer therapy that mainly relies on drugs inhibiting tumor cell growth, anticancer agents must be delivered to the tumor cell nucleus. Therefore, either drug-loaded carriers must be transported intact inside cells, then carriers must release their cargo or carriers must release their cargo at the targeted-cell surface and free drug must be transported inside the cells. Nanoparticles are generally internalized into cells via fluid phase endocytosis, receptor-mediated endocytosis or phagocytosis (Figure 18.2), resulting in the potential delivery of the nanoparticles in different cell compartments.[26,29–33]

Nanoparticle surface modification with a protein-transduction domain of cationic peptides and molecules[34–37] improves cell uptake. Colloids and nanoparticles are mostly taken up by endocytosis in cells via the endosomal-lysosomal pathway. Therefore, intact drug must be released into the cytosol from the lysosomal compartment. Most approaches have used the acidic characteristics of this compartment to dissociate the drug from its carrier, for example, HPMA copolymer, liposomes, polymeric micelles, cationic lipids, and photosensitizers,[38–41] and release into the cytosol to achieve this step. More recently, the activity of lysosomal enzymes has been investigated to release covalently bound drugs from a carrier system. Nuclear delivery is also necessary for many drugs, mainly nucleic acid or protein drugs. In this case, tagging with a nuclear location signal is necessary.

18.2.6 POLYMER FUNCTIONALIZATION

As stated above, therapeutic agents including chemically synthesized therapeutic small or large drugs, therapeutic peptides or proteins, and nucleic acids for gene therapy can be entrapped, encapsulated, adsorbed, and covalently bound either to the surface or at the interior of biodegradable and biocompatible polymeric nanoparticles. These approaches can improve drug solubility problems, and also achieve better drug selectivity. Drugs can be made to form small aggregates, surrounded by a water- and biocompatible, biodegradable polymeric thin layer improving the bio-distribution and bioavailability of drugs. Surface or polymer functionalization with appropriate ligands can allow the targeting of these nanostructures to defined cells, tissues, or body locations depending on the specificity and selectivity of the chosen ligand, improving therapeutic efficacy and decreasing the side effects of the drugs. Finally, the polymer properties may also be defined to respond to changes in pH or redox state, chemical environment, heat (either internal or external), or an external physical stimulus, therefore, allowing the choice for the rate and location of drug release, for example, acidic intracellular organelles, such as the lysosomes. Polymer gels have been designed as controlled release systems for local delivery. The hydrophobic and hydrophilic balance of a gel carrier can be modulated to provide useful diffusion characteristics for periods up to months. The current polymer network drug delivery systems incorporate the pharmaceutical agent by imbibition and equilibrium partitioning after the network is formed before or after polymerization, depending on the drug stability to polymerization pathways. For a more extensive review of the features of the devices, see the article by Hilt and Byrne.[42]

Chemical derivatization[11,21,43] or encapsulation in polymeric micro/nanoparticles[4,7,8,19,20,22,23,44–48] has been evaluated as a possibility for enhancing drug selectivity and biocompatibility (Table 18.1). For hydrophobic or hydrophilic polymers physically entrapping drugs, the biophysical and chemical characteristics of the drugs determine the chemical composition of the system. The structure of the polymer, the methods of entrapping the drugs in the nanoparticles or drug conjugation to the polymers, such as PEGgylation of drugs, will define the drug release kinetics and targeting characteristics.[49,50] Some of these structures are being used clinically or are under clinical evaluation.

Biodegradable polymers are preferred for controlled drug delivery systems as they solve the issue of the removal of the device after delivery of the drug. Commonly used biodegradable polymers for biomedical applications, nonexclusively, include polyglycolic acid, L-, D-, DL-polylactic acid, polycaprolactone, poly(DL-lactide-co-glycolide), poly(vinyl alcohol), or hemiesters of alternating copolymers of maleic anhydride with alkyl vinyl ethers of oligo(ethylene glycol).[7,51–57] The most commonly incorporated polymer, PEG, is a flexible water-soluble molecule that can be end-functionalized to obtain aldehyde, methacryloyl, hydroxyl, primary amine, acetal, or mercapto groups for drug functionalization and copolymerization with other polymers. These polymeric systems have interesting features such as controllable mechanical properties and degradation rates, minimal toxicity, and immune responses.[2]

When drugs are covalently bound to one of the polymeric structures, the necessary chemically reactive groups must be available on both the drugs and the polymers. In many situations, drugs have been linked to the nanocarriers via linkers using various chemical coupling routes (Table 18.2), of which several enzyme-specific releasing linkers have been evaluated.

The preparation and characterization of "intelligent" core-shell nanoparticles able to selectively recognize their targets has been described (for a more extensive review, see the article by Brannon-Peppas and Blanchette[58]) and includes, for example, covalently linked antibodies and ligands for angiogenesis-associated molecules. Active targeting requires that selective ligands for defined cell

---

TABLE 18.1

Characteristics of the Polymer for Biological Compatibility

Polymer	Biological Interest
PVP, PVA, PEG	Decreased aggregation
PEG, PVP, dextrans	Decreased uptake by the RES
PEG, polyacrylates, poly (DL-lactides), chitosan	Biocompatibility
Fatty acids (–COOH), peptides (–NH$_2$), PVA	Chemically functionalizable
Dextrans, PVP	Stabilization

Note: PVP, polyvinylpyrrolidone; PVA, polyvinyl alcohol; PEG, polyethylene glycol.

TABLE 18.2
Design Criteria for Linker-Drug Entities

Polymer-Conjugate System	Criteria	Examples
Polymer backbone	Biocompatible Biodegradable Ability to lower total body clearance	
Linker side chain bonds in polymer drug-nanocarriers	A substrate sensitive to tumor-associated enzymes; ability to increase tumor clearance	*Hydrolytic*: ester, anhydride, orthoester, acetal, hydrazone *Enzymatic*: esters, peptide/saccharide sequences: esterases/lipases, peptidases, glycosidases *Redox*: –S–S– bonds: cellular thiols *Electrostatic*: polycation carrier/polyanionic drug
Drug	Potent chemotherapeutics with undesirable side effects that have sites for covalent attachment, drugs with poor stability in biological environment	Doxorubicin Methotrexate 5-FU Cisplatin

markers are presented in an adequate configuration and concentration at the surface of nanoparticles and that reactive groups must exist at the surface of nanoparticles and in the drug for chemical coupling. Such active targeting strategies also require that selective ligands for defined tumor or tumor-associated cell markers are presented in an adequate configuration and concentration at the surface of nanoparticles. Therefore, a targeting drug-conjugate polymer should be a complex structure (Figure 18.3).

The manipulation of the active surface of polymers and nanoparticles may be performed to increase cytoplasmic drug delivery, for example, with protein-transduction domain peptides[34,59,60] such as HIV-TAT peptides or poly-Arg. These effects are receptor-independent and are related to the interaction of positively charged peptides with negatively charged cell-membrane heparan sulfate proteoglycans and sialic acid-containing glycoproteins, resulting in cell internalization of the complex.[36] Destabilization of the complex and release into the cytoplasm of the nanoparticle payload then arises without fusion with lysosomes. However, cytotoxicity issues of the carrier have been raised. These approaches require that the molecular differences expressed by either diseased cells or by disease-associated cells such as the neo-angiogenic endothelium of cancer tissue[1,42,45,61-66]

Chemical derivatization or encapsulation in polymeric micro/nanoparticles can enhance drug selectivity and biocompatibility. For hydrophobic or hydrophilic polymers physically entrapping drugs, the biophysical and chemical characteristics of the drugs determine the chemical composition of the system. The structure of the polymer and the methods of entrapping the drugs in the nanoparticles or drug conjugation to the polymers, such as PEGgylation of drugs, will define the drug release kinetics and targeting characteristics.

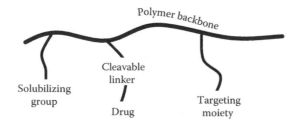

FIGURE 18.3 Structural feature of a targeting drug–polymer conjugate.

are defined. Thus, active targeting approaches involve modified forms of carriers for drugs that are prepared by exploiting the differences between diseased tissues and their normal counterparts[5,18,40,41,67–69] The targeting agents for the recognition molecules of the target cells, include antibodies, ligands for receptors, etc., and can be covalently coupled via an appropriate linker to the polymers incorporating the therapeutic agent. Major obstacles for the delivery of therapeutic drugs include the definition of selective cell-specific targets; the passages of physiological barriers, in particular the epithelial barrier and the BBB; and the chemical synthetic steps able to maintain both the polymer properties and the drug therapeutic efficacy.

18.2.7 LINKERS

To achieve the goals of targeted drug delivery, the methods to assemble on polymers or on the surface of nanoparticles defined recognition molecules, through adsorption or chemicals linkages, must be developed and validated. The surface density, orientation, presentation, spacing, and conformation of these molecules are crucial issues for the success of the ligand-receptor binding and therefore for targeting and drug delivery. Particle and polymer stability, aggregation, and degradability may become a problem. If the intracellular delivery of therapeutics is the goal, the choice of the pair ligand-target molecule is of utmost importance, resulting in different uptake mechanisms and in the potential delivery of the nanoparticles to different cell compartments, depending also on the size of the drug-delivery vector.[26,29,32,33] Uptake mechanisms include receptor-mediated endocytosis, phagocytosis, lipid rafts, etc., and will also determine the efficiency of the internalization and cellular localization of the payload, as well as the pattern of activation of cell signaling pathways. A therapeutic advantage resides in the fact that such structures may bypass multidrug resistance systems, but the major problem of drug release from the carrier in the biological situation remains. The efficient cytoplasmic delivery of drugs is important for drugs whose action is intracellular, and sustained cytoplasmic delivery of drugs with intracellular receptors can only be envisioned using biodegradable nanoparticles.[3] For example, polymeric nanoparticles made from poly(DL-lactide-co-glycolide) can rapidly (of the order of min) escape the endo-lysosomal compartment, in intact form after internalization, and reach the cytoplasm.[30] This escape mechanism is related to the anionic to cationic surface charge in the acidic environment of endosomes-lysosomes. pH-sensitive liposomes have been designed using phospholipids/pH-sensitive polymethacrylate,[70,71] which become unstable at the acidic pH of lysosomes. Therefore, up to now most approaches have involved pH-effects between cellular compartments and surface-functionalized drug-loaded nanoparticles. The chitosan nanoparticles uptake was inhibited by chlorpromazine, suggesting clathrin-mediated endocytosis.[72] Wheat-germ agglutinin-PLGA nanoparticles were taken up by lung carcinoma cells according to a receptor-mediated, caveolae-dependent mechanism.[73] Exocytosis and intracellular retention are also a factor that may control the efficacy of cellular delivery. In a study using PLGA nanoparticles, it was shown that uptake was an endocytic, concentration-, time-, and energy-dependent process;[31] however, a large proportion of the endocytosed nanoparticles were excreted from cells by an energy-dependent exocytic process in as soon as 30 min.[31] The covalent attachment of methotrexate at the surface of the ultrasmall superparamagnetic iron oxide nanoparticles (USPIOs) and its release *in vivo* by lysosomal proteases has led to a study of its therapeutic potential.[74–76] However, to the best of our knowledge, the attachment and delivery of ester-linked anticancer agents to USPIOs has not been exploited to advantage.

The surface modification of polymer (synthetic or natural) aggregates to which the drug is covalently attached is possible. Drugs have been attached to their vector carriers via *linkers*. The design of the chemical bonds linking the drugs to their carriers and the characteristics of the polymers have to be considered together (Table 18.2) and are also of interest for the selective release of the therapeutic agents.[77,78]

The necessary synthesis routes and the design of linkers for conjugation that are appropriate and biocompatible must be developed. Drug-loaded targeting and transport-enhancing nanoparticles must match the mechanical properties and degradation rates that are needed for the application.[54,56] The most commonly used polymer, PEG, is a flexible water-soluble molecule that can be end-functionalized for chemical modification as well as for copolymerization with other polymers.[79] These polymers have features such as controllable mechanical properties and degradation rates, minimal toxicity, and immune responses.[2]

In summary, an optimal nanoparticulate drug carrier should be a device capable of residing *in vivo* for long periods of time, targeting particular cell types, compartmentalizing a large set of molecules, and releasing them in the appropriate environment at the appropriate rate and dose with minimal cytotoxicity for normal cells.

18.2.8 TOXICITY ISSUES AND BIOCOMPATIBILITY CONSIDERATIONS

Nanoparticles interact differently with organs, tissues, and cells as compared with larger particles made of the same components. Therefore, the evaluation of toxicity performed with larger particles cannot be extrapolated to nanoparticles without control. The hazards of inhaled micro- and nanoparticles in air pollution are well established. Epidemiological and toxicological studies have coherently demonstrated their pro-inflammatory and prothrombotic adverse effects in diverse organs. There is virtually no toxicological data available for patients, researchers, or medical workers concerning the new types of nanoparticles under development for drug delivery. Size and surface modification may modify the biocompatibility and biodistribution; and a combination of drugs, devices, and biological agents may behave differently than each agent separately, therefore, combination approval must be obtained by drug control agencies. The exact mechanisms of interaction of nanovectors and cells have been determined in only a very limited number of situations. Therefore, coordinated studies will be rapidly needed to address these issues. Nanostructures can minimize solubility and stability problems and can improve the negative impact of drugs on collateral nontumoral tissues and organs. However, nanomaterials themselves may be cytotoxic[80,81] or induce and/or potentiate cell death[82,83] or immunogenic reactions or nanoparticle aggregates may clog small blood vessels. For example, micelles of cisplatin differently induced gene expression than cisplatin alone,[82] degradation products from poly-(L-lactic acid) were cytotoxic for immune cells.[83]

Gene therapy with viruses had poor success and many problems were linked to the immunogenic reactions to the viral vector constituents and random integration in the genome. Therefore, cationic nanoparticle vectors have been designed to complete viral vectors. Polycations are cytotoxic for cells, inducing mitochondria-mediated necrosis, apoptosis, or membrane destabilization and pore-formation meditated by the interactions of polycations with negatively charged cell-surface glycoproteins or actin.[84] The interactions of cationic polymers with mitochondria need to be better understood, in particular with the proteins of the bcl-2 family. Hypersensitivity reactions secondary to complement activation and induced by the infusion of PEG-modified liposomes[85] may be a potential problem with these materials. To reduce these side effects, it will be necessary to carefully design the polymer formulation and surface functionalization. Therefore, nanoparticle design and polymer formulation and functionalization for gene therapy *in vivo* must be carefully optimized before such treatments can be envisioned.

To gain wide acceptance of nanovectors as anticancer delivery agents, the following toxicity issues need to be addressed:

- The ultimate biological fate of nanomaterials and their degradation products, particularly the nonbiodegradable nanomaterials such as functionalized PEG
- The immunological and pharmacological activities and toxicities
- The possible interferences with cellular machineries, gene expression, and protein processing
- The short- and long-term consequences of exposure to nanovectors
- The translation of *in vitro* studies to *in vivo* application

Another issue with drug-functionalized polymers, whether micro- or nanoparticulate systems, is their biocompatibility. This means that we must understand how tissue or cell exposure to drug-functionalized polymers will affect the functions of these tissues and cells. For example, it might be an inflammatory reaction, a blockade or modification of the filtration machinery in the kidney, modifications in the (re)-absorption processes of the nutriments, ions, etc.

The properties that will affect the biocompatibility of engineered polymers include the following:

- Surface properties (area, charge, molecular structure, etc.)
- the Type of material and especially the change of material properties induced by size, composition, and induction of oxidative stress
- Mechanisms linking particle composition, size, and surface properties to tissue response
- Mechanisms of uptake and intake of particles by organs
- Modification of polymers by living material and their derived molecules

This latter point means that not only must the effect of the drugs and the original polymer(s) to which it was conjugated be analyzed, but we must also evaluate the effects of the degradation products of these man-made entities, following metabolic processing by the exposed living tissue. Presently, very scarce information exists concerning this metabolic processing and the resulting degradation products. Clearly, there is a pressing need to understand how engineered polymers can interact with the human body following exposure. In this context, both the United States and the European Community have launched major programs to solve these issues.

In Section 18.3, we will describe some of the drug-delivery systems that have been developed, exemplifying the possibilities of these approaches for human therapy. However, most of the principles can apply to other forms of drug–polymer conjugates, such as functionalized implant materials.

18.3 DRUG CONJUGATION TO POLYMERS FOR EFFICIENT AND SELECTIVE DRUG RELEASE AND DELIVERY: A FEW EXAMPLES

18.3.1 DEFINITION OF THE OPTIMIZED CHARACTERISTICS OF DRUG–POLYMER CONJUGATES FOR THERAPY

As previously defined, drug-polymeric carriers and nanoparticles[86–88] are defined as submicroscopic colloidal systems, which may act as drug vehicles either as nanospheres (a matrix system in which the drug is dispersed), nanocapsules (reservoirs in which the drug is confined in a hydrophobic or hydrophilic core surrounded by a single polymeric membrane), or micelles (self-assembling amphipathic colloidal aggregates of hydrophilic and hydrophobic block copolymers in which hydrophobic or hydrophilic drugs are physically trapped or covalently bound). Some of these systems are being used clinically or are under evaluation (Table 18.3).

For polymeric nanoparticulate systems, the characteristics, either chemical, biophysical, and biological, of the polymeric part of the drug-delivery device are of utmost importance. Therefore, improvement of the biological characteristics must be considered to achieve viable systems (Table 18.4).

Conventional drug-loaded nanoparticles that are rapidly opsonized in the circulation and cleared by the reticulo-endothelial system may also induce some cytotoxicity against phagocytes, and drugs accumulate in bone marrow resulting in myelosuppression, an unfavorable event. However, the drug-nanoparticle toxicity profile is more favorable than the free drug toxicity profile, for example, the decrease of cardiotoxicity of particulate-doxorubicin under clinical application. The accumulation in cells of the reticulo-endothelial system may also be used as a therapeutic favoring approach.

TABLE 18.3

Some Examples of Nanoparticulate Drugs in Clinical Use for Cancer

Polymer Platform	Development Stage	Drug
Liposomes	Approved	Doxorubicin, amphotericin B, Daunorubicin
PEGylated proteins	Approved	Asparaginase
Biodegradable polymer–drug composites	Clinical trials	Doxorubicin
Polymer–drug conjugate-based particles	Clinical trials	Camptothecin analogs

TABLE 18.4

Advantages and Limitation of Polymers

Polymer	Advantages	Limitations
PEG/dextrans/PVP/ PVA	Improved biocompatibility Decreased uptake by the reticulo-endothelial system Enhanced blood circulation time	Low opportunities for chemical functionalization
Lipids	Enhanced colloidal stability Carboxylate groups for chemical functionalization	Hydrophobicity
Peptides/saccharides	Biocompatibility existing receptors for cell binding Chemical functionalization possible under some limitations	Poor bio-stability due to proteases and glycosidases
Chitosan	Cationic linear polymer Enhanced cell uptake due to positive charges, Reactive groups for chemical functionalization	May be cytotoxic at high level of positive charges
Polyacrylic acid/ poly(D,L-lactide)	Increased stability Biocompatibility of the particles Enhanced adhesion to cells A lot of experience already gained	

Source: Adapted from Koo, Y.E. et al., *Adv. Drug Deliv.*, 85, 1556, 2006.

For example, the accumulation of nanoparticle-doxorubicin in the lysosomes of Kupfer cells in the liver, but not in tumor cells, acts as a long-term active drug delivery system;[89,90] in mice treated with doxorubicin-poly(isohexylcyanoacrylate) (PIHCA) nanospheres,[91] drug accumulates in the liver, spleen, and lungs, but a reduction of hepatic metastasis and a longer life span were also observed[90] compared with free doxorubicin. The same observation was shown for actinomycin D adsorbed on poly(methylcyanoacrylate) (PMCA) and lung accumulation.[92] Actinomycin D adsorbed on the slowly degradable poly(ethylcyanoacrylate) (PECA) accumulated in the small intestine or vinblastine incorporated into PECA accumulated in the spleen,[93] but both systems were efficient anticancer agents. Therefore, both the polymer composition and the drug chemical characteristics and tissue localization are important factors that can be modified to optimize the systems. The preparation and characterization of biodegradable/bioerodible polymers for the controlled-targeted release of proteic drugs (inteferons or growth factors for tissue engineering) have been described. *Bioerodible polymeric matrices* are hemiesters of alternating copolymers of maleic anhydride with alkyl vinyl ethers of oligo(ethylene glycol). Hydrophilic shell coating to minimize opsonization was achieved by grafted β-cyclodextrins. Coprecipitation was used for formulation, based on the dropwise addition of synthetic polymer in the water-miscible organic solvent to aqueous protein solution under stirring, followed by the addition of the glycolipid. A total of 130–150 nm diameter particles were obtained, with β-galactose residues exposed at the surface. *Biodegradable polymer matrices* solve the issue of removal of the device after delivery of the drug. Among them, poly(malolactonates) are biocompatible, degrading to malic acid, and contain reactive side-chain carboxyl groups that can be esterified for the adjustment of the hydrophilic/hydrophobic balance.[52–57] The starting components are commercially available and nanoparticles of 100–150 nm can be obtained by coprecipitation (reviewed[7]).

Some basic rules can be drawn for polymeric carrier systems. An ideal drug carrier should be a system that is capable of residing *in vivo* for long periods of time, targeting particular cell types, compartmentalizing a large set of molecules and releasing them in the appropriate environment at the appropriate rate and dose. The formation of a di- or tri-block copolymer with low polydispersity can be obtained via anionic polymerization, then subsequent self assembly at concentrations favoring spherical micelles, controlled cross-linking using radical chemistry to obtain a hydrogel shell and polymer micelle architecture, followed by conjugation with a biological molecule to achieve targeting, such as peptides via a carboxyl end group on the polymer. The most commonly incorporated polymer, PEG, is a flexible water-soluble molecule that can be end-functionalized to obtain aldehyde, methacryloyl, hydroxyl, primary amine, acetal, mercapto groups, and copolymerization with other polymers.[79,94,95] For covalent binding, most systems use linkers to couple drugs to polymers. Creating a toolbox of molecules that hierarchically assemble in ordered structures spatially and chemically controlled is the requisite for making them attractive and efficient for encapsulating and delivering drugs. Chemistry and chemical routes to achieve biomimetic assemblies comprising the polymer, a linker, and a bioactive molecule have been reviewed.[96] The characteristics of the linkers may be adjusted to allow specific release of therapeutic agents from their carriers. These systems are, for most of them, still experimental.

In the following paragraphs, we will examine in more detail three situations to illustrate the strategies that can be used to achieve drug targeting in *cancer* relying on the use of nanostructures to take advantage of vascular structures for therapy of some human diseases; then the targeting of drugs across a biological barrier, the BBB, for the treatment of brain diseases; and finally the development of imaging agents for *cancer imaging in vivo*.

> *Biodegradable polymer matrices* solve the issue of removal of the device after drug delivery. Poly(malolactonates) are biocompatible, degrading to malic acid, and contain reactive side-chain carboxyl groups that can be esterified for adjustment of the hydrophilic/hydrophobic balance. Nanoparticles of 100–150 nm can be obtained by the coprecipitation of poly(malolactonates).

18.3.2 Anticancer Drug-Delivery Systems

The vast majority of presently used therapies for cancer (for more extensive reviews, see[97,98] and references herein) capitalize on the differences in the rate of cell replication between tumoral and nontumoral cells, which results in general toxicity, suboptimal concentration of the therapeutic agent in the tumor, and poor therapeutic response.[99] Therefore, in order to improve cancer treatments, it is necessary to optimize the delivery and bio-distribution of drugs to diseased organs, tissues, or cells, by devising therapeutic formulations allowing increased localized concentrations of the therapeutic agents in the target tissues. Both tissue- and cell-distribution of anticancer drugs can be controlled and improved by their entrapment in colloidal systems, increasing antitumor efficacy, reversing resistance mechanisms and decreasing side effects. The most promising features of drug–polymer conjugates in targeted drug delivery in cancer are related to the possibility of modifying their properties, mainly their surface to achieve organ-, tissue-, or cell-specific and -selective delivery of therapeutic drugs, to increase drug efficacy and to decrease side effects. Nanoparticles present a large surface for functionalization with drugs when compared with larger particles made of the same materials and can pass epithelial and vascular barriers. Therapeutic agents can be entrapped, encapsulated, adsorbed, and covalently bound either to the surface or at the interior of biodegradable polymeric nanoparticles. The technical problems of developing targeting nanoparticles include the increased complexity/size of the nanoparticles as well as the increased risks of adverse reactions, while the advantages include the fact that more drugs will reach the targets and that increased selectivity and the delivery of multiple agents at the same site will become possible for targeted combination therapies.

The growth of tumors results in the development of their own neo-vascularization. Tumor vasculature is highly abnormal, proliferating, activated, tortuous, and presents with increased permeability and gaps, with pores between 350 and 800 nm and a cutoff around 400 nm. Most solid tumors possess defective vascular architecture, increased vascular permeability, and leaky vessels.[3–6,8,51] This EPR effect allows the passage and distribution of micro/nanoparticulate devices, offering therapeutic windows for the delivery of drug substances. To take advantages of these defects of the tumor vasculature, drugs have been linked to macromolecular structures, polymers, or micro/nanocarriers as vectors[89–106] achieving clinical use. However, the local time of residence in diseased tissue is generally low. Therefore, it is imperative to design drug carriers capable of residing in defined locations for longer periods of time, while releasing therapeutic agents in the appropriate environment at the requisite rate and dose. Several polymer-drug conjugates are in clinical use or under clinical evaluation as anticancer agents (Table 18.5; for more extensive reviews, see[22,23,58]).

Historically, liposomes encapsulating doxorubicin are the archetype of the simplest and initial form of nanoparticles for cancer therapy and will be the only system described in detail here. Doxorubicin-liposomes were the first to be used clinically and ameliorated versions, such as PEGylated doxorubicin liposomes, have been in clinical use for breast and other cancers for several years. Hydrophilic drugs can be easily entrapped with high efficiency in the aqueous core of liposomes whereas hydrophobic weak bases, such as doxorubicin or vincristine are loaded by pH and chemical gradients across the liposome bilayer. Consequently, as many of the agents active against cancer are hydrophobic molecules, current drug delivery systems used in clinics are liposomes, and many have been decorated with PEG to increase their bioavailability (decreased opsonization, decreased clearance by the reticuloendothelial system, increased circulation time), for example, PEGylated doxorubicin-liposomes. Doxorubicin-liposomes of phosphatidylcholinum-carbamoyl-cholesterol (100 nm size particles) have been coated with methoxypolyethyleneglycol (MPEG) to form a hydrophilic layer and for protection against phagocytosis by macrophages, and thus increasing the blood circulation half-life of the particles. Extravasation of nanoparticles via the defective tumor vessels of high permeability allows the release of the doxorubicin in the vicinity of the tumors. Such peggylated doxorubicin-liposomes are in clinical use. Conjugates of doxorubicin and dextran have been encapsulated with chitosan (100 nm size particles) or conjugated to PLGA, PCAA, or poly(gamma-benzyl-L-glutamate)/poly(ethylene oxide) nanoparticles (200–250 nm), resulting in the long-term *in vitro* release of the drug[107] and suppression of tumor growth in *in vivo* experimental models,[108,116] proving efficacy. Efficacy was also suggested to be macrophage-mediated.[117] Brain

TABLE 18.5
Nanoparticulate Drugs under Clinical Use or Evaluation

Drug	Polymer Platform	Biological Advantages	References
Doxorubicin	PEG-liposomes Chitosan, PLGA, etc.	Decreased cardiotoxicity	[48,102,107–109]
5-Fluorouracil	PEG-dendrimers PEG-micelles	Increased half-life	[110,111]
Tamoxifen	PEG-nanospheres	Increased half-life and solubility	[6,101,112]
Cisplatin/carboplatin	Liposomes	Increased half-life	[45,71,113,114]
Methotrexate	PEG-copolymers, folic acid-PANAM	Decreased toxicity	[45,115]
Camptothecins	Liposomes	Increased solubility and stability	[58]

delivery of doxorubicin was also obtained by biodegradable poly(butyl cyanoacrylate)-polysorbate 80-coated nanoparticles.[27,116] Recent developments of nanoparticles for doxorubicin include the development of lecithin lipid core-drug/pluronic (poly-(ethylene oxide)-poly-(propylene oxide)-poly-(ethylene oxide) triblock copolymer)-shell nanoparticles, obtained by the freeze drying procedure,[48] of solid lipid nanoparticles of cholesteryl butyrate of doxorubicine with paclitaxel, which had additive effects[118] and of nanoparticles of poly-isohexylcyano-acrylate able to increase sensitivity to doxorubicin.[119]

The design of long-circulating nanoparticles decorated with targeting agents must be developed to achieve efficient active tumor targeting. Issues to consider in targeting tumor vasculature include the facts that tumors are poorly perfused, tumor vasculature destruction is not enough to totally destroy tumors, high intratumoral osmotic pressure will result from antiangiogenic therapies, and it has to be considered that the destruction of tumor vasculature will also result in the loss of access to the tumors.

Most of the presently investigated systems involve the targeting of the tumor-associated vascular expression of specific angiogenic molecules, including VEGF receptors, integrins, in particular $\alpha_v\beta_3$ and $\alpha_v\beta_5$ integrins via the Arg-Gly-Asp (RGD) recognition motif or cell-adhesion molecules.[62,65]

18.3.3 TRANSPORT ACROSS THE BBB

The endothelium of any organ is a very attractive tissue for targeted drug delivery using drug–polymer conjugates. This is especially true for the delivery of therapeutic agents to the CNS across the brain vascular tree. The specialized vascular system of the CNS, formed by endothelial cells, pericytes, and astrocyte endfeet (Figure 18.4) presents with specific properties that collectively are called the BBB. The BBB is made of tight junctions between endothelial cells and an ensemble of enzymes, receptors, efflux pumps for many therapeutic agents, and transporter systems[120,121] that control and limit the access of molecules to the brain, either by paracellular or transcellular pathways.

The cerebral vascular system is very dense, which means that once a drug has traversed the BBB its brain distribution is immediate. For chronic diseases of the CNS, whether tumoral or

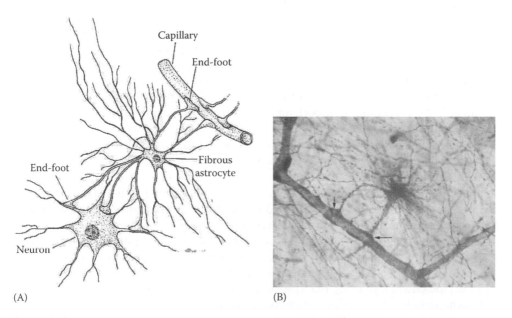

(A)   (B)

FIGURE 18.4 Schematic structure (A) of the BBB, showing the interaction of cells of the CNS with the cerebral capillary, in particular the close interactions of astrocyte end-feet (B) with the BBB capillaries.

neurological, the transvascular route following systemic injection is the limiting step, but the only possibility to envision. Many chronic neurological diseases do not respond to small molecule therapeutics, requesting the use of large molecules, therapeutic peptides, inhibitors, etc.

The surface properties of the nanocarrier may provide passive or active targeting to the endothelium. For example, cationic liposomes are internalized within 1 h in endothelial cells according to an organ- and vessel-specific manner[122] and these effects are likely mediated by vessel-type specific properties. Polystyrene nanoparticles arrest in the bone marrow endothelium where they are internalized by receptor-mediated endocytosis,[123] while polysorbate 80-coated nanoparticles arrest in the BBB endothelium.[27,109] Hydrophilic drugs and the overwhelming majority of all molecules are excluded by the BBB, whereas some, but not all, small (<300 Da) lipophilic molecules may find their way through the BBB mainly by diffusion. A lipophilic drug may be transported to the brain, but increased lipophilicity generally results in a larger biodistribution. Therefore, the utilization of means, including drug–polymer conjugate nanoparticles, which are able to ferry drugs across the BBB, is necessary for drug delivery to the brain. The combination of a drug with a molecule recognized by a luminal blood-to-brain carrier system is mandatory, of which glucose, amino acids, monocarboxylic acid, oligonucleotides, cationic peptides, antibodies to transferrin receptors, or transferrin conjugates represent potential transport systems to the brain (reviews in[124–126]). To be successful, this approach needs the drug to mimic the endogenous ligand, since most transporters are selective. The expression of enzymatic activities at the BBB is also important, and for delivering intact molecules to the brain, chemical modifications, such as cyclization, halogenation, methylation, pegylation, or the introduction of un-natural bonds, may be necessary. However, if the drug needs to be released by specific enzymatic hydrolysis, release may become a problem; therefore, systems allowing diffusion of drugs out of the device may be more favorable. Under these conditions, the structure of the polymer and the method of trapping the drugs in the nanoparticles will define the drug release kinetics and characteristics. However, to achieve these goals, it is necessary to design vectors able to entrap and release the drugs at the right place and time. In addition, the delivery systems and the therapeutic agents must resist hydrostatic, hydrophilic/hydrophobic and biophysical/biochemical barriers, biotransformation, degradation, and clearance mechanisms. It must be noted that the use of biodegradable polymeric matrices solve the issue of removal of the device after delivery of the drug. The conjugation of ligands targeting the BBB on the surface of colloidal carriers, either by covalent or noncovalent linkage, increases selectivity for brain cancers.

The future of development for transporting therapeutic agents across the BBB for treatment of brain diseases likely relies on the development of targeting transport-enhancing nanocarriers. Active targeting requires that reactive groups exist at the surface of nanoparticles for chemical coupling and that selective ligands for defined cell markers are presented in adequate configurations and concentrations at the surface of nanoparticles. Drug release by the carrier must follow extravasation and transvascular transport, and drug therapeutic dosages must be attained.

Some examples of nanoparticles that are able to ferry drugs across the BBB to the CNS have been reported. Nanocontainers have been decorated with ligands for BBB transporters. The anticancer agent 5-fluorouracil[127] for tumors of the CNS have been loaded in Tf-coated nanoparticles, for example. However, the size of even a small protein, such as Tf or an antibody is of the same order of magnitude than that of the container, which will not allow a large number of molecules to decorate the nanocontainer, limits a favorable binding equilibrium. Adsorptive-mediated endocytosis, involving an electrostatic interaction between a positively charged ligand and the negatively charged membrane of cells at the BBB,[128] mainly sialic acid, may also be of interest. Cationized albumin was efficiently transported across the BBB.[46] However, the immunogenic properties of proteins may be an issue in long-term treatments. Attempts using carrier-mediated systems to transport nanoparticles included the GLUT1, showing that α-mannose or choline derivatives incorporated on the surface of nanoparticles were better transported across brain-derived endothelial cells than unfunctionalized particles.[129,130] The folic acid receptor specifically expressed at the BBB was shown to be able to transport doxorubicin-loaded folic acid-decorated nanoparticles.[131] Some hydrophilic surfactants, in particular polysorbates, interact with the surface of the BBB.[27,132,133] Polysorbate-coated doxorubicin nanoparticles,[133,134] but not PEG-coated nanoparticles,[102] may be promising for nanoparticulate drug delivery to the brain. The adsorption of apolipoproteins onto the surfactant-coated nanoparticles may also favor receptor-mediated processes.[133] However, toxicity issues, nonbiocompatibility of the surfactant, increased perme-ability, and tight junction disruption of the BBB by these surfactants may be an important issue, rejoining inva-sive procedures and nonspecific procedures, such as EPR effects. In addition, active brain-to-blood transport efflux transporters expressed at the BBB may also limit transport.

> The treatment of brain diseases can be greatly enhanced by the development of nanocarriers carrying targeting ligand to facilitate active tar-geting. The conjugation of these targeting ligands requires reactive groups at the surface of nano-particles for chemical coupling.

18.3.4 IMAGING AGENTS FOR CANCER OR THE ATHEROMATOUS PLAQUES AND DRUG-DELIVERY SYSTEMS

Colloidal dispersions of USPIOs add a unique function to nanoparticles due to their magnetic properties.[135–138] Biocompatible superparamagnetic nanoparticles have been developed for *in vivo* biomedical applications mainly in MRI[137,139,140] and have been only preclinically evaluated in the tis-sue-specific release of therapeutic agents.[141,142] A strategically interesting way to achieve long-term site-selective delivery is by the chemical attachment of therapeutic agents to USPIOs via a cell-spe-cific labile linkage (Figure 18.5) and steering the drug-USPIO assembly to specific diseased areas in the body under the influence of an external magnetic field. This implies that, subsequently, drugs are released from USPIOs either extracellularly or intracellularly to exert their expected therapeutic effects. The potential of drug delivery based on magnetically activated nanoparticles has been evalu-ated *in vivo* with significant advantages, including the possibility of achieving targeted delivery and decreased off-target effects.[143–149] However, the design of a hierarchical assembly into an ordered, spatially and chemically defined architecture at the surface of magnetically active nanoparticles and the evaluation of magnetic nanoparticles displaying drugs at their surface are only in the early phase of development. The attachment of drugs to the biocompatible polymers coating USPIO nanopar-ticles through ester or peptide bonds would offer the possibility that drugs can be cleaved off the polymer by intracellular esterases or peptidases once inside cells, as a possible solution to selective

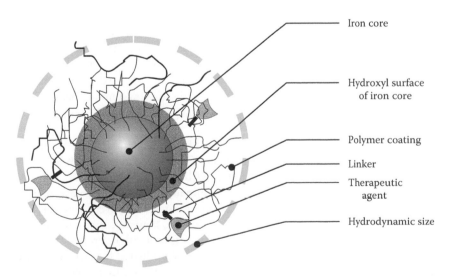

FIGURE 18.5 Schematic representation of iron core stabilized by a polymeric coating.

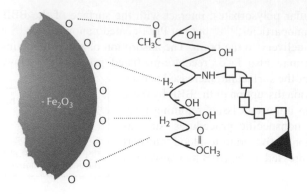

FIGURE 18.6 Structure of a drug-functionalized USPIO. -□-: Linker and ▲: drugs: 5-fluorouridine, doxorubicin, and camptothecin.

drug delivery.[78,150,151] In addition, MRI contrast enhancement allows for noninvasive detection of the sites of localization in the body.

Previous experiments using this approach have been performed by some groups with magnetic particles or magnetic liposomes ranging from 10 μm to 100 nm, loaded with chemotherapeutic agents.[35,143–148] Dextran-USPIOs have been used in gene transfer experiments in a human bladder cancer cells line.[152] USPIOs combined with albumin[153,154] or as liposomes with antibodies targeting Her2 were used for the combination of antibody therapy with hyperthermia.[155] The surface modification of the PEG film of USPIOs with folic acid increased their uptake by human cancer cells.[156]

Very few studies have examined the effects of the surface functionalization of USPIOs. In human cells, we have prepared and evaluated cationic USPIOs chemically functionalized with hydrophilic or hydrophobic drugs[150,151] (Figure 18.6).

Using this system and human melanoma cells, we have observed that the character of the drug is important for the cellular localization of the drug–polymer conjugate. This observation has important implications for drug release from its carrier when specific enzymatic activities are necessary to hydrolyze the drug-linker bond.

18.4 CONCLUDING REMARKS

An ideal therapeutics-polymeric delivery system would be one that selectively targets diseased cells, is nontoxic to normal cells, and is biocompatible. Therefore, for drug delivery, the biophysical, bio-chemical, and biological mechanisms associated with the interaction of drug-functionalized poly-mers with living tissue, at large, must be understood in detail in order to design optimized materials for defined therapeutic goals. The future of such drug-delivery systems depends on the rational design of smart materials combining drug–polymer conjugates. The challenges facing such devel-opments include carrier stability in the living environment and the means to achieve extracellular or intracellular drug release and to overcome biological barriers. Challenges will also include the controlled release of drugs from their vector to achieve efficient delivery, high local drug concen-tration, and drug bioavailability at the disease site, together with acceptable toxicological hazards, including potential immunogenic risks. But the determination of reliable disease-selective markers for targeting such devices must be disclosed. To achieve targeted delivery, several considerations are important. Antibodies have the potential to be selective, however, their size is a limitation to their diffusion into tissue, and the immunogenic potential risks are high. Protein ligands, such as the transferrin and its receptor system, which have been widely evaluated for targeting suffer from the same problem. One possibility would be to release the drug to diffuse freely once its has been trans-ported across the vasculature of the target tissue. This means that the vehicle contains the tissue/cell "address" and the cargo represents the therapeutic agent. The diversity of cellular mechanisms will allow the refining of existing targeting tools and the discovery of new targets. However, it is unrealistic to hope to design a general and unique vector for all situations and purposes. It is more realistic to adapt the vectorization of drugs to defined diseases. There are plenty of possibilities to explore, however, in our opinion, the most promising vectors are vectors involving small molecules as targeting agents and biodegradable and versatile polymers for synthesis purposes.

Viable synthetic routes to construct assemblies comprising a polymer, a linker, and a covalently linked anticancer drug, followed by a hierarchical building of a covalent drug–polymer assembly are possible. Several examples have now been published (Figure 18.7). For example, synthesis

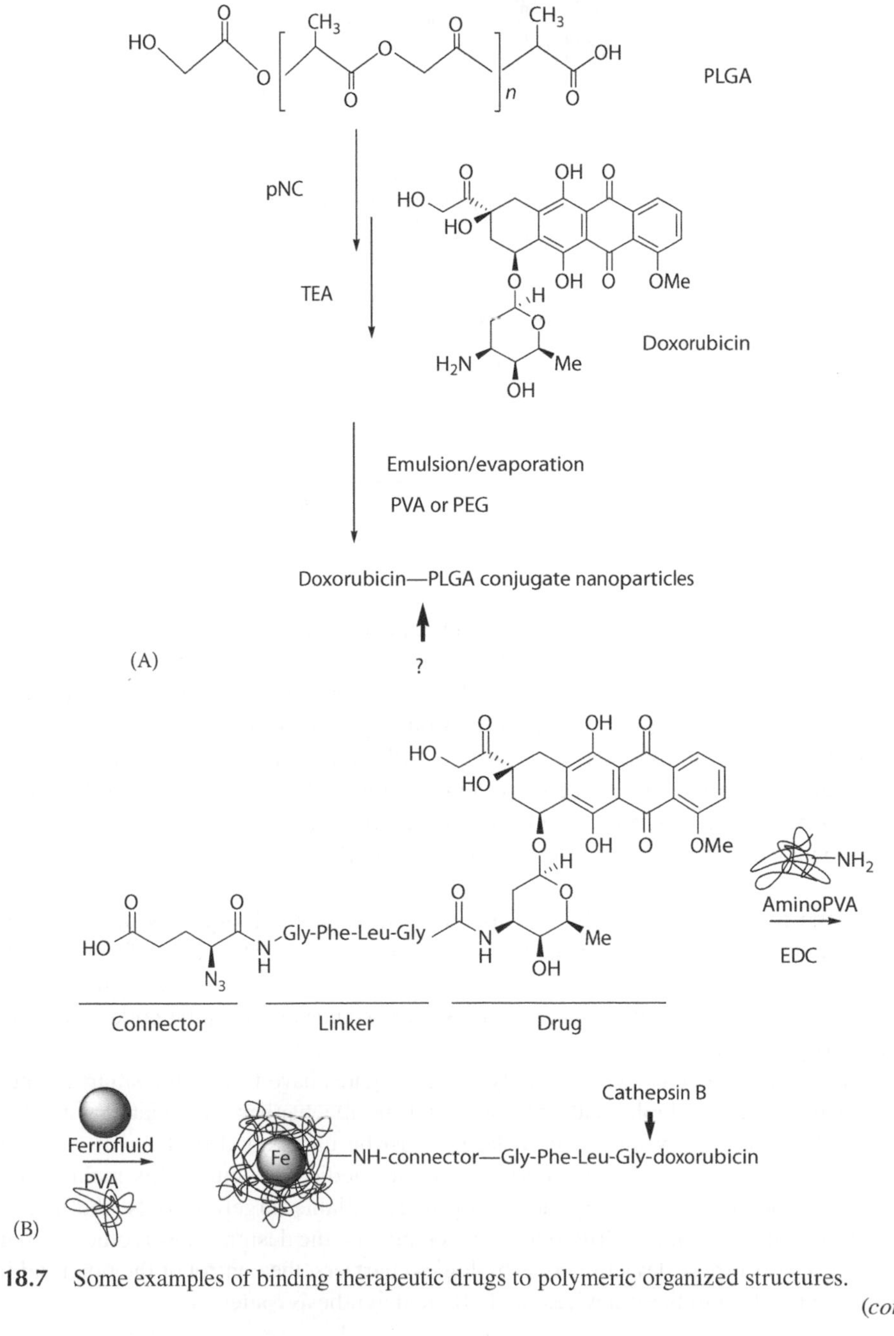

FIGURE 18.7 Some examples of binding therapeutic drugs to polymeric organized structures.

(continued)

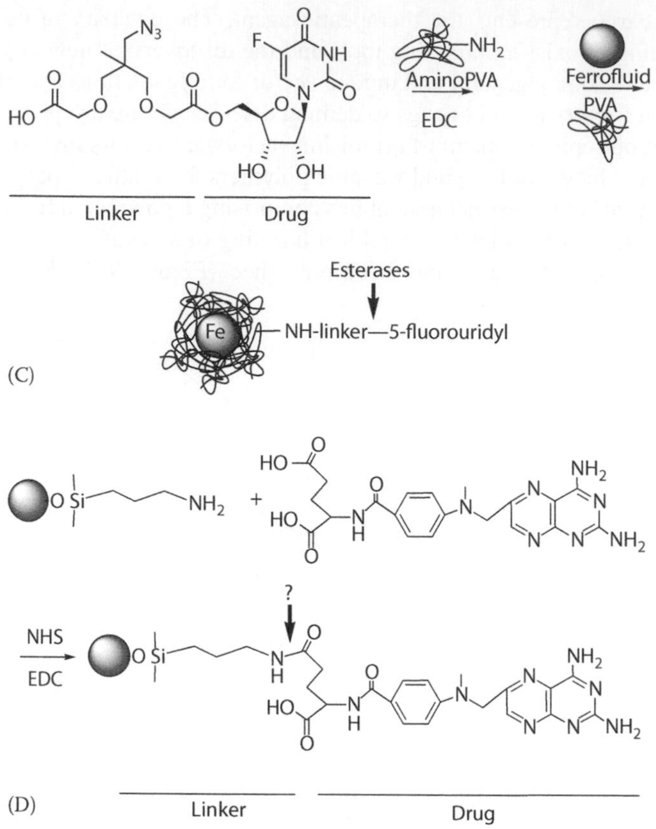

FIGURE 18.7 (continued)

routes have been developed to covalently bind anticancer agents, such as doxorubicin, to polymeric material (see Figure 18.7a) via a linker and a cathepsin B-sensitive bond,[157] since this lysosomal protease is over-expressed in cancer cells and located in the lysosomes, which are the cell organelles where endocytosed material will be routed into by cells. Using a comparable approach, we have linked doxorubicin to the polymer coating USPIO nanoparticles (see Figure 18.7b). Using a different linker, 5-fluorouracyl has been covalently bound to the polymer coating USPIO nanoparticles via an esterase-sensitive bond (see Figure 18.7c) linker as a substrate for cellular esterases.[150] But the therapeutic agent has also been directly linked to the iron oxide core via an aminated silyl-linker.[75]

However, the rate-limiting step for therapeutic efficacy is the bio-processing of these vectors, whether magnetic or not, by cellular mechanisms, releasing the active agent from its carrier. The cell uptake mechanisms and the accessibility to hydrolytic activities for releasing the drugs from the drug–polymer conjugate assemblies are of utmost importance and must be collectively considered for efficient drug delivery.

In summary, for drug delivery, drug–polymer conjugates have to become smarter, and the bio-physical, biochemical, and biological processes and the mechanisms associated with the interaction of these devices with living tissue, at large, must be understood in detail in order to design optimized materials for defined therapeutic goals and medical benefits. This includes improving carrier stability and biocompatibility, designing more reliable targeting tools, the understanding of extracellular and intracellular drug release mechanisms, the design to overcome mechanisms of resistance to transport these devices across biological barriers, the control of the potential immunogenic and toxic reaction to these devices, and efficient synthesis routes.

ACKNOWLEDGMENT

The author thank the Swiss National Science Foundation and the EC FP7 call, NanoImpactNet and NanoTest projects, for financial support.

REFERENCES

1. Lu, Z.R., Shiah, J.G., Sakuma, S., Kopechova, P., and J. Kopechek. 2002. Design of novel bioconjugates for targeted drug delivery. *J. Control. Release* 78:165–173.
2. Lu, Y. and S.C. Chen. 2004. Micro- and nano-fabrication of biodegradable polymers for drug delivery. *Adv. Drug Deliv. Rev.* 56:1621–1633.
3. Moghimi, S.M., Hunter, A.C., and J.C. Murray. 2005. Nanomedicine: Current status and future prospects. *FASEB J.* 19:311–330.
4. Rabinow, B.E. 2005. Nanosuspensions in drug delivery. *Nat. Rev. Drug Discov.* 3:785–796.
5. Satchi-Fainaro, R., Puder, M., Davies, J.W., Tran, H.T., Sampson, D.A., Greene, A.K., Corfas, G., and J. Folkman. 2004. Targeting angiogenesis with a conjugate of HPMA copolymer and TNP-470. *Nat. Med.* 10:255–261.
6. Shenoy, V.S., Vijay, I.K., and R.S. Murthy. 2005. Tumour targeting: Biological factors and formulation advances in injectable lipid nanoparticles. *J. Pharm. Pharmacol.* 57:411–422.
7. Solaro, R., Chiellini, F., Signori, F., Fiumi, C., Bizzarri, R., and E. Chiellini. 2003. Nanoparticle systems for the targeted release of active principles of proteic nature. *J. Mater. Sci. Mater. Med.* 14:705–711.
8. Torchilin, V.P. 2005. Recent advances with liposomes as pharmaceutical carriers. *Nat. Rev. Drug Discov.* 4:145–160.
9. Win, K.Y. and S.S. Feng. 2005. Effects of particle size and surface coating on cellular uptake of polymeric nanoparticles for oral delivery of anticancer drugs. *Biomaterials* 26:2713–2722.
10. Duncan, R. 2003. The dawning era of polymer therapeutics. *Nat. Rev. Drug Discov.* 2:347–360.
11. Duncan, R. 2006. Polymer conjugates as anticancer nanomedicines. *Nat. Rev. Cancer* 6:688–701.
12. Suzawa, T., Nagamura, S., Saito, H., Ohta, S., Hanai, N., Kanazawa, J., Okabe, M., and M. Yamasake. 2002. Enhanced tumor cell selectivity of adriamycin monoclonal antibody conjugate via a poly(ethylene glycol)based cleavable linker. *J. Control. Release* 79:229–242.
13. Lemarchand, C., Gref, R., and P. Couvreur. 2004. Polysaccharide-decorated nanoparticles. *Eur. J. Pharm. Biopharm.* 58:327–341.
14. Batrakova, E.V., Dorodnych, T.Y., Klinskii, E.Y., Kliushnenkova, E.N., Shemchukova, O.B., Goncharova, O.N., Arjakov, S.A., Alakhov, V.Y., and A.V. Kabanov. 1996. Anthracyclin antibiotics noncovalently incorporated into block copolymer micelles: In vivo evaluation of anticancer activity. *Br. J. Cancer* 74:1545–1552.
15. Yasugi, K., Nagasaki, Y., Kato, M., and K. Kataoka, K. 1999. Preparation and characterization of polymer micelles from poly(ethylene glycol)-poly(D,L-lactide) block copolymers as potential drug carrier. *J. Control. Release* 62:89–100.
16. Lo, C.L., Lin, K.M., and G.H. Hsiue. 2005. Preparation and characterization of intelligent core-shell nanoparticles based on poly(D,L-lactide)-g-poly(*N*-isopropyl acrylamide-*co*-methacrylic acid). *J. Control. Release* 104:477–488.
17. Chen, G. and A.S. Hoffman. 1993. Preparation and properties of thermoreversible, phase separating enzyme-oligo(*N*-isopropylacrylamide) conjugates. *Bioconjug. Chem.* 4:509–514.
18. Rehor, A., Hubbell, J.A., and N. Tirelli. 2005. Oxidation-sensitive polymeric nanoparticles. *Langmuir* 21:411–417.
19. Davis, S.S. 1997. Biomedical applications of nanotechnology—Implications for drug targeting and gene therapy. *Trends Biotechnol.* 15:217–224.
20. Davis, M.E., Chen, Z.G., and D.M. Shin. 2008. Nanoparticle therapeutics: An emerging treatment modality for cancer. *Nat. Rev. Drug Discov.* 7:771–782.
21. Duncan, R., Gac-Breton, S., Keane, R., Musila, R., Sat, Y.N., Satchi, R., and F. Searle. 2001. Polymer-drug conjugates, PDEPT and PELT: Basic principles for design and transfer from the laboratory to clinic. *J. Control. Release* 74:135–146.
22. Allen, T.M. and P.R. Cullis. 2004. Drug delivery systems: Entering the mainstream. *Science* 303:1818–1822.
23. Ferrari, M. 2005. Cancer nanotechnology: Opportunities and challenges. *Nat. Rev. Cancer* 5:161–171.
24. Kim, C.K. and S.J. Lim. 2002. Recent progress in drug delivery systems for anticancer agents. *Arch. Pharm. Res.* 25:229–239.

25. Torchilin, V.P. 2000. Drug targeting. *Eur. J. Pharm. Sci.* 11:S81–S91.
26. Dubowchik, G.M. and M.A. Walker. 1999. Receptor-mediated and enzyme-dependent targeting of cytotoxic anticancer drugs. *Pharm. Ther.* 83:67–123.
27. Kreuter, J. 2004. Influence of the surface properties on nanoparticle-mediated transport of drugs to the brain. *J. Nanosci. Nanotechnol.* 4:484–488.
29. Inuma, H., Maruyama, K., Okinaga, K., Sasaki, K., Sekine, T., Ishida, O., Ogiwara, N., Johkura, K., and Y. Yonemura. 2002. Intracellular targeting therapy of cisplatin-encapsulated transferrin-polyethylene glycol liposome on peritoneal dissemination of gastric cancer. *Int. J. Cancer* 99:130–137.
30. Panyam, J., Zhou, W.Z., Prabha, S., Sahoo, S.K., and V. Labhasetwar. 2002. Rapid endo-lysosomal escape of poly(D,L-lactide-*co*-glycolide) nanoparticles: Implications for drug and gene delivery. *FASEB J.* 16:1217–1226.
31. Panyam, J. and V. Labhsetwar. 2003. Dynamics of endocytosis and exocytosis of poly(D,L-lactide-*co*-glycolide) nanoparticles in vascular smooth muscle cells. *Pharm. Res.* 20:212–220.
32. Panyam, J. and V. Labhasetwar. 2004. Sustained cytoplasmic delivery of drugs with intracellular receptors using biodegradable nanoparticles. *Mol. Pharm.* 1:77–84.
33. Savic, R., Luo, L., Eisenberg A., and D. Maysinger. 2003. Micellar nanocontainers distribute to defined cytoplasmic organelles. *Science* 300:615–618.
34. Koch, A.M., Reynolds, F., Merkle, H.P., Weissleder, R., and L. Josephson. 2005. Transport of surface-modified nanoparticles through cell monolayers. *ChemBioChem* 6:337–345.
35. Petri-Fink, A., Chastellain, M., Juillerat-Jeanneret, L., Ferrari, A., and Hofmann, H. 2005. Development of functionalized superparamagnetic iron oxide nanoparticles for interaction with human cancer cells. *Biomaterials* 26:2685–2694.
36. Wadia, J.S., Stan, R.V., and S.F. Dowdy. 2004. Transducible TAT-HA fusogenic peptide enhances escape of TAT-fusion proteins after lipid raft macropinocytosis. *Nat. Med.* 10:310–315.
37. Wyman, T.B., Nicol, F., Zelphati, O., Scaria, P.V., Plank, C., and F.C. Szoka. 1997. Design, synthesis and characterization of a cationic peptide that binds to nucleic acids and permeabilize bilayers. *Biochemistry* 36:3008–3017.
38. Straubinger, R.M. 1993. pH-sensitive liposomes for delivery of macromolecules into cytoplasm of culture cells. *Methods Enzymol.* 221:361–376.
39. Prasmickaite, L., Hogset, A., and K. Berg. 2001. Evaluation of different photosensitizers for use in photochemical gene transfection. *Photochem. Photobiol.* 73:388–395.
40. Leroux, J.C., Roux, E., LeGarrec, D., Hong, K., and D.C. Drummond. 2001. *N*-isopropylacrylamide copolymers for the preparation of pH-sensitive liposomes and polymeric micelles. *J. Control. Release* 72:71–84.
41. Etrych, T., Jelinkova, M., Lhova, B., and K. Ulbrich. 2001. New HPMA copolymers containing doxorubicin bound via pH-sensitive linkage: Synthesis and preliminary in vitro and in vivo biological properties. *J. Control. Release* 73:89–102.
42. Hilt, J.Z. and M.E. Byrne. 2004. Configurational biomimesis in drug delivery: Molecular imprinting of biologically significant molecules. *Adv. Drug Deliv. Rev.* 56:1599–1620.
43. Kukowska-Latallo, J.F., Candido, K.A., Cao, Z., Nigavekar, S.S., Majoros, I.J., Thomas, T.P., Balogh, L.P., Khan, M.K., and J.R. Baker. 2005. Nanoparticles targeting of anticancer drug improves therapeutic response in animal model of human epithelial cancer. *Cancer Res.* 65:5317–5324.
44. Xia, X., Hu, Z., and M. Marquez. 2005. Physically bonded nanoparticle networks: A novel drug delivery system. *J. Control. Release* 103:21–30.
45. Lu, C., Perez-Soler, R., Piperdi, B., Walsh, G.L., Swisher, S.G., Smythe, W.R., Shin, H.J., Ro, J.Y., Feng, L., Truong, M., Yalamanchili, A., Lopez-Berestein, G., Hong, W.K., Khobar, A.R., and D.M. Shin. 2005. Phase II study of a liposome-entrapped cisplatin analog (L-NDDP) administered intrapleurally and pathologic response rates in patients with malignant pleural mesothelioma. *J. Clin. Oncol.* 23:3495–3501.
46. Lu, W., Wan, J., She, Z., and X. Jiang. 2007. Brain delivery property and accelerated blood clearance of cationic albumin conjugated pegylated nanoparticle. *J. Control. Release* 118:38–53.
47. Feng, S.S., Mu, L., Win, K.Y., and G. Huang. 2004. Nanoparticles of biodegradable polymers for clinical administration of paclitaxel. *Curr. Med. Chem.* 11:413–424.
48. Oh, K.S., Lee, K.E., Han, S.S., Cho, S.H., Kim, D., and S.H. Yuk. 2005. Formation of core/shell nanoparticles with a lipid core and their application as a drug delivery system. *Biomacromolecules* 6:1062–1067.
49. van Nostrum, C.F. 2004. Polymeric micelles to deliver photosensitizers for photodynamic therapy. *Adv. Drug Deliv. Rev.* 56:9–16.
50. Derycke, A.S. and P.A. de Witte. 2004. Liposomes for photodynamic therapy. *Adv. Drug Deliv. Rev.* 56:17–30.

51. Moghimi, S.M., Hunter, A.C., and J.C. Murray. 2001. Long-circulating and target-specific nanoparticles: Theory to practice. *Pharm. Rev.* 53:283–318.

52. Cammas, S., Bear, M.M., Moine, L., Escalup, R., Ponchel, G., Kataoka, K., and P. Guerin. 1999. Polymers of malic acid and 3-alkylmalic acid as synthetic PHAs in the design of biocompatible hydrolyzable devices. *Int. J. Biol. Macromol.* 25:273–282.

53. Cammas, S., Nagasaki, Y., and K. Kataoka. 1995. Heterobifunctional poly(ethylene oxide): Synthesis of alpha-methoxy-omega-amino and alpha-hydroxy-omega-amino PEOs with the same molecular weights. *Bioconjug. Chem.* 6:226–230.

54. Grazia Cascone, M., Zhu, Z., Borselli, F., and L. Lazzeri. 2002. Poly(vinyl alcohol) hydrogels as hydrophilic matrices for the release of lipophilic drugs loaded in PLGA nanoparticles. *J. Mater. Sci. Mater. Med.* 13:29–32.

55. Martinez Barbosa, M.E., Cammas S., Appel M., and G. Ponchel. 2004. Investigation of the degradation mechanisms of poly(malic acid) esters in vitro and their related cytotoxicities on J774 macrophages. *Biomacromolecules* 5:137–143.

56. Missirlis, D., Tirelli, N., and J.A. Hubbell. 2005. Amphiphilic hydrogel nanoparticles. Preparation, characterization, and preliminary assessment as new colloidal drug carriers. *Langmuir* 21:2605–2613.

57. Rossignol, H., Bousta, M., and M. Vert. 1999. Synthetic poly(beta-hydroxyalkanoates) with carboxylic acid or primary amine pendent groups and their complexes. *Int. J. Biol. Macromol.* 25:255–264.

58. Brannon-Peppas, L., and J.O. Blanchette. 2004. Nanoparticle and targeted systems for cancer therapy. *Adv. Drug Deliv. Rev.* 56:1649–1659.

59. Console, S., Marty, C., Garcia-Echeverria, C., Schwendener, R., and K. Ballmer-Hofer. 2003. Antennapedia and HIV transactivator of transcription (TAT), protein transduction domains"promote endocytosis of high molecular weight cargo upon binding to cell surface glycosaminoglycans. *J. Biol. Chem.* 278:35109–35114.

60. Silhol, M., Tyagi, M., Giacca, M., Lebleu, B., and E. Vives. 2002. Different mechanisms for cellular internalization of the HIV-1 Tat-derived cell penetrating peptide and recombinant proteins fused to Tat. *Eur. J. Biochem.* 269:494–501.

61. ten Tije, A.J., Verweij, J., Loos, W.J., and A. Sparreboom. 2003. Pharmacological effects of formulation vehicles: Implications for cancer chemotherapy. *Clin. Pharmacokin.* 42:665–685.

62. Arap, W., Pasqualini, R., and E. Ruoshlati. 1998. Cancer treatment by targeted drug delivery to tumor vasculature in a mouse model. *Science* 279:377–380.

63. Molema, G., Meijer, D.K.F., and L.F.M.H de Leij. 1998. Tumor vasculature targeted therapies. *Biochem. Pharm.* 55:1939–1945.

64. Olson, T.A., Mohanraj, D., Roy, S., and S. Ramakrishnan. 1997. Targeting the tumor vasculature: Inhibition of tumor growth by a vascular endothelial growth factor-toxin conjugate. *Int. J. Cancer* 73:865–870.

65. Pasqualini, R., Koivunen, E., and E. Ruoshlati. 1997. Alpha v integrins as receptors for tumor targeting by circulating ligands. *Nat. Biotechnol.* 15:542–546.

66. Reynolds, A.R., Moghimi, S.M., and K. Hodivala-Dilke. 2003. Nanoparticle-mediated gene delivery to tumor vasculature. *Trends Mol. Med.* 9:2–4.

67. Ulbrich, K. and V. Šubr. 2004. Polymeric anticancer drugs with pH-controlled activation. *Adv. Drug Deliv. Rev.* 56:1023–1050.

68. Ulbrich, K., Šubr, V., Strohalm, J., Plocová, D., Jelínková, M., and B. Říhová. 2000. Polymeric drugs based on conjugates of synthetic and natural macromolecules. I. Synthesis and physico-chemical characterisation. *J. Control. Release* 64:63–79.

69. De Groot, F.M., Damen, E.W., and H.W. Scheeren. 2001. Anticancer prodrug for application in monotherapy: Targeting hypoxia, tumor-associated enzymes, and receptors. *Curr. Med. Chem.* 8:1093–1122.

70. Drummond, D.C., Zignani, M., and J.C. Leroux. 2000. Current status of pH-sensitive liposomes in drug delivery. *Prog. Lipid Res.* 39:409–460.

71. Haining, W.N., Anderson, D.G., Little, S.R., von Berwelt-Baildon, M.S., Cardoso, A.A., Alves, P., Kosmatopoulos, K., Nadler, L.M., Langer, R., and D.S. Kohane. 2004. pH-sensitive microparticles for peptide vaccination. *J. Immunol.* 173:2578–2585.

72. Ma, Z. and L.Y. Lim. 2003. Uptake of chitosan and associated insulin in Caco-2 cell monolayers: A comparison between chitosan molecules and chitosan nanoparticles. *Pharm. Res.* 20:1812–1819.

73. Mo, Y. and L.Y. Lin. 2004. Mechanistic study of the uptake of wheat germ agglutinin-conjugated nanoparticles by A549 cells, *J. Pharm. Sci.* 93:20–28.

74. Devineni, D., Blanton, C.D., and J.M. Gallo. 1995. Preparation and in vitro evaluation of magnetic microsphere-methotrexate conjugate drug delivery systems. *Bioconjug. Chem.* **6**:203–210.

75. Kohler, N., Sun, C., Wang, J., and M. Zhang. 2005. Methotrexate-modified superparamagnetic nanoparticles and their intracellular uptake into human cancer cells. *Langmuir* 21: 8858–8864.

76. Kohler, N., Sun, C., Fichtenholtz, A., Gunn, J., Fang, C., and M. Zhang. 2006. Methotrexate-immobilized poly(ethylene glycol) magnetic nanoparticles for MR imaging and drug delivery. *Small* 2:785–792.

77. Reents, R., Jeyaraj, D.A., and H. Waldmann. 2002. Enzymatically cleavable linker groups in polymer-supported synthesis. *Drug Discov. Today* 7:71–76.

78. Schoenmakers, R.G., van de Wetering, P., Elbert, D.L., and J.A. Hubbell JA. 2004. The effect of the linker on the hydrolysis rate of drug-linked ester bonds. *J. Control. Release* 95:291–300.

79. Lee, K.B., Yoon, K.R., Woo, S.I., and I.S. Choi. 2003. Surface modification of poly(glycolic acid) (PGA) for biomedical applications. *J. Pharm. Sci.* 92:933–937.

80. Colvin, V.L. 2003. The potential environmental impact of engineered nanomaterials. *Nat. Biotechnol.* 21:1166–1170.

81. Hunter, A.C. and S.M. Moghimi. 2002. Therapeutic synthetic polymers: A game of Russian roulette? *Drug Discov. Today* 7:998–1001.

82. Nishiyama, N., Kiozumi, F., Okazaki, S., Matsumura, Y., Nishio, K., and K. Kataoka. 2003. Differential gene expression profile between PC14 cells treated with free cisplatin and cisplatin-incorporated polymeric micelles. *Bioconjug. Chem.* 14:449–457.

83. Lam, K.H., Schakenraad, J.M., Esselbrugge, H., Feijen, J., and P. Nieuwehuis. 1993. The effect of phagocytosis of poly(L-lactic acid) fragments on cellular morphology and viability. *J. Biomed. Mater. Res.* 27:1569–1577.

84. Murray, J.C., Moghimi, S.M., Hunter, A.C., Symonds, P., Debska, G., and A. Szewczyk. 2004. Lymphocytic death by cationic polymers: A role for mitochondrion and implications in gene therapy. *Br. J. Cancer* 91:S75.

85. Szebeni, J. 2001. Complement activation-related pseudoallergy caused by liposomes, micellar carriers of intravenous drugs, and radiocontrast agents. *Crit. Rev. Ther. Drug Carr. Syst.* 18:587–606.

86. Beduneau, A., Saulnier, P., and J.P. Benoit. 2007. Active targeting of brain tumors using nanocarriers. *Biomaterials* 28:4947–4967.

87. Chiannikulchai, N., Ammoury, N., Caillou, B., Devissaguet, J.P., and P. Couvreur. 1990. Hepatic tissue distribution of doxorubicin-loaded particles after i.v. administration in reticulosarcoma M 5076 metastasis-bearing mice. *Cancer Chemother. Pharmacol.* 26:122–126.

88. Koo, Y.E., Reddy, G.R., Bhojani, M., Schneider, R., Philbert M.A., Rehemtulla, A., Ross, B.D., and R. Kopelman. 2006. Brain cancer diagnosis and therapy with nanoplatforms. *Adv. Drug Deliv. Rev.* 85:1556–1577.

89. Juillerat-Jeanneret, L. 2006. Critical analysis of cancer therapy using nanomaterials. Series: *Nanotechnologies for Life Sciences. Volume 6: Nanomaterials for Cancer Therapy and Diagnosis.* C.S.S.R. Kumar (Ed.), Wiley-VCH, Weinheim, Germany, pp. 199–232.

90. Chiannikulchai, N., Driouch, Z., Benoit, J.P., Parodi, A.L., and P. Couvreur. 1989. Doxorubicin-loaded nanoparticles: Increased efficiency in murine hepatic metastasis. *Sel. Cancer Ther.* 5:1–11.

91. Verdun, C., Brasseur, F., Vrancks, H., Couvreur, P., and M. Roland. 1990. Tissue distribution of doxorubicin associated with polyhexylcyanoacrylate nanoparticles. *Cancer Chemother. Pharmacol.* 26:13–18.

92. Brasseur, F., Couvreur, P., Kante, B., Deckers-Passau, L., Roland, M., Deckers, C., and P. Speiser. 1980. Actinomycin D adsorbed on polymethylcyanoacrylate nanoparticles: Increased efficiency against an experimental tumor. *Eur. J. Cancer* 10:1441–1445.

93. Couvreur, P., Kante, B., Lenaerts, V., Scailteur, V., Roland, M., and P. Speiser. 1980. Tissue distribution of antitumor drugs associated with polyalykylcyanoacrylate nanoparticles. *J. Pharm. Sci.* 69:199–202.

94. Nagasaki, Y., Kutsuna, T., Iijima, M., Kato, M., Kataoka, K., Kitano, S., and Y. Kadoma. 1996. Formyl-ended heterobifunctional poly(ethylene oxide) synthesis of poly(ethylene oxide) with a formyl group at one end and a hydroxyl group at the other end. *Bioconjug. Chem.* 6:231–233.

95. Shao, H., Zhang, Q., Goodnow, R., Chen, L., and S. Tam. 2000. A new polymer-bound N-hydroxysuccinimidyl active ester linker. *Tetrahedron Lett.* 41:4257–4260.

96. Tu, R.S. and M. Tirrell. 2004. Bottom-up design of biomimetic assemblies. *Adv. Drug Deliv. Rev.* 56:1537–1563.

97. Couvreur, P., Gref, R., Andrieux, K., and C. Malvy. 2006. Nanotechnologies for drug delivery: Application to cancer and autoimmune diseases. *Progr. Solid State Chem.* 34:231–235.

98. Gordon, E.M. and F.L. Hall. 2005. Nanotechnology blooms, at last. *Oncol. Rep.* 13:1003–1007.

99. Ross, J.S., Schenkein, D.P., Pietrusko, R., Rolfe, M., Linette, G.P., Stec, J., Stagliano, N.E., Ginsburg, G.S., Symmans, W.F., Pusztai, L., and G.N. Hortobagyi. 2004. Targeted therapies for cancer 2004. *Am. J. Clin. Pathol.* 122:598–609.

100. Haag, R. and F. Kratz. 2006. Polymer therapeutics: Concepts and applications. *Angew. Chem. Int. Ed.* 45:1198–1215.

101. Brigger, I., Chaminade, P., Marsaud, V., Appel, M., Besnard, M., Gurny, R., Renoir, M., and P. Couvreur. 2001. Tamoxifen encapsulation within polyethylene glycol-coated nanospheres. A new antiestrogen formulation. *Int. J. Pharm.* 214:37–42.

102. Brigger, I., Morizet, J., Laudani, L., Aubert, G., Appel, M., Velasco, V., Terrier-Lacombe, M.J., Desmaele, D., d'Angelo, J., Couvreur, P., and G. Vassal. 2004. Negative preclinical results with stealth® nanospheres-encapsulated doxorubicin in an orthopic murine brain tumor model. *J. Control. Release* 100:29–40.

103. Brigger, I., Dubernet, C., and P. Couvreur. 2002. Nanoparticles in cancer therapy and diagnosis. *Adv. Drug Deliv. Rev.* 54:631–651.

104. Juillerat-Jeanneret, L. and F. Schmitt. 2007. Chemical modification of therapeutic drugs or drug vector systems to achieve targeted therapy: Looking for the Grail. *Med. Res. Rev.* 27:574–590.

105. Parveen, S. and S. K. Sahoo. 2008. Polymeric nanoparticles for cancer therapy. *J. Drug Target.* 16:108–123.

106. Cho, K., Wang, X., Nie, S., Chen, Z., and D.M. Shin. 2008. Therapeutic nanoparticles for drug delivery in cancer. *Clin. Cancer Res.* 14:1310–1316.

107. Oh, I., Lee, K., Kwon, H.Y., Lee, Y.B., Shin, S.C., Cho, C.S., and C.K. Kim. 1999. Release of adriamycin from poly(gamma-benzyl-L-glutamate)/poly(ethylene oxide) nanoparticles. *Int. J. Pharm.* 181:107–115.

108. Chen, J.H., Ling, R., Yao, Q., Wang, L., Ma, Z., Li, Y., Wang, Z., and H. Xu. 2004. Enhanced antitumor efficacy on hepatoma-bearing rats with adriamycin-loaded nanoparticles administered into hepatic artery. *World J. Gastroenterol.* 10:1989–1991.

109. Gulyaev, A.E., Gelperina, S.E., Skidan, I.N., Antropov, A.S., Kivman, G.Y., and J. Kreuter. 1999. Significant transport of doxorubicin into the brain with polysorbate 80-coated nanoparticles. *Pharm. Res.* 16:1564–1569.

110. Li, S., Jiang, W.Q., Wang, A.X., Guan, Z.Z., and S.R. Pan. 2004. Studies on 5-FU/PEG-PBLG nano-micelles: Preparation, characteristics, and drug releasing in vivo, *Aizheng* 23:381–385.

112. Maillard, S., Ameller, T., Gauduchon, J., Gougelet, A., Gouilleux, F., Legrand, P., Marsaud, V., Fattal, E., Sola, B., and J.M. Renoir. 2005. Innovative drug delivery nanosystems improve the anti-tumor activity in vitro and in vivo of anti-estrogens in human breast cancer and multiple myeloma. *J. Steroid Biochem. Mol. Biol.* 94:111–121.

113. Marr, A.K., Kurzman, I.D., and D.M. Vail. 2004. Preclinical evaluation of a liposome-encapsulated formulation of cisplatin in clinically normal dogs. *Am. J. Vet. Res.* 65:1474–1478.

114. Avgoustakis, K., Beletsi, A., Panagi, Z., Kleptsanis, P., Karydas, A.G., and D.S. Ithakissios. 2002. PLGA-mPEG nanoparticles of cisplatin: In vitro nanoparticles degradation, in vitro drug release and in vivo drug residence in blood properties. *J. Control. Release* 79:123–135.

115. Zhang, Z., Lee, S.H., and S.S. Feng. 2007. Folate-decorated poly(lactide-*co*-glycolide)-vitamin E TPGS nanoparticles for targeted drug delivery. *Biomaterials* 28:1889–1899.

116. Chen, D.B., Yang, T.Z., Lu, W.L., and Q. Zhang. 2001. In vitro and in vivo study of two types of long-circulating solid lipid nanoparticles containing paclitaxel. *Chem. Pharm. Bull.* 49:1444–1447.

117. Soma, C.E., Dubernet, C., Barratt, G., Benita, S., and P. Couvreur. 2000. Investigation of the role of macrophages on the cytotoxicity of doxorubicin and doxorubicin-loaded nanoparticles on M5076 cells in vitro. *J. Control. Release* 68:283–289.

118. Serpe, L., Catalano, M.G., Cavalli, R., Ugazio, E., Bosco, O., Canaparo, R., Muntoni, E., Frairia, R., Gasco, M.R., Eandi, M., and G.P. Zara. 2004. Cytotoxicity of anticancer drugs incorporated in solid lipid nanoparticles on HT-29 colorectal cancer cell line. *Eur. J. Pharm. Biopharm.* 58:673–680.

119. Barraud, L., Merle, P., Soma, E., Lefrancois, L., Guerret, S., Chevallier, M., Dubernet, C., Couvreur, P., Trepo, C., and L. Vitvitski. 2005. Increase of doxorubicin sensitivity by doxorubicin-loading into nanoparticles for hepatocellular carcinoma cells in vitro and in vivo. *J. Hepatol.* 42:736–743.

120. Begley, D.J. and M.W. Brightman. 2003. Structural and functional aspects of the blood–brain barrier. *Progr. Drug Res.* 61:39–78.

121. Tamai, I. and A. Tsuji. 2000. Transporter-mediated permeation of drugs across the blood–brain barrier. *J. Pharm. Sci.* 89:1371–1388.

122. McLean, J.W., Fox, E.A., Baluk, P., Bolton, P.B., Pearlman, R., Thurston, C., Unemoto, E.Y., and D.M. McDonald. 1997. Organ-specific endothelial uptake of cationoic liposome–DNA complexes in mice. *Am. J. Physiol.* 273:H387–H404.

123. Porter, C.J.H., Moghimi, S.M., Illum, L., and S.S. Davis. 1992. The polyoxoethylene/polyoxopropylene block copolymer poloxamer-407 selectively redirects intravenously injected microspheres to sinusoidal endothelial cells of rabbit bone-marrow. *FEBS Lett.* 305:62–66.

124. Mizuno, N., Niwa, T., Yotsumoto, Y., and Y. Sugiyama. 2003. Impact of drug transporter studies on drug discovery and development. *Pharmacol. Rev.* 55:425–461.
125. Schally, A.V. and A. Nagy. 2004. Chemotherapy targeted to cancers through tumoral hormone receptors. *Trends Endocrinol. Metab.* 15:300–310.
126. Pardridge W.M. 2003. Blood–brain barrier drug targeting: The future of brain drug development. *Mol. Interv.* 3:90–105.
127. Soni, V., Kohli, D.V., and S.K. Jain. 2005. Transferrin coupled liposomes as drug delivery carriers for brain targeting of 5-fluorouracil. *J. Drug Target.* 13:245–250.
128. Jallouli, Y., Paillard, A., Chang, J., Sevin, E., and D. Betbeder. 2007. Influence of surface charge and inner composition of porous nanoparticles to cross blood–brain barrier in vitro. *Int. J. Pharmaceutics* 344:103–109.
129. Fenart, L., Casanova, A., Dehouck, B., Duhem, C., Slupek, S., Cecchelli, R., and D. Betbeder. 1999. Evaluation of effect of charge and lipid coating on ability of 60 nm nanoparticles to cross an in vitro model of the blood–brain barrier. *J. Pharm. Exp. Ther.* 29:1017–1022.
130. Umezawa, F. and Y. Eto. 1988. Liposomes targeting to mouse brain: Mannose as a recognition marker. *Biochem. Biophys. Res. Commun.* 153:1038–1044.
131. Wu, D. and W.M. Pardridge. 1999. Blood–brain barrier transport of reduced folic acid. *Pharm. Res.* 16:415–419.
132. Petri, B., Bootz, A., Khalansky, A., Hekmatara, T., Muller, R., Uhl, R., Kreuter, J., and S. Gelperina. 2007. Chemotherapy of brain tumour using doxorubicin bound to surfactant-coated poly(butyl cynoacrylate) nanoparticles. Revisiting the role of surfactants. *J. Control. Release* 117:51–58.
133. Steiniger, S.C., Kreuter, J., Khalansky, A.S., Skidan, I.N., Bobruskin, A.I.M, Smirnovam, Z.S., Severin, S.E., Uhl, R., Kock, M., Geiger, K.D., and S.E. Gelperina. 2004. Chemotherapy of glioblastoma in rats using doxorubicin-loaded nanoparticles. *Int. J. Cancer* 109:759–767.
134. Ambruosi, A. et al. 2006. Influence of surfactants, polymer and doxorubicin loading on the anti-tumour effects of poly(butyl cyanoacrylate) nanoparticles in a rat glioma model. *J. Microencaps.* 23:582–592.
135. Goya, G.F., Grazú, V., and M.R. Ibarra. 2008. Magnetic nanoparticles for cancer therapy. *Curr. Nanosci.* 4:1–16.
136. Arruebo, M., Fernández-Pacheco, R., Ibarra, M.R., and J. Santamaria. 2007. *Nano Today* 2:22–32.
137. Gupta, A.K. and Gupta, M. 2005. Synthesis and surface engineering of iron oxide nanoparticles for biomedical applications. *Biomaterials* 26:3995–4021.
138. Neuberger, T., Schöpf, B., Hofmann, H., Hofmann, M., and B. von Rechenberg. 2005. Superparamagnetic nanoparticles for biomedical applications: Possibilities and limitations of a new drug delivery system. *J. Magn. Magn. Mater.* 293:483–496.
139. Cao, Z.G., Zhou, S.W., Sun, K., Lu, X.B., Luo, G., and J.H. Liu. 2004. Preparation and feasibility of superparamagnetic dextran iron oxide nanoparticles as gene carrier. *Aizheng*, 23:1105–1109.
140. Corot, C., Robert, P., Idee, J.M., and M. Port. 2006. Recent advances in iron oxide nanocrystal technology for medical imaging. *Adv. Drug Deliv. Rev.* 58:1471–1504.
141. Lübbe, A.S., Bergemann, C., Huhnt, W., Fricke, T., Riess, H., Brock, J.W., and D. Huhn. 1996. Preclinical experiences with magnetic drug targeting: Tolerance, and efficacy. *Cancer Res.* 56:4694–4701.
142. Lübbe, A.S., Alexiou, C., and C. Bergemann. 2001. Clinical applications of magnetic drug targeting. *J. Surg. Res.* 95:200–206.
143. Alexiou, C., Arnold, W., Klein, R.J., Parak, F.G., Hulin, P., Bergemann, C., Erhardt, W., Wagenpfeil, S., and A.S. Lübbe. 2000. Locoregional cancer treatment with magnetic drug targeting. *Cancer Res.* 60:6641–6648.
144. Alexiou, C., Jurgons, R.J., Schmid, C., Bergemann, J., Henke, W., Erhardt, E., Huenges, F., and F.G. Parak. 2003. Targeting cancer cells: Magnetic nanoparticles as drug carriers. *J. Drug Target.* 11:139–149.
145. Jain, T.K., Morales, M.A., Sahoo, S.K., Leslie-Pelecki, D.L., and V. Labhasetwar. 2005. Iron oxide nanoparticles for sustained delivery of anticancer agents. *Mol. Pharm.* 2:194–205.
146. Jain, K.K. 2007. Use of nanoparticles for drug delivery in glioblastoma multiforme. *Exp. Rev. Neurother.* 7:363–372.
147. Nasongkla, N., Bey, E., Ren, J., Ai, H., Khemtong, C., Guthi, J.S., Chin, S.F., Sherry, A.D., Boothman, D.A., and J. Gao. 2006. Multifunctional polymeric micelles as cancer-targeted, MRI-ultrasensitive drug delivery systems. *Nano Lett.* 6:2427–2430.
148. Rudge, S., Peterson, C., Vessely, C., Koda, J., Stevens, S., and L. Catterall. 2001. Adsorption and desorption of chemotherapeutic drugs from a magnetically targeted carrier (MTC). *J. Control. Release* 74:335–340.

149. Weissleder, R., Kelly, K., Sun, E.Y., Shtatland, T., and L. Josephson. 2005. Cell-specific targeting of nanoparticles by multivalent attachment of small molecules. *Nat. Biotechnol.* 23:1418–1423.
150. Hanessian, S., Grzyb, J. A., Cengelli, F., and L. Juillerat-Jeanneret. 2008. Synthesis of chemically functionalized superparamagnetic nanoparticles as delivery vectors for chemotherapeutic drugs. *Bioorg. Med. Chem.* 16:2921–2931.
151. Cengelli, F., Maysinger, D., Tschudi-Monnet, F., Montet, X., Corot, C., Petri-Fink, A., Hofmann, H., and L. Juillerat-Jeanneret, L. 2006. Interaction of functionalized superparamagnetic iron oxide nanoparticles with brain structures. *J. Pharm. Exp. Ther.* 318: 108–116.
152. Flynn, E.R. and H.C. Bryant. 2005. A biomagnetic system for in vivo cancer imaging. *Physics. Med. Biol.* 50:1273–1293.
153. Wilhelm, C., Billotey, C., Roger, J., Pons, J.N., Bacri, J.C., and F. Gazeau. 2003. Intracellular uptake of anionoic superparamagnetic nanoparticles as a function of their surface coating. *Biomaterials* 24:1001–1011.
154. Gong, L.S., Zhang, Y.D., and S. Liu. 2004. Target distribution of magnetic albumin nanoparticles containing adriamycin in transplanted rat liver cancer model. *Hepatobil. Pancr. Dis. Int.* 3:365–368.
155. Ito, A., Kuga, Y., Honda, H., Kikkawa, H., Horiuchi, A., Watanabe, Y., and T. Kobayashi. 2004. Magnetite nanoparticle-loaded anti-HER2 immunoliposomes for combination of antibody therapy with hyperthermia. *Cancer Lett.* 212:167–1675.
156. Zhang, Y., Kohler, N., and M. Zhang. 2002. Surface modification of superparamagnetic magnetite nanoparticles and their intracellular uptake. *Biomaterials* 23:1553–1561.
157. Sengupta, S., Eavarone, D., Capila, I., Zhao, G., Watson, N., Kiziltepe, T., and R. Sasisekharan. 2005. Temporal targeting of tumour cells and neovasculature with a nanoscale delivery system. *Nature* 436:568–572.

19 Polymer Micelles for Drug Delivery

Sungwon Kim and Kinam Park

CONTENTS

19.1 INTRODUCTION

Polymer micelles have been used widely in the delivery of various therapeutic drugs, which are also known as active pharmaceutical ingredients (APIs). Recent advances in drug discovery technology, including an accumulated database on therapeutic targets, combinational chemistry, and high-throughput screening (HTS), have further increased the number of candidate compounds and constructed a huge pipeline for the discovery and development of new chemical entities (NCEs).[1,2] A very large number of chemicals are hailed as new drug candidates, but almost one-third of them are poorly water soluble.[3] Polymer micelles consisting of amphiphilic

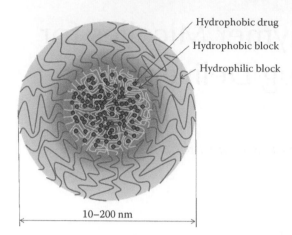

FIGURE 19.1   A typical structure of a polymer micelle in water. Amphiphilic diblock copolymers spontaneously produce a core-shell structure and lipophilic drugs are physically entrapped in the hydrophobic core.
The size of a micelle is usually ranged from 10 to 200 nm.

block copolymers or lipids form a hydrophobic core, in which lipophilic drugs can be physically
incorporated. Hydrophilic blocks or segments generate water-friendly corona and encapsulate the
hydrophobic core. In this way, poorly soluble drugs can be successfully solubilized in aqueous
media (Figure 19.1).

The size of polymer micelles loaded with hydrophobic drugs typically ranges from 10 to 200 nm
in pure water. Nanosized particles dispersed in aqueous media might have a chance of intravenous
(i.v.) injection. In certain inflammatory diseases, such as cancer, vascular structures become leaky,
and thus, nanoparticles can extravasate into the disease site easily. This phenomenon is known as
the "enhanced permeation and retention (EPR)" effect.[4–6] During circulation in blood, nanoparticles
can avoid phagocytotic clearance of the reticuloendothelial system (RES) in the spleen and the
liver.[7,8] Especially, the supramolecular structure of micelles and hydrophilic shells facilitate prolonged circulation in the bloodstream. The hydrophobic core of polymer micelles releases drug in a
sustained manner, but the release pattern is tunable by controlling the hydrophobic block length and
the monomer species. All those features are generally accepted as advantages of polymer micelles
in drug delivery.

In spite of such advantages, only few polymer micelles are used in clinical applications.
Table 19.1 lists polymer micelles used in current clinical trials. Block copolymer of monomethoxy
poly(ethylene glycol) and poly(D,L-lactide) (MPEG-b-PDLLA) has been a popular material used to
prepare polymer micelles, and is now under clinical phase I/II studies.[9–11] MPEG-b-poly(aspartic
acid) (PAsp) has been suggested as another possible micelle system for anticancer drug delivery,
which is now in clinical phase I.[12,13] Pluronic® block copolymers have been widely used in the
pharmaceutical field, but only one case of clinical study has been reported.[14] The first two polymers
are biodegradable due to hydrolyzable ester and peptide bonds, but Pluronics are not. The chemical
structures of polymers and drugs are shown in Figure 19.2.

Researchers have developed many types of micelle systems utilizing new monomers and polymers, stimuli-sensitive moieties, targeting ligands, and different therapeutic drugs. However, only a
few formulations have been reported in clinical studies. Then, what are the major hurdles to developing an effective polymer micelle system that carries and delivers therapeutic drugs? The primary
aim of this chapter is to answer that question. Effort will be made to discuss two important criteria:
the drug loading capacity and the *in vivo* stability of polymer micelles. Polymer micelles currently
under development vary in polymer topology, the nature of core-forming blocks, and the type of
therapeutic drugs. This chapter focuses on diblock copolymer-based polymer micelles and their
ability to solubilize hydrophobic drugs.

TABLE 19.1
Polymer Micelles in Clinical Studies

Polymer	Drug	Particle Size (nm)	Status	Maximum Tolerated Dose	References
MPEG-*b*-PDLLA (2000–1750)[a]	Paclitaxel (Genexol-PM)	30–60	Phase I/II	300 mg/m^2 intravenous infusion for 3 h, once every 3 weeks	[9–11]
Pluronic L61/F127 (~2,000/~12,600)	Doxorubicin	~25	Phase I	70 mg/m^2 intravenous infusion for 12.5 min, once every 3 weeks, six cycles	[14]
NK911					
MPEG-*b*-PAsp-Doxorubicin (5000–4000–543)	Doxorubicin	30–50	Phase I	67 mg/m^2 intravenous infusion for 58 s –12.25 min, once every 3 weeks	[12]
NK105					
MPEG-*b*-PAsp (12,000–8,000)	Paclitaxel	~85	Phase I	180 mg/m^2 intravenous infusion for 1 h, once every 3 weeks	[13,15]

Abbreviations: MPEG, methoxy poly(ethylene glycol); PDLLA, poly(D,L-lactic acid); PAsp, poly(aspartic acid).
[a] Molecular weight of each block (i.e., 2000 and 1750 Da for MPEG and PDLLA, respectively).

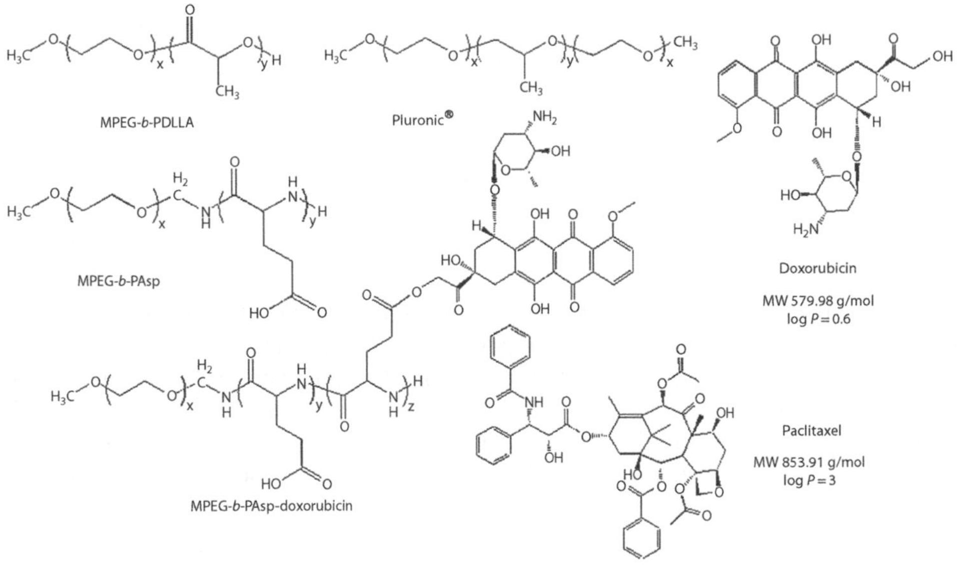

FIGURE 19.2 Structures of block copolymers and drugs examined in clinical phases. Particle size, clinical phase, and maximum tolerated dose are listed in Table 19.1.

19.2 DRUG SOLUBILIZATION METHODS

One of the primary difficulties in the formulation of pharmaceutical drugs is the poor solubility of drug candidates in water. Several methods to formulate poorly soluble drugs have been developed, but there is no standard protocol that can be applied to all drugs. Thus, development of a suitable formulation for an NCE has been a rate-limiting step in the process from drug discovery to

TABLE 19.2
Representative Methods to Solubilize Poorly Water-Soluble Drugs

Method	Advantages	Disadvantages
Salt formation	Simple and relatively easy formulation	Only drugs containing ionizable groups
	Applicable to protein formulation	Common-ion effect
		Prone to be self-aggregated
Nanosizing	Relatively good drug stability	Relatively difficult to prepare
	Injectable	Time-consuming
	Applicable to protein formulation	Drug loss
Solubilizing excipient	Simple	Body toxicity
	Easy and injectable formulation	Drug precipitation by dilution in body
	Applicable to protein formulation	
Solid dispersion	Relatively easy	Conditioning for good reproducibility
	Ready-to-dose form	Drug decomposition
		Difficult to find common solvent
Lipid emulsification	Enhancing oral adsorption	Frequently low drug solubility in lipid
	Relatively easy preparation methods	Difficulty in lipid selection
Liposome	Injectable	Very limited loading capacity
	Versatility in surface modification	Low carrier stability
	Multifunctionality	Cost of phospholipids
	Applicable to protein and gene delivery	
Polymer–drug conjugate	Injectable	Chemical modification of drug
	Versatility in backbone modification	Only drugs with reactive side groups
	Multifunctionality	Purification
	Applicable to protein and gene delivery	
Polymer micelle	Injectable	Low loading capacity
	Versatility in monomer species	Carrier stability
	Well-defined polymer structure	
	Surface modification	
	Multifunctionality	
	Applicable to protein and gene delivery	
	Relatively easy preparation method	

preclinical animal studies. Failure in achieving a suitable formulation often leads to trouble with *in vitro* efficacy/safety evaluation, precipitation, poor bioavailability, and lack of dose-response proportionality after administration.[16] Each formulation method for poorly soluble drugs has advantages and disadvantages as listed in Table 19.2. Understanding the basic principle and limitation of these methods is important to the development of an effective polymer micelle. In this section, representative methods for formulating poorly soluble drugs and for increasing their solubility are briefly reviewed.

19.2.1 SALT FORMATION

One of the simplest ways to increase drug solubility and dissolution rate is salt formation. It is a common, effective, and relatively easy way to increase solubility and dissolution rates of drugs with ionizable groups by the addition of counter ions. Approximately 300 drugs had been approved by Food and Drug Administration (FDA) during the period of 1995–2006, and 120 of them were in the salt form.[17] Typically, solubility of a salt drug depends on the pH of media. There exists a certain pH to achieve the maximal solubility (pH_{max}). For example, the total solubility (S_T) of a basic drug (B) is expressed by

$$\text{if } pH > pH_{max}, \quad S_T = [B]_s(1 + 10^{pK_a - pH}) \tag{19.1}$$

$$\text{if } pH < pH_{max}, \quad S_T = [BH^+]_s(1 + 10^{pH - pK_a}) \tag{19.2}$$

where $[B]_s$ and $[BH^+]_s$ are the solubility of the free drug and the protonated drug (salt), respectively. In Equation 19.1, the saturation species is B, while BH^+ is the saturation species in Equation 19.2. The intersection of two equations gives the pH_{max}. However, the drug solubility is highly influenced by ionic species in media (common-ion effect). At a given pH, for instance, the apparent solubility of the basic drug (K'_{sp}) in the presence of a counter ion (X^-) can be determined by

$$K'_{sp} = [BH^+]_s[X^-] \tag{19.3}$$

Equation 19.3 demonstrates that the maximal solubility of salt may decrease as the concentration of the counter ion increases. As a result, the dissolution rate of salt drug is significantly decreased by excess concentration of common ions. Another possible problem is self-aggregation due to the amphiphilic nature of the hydrophobic drug.[18] The aggregation is generally provoked at the saturation point of ionic drugs near pH_{max}, which makes actual solubility unpredictable. The salt formation method, of course, is not useful for poorly soluble drugs without any ionizable group.

19.2.2 Nanosizing

The nanosizing method, or nanocrystallization, reduces the size of drug particles down to the submicron scale.[16,19] Until 2006, 14 formulations employing this method were examined in clinical studies.[20] Dissolution rate of a nanosized drug follows the Nernst–Brunner equation that was refined later by Noyes and Whitney. If a perfect sink condition is accomplished, that is, the actual concentration of a drug in aqueous medium at time t (C_t) is much less than the saturation concentration (C_s), the equation is expressed by

$$C_t = \frac{D}{h} \times A \times C_s \tag{19.4}$$

where D, A, and h are the diffusion coefficient, the effective surface area, and the effective boundary layer thickness, respectively. Even though the drug solubility remains constant, increase of the surface area by size reduction facilitates drug dissolution in medium. The dissolution rate is important in bioavailability after oral administration of a drug formulation. Faster dissolution results in better bioavailability because of the limited locations of high drug permeation/absorption (window of adsorption) in the gastrointestinal tract for many drugs.[16] At constant drug solubility, C_s can be increased by changing pH using the principle of salt formation, as discussed previously.

Nanosizing of a drug can be accomplished by either top-down or bottom-up methods.[21] Wet-milling and high-pressure homogenization technologies break microparticles down, while precipitation and crystallization build nanoparticles up from individual drug molecules. Regardless of nanosizing methods, a new surface area (ΔA) is generated. The free energy (ΔG) associated with this surface area is defined by

$$\Delta G = \gamma \cdot \Delta A \tag{19.5}$$

where γ represents the surface or interfacial tension. Because of the higher free energy with smaller drug particles, the nanosizing technology requires excipients that can reduce the interfacial tension (γ).

Advantages of nanosizing methods are the relatively good stability of drugs and the opportunity of intravenous injection with reduced toxicity.[20] Therefore, selection of appropriate excipients is important in this method to prevent nanosized drug particles from aggregation and to minimize the dissolution rate. Typically, hydroxypropylcellulose (HPC), hydroxypropylmethylcellulose (HPMC), polyvinylpyrrolidone (PVP), and Pluronic have been used as polymeric excipients, which are well summarized elsewhere.[19] In addition, these methods can be applied to formulate protein drugs because no organic solvent is utilized.[20] However, drug loss during the time-consuming nanosizing process cannot be avoided.

> Advantages of nanosizing methods are relatively good stability of drugs and opportunity of intravenous injection with reduced toxicity. Therefore, selection of appropriate excipients is important to prevent nanosized drug particles from aggregation and to control the dissolution rate. Typically, hydroxypropylcellulose (HPC), hydroxypropylmethylcellulose (HPMC), polyvinylpyrrolidone (PVP), and Pluronic® have been used as polymeric excipients.

19.2.3 SOLUBILIZING EXCIPIENTS

If the free energy of a drug in solution is less than the free energy of the drug in solid state at constant pressure and temperature, the drug dissolves in an aqueous medium until it reaches the saturation solubility. The methods described above, salt formation and nanosizing, increase the free energy of the solid-state drug in order to move the equilibrium toward the solution-state drug. One problem that these methods frequently face is that the free energy of initial solids (salts or nanoparticles) is usually not maintained for a long time, because of salt dissociation or increase/decrease in the particle agglomeration/association/growth leading to increased size. An alternative technique is the use of solubilizing excipients. These excipients are designed to reduce the chemical potential of hydrophobic drugs in solution. At a given solubility, decrease in the chemical potential leads to the lowering of the free energy of a drug in solution.

In a cosolvent system composed of solvent and water, the total free energy of the system is the sum of the free energies of individual components. Accordingly, total drug solubility is the sum of the drug solubilities in the individual components of the system:

$$\log S_m = f \log S_c + (1 - f) \log S_w \tag{19.6}$$

where
S_m is the total solubility in the cosolvent system
S_c is the solubility of a drug in pure organic solvent
S_w is the solubility of a drug in pure water
f is the fraction of the organic solvent in the system[22]

The total solubility of drug is enhanced as the cosolvent fraction increases. In addition, excipients can be used as ligands to form a complex with drug or lipids to make an emulsion.

Various cosolvents (e.g., dimethyl sulfoxide (DMSO), ethanol, propylene glycol (PG), PEG, and dimethylacetamide (DMA)) and surfactants (such as Cremophor®, Tween®, and Solutol®) have been commonly used to improve the solubility of poorly soluble drugs.[23] Cyclodextrin is a popular ligand, and currently, there exist eight different derivatives. Since 1976, more than 35 pharmaceutical products have been developed worldwide.[24] A representative product is Brexin®, a formulation of piroxicam complexed β-cyclodextrin in the molar ratio of 1:2.5. Since launched by Chiesi Farmaceutici (Italy) in 1988, it has been a worldwide drug to control inflammation.[25] Excipients to enhance the drug solubility, however, are chemicals that may possess potential toxicity.[26] For example, the mixture of Cremophor® EL and ethanol for paclitaxel formulation is known to frequently induce significant hypersensitivity, originating from the polyoxyl 35 castor oil.[27,28] Toxicity of diethylene glycol (DEG), used to formulate sulfanilamide, an antibacterial agent, led to a tragic accident in 1937, when more than 100 children died from kidney failure caused by DEG.[26] Cyclodextrin also shows subchronic and chronic toxicity.[29-31] To prevent such untoward incidents, the Center for Drug Evaluation and Research (CDER) of the FDA of the United States now requests industry to demonstrate suitable safety data on excipients for pharmaceutical formulation.

The solid dispersion method can also be considered as a solubilization method using excipients. In solid dispersion, poorly soluble drugs are physically mixed with water-soluble carriers to form an eutectic mixture.[32] Because drugs are dispersed in the carrier matrix, the surface area is very large, and thus, the dissolution rate becomes very high (Equation 19.4). When the dispersed phase is molecularly dispersed in the carrier matrix, the eutectic mixture is called a "solid solution." For example, Chawla and Bansal formulate irbesartan, an angiotensin II receptor agonist to treat hypertension, by the solid dispersion method (heating and quench cooling) using tartaric acid, mannitol, PVP, and HPMC as excipients.[33] Among them, tartaric acid and PVP showed significant enhancement in the solubility of irbesartan up to 9.5 and 7 fold, respectively. However, small molecular carriers frequently require high melting temperature, resulting in drug decomposition. To avoid the melting process, solvents are usually employed. Drug and carrier are dissolved in a common solvent together followed by evaporating the solvent.[34] Because drugs are hydrophobic and carriers are usually hydrophilic, it is difficult to find a common solvent. Moreover, the extent of dispersion of a hydrophobic drug depends on the ratio of drug to carrier, which also determines the crystalline or amorphous state of the dispersed drug.

19.2.4 LIPOSOMES

Biomembrane is mainly composed of phospholipids that have a polar head group and long lipid chains. In water, they get assembled into a bilayer structure. For a pure lipid bilayer without any other biomolecules, interaction of a hydrophobic drug with the membrane might be governed by simple partitioning, which will be discussed later. The liposome is a kind of phospholipid bilayer with unique structure and properties.[35] Spherical, nanosized structure of closed bilayer membrane can hold not only lipophilic compounds in the lipid layer but also hydrophilic drugs at the aqueous core (Figure 19.3). Since first introduced in 1964,[36] liposomes have been a major tool used for drug

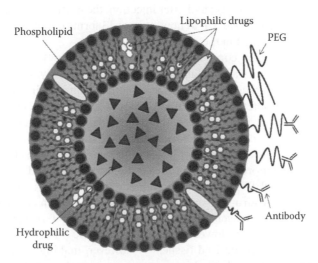

FIGURE 19.3 Representative structure of liposome. Phospholipid molecules form a bilayer in water. Lipophilic drugs are intercalated in the layer while hydrophilic drugs are encapsulated by the lipid membrane. PEG and antibodies are used to lower the RES clearance and to target liposome at specific site, respectively.

delivery. Currently there are at least 14 liposomal formulations under clinical evaluation.[37] The concept of drug delivery includes solubilizing poorly soluble drugs as well as delivering the drugs to a desired target site. Liposomes satisfy those requirements and also take advantages of versatility in the surface properties.[37,38]

An early form of liposomes consisting of bare phospholipids showed opsonin- and complement-mediated clearance after intravenous administration. Liu et al. observed that liver uptake of a liposome composed of phosphatidylcholine, cholesterol, and phosphatidylserine (10:5:1) was promoted by adding serum or whole blood.[39] Primary parameters that influence such a clearance mechanism are the size, the surface charge, and the composition of liposomes.[40] The size of liposomes increased by adsorption of serum proteins and opsonization, which can be mediated by the phosphatidylserine.[39] Cholesterols in the bilayer of a liposome interact with serum antibodies and complements resulting in blood clearance. Opsonization of liposomes can be significantly improved by surface modification. For example, PEG conjugation increases hydrophilicity by providing prolonged circulation in blood, better biocompatibility, and reduced opsonization by RES.[41]

Chiu et al. found that the incorporation of 15 mol% of 1,2-distearoyl-*sn*-glycero-3-phosphoethanolamine (DSPE)-$PEG_{2,000}$ into liposomes of phosphatidylserine significantly improved the blood circulation time of the liposomes.[42] In addition, targeting moieties, such as ligands or antibodies (of immunoliposomes), for an active targeting strategy is used over passive accumulation at leaky tissues by the EPR effect. Recent advances in liposome technology have brought multifunctional liposomes with multiple add-ons of stealth coating, targeting ligands, stimuli sensitivity, and imaging agents in a single carrier.[43] Nevertheless, liposomes have inherent drawbacks of low blood stability, limited drug loading capacity, and expensive starting materials.

19.2.5 POLYMER–DRUG CONJUGATES

Chemical derivatives of therapeutic drugs have provided another opportunity to enhance the aqueous solubility. Such prodrugs are pharmacologically inactive compounds by themselves, but they can be converted to active forms by chemical modification after administration. Usually, change in the redox state,[44] acid-/base-catalyzed hydrolysis,[45,46] or enzymatic metabolism[47,48] are the major mechanisms to restore the drug activity. The pilot study was reported in 1975, in which Ferruti introduced a pharmacologically active polymer for the first time, called "macromolecular drug."[49] He conjugated nicotinic acid, a hydrolipidemizing agent with fast excretion rate from blood, to starch backbone via hydrolyzable ester linkage; and after injection, the macromolecular drug showed good bioactivity with delayed excretion rate. Up to now, at least 13 forms of polymer–drug conjugates for cancer therapy have been evaluated in the clinical trials.[50,51]

A representative polymer is a copolymer of N-(2-hydroxypropyl) methacrylamide (HPMA) and methacrylic acid. Excellent water solubility of the HPMA copolymers is good to solubilize various hydrophobic drugs, such as paclitaxel, doxorubicin, camptothecin, or palatinate. Polymer–drug conjugates in the nanometer size take all advantages of nanomedicine, including solubility enhancement of hydrophobic drugs, prolonged blood circulation, and accumulation at leaky tissues by the EPR effect. Moreover, polymer backbone can be further modified by adding targeting ligands and imaging agents. Recent progress in genomics and proteomics has provided a unique chance to develop novel and more effective prodrugs, such as antibody-directed enzyme prodrug therapy (ADEPT) and gene-DEPT (GDEPT). Both methods aim to increase sensitivity of a target tissue (e.g., tumor) toward a prodrug. To accomplish the goal, either an enzyme directly linked to the antibody in the ADEPT or the sensitization gene in the GDEPT is injected through systematic or local administration route, followed by injecting nontoxic prodrugs. Inactive prodrugs are converted into active drugs at the desired tissue.[47,48] However, making prodrugs requires chemical modification of APIs, causing difficulties in purification and permanent loss of drug activity. Furthermore, a prodrug is considered a new chemical entity, resulting in stringent regulatory requirements.

19.3 POLYMER MICELLES AS A DRUG CARRIER

Polymer micelles used for solubilizing poorly soluble drugs possess all advantages of other formulation methods discussed above. Amphiphilic block copolymers function as excipients to solubilize hydrophobic drugs, but polymer micelles act as drug delivery systems. Versatility in monomer species, block length ratio, and surface modification provide polymer micelles with multifunctionality. Unfortunately, however, polymer micelles have two major drawbacks: low drug loading capacity and low stability in aqueous media. This section deals with the drug loading property of polymer micelles.

19.3.1 Micellar Drug Solubilization Theory

Hydrophobic interaction is the often cited mechanism to explain the loading of poorly water-soluble drugs in polymer micelles. The hydrophobic interaction, however, is based on the London dispersive force that occurs between all molecules. For example, aliphatic polyester blocks in an aqueous medium have a stronger London dispersive force between themselves than to polar water molecules. Likewise, the dispersive force between water molecules is much stronger than that between water and hydrophobic polymer molecules. Hydrophobic molecules become aggregated together in water to produce minimal surface contact with water molecules. Such a microscopic process looks like hydrophobic molecules hiding from water molecules. If poorly soluble drugs coexist in a polymer/water mixture system, drug molecules form aggregates with other drug molecules as well as hydrophobic polymer molecules due to their relatively stronger dispersive force toward polymers than water molecules. This, the driving force for loading a poorly soluble drug in a micelle core, is not the hydrophobic interaction, but an overall effect (hydrophobic effect) of the London dispersive force on aggregation of water-immiscible molecules in an aqueous environment. The London dispersive force is the weakest intermolecular force, but the only interaction force between nonpolar molecules. This force is based on the temporary dipole (or multipole) of nonpolar molecules and depends on the size of molecules.

In a sense, the drug loading process is a process of solubilizing drug in a polymer matrix. Therefore, it is more reasonable to explain the drug loading mechanism in terms of the solubility parameters.

Hildebrand suggested that solubility of a solute in a solvent can be expressed by the Hildebrand–Scatchard solubility parameter (δ):

$$\delta = \sqrt{\frac{\Delta E_{vap}}{V}} \tag{19.7}$$

where
ΔE_{vap} is the energy of vaporization
V is the molar volume of the solvent[52]

The relationship was derived from Polak's equation,

$$-U = {}_l\Delta_g U + {}_g\Delta_\infty U \tag{19.8}$$

where
U is the molar internal energy
${}_l\Delta_g U$ ($=\Delta E_{vap}$) is the molar vaporization energy
${}_g\Delta_\infty U$ is the energy required to expand the saturated vapor to infinite volume at constant temperature[53]

In a system of nonpolar solvent, $_g\Delta_\infty U$ becomes zero $(-U =_l\Delta_g U)$. The cohesive energy density (c) defining cohesive effect in condensed phases such as solvent is expressed by

$$c = -\frac{U}{V} \tag{19.9}$$

The Hildebrand–Scatchard solubility parameter is defined by the square root of c.[52,53]

This model also has been a very useful method to explain the thermodynamics of polymer solutions.[54] The Flory–Huggins interaction parameter (χ_{12}) of two components, solvent and polymer, is defined by

$$\chi_{12} = \frac{V_1}{RT}(\delta_1 - \delta_2)^2 \tag{19.10}$$

where

V_1 is the volume of the solvent
δ_1 and δ_2 are the solubility parameters of the solvent and polymer, respectively
R is the ideal gas constant
T is the temperature

According to Equation 19.10, χ_{12} is always positive, and if $\chi_{12} < 0.5$, then the solvent is a good solvent for the polymer.

Equation 19.10, which expresses the compatibility of polymers and solvents, can be expanded to the miscibility of drugs and polymers, as follows:

$$\chi_{drug-polymer} = \frac{V_{drug}}{RT}(\delta_{drug} - \delta_{polymer})^2 \tag{19.11}$$

where

$\chi_{drug-polymer}$ is the Flory–Huggins interaction parameter between the drug and the polymer
V_{drug} is the volume of drug
δ_{drug} and $\delta_{polymer}$ are the solubility parameters of the drug and the polymer repeating unit, respectively[55]

Since the Hildebrand–Scatchard solubility parameter was applied only for regular solution, an extended form of the solubility parameter, e.g., in polar solvent, was developed by Hansen.[53,56] The Hansen solubility parameter (HSP) consists of three different interactions of dispersion (δ_d), polar (δ_p), and hydrogen bonding (δ_h) components and is expressed by

$$\delta^2 = \delta_d^2 + \delta_p^2 + \delta_h^2 \tag{19.12}$$

Each component can be calculated by following equations:

$$\delta_d = \sum \frac{F_{di}}{V} \tag{19.13}$$

$$\delta_p = \frac{\sqrt{\sum F_{pi}^2}}{V} \tag{19.14}$$

$$\delta_h = \sqrt{\sum \frac{E_{hi}}{V}} \qquad (19.15)$$

where

F_{di} is the molar dispersion constant

F_{pi} is the molar dipole–dipole interaction constant

E_{hi} is the hydrogen bonding energy

V is the molar volume of drugs or polymers[57,58]

Liu et al. estimated the heat of mixing (ΔH_m) between 15 homopolymers and 1 anticancer drug, ellipticine.[57] The ΔH_m can be calculated by

$$\Delta H_m = \varphi_{drug}\varphi_{polymer}(\delta_{drug} - \delta_{polymer})^2 \qquad (19.16)$$

where ϕ_{drug} and $\phi_{polymer}$ are the volume fraction of the drug and the polymer, respectively. The dispersion, polar, and hydrogen bonding forces can be calculated from Equations 19.13 through 19.15 using the group contribution method as discussed later (Section 19.3.2.3), which leads to the total solubility parameters of drug and polymer from Equation 19.12. If they equal to zero, it means that the drug and the polymer are completely miscible. Based on the ΔH_m value of each polymer–drug pair, the solubility order of polymers with ellipticine was found to be poly(β-benzyl-L-aspartate) (PBLA$_{11,500}$) > poly(ε-caprolactone) (PCL$_{14,000}$) > poly(D,L-lactide) (PDLLA$_{75,000-120,000}$) > polyglycolide (PGA$_{100,000-125,000}$), where the subscript is the molecular weight (MW) of each polymer. They also evaluated the ellipticine loading efficiency of PEG$_{5000}$-b-PCL$_{4000}$ and PEG$_{5000}$-b-PDLLA$_{4200}$. The drug loading efficiency was slightly changed by the polymer-to-drug ratio, but was highly dependent on species of the micelle core-forming block. The PEG-b-PCL micelles loaded more than 20% (w/w) ellipticine with 76% (w/w) loading efficiency, while PEG-b-PDLLA micelles showed only 0.1% (w/w) loading capacity and 1.9% (w/w) loading efficiency.

In another study, Letchford et al. investigated the compatibility of five drugs (curcumin, paclitaxel, etoposide, plumbagin, and indomethacin; in the order of their aqueous solubility from low to high) with PEG$_{5000}$-b-PCL$_{2143}$ micelle.[58] The order of Flory–Huggins parameter, $\chi_{drug-polymer}$, was etoposide > paclitaxel > plumbagin > curcumin > indomethacin, which did not follow the aqueous solubility of each drug. However, the micellar drug solubilization exactly reflected the $\chi_{drug-polymer}$ values. Indomethacin showed the best solubility in micelle, while the micelle poorly solubilized etoposide. Furthermore, they determined the partition coefficient of each drug into PEG-b-PCL copolymers with different block lengths by the following equations:

$$\frac{[drug]_{micelle}}{[drug]_{aqueous}} = KX_{PCL}\frac{C}{\rho} \qquad (19.17)$$

where

$[drug]_{micelle}$ and $[drug]_{aqueous}$ are the concentrations of drug in micelle and water, respectively

K is the partition coefficient of the drug

X_{PCL} is the mole fraction of PCL in the copolymer

C is the concentration of the copolymer

ρ is the density of PCL

The results demonstrated that the longer PCL chain provided the better drug loading. Additionally, it was confirmed that the longer PEG chain hindered the drug partition into hydrophobic core, as they reported elsewhere.[59]

The solubility and Flory–Huggins parameters can be a good index to predict the polymer–drug compatibility. By combination of Flory–Huggins theory and Hansen solubility parameters, multiple interactive forces influencing the drug loading in micelles can be explained. In addition to the dispersive intermolecular force, dipole–dipole interaction and hydrogen bonding are important in micellar drug solubilization. Lipinski also stressed the importance of hydrogen bonding to understand solubility of a drug in addition to its size and lipophilicity. From the turbidimetric aqueous solubility screening, more than half of the drugs showed poor solubility in water (≤20 μg/mL in phosphate buffer, pH 7) due to the hydrogen bonding.[3] The hydrogen bonding is known as a major force responsible for drug crystallization.[60] According to the theory, presence of hydrogen bonding donors and acceptors in the micelle core-forming polymer block may improve the loading capacity for drugs with hydrogen bonding moieties.

> The solubility and Flory–Huggins parameters can be a good index to predict the polymer–drug compatibility. By combination of Flory–Huggins theory and Hansen solubility parameters, multiple interactive forces influencing the drug loading in micelles can be explained. In addition to dispersive intermolecular force, dipole–dipole interaction and hydrogen bonding are important in micellar drug solubilization.

19.3.2 Hydrotropy

19.3.2.1 Hydrotropes and Their Mechanism of Drug Solubilization

The term "hydrotropy" means the increased solubility of a lipophilic organic compound in water by the addition of large amounts of a second organic compound, hydrotrope (or hydrotropic agent).[61] The hydrotrope was first used to describe an anionic short-chain molecule that induced significant enhancement of solubility of other organic compounds in water.[62] The hydrotrope has several features that are either similar to or distinct from surfactants, as listed in Table 19.3.[62,63]

First, most hydrotropes have aromatic structure, although some of them have a linear alkyl chain. Typically, the aromatic ring is substituted by anionic or cationic side groups. Therefore, hydrotropes are amphiphiles with small MW. Some of the representative hydrotropes are shown in Figure 19.4. Second, hydrotropes are surface active, similar to surfactants, in that the surface tension of water decreases as the hydrotrope concentration increases. However, high concentration of hydrotropes is generally required to solubilize hydrophobic molecules. Also, there exists the minimal hydrotropic concentration (MHC) over which hydrotropes effectively solubilize hydrophobic compounds. While the critical micelle concentration (CMC) of a surfactant is usually a few moles, the MHC is

TABLE 19.3
Characteristic Features of Hydrotropes in Comparison to Surfactants

Difference

Hydrotrope	Surfactant
High concentration for hydrotropic effect	Low effective concentration
Usually, aromatic structure with ionizable groups	Usually, aliphatic structure with polar head groups
Multiple mechanisms to induce hydrotropic drug solubilization (e.g., π–π stacking)	
Compound (drug) selectivity	

Similarity

Amphiphilicity
Surface activity
Aggregation-induced solubilization of lipophilic molecules

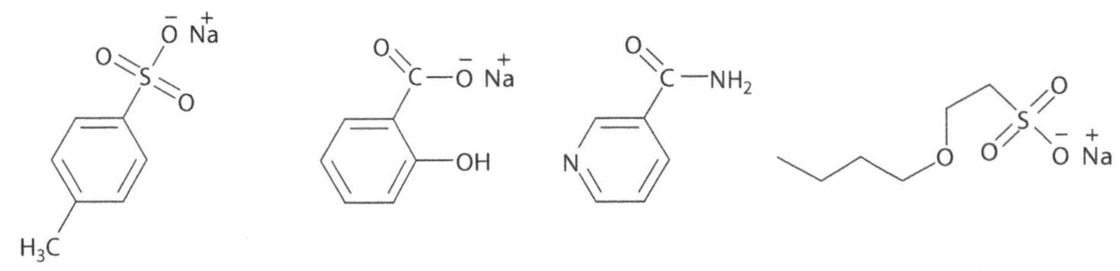

FIGURE 19.4 Structure of some hydrotropes. Typically, hydrotropes consist of an aromatic ring and a hydrophilic side group. However, some hydrotropes have a short lipid chain instead of benzene ring.

generated around 1 M.[64] The MHC of a certain hydrotrope is the same regardless of compounds to be solubilized, but is a specific nature depending on each hydrotrope. For instance, MHCs of sodium p-toluenesulfonate (NaPTS), sodium butyl monoglycol sulfate (NaBMGS), and sodium salicylate (NaS) are approximately 0.3, 0.7, and 0.8 M. However, hydrotropic effect of NaBMGS was shown at 0.7 M regardless of solutes such as fluorescein diacetate, perlyene, or ethyl p-nitrobenzoate.[65] The MHC can be determined by fluorospectrometry using a hydrophobic dye.[66] Third, hydrotropes more selectively solubilize hydrophobic compounds than surfactants. For example, Sanghvi et al. examined hydrotropic solubilization using nicotinamide, a famous hydrotrope, against 11 hydrophobic drugs.[67] It was found that the solubility-enhancement power of nicotinamide was not proportional to the intrinsic solubility of each drug. Furthermore, they suggested that one nicotinamide molecule formed 1:1 (drug:nicotinamide, [nicotinamide] <10%, w/v) or 1:2 (>10%, w/v) stacking complexes with hydrophobic drugs. On the other hand, it was found that the average aggregation number of the nicotinamide for self-association was 4.37 by dynamic light scattering and vapor pressure osmometry measurements.[68] Finally, the hydrotropic activity of a hydrotrope can be improved by adding water-miscible cosolvent(s), which is called as the "facilitated hydrotropy."[63] For example, Simamora et al. showed that the aqueous solubility of rapamycin (in water: 2.6 μg/mL) was enhanced up to 11.26 mg/mL by mixing 5% benzyl alcohol, 10% ethanol, 40% propylene glycol, and 5% benzoate buffer.[69] The primary hydrotrope was benzyl alcohol, but its solubility in water was less than 40 mg/mL. By adding multiple cosolvents, the solubility of benzyl alcohol could be increased, which led to significant enhancement of rapamycin solubility in water. However, the facilitated hydrotropy can be induced by mixing two different hydrotropes. Evstigneev et al. found that the mixture of nicotinamide and caffeine could synergistically increase the aqueous solubility of flavin-mononuclotide.[70]

The mechanism of hydrotropic solubilization is not clearly understood (Table 19.4). It is generally agreed that aromatic stacking is primarily attributed to the hydrotropic effect. The aromatic interaction is usually based on the charge transfer of π electrons. The sp^2 hybridized atom is composed of σ framework sandwiched by two π-electrons. The π-electron density is highly dependent on substituted heteroatoms. As shown in Figure 19.5, for example, an NH_2-substituted ring (e.g., aniline) has more π-electrons than a NO_2-substituted one (e.g., nitrobenzene). As a result, aniline acts as a π-electron donor while nitrobenzene is a π-electron acceptor.[71] In 1950, Mulliken suggested that charge transfer between two aromatic rings formed 1:1 complex.[72] The complex generates an absorption band in the UV-VIS spectra, typically in longer wavelength region.[71,73] However, the charge transfer band is not always observed in aromatic complexes. Therefore, charge transfer alone cannot explain the aromatic stacking phenomena. Other mechanisms for the aromatic stacking have also been suggested, which include van der Waals interaction, electrostatic interaction, induction, and desolvation.[74]

Van der Waals force, especially London dispersive force, just like in surfactants, takes part in the hydrotropic solubilization mechanism. Several reports describe that the hydrophobic moieties

TABLE 19.4

Possible Mechanisms to Explain Hydrotropic Solubilization

Mechanism/Forces	Cases Where Typically Predominant	References
London dispersive force (hydrophobic effect)	An aromatic ring or an aliphatic chain in the structure	[62,64,65]
π–π stacking complex	An aromatic ring (benzene, pyridine) in the structure	[63,71]
Self-aggregation	Minimum hydrotropic concentration and stacking complexation	[63,71,73]
Hydrogen bonding	Hydrogen bonding donors/acceptors in the structure	[75]

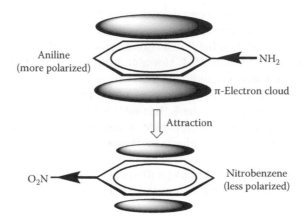

FIGURE 19.5   A simple example of π–π stacking between π-electron rich aniline and π-electron deficient nitrobenzene. Electrostatic interaction between aniline and nitrobenzene leads to stacking of both molecules.

are essential for the hydrotropic effect.[62,64,65] Aromatic rings and aliphatic hydrocarbons are basic structures of hydrotropes. Another possible mechanism is the ionic interaction or hydrogen bonding. Heteroatoms substituting aromatic rings are mostly charged. Since hydrotropes solubilize non-electrolytes, the ionic interaction may not be a major mechanism. As described earlier, hydrogen bonding is one of the important parameters responsible for the poor solubility of many drugs. Sulfonyl or carbonyl groups in hydrotropes can be hydrogen bond acceptors, while amino or hydroxyl group can be hydrogen bond donors. For example, nicotinamide, based on a pyridine ring, has an amide bond. The amide bond is not only a hydrogen bond donor, but also an acceptor, so that nicotinamide shows self-aggregation via hydrogen bonding.[75] Hydrogen bonding may not be the only force generating self-aggregates of hydrotropes, but π–π stacking as well as dispersive force also take part in producing the aggregation. Since a hydrotrope has effective solubilization effect only at concentrations over the MHC, aggregation of hydrotropes may be one of the mechanisms to explain the enhanced solubility of poorly soluble drugs. However, the aggregation is a necessary condition for hydrotropy, but not a sufficient condition. Therefore, it might be considerable that the hydrotropic solubilization power is maximized by the aggregation effect that is derived from various intermolecular interactions.

19.3.2.2   Hydrotropic Polymer Micelles

It is through the hydrotropic polymer micelle that the concept of hydrotropy was introduced to the polymer micelle. Earlier work on hydrotropic polymers was done in 2003.[76] Because a hydrotrope has selectivity in drug solubilization as described above, Lee et al. attempted to solubilize paclitaxel as a target drug using various hydrotropes. Paclitaxel is an anticancer drug having therapeutic effect on a wide range of cancers including breast, ovarian, colon, and non-small cell lung carcinomas.[77] However, the poor solubility of paclitaxel in water has limited its use in clinical applications. Solubility enhancement power of more than 60 candidates of potential hydrotropes was initially examined.[78] The intrinsic solubility of paclitaxel was 0.3 μg/mL, and hydrotropes, mostly derivatives of nicotinamide, effectively enhanced the solubility up to the mg/mL ranges (Table 19.5).

Nicotinamide is a well-known hydrotrope to solubilize various hydrophobic drugs.[67,79,80] With other organic compounds such as caffeine, it synergistically increases the aqueous solubility of hydrophobic solutes.[70,81] As shown in Table 19.5, it is obvious that hydrotropic effect on paclitaxel highly depends on the structure of hydrotropes. At the concentration of 3.5 M in water, N,N-diethylnicotinamide (DENA) and N-picolylnicotinamide (PNA) enhanced the aqueous solubility of paclitaxel up to ~39 and ~29 mg/mL, respectively. However, other compounds such as NaS or N,N-dimethylnicotinamide (DMNA) did not achieve as much enhancement of paclitaxel solubility as DENA or PNA. It is noteworthy that the DMNA showed only ~1.8 mg/mL of drug solubility, which is much lower than that achieved by DENA.

TABLE 19.5
Some Hydrotropes Used to Solubilize Paclitaxel

Hydrotrope	Structure	Paclitaxel Solubility[a] (mg/mL)
None (pure water)		0.0003
N,N-Diethylnicotinamide (DENA)		39.071
N-Picolylnicotinamide (PNA)		29.435
N-Allylnicotinamide (ANA)		14.184
Sodium salicylate (NaS)		5.542
N,N-Dimethylnicotinamide (DMNA)		1.771

[a] At the hydrotrope concentration of 3.5 M in water.

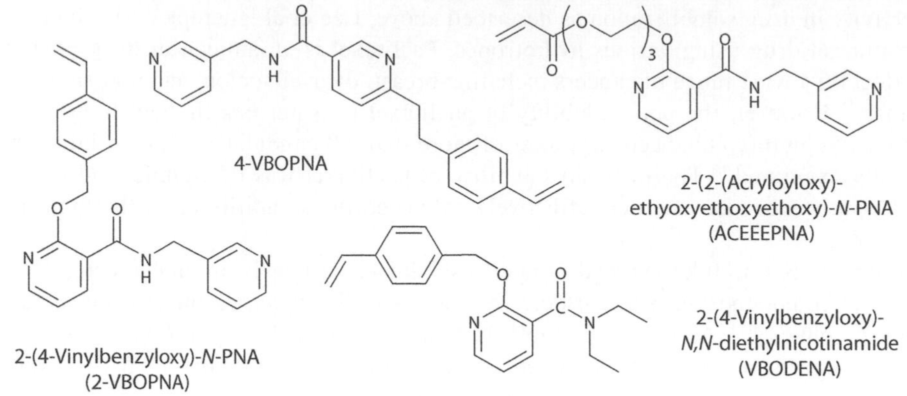

FIGURE 19.6 Hydrotropic monomers utilized for hydrotropic polymers.

To prepare polymeric hydrotropes, vinyl derivatives of the PNA, 2-(2-(acryloyloxy)-ethyoxyethoxyethoxy)-*N*-PNA (ACEEEPNA), 2-(4-vinylbenzyloxy)-*N*-PNA (2-VBOPNA), and 6-VBOPNA were synthesized (Figure 19.6). As a result, the polymerized poly(ACEEEPNA) enhanced the aqueous solubility of paclitaxel up to 0.32 mg/mL at the hydrotrope concentration of 290 mg/mL. In addition, poly(2-(VBOPNA)) and poly(6-(VBOPNA)) retained the hydrotropic effect of PNA by increasing the paclitaxel solubility to 0.56 and 0.13 mg/mL, respectively, at the hydrotrope concentration of 165 mg/mL. Hydrotropic polymers significantly solubilized paclitaxel even at low concentrations (<50 mg/mL), in contrast to the PNA or its vinyl derivatives. Moreover, structure of PNA derivatives also influenced the solubility enhancement power even after polymerization. 2-VBOPNA with hydrophobic substitution at 2-position of pyridine ring showed the highest solubility enhancement power, while 6-substituted monomer (6-(VBOPNA)) significantly lowered the hydrotropic effect. The hydrophilic side group at the 2-position of the pyridine ring also decreased the solubility enhancement power. Structural importance of hydrotropes was also reported elsewhere.[82]

The hydrotropic polymer micelle was prepared from a vinyl derivative of DENA.[83] Using a macroinitiator, brominated PEG, an amphiphilic block copolymer was synthesized from 4-(2-vinylbenzyloxy)-*N,N*-DENA (VBODENA, Figure 19.6) with a hydrophobic substitution at 4-position of pyridine ring by atom transfer radical polymerization (ATRP). It was found that PEG_{5000}-*b*-poly(VBODENA)$_{4350}$ loaded paclitaxel up to ~37% (w/w), which was much higher than the loading capacity of PEG_{2000}-*b*-PLA_{2000} (~28%, w/w). Also, the paclitaxel-containing hydrotropic polymer micelle did not show any precipitation for a month when kept in water at 37°C, indicating high aqueous stability. Lee et al. confirmed the aqueous stability by measuring particle size, and reported that the hydrotropic polymer micelle had low cytotoxicity in cell culture tests.[84] Kim et al. suggested that the incorporation of acrylic acid moieties into the poly(VBODENA) block could modulate the drug release kinetics.[85] Because the acrylic acid moiety is hydrophilic and pH sensitive, the release profile of paclitaxel was tunable by varying the molar feed ration of VBODENA-to-acrylic acid. Introduction of more than 20% (mole) acrylic acids completely released paclitaxel within 12 h. Hydrotropic micelles containing acrylic acid did not significantly lower the paclitaxel loading capacity.

Nicotinamide is a well-known hydrotrope to solubilize various hydrophobic drugs. With other organic compounds such as caffeine, it synergistically increases aqueous solubility of hydrophobic solutes.

Another interesting feature of hydrotropic polymer micelles is the spontaneous formation of the micelle structure simply by adding a drug. It was demonstrated that a block copolymer of PEG and 2-VBOPNA successfully produced micelle structure simply by adding paclitaxel into the polymer solution.[86] Although the hydrotropic micelle was developed to solubilize only paclitaxel, it has opened a new opportunity to improve the drug loading capacity and the aqueous stability of polymer micelles.

19.3.2.3 A Theory to Explain Hydrotropy

Conventional polymer micelles have suffered from low drug loading capacity (generally, less than 20%). However, the hydrotropic polymer micelles exhibit relatively high capacity for drug loading (up to 37%). The aqueous stability of drug-containing hydrotropic micelles was maintained for a long time. Therefore, insights into the drug loading mechanism of hydrotropic polymer micelles may suggest clues to the long-lasting questions in the field of polymer micelles—how to increase the drug loading amount and how to maintain the micelle stability after administration.

According to the theories about drug loading in polymer micelle, the maximal drug loading can be achieved by good miscibility between the drug and the polymer, as described in the previous section. However, these theories cannot fully explain the mechanism of drug solubilization by hydrotropic polymer micelles. The Flory–Huggins interaction parameter from the regular solution theory does not consider the specific interactions between drugs and polymers. Moreover, it is very difficult to obtain each component of the Hildebrand–Scatchard solubility parameter for a certain polymer. Each individual component can be calculated by the group contribution method (GCM), a kind of classical approach to predict solubility and partition coefficient.[57,58,87] In the GCM, a mixture of two liquids is regarded as a mixture of the functional groups on each liquid. Because the GCM is based on the vapor–liquid equilibrium data, it has its limitations in predicting the polymer–drug interaction.[88]

Recently, Mokrushina et al. reported a modified universal quasi-chemical functional-group activity coefficient (UNIFAC), similar to GCM, to predict the partition coefficient of organic compounds between water and micelles.[89] The classical UNIFAC model consists of two contributions: a combinatorial part responsible for the difference in molecular size and shape ($\gamma_i^{\text{combinatorial}}$), and a residual part accounting for group–group interactions ($\gamma_i^{\text{residual}}$). In the modified UNIFAC, a new contribution of the interfacial part ($\gamma_i^{\text{interfacial}}$) was introduced. As a result, the activity coefficient of the modified UNIFAC with an interfacial (IF) contribution is expressed by

$$\ln \gamma_i^{\text{UNIFAC-IF}} = \ln \gamma_i^{\text{combinatorial}} + \ln \gamma_i^{\text{residual}} + \ln \gamma_i^{\text{interfacial}} \qquad (19.18)$$

$$\ln \gamma_i^{\text{interfacial}} = \frac{2\sigma \upsilon_i \sqrt[3]{(1-\phi_i)}}{RTr} \qquad (19.19)$$

where
σ is the interfacial tension on micelle/water interface
υ_i is the molar volume of the solute i
ϕ_i is the volume fraction of the solute i
r is the radius of the micelle

However, the modified UNIFAC-IF model still lacks a term of specific interactions between drugs and polymers.

The octanol–water partition coefficient (log P) has been widely used to estimate the lipophilicity of a drug. It was first proposed by Hansch et al. to explain the relationship between the aqueous solubility of organic liquids and log P,[90] which is expressed by

$$\log\left(\frac{1}{S}\right) = \log P + \frac{\mu_i^{\circ}(\text{oct}) - \mu(l)}{2.302RT} \qquad (19.20)$$

where

    S is the molar solubility of the organic liquid in water

    P is its partition coefficient between 1-octanol and water

    $\mu_i^0(\text{oct})$ is the chemical potential of the pure liquid solute in a 1 M ideal 1-octanol solution

    $\mu(l)$ is the chemical potential of the pure liquid solute

The log P can be experimentally measured or calculated from structural features of a compound, using commercially available software.

    Yalkowsky et al. expanded the application of octanol–water partition coefficient to the solubility of solid solutes. The activity coefficient of a solid solute (log γ^P) is calculated from the equation

$$\log \gamma^P = \log P + 0.94 \tag{19.21}$$

In 1980, Yalkowski and Valvani proposed the general solubility equation (GSE) in which the crystallinity of a solute as well as the interaction of the solute with water are connected to the log P concept.[91] The GSE is

$$\log S_w = 0.5 - 0.01(\text{MP} - 25)\log K_{ow} \tag{19.22}$$

where

    S_w is the molar aqueous solubility of a solute

    MP is the melting point (°C)

    K_{ow} is the octanol–water partition coefficient (=log P)

The GES reasonably predicted the solubility of numerous compounds.[92] However, log P and log S_w still fail to explain the polymer–drug miscibility and the specific interactions between them.

    Recently, the linear solvent free energy relationship (LSER) equation was employed to explain partition of solid solutes into micelles.[93,94] The LSER assumes that drug partitioning between two immiscible phases is directly related to the transfer of free energy from water to the other phase (solvent or micelle). This free energy is the sum of independent and additive contributions of various drug–polymer interactions. Therefore, the LSER equation is expressed by

$$\log \text{SP} = c + rR_2 + s\pi_2 + a\sum\alpha_2 + b\sum\beta_2 + vV_x \tag{19.23}$$

where

    SP is the property of interest for a solute or drug, i.e., partition coefficient

    R_2 is the excess molar refraction of the solute (derived from the dispersion force)

    π_2 is the solute dipolarity/polarizability

    $\sum\alpha_2$ is the solute overall or effective hydrogen bond acidity

    $\sum\beta_2$ is the solute overall or effective hydrogen bond basicity

    V_x is the McGowan's characteristic volume calculated from molecular structure ((cm^3 mol^{-1})/100)

The c, r, s, a, b, and v refer to the regression coefficients obtained by compilation from database. Each individual component is determined either by multiple regression analysis based on measurement of partition coefficients (K in Equation 19.17)[58,93–95] or by direct measurement.[96–100] The LSER model contains various terms responsible for the drug–polymer interactions. In addition, the equation describes the miscibility of the polymer and the drug, which is applicable to polymer micelles. Therefore, LSER might be a good theory to explain the drug loading/solubilization mechanism of hydrotropic polymer micelles or even of conventional micelles. Also, the equation can be used to design an efficient polymer micelle for a given drug.

19.4 STABILITY OF POLYMER MICELLE

The aqueous stability is another big issue to develop effective polymer micelles. Because a polymer micelle is a physically assembled structure in water, thermodynamic equilibrium and kinetic stability should be considered for practical application. Especially, the stability under biological condition is very important to accomplish successful delivery of therapeutic drugs. In this section, the stability of polymer micelles will be discussed from various angles.

19.4.1 STABILITY OF POLYMER MICELLE IN WATER AND BUFFERS

19.4.1.1 Thermodynamic Stability

Micelle is a structure in thermodynamic equilibrium, and in general, a closed association model is employed to explain micelle formation.[101] The strict closed association model is based on an all-or-none process, in which block copolymers (unimers) generate homogeneous micelles in size. As a result, an aqueous medium contains only unimers and monodisperse micelles. In pure water, the standard free energy change of micellization is

$$\Delta G^\circ = RT \ln(\text{CMC}) \tag{19.24}$$

where CMC is the critical micelle concentration.[55,102,103] The CMC, that is the lowest polymer concentration to generate micelles by unimer aggregation, has significance in micelle stability. It may be reasonable, therefore, that micelles at equilibrium state will be destabilized (i.e., dissociated into unimers) when diluted. In general, higher MW of hydrophobic block provides the lower CMC value, which means more "stable."[102]

Attwood et al. scored hydrophobicity of core-forming polymer blocks based on the analysis of CMC change as a function of the degree of polymerization (DP). For example, the hydrophobic ratio of propylene oxide:lactic acid:ε-caprolactone is 1:4:12.[104] Logarithm curve of CMC vs. DP of a polyester (=block length) shows two transition points. As the DP increases, it is hypothesized that a long and linear chain of hydrophobic block spontaneously collapses, leading block copolymers to form unimeric or oligomeric micelles. Figure 19.7 shows a hypothetical mechanism to explain the relationship between log CMC and the DP of hydrophobic block. Line I (short dot, Figure 19.7A) shows Pluronic micelles, which are relatively hydrophilic block copolymers. Lines II and III show block copolymers containing lactic acid and ε-caprolactone as repeating units of their hydrophobic blocks, respectively. When the DP of the hydrophobic block is ranged in B section, unimers are assembled to micelles above CMC (general closed association model, Figure 19.7B). Before the second transition point of DP, unimers and unimolecular micelles are equilibrated under a CMC, while they form a micelle over CMC (Figure 19.7C). High DP possibly makes all unimers to unimolecular micelles below CMC, which can be further aggregated as polymer concentration increases. Yamamoto et al. reported a similar description to explain a temperature-dependent change in CMC of PEG-b-PDLLA micelles.[105]

These reports support the "bunchy micelle" model, in which the micellization occurs by aggregation of unimers with collapsed hydrophobic segments.[106] Since the stable geometry of the collapsed segments is a sphere, the micelle core may have many pores that are filled with solvents or drugs. However, it has been considered that the micelle core is a molten globule.[55] Usually, micelles are prepared from polymer solution of high concentration followed by removal of the solvent. Even though the preparation method is a thermodynamically quenching process, long polymer chains, especially hydrophobic polymer chains, are liable to be entangled together. If the time scale is

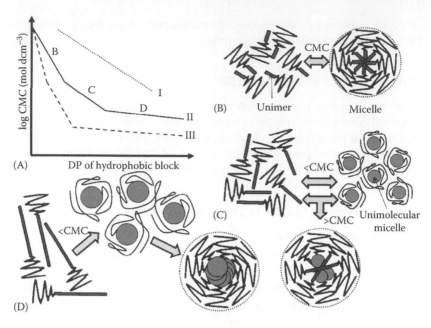

FIGURE 19.7 A hypothesis to explain unimolecular and multimolecular micelles. (A) Relationship between log CMC and the degree of polymerization (DP) of the hydrophobic block. The log CMC decreases as the hydrophobicity of the core-forming block increases (e.g., I: polypropylene, II: poly(D,L-lactide), and III: poly(ε-caprolactone)). (B) If the block length is short, there exists only unimer–micelle equilibrium. (C) As DP of the hydrophobic block increases, unimers collapse to unimolecular micelles. Over the CMC, multimolecular micelles are generated. (D) Hydrophobic block with high DP is spontaneously collapsed, and most of the unimers exist as unimolecular micelles. At higher polymer concentration, the unimolecular micelles aggregate further to form multimolecular micelles.

infinite, then all hydrophobic polymer chains can be converted to globular structures. As a result, micellization may be explained by combining the molten liquid core model and the bunchy micelle model together (Figure 19.8).

As described above, the CMC depends on the hydrophobicity of the core-forming block. However, it is also influenced by the crystallinity of hydrophobic blocks.[107,108] For instance, the PDLLA, a kind of polyester, is an amorphous polymer, which has its glass transition temperature (T_g) around 55°C. Likewise, poly(lactide-*co*-glycolide) (PLGA) is an amorphous polymer (T_g ~50–60°C). However, poly(L-lactide) (PLLA) has high crystallinity with melting temperature (T_m) and T_g around 130°C and 60°C, respectively. Poly(ε-caprolactone) (PCL) is a semicrystalline polymer. T_m and T_g of PCL are ~55–65°C and −60°C, respectively.[87,104,109] Isomers of D- and L-lactic acid in PDLLA influence the molecular configuration, which makes packing structure more spacey, i.e., more mobility of each PDLLA molecule. Glycolic acid, which loses a methyl group from lactic acid, is more hydrophilic, and also provides more space for the packing structure of PLGA.[110] Therefore, D-lactic acid and glycolic acid play the role of crystal structure breakers. Void volume at the micelle core is possessed by water molecules during micelle preparation. Therefore, micelle dissociation (relaxation) process can be more facilitated in short-term application to a diluted environment.

Block length ratio of diblock copolymers also controls CMC.[102,104,111] The hydrophilic–lipophilic balance (HLB) is another expression of the block length ratio. For surfactant molecules containing PEG block, the HLB is equivalent to the mass percentage of oxyethylene content (E) divided by 5 (HLB = $E/5$).[112] Block copolymer with higher HLB value (more hydrophilic) generally decreases the CMC and increases the micelle size due to loose packing density.[102] Diblock copolymer with HLB < 10 has a conical shape in water, which produces micellar structure by assembly. Polymers

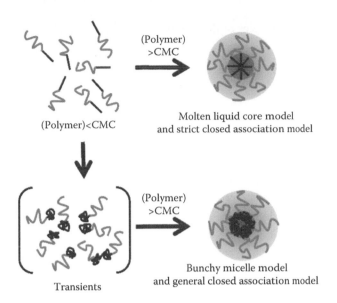

FIGURE 19.8 Two examples of micellization models. In relation to Figure 19.7, the molten liquid core model adopts a closed association model, in which only unimers and micelles are present in a system. In the bunchy micelle model, unimers are changed to unimolecular micelles by the collapsed hydrophobic block, which in turn produce multimolecular micelles.

with HLB > 10 can generate different shapes of supramolecular structure.[113–115] If the hydrophobic block is long enough to be of cylinder shape in water, copolymer generates polymersome, which is very similar to the conformation of phospholipids.[114]

19.4.1.2 Kinetic Stability

Micelle association is a kinetic process, and similarly, micelle dissociation is the same. Aniansson and Wall (A–W) interpreted the dynamic mechanism of micelle relaxation.[116] The A–W equations show that the exchange of unimers between micelles is a fast process and the decomposition of micelles into unimers is a slow process. The relationship between the number of unimers in a micelle and the concentration of micelles shows three continuous regions: the initial association (unimer-abundant) region, the intermediate region with unimer aggregates, and the micelle-abundant region. Because the aggregation process is very fast, micelle-containing solution will show a sharp bimodal distribution of the micelle size (either unimer- or micelle-dominant distribution). And, dissociation of unimers from micelles is governed by the internal free energy of micelles that is proportional to the length of hydrophobic blocks. However, experimental data have showed that this model (A–W model) of micelle relaxation was not always well-fit. This was because drastically simplified assumptions were made to explain the micelle relaxation process. The A–W model did not consider the micelle–micelle interaction, but only the fission mechanism was evaluated. A modified model, Gaussian model, suggests that the micelle relaxation depends on the fusion as well as the fission of micelles. By this model, the size distribution of micelles observed in experiments could be better explained.[117]

The A–W equations explain micelle relaxation by unimer dissociation and exchange between micelles, while the Gaussian model further suggests the size distribution of micelles by the fission–fusion mechanism. Studies on the exchange of unimers between micelles at equilibrium state supported the importance of fusion mechanism in micelle relaxation.[118–120] To monitor the unimers exchange, nonradiative energy transfer (NET) was employed, which is known as the fluorescence (or Förster) resonance energy transfer (FRET). FRET is a physical process of transferring nonradiative energy from a donor fluorophore to an acceptor molecule.[121] This type of energy transfer is also achievable between the same species of fluorophores (self-quenching). The transfer efficiency (E) is expressed as

$$E = k_T(\tau_D^{-1} + k_T)$$ (19.25)

where
  k_T is the transfer rate
  τ_D is the lifetime of donor in the absence of acceptors or self-quenching effect[121]

For effective FRET, a donor molecule should be close enough to transfer its emission energy to an acceptor (Figure 19.9). The transfer efficiency is inversely proportional to the sixth power of the distance (r) between donor and acceptor molecules:

$$E = \frac{R_0^6}{R_0^6 + r^6}$$ (19.26)

R_0 is known as the Förster distance at which a FRET pair of donor and acceptor shows 50% of transfer efficiency. The initial study was performed by Prochazka et al.[118] They conjugated anthracene (FRET acceptor) or carbazole (FRET donor) to a block copolymer Kraton G-1701. By mixing micelles separately prepared from each dye-conjugated polymer, increase in fluorescence intensity from the anthracene was observed, while carbazole lowered its fluorescence emission.

Haliloglu et al. identified that the predominant mechanisms in the unimer exchange were insertion/expulsion and merger/splitting.[120] The former mechanism is dominant at low polymer concentration and at high interaction energy between core-forming blocks (e.g., block length), while the latter mainly acts at high polymer concentration.

Insertion and expulsion of unimers during aggregation (oligomers or micelles) are governed by entropic free energy barrier. Therefore, either micellization or micelle decomposition is an activation process involving collective energy barriers, which can be explained by the internal free energy of micelle.[101,122] The internal free energy of micelle suppresses association of too many unimers in a micelle (internal free energy of association, F_a) and dissociation of unimers from a micelle (internal free energy of dissociation, F_d). Due to F_a, a thermodynamic equilibrium of the micellization requires a very long time, which is not achievable in practical situations. As a result, micelles are

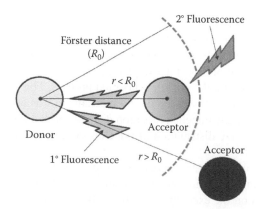

FIGURE 19.9 Fluorescence resonance energy transfer (FRET). If an acceptor dye exists within the Förster distance ($r < R_0$), fluorescence emission from a donor dye (1° fluorescence) will be used as excitation energy of the acceptor dye. As a result, fluorescence emission from acceptor (2° fluorescence) increases with decreased donor dye emission.

loosely aggregated under experimental conditions. The F_d tends to prevent micelle disintegration. However, a "jump" condition, such as either dilution or increased temperature, provides enough energy for micelles to overcome the energy barrier, resulting in increased micelle disintegration.

> While insertion/expulsion as a mechanism of unimer exchange is dominant at low polymer concentration and at high interaction energy between core-forming blocks (e.g., block length), merger/splitting acts as a mechanism mainly at high polymer concentration.

19.4.1.3 Drug Effect

Drugs loaded in polymer micelles can act as either plasticizers or fillers for the hydrophobic core. If the drug acts as a plasticizer, the friction of polymer chains will be reduced enough to decrease T_g of the hydrophobic core. In other words, addition of drug (plasticizer) will create more free volume in the micelle core. In contrast, filler effect will remove free volume from the polymer core.

The Kelley–Bueche equation expresses the effect of additives on effective T_g:

$$T_g = \frac{\varphi_2 \alpha_2 T_{g2} + \varphi_1 \alpha_1 T_{g1}}{\varphi_2 \alpha_2 + \varphi_1 \alpha_1} \tag{19.27}$$

where
  φ is the volume fraction
  α is the difference between volume extension factors above and below T_g
  numerals 1 and 2, refer to the polymer and the drug, respectively[123]

Although the above equation assumes diluted concentration of the additive, there exist some data showing that the drug acts as a plasticizer. For example, ketoprofen in PLGA polymer, microsphere in this case, decreased T_g of the polymer proportional to the drug loading amount.[124] On the contrary, there also exists some evidence that drug loading increases T_g. Quercetin effectively increased T_g of PCL block in PEG-b-PCL micelles, which proportionally depended on the drug loading amount.[125] Authors demonstrated that the increased T_g would be due to the hydrogen bonds between drug and carbonyl groups of PCL. Also, a poly(N-isopropylacrylamide-co-N,N-dimethylacrylamide)-b-PLGA (P(NIPAAm-co-DMAAm)-b-PLGA) micelle increased T_g of PLGA block by addition of paclitaxel.[126] As discussed previously, T_g of core-forming polymers should be important for micelle stability.

It has been believed that hydrophobic drugs may enhance the micelle stability primarily due to the hydrophobic effect, but there is not enough evidence to support this. It is more reasonable that the role of drugs is determined by the miscibility with hydrophobic polymer block. Actually, one unsolved problem of drug-loaded polymer micelles is the aqueous stability. Frequently, drug precipitation is observed when the micelles are stored in an aqueous medium, even though the micelle structure is not disrupted.[83,84] It is explained by phase separation out of poor miscibility between the drug and the polymer.

19.4.2 Stability of Polymer Micelle in Biological Environments

19.4.2.1 Micelle–Protein Interaction

Recently, Chen et al. clarified that a polymer micelle composed of PEG-b-PDLLA diblock copolymer was not stable in blood.[127] To investigate the stability of the micelle, a pair of FRET dyes (red and green) was loaded into the PEG-b-PDLLA micelles and injected into the bloodstream via tail vein. It was observed that the initial high FRET signal (0.886) significantly decreased in 15 min after injection down to 0.463. The FRET ratio was simply defined as

$$-FRET = \frac{I_R}{I_R + I_G} \tag{19.28}$$

where

   I is the fluorescence intensity with arbitrary unit

   R and G refer to the red and green dyes, respectively

In the experiments to examine the effect of blood components on the micelle stability, red blood cells did not show any significant interaction with the micelle. However, α- and β-globulins significantly destabilized the micelle, while albumin or γ-globulin was not responsible for decrease in the FRET ratio. Although they demonstrated the micelle stability in blood by an indirect method of loading FRET dyes, it was revealed that blood components, especially proteins, play a key role in micelle destabilization.

Polymer micelles have a similar property to amphiphilic surfactants in terms of micellization. Therefore, it is meaningful to predict the polymer micelle–protein interaction from surfactant–protein interaction. Interaction between surfactants and proteins has been extensively studied. In general, anionic surfactants exhibit relatively strong interaction leading to protein unfolding, while cationic surfactants weakly interact with proteins. For example, both cationic decyltriethylammonium bromide (DTAB) or anionic sodium decyl sulfonate (SDS) bind to bovine serum albumin (BSA), but a mixture of both surfactants, that made the net charge neutral, diminished interaction with BSA.[128] However, increase of hydrophobic parts in a cationic surfactant can significantly increase binding to proteins and their denaturation. For example, alkylenediyl-α,ω-bis(DTAB)s with hydrophobic alkyl chains showed BSA unfolding effect, which increased with alkyl chain length.[129]

Nonionic surfactants have the weakest interactions with proteins, which is possibly explained by the lack of electrostatic interactions with proteins and their low CMC values.[130] It was reported that PEG-containing diblock copolymers also had interaction with BSA.[131] The HLB of all copolymers used exceeded 10, so that at the CMC value the polymers formed 100–200 mM range micelles. As a result, interaction of block copolymers with BSA increased proportionally with the HLB value. This indicates that the major driving force of BSA–micelle (or block copolymer) interaction is the hydrophobic aggregation. Likewise, a micelle consisting of PEG-conjugated phospholipid (PEG_{2000}-b-PE) is destabilized in the presence of BSA.[132] At a high concentration of BSA (1%, w/v), the micelle structure was disrupted and BSA/PEG-b-PE aggregates were generated with increased particle size. A circular dichromism (CD) study showed that Trp in BSA structure was exposed to water at high concentration of BSA, but it was buried into a hydrophobic part of BSA as the BSA concentration increased. In a further study, it was found that the PEG-b-PE molecules were in contact with the Trp groups of BSA, leading to BSA unfolding and BSA/PEG-b-PE complexation.[133]

19.4.2.2 PEG–Protein Interactions

PEG is a common and popular polymer used for micelle corona formation. PEG is nontoxic and biocompatible, but not totally inert under biological environments. The term biocompatibility is defined as the ability of a material to perform with an appropriate host response,[134] and does not necessarily mean the biological inertness. According to this definition, it can be considered that polymer micelles with the PEG shell are biocompatible rather than biologically inactive. However, polymer micelles have been described as stealth nanocarriers primarily due to the PEG outer shell. Because PEG has been used as a crystallizing agent for proteins instead of solvents or high concentration salts,[135,136] it was considered that PEG has unfavorable interaction with proteins leading to precipitation or crystallization.[137] Paradoxically, an aqueous two-phase partition system (ATPS) consisting of polymer and salt solution phases has been also used to extract proteins, in which proteins are dominantly located at the polymer (PEG) phase.[138] In addition, many evidences have shown that PEG does interact with biomolecules, especially proteins or lipids. As listed in Table 19.6,

---

PEG interacts with biomolecules, especially proteins or lipids via the repulsive (primarily due to the chain flexibility and strong hydrogen bonding to water molecules) and attractive forces (hydrogen bonding, electrostatic, and van der Waals interactions). PEG directly interacts with proteins including lysozyme, fibronectin, serum albumin, pepsin, and α-chymotrypsin.

TABLE 19.6
Repulsive and Attractive Forces of PEG toward Serum Proteins

Repulsive	Attractive
Strong hydrogen bonding to water molecules	Hydrogen bonding
Entalpy restoration[a]	Electrostatic interaction[c]
Steric force due to the chain flexibility	van der Waals interaction (hydrophobic effect)
Hydrodynamic lubrication force[b]	

[a] Incoming protein toward end-grafted PEG layer (e.g., micelle) may squeeze out water molecules from the layer, which is not entropically favorable.

[b] Imposed motion of proteins toward PEG layer sets up a transverse pressure gradient.[139]

[c] Oxygen atoms in PEG backbone have ability to chelate some cations such as Li$^+$ or possibly Ca^{2+}, which may electrostatistically interact with charged proteins.[140–142]

Rixman et al. well summarized the repulsive (primarily due to the chain flexibility and strong hydrogen bonding to water molecules) and attractive forces (hydrogen bonding, electrostatic, and van der Waals interactions) of PEG to proteins in water.[142]

Several reports elucidate that the PEG has direct interaction with proteins including lysozyme, fibronectin, serum albumin, pepsin,[143] and α-chymotrypsin.[144] Furness et al. examined the interaction between PEG and hen-egg-white lysozyme by proton nuclear magnetic resonance (^{1}H-NMR) spectroscopy.[145] By calculating maximal chemical shift change of amino acids upon PEG binding, it was found that six amino acids of the lysozyme Arg-61, Trp-62, Trp-63, Arg-73, Lys-96, and Asp-101 are selectively perturbed by PEG. The chemical shift change induced by PEG-poly(propylene oxide) block copolymer did not much differ from that observed by PEG treatment. However, a more hydrophilic polymer, poly(dihydroxypropyl methacrylate), significantly reduced change in the chemical shift. Based on these results, they concluded that the PEG–lysozyme binding was probably due to the hydrophobic interaction of the ethylene moieties of PEG.

Actually, PEG was a useful tool to detect soluble immune complexes from serum in systemic lupus erythematosus (SLE) and rheumatoid arthritis (RA).[146] Hurbert et al. found that fibronectin directly bound to the circulating immune complexes and in turn PEG could precipitate the immune complex.[147] Further, Robinson et al. demonstrated that many other non-immunoglobulin proteins such as fibronectin, haptoglobin, albumin, transferrin, and α-antitrypsin were also precipitated by 4% (w/v) PEG, and that the interaction between PEG and proteins was not specific.[148]

As described above, BSA binding to PEG-containing diblock copolymers was reduced proportional to the PEG length (or polymer HLB).[131] However, it was disproved that the BSA could bind to the micelles to some extent. There are some evidences to show that serum albumin directly binds to PEG. Cocke et al. examined the interaction between PEG and human serum albumin (HSA) by affinity capillary electrophoresis (ACE).[149] Upon PEG binding with HSA, the enthalpy change was 19.1 kJ/mol and the entropy change was 16.6 J/mol · K, which led to the total free energy change of −31.4 kJ/mol. The negative but small change of the free energy implies that binding of HSA to PEG is a thermodynamically favorable (or spontaneous) reaction, and that the HSA–PEG interaction is forced primarily by entropy change.

Similar phenomenon was observed from isothermal titration calorimetry (ITC) of lysozyme and ovalbumin.[150] Rixman et al. directly measured the force between PEG and HSA using HSA-coated molecular force probe.[142] The binding force of HSA-coated probe to individual PEG chain was determined as 0.06 ± 0.1 nN, which was primarily attributed to hydrogen bonding and van der Waals interaction (or hydrophobic effect) between PEGs and HSAs. Hydrogen bond between PEG and HSA was also confirmed by Fourier transform-infrared (FT-IR) spectroscopy.[151] CD spectra revealed that PEG forming a complex with HSA denatured the secondary structure of the albumin.

Based on a database for protein crystal structures in the presence of PEG, Hasek found four modes of the interaction between PEG and proteins: (1) multiple coordination via positively charged amino acids, i.e., Lys, Arg, His; (2) hydrogen bonding of amino acid side groups; (3) hydrogen bonding of backbone amide group; and (4) cation coordination.[152]

In summary, it is highly possible that polymer micelles composed of PEG-containing block copolymers are not completely inert in a body. Interactions between serum proteins and PEG corona of micelles have been frequently observed. The PEG shell of a micelle is known to expel serum proteins by hydrated chain mobility. However, the protein penetration into micelle has been also observed as described in the following section.

19.4.2.3 Protein Penetration into Micelles

Exposure of hydrophobic segments of micelles should eventually induce protein adsorption and denaturation because poor biocompatibility of a certain material mostly originates from its hydrophobicity.[153] In polymer micelles, the hydrophilic PEG shell has been considered as a shield preventing the hydrophobic micelle core from direct contact to biological constituents. As described above, however, the PEG molecule apparently has activities in blood that may provoke micelle destabilization. In contrast, there is another possibility that unimers from destabilized micelles interact with proteins or lipid membranes, even though no evidence has been found.

Protein penetration into micelles can also reduce micelle stability in blood. Li et al. observed that lipase slowly degraded the PCL block of PEG-b-PCL micelles, although the degradation rate was slower than the PCL-b-PEG-b-PCL triblock copolymer or the PCL homopolymer.[154] The mechanism of action of lipase K is to hydrolyze fatty acids, but it is also able to cleave the polyester backbone such as PCL. Adsorption of lipase onto PCL surface was the necessary condition for enzymatic activity.[155] Hydrolysis of the ester backbone catalyzed by lipase is limited to the amorphous region of PCL polymer matrix because PCL is a semicrystalline polymer, as mentioned previously.[155,156]

Carstens et al. investigated the kinetics of enzymatic hydrolysis of a micelle consisting of PEG_{750} and oligo-PCL (degree of polymerization, DP, ~5).[157] According to the Michaelis–Menten equation, the Michaelis constant, V_m, representing the maximal rate of enzymatic activity was $4.4 \pm 0.2\,\mu mol/min$, and K_m of the maximal binding affinity of lipase to PCL was $2.2 \pm 0.3\,mg/mL$ at an enzyme concentration of 19 mU/mL. Also, they proposed that there were two possibilities of lipase-catalyzed PCL degradation, viz., hydrolysis of unimers dissociated from micelles and degradation of micelle core via lipase penetration. In experiments examining biodegradation of a polymer micelle composed of a triblock copolymer, PEG-b-poly(3-hydroxybutyrate)-b-PEG (PEG-b-PHB-b-PEG), hydrolysis of the PHB polymer block by extracellular PHB depolymerase depended on the enzyme concentration, initial polymer concentration, and PHB block length.[158] Authors demonstrated that the amorphous core of micelles was enzyme penetrable. Hence, it is highly probable that protein penetration induces micelle instability under a biological condition.

19.4.3 Micelle–Cell Interaction

Two possible interactions exist between polymer micelles and cells, viz., cellular uptake and cell membrane perturbation, although mechanisms of these events are not clear yet. As described in the previous section, PEGs or micelles can interact with proteins, which is a possible mechanism. Cellular internalization, or endocytosis, can be accomplished by either phagocytosis or pinocytosis.[159,160] Relatively large particles are engulfed by phagocytosis, which is mediated by pseudopods extended from cell surface. Pinocytosis is frequently mediated by clathrin[161,162] and caveolae.[163] Both these pathways include dynamin polymerization for vesicle budding. There exist many nonspecific pathways of endocytosis, including a clathrin- and dynamin-independent pathway.[159] Recently, Stephanie et al. demonstrated that polymer particles with high homogeneity in size are endocytosed either by phagocytosis and clathrin-medicated endocytosis.[164] The endocytosis depended on the particle size: particles with submicron size showed faster uptake than few micron-sized particles.

If the hydrophilic shell is a stealth coat of polymer micelles, their internalization will be much inhibited. Recently, Chen et al. showed that a polymer micelle composed of PEG-*b*-PDLLA and fluorescein isothiocyanate (FTIC-PEG-*b*-PDLLA) did not enter into cultured HeLa cells.[165] When the cancer cells were incubated with polymer micelles of PEG-*b*-PDLLA loading a FRET dye pair, the hydrophobic dyes were observed in the cytoplasmic compartment. These results demonstrate the diffusion of hydrophobic molecules (e.g., drugs) across the cell membrane, rather than the internalization of whole micelle.

Nevertheless, evidence of micelle internalization has been reported. A polymer micelle of Pluronic P85 effectively accumulated a hydrophobic fluorescent probe inside living cells. At lower concentration, effect of the P85 on cellular accumulation of the dye was mediated by preventing the pump-out mechanism of P-glycoprotein (P-gp), but at higher concentration, vesicular transport was facilitated by the Pluronic.[166] In another experiment, pH-sensitive dye-labeled Pluronic (P105) was also observed inside various cancer cells, including multidrug resistance (MDR) cell lines.[167] P105 internalization increased the membrane permeability resulting in effective drug uptake by MDR cells. Later, Sahay et al. revealed that internalization of the P85 had two different pathways: caveolae-mediated endocytosis at lower concentration (<CMC) and clathrin-mediated endocytosis at higher concentration (>CMC).[160] The authors suggested a possibility that the interaction of the hydrophobic polymer block with caveolin may cause P-gp inhibition as well as other intracellular events, including gene expression. It was revealed that the most effective structure of Pluronic has HLB < 20.[168] Similarly, P-gp inhibition was also induced by the PEG-*b*-PCL block copolymer at a concentration below the CMC.[169] It is highly probable that the PEG-*b*-PCL has the same mechanism, viz., unimer-mediated lipid raft (e.g., caveolae) interruption, as Pluronics inhibit P-gp.

It has been often reported that polymer micelles consisting of PEG-*b*-PCL at high concentration (>CMC) can be internalized. Allen et al. showed that a PEG-*b*-PCL micelle loading a fluorescent probe was effectively localized inside PC12 cells.[170] Also, the cellular uptake of ^{3}H-labeled FK506 was much improved by the micelle carrier comparing to free FK506. However, internalization of either fluorescent dye or isotope-labeled drug may not exactly reflect the micelle endocytosis. Later, they visualized internalization of blank polymer micelle using rhodamine-labeled PEG-*b*-PCL (PEG-*b*-PCL-Rh)[171] and endocytosis of a drug-containing polymer micelle.[172] Moghimi et al. suggested a refutation that stressed the role of fluorescent dye.[173] Because rhodamine is positively charged, electrostatic attraction is possibly responsible for cellular uptake of the micelle. Also, PEG-*b*-PCL micelle endocytosis might depend on characteristics of used cells[174] and the MW of the hydrophobic or the hydrophilic block.[175]

The micelle endocytosis observed in cultured cells cannot provide enough evidence to clarify whether the internalization process really happens *in vivo*. *In vitro* experiments are usually performed in a static culture of cancer cell lines incubated with a high concentration of polymer micelles. Limitations of the *in vitro* culture systems arise from the deficiency of whole blood components and various cell types, the monolayer of cultured cells exposing maximum surface area to the environment, the lack of biochemical dynamics present in a living organism, and the localization of high concentration of polymers.

On the other hand, membrane perturbation by unimers dissociated from micelles is another possible interaction mechanism between micelles and cells. As discussed above, Pluronic and PEG-*b*-PCL block copolymers showed an interesting activity on P-gp inhibition at concentrations below their CMCs. Discher and Ahmed suggested that hemolytic activity of block copolymers are highly related to their HLB and MW.[114] A high value of HLB may generate a cylinder-like unimer structure, similar to the shape of phospholipids, which possibly facilitates membrane disruption. Additional activity of Pluronic (poloxamer 188; P188) on cells is the membrane-sealing effect. It was first demonstrated in electropermeabilized skeletal muscle cells,[176] which was recently confirmed by the magnetic resonance imaging (MRI) technique.[177] Numerous reports indicate that P188 is very effective in healing damaged plasma membrane *in vitro* and *in vivo*.[178] P188 binds to the lipid bilayer where the packing density is locally low. It is also possible that the PEG shell of polymer micelles mediates the membrane sealing. It is well known that the PEG provokes lipid membrane fusion and a critical PEG concentration is required for membrane fusion.[179] Due to the water-trapping ability of PEG, free water content around cells might be reduced. This is believed as one mechanism inducing lipid molecule exchange between phospholipid vesicles.[180,181]

Membrane curvature, which alters outer leaflet packing density, and the small impurities in membrane vesicles (e.g., unsaturated acryl chain of phospholipids) effectively lower the threshold concentration of PEG for membrane fusion.[182,183] For this reason, PEG is a potential therapeutic material to restore the damaged membrane. For example, PEG has excellent healing effect on injured spinal cords via the membrane-sealing mechanism.[184,185] If PEG induces local dehydration around cell membrane and block copolymers nonspecifically bind to lipid rafts, as mentioned above, then the insertion of unimers dissociated from micelles, the disruption of plasma membrane, or cell–cell fusion are highly possible.

19.4.4 *In Vivo* Stability of Polymer Micelles

Polymer micelles as drug carriers should be stable in the bloodstream to deliver drugs to target sites or to improve the pharmacokinetics of the drug. However, prediction about *in vivo* stability of polymer micelles is very difficult because of the biological and the physiological complexity of a living organism. In addition to the thermodynamic and kinetic stability issues in an aqueous medium and the interaction of polymer micelles with biomolecules, continuous flow of blood, the presence of many kinds of cell types, organ-specific physiological function, and diversity of individuals produce a totally complicated biological barrier. Although *in vitro* characterization methods for micelle stability may provide an insight to design carrier systems and appropriate *in vivo* experimental setups, there is no practical method to evaluate micelle stability *in vivo*.

The fate of micelles after intravenous administration has been frequently monitored by labeling with radioisotopes, as summarized in Table 19.7. Valuable information was obtained about the *in vivo* fate of polymer micelles. In the study using ^{3}H-labeled Pluronic P85, higher concentration of polymers, especially over the CMC, showed much longer circulation time.[186] It indicated that the polymer micelle is not immediately dissociated in bloodstream. The primary location of polymers was in blood. However, polymer micelles are likely to end up in liver and spleen, where the RES system is working. In other words, the stealth hydrophilic shell of micelles might not be good enough to escape the host defense system. However, radioisotope labeling studies lack direct evidence for *in vivo* micelle stability, because unimers dissociated from micelles and even their degraded products show radioactivity.

19.5 PERSPECTIVES AND CONCLUSIVE REMARKS

Polymer micelles present a great potential to formulate and deliver poorly soluble drugs. However, their two major limitations, low drug loading capacity and aqueous instability, remain unresolved. Hydrotropy is a potential solution alleviating the problems associated with drug loading. To obtain an efficient polymeric micelle carrier, extensive research on polymer–drug compatibility should be carried out. Based on understanding about interactions between polymers and drugs, strategies can be developed to improve micelle stability.

Optical imaging techniques, including FRET, opened a new possibility to examine the *in vitro* and *in vivo* stability of micelles. The radio-labeling method to determine the biodistribution of polymer micelles could not fully reflect the micelle stability *in vivo*. Also, it is an invasive method inducing damage to cells and tissues. Tissue damage may alter physiological response to polymer micelles. Recent advances in molecular imaging techniques allow noninvasive imaging at molecular and subcellular levels. In particular, fluorescence imaging techniques can provide useful tools to observe micelle stability due to easy accessibility at a lab scale and moderate cost of imaging instruments.[187] In addition to *in vivo* stability monitoring, micelles loaded with imaging agents can be applied as

TABLE 19.7
Studies on Biodistribution of Polymer Micelles

Polymer	Building Blocks Block Length (kDa)	Drug	Micelle Size (nm)	Label	Biodistribution	Reference
PEG_x-b-PCL_y	$x=6.0$, $y=1.0$	N/A	60	^{125}I-PEG	In 1 and 24 h after tail vein injection, blood>bone>kidney>liver>lung>brain	[188]
	$x=5.0$, $y=5.0$	N/A	56	^{3}H-PCL	Liver>kidney>spleen, lung>heart; biodistribution profile did not change much up to 48 after tail vein injection regardless of initial dose	[189]
	$x=2.0$, $y=2.4$	N/A	~25	F-5-CADA (fluorescent)	In 1 h after intramuscular or subcutaneous injection, micelle disintegration was observed; Too bright background fluorescence from mice	[190]
PEG_x-b-PLA_y	$x=5.0$, $y=7.0$	N/A	300	^{125}I-PLA	Micelle with smaller size was cleared faster in spite of longer PEG. In 2 h after tail vein injection, blood>bowel (inflamed site)>liver>kidney>spleen	[191]
	$x=14.0$, $y=6.0$	N/A	72		Blood>liver>kidney>lung, heart, spleen; With time, radioactivity gradually decreased without changing the organ distribution	[192]
	$x=5.0$, $y=5.0$	N/A	300	^{125}I-PLA		
	$x=5.1$, $y=5.3$	N/A	37–38	^{125}I-Tyr; ^{125}I-Tyr-Glu	Liver>kidney>lung, spleen; With time, liver and spleen showed more radioactivity while kidney and lung decreased it; No significant effect of anionic amino acid (Glu)	[193]
	$x=2.0$, $y=2.0$	Ptx	—	^{14}C-PDLLA or ^{14}C-PEG	Plasma elimination half life was 2.6–2.9 h	[59]
PEG_x-b-$PAsp_y$-Dox	$x=4.3$, $y=1.9$	Dox	~50	^{125}I-PEG	In 1 h after tail vein injection, blood ($17.1\% \pm 2.3\%$ dose/g)>spleen>kidney>liver>lung>heart	[194]

(continued)

TABLE 19.7 (continued)
Studies on Biodistribution of Polymer Micelles

Polymer	Building Blocks Block Length (kDa)	Drug	Micelle Size (nm)	Label	Biodistribution	Reference
PAA$_x$-b-PMAA$_y$	$x=4.8$, $y=18.6$	N/A	~24	^{64}Cu (PET)	Shell crosslinked by a bifunctional amine and coated with PEG$_{5,400}$;	[195]
	$x=6.0$, $y=7.0$	N/A	~37		Spleen>liver>kidney>blood>lung regardless of polymer block length; No PEG effect	
	$x=6.0$, $y=7.0$	N/A	19–22	^{64}Cu (PET)	Shell crosslinked by a bifunctional amine and coated with PEG$_{2,000}$; Micelles with lower PEG density showed spleen>liver>kidney>lung>blood; micelles with higher PEG density showed spleen>liver, blood>lung>kidney	[196]
PAA$_x$-b-PS$_y$	$x=8.7$, $y=7.4$	N/A	~18	^{64}Cu (PET)	Shell crosslinked by a bifunctional amine and coated with PEG$_{5,400}$; random distribution	[195]
	$x=6.0$, $y=15.4$	N/A	~37			
PEO$_x$-b-PPO$_y$-b-PEO$_x$ (P85)	$x=1.2$, $y=2.3$	N/A	1.5 [197]	^{3}H	The higher dose led to the larger AUC; Only over the CMC, the circulation time was prolonged; Liver>spleen>kidney>lung>brain	[186]

Note: AUC, area under curve; Dox, doxorubicin; F-5-CADA, fluorecein-5-carbonyl azide diacetate; Glu, glutamic acid; N/A, not applied; PAA, poly(acrylic acid); PAsp, poly(aspartic acid); PCL, poly(ε-caprolactone); PE, phosphatidylethanolamine; PEG, poly(ethylene glycol); PEO, poly(ethylene oxide); PET, Positron emission tomography; PLA, poly(D,L-lactide); PMAA, poly(methacrylate); PPO, poly(propylene oxide); PS, poly(styrene); Ptx, paclitaxel; Tyr, tyrosine.

molecular imaging probes. Multifunctional micelles performing drug delivery and molecular imaging allow simultaneous therapy and imaging by the same system.[43,198]

The poor stability of micelles in water and biological media originates from the physical association of unimers. Chemical crosslinking between unimers can improve micelle stability. The CMC is no more valid in crosslinked micelles, so that aqueous instability upon dilution is obviated as an issue. Various versions of crosslinked micelles have been developed.[199,200] In Table 19.7, PAA-*b*-PMAAs and PAA-*b*-PS are examples for shell-crosslinked micelles. In those micelles, an additional layer of PEG was coated to improve the biocompatibility.[195,196] A macromonomer of PEG-*b*-PCL with a polymerizable vinyl group at the PCL end led to a core-crosslinked micelle mediated by a radical initiator.[201] The crosslinked PEG-*b*-PCL micelle showed fair efficiency in paclitaxel loading property. Although such crosslinked micelles are expected to improve aqueous stability, additional modification steps with highly reactive chemicals as well as no or slow degradation of block copolymers may be unfavorable for a drug delivery system. An interesting example of crosslinked micelles is the interfacial crosslinking with reversible disulfide bridges.[202] Disulfide bonds can be reduced by glutathione that exists in cells. Application of crosslinked micelles in the drug delivery field is still limited, but due to the advantage of structural integrity, they have a great potential to improve the micellar drug delivery system.

Since the assembly/disassembly of micelles highly depends on the structure of block copolymer, it is also important to design and prepare polymers with well-controlled structure. The combinatorial synthetic strategy in polymerization (parallel synthesis) now provides a great chance to prepare numerous polymers in a simple manner.[203,204] In addition to the high-throughput synthetic method, controlled radical polymerization (CRP) methods, including atom transfer radical polymerization (ATRP), reversible addition fragmentation chain transfer (RAFT) polymerization, and nitroxide-mediated polymerization (NMP), are useful in synthesizing well-defined block copolymers.[205–207] The CRP methods provide not only controllability of polymer structure/topology, but also functionality of block copolymers to conjugate ligands or imaging agents. Micelle stability under physiological conditions can also be improved by polymer chemistry.

The disintegration of polymer micelles depending on a certain stimulus is now an important strategy in the micellar drug delivery system. Smart materials actively change their physicochemical properties responding to the environmental signals. Such smart polymers have been aggressively employed to improve therapeutic efficacy and to reduce undesirable side effects of drugs.[208]

In conclusion, two limitations of polymer micelles in drug delivery, the low drug loading capacity and aqueous instability, need to be overcome. These limitations also provide a new opportunity to improve the micellar drug delivery system, via advanced technologies in polymer chemistry and molecular imaging. Polymer micelles are currently undergoing evolution to become a useful tool for clinical applications. Increasing research interest is expected in the mechanisms on micellar interaction with drug, biomolecules, or cells.

REFERENCES

1. Lombardino JG, Lowe JA, 3rd, The role of the medicinal chemist in drug discovery—Then and now. *Nat Rev Drug Discov* 2004; **3:** 853–862.
2. Kramer JA, Sagartz JE, Morris DL, The application of discovery toxicology and pathology towards the design of safer pharmaceutical lead candidates. *Nat Rev Drug Discov* 2007; **6:** 636–649.
3. Lipinski CA, Drug-like properties and the causes of poor solubility and poor permeability. *J Pharmacol Toxicol Methods* 2000; **44:** 235–249.
4. Maeda H, Wu J, Sawa T, Matsumura Y, Hori K, Tumor vascular permeability and the EPR effect in macromolecular therapeutics: A review. *J Control Release* 2000; **65:** 271–284.
5. Maeda H, Sawa T, Konno T, Mechanism of tumor-targeted delivery of macromolecular drugs, including the EPR effect in solid tumor and clinical overview of the prototype polymeric drug SMANCS. *J Control Release* 2001; **74:** 47–61.

6. Iyer AK, Greish K, Seki T, Okazaki S, Fang J, Takeshita K, Maeda H, Polymeric micelles of zinc proto-porphyrin for tumor targeted delivery based on EPR effect and singlet oxygen generation. *J Drug Target* 2007; **15:** 496–506.

7. Paciotti GF, Myer L, Weinreich D, Goia D, Pavel N, McLaughlin RE, Tamarkin L, Colloidal gold: A novel nanoparticle vector for tumor directed drug delivery. *Drug Deliv* 2004; **11:** 169–183.

8. Dobrovolskaia MA, Aggarwal P, Hall JB, McNeil SE, Preclinical studies to understand nanoparticle interaction with the immune system and its potential effects on nanoparticle biodistribution. *Mol Pharm* 2008; **5:** 487–495.

9. Kim TY, Kim DW, Chung JY, Shin SG, Kim SC, Heo DS, Kim NK, Bang YJ, Phase I and pharmacoki-netic study of Genexol-PM, a cremophor-free, polymeric micelle-formulated paclitaxel, in patients with advanced malignancies. *Clin Cancer Res* 2004; **10:** 3708–3716.

10. Kim DW, Kim SY, Kim HK, Kim SW, Shin SW, Kim JS, Park K, Lee MY, Heo DS, Multicenter phase II trial of Genexol-PM, a novel Cremophor-free, polymeric micelle formulation of paclitaxel, with cisplatin in patients with advanced non-small-cell lung cancer. *Ann Oncol* 2007; **18:** 2009–2014.

11. Lee KS, Chung HC, Im SA, Park YH, Kim CS, Kim SB, Rha SY, Lee MY, Ro J, Multicenter phase II trial of Genexol-PM, a Cremophor-free, polymeric micelle formulation of paclitaxel, in patients with metastatic breast cancer. *Breast Cancer Res Treat* 2008; **108:** 241–250.

12. Matsumura Y, Hamaguchi T, Ura T, Muro K, Yamada Y, Shimada Y, Shirao K et al., Phase I clinical trial and pharmacokinetic evaluation of NK911, a micelle-encapsulated doxorubicin. *Br J Cancer* 2004; **91:** 1775–1781.

13. Negishi T, Koizumi F, Uchino H, Kuroda J, Kawaguchi T, Naito S, Matsumura Y, NK105, a paclitaxel-incorporating micellar nanoparticle, is a more potent radiosensitising agent compared to free paclitaxel. *Br J Cancer* 2006; **95:** 601–606.

14. Danson S, Ferry D, Alakhov V, Margison J, Kerr D, Jowle D, Brampton M, Halbert G, Ranson M, Phase I dose escalation and pharmacokinetic study of pluronic polymer-bound doxorubicin (SP1049C) in patients with advanced cancer. *Br J Cancer* 2004; **90:** 2085–2091.

15. Hamaguchi T, Kato K, Yasui H, Morizane C, Ikeda M, Ueno H, Muro K et al., A phase I and pharmacoki-netic study of NK105, a paclitaxel-incorporating micellar nanoparticle formulation. *Br J Cancer* 2007; **97:** 170–176.

16. Merisko-Liversidge EM, Liversidge GG, Drug nanoparticles: Formulating poorly water-soluble com-pounds. *Toxicol Pathol* 2008; **36:** 43–48.

17. Serajuddin AT, Salt formation to improve drug solubility. *Adv Drug Deliv Rev* 2007; **59:** 603–616.

18. Attwood D, Thermodynamic properties of amphiphilic drugs in aqueous solution. *J Chem Soc Faraday Trans I* 1989; **85:** 3011–3017.

19. Kesisoglou F, Panmai S, Wu Y, Nanosizing–oral formulation development and biopharmaceutical evalu-ation. *Adv Drug Deliv Rev* 2007; **59:** 631–644.

20. Rabinow BE, Nanosuspensions in drug delivery. *Nat Rev Drug Discov* 2004; **3:** 785–796.

21. Keck CM, Muller RH, Drug nanocrystals of poorly soluble drugs produced by high pressure homogeni-sation. *Eur J Pharm Biopharm* 2006; **62:** 3–16.

22. Strickley RG, Solubilizing excipients in oral and injectable formulations. *Pharm Res* 2004; **21:** 201–230.

23. Buggins TR, Dickinson PA, Taylor G, The effects of pharmaceutical excipients on drug disposition. *Adv Drug Deliv Rev* 2007; **59:** 1482–1503.

24. Brewster ME, Loftsson T, Cyclodextrins as pharmaceutical solubilizers. *Adv Drug Deliv Rev* 2007; **59:** 645–666.

25. Loftsson T, Duchene D, Cyclodextrins and their pharmaceutical applications. *Int J Pharm* 2007; **329:** 1–11.

26. Osterberg RE, See NA, Toxicity of excipients–a Food and Drug Administration perspective. *Int J Toxicol* 2003; **22:** 377–380.

27. Dye D, Watkins J, Suspected anaphylactic reaction to Cremophor EL. *Br Med J* 1980; **280:** 1353.

28. Strachan EB, Case report–suspected anaphylactic reaction to Cremophor El. *SAAD Dig* 1981; **4:** 209.

29. Barrow PC, Olivier P, Marzin D, The reproductive and developmental toxicity profile of beta-cyclodex-trin in rodents. *Reprod Toxicol* 1995; **9:** 389–398.

30. Lina BA, Bar A, Subchronic (13-week) oral toxicity study of alpha-cyclodextrin in dogs. *Regul Toxicol Pharmacol* 2004; **39**(Suppl 1)**:** S27–S33.

31. Ulloth JE, Almaguel FG, Padilla A, Bu L, Liu JW, De Leon M, Characterization of methyl-beta-cyclo-dextrin toxicity in NGF-differentiated PC12 cell death. *Neurotoxicology* 2007; **28:** 613–621.

32. Serajuddin AT, Solid dispersion of poorly water-soluble drugs: Early promises, subsequent problems, and recent breakthroughs. *J Pharm Sci* 1999; **88:** 1058–1066.

33. Chawla G, Bansal AK, Improved dissolution of a poorly water soluble drug in solid dispersions with polymeric and non-polymeric hydrophilic additives. *Acta Pharm* 2008; **58:** 257–274.

34. Chiou WL, Riegelman S, Preparation and dissolution characteristics of several fast-release solid dispersions of griseofulvin. *J Pharm Sci* 1969; **58:** 1505–1510.

35. Van Balen GP, Martinet GM, Caron G, Bouchard G, Reist M, Carrupt PA, Fruttero R, Gasco A, Testa B, Liposome/water lipophilicity: Methods, information content, and pharmaceutical applications. *Med Res Rev* 2004; **24:** 299–324.

36. Bangham AD, Horne RW, Negative staining of phospholipids and their structural modification by surface-active agents as observed in the electron microscope. *J Mol Biol* 1964; **8:** 660–668.

37. Torchilin VP, Recent advances with liposomes as pharmaceutical carriers. *Nat Rev Drug Discov* 2005; **4:** 145–160.

38. Gabizon AA, Shmeeda H, Zalipsky S, Pros and cons of the liposome platform in cancer drug targeting. *J Liposome Res* 2006; **16:** 175–183.

39. Liu D, Liu F, Song YK, Recognition and clearance of liposomes containing phosphatidylserine are mediated by serum opsonin. *Biochim Biophys Acta* 1995; **1235:** 140–146.

40. Yan X, Scherphof GL, Kamps JA, Liposome opsonization. *J Liposome Res* 2005; **15:** 109–139.

41. Papisov MI, Theoretical considerations of RES-avoiding liposomes: Molecular mechanics and chemistry of liposome interactions. *Adv Drug Deliv Rev* 1998; **32:** 119–138.

42. Chiu GN, Bally MB, Mayer LD, Selective protein interactions with phosphatidylserine containing liposomes alter the steric stabilization properties of poly(ethylene glycol). *Biochim Biophys Acta* 2001; **1510:** 56–69.

43. Torchilin V, Multifunctional and stimuli-sensitive pharmaceutical nanocarriers. *Eur J Pharm Biopharm* 2009; **71:** 431–444.

44. Amsberry KL, Borchardt RT, Amine prodrugs which utilize hydroxy amide lactonization. I. A potential redox-sensitive amide prodrug. *Pharm Res* 1991; **8:** 323–330.

45. Cook CS, Karabatsos PJ, Schoenhard GL, Karim A, Species dependent esterase activities for hydrolysis of an anti-HIV prodrug glycovir and bioavailability of active SC-48334. *Pharm Res* 1995; **12:** 1158–1164.

46. Riley CM, Mummert MA, Zhou J, Schowen RL, Vander Velde DG, Morton MD, Slavik M, Hydrolysis of the prodrug, 2′,3′,5′-triacetyl-6-azauridine. *Pharm Res* 1995; **12:** 1361–1370.

47. Springer CJ, Niculescu-Duvaz II, Antibody-directed enzyme prodrug therapy (ADEPT): A review. *Adv Drug Deliv Rev* 1997; **26:** 151–172.

48. Chen L, Waxman DJ, Cytochrome P450 gene-directed enzyme prodrug therapy (GDEPT) for cancer. *Curr Pharm Des* 2002; **8:** 1405–1416.

49. Ringsdorf H, Structure and properties of pharmacologically active polymers. *J Polym Sci Polym Symp* 1975; **51:** 135–153.

50. Li C, Wallace S, Polymer-drug conjugates: Recent development in clinical oncology. *Adv Drug Deliv Rev* 2008; **60:** 886–898.

51. Kratz F, Muller IA, Ryppa C, Warnecke A, Prodrug strategies in anticancer chemotherapy. *Chem Med Chem* 2008; **3:** 20–53.

52. Hildebrand JH, A critique of the theory of solubility of non-electrolytes. *Chem Rev* 1949; **44:** 37–45.

53. Zeng W, Du Y, Xue Y, Frish HL, in *Physical Properties of Polymer Handbook*. E. M. James (Ed.) (Springer-Verlag New York, LLC, New York, 2006).

54. Flory PJ, *Principle of Polymer Chemistry* (Cornell University Press, Ithaca, NY, 1953).

55. Liu R, Forrest ML, Kwon GS, in *Water-Insoluble Drug Formulation*. R. Liu (Ed.) (CRS Press, Taylor & Francis Group, New York, 2008).

56. Adamska K, Voelkel A, Inverse gas chromatographic determination of solubility parameters of excipients. *Int J Pharm* 2005; **304:** 11–17.

57. Liu J, Xiao Y, Allen C, Polymer–drug compatibility: A guide to the development of delivery systems for the anticancer agent, ellipticine. *J Pharm Sci* 2004; **93:** 132–143.

58. Letchford K, Liggins R, Burt H, Solubilization of hydrophobic drugs by methoxy poly(ethylene glycol)-block-polycaprolactone diblock copolymer micelles: Theoretical and experimental data and correlations. *J Pharm Sci* 2008; **97:** 1179–1190.

59. Burt HM, Zhang XC, Toleikis P, Embree L, Hunter WL, Development of copolymers of poly(D,L-lactide) and methoxypolyethylene glycol as micellar carriers of paclitaxel. *Colloids Surf B Biointerfaces* 1999; **16:** 161–171.

60. Vippagunta SR, Brittain HG, Grant DJ, Crystalline solids. *Adv Drug Deliv Rev* 2001; **48:** 3–26.
61. Coffman RE, Kildsig DO, Hydrotropic solubilization—Mechanistic studies. *Pharm Res* 1996; **13:** 1460–1463.
62. Matero A, in *Handbook of Applied Surface and Colloid Chemistry.* K. Holmberg (Ed.) (John Wiley & Sons, New York, 2001).
63. Ooya T, Lee S, Huh KM, Park K, in *Nanocarrier Technologies: Frontiers of Nanotherapy.* M. R. Mozafari (Ed.) (Springer, Amsterdam, the Netherlands, 2006).
64. Bauduin P, Renoncourt A, Kopf A, Touraud D, Kunz W, Unified concept of solubilization in water by hydrotropes and cosolvents. *Langmuir* 2005; **21:** 6769–6775.
65. Balasubramanian D, Srinivas V, Gaikar VG, Sharma MM, Aggregation behavior of hydrotropic compounds in aqueous solution. *J Phys Chem B* 1989; **93:** 3865–3870.
66. Neumann MG, Schmitt CC, Prieto KR, Goi BE, The photophysical determination of the minimum hydrotrope concentration of aromatic hydrotropes. *J Colloid Interface Sci* 2007; **315:** 810–813.
67. Sanghvi R, Evans D, Yalkowsky SH, Stacking complexation by nicotinamide: A useful way of enhancing drug solubility. *Int J Pharm* 2007; **336:** 35–41.
68. Coffman RE, Kildsig DO, Self-association of nicotinamide in aqueous solution: Light-scattering and vapor pressure osmometry studies. *J Pharm Sci* 1996; **85:** 848–853.
69. Simamora P, Alvarez JM, Yalkowsky SH, Solubilization of rapamycin. *Int J Pharm* 2001; **213:** 25–29.
70. Evstigneev MP, Evstigneev VP, Santiago AA, Davies DB, Effect of a mixture of caffeine and nicotin-amide on the solubility of vitamin (B2) in aqueous solution. *Eur J Pharm Sci* 2006; **28:** 59–66.
71. Landaur J, McConnell H, A study of molecular complexes formed by aniline and aromatic nitrohydro-carbons. *J Am Chem Soc* 1952; **74:** 1221–1224.
72. Mulliken RS, Structures of complexes formed by halogen molecules with aromatic and oxygenated solvent. *J Am Chem Soc* 1950; **72:** 600–608.
73. Lawrey DMG, McConnell H, A spectroscopic study of the benzene—s-Trinitrobenzene molecular complex. *J Am Chem Soc* 1952; **74:** 6175–6177.
74. Hunter CA, Lawson KR, Perkins J, Urch CJ, Aromatic interactions. *J Chem Soc Perkin Trans* 2001; **2:** 651–669.
75. Charman WN, Lai CSC, Craik DJ, Finnin BC, Reed BL, Self-association of nicotinamide in aqueous solution: N.M.R. studies of nicotinamide and the mono- and di-methyl-substituted amide analogues. *Aust J Chem* 1993; **46:** 377–385.
76. Lee SC, Acharya G, Lee J, Park K, Hydrotropic polymers: Synthesis and characterization of polymers containing picolylnicotinamide moieties. *Macromolecules* 2003; **36:** 2248–2255.
77. Rowinsky EK, Donehower RC, Paclitaxel (taxol). *N Engl J Med* 1995; **332:** 1004–1014.
78. Lee J, Lee SC, Acharya G, Chang CJ, Park K, Hydrotropic solubilization of paclitaxel: Analysis of chemical structures for hydrotropic property. *Pharm Res* 2003; **20:** 1022–1030.
79. Rasool AA, Hussain AA, Dittert LW, Solubility enhancement of some water-insoluble drugs in the pres-ence of nicotinamide and related compounds. *J Pharm Sci* 1991; **80:** 387–393.
80. Agrawal S, Pancholi SS, Jain NK, Agrawal GP, Hydrotropic solubilization of nimesulide for parenteral administration. *Int J Pharm* 2004; **274:** 149–155.
81. Nicoli S, Zani F, Bilzi S, Bettini R, Santi P, Association of nicotinamide with parabens: Effect on solubil-ity, partition and transdermal permeation. *Eur J Pharm Biopharm* 2008; **69:** 613–621.
82. Mansur CR, Pires RV, Gonzalez G, Lucas EF, Influence of the hydrotrope structure on the physical chemical properties of polyoxide aqueous solutions. *Langmuir* 2005; **21:** 2696–2703.
83. Huh KM, Lee SC, Cho YW, Lee J, Jeong JH, Park K, Hydrotropic polymer micelle system for delivery of paclitaxel. *J Control Release* 2005; **101:** 59–68.
84. Lee SC, Huh KM, Lee J, Cho YW, Galinsky RE, Park K, Hydrotropic polymeric micelles for enhanced paclitaxel solubility: In vitro and in vivo characterization. *Biomacromolecules* 2007; **8:** 202–208.
85. Kim S, Kim JY, Huh KM, Acharya G, Park K, Hydrotropic polymer micelles containing acrylic acid moieties for oral delivery of paclitaxel. *J Control Release* 2008; **132:** 222–229.
86. Huh KM, Min HS, Lee SC, Lee HJ, Kim S, Park K, A new hydrotropic block copolymer micelle system for aqueous solubilization of paclitaxel. *J Control Release* 2008; **126:** 122–129.
87. Huang JC, Lin KT, Deanin RD, Three-dimensional solubility parameters of poly(εcaprolactone). *J Appl Polym Sci* 2006; **100:** 2002–2009.
88. Nair R, Nyamweya N, Gonen S, Martinez-Miranda LJ, Hoag SW, Influence of various drugs on the glass transition temperature of poly(vinylpyrrolidone): A thermodynamic and spectroscopic investigation. *Int J Pharm* 2001; **225:** 83–96.

89. Mokrushina L, Buggert M, Smirnova I, Arlt W, Schomcker R, COSMO-RS and UNIFAC in prediction of micelle/water partition coefficients. *Ind Eng Chem Res* 2007; **46:** 6501–6509.

90. Hansch C, Quinlan JE, Lawrence GL, The linear free-energy relationship between partition coefficients and the aqueous solubility of organic liquids. *J Org Chem* 1968; **33:** 347–350.

91. Yalkowsky SH, Valvani SC, Solubility and partitioning. I: Solubility of nonelectrolytes in water. *J Pharm Sci* 1980; **69:** 912–922.

92. Yalkowsky SH, He Y, *Handbook of Aqueous Solubility Data* (CRC Press, New York, 2003).

93. Quina FH, Alonso EO, Farah JPS, Incorporation of nonionic solutes into aqueous micelles: A linear solvation free energy relationship analysis. *J Phys Chem* 1995; **99:** 11708–11714.

94. Abraham MH, Chadha HS, Dixon JP, Rafols C, Treiner C, Hydrogen bonding. Part 41. Factors that influence the distribution of solutes between water and hexadecylpyridinium chloride micelles. *J Chem Soc Perkin Trans* 1997; **2:** 19–24.

95. Rodrigues MA, Alonso EO, Yihwa C, Farah JPS, Quina FH, A linear solvent free energy relationship analysis of solubilization in mixed cationic-nonionic micelles. *Langmuir* 1999; **15:** 6770–6774.

96. Kamlet MJ, Taft RW, Solvatochromic comparison method. 1. Beta-scale of solvent hydrogen-bond acceptor (Hba) basicities. *J Am Chem Soc* 1976; **98:** 377–383.

97. Taft RW, Kamlet MJ, Solvatochromic comparison method. 2. Alpha-scale of solvent hydrogen-bond donor (Hbd) acidities. *J Am Chem Soc* 1976; **98:** 2886–2894.

98. Yokoyama T, Taft RW, Kamlet MJ, Solvatochromic comparison method. 3. Hydrogen-bonding by some 2-nitroaniline derivatives. *J Am Chem Soc* 1976; **98:** 3233–3237.

99. Kamlet MJ, Abboud JL, Taft RW, Solvatochromic comparison method. 6. Pi-star scale of solvent polarities. *J Am Chem Soc* 1977; **99:** 6027–6038.

100. Kim IW, Jang MD, Ryu YK, Cho EH, Lee YK, Park JH, Dipolarity, hydrogen-bond basicity and hydrogen-bond acidity of aqueous poly(ethylene glycol) solutions. *Anal Sci* 2002; **18:** 1357–1360.

101. Nyrkova IA, Semenov AN, Multimerization: Closed or open association model? *Eur Phys J E* 2005; **17:** 327–337.

102. Croy SR, Kwon GS, Polymeric micelles for drug delivery. *Curr Pharm Des* 2006; **12:** 4669–4684.

103. Liu R, Dannenfelser RM, Li S, in *Water-Insoluble Drug Formulation*. R. Liu (Ed.) (CRC Press, Taylor & Francis Group, New York, 2008).

104. Attwood D, Booth C, Yeates SG, Chaibundit C, Ricardo NM, Block copolymers for drug solubilisation: Relative hydrophobicities of polyether and polyester micelle-core-forming blocks. *Int J Pharm* 2007; **345:** 35–41.

105. Yamamoto Y, Yasugi K, Harada A, Nagasaki Y, Kataoka K, Temperature-related change in the properties relevant to drug delivery of poly(ethylene glycol)–poly(D,L-lactide) block copolymer micelles in aqueous milieu. *J Control Release* 2002; **82:** 359–371.

106. Marques CM, Bunchy micelles. *Langmuir* 1997; **13:** 1430–1433.

107. Allen C, Maysinger D, Eisenberg A, Nano-engineering block copolymer aggregates for drug delivery. *Adv Drug Deliv Rev* 1999; **16:** 3–27.

108. Gaucher G, Dufresne MH, Sant VP, Kang N, Maysinger D, Leroux JC, Block copolymer micelles: Preparation, characterization and application in drug delivery. *J Control Release* 2005; **109:** 169–188.

109. Kissel T, Li Y, Unger F, ABA-triblock copolymers from biodegradable polyester A-blocks and hydrophilic poly(ethylene oxide) B-blocks as a candidate for in situ forming hydrogel delivery systems for proteins. *Adv Drug Deliv Rev* 2002; **54:** 99–134.

110. Lan P, Jia L, Thermal properties of copoly(L-lactic acid/glycolic acid) by direct melt polycondensation. *J Macromol Sci Pure Appl Chem* 2006; **43:** 1887–1894.

111. Letchford K, Burt H, A review of the formation and classification of amphiphilic block copolymer nanoparticulate structures: Micelles, nanospheres, nanocapsules and polymersomes. *Eur J Pharm Biopharm* 2007; **65:** 259–269.

112. Pasquali RC, Taurozzi MP, Bregni C, Some considerations about the hydrophilic-lipophilic balance system. *Int J Pharm* 2008; **356:** 44–51.

113. Ahmed F, Pakunlu RI, Brannan A, Bates F, Minko T, Discher DE, Biodegradable polymersomes loaded with both paclitaxel and doxorubicin permeate and shrink tumors, inducing apoptosis in proportion to accumulated drug. *J Control Release* 2006; **116:** 150–158.

114. Discher DE, Ahmed F, Polymersomes. *Annu Rev Biomed Eng* 2006; **8:** 323–341.

115. Geng Y, Dalhaimer P, Cai S, Tsai R, Tewari M, Minko T, Discher DE, Shape effects of filaments versus spherical particles in flow and drug delivery. *Nat Nanotechnol* 2007; **2:** 249–255.

116. Aniansson EAG, Wall SN, On the kinetics of step-wise micelle association. *J Phys Chem* 1974; **78:** 1024–1030.

117. Halperin A, Alexander S, Polymer micelles: The relaxation kinetics. *Macromolecules* 1989; **22:** 2403–2412.

118. Prochazka K, Bednar B, Mukhtar E, Svoboda P, Trnena J, Almgren M, Nonradiative energy transfer in block copolymer micelles. *J Phys Chem* 1991; **95:** 4563–4568.

119. Wang Y, Kausch CM, Chun M, Quirk RP, Mattice WL, Exchange of chains between micelles labeled polystyrene-block-poly(oxyethylene) as monitored by nonradiative single energy transfer. *Macromolecules* 1995; **28:** 904–911.

120. Haliloglu T, Bahar I, Erman B, Mattice WL, Mechanisms of the exchange of diblock copolymers between dynamic equilibrium. *Macromolecules* 1996; **29:** 4764–4771.

121. Berney C, Danuser G, FRET or no FRET: A quantitative comparison. *Biophys J* 2003; **84:** 3992–4010.

122. Nyrkova IA, Semenov AN, On the theory of micellization kinetics. *Macromol Theory Simul* 2005; **14:** 569–585.

123. Senichev VY, Tereshatov VV, in *Handbook of Plasticizers*. G. Wypych (Ed.), (William Andrew Publishing, Norwich, NY, 2004), pp. 218–227.

124. Blasi P, Schoubben A, Giovagnoli S, Perioli L, Ricci M, Rossi C, Ketoprofen poly(lactide-co-glycolide) physical interaction. *AAPS Pharm Sci Tech* 2007; **8:** Article 37.

125. Yang X, Zhu B, Dong T, Pan P, Shuai X, Inoue Y, Interactions between an anticancer drug and polymeric micelles based on biodegradable polyesters. *Macromol Biosci* 2008; **8:** 1116–1125.

126. Liu SQ, Tong YW, Yang YY, Thermally sensitive micelles self-assembled from poly(*N*-isopropylacrylamide-*co*-N,N-dimethylacrylamide)-*b*-poly(D,L-lactide-*co*-glycolide) for controlled delivery of paclitaxel. *Mol Biosyst* 2005; **1:** 158–165.

127. Chen H, Kim S, He W, Wang H, Low PS, Park K, Cheng JX, Fast release of lipophilic agents from circulating PEG-PDLLA micelles revealed by in vivo Forster resonance energy transfer imaging. *Langmuir* 2008; **24:** 5213–5217.

128. Lu RC, Cao AN, Lai LH, Zhu BY, Zhao GX, Xiao JX, Interaction between bovine serum albumin and equimolarly mixed cationic-anionic surfactants decyltriethylammonium bromide-sodium decyl sulfonate. *Colloids Surf B Biointerfaces* 2005; **41:** 139–143.

129. Pi Y, Shang Y, Peng C, Liu H, Hu Y, Jiang J, Interactions between bovine serum albumin and gemini surfactant alkanediyl-alpha, omega-bis(dimethyldodecyl-ammonium bromide). *Biopolymers* 2006; **83:** 243–249.

130. Moore PN, Puvvada S, Blackschtein D, Role of the surfactant polar head structure in protein–surfactant complexation: Zein protein solubilization by SDS and by SDS/C12En surfactant solutions. *Langmuir* 2003; **19:** 1009–1016.

131. Asadi A, Saboury AA, Moosavi-Movahedi AA, Divsalar A, Sarbolouki MN, Interaction of bovine serum albumin with some novel PEG-containing diblock copolymers. *Int J Biol Macromol* 2008; **43:** 262–270.

132. Castelletto V, Krysmann M, Kelarakis A, Jauregi P, Complex formation of bovine serum albumin with a poly(ethylene glycol) lipid conjugate. *Biomacromolecules* 2007; **8:** 2244–2249.

133. Kelarakis A, Castelletto V, Krysmann MJ, Havredaki V, Viras K, Hamley IW, Interactions of bovine serum albumin with ethylene oxide/butylene oxide copolymers in aqueous solution. *Biomacromolecules* 2008; **9:** 1366–1371.

134. Ratner BD, Hoffman A, Schoen F, Lemons J, *Biomaterials Science: An Introduction to Materials in Medicine*, 2nd edn. (Academic Press, New York, 2004).

135. Amiconi G, Bonaventura C, Bonaventura J, Antonini E, Functional properties of normal and sickle cell hemoglobins in polyethylene glycol 6000. *Biochim Biophys Acta* 1977; **495:** 279–286.

136. McPherson A, Jr., Crystallization of proteins from polyethylene glycol. *J Biol Chem* 1976; **251:** 6300–6303.

137. Lee JC, Lee LL, Preferential solvent interactions between proteins and polyethylene glycols. *J Biol Chem* 1981; **256:** 625–631.

138. Rito-Palomares M, Practical application of aqueous two-phase partition to process development for the recovery of biological products. *J Chromatogr B Analyt Technol Biomed Life Sci* 2004; **807:** 3–11.

139. Fredrickson GH, Pincus P, Drainage of compressed polymer layers - dynamics of a squeezed sponge. *Langmuir* 1991; **7:** 786–795.

140. Yokoyama M, Okano T, Sakurai Y, Fukushima S, Okamoto K, Kataoka K, Selective delivery of adriamycin to a solid tumor using a polymeric micelle carrier system. *J Drug Target* 1999; **7:** 171–186.

141. Armstrong JK, Leharne SA, Stuart BH, Snowden MJ, Chowdhry BZ, Phase transition properties of poly(ethylene oxide) in aqueous solutions of sodium chloride. *Langmuir* 2001; **17:** 4482–4485.

142. Rixman MA, Dean D, Ortiz C, Nanoscale intermolecular interactions between human serum albumin and low grafting density surfaces of poly(ethylene oxide). *Langmuir* 2003; **19:** 9357–9372.

143. Xia JL, Dubin PL, Kokufuta E, Dynamic and electrophoretic light-scattering of a water-soluble complex formed between pepsin and poly(ethylene glycol). *Macromolecules* 1993; **26:** 6688–6690.

144. Topchieva IN, Sorokina EM, Efremova NV, Ksenofontov AL, Kurganov BI, Noncovalent adducts of poly(ethylene glycols) with proteins. *Bioconjug Chem* 2000; **11:** 22–29.

145. Furness EL, Ross A, Davis TP, King GC, A hydrophobic interaction site for lysozyme binding to poly-ethylene glycol and model contact lens polymers. *Biomaterials* 1998; **19:** 1361–1369.

146. Chia D, Barnett EV, Yamagata J, Knutson D, Restivo C, Furst D, Quantitation and characterization of soluble immune complexes precipitated from sera by polyethylene glycol (PEG). *Clin Exp Immunol* 1979; **37:** 399–407.

147. Herbert KE, Coppock JS, Griffiths AM, Williams A, Robinson MW, Scott DL, Fibronectin and immune complexes in rheumatic diseases. *Ann Rheum Dis* 1987; **46:** 734–740.

148. Robinson MW, Scott DG, Bacon PA, Walton KW, Coppock JS, Scott DL, What proteins are present in polyethylene glycol precipitates from rheumatic sera? *Ann Rheum Dis* 1989; **48:** 496–501.

149. Cocke DL, Wang HJ, Chen JJ, Interaction between poly(ethylene glycol) and human serum albumin. *Chem Commun* 1997; 2331–2332.

150. Pico G, Bassani G, Farruggia B, Nerli B, Calorimetric investigation of the protein-flexible chain polymer interactions and its relationship with protein partition in aqueous two-phase systems. *Int J Biol Macromol* 2007; **40:** 268–275.

151. Ragi C, Sedaghat-Herati MR, Ouameur AA, Tajmir-Riahi HA, The effects of poly(ethylene glycol) on the solution structure of human serum albumin. *Biopolymers* 2005; **78:** 231–236.

152. Hasek J, Poly(ethylene glycol) interactions with proteins. *Zeitschrift Fur Kristallographie* 2006; 613–618.

153. Baier RE, Surface behaviour of biomaterials: The theta surface for biocompatibility. *J Mater Sci Mater Med* 2006; **17:** 1057–1062.

154. Li S, Garreau H, Pauvert B, McGrath J, Toniolo A, Vert M, Enzymatic degradation of block copolymers prepared from epsilon-caprolactone and poly(ethylene glycol). *Biomacromolecules* 2002; **3:** 525–530.

155. Herzog K, Muller RJ, Deckwer WD, Mechanism and kinetics of the enzymatic hydrolysis of polyester nanoparticles by lipases. *Polym Degrad Stabil* 2006; **91:** 2486–2498.

156. Chen DR, Bei JZ, Wang SG, Polycaprolactone microparticles and their biodegradation. *Polym Degrad Stabil* 2000; **67:** 455–459.

157. Carstens MG, van Nostrum CF, Verrijk R, de Leede LG, Crommelin DJ, Hennink WE, A mechanistic study on the chemical and enzymatic degradation of PEG-oligo(epsilon-caprolactone) micelles. *J Pharm Sci* 2008; **97:** 506–518.

158. Chen C, Yu CH, Cheng YC, Yu PH, Cheung MK, Biodegradable nanoparticles of amphiphilic triblock copolymers based on poly(3-hydroxybutyrate) and poly(ethylene glycol) as drug carriers. *Biomaterials* 2006; **27:** 4804–4814.

159. Mayor S, Pagano RE, Pathways of clathrin-independent endocytosis. *Nat Rev Mol Cell Biol* 2007; **8:** 603–612.

160. Sahay G, Batrakova EV, Kabanov AV, Different internalization pathways of polymeric micelles and unimers and their effects on vesicular transport. *Bioconjug Chem* 2008; **19:** 2023–2029.

161. Edeling MA, Smith C, Owen D, Life of a clathrin coat: Insights from clathrin and AP structures. *Nat Rev Mol Cell Biol* 2006; **7:** 32–44.

162. Rappoport JZ, Focusing on clathrin-mediated endocytosis. *Biochem J* 2008; **412:** 415–423.

163. Carver LA, Schnitzer JE, Caveolae: Mining little caves for new cancer targets. *Nat Rev Cancer* 2003; **3:** 571–581.

164. Gratton SE, Ropp PA, Pohlhaus PD, Luft JC, Madden VJ, Napier ME, DeSimone JM, The effect of particle design on cellular internalization pathways. *Proc Natl Acad Sci USA* 2008; **105:** 11613–11618.

165. Chen H, Kim S, Li L, Wang S, Park K, Cheng JX, Release of hydrophobic molecules from polymer micelles into cell membranes revealed by Forster resonance energy transfer imaging. *Proc Natl Acad Sci USA* 2008; **105:** 6596–6601.

166. Miller DW, Batrakova EV, Waltner TO, Alakhov V, Kabanov AV, Interactions of pluronic block copolymers with brain microvessel endothelial cells: Evidence of two potential pathways for drug absorption. *Bioconjug Chem* 1997; **8:** 649–657.

167. Rapoport N, Marin A, Luo Y, Prestwich GD, Muniruzzaman MD, Intracellular uptake and trafficking of pluronic micelles in drug-sensitive and MDR cells: Effect on the intracellular drug localization. *J Pharm Sci* 2002; **91:** 157–170.

168. Batrakova EV, Li S, Alakhov VY, Miller DW, Kabanov AV, Optimal structure requirements for pluronic block copolymers in modifying P-glycoprotein drug efflux transporter activity in bovine brain microvessel endothelial cells. *J Pharmacol Exp Ther* 2003; **304:** 845–854.

169. Zastre JA, Jackson JK, Wong W, Burt HM, P-glycoprotein efflux inhibition by amphiphilic diblock copolymers: Relationship between copolymer concentration and substrate hydrophobicity. *Mol Pharm* 2008; **5:** 643–653.

170. Allen C, Yu Y, Eisenberg A, Maysinger D, Cellular internalization of PCL(20)-b-PEO(44) block copolymer micelles. *Biochim Biophys Acta* 1999; **1421:** 32–38.

171. Luo L, Tam J, Maysinger D, Eisenberg A, Cellular internalization of poly(ethylene oxide)-b-poly(epsilon-caprolactone) diblock copolymer micelles. *Bioconjug Chem* 2002; **13:** 1259–1265.

172. Savic R, Luo L, Eisenberg A, Maysinger D, Micellar nanocontainers distribute to defined cytoplasmic organelles. *Science* 2003; **300:** 615–618.

173. Moghimi SM, Hunter AC, Murray JC, Szewczyk A, Cellular distribution of nonionic micelles. *Science* 2004; **303:** 626–628.

174. Maysinger D, Berezovska O, Savic R, Soo PL, Eisenberg A, Block copolymers modify the internalization of micelle-incorporated probes into neural cells. *Biochim Biophys Acta* 2001; **1539:** 205–217.

175. Mahmud A, Lavasanifar A, The effect of block copolymer structure on the internalization of polymeric micelles by human breast cancer cells. *Colloids Surf B Biointerfaces* 2005; **45:** 82–89.

176. Lee RC, River LP, Pan FS, Ji L, Wollmann RL, Surfactant-induced sealing of electropermeabilized skeletal muscle membranes in vivo. *Proc Natl Acad Sci USA* 1992; **89:** 4524–4528.

177. Collins JM, Despa F, Lee RC, Structural and functional recovery of electropermeabilized skeletal muscle in-vivo after treatment with surfactant poloxamer 188. *Biochim Biophys Acta* 2007; **1768:** 1238–1246.

178. Maskarinec SA, Wu G, Lee KY, Membrane sealing by polymers. *Ann NY Acad Sci* 2005; **1066:** 310–320.

179. Lentz BR, PEG as a tool to gain insight into membrane fusion. *Eur Biophys J* 2007; **36:** 315–326.

180. Blow AM, Botham GM, Fisher D, Goodall AH, Tilcock CP, Lucy JA, Water and calcium ions in cell fusion induced by poly(ethylene glycol). *FEBS Lett* 1978; **94:** 305–310.

181. Wu JR, Lentz BR, Mechanism of poly(ethylene glycol)-induced lipid transfer between phosphatidylcholine large unilamellar vesicles: A fluorescent probe study. *Biochemistry* 1991; **30:** 6780–6787.

182. Burgess SW, Massenburg D, Yates J, Lentz BR, Poly(ethylene glycol)-induced lipid mixing but not fusion between synthetic phosphatidylcholine large unilamellar vesicles. *Biochemistry* 1991; **30:** 4193–4200.

183. Talbot WA, Zheng LX, Lentz BR, Acyl chain unsaturation and vesicle curvature alter outer leaflet packing and promote poly(ethylene glycol)-mediated membrane fusion. *Biochemistry* 1997; **36:** 5827–5836.

184. Shi R, Borgens RB, Acute repair of crushed guinea pig spinal cord by polyethylene glycol. *J Neurophysiol* 1999; **81:** 2406–2414.

185. Liu-Snyder P, Logan MP, Shi R, Smith DT, Borgens RB, Neuroprotection from secondary injury by polyethylene glycol requires its internalization. *J Exp Biol* 2007; **210:** 1455–1462.

186. Batrakova EV, Li S, Li Y, Alakhov VY, Elmquist WF, Kabanov AV, Distribution kinetics of a micelle-forming block copolymer Pluronic P85. *J Control Release* 2004; **100:** 389–397.

187. Rudin M, Weissleder R, Molecular imaging in drug discovery and development. *Nat Rev Drug Discov* 2003; **2:** 123–131.

188. Park YJ, Lee JY, Chang YS, Jeong JM, Chung JK, Lee MC, Park KB, Lee SJ, Radioisotope carrying polyethylene oxide-polycaprolactone copolymer micelles for targetable bone imaging. *Biomaterials* 2002; **23:** 873–879.

189. Liu J, Zeng F, Allen C, In vivo fate of unimers and micelles of a poly(ethylene glycol)-block-poly(caprolactone) copolymer in mice following intravenous administration. *Eur J Pharm Biopharm* 2007; **65:** 309–319.

190. Savic R, Azzam T, Eisenberg A, Maysinger D, Assessment of the integrity of poly(caprolactone)-*b*-poly(ethylene oxide) micelles under biological conditions: A fluorogenic-based approach. *Langmuir* 2006; **22:** 3570–3578.

191. Novakova K, Laznicek M, Rypacek F, Machova L, Pharmacokinetics and distribution of 125I-PLA-b-PEO block copolymers in rats. *Pharm Dev Technol* 2003; **8:** 153–161.

192. Novakova K, Laznicek M, ^{125}I-labeled PLA/PEO block copolymer: Biodistribution studies in rats. *J Bioact Compat Polym* 2002; **17:** 285–296.

193. Yamamoto Y, Nagasaki Y, Kato Y, Sugiyama Y, Kataoka K, Long-circulating poly(ethylene glycol)-poly(D,L-lactide) block copolymer micelles with modulated surface charge. *J Control Release* 2001; **77:** 27–38.

194. Yokoyama M, Okano T, Sakurai Y, Ekimoto H, Shibazaki C, Kataoka K, Toxicity and antitumor activity against solid tumors of micelle-forming polymeric anticancer drug and its extremely long circulation in blood. *Cancer Res* 1991; **51:** 3229–3236.

195. Sun X, Rossin R, Turner JL, Becker ML, Joralemon MJ, Welch MJ, Wooley KL, An assessment of the effects of shell cross-linked nanoparticle size, core composition, and surface PEGylation on in vivo biodistribution. *Biomacromolecules* 2005; **6:** 2541–2554.

196. Sun G, Hagooly A, Xu J, Nystrom AM, Li Z, Rossin R, Moore DA, Wooley KL, Welch MJ, Facile, efficient approach to accomplish tunable chemistries and variable biodistributions for shell cross-linked nanoparticles. *Biomacromolecules* 2008; **9:** 1997–2006.

197. Sezgin Z, Yuksel N, Baykara T, Preparation and characterization of polymeric micelles for solubilization of poorly soluble anticancer drugs. *Eur J Pharm Biopharm* 2006; **64:** 261–268.

198. Torchilin VP, Micellar nanocarriers: Pharmaceutical perspectives. *Pharm Res* 2007; **24:** 1–16.

199. Wooley KL, Shell crosslinked polymer assemblies: Nanoscale constructs inspired from biological systems. *J Polym Sci A: Polym Chem* 2000; **38:** 1397–1407.

200. O'Reilly RK, Hawker CJ, Wooley KL, Cross-linked block copolymer micelles: Functional nanostructures of great potential and versatility. *Chem Soc Rev* 2006; **35:** 1068–1083.

201. Shuai X, Merdan T, Schaper AK, Xi F, Kissel T, Core-cross-linked polymeric micelles as paclitaxel carriers. *Bioconjug Chem* 2004; **15:** 441–448.

202. Li Y, Lokitz BS, Armes SP, McCormick CL, Synthesis of reversible shell cross-linked micelles for controlled release of bioactive agents. *Macromolecules* 2006; **39:** 2726–2728.

203. Kohn J, New approaches to biomaterials design. *Nat Mater* 2004; **3:** 745–747.

204. Kohn J, Welsh WJ, Knight D, A new approach to the rationale discovery of polymeric biomaterials. *Biomaterials* 2007; **28:** 4171–4177.

205. Matyjaszewski K, Xia J, Atom transfer radical polymerization. *Chem Rev* 2001; **101:** 2921–2990.

206. Stenzel MH, RAFT polymerization: An avenue to functional polymeric micelles for drug delivery. *Chem Commun* 2008; **14:** 3486–3503.

207. Hawker CJ, Bosman AW, Harth E, New polymer synthesis by nitroxide mediated living radical polymerizations. *Chem Rev* 2001; **101:** 3661–3688.

208. Kwon IK, Kim SW, Chaterji S, Vedantham K, Park K, in *Smart Materials*, M. Schwartz (Ed.) (Taylor & Francis Group, LLC, Boca Raton, FL, 2009), pp. 13-1–13-10.

Part VII

Stimuli-Responsive Systems

20 Multifunctional Stimuli–Responsive Nanoparticles for Targeted Delivery of Small and Macromolecular Therapeutics

Srinivas Ganta, Arun Iyer, and Mansoor Amiji

CONTENTS

20.1 INTRODUCTION

20.1.1 BARRIERS IN SMALL AND MACROMOLECULAR DRUG DELIVERY

Many small and macromolecular therapeutics fail to treat diseases because of anatomical and physiological barriers that limit their direct entry into the target extracellular or intracellular compartments.[1,2] The major hurdles for these therapeutic molecules reaching the target compartment are poor aqueous solubility, permeability, stability, and limited transport across epithelial layers in the biological environment.[1] These problems are particularly significant in the case of macromolecular therapeutic agents such as nucleic acids (plasmid DNA, oligonucleotides, small interfering double-stranded RNA), peptides, and proteins.

In order to overcome these challenges, it is critical to develop drug delivery strategies that protect the payload from degradation in the biological environment, while facilitating their transport through anatomic and physiological barriers to increase their availability at the target site. During the last decade, the remarkable growth of nanotechnology has opened the doors to challenging innovations in drug delivery, which are in the process of revolutionizing the delivery of biologically active molecules. Nanoparticles, an evolvement of nanotechnology, are exploited for therapeutic purpose to carry the drug in the body in a controlled manner from the site of administration to the target compartment. These particles are colloidal carriers with a diameter smaller than 1000 nm and can safely carry therapeutic agents through the small capillaries into a targeted compartment in an organ, a particular tissue, or a cell.[3] This implies the passage of the therapeutic molecules and nanoparticle systems across various physiological barriers, which represent the most challenging objective in drug targeting.

For nanoparticles administered intravenously, the first limiting physiological barrier is that of the vascular endothelium and the basement membrane.[4] The transport of drug delivery systems (DDS) and released drug molecules across the vascular endothelium is determined by the size of the DDS and the molecular weight as well as the hydrophilicity–hydrophobicity of the molecule.[5] The blood–brain barrier (BBB), constituted of tight endothelial cells in the brain, can prevent the entry of most drugs and DDS. However, the altered vascular endothelia in tumors and inflammatory sites allows the extravasation of macromolecules and the nanoparticulate DDS.[6] Surface properties are also a key determinant in the biodistribution of the nanoparticles. The hydrophobic surface of the nanoparticles favors their binding to plasma proteins, resulting in subsequent clearance by the reticulo-endothelial system (RES). For the nanoparticles to remain in blood circulation for a long time, the major problem is to avoid its opsonization and subsequent uptake by the RES.[5] The hydrophilic modification of nanoparticles with poly(ethylene glycol) (PEG) or poly(ethylene oxide) (PEO) avoids opsonization and uptake by the RES. Another physiological barrier to nanoparticulate delivery is the extracellular matrix, which should be overcome in order to reach the target cells in a tissue. If the whole tissue constitutes a target site, then the uniform distribution of drug throughout the tissue is another barrier.[4] If the drug targets are present in the cytoplasm/nucleus of a cell, an additional barrier needs to be overcome to achieve internalization and exhibit the desired therapeutic effect.

A nanoparticle with targeting ability to specific cell receptors provides the driving force for the diffusion of the carrier to specific cells. For example, with macromolecular therapeutics, there is a need for the molecules to enter into subcellular sites in an effective manner to produce the required cellular events.[7] This is also important for many anticancer drugs whose primary site of action is the mitochondrial membrane.[7] Taken together, the function of the nanoparticle is to (1) protect a drug from degradation, (2) facilitate drug diffusion through the epithelium, (3) modulate the pharmacokinetic and biodistribution profiles, and/or (4) enhance intracellular distribution. Many types of nanoparticle DDS evaluated for their prospective therapeutic applications are in various stages of development. The application of a stimuli-responsive nanoparticle DDS offers an interesting opportunity for small and macromolecular drug delivery where the nanoparticles become an active

TABLE 20.1
Summary of Stimuli Properties That Can Be Utilized to Control the Behavior of Stimuli-Responsive Nanoparticles for Small and Macromolecular Delivery

Stimuli Type	Stimuli Origin	Remarks
Internal stimuli		
pH	Decreased pH in pathological sites, such as tumors, infection, and inflammation because of hypoxia and massive cell death	Can be utilized for the controlled release of therapeutics at target tissue from the pH-responsive nanoparticles
Temperature	Hyperthermia associated with inflammation	Can cause enhanced permeability of microvasculature to nanoparticles and heat release
Redox potential	Increased intracellular glutathione levels in many pathological cells compared with its extracellular concentration	Can be exploited for nanoparticles coupled with –S–S– bonds that will release payload inside the target cell
External stimuli		
Temperature	Locally applied hyperthermia by means of high frequency magnetic energy, ultrasound or light	Can facilitate inside target tissue accumulation of nanoparticles and heat release
Magnetic energy	Magnetic energy applied with extracorporeal magnet movement with different energy profiles	Can concentrate magneto-responsive nanoparticles in tissue, facilitate hyperthermia and imaging at target tissue
Ultrasound	Sonication can be applied to the body to get a diagnostic signal from contrast agents	Can facilitate ultrasound-responsive nanoparticles penetration into tissue
Light	Light irradiation at the target site induces heating of metal nanoparticles	Can control the release of drugs in the target area

participant in the optimization of therapy.[8] The main properties of stimuli-responsive nanoparticles are their ability to reach the target compartment and deliver the payload to the subcellular compartment in response to external (magnetic field, light, and heat) or biological stimulus (pH gradient and redox potential).[8] The following sections will address the stimuli-responsive nanoparticle's targeting potential, subcellular distribution ability, and their fabrication to respond to biological or external stimuli (Table 20.1).

20.1.2 TARGET-SPECIFIC DELIVERY TO IMPROVE THERAPEUTIC PROFILE

Conventional pharmaceutical formulations do not differentiate the disease sites from the normal sites. This causes the nonspecific distribution of its active compounds resulting in undesired toxic effects on normal tissue. For example, the treatment of cancer, human immune deficiency virus (HIV) infection, leishmaniasis, and malaria generally involves highly toxic compounds, and their use is considerably restricted by the occurrence of side effects. The application of nanotechnology in pharmacotherapy allows for temporal and spatial site-specific delivery.[9] The nanotechnology-based DDSs have the ability to deliver the therapeutics directly into the disease site. A site-specific delivery approach would not only enhance the therapeutic response of drugs, but will also reduce the toxicity and allow lower/optimum doses of the drug to be used in therapy.[5]

The methods to achieve drug targeting are mainly classified into passive and active targeting. Passive targeting refers to the accumulation of the drug or delivery system at the site of interest due to physicochemical or pharmacological properties.[4] Small or macromolecule drug-loaded nanoparticles can be passively targeted by exploiting the anatomical and pathophysiological abnormalities of disease sites. For instance, the defective vasculature and lack of effective lymphatic drainage from the tumor results in the extravasation and accumulation of nanoparticles, plasma proteins, and macromolecules.[10] This phenomenon of exploiting the "leaky" vasculature of tumor tissues for macromolecular drug targeting has been termed the "enhanced permeability and retention" (EPR) effect, schematically shown in Figure 20.1. The EPR effect was first described in murine solid tumors for macromolecules accumulation by Maeda and colleagues.[11] The EPR effect is now thought to contribute to the effects of many anticancer drugs delivered as conjugates with synthetic polymers[12] or in liposomes.[13] The tumor uptake of highly protein bound drugs (e.g., anthracyclines, paclitaxel, etoposide) also seems to be mediated through the EPR effect.[14]

Enhanced drug permeation associated with drug delivery carriers to tumors through the leaky vasculature is termed passive tumor targeting.[15,16] The particles in the range of 10–500 nm in size can extravasate and accumulate inside the tumor tissue. However, the cut-off size of the permeable vasculature varies from tumor to tumor, and the size of a drug-carrying particle may be used to control the passive drug delivery.[16] Apart from the nanosize of the drug carrier, the ability of the particle to circulate long enough in the blood to provide sufficient time for accumulation into tumors is important. For example, PEG-modified nanoparticles can preferentially accumulate in the tumor tissue upon systemic delivery based on the EPR effect. Doxorubicin incorporated into long circulating PEG-modified liposomes showed excellent tumor accumulation through the EPR effect and reduced the side effects of doxorubicin.[17] The EPR effect has also been observed in other diseases such as infections and chronic inflammations. Thus, the application of nanoparticles is expected to have therapeutic benefits for treating these diseases as well.[18]

The tendency of nanoparticles to localize in the RES also presents an opportunity for the passive targeting of drugs to the macrophages present in the liver and spleen. For example, macrophages are directly associated with certain intracellular infections like candidiasis, leishmaniasis, and listeria.[19] The drug-loaded nanoparticles can be passively targeted to these sites for treating the infections.

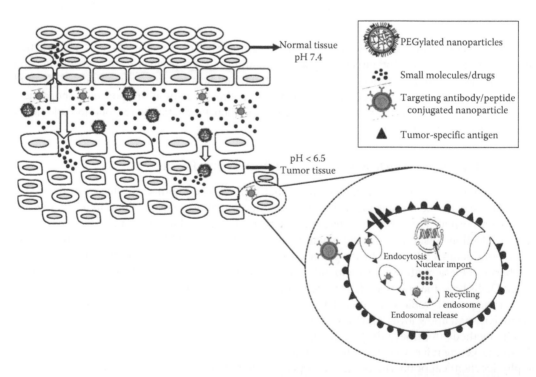

FIGURE 20.1 Localization of stimuli-responsive nanoparticles at tumor site through the EPR effect, and involvement of passive and active targeting strategies.

Other methods for passive targeting involve the use of stimuli-responsive nanoparticles that can release the encapsulated therapeutics only when the appropriate stimulus is present. Such multifunctional nanoparticles have the ability to localize by passive targeting and release their payload to subcellular compartments in response to external (magnetic, light, or heat) or biological (pH or redox potential) stimuli. For example, the pH level around tumor and other hypoxic disease tissues in the body tends to be more acidic (i.e., ~5.5–6.5) relative to physiological pH levels (i.e., 7.4). This change in pH condition can be utilized for controlled delivery of therapeutics. Other approaches for passive targeting involve the surface charge modulation of nanoparticles. Nanoparticles of <200 nm in diameter and those with positive surface charge are known to preferentially accumulate and reside in the tumor mass for a longer duration than either neutral or negatively charged nanoparticles.

Gelatin is one of the widely investigated natural and biocompatible polymers for gene delivery. It is produced from collagen by alkaline or acidic pretreatment and thermal denaturation. Depending on this pretreatment, two types of gelatin can be distinguished: A and B. Gelatin A is processed by acidic pretreatment, while gelatin B is processed by alkaline pretreatment. The alkaline pretreatment converts glutamine and asparagine residues into glutamic acid and aspartic acid, which results in higher carboxylic acid content for gelatin B than for gelatin A.[20] We have investigated the passively-targeted delivery of type B gelatin-based nanoparticles that have been very effective in systemic gene delivery to solid tumors.[21] The DNA delivered in PEG-modified gelatin nanoparticles was more effective *in vitro* and *in vivo* in the transfection of reporter plasmid DNA expressing green fluorescent protein (GFP) and beta-galactosidase.[22,23]

The other targeting strategy is active targeting, in which nanoparticles are coupled with ligands that bind to specific receptors or antigens over-expressed on target cells,[24] schematically shown in Figure 20.1, thus maximizing the therapeutic efficacy of the drug and reducing its side effects. The coupling of targeting ligands to nanoparticles would allow the import of a multitude of drug molecules compared with the direct coupling of targeting ligands with drug molecules.[5] The target receptors and surface bound antigens may be either differentially over-expressed in diseased cells or expressed uniquely in diseased cells only as compared with the normal cells. For example, rapidly proliferating tumor cells over-express certain receptors for the enhanced uptake of nutrients, including folic acid, vitamins, and sugars. The nanoparticles attached with folic acid can be targeted to the tumor cells that over-express folate receptors.[25] In addition, the folate bound nanoparticles can be made to be stimuli-responsive. Such multifunctional nanoparticles internalize via folate-receptor mediated endocytosis[25] and release their contents in response to internal stimuli. Tumor and vascular endothelial cells over-express specific integrin receptors, such as $\alpha_v\beta_5$ or $\alpha_v\beta_3$, that can bind to the arginine-glycine-aspartic acid (RGD) tripeptide sequence. RGD-modification, therefore, has been used to target nanoparticles to tumor cells and vascular endothelial cells of the angiogenic blood vessels. Aptamer, a nucleic acid construct that specifically recognizes prostate membrane antigen on prostate tumor cells,[26] provides an additional strategy for active targeting. Low density lipoprotein (LDL) receptors that transport cholesterol rich lipoproteins into cells through receptor-mediated endocytosis can be used as targets for lipid-based systems, such as liposomes and cholesterol rich emulsions.[27] Apolipoprotein enriched liposomes[28] and anionic liposomes[29] were found to mimic LDL protein and provide targeted delivery of anticancer agents to tumor cells through the LDL receptors.

The discovery of hybridoma technology has provided extensive use of antibodies as targeting ligands against specific antigens/proteins expressed on the surface of cells. The use of monoclonal antibodies against surface bound antigens present only on tumor cells allows for other targeting strategies. For example, human epithelial growth factor receptor 2 (HER2)-antibody anchored nanoparticles were able to deliver the therapeutic agents specifically in HER2 expressing tumor cells.[30] Transferrin, an iron-binding protein, can also be used as a site-specific ligand for directing nanoparticles to the tumor cells.[31] Epidermal growth factor receptors are over-expressed in breast or prostate cancers, making it a good site for targeting gene-delivery complexes.[32] The endothelial cells lining the blood vessels, epithelial surfaces of the lungs and gastrointestinal tract, muscle myoblasts, and skin fibroblasts are also potential targets for gene delivery.[33] Apart from the

The EPR effect greatly influences the delivery of many anticancer drugs when formulated as conjugates with synthetic polymers or in liposomes. The tumor uptake of highly protein bound drugs (e.g., anthracyclines, paclitaxel, and etoposide) also seems to be mediated through the EPR effect.

targeting potential, the nanoparticles can also be made stimuli-responsive to enhance the transfection ability of the nanoparticles. Oishi and Nagasaki[34] showed that pH-responsive and PEG-modified nanogels bearing a lactose group at the PEG end display endosomolytic abilities and have enhanced transfection efficiency.

20.1.3 INTRACELLULAR DRUG AVAILABILITY AND DISTRIBUTION

Intracellular distribution is desirable for drugs whose site of action is located in the intracellular compartments. Intracellular targeting is also important for drugs that are effluxed from the cell by the efflux transporters such as P-glycoproteins (Pgp) and multi-drug resistance proteins (MRP).[35] For example, with macromolecular therapeutics (proteins and plasmid DNA), there is a need for the molecules to enter into the cytoplasm or nucleus intact to produce the required cellular events.[7] This is also important for many anticancer drugs whose primary action site is the mitochondrial membrane.[7] Proteins and plasmid DNA are prone to degradation by the nucleases or the endolysosomal enzymes while delivering them into the cytoplasm or the nucleus.[5]

Nanoparticulate systems have been explored for specific intracellular delivery of small and macromolecular drugs, they are expected to enter the target cells and deliver the therapeutics in its stable form to subcellular compartments. The intracellular distribution of small and macromolecules using nanoparticles is schematically shown in Figure 20.2. The mode of nanoparticle internalization is by either nonspecific or specific cellular uptake.[7] Following the nonspecific cellular uptake of a nanoparticle, the cell membrane envelops the nanoparticle to form a vesicle in the cell, called an endosome. Then, the endosome fuses with lysosomes, which are highly acidic organelles rich in degrading enzymes. This acidic environment is deterrent to therapeutic molecules encapsulated

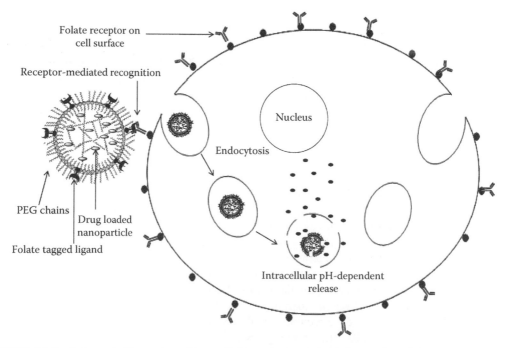

FIGURE 20.2 Schematic illustration of intracellular and subcellular delivery of small and macromolecular therapeutics using surface-functionalized nanoparticles. It shows the intracellular delivery of folate anchored nanoparticles through endocytosis process and releasing its content in response to internal pH stimuli.

in the nanoparticles. This bottleneck in gene delivery can be responsible for the degradation of most (~99%) of the internalized DNA molecules. Endosomes can be buffered to effect the safer release of its contents into the cytoplasm. For example, the buffering property of the polycationic carriers can reduce the acidification of the endosomes, resulting in the swelling and bursting of endosomes before they fuse with lysosomes, resulting in a safe release of the trapped contents.[36,37]

The specific cellular uptake involves receptor-mediated endocytosis of ligand-modified nanoparticles. The ligand-modified nanoparticle forms a complex with the receptor, internalizes, and undergoes vesicular transport through the endosomes. Following the dissociation of the nanoparticle-receptor complex, the receptor is re-cycled back to the cell membrane.

In addition, cell penetrating peptides (CPPs) including synthetic peptides, protein transduction domains, and membrane-translocating sequences have been described for the intracellular delivery of small and macromolecular therapeutics.[38] These CPPs consist of a short sequence of amino acids (<30 amino acids), are positively charged, and have the ability to translocate the cell membrane and deliver therapeutics into the cytoplasm or nucleus. Recently, HIV-protein derived trans-activating regulatory peptide (HIV TAT) was identified to promote the nonspecific intracellular localization of various molecules upon systemic delivery.[39] An efficient gene transfection was achieved by means of TAT-modified liposomes.[40] For efficient systemic gene therapy using nonviral vectors, Weissig's group has investigated various nanoparticle delivery systems to target mitochondria using delocalized cationic amphiphiles and other mitochondriotropic vector systems.[41]

20.1.4 Multifunctional and Targeted Delivery with Stimuli-Responsive Nanoparticles

The main goal of multifunctional nanoparticles is to achieve a compound effect using one system. Ferrari has elegantly described the strategies to be adopted by these systems to attain a combination of effects such as the delivery of multiple therapeutic agents, diagnostic and imaging capability, target-specificity, and internalization property.[42] The multifunctional property of the nanoparticle is schematically illustrated in Figure 20.3. Multifunctional nanoparticles in general have three key constituents in the optimal delivery of drug or imaging agents:[43] (1) they can evade RES clearance mechanisms with PEG-modification, which allows longer *in vivo* residence and enhanced specific uptake of nanoparticles; (2) they allow specific targeting and facilitated uptake through surface modification with targeting ligands; and (3) they are loaded with a combination of therapeutic/imaging agents that can augment a therapeutic activity. Apart from the above functionalities, the multifunctional nanoparticles could also have the capability to deliver the therapeutics to subcellular

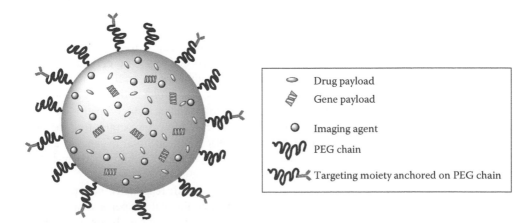

	Drug payload
	Gene payload
	Imaging agent
	PEG chain
	Targeting moiety anchored on PEG chain

FIGURE 20.3 A conceptual model of multifunctional nanoparticle used for simultaneous targeted delivery of therapeutic drugs/genes and imaging agents for compound effect.

compartments. For example, genes and certain anticancer drugs have their site of action located in the cytoplasm, nucleus, or mitochondrial membrane. Adopting the stimuli-responsive property to the multifunctional nanoparticle further improves its delivery capabilities to the subcellular organelles. For example, these multifunctional systems can cause disruption of the endosomal membrane in response to acidic endosomal pH and release its payload in the cytoplasm.[8]

The multifunctional nanoparticles have been investigated for the enhancement of magnetic resonance imaging (MRI) contrast used clinically and in research protocols. These include gadolinium and iron oxide-based nanoparticles and multiple-mode imaging contrast nano-agents that combine magnetic resonance with biological targeting and detection.[44] Feldherr and colleagues investigated the nuclear translocation of gold nanoparticles carrying peptides from the simian virus-40 (SV-40) large T-antigen.[45] This colloidal gold tracer was microinjected into the cytoplasm, and their subsequent nuclear uptake was analyzed by electron microscopy. Weissleder and colleagues prepared super-paramagnetic nanoparticles with the HIV TAT peptide,[46] which produced efficient nuclear targeting in HeLa cells. Gao and coworkers synthesized multifunctional polymeric micelles that can image and treat tumors simultaneously.[47] Doxorubicin and clusters of iron oxide were loaded inside the micelle core and the surface of the micelle was modified with cyclic arginine-guanine-aspartate peptide (cRGD), resulting in tumor targeting via $\alpha_v\beta_3$-expressing tumor cells. These nanoparticles are detected using MRI and release their drug payload only inside the acidic environment of a tumor cell.

20.2 PHYSIOLOGICAL AND ENVIRONMENTAL STIMULI

Several pathological conditions alter the chemical, physical, and biological properties of the target environment. The properties of nanoparticle DDS can be tuned to respond to these changes specifically at the diseased site. Stimuli-responsive materials that are able to alter their conformation, and as a result their properties, in response to changes in different physiological variables are receiving greater attention as components of nanoparticulate systems for various biomedical applications.

20.2.1 pH Differences

Changes in pH profile in pathological tissues could be used as potential stimuli for the pH-responsive material. The pH profile of the infectious, inflammatory, and tumor tissue is remarkably different compared with the normal tissue.[48] Primary and secondary tumors as well as certain infectious sites in the body exhibit significantly lower pH values as compared with healthy tissue. For example, the pH values of the region drops from 7.4 under normal conditions to 6.5 after 60 h following onset of inflammatory reaction.[49]

This altered pH condition at the site of the diseased tissue can be utilized for the fabrication of stimuli-responsive nanoparticles for small and macromolecular drug delivery, which can exploit the biochemical properties of the diseased tissue for targeted delivery. The cellular components exhibit a trans-membrane pH gradient in normal as well as pathological conditions, which can also be a potential trigger for stimuli-responsive nanoparticles. For the targeted delivery of peptide and gene macromolecules, such as antigenic peptides directed to the major histocompatibility complex-I pathway, antisense oligonucleotides targeting mRNA, or corrective genes targeting the nucleus, delivery to the cytosol becomes essential for therapeutic effect. Intracellular organelles are known to maintain their pH values. The pH values range from 4.5 in the lysosome to about 8.0 in the mitochondria.[48]

As evident from a survey of current literature,[8,50–54] the stimuli-responsive nanoparticles have been widely investigated for cancer therapeutics as the physiological properties and microenvironment of tumor tissue are well defined. Cancer chemotherapy is normally linked with severe toxic side effects, mainly due to the nonspecific distribution of drugs into healthy tissue. The site-specific delivery of cytotoxic drugs or macromolecules in tumor tissue is of high interest in cancer therapy. The pH and density of LDL receptors show remarkable differences between the normal and tumor tissues.[48,55] These properties could be exploited for the targeted delivery of anticancer therapeutics.

Solid tumor tissue exhibits lower pH values (<6.5) than normal tissue (pH 7.5).[56] Tumor cells divide very rapidly but not the tumor vasculature, leading to an insufficient supply of nutrients and oxygen for the expanding population of tumor cells. The oxygen stress in tumor tissue leads to hypoxia and the formation of lactic acid. The hydrolysis of ATP in an energy-deficient environment adds to an acidic microenvironment. The pH is compartmentalized in the tumor tissue into an intracellular component (pHi) and extracellular component (pHe). The intracellular component is similar in tumor and normal tissue, but the extracellular component is relatively acidic in tumor tissue.[57] This variation gives rise to the cellular trans-membrane pH gradient between normal tissue and tumor tissue. The low pH can be exploited for the delivery of drugs that are weak electrolytes with the appropriate dissociation constant (pK_a).[48] The nonionized form of weakly acidic drugs can diffuse freely across the cell membrane. Upon reaching a relatively basic intracellular compartment, it can become ionized and trapped within a cell, leading to a substantial difference in drug concentration between normal and tumor tissue. For example, therapeutic compounds with pK_a between 5.0 and 8.0 can display dramatic changes in physicochemical properties due to a change in pH gradients. These pH-responsive compounds can be incorporated into nanoparticles or conjugated to macromolecules to achieve enhanced intracellular delivery and subcellular localization.

> Solid tumor tissue exhibits lower pH values (<6.5) than normal tissue (pH 7.5). Tumor cells divide rapidly but not the tumor vasculature, leading to insufficient supply of nutrients and oxygen for the expanding population of tumor cells. The oxygen stress in tumor tissue leads to hypoxia and the formation of lactic acid. The pH is compartmentalized in tumor tissue into an intracellular component (pHi) and extracellular component (pHe). The intracellular component is similar in tumor and normal tissue, but the extracellular component is relatively acidic in tumor tissue. This variation gives rise to a cellular trans-membrane pH gradient between normal tissue and tumor tissue.

20.2.2 TEMPERATURE DIFFERENCES

Temperature responsiveness is one of the most interesting properties in stimuli-responsive nanoparticulate DDS. The use of externally applied hyperthermia can cause the accumulation of the thermo-responsive nanoparticles in the target region. This strategy has the potential to both control and deliver the therapeutics to externally targeted sites in the body. Hyperthermia has been clinically used in the management of solid tumors because it can synergistically enhance tumor-kill efficiency when combined with radiation or chemotherapy.[58] Furthermore, hyperthermia preferentially increases the permeability of the tumor vasculature when compared with normal tissue vasculature, which can further increase the passive targeting of nanoparticles to the tumors.[59] In addition, tumor cells seem to be more sensitive to heat-induced damage than normal cells. Combined, these facts suggest that the thermal targeting of thermo-responsive nanoparticles may offer potential benefits in therapy.

In recent clinical studies, super-paramagnetic iron oxide-containing liposomes or nanoparticles have been used to produce hyperthermia under an externally applied magnetic field.[60] Magnetic hyperthermia is appealing because it offers a way to ensure that only the intended target is heated. A typical dose of 100–120 kHz magnetic field is applied to experimental tumor models for about 30 min to elevate temperatures between 40°C and 45°C. For example, liposomal doxorubicin in combination with radiofrequency ablation has been investigated as an approach to promote the doxorubicin accumulation in highly refractory tumors.[61]

Hyperthermia preferentially increases the permeability of the tumor vasculature. This can act as a driving force for the extravasation of nanoparticles into the tumor region. Dewhirst and coworkers[62] have shown that a greater amount of the intravenously administered liposomes and other nanocarriers of up to 400 nm in diameter were able to extravasate into the tumor mass upon heating to 42°C in a human ovarian (SKOV-3) tumor model. The higher tumor concentration and enhanced efficacy of doxorubicin were noted in the tumor tissue upon delivery in heat-sensitive liposomal formulations.[63]

20.2.3 ALTERATIONS IN REDOX POTENTIAL

The change in intracellular and extracellular glutathione (GSH) levels in a diseased condition alters the redox potential. Intracellular GSH levels in tumor cells are 100- to 1000-fold higher than the extracellular levels.[64] This concentration gradient can be exploited for stimuli-responsive nanoparticles coupled with disulfide bonds that will release the payload inside the cell. Nanoparticle DDSs, which are responsive to redox potential, are highly useful in the delivery of macromolecular drugs such as plasmid DNA, small interference RNA, or oligonucleotides, since these molecules have to reach the nucleus in a stable form for efficient therapeutic effect.

The potential for gene therapeutics has grown rapidly over the past decade to treat genetic and acquired diseases. Redox potential as a stimuli mechanism has been put forward in gene delivery apart from other stimuli mechanisms like pH change and temperature. Redox-responsive systems containing disulfide linkages that are taken up by endocytosis may undergo disulfide cleavage in the lysosomes.[65] The GSH pathway that controls the intracellular redox potential is significantly involved in this stimuli mechanism.

20.2.4 ELECTROMAGNETIC ENERGY

The physical targeting of drugs and genes can also be achieved by applying external stimuli like a magnetic field, ultrasound, and light. Super-paramagnetic iron oxide crystals incorporated in nanoparticles are designed for delivery by induction with extracorporeal magnet movement. Additionally, these nanoparticles provide a source of heat induced by an external alternating magnetic field.[60] Tumor tissue seems to be more sensitive to heat-induced damage than normal cells.[66] This suggests that the magnetite-loaded nanoparticles can be used as a localized heating mediator for hyperthermia or for direct ablation of tumor tissue.[61] Alternatively, magnetite nanoparticles can be used as MRI contrast agents for the monitoring of therapy.[67]

Ultrasound can also be used effectively to ablate the tumor tissue. It can be coupled with the DDS for targeted delivery of small and macromolecular therapeutics.[68] The advantage of using ultrasound-mediated DDS is the ability to trigger drug release only at the region of interest. In addition, ultrasound imaging may aid the guidance and monitoring of therapy.

Light as an external stimulus to induce the heating of metal nanoparticles has been used to produce cell damage in nanoparticle-labeled cells.[69] For example, the liposomes loaded with gold nanoparticles could prove useful in the controlled release of drugs in targeted areas such as the eye and skin, which are easily accessible to light irradiation.[70]

20.3 ILLUSTRATIVE EXAMPLES

20.3.1 pH-RESPONSIVE NANOPARTICLES

20.3.1.1 pH-Responsive Polymeric Nanoparticles

The pH-responsive nanoparticles are one of the most widely investigated responsive systems, for reasons of wide applicability and faster response. Tumor tissues are more acidic than normal tissue, the bacterial infection generally lowers pH, and protonation and deprotonation reactions occur during a change in pH gradient—these events would help in triggering the pH-responsive nanoparticles for the discharge of their payload at target sites. A number of recent stimuli-responsive nanoparticle systems feature combined responses to pH and temperature, which is obtained by using stimuli-responsive cores based on cross-linked poly(*N*-isopropyl acrylamide-*co*-(methyl) acrylic acid) (NIPAAm).[71] This gives an opportunity for modulating the lower critical solution temperature (LCST) of the stimuli-responsive material through its protonation/deprotonation, allowing greater control on the release of the encapsulated drug. Apart from combined property, attaching targeting moieties on these systems would allow multifunctional ability. For example, pH-responsive nanoparticles that selectively release doxorubicin, under a reduced pH (of ~4–5) in endosomes and/or lysosomes, were functionalized by conjugating tumor targetable ligand folic acid.[72] These folate-conjugated and pH-sensitive nanoparticles showed lower *in vivo* toxicity and higher antitumor activity compared with the free drug.

A novel pH-responsive cationic polymer, poly(β-amino ester) (PbAE) has been used in small and macromolecular drug delivery. In the tumor microenvironment (pH<6.5), PbAE undergoes rapid dissolution and releases its contents. We have prepared paclitaxel-loaded PbAE nanoparticles, which remarkably enhanced the tumor bioavailability of paclitaxel as compared with paclitaxel loaded poly (ε-caprolactone) PCL nanoparticles, a non-pH-sensitive polymer, and paclitaxel solution, see Figure 20.4.[73–76] In another study, pullulan acetate, a linear polysaccharide, has been conjugated with sulfadimethoxine (pK_a 6.1) to prepare pH-sensitive and self-assembled hydrogel nanoparticles. These showed increased doxorubicin release in response to lower pH values.[77]

The pH-responsiveness of nanoparticles can be manipulated by controlling the length of hydrophobic alkyl segments. For example, the pH sensitivity of poly(alkyl acrylic acid) polymers is controlled by the choice of the alkylacrylic acid monomer and by the ratio of the carboxylate-containing alkylacrylic acid monomer to alkylacrylate monomer.[78] Poly(propylacrylic acid) is from the family of poly(alkyl acrylic acid) polymers, which are very effective at membrane disruption at pH values below 6.5 and significantly increase the *in vitro* transfection efficiency of lipoplexes.[78] Representative chemical blocks of pH-responsive polymers are shown in Figure 20.5A.

Macrophage targeting has gained recent attention mainly due to its association in inflammatory and immune reactions. However, the intracellular delivery of small or macromolecular drugs to macrophages is a particular challenge mainly because of the high degradative activities of the endosomal/phagosomal components. pH-responsive nanoparticles can increase the intracellular delivery of genes in macrophages. Murthy and colleagues[79] have described the multifunctional nanoparticles that can present three functionalities of viruses: (1) a targeting molecule that directs receptor-mediated endocytosis, (2) a pH-responsive component that selectively disrupts the endosomal membrane, and (3) the therapeutic agent.

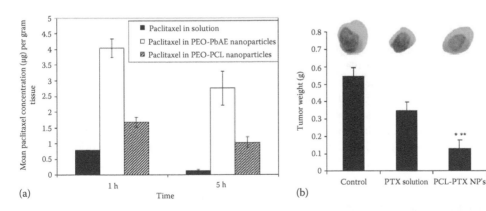

FIGURE 20.4 Tumor bioavailability of paclitaxel following intravenous administration in aqueous solution or in poly(ethylene oxide)-modified poly(ε-caprolactone) (PEO-PCL) and PEO-modified poly(β-amino ester) (PEO-PbAE) nanoparticles at 1 and 5 h after intravenous administration in SKOV-3 human ovarian adenocarcinoma-bearing female nu/nu mice (a) and the anticancer efficacy as measured by the weights of excised tumors 25 days post-administration of single dose of paclitaxel in aqueous solution or in PEO-PCL and PEO-PbAE nanoparticle formulations (b). The dose of paclitaxel was administered at 20 mg/kg body weight and control represents a group of untreated animals. (Adapted from Devalapally, H. et al., *Cancer Chemother. Pharmacol.*, 59, 477, 2007; Shenoy, D. et al., *Pharm. Res.*, 22, 2107, 2005.)

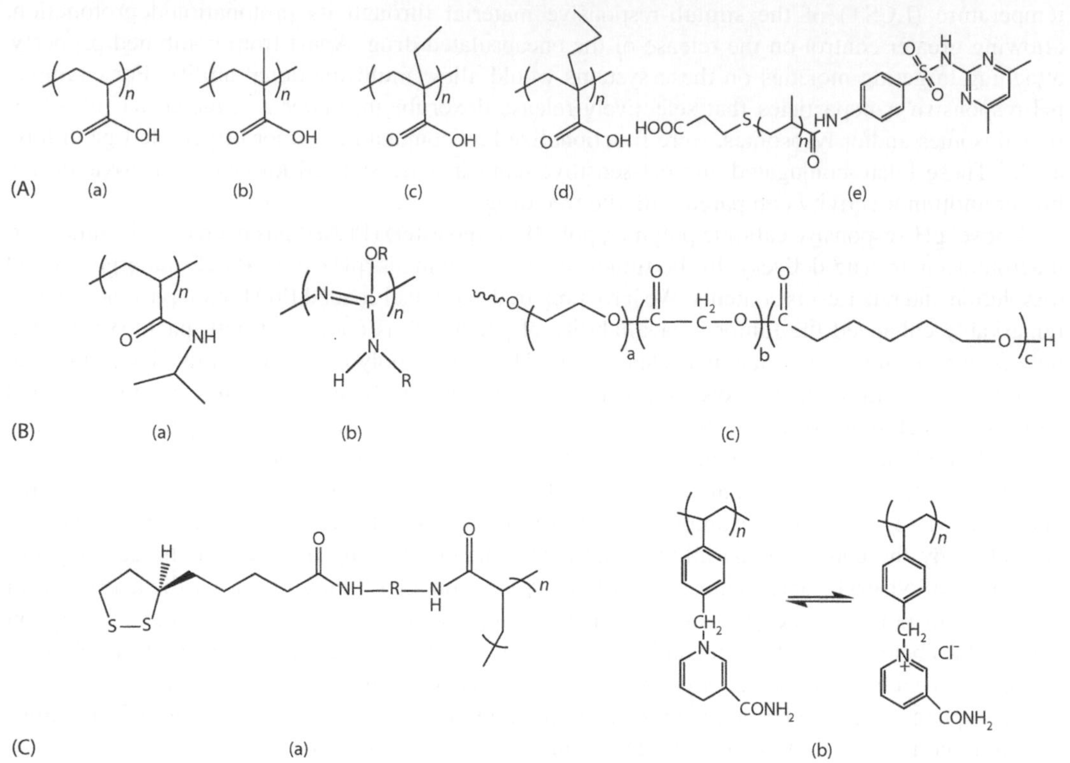

FIGURE 20.5 Representative chemical blocks of stimuli-responsive polymers. (A) pH-responsive polymer blocks: (a) poly(acrylic acid), (b) poly(methacrylic acid), (c) poly(2-ethyl acrylic acid, (d) poly(2-propyl acrylic acid), (e) sulfamethazine oligomer. (B) Temperature-responsive polymer blocks: (a) *N*-isopropylacrylamide, (b) poly(organophosphazenes), (c) poly ethylene glycol)–poly (caprolactone-glycolic acid) (PEG–PCGA). (C) Redox-responsive polymer blocks: (a) compounds containing the five-membered disulfide ring of lipoic acid and its derivatives, (b) the reversible redox reaction of the nicotinamide containing polymer, poly[3-carbamoyl-1-(*p*-vinylbenzyl)pyridinium chloride (CVPy) involves the species shown in redox system.

The encrypted system is made pH-responsive through the linking of acid-cleavable groups.[79] For example, the pH-sensitivity can be achieved through acid-cleavable acetal bonds that link the PEGs and PEG-modified drugs or targeting ligands to the polymer backbone. These systems can be internalized into cells through a specific uptake mechanism and display enhanced cytosolic delivery by disrupting endosomal membranes in a pH-dependent manner. A functionalized monomer, pyridyl disulfide acrylate, incorporated into an amphiphilic copolymer of methacrylic acid and butyl acrylate resulted in a pH-sensitive and glutathione-membrane disruptive terpolymer with thiol functional groups that can allow the conjugation of peptide moieties. Oligonucleotides and peptides conjugated to this polymer showed significant enhancement in cytoplasmic delivery.[80]

20.3.1.2 pH-Responsive Liposomes

The use of pH-responsive liposomes as a nanoparticle system has been an area of interest in the targeted delivery of small and macromolecular therapeutics. Liposomes are bilayered phospholipid vesicles that can be fabricated to achieve pH-responsiveness using pH-responsive materials. Upon reaching the target cells, pH-responsive liposomes can be endocytosed in intact form and fuse with the endovascular membrane. Due to the acidic pH inside the endosomes, the pH-responsive nanoparticles undergo phase transitions. This results in liposomal destabilization and release of its payload into the cytoplasm.[81]

Effective localization at a desired site and cellular uptake are dictated by various properties of liposomes. The targeting moieties anchored on liposomes will guide the liposomes toward the desired site. The PEG-modification could evade RES uptake and enhance longer blood circulation times. These multifunctional characteristics—longevity, targeting ability, and pH-sensitivity of liposomes—can help effectively deliver their contents into the cytoplasm.[82] Liposomes with pH-responsive and targeting property (folate or transferrin (Tf)-anchored) have been proposed for cytosolic drug delivery.[83] Making the liposomal surface hydrophilic by covalent linking or physical coating of PEG prolongs the residence time of liposomes during circulation in blood by avoiding opsonization and thus minimizing RES uptake. In addition, prolonged blood circulation promotes the accumulation of liposomes at the desired site through the EPR effect. This is highly valuable in the passive targeting of small and macromolecules for cancer therapy. PEG-modified pH-responsive liposomes have been made using a combination of PEG and a pH-sensitive NIPAAm and methacrylic acid.[84]

The widely investigated class of pH-responsive liposomes is composed of polymorphic lipids such as unsaturated phosphatidylethanolamine (PE) with mildly acidic amphiphiles that act as stabilizers at neutral pH values.[85] Amphiphile head groups are protonated in acidic conditions and cause the destabilization of the liposomal bilayer, usually accompanied by the release of liposomal contents.[86] pH-responsive liposomes have been successfully applied for the *in vitro* cytoplasmic delivery of antitumor drugs, proteins, antigens, antisense oligonucleotides, and plasmid DNA.[87,88] NIPAAm bearing pH-sensitive moiety has been studied for the release of water soluble fluorescent markers and doxorubicin. The release from the NIPAAm modified liposomes was found to be pH-dependent.[89]

Dioleoyl phosphatidyl ethanolamine (DOPE) forms a nonbilayer structure in an aqueous medium at neutral pH values. When combined with stabilizing agents such as cholesteryl hemisuccinate (CHEMS), it can assemble into a bilayer.[90] Liposomes prepared using DOPE and CHEMS are destabilized in the acidic pH of the endosomes thus releasing their contents.[90] DOPE liposomes stabilized with a cleavable lipid derivative of PEG (mPEG–S–S–DSPE) improved the doxorubicin delivery into the nuclei of the CD19 epitope expressing B-lymphoma cells, resulting in increased cytotoxicity compared with non-pH-sensitive liposomes.[91]

The pH-dependent release of drugs from liposomes can be achieved both with drugs that increase as well as decrease membrane permeabilities upon reduction in pH values, as long as the intraliposomal buffer strength and pH is rationally selected. Lee et al.[92] studied the folate receptor-targeted liposomes with three model compounds whose pK_a were dependent on pH. Anionic 5[6]-carboxyfluorescein converts into its nonionic form at endosomal pH and is released in endosomes following internalization by cells, since only its nonionic form is membrane permeable. The endocytosis-triggered unloading of drugs of this sort is enhanced by encapsulating the drug in a weak buffer at neutral pH values, so that acidification of the intraliposomal compartment following cellular uptake can occur rapidly. Sulforhodamine B, in contrast, retains both anionic and cationic charges at the endosomal pH value (approximately 5), and as a result they remained in endosomes for long time. Another category of compounds are those that exist in cationic form and still display endocytosis-triggered release. For example, doxorubicin is in its cationic (membrane-impermeable) form in strong acidic buffer when loaded into liposomes. It displays an endocytosis-triggered release, since sufficient uncharged doxorubicin remains at the endosomal pH to allow rapid re-equilibration of the drug according to the new proton gradient across the membrane.

> pH-responsive liposomes are composed of polymorphic lipids such as unsaturated PE with mildly acidic amphiphiles that act as stabilizers at neutral pH values. Amphiphile head groups are protonated in acidic conditions and cause the destabilization of liposomal bilayers, usually accompanied by the release of liposomal contents. pH-responsive liposomes have been successfully applied for the *in vitro* cytoplasmic delivery of antitumor drugs, proteins, antigens, antisense oligonucleotides, and plasmid DNA.

20.3.1.3   pH-Responsive Micelles

The supramolecular block copolymer networks composed of cross-linked combinations of hydrophilic and hydrophobic monomers are called polymeric micelles. Micelles are spherical nanoassemblies ranging from 20 to 100 nm in diameter. They self-arrange in shell-like structures with their hydrophilic and hydrophobic ligands aligned on opposing sides. In an aqueous medium, the hydrophilic portions form the outer shell.

Micelles have attracted considerable interest as potential drug carriers due to their unique properties such as high solubility, high drug-loading capacity, and low toxicity.[93] Furthermore, their hydrophilic outer shells help protect the cores and their contents from chemical attack by the aqueous medium, in which they must travel. In addition, drug release is controlled via common polymer degradation mechanisms, with the selectivity of the delivery achieved by the micelle synthetic design. For example, polymeric network of micelles attached with sugar-group ligands have been shown to target glycol-receptors in cellular plasma membranes. The micelles, only tens of nanometer in diameter, prevent rapid renal exclusion and uptake by the RES.[94] As a consequence, the micelles circulate for a prolonged time in blood. This can facilitate their passive accumulation in tumor tissue.

Recent studies have focused on pH-responsive micelles that can exploit the acidic conditions in tumor tissue to release its contents.[95] Linking of titrable groups such as amines or carboxylic acids into the block copolymers can control the micelle formation by the protonation of these groups. However, only a few of these undergo transitions in the physiologically relevant pH range of 5.0–7.4 and efficiently encapsulate drugs.[89] Shim and coworkers have explored block copolymer micelles for the delivery of paclitaxel, in which micelle-unimer transition takes place due to the inonization-non-ionization of sulfamethazine oligomer in the pH range (7.2–8.4) above the CMC.[96] Due to the pH responsive properties of the block copolymer, the hydrophobic drug paclitaxel was incorporated into a pH responsive block copolymer micelle by the pH-induced micellization method, without using an organic solvent. A polyamine, poly(L-histidine), was investigated in pH-sensitive micellar systems because of its amphoteric property and fusogenic activity due to the imidazole group and the interaction between the endosomal membrane and poly(L-histidine).[97] Recently, Bae and coworkers have demonstrated that the pH-responsive polymeric micelles can release doxorubicin in response to the acidic environment of endosomes (pH 5.0–6.0) and lysosomes (pH 4.0–5.0), which can enhance the drug delivery efficiency to the tumor site.[98]

Hydrophilic block copolymers have attracted recent attention for drug delivery, as these polymers exhibit different forms in aqueous pH. For example, block copolymers based on poly[4-vinylbenzoic acid] (VBA) is soluble above pH 6.0. However, VBA forms micelles if the pH is below 6.0.[99] Triblock-based copolymers such as poly(acrylic acid)-b-polystyrene-b-poly(4-vinyl pyridine) (PAA-b-PS-b-P4VP) exist in different forms as a function of the aqueous pH. Poly[2-(dimethylamino) ethylmethacrylate]-block-poly[2-(N-morpholino)ethyl methacrylate] (DEA-MEMA) forms MEMA-core micelles at a pH value of 6.5 in the presence of 1.0 M Na_2SO_4, whereas the DEA block forms a micellar core at a pH value of 1.0.[100] These unique properties of amphiphilic block copolymers are responsible for the special advantage of using micelles for various drug delivery applications.

NIPAAm has been widely investigated for the preparation of stimuli-responsive nanoparticles.[101] It exhibits a LCST of 32°C, below which the polymer is soluble. It precipitates if the temperature is raised above the LCST.[71,101] A hydrophilic titrable monomer on NIPAAm can result in a higher LCST, making the polymer pH-sensitive.[102] Polymeric micelles prepared from random copolymers of NIPAAm, methacrylic acid, and octadecyl acrylate[103] with the hydrophilic monomer N-vinyl-2-pyrrolidone (VP) decreased the RES uptake and enhanced accumulation in tumors.[104] Polymeric micelles based on poly(L-lactide)-b-poly(2-ethyl-2-oxazoline)-b-poly(L-lactide) (PLLA-PEOz-PLLA) ABA-type triblock copolymers and diblock copolymers (PEOz-PLLA) have been successfully used for the tumor targeting of doxorubicin.[105] Interesting reviews on types of block copolymers are published elsewhere.[93,106–108]

Polymeric micelles can be made multifunctional by incorporating targeting ligands. For example, poly(L-histidine)-based micelles were conjugated to either folic acid or biotin to enhance the tumor uptake by folate biotin receptor-mediated endocytosis.[109] Tumor uptake could be further augmented by preparing the mixed micelles [poly(L-histidine)/PEG and poly(L-lactic acid)/PEG block copolymer] conjugated with folic acid. However, significantly enhanced cytotoxicity was noted *in vitro* using these mixed micelles systems.

20.3.1.4 pH-Responsive Dendrimers

Dendrimers have emerged as one of the most interesting polymeric nanoparticles as a result of their well-defined molecular architecture and macromolecular characteristics. They are monodispersed, highly branched macromolecules in nanometer dimensions. They were developed as a result of the pioneering work of Tomalia and coworkers.[110] Dendrimers are water soluble and have the ability to display a high surface functionality. These characteristics make them attractive for drug delivery and biomedical applications.[111]

A variety of physical properties can be imparted in dendrimer structures through functional group modifications at the core, branches, and the periphery. For example, a pH-responsive component in its structure widens its scope for drug delivery applications. Doxorubicin linked via a pH-sensitive component to the dendritic polyester system based on the monomer unit 2,2-bis(hydroxymethyl) propanoic acid demonstrated the feasibility of making a dendritic polymer-drug conjugate that has pH-responsive properties.[112] The dendritic polymer system can be attached to doxorubicin through several functional groups of doxorubicin. The hydrolyzable amide linkage with the polymer may be too stable toward acid catalyzed hydrolysis. On the other hand, the keto group of doxorubicin can be used to form an acid labile hydrazone linkage. The resulting compound exhibited excellent water solubility, making it a good candidate for biological evaluation.[112]

Recently, Gillies and coworkers developed a new approach using PEO-dendrimer hybrids as backbones for pH-sensitive micelles.[113] This approach involves the incorporation of hydrophobic groups to the periphery of the core forming a dendrimer block using an acid-sensitive acetal linkage. These micelles are stable in aqueous solution at neutral pH values but disintegrate into unimers at mildly acidic pH values following the loss of the hydrophobic groups upon acetal hydrolysis. Then, the core-forming block becomes hydrophilic. This destabilizes the micelle and allows the release of the drug from its core. The stepwise synthesis of the PEO-dendrimer backbone allows a high degree of control over the polymer structures. This, in turn, controls its properties such as the rate of micelle disruption, the critical micelle concentration, and the size of the micelles.[113] This approach has been investigated for the tumor-specific delivery of doxorubicin.[113] Hui et al. synthesized a novel dendrimer derivative combining the pH and temperature responsiveness.[114] In another study, Kono and coworkers prepared poly(amidoamine) (PAMAM) dendrimers that incorporated PEG chains through a glutamic acid linker at every chain end of the dendrimer.[115] Then, the doxorubicin was attached to glutamic acid using an amide bond or hydrazone bond. The dendrimer bearing doxorubicin through hydrazone linkage showed a significant drug release at pH 5.5, which corresponds to the pH values of late endosomes.

20.3.2 TEMPERATURE-RESPONSIVE NANOPARTICLES

20.3.2.1 Temperature-Responsive Polymeric Nanoparticles

The majority of temperature-responsive nanoparticles utilize polymer derivatives. Their physical properties, such as swelling/deswelling, particle disruption, and aggregation change in response to the changes in the environmental condition.[101] These properties, in turn, alter the interactions of the nanoparticles with the cells and allow the release of active contents at the target sites. Temperature-responsive polymers exhibit a LCST in aqueous solution, below which the polymers are water soluble and above which they become water-insoluble.[71]

Temperature-responsive amphiphilic polymers generally have temperature-sensitive hydrophilic segments and a suitable hydrophobic segment in its structure. For example, NIPAAm and its random copolymers[101] utilize block copolymers of PEG as a hydrophilic segment and NIPAAm or poly(*N*-isopropylacrylamide)-*co*-*N*-(2-hydroxypropyl) methacrylamide-dilactate as a temperature-responsive segment. They self-assemble in water into temperature-responsive nanoparticles above the LCST of the temperature-responsive segment.[116] The hydrophobic blocks, poly(L-lactide), cholic acid, alkyl, and poly(γ-benzyl-L-glutamate), have also been used in diblock polymers with the temperature-sensitive polyacrylamide derivatives being the hydrophilic blocks.

Temperature-responsive block copolymeric nanoparticles were also prepared from poloxamer and poly(ε-caprolactone). They were used to encapsulate indomethacin.[116] These systems displayed a reversible change of size depending on the temperature. They were able to reduce cell damage to a greater extent than free indomethacin, when evaluated by a cell viability assay. In another study, gold nanoparticles prepared from cross-linked poloxamer micelles showed reversibly temperature-responsive swelling/deswelling.[117] This behavior of the micelles was caused by the hydrophobic interactions of cross-linked poloxamer copolymer chains in the micelle structure with rising temperatures.[117] Representative chemical blocks of temperature-responsive polymers are shown in Figure 20.5B. An interesting review on the triggered destabilization of polymeric micelles by changing polymer polarity was published recently.[118]

NIPAAm displays a very sharp change in hydrophilicity and hydrophobicity at its phase-transition temperature (or LCST) around 32°C.[101] The LCST of NIPAAm can be altered to reach above 37°C using copolymers with varying hydrophilicity or hydrophobicity. The most commonly used hydrophilic segment of the copolymers forming the micelles is the PEG, because of its biocompatibility and good "stealth" properties.[119] The micelle's hydrophobic inner core offers an important control point for temperature-responsive drug release. Both inner cores and outer shell polymer chemistries were studied to modify the temperature responsive behavior of micelles for targeted drug delivery.[120] AB type block copolymers composed of a NIPAAm block and hydrophobic block can form core-shell micelle structures below the NIPAAm LCST. The inner hydrophobic core can incorporate water-insoluble drugs, while the NIPAAm outer shell plays the role of temperature-responsiveness and aqueous solubilization.

Temperature-sensitive polymers were extensively studied for macromolecular (plasmid DNA, siRNA, oligonucleotides, proteins, and peptides) delivery.[121] These included various molecular weights of cationic polyethylene imines (PEI) and their copolymers with NIPAAm segments as temperature-responsive nanoparticles for the *in vitro* and *in vivo* transfection of plasmid DNA.[122] Incorporating PEI units into NIPAAm chains increased its LCST up to 37°C.[122,123] A GFP expressing plasmid was linked to PEIs and NIPAAm copolymers. The copolymerization resulted in the reduced cytotoxicity of PEI, when used to transfect HeLa cells. Efficient GFP expression without any significant toxicity was achieved with the complex prepared with NIPAAm/PEI25k. These investigators also showed the release of plasmid DNA from polycationic polymers in response to temperature responsiveness and enhanced *in vivo* transfection efficiency.[123] Reviews on gene therapy with a main emphasis on poly cationic stimuli-responsive carriers as nonviral gene vectors are available.[124,125]

> Temperature-sensitive polymers were extensively studied for macromolecular (plasmid DNA, siRNA, oligonucleotides, proteins, and peptides) delivery. These included various molecular weights of cationic PEI and their copolymers with NIPAAm segments as temperature-responsive nanoparticles for the *in vitro* and *in vivo* transfection of plasmid DNA. Incorporating PEI units into NIPAAm chains increased its LCST up to 37°C.

20.3.2.2 Temperature-Responsive Liposomes

Temperature-responsive drug release from the thermo-sensitive liposomes was first described in 1978 by Yatvin et al.[126] These systems release their contents to the target site where the heat is applied due to liposomal membrane instability at the phase transition temperature (T_m) of the lipids. The liposomal membrane containing various types of phospholipids undergoes phase transitions at temperatures around 41°C, such as gel-to-liquid crystalline and lamellar-to-hexagonal transition, and becomes highly leaky to small water-soluble molecules. Dipalmitoylphosphatidylcholine (DPPC) as a primary lipid-based liposome exhibits a gel-to-liquid crystalline membrane transition at the clinically achievable temperature of 41°C.[126] The liposomal membrane T_m can be altered by incorporating a small amount of a co-lipid such as distearoylphosphatidylcholine (DSPC). An interesting example of temperature-responsive liposome is ThermoDox®, which has demonstrated an enhanced antitumor efficacy at 42°C in the murine tumor model.[127] Currently, ThermoDox® is in a Phase I trial in humans to treat liver cancer.

Recently, temperature-responsive polymers that display a LCST have been used in sensitizing the liposomes to a change in temperature. These polymers exhibit a coil-to-globule transition in response to a change in temperature. They can provide the liposomes with temperature-controlled functionalities. For example, highly hydrated polymer chains attached to the liposomes stabilize the liposomes below the LCST. Above the LCST, the dehydrated polymer chains cause destabilization of the liposomes, resulting in the release of its contents.[128] In addition, the change in temperature can alter the polymer chain conformation and the change in liposomal surface properties, which in turn exhibit temperature-controlled fusion or an affinity to cells.[129] NIPAAm is the widely investigated copolymer used to obtain liposomes with temperature-sensitivity.[130] Liposomes modified with poly(N-isopropylacrylamide-co-acrylamide) (NIPAAm-AAM) and PEG showed enhanced release of doxorubicin around the transition temperature of the polymer.[131] Furthermore, these liposomes were found to be stable in the plasma in comparison with unmodified liposomes, suggesting that NIPAAm-AAM/PEG modified liposomes are suitable for targeted drug delivery. An interesting review on thermo-responsive polymer-modified liposomes was published recently.[132]

20.3.3 Redox-Responsive Nanoparticles

20.3.3.1 Redox-Responsive Polymeric Nanoparticles

The intracellular release of free DNA from the polymeric nanoparticles is one of the critical steps limiting the efficiency of nonviral gene delivery. The complex should be stable enough to prevent DNA degradation outside, but it should be destabilized inside the cell to allow DNA release and transcription. The difference in intracellular and extracellular redox potential due to higher GSH levels in diseased cells could provide an opportunity for the targeted delivery of drug and gene therapeutics. The disulfide bonds of redox-responsive polymeric nanoparticles will reduce in the presence of high GSH levels inside the cell. This would facilitate the release of its payload to intracellular sites.

A disulfide bond (–S–S–) is a covalent linkage that forms as a result of the oxidation of two sulfhydryl (SH) groups of cysteines or other SH-containing material. The high plasma stability of nanoparticles that prevents the premature release of its contents can be achieved by introducing the covalent linkages between polymer chains of the nanoparticle, i.e., intramolecular and intermolecular cross-linking. This could stabilize the polymeric nanoparticles during its blood circulation and inhibit the premature release of DNA.[133] Polyaspartamide nanoparticles have been proposed as nonviral vectors for DNA delivery based on polycation strategy.[134] In these nanoparticles, positively charged groups are introduced on the polymer backbone for electrostatic interactions with DNA and thiol groups for the formation of disulfide bridges between polymer chains. This arrangement produced stable thiopolyplexes. Incorporating disulfide bridges between polymer chains can prevent the dissociation of polyplexes in the blood, but allow an intracellular DNA release.[64] An interesting example is the U.S. Food and Drug Administration (FDA)-approved calicheamicin-anti-CD33 antibody-conjugate (Mylotarg®) for the treatment of acute myeloid leukemia. This consists of two cleavable sites in the linker, a disulfide bond, and an acylhydrazone bond. Once Mylotarg® binds to CD33, the receptor-antibody conjugate complex is internalized and hydrolyzed. The resulting hydrolysis of the hydrazone bond in the lysosomes, where the pH is low, releases calicheamicin, which freely localizes in the nucleus, initiating DNA alkylation and promoting cell death.[135] Representative chemical blocks of redox-responsive polymers are shown in Figure 20.5C.

We have prepared gelatin thiopolyplexes for the intracellular delivery of plasmid DNA.[21–23,136,137] These redox-responsive nanoparticles could exploit the highly reducing environment present in diseased tissue, schematically illustrated in Figure 20.6. Thiolated gelatin was prepared by covalent

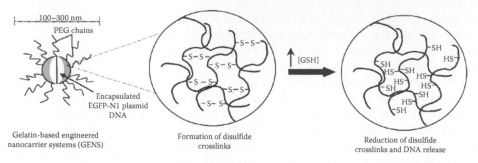

FIGURE 20.6 Schematic illustration of intracellular DNA delivery with thiolated gelatin nanoparticles (thiopolyplexes) in the presence of higher glutathione (GSH) concentrations. (Adapted from Kommareddy, S. and Amiji, M., *Nanomed. Nanotechnol. Biol. Med.*, 3, 32, 2007.)

modification of the primary amino groups of Type B gelatin using 2-iminothiolane. The *in vitro* evaluation of gelatin thiopolyplexes for plasmid DNA transfection in NIH-3T3 murine fibroblast cells for enhanced green fluorescent protein (EGFP-N1) expression was done by fluorescence confocal microscopy and fluorescence-activated cell sorting (FACS). Qualitative results showed a highly efficient expression of GFP that remained stable for up to 96 h. The thiolated gelatin nanoparticles (SHGel-20) were remarkably more effective in transfecting NIH-3T3 cells than other carrier systems investigated. This study suggests that thiolated gelatin nanoparticles would serve as a biocompatible intracellular delivery system that can release the payload in a highly reducing environment. Recently, we have demonstrated that long circulating PEG-modified thiolated gelatin nanoparticles could also deliver DNA and transfect tumor cells in response to higher intracellular GSH concentrations.[136,137] These nanoparticles loaded with plasmid DNA encoding for soluble vascular endothelial growth factor receptor 1 (sVEGFR-1 or sFlt-1) exhibited a highly efficient transgene expression in human breast cancer cells in an *in vivo* tumor model.[138] In addition, the expressed sFlt-1 was very effective in suppressing tumor growth and angiogenesis,[138] as shown in Figure 20.7.

Currently, one of the widely investigated polymers for gene delivery is PEI. The PEI with a molecular weight of 25 kDa exhibits high transfection efficiency, probably due to efficient endosomal escape, but also considerable toxicity, whereas low molecular weight PEI is less toxic but shows no transfection.[139] The use of reducible polymers for gene delivery achieves efficient gene transfection *in vivo* while limiting toxicity. For example, the PEI/DNA polyplex formed by disulfide cross-linking enhanced the transfection efficiency, as shown in Figure 20.8.[140] Nanoparticles of plasmid DNA condensed with thiolated PEI and coated with thiol-reactive poly[*N*-(2-hydroxypropyl)methacrylamide] with 2-pyridyldisulfanyl or maleimide groups formed reducible disulfide-linked or stable thioether-linked coatings.[141] Disulfide-linked complexes showed 40- to 100-fold higher transfection efficiency than thioether-linked ones. Reduction with dithiothreitol allowed the complete release of DNA from disulfide-linked complexes. In another method, thiol groups prone to oxidation were immobilized on the polymeric backbone of chitosan. These showed extracellular stability and intracellular gene release due to reversible disulfide bonds.[142] The chitosan-thiobutylamidine conjugate, exhibiting 299.1 ± 11.5 μmol of free thiol groups per gram polymer, formed coacervates with pDNA. The highest transfection efficiency was observed in Caco-2 cells. RGD was noncovalently introduced into the disulfide linked PEI (SS-PEI)/DNA complex to impart the targeting ability and enhance the biological activities.[143] *In vitro* transfection study showed that SS-PEI/DNA displayed comparable transfection efficiency, but reduced cytotoxicity in comparison with PEI 25 kDa.

20.3.3.2 Redox-Responsive Liposomes

The reversible nature of the disulfide (–S–S–) bond is exploited in liposomal targeted delivery. Disulfide bonds can be used as linkers to prepare lipids with –S–S– bridges, where the disulfide

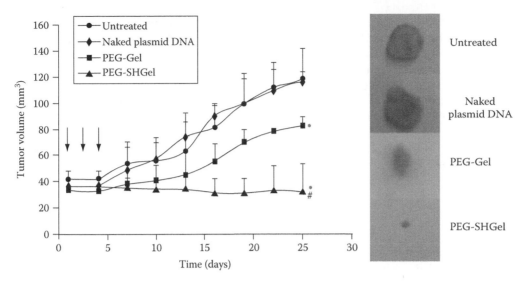

FIGURE 20.7 Antitumor efficacy studies in MDA-MB-435 human breast adenocarcinoma-bearing female nu/nu mice upon intravenous administration of sFlt-1 (VEGFR-1) encoding plasmid DNA encapsulated in poly(ethylene glycol) (PEG)-modified type B gelatin (PEG-Gel) and PEG-modified thiolated gelatin (PEG-SHGel) nanoparticles. A total 60 μg dose of plasmid DNA was given per animal in different formulations. The naked plasmid DNA treated and untreated animals were served as controls. (Adapted from Kommareddy, S. and Amiji, M., *Cancer Gene Ther.*, 14, 488, 2007.)

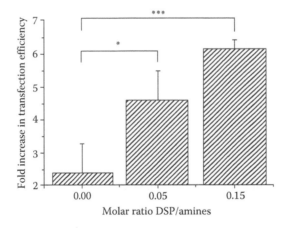

FIGURE 20.8 Transfection efficiency in NIH-3T3 fibroblasts for PEI/DNA polyplexes with different degree of cross linking with dithiobis(succinimidyl propionate) (DSP) and reconstitution of the transfection by reduction with DTT. Differences between uncrosslinked and cross linked PEI/DNA polyplexes are marked with an asterisk, $^*p < 0.05$, $^{***}p < 0.001$. (Adapted from Neu, M. et al., *J. Control. Release*, 118, 370, 2007.)

bond is important to maintaining the stability of liposomes. These disulfide-linked liposomes destabilize in a reducing environment, where the higher GSH levels are present. This destabilizing effect is attributed to the reducing of –S–S– bridges of liposomes. Liposomal destabilization promotes the release of its active contents. Therefore, genes encapsulated in redox-responsive liposomes release intracellularly and produce efficient transfection. Redox-responsive liposomes are prepared using phospholipids and a small portion of another lipid in which the hydrophobic and hydrophilic parts are linked through a disulfide bond. Such liposomal systems demonstrated stability until reaching a reducing environment that cleaves the disulfide bonds, disrupting the liposomal membrane, and releasing the liposomal contents.[144] Redox-responsive liposomes prepared using thiocholesterol-based cationic lipids exhibited DNA release in a reducing environment.[145] Disulfide-linked PEG-modified liposomes demonstrated longer circulation. These showed enhanced accumulation at the tumor site, and release of its contents into target cells in response to redox stimulus.[146] A lipid-based mitomycin C conjugate with cleavable disulfide bonds were encapsulated in PEGylated liposomes.[147] They exhibited superior therapeutic activity and less toxicity compared with free mitomycin C. The multifunctional ability of liposomes can further enhance the efficacy of small and macromolecular therapeutics. For example, sterically stabilized methoxy poly(ethylene glycol)-dithio propionyl-distearoylphosphatidylethanolamine (mPEG-DTP-DSPE) anti-CD19 liposomes were effective in delivering doxorubicin into B-lymphoma cell cytoplasm.[91] This DDS showed a modest increase in therapeutic activity *in vivo*.

20.3.4 NANOPARTICLES RESPONSIVE TO ELECTROMAGNETIC ENERGY

External stimuli-targeted nanoparticle DDSs can allow nanoparticles to navigate and accumulate at the local diseased site inside the body by controlling the external stimuli, like a magnetic field, ultrasound, or light. An interesting example is the targeted delivery of super-paramagnetic iron oxide nanoparticles using an externally applied magnetic field. Super-paramagnetic iron oxide nanoparticles possess the ability to function at the cellular and molecular level of biological interactions, thus making them an attractive platform as a contrast agent for MRI and as vehicles for small and macromolecular delivery. These nanoparticles are being developed as multifunctional carriers for specific biomedical applications through the incorporation of highly specific targeting agents and permeation enhancers.[148]

Polymeric modification or liposomal loading is essential for iron oxide nanoparticles for biomedical application. A variety of natural and synthetic polymers have been investigated for use as surface modifications of iron oxide crystals.[60,149] The polymeric or liposomal-loaded magnetite nanoparticles have demonstrated their ability to accumulate at the tumor site in several studies. For example, early clinical trials of iron oxide nanoparticles loaded with epirubicin and directed toward solid tumors have shown enhanced accumulation in the target site in about half the patients.[150] In another study, starch-coated magnetite nanoparticles loaded with mitoxantrone were completely eliminated to VX2-squamous cell tumors in rabbits after approximately 35 days of treatment.[151] In addition to small drug molecules, magnetite nanoparticles were also investigated as carriers for proteins and peptides. Herceptin incorporated in magnetite nanoparticle-loaded liposomes showed an enhanced antiproliferative effect on breast tumor cells.[152] Furthermore, magnetite nanoparticles can enhance the macromolecular therapeutics (siRNA, plasmid DNA, oligonucleotides) transfection efficiencies.[153] This combination is referred to as magnetofection.

Ultrasound has been used effectively to ablate solid tumors. A variety of cancers are currently being treated in clinics using these types of ultrasound exposure. Recently, ultrasound has been proposed as a targeting modality for small and macromolecular therapeutics for the delivery of drugs and genes and opening the BBB.[154] Rapoport and coworkers have demonstrated the enhanced accumulation of ultrasound-responsive micellar encapsulated drugs after the local sonication of tumor tissue.[155] In addition to enhanced tumor uptake, this technique also allowed the uniform distribution of micelles and drug throughout the tumor tissue. An interesting review describing the mechanism and application of ultrasound was published recently.[154] Light-responsive nanoparticles have gained recent attention for numerous therapeutic applications.[69] The development of light-responsive polymeric carriers that undergo reverse micellization/disruption under exposure to light is an attractive idea that would allow the external control of drug release.[156] In another strategy, light is used to induce the heating of metal nanoparticles to control the drug release in targeted areas.[69,70]

20.4 ISSUES TO CONSIDER IN THE DEVELOPMENT OF NANOPARTICLE DELIVERY SYSTEMS

20.4.1 MATERIAL SAFETY

Targeted drug delivery using nanoparticles aims at increasing the therapeutic index by making more drug molecules available at the diseased sites, while reducing systemic drug exposure and toxicity. The choice of materials used for designing such delivery vehicles poses a big challenge. Despite increased interest in the development of nanoparticles for drug delivery, few studies address their potential toxicity. Regulatory agencies place significant emphasis on how nanoparticle materials affect human health and the environment. This is more so in the application of nanotechnology in medicine because of its serious implications to human health.

Although major advances have been made in polymeric nanoparticulate technologies in drug delivery and diagnostic imaging, much of the work lies ahead in terms of accessing their safety and long-term effects. For example, the kind of hazards that are introduced by using nanoparticles for drug delivery are beyond those posed by chemicals in classical delivery systems.[157] Several recent reports have shown that exposure to nanoparticles pose serious safety issues to biological systems.[158,159] For example, the incubation of single-walled nanotubes (SWNTs) with keratinocytes and bronchial epithelial cells resulted in the generation of reactive oxygen species (ROS), lipid peroxidation, oxidative stress, mitochondrial dysfunction, and changes in cell morphology.[160,161] The metabolic constituents from poly(L lactic acid) particles show cytotoxicity,[162] thus raising concern over their use for sustained cytosolic drug release. Depending on the nature of the monomers used for engineering polymeric micelles, some systems induce immune response, produce cytotoxicity via apoptosis or necrosis,[163] or alter gene expression in certain cells.[164] Another problem is the entrapment in the RES, as present in the liver and spleen, and producing toxicity to these organs.[165]

Nevertheless, biocompatible polymeric materials like PEG, poly(lactic-co-glycolic acid) (PLGA), and poloxamers have been used in a number of approved DDSs and have a proven safety record. In addition, there are many natural and synthetic polymers that are classified as "generally regarded as safe" (GRAS) by the U.S. FDA. Cationic nanoparticles, including gold and polystyrene, cause hemolysis and blood clotting, while anionic particles are known to be usually less toxic. This conceptual understanding may be used to engineer nanoparticles with preferred surface characteristics. This is geared toward reducing side-effects and having desirable properties, while also being biocompatible.[149]

Despite an increasing interest in the use and choice of these materials in small and macromolecular delivery, there are areas of research that are largely neglected including pharmacological activity, immunotoxicity, and cytotoxicity.[159] The material safety issues become even more serious for parenterally injected polymeric nanoparticles, as nanocarrier size partly determines biodistribution.[166] Also, the processing parameters for nanoparticle formulation, such as the use of organic solvents, are important criteria for evaluation before systemic administration. For example, most of the conventional methods for nanoparticle preparation involve the use of harsh organic solvents, which are hazardous to the environment as well as to the physiological system.[167] The U.S. FDA has issued guidance on the acceptable amounts of residual organic solvents in injectable colloidal systems.[168,169] It is, thus, not only important and imperative to maintain the tolerable toxicity levels during manufacturing but also essential to realize the full potential of such nanoparticulate DDSs from the lab to the clinic.

When evaluating the efficacy or testing nanoparticles in model systems, caution must be employed with regard to the choice of model system used to assess polymeric and nanoparticle material safety. In many cases, researchers use *in vitro* cell viability assays. These can reveal some vital information about toxicity profiles of the drugs and nanoparticles of interest. However, these tests are often inconclusive in determining the biocompatibility of the polymeric nanoparticles. This is because of absence of a true dynamic environment and functional immunizing systems in *in vitro* settings.

> Although major advances have been made in polymeric nanoparticulate technologies in drug delivery and diagnostic imaging, much of the work lies ahead in terms of accessing their safety and long-term effects. For example, the kind of hazards that are introduced by using nanoparticles for drug delivery are beyond those posed by chemicals in classical delivery systems.

Also, care must be taken when evaluating and translating data obtained from animal models. There is always a possibility of variability or alteration in the results due to intra and inter-species variation. Moreover, the time scale and residence time of drugs in animal settings, such as mice, rats, and rabbits, usually are different than for human clinical settings. Regulatory guidelines are not yet fully available regarding the use of nanoparticles in biological application. This is mainly because the area of nanotechnology in drug delivery and imaging is too broad. Regulatory aspects are, therefore, handled on a case-by-case basis.

20.4.2 Scale-Up and GMP Manufacturing

Scale-up can be broadly defined as the technology transfer of a product from research to the production scale with a simultaneous increase in production output. These pose a significant challenge in terms of engineering design complexity and production. It is important to maintain all the parameters within tolerable limits, such as the particle size, loading, and drug stability. The technological challenge in reproducing nanoparticle formulations from the ones obtained in a lab scale with negligible batch-to-batch variation in bulk manufacturing is more complex than the conventional drugs and formulations.

One of the basic reasons for this complexity is the multiple steps involved in the preparation of nanoparticles. Another major hurdle, which applies to all scale-up operations, is the difference in processing equipment employed in a lab scale and industrial production scale. Moreover, insufficient information or a lack of information about the equipment, requirements of process control, complexity of the process involving several unit operations, and behavior of ingredients/components at different scales also add significantly to scale-up issues. This highlights the importance and complexity involved in technology transfer and scale-up in the product development process.

Recent developments in the nanoparticulate DDS and their potential for successful application has the involvement and support of pharmaceutical and biotechnology companies, which have significant interest in addressing some of the scale-up and regulatory issues. However, concrete steps to address these issues have not yet fully evolved.

Apart from the scale-up, the nanoparticles processing also need to meet regulatory guidelines to translate them successfully from the bench to clinical use. The U.S. FDA recommends Current Good Laboratory Practice (cGLP) and Current Good Manufacturing Practice (cGMP) guidelines for products that are used for human administration. These are mainly focused on reproducible manufacturing under controlled quality control systems. The Good Laboratory Practice (GLP) guidelines are essential for validating analytical techniques to confirm the identity, strength, and stability of nanoparticles. These help ensure the complete and thorough characterization of nanoparticles. Furthermore, the GLP guidelines must also be implemented for new screening models in order to establish pharmacological and toxicological properties of the nanoparticles.

Along these lines, the National Cancer Institute's Alliance for Nanotechnology in Cancer (http://nano.cancer.gov) has setup the Nanotechnology Characterization Laboratory (NCL) for providing complete preclinical characterization of nanosystems intended for cancer prevention, diagnosis, and therapy. NCL works in collaboration with the National Institute of Standards and Technology (NIST) and the FDA to develop appropriate standards for quality control as well as *in vitro* and *in vivo* preclinical testing methodologies for safety and efficacy evaluation. At the end, FDA review ensures that only those nanotechnology products are approved that are deemed to be safe and efficacious. Because of the complexity involved in the production of a nanoparticulate DDS, the most appropriate way to deal with multifunctional nanoparticles will be to evaluate them on a case-by-case basis and on the nature of its intended use.

20.4.3 Quality Control Issues

The control on the manufacturing of nanoparticulate DDSs is important to their clinical application. This calls for stringent quality control norms and precise characterization of the nanoparticles. The prerequisite for clinical development requires physicochemical characterization (the chemical structure and molecular weight of the polymer used and the size, charge, and morphology of nanoparticles), *in vivo* fate (absorption, distribution, metabolism, and elimination), and safety evaluation in the biological setting (hemolysis, complement activation, and interaction with immune system). These studies in general should involve a complete study of all parameters in both *in vitro* and *in vivo* settings. Also, the optimization of parameters and precise control on the methods of manufacturing are of paramount importance.

Physicochemical properties resulting from the nature of the polymer used for the preparation of nanoparticles and their surface properties, such as size and charge, influence their behavior dramatically in the biological setting.[170,171] Size and charge are major factors that dictate the biodistribution and safety of nanoparticles in the body. These characteristics can be easily and reliably determined by using dynamic light-scattering techniques. The traditional techniques such as atomic force microscopy, scanning electron microscopy, and transmission electron microscopy can also be used to characterize the size and size distribution of nanoparticles. However, these microscopic techniques are mainly useful in morphological evaluation. The surface charge of the nanoparticle also partly determines the biodistribution, safety, and efficacy of nanoparticles. The surface charge of nanoparticles is normally determined by calculating their electrophoretic mobility using the light-scattering technique. X-ray photoelectron spectroscopy can also be used to study the surface chemistry of nanoparticles.[172] These techniques are important for assessing the characteristics of nanoparticles in order to fulfill the quality control requirements for their bulk manufacturing and eventual clinical application.

Quality control involving the biodistribution and safety of nanoparticles for clinical development requires both *in vitro* and *in vivo* evaluation. *In vitro* cytotoxicity testing can be done using various cell lines. *In vitro* assays are often used to provide meaningful efficacy and safety data on nanoparticles.[173] However, *in vivo* biodistribution and toxicity evaluation are more important in determining safety and efficacy for clinical trials. Thus, preclinical characterization must include *in vivo* biodistribution and toxicity in animal models. The U.S. FDA provides detailed guidelines for biodistribution and safety assessment of drug formulations *in vivo* using animal models[174,175] with specific considerations for nanoparticles.[173]

20.5 CONCLUDING REMARKS

The tremendous interest in multifunctional stimuli-responsive nanoparticles for targeted delivery of small and macromolecular therapeutics suggests that this approach could become a potential application in the treatment of cancer and infectious diseases. Stimuli-responsive nanoparticles can be made to respond to a variety of local stimuli such as pH, temperature, and redox-potential. These stimuli can exist inherently at the disease site or upon application of external electromagnetic energy (e.g., light, magnetic field, or ultrasound). These help control the payload delivery and release at the site of interest. Additionally, the multifunctional ability of these systems could enhance the intracellular distribution of therapeutics and enhance the efficacy.

In this review, we have discussed the role of multifunctional stimuli-responsive delivery systems such as polymeric nanoparticles, liposomes, and dendrimers. Passive- and active-targeted nanoparticle systems can efficiently package the payload and deliver specifically to tissue and cellular targets and enhance intracellular availability. Based on advances in material sciences and especially the opportunity to custom-synthesize polymers and other functional materials for the intended biological application, newer generations of multifunctional nanoparticles that respond to specific biologically-relevant stimuli are being produced. However, those involved in this effort should place special emphasis on the selection of material that is safe for chronic *in vivo* administration and pay attention to the regulatory issues such as manufacturing and quality in order to facilitate the translation of these experimental technologies into clinically relevant therapeutic options that benefit patients.

REFERENCES

1. Alonso MJ. Nanomedicines for overcoming biological barriers. *Biomedicine & Pharmacotherapy.* 2004;58(3):168–172.
2. Belting M, Sandgren S, Wittrup A. Nuclear delivery of macromolecules: Barriers and carriers. *Advanced Drug Delivery Reviews.* 2005;57(4):505–527.
3. Yih TC, Al-Fandi M. Engineered nanoparticles as precise drug delivery systems. *Journal of Cellular Biochemistry.* 2006;97(6):1184–1190.
4. Garnett MC. Targeted drug conjugates: Principles and progress. *Advanced Drug Delivery Reviews.* 2001;53(2):171–216.
5. Vasir JK, Reddy MK, Labhasetwar VD. Nanosystems in drug targeting: Opportunities and challenges. *Current Nanoscience.* 2005;1:47–64.
6. Maeda H, Wu J, Sawa T, Matsumura Y, Hori K. Tumor vascular permeability and the EPR effect in macromolecular therapeutics: A review. *Journal of Controlled Release.* 2000;65(1–2):271–284.
7. Torchilin VP. Recent approaches to intracellular delivery of drugs and DNA and organelle targeting. *Annual Review of Biomedical Engineering.* 2006;8(1):343–375.
8. Ganta S, Devalapally H, Shahiwala A, Amiji M. A review of stimuli-responsive nanocarriers for drug and gene delivery. *Journal of Controlled Release.* 2008;126:187–204.
9. Couvreur P, Vauthier C. Nanotechnology: Intelligent design to treat complex disease. *Pharmaceutical Research.* 2006;23(7):1417–1450.
10. Jain RK. Vascular and interstitial barriers to delivery of therapeutic agents in tumors. *Cancer and Metastasis Reviews.* 1990;9(3):253–266.
11. Maeda H, Matsumura Y. Tumoritropic and lymphotropic principles of macromolecular drugs. *Critical Reviews in Therapeutic Drug Carrier Systems.* 1989;6(3):193–210.
12. Seymour LW. Passive tumor targeting of soluble macromolecules and drug conjugates. *Critical Reviews in Therapeutic Drug Carrier Systems.* 1992;9(2):135–187.
13. Yuan F. Microvascular permeability and interstitial penetration of sterically stabilized (stealth) liposomes in a human tumor xenograft. *Cancer Research.* 1994;54(13):3352–3356.
14. Baban DF, Seymour LW. Control of tumour vascular permeability. *Advanced Drug Delivery Reviews.* 1998;34(1):109–119.
15. Brannon-Peppas L, Blanchette JO. Nanoparticle and targeted systems for cancer therapy. *Advanced Drug Delivery Reviews.* 2004;56(11):1649–1659.
16. Torchilin VP. Drug targeting. *European Journal of Pharmaceutical Sciences.* 2000;11:81–91.
17. Gabizon AA. Selective tumor localization and improved therapeutic index of anthracyclines encapsulated in long-circulating liposomes. *Cancer Research.* 1992;52(4):891–896.
18. Allen TM, Cullis PR. Drug delivery systems: Entering the mainstream. *Science.* 2004;303(5665):1818.
19. Davis SS. Biomédical applications of nanotechnology—Implications for drug targeting and gene therapy. *Trends in Biotechnology.* 1997;15(6):217–224.
20. Johns P, Courts A. Relationship between collagen and gelatin. In AGW, Courts A, eds., *The Science and Technology of Gelatin*, London, U.K.: Academic Press; 1977.
21. Kommareddy S, Tiwari SB, Amiji MM. Long-circulating polymeric nanovectors for tumor-selective gene delivery. *Technology in Cancer Research and Treatment.* 2005;4(6):615–625.
22. Kaul G, Amiji M. Tumor-targeted gene delivery using poly (ethylene glycol)-modified gelatin nanoparticles: In vitro and in vivo studies. *Pharmaceutical Research.* 2005;22(6):951.
23. Kaul G, Amiji M. Cellular interactions and in vitro DNA transfection studies with poly (ethylene glycol)-modified gelatin nanoparticles. *Journal of Pharmaceutical Sciences.* 2005;94(1):184–198.
24. Marcucci F, Lefoulon F. Active targeting with particulate drug carriers in tumor therapy: Fundamentals and recent progress. *Drug Discovery Today.* 2004;9(5):219–228.
25. Ríhová B. Receptor-mediated targeted drug or toxin delivery. *Advanced Drug Delivery Reviews.* 1998;29(3):273–289.
26. Farokhzad OC, Karp JM, Langer R. Nanoparticle-aptamer bioconjugates for cancer targeting. *Expert Opinion on Drug Delivery.* 2006;3(3):311–324.

27. Chung NS, Wasan KM. Potential role of the low-density lipoprotein receptor family as mediators of cellular drug uptake. *Advanced Drug Delivery Reviews.* 2004;56(9):1315–1334.

28. Rensen PCN, Schiffelers RM, Versluis AJ, Bijsterbosch MK, Van Kuijk-Meuwissen MEMJ, Van Berkel TJC. Human recombinant apolipoprotein E-enriched liposomes can mimic low-density lipoproteins as carriers for the site-specific delivery of antitumor agents. *Molecular Pharmacology.* 1997 September 1, 1997;52(3):445–455.

29. Amin K, Ng KY, Brown CS, Bruno MS, Heath TD. LDL induced association of anionic liposomes with cells and delivery of contents as shown by the increase in potency of liposome dependent drugs. *Pharmaceutical Research.* 2001;18(7):914–921.

30. Kirpotin DB, Drummond DC, Shao Y, Shalaby MR, Hong K, Nielsen UB et al. Antibody targeting of long-circulating lipidic nanoparticles does not increase tumor localization but does increase internalization in animal models. *Cancer Research.* 2006 July 1, 2006;66(13):6732–6740.

31. Sahoo SK, Labhasetwar V. Enhanced antiproliferative activity of transferrin-conjugated paclitaxel-loaded nanoparticles is mediated via sustained intracellular drug retention. *Molecular Pharmaceutics.* 2005;2(5):373–383.

32. Blessing T, Kursa M, Holzhauser R, Kircheis R, Wagner E. Different strategies for formation of PEGylated EGF-conjugated PEI/DNA complexes for targeted gene delivery. *Bioconjugate Chemistry.* 2001;12(4):529–537.

33. Leiden JM. Gene therapy-promise, pitfalls, and prognosis. *The New England Journal of Medicine.* 1995;333(13):871–873.

34. Oishi M, Nagasaki Y. Synthesis, characterization, and biomedical applications of core–shell-type stimuli-responsive nanogels—Nanogel composed of poly [2-(N,N-diethylamino) ethyl methacrylate] core and PEG tethered chains. *Reactive and Functional Polymers.* 2007;67(11):1311–1329.

35. Panyam J, Labhasetwar V. Targeting intracellular targets. *Current Drug Delivery.* 2004;1:235–247.

36. Kichler A, Leborgne C, Coeytaux E, Danos O. Polyethylenimine-mediated gene delivery: A mechanistic study. *Journal of Gene Medicine.* 2001;3(2):135–144.

37. Ogris M, Wagner E. Targeting tumors with non-viral gene delivery systems. *Drug Discovery Today.* 2002;7(8):479–485.

38. Järver P, Langel Ü. The use of cell-penetrating peptides as a tool for gene regulation. *Drug Discovery Today.* 2004;9(9):395–402.

39. Snyder EL, Dowdy SF. Protein/peptide transduction domains: Potential to deliver large DNA molecules into cells. *Current Opinion in Molecular Therapeutics.* 2001;3(2):147–152.

40. Torchilin VP, Rammohan R, Weissig V, Levchenko TS. TAT peptide on the surface of liposomes affords their efficient intracellular delivery even at low temperature and in the presence of metabolic inhibitors. *Proceedings of the National Academy of Sciences.* 2001;98(15):8786.

41. Weissig V, Torchilin VP. Drug and DNA delivery to mitochondria. *Advanced Drug Delivery Reviews.* 2001;49(1–2):1–2.

42. Ferrari M. Cancer nanotechnology: Opportunities and challenges. *Nature Reviews Cancer.* 2005;5(3):161–171.

43. Jabr-Milane LS, van Vlerken LE, Yadav S, Amiji MM. Multi-functional nanocarriers to overcome tumor drug resistance. *Cancer Treatment Reviews.* 2008;34:592–602.

44. Levy L, Sahoo Y, Kim KS, Bergey EJ, Prasad PN. Nanochemistry: Synthesis and characterization of multifunctional nanoclinics for biological applications. *Chemistry of Materials.* 2002;14(9):3715–3721.

45. Feldherr CM, Akin D. The permeability of the nuclear envelope in dividing and nondividing cell cultures. *The Journal of Cell Biology.* 1990;111(1):1–8.

46. Hogemann D, Ntziachristos V, Josephson L, Weissleder R. High throughput magnetic resonance imaging for evaluating targeted nanoparticle probes. *Bioconjugate Chemistry.* 2002;13(1):116–121.

47. Nasongkla N, Bey E, Ren J, Ai H, Khemtong C, Guthi JS et al. Multifunctional polymeric micelles as cancer-targeted, MRI-ultrasensitive drug delivery systems. *Nano Letters.* 2006;6(11):2427–2430.

48. Gerweck LE. Cellular pH gradient in tumor versus normal tissue: Potential exploitation for the treatment of cancer. *Cancer Research.* 1996;56(6):1194–1198.

49. Hunt CA, MacGregor RD, Siegel RA. Engineering targeted in vivo drug delivery. I. The physiological and physicochemical principles governing opportunities and limitations. *Pharmaceutical Research.* 1986;3(6):333–344.

50. Lee ES, Gao Z, Bae YH. Recent progress in tumor pH targeting nanotechnology. *Journal of Controlled Release.* 2008;132(3):164–710.

51. You J-O, Auguste DT. Feedback-regulated paclitaxel delivery based on poly(N,N-dimethylaminoethyl methacrylate-co-2-hydroxyethyl methacrylate) nanoparticles. *Biomaterials.* 2008;29(12):1950–1957.

52. Torchilin V. Multifunctional and stimuli-sensitive pharmaceutical nanocarriers. *European Journal of Pharmaceutics and Biopharmaceutics* 2009;71(3):431–444.

53. Fan L, Wu H, Zhang H, Li F, Yang T-h, Gu C-h et al. Novel super pH-sensitive nanoparticles responsive to tumor extracellular pH. *Carbohydrate Polymers*. 2008;73(3):390–400.

54. Stover TC, Kim YS, Lowe TL, Kester M. Thermoresponsive and biodegradable linear-dendritic nanoparticles for targeted and sustained release of a pro-apoptotic drug. *Biomaterials*. 2008;29(3):359–369.

55. Gal D, MacDonald PC, Porter JC, Simpson ER. Cholesterol metabolism in cancer cells in monolayer culture. III. Low-density lipoprotein metabolism. *International Journal of Cancer*. 1981;28(3):315–319.

56. Wike-Hooley JL, Haveman J, Reinhold HS. The relevance of tumour pH to the treatment of malignant disease. *Radiotherapy and Oncology*. 1984;2(4):343–366.

57. Vaupel P. Blood flow, oxygen and nutrient supply, and metabolic microenvironment of human tumors: A review. *Cancer Research*. 1989;49(23):6449–6465.

58. Dewhirst MW, Prosnitz L, Thrall D, Prescott D, Clegg S, Charles C et al. Hyperthermic treatment of malignant diseases: Current status and a view toward the future. *Seminars in Oncology*. 1997;24(6):616–625.

59. Engin K. Biological rationale and clinical experience with hyperthermia. *Controlled Clinical Trials*. 1996;17(4):316–342.

60. Gupta AK, Naregalkar RR, Vaidya VD, Gupta M. Recent advances on surface engineering of magnetic iron oxide nanoparticles and their biomedical applications. *Nanomedicine*. 2007;2(1):23–39.

61. Ahmed M, Lukyanov AN, Torchilin V, Tournier H, Schneider AN, Goldberg SN. Combined radiofrequency ablation and adjuvant liposomal chemotherapy: Effect of chemotherapeutic agent, nanoparticle size, and circulation time. *Journal of Vascular and Interventional Radiology*. 2005;16(10):1365–1371.

62. Meyer DE, Shin BC, Kong GA, Dewhirst MW, Chilkoti A. Drug targeting using thermally responsive polymers and local hyperthermia. *Journal of Controlled Release*. 2001;74(1–3):213–224.

63. Ponce AM, Vujaskovic Z, Yuan F, Needham D, Dewhirst MW. Hyperthermia mediated liposomal drug delivery. *International Journal of Hyperthermia*. 2006;22(3):205–213.

64. Saito G, Swanson JA, Lee KD. Drug delivery strategy utilizing conjugation via reversible disulfide linkages: Role and site of cellular reducing activities. *Advanced Drug Delivery Reviews*. 2003;55(2):199–215.

65. Noss EH, Pai RK, Sellati TJ, Radolf JD, Belisle J, Golenbock DT et al. Toll-like receptor 2-dependent inhibition of macrophage class II MHC expression and antigen processing by 19-kDa lipoprotein of Mycobacterium tuberculosis 1. *The Journal of Immunology*. 2001;167(2):910–918.

66. Kawai N, Ito A, Nakahara Y, Futakuchi M, Shirai T, Honda H et al. Anticancer effect of hyperthermia on prostate cancer mediated by magnetite cationic liposomes and immune-response induction in transplanted syngeneic rats. *The Prostate*. 2005;64:373–381.

67. Anderson SA, Glod J, Arbab AS, Noel M, Ashari P, Fine HA et al. Noninvasive MR imaging of magnetically labeled stem cells to directly identify neovasculature in a glioma model. *Blood*. 2005;105(1):420.

68. Pitt WG, Husseini GA, Staples BJ. Ultrasonic drug delivery—A general review. *Expert Opinion on Drug Delivery*. 2004;1(1):37.

69. Pissuwan D, Valenzuela SM, Cortie MB. Therapeutic possibilities of plasmonically heated gold nanoparticles. *Trends in Biotechnology*. 2006;24(2):62–67.

70. Paasonen L, Laaksonen T, Johans C, Yliperttula M, Kontturi K, Urtti A. Gold nanoparticles enable selective light-induced contents release from liposomes. *Journal of Controlled Release*. 2007;122(1):86–93.

71. Soppimath KS, Tan DCW, Yang YY. pH-triggered thermally responsive polymer core-shell nanoparticles for drug delivery. *Advanced Materials (Weinheim)*. 2005;17(3):318–323.

72. Bae Y, Nishiyama N, Kataoka K. In vivo antitumor activity of the folate-conjugated pH-sensitive polymeric micelle selectively releasing adriamycin in the intracellular acidic compartments. *Bioconjugate Chemistry*. 2007;18:1131–1139.

73. Shenoy D, Little S, Langer R, Amiji M. Poly (ethylene oxide)-modified poly(ß-amino ester) nanoparticles as a pH-sensitive system for tumor-targeted delivery of hydrophobic drugs: Part I. In vitro evaluations. *Molecular Pharmaceutics*. 2005;2(5):357.

74. Shenoy DB, Amiji MM. Poly (ethylene oxide)-modified poly (epsilon-caprolactone) nanoparticles for targeted delivery of tamoxifen in breast cancer. *International Journal of Pharmaceutics*. 2005;293(1–2):261–270.

75. Devalapally H, Shenoy D, Little S, Langer R, Amiji M. Poly (ethylene oxide)-modified poly (beta-amino ester) nanoparticles as a pH-sensitive system for tumor-targeted delivery of hydrophobic drugs: Part 3. Therapeutic efficacy and safety studies in ovarian cancer xenograft model. *Cancer Chemotherapy and Pharmacology*. 2007;59(4):477–484.

76. Shenoy D, Little S, Langer R, Amiji M. Poly(ethylene oxide)-modified poly(β-amino ester) nanoparticles as a pH-sensitive system for tumor-targeted delivery of hydrophobic drugs: Part 2. In vivo distribution and tumor localization studies. *Pharmaceutical Research*. 2005;22(12):2107–2114.

77. Na K, Seong Lee E, Bae YH. Adriamycin loaded pullulan acetate/sulfonamide conjugate nanoparticles responding to tumor pH: pH-dependent cell interaction, internalization and cytotoxicity in vitro. *Journal of Controlled Release*. 2003;87(1–3):3–13.

78. Stayton PS, El-Sayed MEH, Murthy N, Bulmus V, Lackey C, Cheung C et al. 'Smart'delivery systems for biomolecular therapeutics. *Orthodontics & Craniofacial Research*. 2005;8(3):219–225.

79. Murthy N, Campbell J, Fausto N, Hoffman AS, Stayton PS. Design and synthesis of pH-responsive polymeric carriers that target uptake and enhance the intracellular delivery of oligonucleotides. *Journal of Controlled Release*. 2003;89(3):365–374.

80. Bulmus V, Woodward M, Lin L, Murthy N, Stayton P, Hoffman A. A new pH-responsive and glutathione-reactive, endosomal membrane-disruptive polymeric carrier for intracellular delivery of biomolecular drugs. *Journal of Controlled Release*. 2003;93(2):105–120.

81. Torchilin VP. Recent advances with liposomes as pharmaceutical carriers. *Nature Reviews Drug Discovery*. 2005;4(2):145–160.

82. Simões S, Moreira JN, Fonseca C, Düzgünes N, Pedroso de Lima MC. On the formulation of pH-sensitive liposomes with long circulation times. *Advanced Drug Delivery Reviews*. 2004;56(7):947–965.

83. Kakudo T, Chaki S, Futaki S, Nakase I, Akaji K, Kawakami T et al. Transferrin-modified liposomes equipped with a pH-sensitive fusogenic peptide: An artificial viral-like delivery system. *Biochemistry*. 2004;43(19):5618–5628.

84. Roux E, Passirani C, Scheffold S, Benoit JP, Leroux JC. Serum-stable and long-circulating, PEGylated, pH-sensitive liposomes. *Journal of Controlled Release*. 2004;94(2–3):447–451.

85. Wang CY, Huang L. Highly efficient DNA delivery mediated by pH-sensitive immunoliposomes. *Biochemistry*. 1989;28(24):9508–9514.

86. Litzinger DC, Huang L. Phosphatodylethanolamine liposomes: Drug delivery, gene transfer and immunodiagnostic applications. *BBA-Reviews on Biomembranes*. 1992;1113(2):201–227.

87. Connor J. pH-sensitive immunoliposomes as an efficient and target-specific carrier for antitumor drugs. *Cancer Research*. 1986;46(7):3431–3435.

88. Couvreu P, Fattal E, Malvy C, Dubernet C. pH-sensitive liposomes: An intelligent system for the delivery of antisense oligonucleotides. *Journal of Liposome Research*. 1997;7(1):1–18.

89. Leroux JC, Roux E, Le Garrec D, Hong K, Drummond DC. N-isopropylacrylamide copolymers for the preparation of pH-sensitive liposomes and polymeric micelles. *Journal of Controlled Release*. 2001;72(1–3):71–84.

90. Ellens H, Bentz J, Szoka FC. pH-Induced destabilization of phosphatidylethanolamine-containing liposomes: Role of bilayer contact. *Biochemistry*. 1984;23(7):1532–1538.

91. Ishida T, Kirchmeier MJ, Moase EH, Zalipsky S, Allen TM. Targeted delivery and triggered release of liposomal doxorubicin enhances cytotoxicity against human B lymphoma cells. *BBA-Biomembranes*. 2001;1515(2):144–158.

92. Lee RJ, Wang S, Turk MJ, Low PS. The effects of pH and intraliposomal buffer strength on the rate of liposome content release and intracellular drug delivery. *Bioscience Reports*. 1998;18(2):69–78.

93. Kataoka K, Harada A, Nagasaki Y. Block copolymer micelles for drug delivery: Design, characterization and biological significance. *Advanced Drug Delivery Reviews*. 2001;47(1):113–131.

94. Kwon GS, Okano T. Polymeric micelles as new drug carriers. *Advanced Drug Delivery Reviews*. 1996;21(2):107–116.

95. Gillies ER, Frechet JMJ. Development of acid-sensitive copolymer micelles for drug delivery. *Pure and Applied Chemistry*. 2004;76:1295–1308.

96. Shim WS, Kim SW, Choi EK, Park HJ, Kim JS, Lee DS. Novel pH sensitive block copolymer micelles for solvent free drug loading. *Macromolecular Bioscience*. 2006;6(2):179.

97. Lee ES, Shin HJ, Na K, Bae YH. Poly (l-histidine)–PEG block copolymer micelles and pH-induced destabilization. *Journal of Controlled Release*. 2003;90(3):363–374.

98. Bae Y, Nishiyama N, Fukushima S, Koyama H, Yasuhiro M, Kataoka K. Preparation and biological characterization of polymeric micelle drug carriers with intracellular pH-triggered drug release property: Tumor permeability, controlled subcellular drug distribution, and enhanced in vivo antitumor efficacy. *Bioconjugate Chemistry*. 2005;16(1):122–130.

99. Liu S, Armes SP. Synthesis and aqueous solution behavior of a pH-responsive schizophrenic diblock copolymer. *Langmuir*. 2003;19(10):4432–4438.

100. Bütün V, Armes SP, Billingham NC, Tuzar Z, Rankin A, Eastoe J et al. The remarkable 'flip-flop'self-assembly of a diblock copolymer in aqueous solution. *Macromolecules*. 2001;34(5):1503–1511.

101. Yoshida R, Uchida K, Kaneko Y, Sakai K, Kikuchi A, Sakurai Y et al. Comb-type grafted hydrogels with rapid de-swelling response to temperature changes. *Nature*. 1995;374(6519):240–242.

102. Beltran S, Baker JP, Hooper HH, Blanch HW, Prausnitz JM. Swelling equilibria for weakly ionizable, temperature-sensitive hydrogels. *Macromolecules*. 1991;24(2):549–551.

103. Taillefer J, Jones MC, Brasseur N, Van Lier JE, Leroux JC. Preparation and characterization of pH-responsive polymeric micelles for the delivery of photosensitizing anticancer drugs. *Journal of Pharmaceutical Sciences*. 2000;89(1):52–62.

104. Le Garrec D, Taillefer J, Van Lier JE, Lenaerts V. Optimizing pH-responsive polymeric micelles for drug delivery in a cancer photodynamic therapy model. *Journal of Drug Targeting*. 2002;10(5):429–437.

105. Hsiue GH, Wang CH, Lo CL, Li JP, Yang JL. Environmental-sensitive micelles based on poly (2-ethyl-2-oxazoline)-b-poly (l-lactide) diblock copolymer for application in drug delivery. *International Journal of Pharmaceutics*. 2006;317(1):69–75.

106. Bajpai AK, Shukla SK, Bhanu S, Kankane S. Responsive polymers in controlled drug delivery. *Progress in Polymer Science*. 2008;33(11):1088–1118.

107. Chiappetta DA, Sosnik A. Poly(ethylene oxide)-poly(propylene oxide) block copolymer micelles as drug delivery agents: Improved hydrosolubility, stability and bioavailability of drugs. *European Journal of Pharmaceutics and Biopharmaceutics*. 2007;66(3):303–317.

108. Harada A, Kataoka K. Supramolecular assemblies of block copolymers in aqueous media as nanocontainers relevant to biological applications. *Progress in Polymer Science*. 2006;31(11):949–982.

109. Lee ES, Na K, Bae YH. Super pH-sensitive multifunctional polymeric micelle. *Nano Letters*. 2005;5(2):325–329.

110. Tomalia DIA, Dvornic PR. What promise for dendrimers. *Nature*. 1994;372(6507):617–618.

111. Esfand R, Tomalia DA. Poly (amidoamine)(PAMAM) dendrimers: From biomimicry to drug delivery and biomedical applications. *Drug Discovery Today*. 2001;6(8):427–436.

112. Ihre HR, De Jesus OLP, Szoka FC, Frechet JMJ. Polyester dendritic systems for drug delivery applications: Design, synthesis, and characterization. *Bioconjugate Chemistry*. 2002;13(3):443–452.

113. Gillies ER, Jonsson TB, Frechet JMJ. Stimuli-responsive supramolecular assemblies of linear-dendritic copolymers. *Journal-American Chemical Society*. 2004;126(38):11936–11943.

114. Hui H, Xiao-dong F, Zhong-lin C. Thermo- and pH-sensitive dendrimer derivatives with a shell of poly(*N,N*-dimethylaminoethyl methacrylate) and study of their controlled drug release behavior. *Polymer*. 2005;46(22):9514–9522.

115. Kono K, Kojima C, Hayashi N, Nishisaka E, Kiura K, Watarai S et al. Preparation and cytotoxic activity of poly(ethylene glycol)-modified poly(amidoamine) dendrimers bearing adriamycin. *Biomaterials*. 2008;29(11):1664–1675.

116. Kim SY, Ha JC, Lee YM. Poly (ethylene oxide)-poly (propylene oxide)-poly (ethylene oxide)/poly (epsilon-caprolactone)(PCL) amphiphilic block copolymeric nanospheres II. Thermo-responsive drug release behaviors. *Journal of Controlled Release*. 2000;65(3):345–358.

117. Bae KH, Choi SH, Park SY, Lee Y, Park TG. Thermosensitive pluronic micelles stabilized by shell cross-linking with gold nanoparticles. *Langmuir*. 2006;22(14):6380–6384.

118. Rijcken CJF, Soga O, Hennink WE, Nostrum CF. Triggered destabilisation of polymeric micelles and vesicles by changing polymers polarity: An attractive tool for drug delivery. *Journal of Controlled Release*. 2007;120(3):131–148.

119. Molineux G. Pegylation: Engineering improved pharmaceuticals for enhanced therapy. *Cancer Treatment Reviews*. 2002;28:13–16.

120. Chung JE, Yokoyama M, Okano T. Inner core segment design for drug delivery control of thermo-responsive polymeric micelles. *Journal of Controlled Release*. 2000;65(1–2):93–103.

121. Yokoyama M. Gene delivery using temperature-responsive polymeric carriers. *Drug Discovery Today*. 2002;7(7):426–432.

122. Türk M, Dinçer S, Yulug IG, Piskin E. In vitro transfection of HeLa cells with temperature sensitive polycationic copolymers. *Journal of Controlled Release*. 2004;96(2):325–340.

123. Turk M, Dincer S, Piskin E. Smart and cationic poly (NIPA)/PEI block copolymers as non-viral vectors: In vitro and in vivo transfection studies. *Journal of Tissue Engineering and Regenerative Medicine*. 2007;5:377–388.

124. Dincer S, Turk M, Piskin E. Intelligent polymers as nonviral vectors. *Gene Therapy*. 2005;12(1):S139–S145.

125. Piskin E. Stimuli-responsive polymers in gene delivery. *Expert Reviews of Medical Devices*. 2005;2(4):501–509.

126. Yatvin MB, Weinstein JN, Dennis WH, Blumenthal R. Design of liposomes for enhanced local release of drugs by hyperthermia. *Science*. 1978;202(4374):1290–1293.

127. Chen Q, Tong S, Dewhirst MW, Yuan F. Targeting tumor microvessels using doxorubicin encapsulated in a novel thermosensitive liposome. *Molecular Cancer Therapeutics*. 2004;3(10):1311–1317.

128. Kono K, Nakai R, Morimoto K, Takagishi T. Thermosensitive polymer-modified liposomes that release contents around physiological temperature. *BBA-Biomembranes*. 1999;1416(1–2):239–250.

129. Kono K, Nakai R, Morimoto K, Takagishi T. Temperature-dependent interaction of thermo-sensitive polymer-modified liposomes with CV1 cells. *FEBS Letters*. 1999;456(2):306–310.

130. Kono K, Yoshino K, Takagishi T. Effect of poly (ethylene glycol) grafts on temperature-sensitivity of thermosensitive polymer-modified liposomes. *Journal of Controlled Release*. 2002;80(1–3):321–332.

131. Han HD, Shin BC, Choi HS. Doxorubicin-encapsulated thermosensitive liposomes modified with poly (*N*-isopropylacrylamide-*co*-acrylamide): Drug release behavior and stability in the presence of serum. *European Journal of Pharmaceutics and Biopharmaceutics*. 2006;62(1):110–116.

132. Kono K. Thermosensitive polymer-modified liposomes. *Advanced Drug Delivery Reviews*. 2001;53(3):307–319.

133. Ward CM, Read ML, Seymour LW. Systemic circulation of poly (L-lysine)/DNA vectors is influenced by polycation molecular weight and type of DNA: Differential circulation in mice and rats and the implications for human gene therapy. *Blood*. 2001;97(8):2221.

134. Cavallaro G, Campisi M, Licciardi M, Ogris M, Giammona G. Reversibly stable thiopolyplexes for intracellular delivery of genes. *Journal of Controlled Release*. 2006;115(3):322–334.

135. Voutsadakis IA. Gemtuzumab ozogamicin (CMA-676, Mylotarg) for the treatment of CD33+ acute myeloid leukemia. *Anticancer Drugs*. 2002;13:685–692.

136. Kommareddy S, Amiji M. Preparation and evaluation of thiol-modified gelatin nanoparticles for intracellular DNA delivery in response to glutathione. *Bioconjugate Chemistry*. 2005;16(6):1423–1432.

137. Kommareddy S, Amiji M. Poly (ethylene glycol)–modified thiolated gelatin nanoparticles for glutathione-responsive intracellular DNA delivery. *Nanomedicine: Nanotechnology, Biology, and Medicine*. 2007;3(1):32–42.

138. Kommareddy S, Amiji M. Antiangiogenic gene therapy with systemically administered sFlt-1 plasmid DNA in engineered gelatin-based nanovectors. *Cancer Gene Therapy*. 2007;14(5):488.

139. Godbey WT, Wu KK, Mikos AG. Poly(ethylenimine) and its role in gene delivery. *Journal of Controlled Release*. 1999;60(2–3):149–160.

140. Neu M, Germershaus O, Mao S, Voigt KH, Behe M, Kissel T. Crosslinked nanocarriers based upon poly (ethylene imine) for systemic plasmid delivery: In vitro characterization and in vivo studies in mice. *Journal of Controlled Release*. 2007;118(3):370–380.

141. Carlisle RC, Etrych T, Briggs SS, Preece JA, Ulbrich K, Seymour LW. Polymer-coated polyethylenimine/DNA complexes designed for triggered activation by intracellular reduction. *Journal of Gene Medicine*. 2004;6(3):337–344.

142. Schmitz T, Bravo-Osuna I, Vauthier C, Ponchel G, Loretz B, Bernkop-Schnürch A. Development and in vitro evaluation of a thiomer-based nanoparticulate gene delivery system. *Biomaterials*. 2007;28(3):524–531.

143. Sun Y-X, Zeng X, Meng Q-F, Zhang X-Z, Cheng S-X, Zhuo R-X. The influence of RGD addition on the gene transfer characteristics of disulfide-containing polyethyleneimine/DNA complexes. *Biomaterials*. 2008;29(32):4356–4365.

144. West KR, Otto S. Reversible covalent chemistry in drug delivery. *Current Drug Discovery Technologies*. 2005;2(3):123.

145. Huang Z, Li W, MacKay JA, Szoka FC Jr. Thiocholesterol-based lipids for ordered assembly of bioresponsive gene carriers. *Molecular Therapy*. 2005;11:409–417.

146. Kirpotin D, Hong K, Mullah N, Papahadjopoulos D, Zalipsky S. Liposomes with detachable polymer coating: Destabilization and fusion of dioleoylphosphatidylethanolamine vesicles triggered by cleavage of surface-grafted poly (ethylene glycol). *FEBS Letters*. 1996;388(2–3):115–118.

147. Gabizon AA, Tzemach D, Horowitz AT, Shmeeda H, Yeh J, Zalipsky S. Reduced toxicity and superior therapeutic activity of a mitomycin C lipid-based prodrug incorporated in pegylated liposomes. *Clinical Cancer Research*. 2006;12(6):1913–1920.

148. Sun C, Lee JSH, Zhang M. Magnetic nanoparticles in MR imaging and drug delivery. *Advanced Drug Delivery Reviews*. 2008;60(11):1252–1265.

149. Gupta AK, Gupta M. Synthesis and surface engineering of iron oxide nanoparticles for biomedical applications. *Biomaterials*. 2005;26(18):3995–4021.

150. Lubbe AS, Bergemann C, Riess H, Schriever F, Reichardt P, Possinger K et al. Clinical experiences with magnetic drug targeting: A phase I study with 4′-epidoxorubicin in 14 patients with advanced solid tumors. *Cancer Research*. 1996;56(20):4686–4693.

151. Alexiou C, Schmid RJ, Jurgons R, Kremer M, Wanner G, Bergemann C et al. Targeting cancer cells: Magnetic nanoparticles as drug carriers. *European Biophysics Journal*. 2006;35(5):446–450.

152. Ito A, Kuga Y, Honda H, Kikkawa H, Horiuchi A, Watanabe Y et al. Magnetite nanoparticle-loaded anti-HER2 immunoliposomes for combination of antibody therapy with hyperthermia. *Cancer Letters*. 2004;212(2):167–175.

153. Dobson J. Gene therapy progress and prospects: Magnetic nanoparticle-based gene delivery. *Gene Therapy*. 2006;13:283–287.

154. Frenkel V. Ultrasound mediated delivery of drugs and genes to solid tumors. *Advanced Drug Delivery Reviews*. 2008;60(10):1193–1208.

155. Rapoport N, Marin A, Christensen DA. Ultrasound-activated drug delivery. *Drug Delivery Systems and Sciences*. 2002;2:37–46.

156. Rapoport N. Physical stimuli-responsive polymeric micelles for anti-cancer drug delivery. *Progress in Polymer Science*. 2007;32(8–9):962–990.

157. De Jong WH, Borm PJA. Drug delivery and nanoparticles: Applications and hazards. *International Journal of Nanomedicine*. 2008;3(2):133.

158. Colvin VL. The potential environmental impact of engineered nanomaterials. *Nature Biotechnology*. 2003;21:1166–1170.

159. Hunter AC, Moghimi SM. Therapeutic synthetic polymers: A game of Russian roulette? *Drug Discovery Today*. 2002;7(19):998–1001.

160. Sayes CM, Liang F, Hudson JL, Mendez J, Guo W, Beach JM et al. Functionalization density dependence of single-walled carbon nanotubes cytotoxicity in vitro. *Toxicology Letters*. 2006;161(2):135–142.

161. Shvedova A, Castranova V, Kisin E, Schwegler-Berry D, Murray A, Gandelsman V et al. Exposure to carbon nanotube material: Assessment of nanotube cytotoxicity using human keratinocyte cells. *Journal of Toxicology and Environmental Health, Part A*. 2003;66(20):1909–1926.

162. Lam KH, Schakenraad JM, Esselbrugge H, Feijen J, Nieuwenhuis P. The effect of phagocytosis of poly(L-lactic acid) fragments on cellular morphology and viability. *Journal of Biomedical Materials Research*. 1993;27(12):1569–1577.

163. Savic R, Luo LB, Eisenberg A, Maysinger D. Nanocontainers distribute to defined cytoplasmic organelles. *Science*. 2003;300:615–618.

164. Nishiyama N, Koizumi F, Okazaki S, Matsumura Y, Nishio K, Kataoka K. Differential gene expression profile between PC-14 cells treated with free cisplatin and cisplatin-incorporated polymeric micelles. *Bioconjugate Chemistry*. 2003;14(2):449–457.

165. Demoy M, Gibaud S, Andreux JP, Weingarten C, Gouritin B, Couvreur P. Splenic trapping of nanoparticles: Complementary approaches for in situ studies. *Pharmaceutical Research*. 1997;14(4):463–468.

166. Moghimi SM, Hunter AC, Murray JC. Nanomedicine: Current status and future prospects. *FASEB Journal*. 2005;19(3):311–330.

167. Birnbaum DT, Kosmala JD, Henthorn DB, Brannon-Peppas L. Controlled release of ß-estradiol from PLAGA microparticles: The effect of organic phase solvent on encapsulation and release. *Journal of Controlled Release*. 2000;65(3):375–387.

168. Bodmeier R, McGinity JW. Solvent selection in the preparation of poly (DL-lactide) microspheres prepared by the solvent evaporation method. *International Journal of Pharmaceutics*. 1988;43(1–2):179–186.

169. Arshady R. Preparation of biodegradable microspheres and microcapsules. II, Polylatides and related polyesters. *Journal of Controlled Release*. 1991;17(1):1–22.

170. Ogawara K-i, Yoshida M, Kubo J-i, Nishikawa M, Takakura Y, Hashida M et al. Mechanisms of hepatic disposition of polystyrene microspheres in rats: Effects of serum depend on the sizes of microspheres. *Journal of Controlled Release*. 1999;61(3):241–250.

171. Kobayashi H, Kawamoto S, Jo SK, Bryant HL, Brechbiel MW, Star RA. Macromolecular MRI contrast agents with small dendrimers: Pharmacokinetic differences between sizes and cores. *Bioconjugate Chemistry*. 2003;14(2):388–394.

172. Pan J, Feng SS. Targeted delivery of paclitaxel using folate-decorated poly (lactide)–vitamin E TPGS nanoparticles. *Biomaterials*. 2008;29(17):2663–2672.

173. Patri A, Dobrovolskaia M, Stern S, McNeil S. Preclinical characterization of engineered nanoparticles intended for cancer therapeutics. In MM Amiji, ed., *Nanotechnology for Cancer Therapy*, Boca Raton, FL: CRC Press/Taylor & Francis; 2006.

174. Anderson DG, Levenberg S, Langer R. Nanoliter-scale synthesis of arrayed biomaterials and application to human embryonic stem cells. *Nature Biotechnology.* 2004 Jul;22(7):863–866.

175. United States. Food and Drug Administration CDER/CBER Guidance for industry ICH S6: Preclinical safety evaluation of biotechnology-derived pharmaceuticals 1997.

21 Physiological Stress Responsive Gene Regulation Systems for Tissue Targeting

Hyun Ah Kim and Minhyung Lee

CONTENTS

21.1 INTRODUCTION

Gene therapy involves the intracellular delivery of genetic materials to treat inherited or acquired diseases. Although gene therapy is not generally applied to clinical settings, it will be a clinical option for many diseases in the near future due to extensive research and development efforts. The barriers and problems experienced in developing gene therapy are being addressed by new technology. The problems include delivery-related issues such as efficiency, specificity, cytotoxicity, and clearance.[1] Also, gene-related issues such as the selection of appropriate genes for a certain disease, immune activation by DNA or RNA, gene expression regulation, and degradation of the gene by endogenous enzymes, should be addressed for safe and efficient gene therapy. Of these, gene expression regulation is related to the production of a therapeutic protein in a timely and localized manner.[2,3]

Most of the genes in our cells are expressed at a specific time and location. Without gene expression specificity, the homeostasis of the cells will be disrupted, which usually results in cell death. Therefore, cells have very sophisticated regulatory systems for gene regulation. With the advance of molecular biology techniques, a lot of information about gene regulation has been elucidated. This information is valuable for the development of gene therapy technology, since an exogenous-delivered gene should not interrupt normal cell processes, and gene expression should be controlled by the cell condition.

Gene expression can be regulated at the transcriptional, translational, or posttranslational level. For transcriptional regulation, various promoters and enhancers have been evaluated for use in gene therapy.[3–5] Tissue-specific promoters have been employed to restrict gene expression to specific tissues, leading to tissue-targeted gene therapy. However, there are still drawbacks, such as leaky expression by basal promoter activity in untargeted tissues[6] and weak promoter activity of the tissue-specific promoter, which are usually inadequate for clinical gene therapy.[7] Therefore, amplification systems such as the two-step transcription amplification (TSTA) system have been designed. The TSTA system contains two expression units. The first unit expresses the sequence-specific transactivator, which induces therapeutic genes in the second expression unit.[7–15]

For translational regulation, the most efficient method is to use small interfering RNA (siRNA) or antisense oligonucleotides. The antisense technique has been employed to reduce gene expression in a sequence-specific manner by the degradation of specific mRNAs or translation inhibition. siRNA is highly effective in knocking down gene expression and is expected to be one of the first gene therapy drugs on the market. Posttranslational regulation is not generally used in therapeutic gene regulation. One of the approaches used involves controlling protein stability and promoting the degradation of the target protein under a specific condition.[6] For example, the oxygen-dependent degradation (ODD) domain has been employed for the stabilization of therapeutic proteins in ischemic tissue.[6,16–18]

The physiological condition of cells is an important regulatory signal of endogenous gene expression. Gene expression in normal cells is tightly regulated in response to subtle changes in the physiological condition of the cells. For example, low oxygen concentration increases angiogenic gene expression to recover blood and oxygen supply to the tissue. However, the unregulated expression of angiogenic genes in normal tissue may induce a deleterious effect such as tumor formation.[19,20] Like natural gene regulation, therapeutic gene expression should also be tightly regulated to avoid any possible problems, such as toxicity and unwanted side effects of gene therapy. Currently, two possible strategies for therapeutic gene regulation are under development. First, an exogenous drug could regulate gene expression.[2,3,21] For example, tetracycline can activate a tetracycline-dependent transcription factor, which has been designed to include tetracycline-binding sites, resulting in an increase or decrease of transcription factor activity. These transcription factors undergo conformational changes upon binding to tetracycline. Therefore, the amount of tetracycline administered is important for gene regulation. Second, gene expression can be regulated by a physiological condition.[22–24] Cells have transcription regulatory enzymes, which regulate gene expression in response to changes in the environmental conditions. Therapeutic gene expression can also be regulated using this endogenous regulatory system.

Self-regulation is one of the advantages of the physiological response system, since it does not require the administration of the activating drug. The commonly used physiological regulation signals include hypoxia, glucose, and heat shock. In this chapter, basic concepts, transcriptional regulation, and examples of applications of physiological signal regulation systems will be introduced. In addition, an important posttranscriptional regulation method, controlling mRNA stability using an untranslated region (UTR), and the posttranslational regulation of proteins will be discussed.

21.2 PHYSIOLOGICAL STATES OF DISEASES

Hypoxia is the most important hallmark of various ischemic diseases. The lack of blood supply, caused by narrowed bloody vessels, reduces oxygen and nutrient concentration in the tissue. The low oxygen condition induces the expression of anti-apoptotic and angiogenic genes to survive the unfavorable condition and recover the normal blood supply. For example, the expression of the vascular endothelial growth factor (VEGF) gene is induced in ischemic myocardium. A similar condition is observed in an ischemic brain, ischemic limb, or injured spinal cord. HIF-1α is accumulated in these disease tissues and induces the transcription of the genes with hypoxia response elements (HREs) in their control region. Therefore, HIf-1α can be utilized for hypoxia regulated therapeutic gene expression.

A low oxygen condition is also observed in solid tumors. Rapidly growing tumors require new blood vessel formation for the supply of nutrients and oxygen. However, new blood formation is often not enough to meet this requirement, which causes the core region of the tumor to undergo hypoxia. Therefore, hypoxia is an important characteristic of a solid tumor. Low blood supply also limits glucose supply, which is another characteristic of a solid tumor. Low glucose supply induces glucose regulated proteins (GRPs), which are required for the survival of the cells under low glucose concentration. GRPs are induced transcriptionally and therefore, the GRP promoters are good candidates for low glucose concentration regulatory gene expression systems.

Diabetes is classified into two groups, type 1 and type 2. The common property of the two diabetes types is high blood glucose concentration. The high glucose concentration may induce oxidative stress to the cells and causes irreversible damage. The high glucose concentration induces gene expressions, which are related to glucose uptake and metabolism. Therefore, therapeutic genes for diabetes may be physiologically induced by using glucose response gene expression systems.

> Self-regulation is one of the advantages of the physiological response system, since it does not require the administration of the activating drug. The commonly used physiological regulation signals include hypoxia, glucose, and heat shock.

21.3 HYPOXIA

21.3.1 Hypoxia-Inducible Factor-1 as a Key Regulator of Gene Expression under Hypoxia

Hypoxia is a state of low oxygen concentration, usually due to the lack of blood supply. Hypoxia is a serious stress condition, which threatens the survival of cells. To survive this stress condition, cells decrease their metabolic rate and increase the expression of protective genes. The key regulator of gene expression under hypoxia is hypoxia-inducible factor (HIF)-1α.[25–28] HIF-1 is composed of two subunits, HIF-1α and HIF-1β (Figure 21.1A).[27] Whereas HIF-1β is constitutively expressed, the expression of HIF-1α changes rapidly in response to oxygen concentration. HIF-1α is regulated at the transcriptional, translational, and posttranslational steps.[29] At the transcriptional step, the HIF-1α promoter is activated and increases the production of HIF-1α mRNA at low oxygen concentrations. At the translational level, the HIF-1α 5′-UTR stabilizes the HIF-1α mRNA in response to low oxygen concentrations, resulting in an increase of the mRNA translation rate. However, the rapid accumulation of HIF-1α under hypoxia is mainly due to the stabilization of the HIF-1α protein.

HIF-1α has a short half-life under normal oxygen concentrations. HIF-1α has a DNA-binding domain (DBD), a transactivation domain (TAD), and an ODD domain.[26,30,31] DBD and TAD are required for sequence-specific DNA binding and transcription activation, respectively. The ODD domain is responsible for the regulation of HIF-1α stability. It has specific proline residues, which are the targets of hydroxylation by prolyl hydroxylases (PHDs) (Figure 21.1B).[32–34] PHDs are activated at low oxygen concentrations and attach hydroxyl groups to the prolines of the ODD domain.[34] The von Hippel Lindau protein (pVHL), which has ubiquitin ligase activity, recognizes the hydroxylated prolines. The ODD domain is then polyubiquitinated by pVHL and degraded via the ubiquitin-proteasome pathway. As a result, HIF-1α is maintained at a low protein level under normoxia. However, as the oxygen concentration decreases, PHD activity rapidly decreases. This leads to a decrease in the hydroxylation level of the ODD domain and HIF-1α degradation via the ubiquitin-proteasome pathway is reduced. Thus, HIF-1α is accumulated under hypoxia. HIF-1 then binds to and activates hypoxia response promoters for the induction of stress-related proteins.

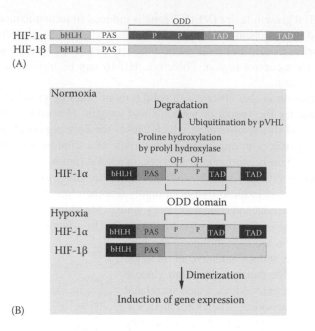

FIGURE 21.1 Structure and regulation of HIF-1. (A) Structure of HIF-1. HIF-1 is composed of HIF-1α and HIF-1β. HIF-1α is stabilized specifically under hypoxia. The ODD domain of HIF-1α has two specific proline residues for hydroxylation under normoxia. Proline hydroxylation triggers the degradation of HIF-1α via ubiquitin-proteasome pathway. bHLH, basic helix loop helix; PAS, per arnt sim; TAD, transactivation domain; P, proline. (B) Posttranslational regulation of HIF-1. The ODD domain has specific proline residues, which are the targets of hydroxylation by PHDs. PHDs are activated at low oxygen concentrations and attach hydroxyl groups to the prolines of the ODD domain. The pVHL, which is an ubiquitin ligase, recognizes the hydroxylated prolines. The ODD domain is then polyubiquitinated by pVHL and degraded via the ubiquitin-proteasome pathway.

21.3.2 Transcriptional Regulation of Gene Expression by Hypoxia

The transcriptional regulation of gene expression under hypoxia is mediated by HIF-1. As described above, HIF-1 is accumulated under hypoxia. For transcriptional regulation, the 5′-regulatory regions of therapeutic genes should contain HIF-1 binding sites, referred to as HREs. HREs have a consensus sequence for the binding of HIF-1. For hypoxia-specific gene induction, HREs were combined with the basal promoters of therapeutic genes as hybrid systems (Figure 21.2).[35–37] The integration of multiple copies of HREs into the regulation system can increase the hypoxia-inducible promoter activity, which increases the specificity of gene expression.

The HREs from several hypoxia response promoters have been investigated for hypoxia-inducible gene therapy. The transcriptional activities of the HREs have been compared with each other in combination with the SV40 basal promoter.[36] For example, the erythropoietin (Epo) enhancer, which contains HREs, was linked to the SV40 basal promoter for hypoxia-inducible transcription.[10,38] The Epo enhancer-SV40 promoter showed higher gene expression under hypoxia than the SV40 promoter (Figure 21.3). Of the tested HREs, the HRE from the phosphoglycerate kinase-1 (PGK-1) had the strongest hypoxia-inducible transactivation. The combination of the HRE from the PGK-1 gene and the SV40 basal promoter was referred to as Oxford Biomedica HRE (OBHRE).

In some studies, the promoters from hypoxia-inducible genes, not just HREs, have been used for hypoxia-inducible expression as a single promoter system (Figure 21.2). These promoters contained HREs and basal promoter elements from the same gene. For example, the glyceraldehyde-3-phosphate dehydrogenase (GAPDH) promoter and the RTP801 promoter show hypoxia-inducible gene expression.[39–44] The activity of the RTP801 promoter was relatively strong and has been used

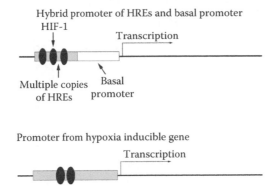

FIGURE 21.2 Hypoxia inducible promoter systems. Hypoxia inducible hybrid promoter systems are composed of HREs and basal promoter. On HIF-1 binding to HREs, the promoter activity is induced and gene expression increases. Promoters from hypoxia inducible genes have their own HREs in the promoter region.

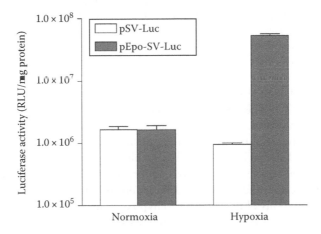

FIGURE 21.3 Inducible gene expression under hypoxia by the Epo enhancer-SV40 promoter. pSV-Luc and pEpo-SV-Luc were transfected into Neuro2A cells. The cells were incubated under normoxia or hypoxia for 20 h and assessed for luciferase activity. The data expressed as mean values ± standard deviation.

without the help of a viral promoter/enhancer. However, the activity of the GAPDH promoter was relatively weak and it was often used in combination with a strong viral enhancer and promoter, such as the cytomegalovirus (CMV) immediate early enhancer and promoter.[39]

21.3.3 Translational Regulation of Gene Expression by Hypoxia

The half-life of mRNA is an important factor that determines the translation rate of a gene. Therefore, gene expression can be regulated at the translational level by adjusting the mRNA stability. The hypoxia-specific regulation of mRNA stability can be achieved by using an UTR. For example, the Epo 3′-UTR stabilizes the Epo mRNA under hypoxia by binding to Epo RNA-binding proteins (ERBPs).[16,45] The binding of ERBPs increased the mRNA half-life by 40%–50%, depending on the hypoxia status. When the Epo 3′-UTR was linked to the luciferase or VEGF mRNA, the Epo 3′-UTR stabilized the mRNA and increased the gene expression in a hypoxia-specific manner (Figure 21.4).[46,47] This suggests that the Epo 3′-UTR can stabilize the mRNA without any sequence specificity of the linked RNA, and therefore, the Epo 3′-UTR can be applied to various therapeutic genes.

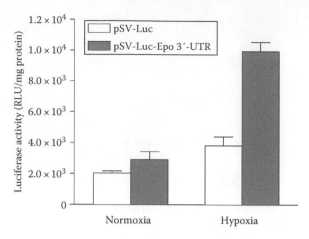

FIGURE 21.4 Inducible gene expression under hypoxia by the Epo 3′-UTR. pSV-Luc and pSV-Luc-Epo 3′-UTR were transfected into Neuro2A cells. The cells were incubated under normoxia or hypoxia for 20 h and assessed for luciferase activity. The data expressed as mean values ± standard deviation.

The VEGF 3′-UTR can also be used for the hypoxia-specific stabilization of mRNA. Under hypoxia, the VEGF 3′-UTR and the Epo 3′-UTR bind to a common protein, suggesting that a common stabilization mechanism is involved.[48] However, the VEGF 3′-UTR has an AT-rich destabilizing region. It was reported that the VEGF 3′-UTR itself did not show a hypoxia-specific stabilization effect on a linked mRNA.[49,50] Therefore, further modification of the VEGF 3′-UTR is required for hypoxia-specific gene expression.

Other UTRs, such as the HIF-1α 3′-UTR,[29] the tyrosine hydroxylase (TH) 3′-UTR,[48] the transferrin receptor 3′-UTR,[51] and the ferritin 3′-UTR,[51] were also suggested to be hypoxia-specific stabilizing UTRs. Specifically, the transferrin receptor and ferritin 3′-UTRs have iron responsive elements (IREs).[51] It was suggested that the IREs might be involved in mRNA stabilization in response to hypoxia. Although applications of these UTRs to hypoxia-inducible gene expression have not been reported, it is highly likely that these RNA elements will be very useful for the development of the hypoxia-specific gene expression systems.

21.3.4 Posttranslational Regulation of Gene Expression by Hypoxia

For hypoxia-specific gene therapy, the stability of therapeutic proteins can be regulated through posttranslational regulation. As described above, the ODD domain regulates HIF-1α stability. Similarly, when the ODD domain is integrated into therapeutic proteins, it can regulate the half-life of these proteins. The ODD domain coding sequence has been located downstream of the luciferase cDNA (Figure 21.5).[6] After gene expression, the luciferase-ODD fusion protein was stabilized in a hypoxia-specific manner. In another example, the ODD domain was linked to diphtheria toxin A (DT-A).[16] After the translation of the gene encoding ODD-DT-A, the fusion protein level was higher under hypoxia than normoxia. In combination with the transcriptional regulation system, the posttranslational regulatory system had high enough specificity to be used with the *in vivo* imaging of HIF-1 activity in tumor xenograft.[18]

The ODD domain was applied to the TSTA system to regulate the stability of an artificial transcription factor,[11] which was composed of the Gal4 DBD and p65 TAD. The Gal4 DBD is derived from the yeast Gal4 gene and enables the transcription factor to be highly specific to the Gal4 upstream activating sequence (UAS) in mammalian cells. Also, the transcription factor has a high transactivation effect, since p65 TAD is from the nuclear factor-κB (NF-κB).

The TSTA system using Gal4DBD-p65TAD is composed of two gene expression units (Figure 21.6). The first unit produces the Gal4DBD-p65TAD artificial transcription factor, which

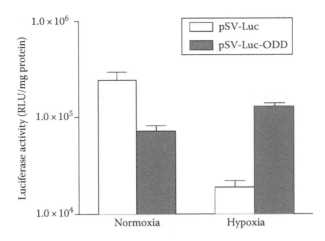

FIGURE 21.5 Posttranslational regulation of gene expression under hypoxia by the ODD domain. pSV-Luc and pSV-Luc-ODD were transfected into Neuro2A cells. The cells were incubated under normoxia or hypoxia for 20 h and assessed for luciferase activity. The data expressed as mean values ± standard deviation.

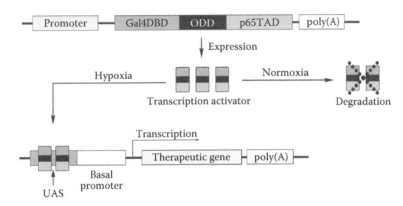

FIGURE 21.6 ODD-mediated gene regulation system. There are two expression units in the ODD-mediated gene regulation system. The first unit produces a transcription activator with the ODD domain. The transcription activator is stabilized under hypoxia and binds to the control region of the second expression unit, while it is rapidly degraded under normoxia.

binds specifically to the UAS sequence and activates the expression of the target gene. Since Gal4DBD-p65TAD is a strong transcriptional activator, the target gene expression level in the TSTA system is much higher than in the single expression system. Therefore, the TSTA system has been used to amplify the weak transcriptional activity of tissue-specific promoters. For hypoxia-specific gene expression, the ODD domain is integrated between Gal4DBD and p65TAD (Figure 21.6). The ODD domain stabilizes the artificial transcription factor and facilitates the expression of the therapeutic gene in a hypoxia-specific manner. Under normoxia, the transcription factor degrades rapidly, showing a basal level of gene expression.

The regulation methods at the transcriptional, translational, and posttranslational steps are independent from each other. Therefore, a combination of the regulatory strategies may have synergistic effects for hypoxia-responsive therapeutic gene expression.

The regulation methods at the transcriptional, translational, and posttranslational steps are independent from each other. Therefore, a combination of the regulatory strategies may have synergistic effects for hypoxia-responsive therapeutic gene expression.

21.3.5 APPLICATION OF HYPOXIA-SPECIFIC GENE EXPRESSION SYSTEMS TO GENE THERAPY

Hypoxic conditions can be found in various disease states. Hypoxia-specific gene expression systems have been applied to gene therapy for ischemic myocardium, ischemic limb, stroke, injured spinal cord, solid tumor, and ischemic corpus cavernosum.

For ischemic myocardium gene therapy, the RTP801 promoter-driven VEGF gene was injected directly into the myocardium.[41] VEGF expression was higher in the myocardium injected with the RTP801-VEGF gene, compared with the SV40 promoter-driven VEGF gene. The RTP801 promoter was reported to have high gene expression in the ischemic cavernosum of an erectile dysfunction animal model.[44] Also, the RTP801 promoter induced gene expression in islet cells, showing its effect in islets protection under the ischemic condition.[52]

The inducibility of a promoter may differ depending on the tissue type. For example, the RTP801 promoter showed lower activity than the Epo enhancer-SV40 hybrid promoter system in neuronal tissue.[43] For spinal cord gene therapy, the VEGF gene with the RTP801 promoter or the Epo enhancer-SV40 hybrid promoter was injected directly into the injured spinal cord. The results showed that the Epo enhancer-SV40 promoter system had higher activity than the RTP801 promoter in the spinal cord. On the contrary, the RTP801 promoter was stronger than the Epo enhancer-SV40 promoter in ischemic cavernosum.[44]

Usually, a tissue-specific or physiological condition response promoter is too weak to express a protein at a high enough level to have a therapeutic effect. Therefore, the TSTA system has been developed with the hypoxia promoter.[9] This hypoxia-specific vigilant human heme oxygenase-1 (hHO-1) expression system was applied to a myocardial infarction model.[11,12] The expression of hHO-1 was detected only in the vigilant hHO-1 plasmids injected into an ischemic heart. Masson trichrome staining showed that fibrotic areas significantly decreased in vigilant hHO-1 plasmids injected into mice, as compared with a saline-injected control.

The hypoxia-inducible system was also applied to cancer therapy. The Epo-early growth response protein (Egr)-tumor necrosis factor-α (TNF-α) plasmid was constructed by inserting the Epo hypoxia-responsive element upstream of the Egr promoter for the expression of TNF-α.[53] When this plasmid was injected into human colon adenocarcinoma in nude mice, tumor growth was significantly delayed when compared with all other groups. Similarly, the ODD-diphtheria toxin A (DT-A/ODD) fusion protein was used for tumor-targeting gene therapy.[16] In a Lewis lung carcinoma model, the DT-A/ODD fusion protein reduced tumor volume in a hypoxia-regulated manner.

Hypoxia regulatory systems are effective in that they can induce gene expression specifically in ischemic tissues. However, the basal level expression in normal tissue and weak promoter activity should be addressed for its clinical applications. The ODD domain is useful for the reduction of the basal level expression. However, modification of the therapeutic genes with the ODD domain may interfere with the normal folding of the proteins and may reduce biological activity after translation. Also, the modification of the genes may induce an immune response against the fusion proteins. Second, the activity of the hypoxia-specific promoter may be induced in combination with the TSTA system or viral enhancer. However, the hypoxia specificity in gene expression may be compromised. Therefore, the gene regulatory systems should be carefully optimized.

21.4 GLUCOSE

21.4.1 GLUCOSE-REGULATED GENE EXPRESSION

Glucose is an important signal in regulating gene expression. Some glucose-responsive genes are induced by high glucose concentrations, such as the glucose metabolism-related genes. A high glucose concentration, usually prevalent in diabetes, is a stress condition, which causes damage in various organs. Therefore, the glucose-inducible genes are tightly regulated to maintain a normal blood glucose level. Other types of glucose-responsive genes are induced by a low glucose concentration.

In ischemic tissues, which are usually found in solid tumors, glucose concentration, as well as oxygen tension, is not enough to maintain normal cellular processes since blood supply to the tissue is low. Therefore, cellular protective genes, such as growth factors and anti-apoptotic genes, are induced for survival of the cells under an ischemic condition.

Gene expression in response to glucose concentration is regulated mainly at the transcriptional level. Glucose-inducible promoters have glucose response elements (GlREs), which are usually combined with insulin response elements.[54–56] Therefore, gene expression by glucose-inducible promoters is induced by high glucose concentrations and inhibited by high insulin concentrations. On the contrary, the GRP promoters have glucose-regulated elements, which are activated at low glucose concentrations.[57–62] The GRP promoters, which also have hypoxia-inducible elements, are induced by oxygen deprivation and glucose starvation. These characteristics of the GRP promoters make them useful for tumor gene therapy.

> Gene expression in response to glucose concentration is regulated mainly at the transcriptional level. Glucose-inducible promoters have GlREs, which are usually combined with insulin response elements.

21.4.2 GLUCOSE-INDUCIBLE PROMOTERS

The promoters induced by high glucose have been used for insulin gene therapy in diabetes. Blood glucose levels change rapidly depending on food intake, and insulin expression should be tightly regulated to maintain blood glucose levels. The transcription and translation of a gene takes substantial time (several hours). Therefore, a rapid response to high glucose concentration, which in a normal pancreas takes minutes, is difficult to achieve with transcriptional regulation. However, it is possible to regulate blood glucose concentration within a reasonable range with a glucose-inducible promoter system, although it is not as perfectly regulated as a normal pancreas. The L-type pyruvate kinase (LPK) promoter has been extensively studied for insulin gene therapy. The insulin gene under the control of the LPK promoter was applied to streptozotocin-induced type 1 diabetes animal models.[63] In this study, three copies of the stimulatory GlREs from the LPK promoter were combined with the insulin-like growth factor binding protein-1 (IGFBP-1) basal promoter. The IGFBP-1 basal promoter has an inhibitory insulin response element and reduces gene expression by increasing insulin concentration in the blood. Therefore, the IGFBP-1 promoter reduced gene expression to inhibit hypoglycemia. Another example of the LPK promoter application was for single chain insulin analog (SIA) expression.[64] In this study, Lee et al. showed that a normal glucose level was maintained over one year after one injection of the adeno-associated viral vector, which carried the LPK-regulated SIA expression unit. Interestingly, it was reported that the GlRE of the LPK promoter was responsive to hypoxia as well as glucose.[65] It was suggested that HIF-1α might bind to GlRE in combination with the upstream stimulating factor-1 (USF-1). The results suggest that HIF-1 may be the dominant transcription regulator of the LPK promoter at a low oxygen concentration, and that HIF-1 binding to the LPK promoter may interfere with the glucose-dependent induction of the LPK promoter. Therefore, the application of the LPK promoter to gene therapy should be carefully optimized to avoid any possible problems caused by the hypoxia and glucose cross-talk.

Another important stimulatory glucose response promoter is the insulin promoter, which is active specifically in pancreatic β cells. In addition to spatial specificity, the insulin promoter increases transcription in response to the blood glucose level. Therefore, the insulin promoter has been used for localized gene expression specifically in the pancreas, and in a glucose-dependent manner. For example, the rat insulin promoter was used to produce antisense glutamic acid dehydrogenase (GAD) mRNA in the pancreas.[66,67] Transgenic mice with the antisense GAD mRNA expression showed low GAD expression in the pancreas and a low incidence of type 1 diabetes. This result suggested that GAD might be an autoantigen responsible for autoimmune inflammation in the pancreas.[66] Also, the rat insulin promoter-controlled antisense GAD plasmid was delivered to the pancreas using a polymeric carrier, which showed the glucose response induction of the antisense GAD mRNA.[67] The rat insulin promoter was also used to induce interleukin-4, luciferase, and insulin in a glucose-dependent manner.[68,69] It was further modified to increase the specificity by multimerization of the promoter. Three copies of the rat insulin promoter increased insulin gene expression in response to a high glucose concentration more effectively than a single copy of the rat insulin promoter.

The glucose-6-phosphatase (G6pase) promoter has also been investigated for insulin gene expression.[54,55,70] The G6pase promoter has glucose-dependent stimulating and insulin-dependent repression activity. Due to self-deactivation activity at high insulin expression, the G6pase promoter is useful for insulin gene therapy. Recently, the glucose response activity of the G6pase promoter was enhanced by combining it with the LPK promoter.[56]

Other glucose response promoters include the spot 14 (S14) and fatty acid synthase promoter. The GlRE from the S14 promoter showed that insulin expression was regulated in a glucose-dependent manner, and that the blood glucose level was reduced in the streptozotocin-induced type 1 diabetes mouse model.[71] Fatty acid synthase expression is induced in adipocytes and hepatocytes by high glucose concentrations, suggesting that the fatty acid synthase promoter is a possible candidate for the glucose response gene expression system.[72]

Glucose-inducible promoters are useful for diabetes gene therapy, inducing therapeutic genes at high glucose concentrations. Especially, insulin gene therapy requires a rapid response to a change of blood glucose level to maintain the glucose level in a normal range without the risk of hypoglycemia. The promoter-mediated transcriptional regulation of the insulin gene expression may not be adequate for rapid response to a change of blood glucose concentration. Therefore, more rapid regulatory strategies may be more useful for insulin gene therapy such as translational or posttranslational regulation. Further research is required for the development of such systems.

21.4.3 GLUCOSE-REGULATED PROMOTERS

GRPs are over-expressed in tissues with low glucose and oxygen concentration.[57–60] They are induced in tissues when there is glucose deprivation, chronic anoxia, and acidic pH. All of these are found in tumor ischemia.[60–62] Grp78 is an evolutionally well-conserved protein, while grp94 is a vertebrate-specific protein. The grp78 promoter has the yeast unfolded protein response element (UPRE)-like sequence,[61] which binds the yeast Hac1. However, homologs of yeast Hac1 have not been identified in mammalian cells. Further study is required to fully identify the transcriptional mechanism of the gene induction. The grp78 promoter has been used to regulate the suicide gene in cancer therapy.[59] For example, the herpes simplex virus-thymidine kinase (HSV-tk) gene expression was regulated by the grp78 promoter in a gene therapy trial for murine fibrosarcomas.[59]

21.5 HEAT SHOCK

21.5.1 HEAT SHOCK–INDUCIBLE GENE EXPRESSION

Molecular chaperons, such as heat shock proteins (HSPs), are induced in response to various stress conditions. HSPs are classified by their molecular weight, which include HSP70, heme oxygenase-1 (HSP32), and HSP27.[73] It was previously reported that these proteins are induced in response to various conditions, such as hypoxia and heat shock.[57,74–78] Under the stress condition, HSPs are over-expressed and protect the cells from ischemic cell death and inflammation.[74–76,79,80] Recently, it was reported that HSPs also protect cells from obesity-induced insulin resistance.[81]

HSP gene expression is controlled at the transcriptional level. The HSP promoters have the heat shock element (HSE), which is recognized by the heat shock factor (HSF). HSFs are activated under stress conditions and bind to the HSEs for transcriptional activation.[22,74] Therefore, the HSP promoters are available for special and temporal gene induction and are possible candidates for heat shock response gene expression. Of these promoters, the HSP70B promoter has been extensively investigated for inducible gene expression.[82–86]

21.5.2 Heat Shock Protein Promoter-Mediated Gene Regulation

The HSP70B promoter has been investigated for spatial and temporal gene expression.[84] In one study, a therapeutic gene under the control of the HSP70B promoter was administered directly to the target organ or intravenously. Then, heat was applied to the target organ to induce gene expression. Without heat shock, the HSP70B promoter has basal promoter activity, which is usually low in various tissues.[84] The local application of heat induced gene expression in the target organ.

The HSP70B promoter is widely used in cancer therapy. The HSV-tk suicide gene under the control of the HSP70B promoter has been extensively studied.[82,87] An Escherichia coli cytosine deaminase (CD)-HSV-tk fusion gene was developed and the HSP70B promoter regulated its gene expression in prostate carcinoma cells.[87] The heating of the transduced prostate carcinoma cells to 41°C increased CD-HSV-tk gene expression several folds.

The HSP70B promoter has also been used for the expression of interleukin-12,[88] green fluorescent protein (GFP),[89,90] and granulocyte-macrophage colony-stimulating factor (GM-CSF).[85] Also, the HSP70B promoter was used for the inducible expression of the insulin gene.[91]

The HSP70B promoter has been further optimized for the highest promoter activity. A small fragment of the promoter, hsp70B' promoter, had higher promoter activity than the full-length promoter.[86] The hsp70B' promoter has HSE for the recognition of HSF. In the tumor-specific gene expression system, the human telomerase reverse transcriptase gene (hTERT) promoter regulates HSF expression (Figure 21.7A).[82] hTERT is over-expressed and active in immortalized tumor cells. Therefore, HSF expression, under the control of the hTERT promoter, is specific to tumor cells. In the second expression unit of this system, the tumor-specific HSF binds to HSE for CD expression. Therefore, the hTERT promoter specifically induces CD expression in tumor cells.

In another application, the hsp70B' promoter was used for dual-specific gene expression (Figure 21.7B). In this system, the hsp70B' promoter drives the expression of a Gal4-DNA binding domain (Gal4DBD)-hormone receptor-VP16 transactivation domain fusion protein.[92] In the first expression unit, hsp70B' promoter induces gene expression in response to heat shock. The expressed fusion protein itself is active in the presence of its ligand. The ligand, mifepristone, is an inducer, which binds to the receptor site of the fusion protein and facilitates the conformational change of the fusion protein, resulting in the activation of the transcription factor. Then, the transcription factor binds to the yeast Gal4 binding sites, UAS sequences, in the second expression unit and induces gene expression.

Various activation methods of the HSP70B promoters have also been developed. The most widely used induction method is the application of heat around 42°C. In addition to heat shock, other activation methods have been developed. High-intensity focused ultrasound (HIFU) was applied to target tissues.[83,84] HIFU could raise tissue temperature locally and it induced expression of the reporter gene, GFP, driven by the HSP70B promoter. Also, photodynamic therapy (PDT) was developed for the activation of the HSP promoter.[90,93] In this approach, photosensitizers were activated by light and produced reactive oxygen species. Then, the PDT-mediated damage induced several cellular responses such as cytokine expression and the induction of glucose-regulated proteins and HSPs. Therefore, genes under the control of the hsp70B promoter are induced by PDT.

Other promoters have also been used for heat shock-inducible gene expression, such as the human MDR1 promoter.[94] In this study, the human MDR1 promoter controlled the expression of TNF-α, which was induced two- to sevenfold by applying heat to the tissue.

Heat shock-inducible gene expression systems are useful for targeting gene expression to disease tissue and are applicable to various diseases. The improvement of the activation method of the heat shock promoter also increased the applicability to targeting gene therapy.

> PDT can be developed for the activation of the HSP promoter. In this approach, photosensitizers are activated by light and produce reactive oxygen species. Then, the PDT-mediated damage induces several cellular responses, such as cytokine expression and the induction of glucose-regulated proteins and HSPs. Therefore, genes under the control of the hsp70B promoter are induced by PDT.

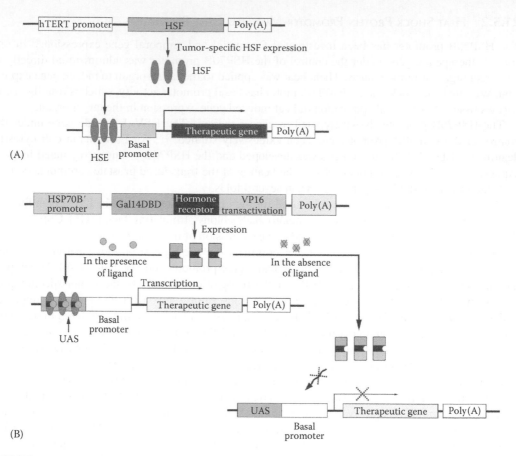

FIGURE 21.7 Dual-specific gene regulation systems. (A) Tumor-specific and heat shock response gene expression. The human telomerase reverse transcriptase promoter induces HSF expression specifically in tumor cells. Then, HSF binds to HSE for therapeutic gene expression. (B) Heat shock response and hormone regulated gene expression. The HSP70B′ promoter induces the expression of the Gal4DBD-hormone receptor-VP16 TAD fusion protein in response to heat shock. The expressed fusion protein is activated in the presence of is ligand and facilitates the expression of the therapeutic gene.

21.6 CONCLUSIONS

Physiological gene expression systems are essential for efficient gene therapy. As discussed above, low oxygen concentration, glucose, and heat shock are important physiological signals that can induce or repress gene expression (Table 21.1). Most of the physiological gene regulation systems are focused on transcriptional regulation. However, posttranscriptional regulation systems should also be developed.

Physiological regulatory systems will be more useful for gene therapy with possible new applications and approaches. First, RNA interference (RNAi) is becoming a central research field for gene regulation in gene therapy. Synthetic siRNA, short hairpin RNA (shRNA), or microRNA (miRNA) are important tools to regulate gene expression. It was previously reported that the nonspecific expression of shRNA had dose-dependent liver toxicity and caused the death of the tested animal.[95] Therefore, shRNA or miRNA expression in a specific tissue may be a useful approach for targeted gene therapy without side effects in untargeted tissues.[96] Therefore, transcriptional regulation of miRNA expression is an important field for therapeutic gene regulation.

Second, some diseases require faster gene induction than is possible with transcriptional regulation. Generally, RNA control and protein stabilization may be faster regulation strategies for gene therapy. For example, insulin gene therapy requires rapid insulin gene expression for the quick

TABLE 21.1
Regulation Strategies for Physiological Condition Response Gene Expression

Physiological Condition	Regulation Strategy	Regulation Element	References
Hypoxia	Transcriptional regulation	Epo promoter, enhancer	[10,38,99]
		PGK-1 promoter	[36,37,99–103]
		Glyderaldehyde-3-phosphate dehydrogenase promoter	[39]
		VEGF promoter	[104]
		RTP801 promoter	[40,42–44]
	Translational regulation	Epo 3′-UTR	[46]
	Posttranslational regulation	HIF-1α ODD domain	[6,16,18,105]
Glucose	Transcription-high glucose response regulation	LPK promoter	[63,64]
		Insulin promoter	[66,67,71]
		G6pase promoter	[54,55]
		Spot14 promoter	[71]
	Transcription-low glucose response regulation	Glucose response protein 78 promoter	[58,59]
Heat shock	Transcriptional regulation	HSP 70B promoter	[83–89,91,106–108]

increase of blood glucose after a meal. RNA stability regulation is one of the important approaches for regulating insulin. It was previously reported that the G6pase mRNA level was increased at high glucose concentrations by posttranscriptional regulation, as well as transcriptional regulation.[97,98] This suggests that gene expression may be induced by high glucose concentrations at the posttranscriptional level.

Third, posttranslational regulation will be an important strategy for gene regulation. For example, the ODD domain-mediated gene regulation can be applied to ischemic disease and ischemic tumor-specific gene therapy. Furthermore, the combination of transcriptional, translational, and posttranslational regulations can achieve a much higher level of specificity than a single regulatory system. For example, combining a hypoxia-specific promoter and the ODD domain showed gene expression that was more than 1000 times higher in hypoxic cells than in normoxic cells (Figure 21.8).[6]

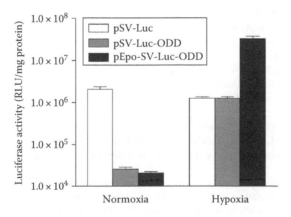

FIGURE 21.8 Transcriptional and posttranslational regulations of gene expression under hypoxia by the Epo enhancer-SV40 promoter and the ODD domain. pSV-Luc, pSV-Luc-ODD and pEpo-SV-Luc-ODD were transfected into Neuro2A cells. The cells were incubated under normoxia or hypoxia for 20 h and assessed for luciferase activity. The data expressed as mean values ± standard deviation.

In conclusion, promoters for physiological condition gene expression are useful tools for targeting gene expression. Synthetic, natural, or hybrid promoters are under investigation for targeting gene therapy. Furthermore, posttranscriptional regulation using UTRs and ODD will increase the efficiency and specificity of gene therapy. In combination with targeted delivery, gene expression systems in response to physiological conditions will be self-regulating, safe gene therapy systems.

REFERENCES

1. Kang HC, Lee M, Bae YH. Polymeric gene carriers. *Crit Rev Eukaryot Gene Expr* 2005; **15**: 317–342.
2. Goverdhana S, Puntel M, Xiong W, Zirger JM, Barcia C, Curtin JF, Soffer EB, Mondkar S, King GD, Hu J, Sciascia SA, Candolfi M, Greengold DS, Lowenstein PR, Castro MG. Regulatable gene expression systems for gene therapy applications: Progress and future challenges. *Mol Ther* 2005; **12**: 189–211.
3. Vilaboa N, Voellmy R. Regulatable gene expression systems for gene therapy. *Curr Gene Ther* 2006; **6**: 421–438.
4. Haviv YS, Curiel DT. Conditional gene targeting for cancer gene therapy. *Adv Drug Deliv Rev* 2001; **53**: 135–154.
5. Miller N, Whelan J. Progress in transcriptionally targeted and regulatable vectors for genetic therapy. *Hum Gene Ther* 1997; **8**: 803–815.
6. Kim HA, Kim K, Kim SW, Lee M. Transcriptional and post-translational regulatory system for hypoxia specific gene expression using the erythropoietin enhancer and the oxygen-dependent degradation domain. *J Control Release* 2007; **121**: 218–224.
7. Zhang L, Adams JY, Billick E, Ilagan R, Iyer M, Le K, Smallwood A, Gambhir SS, Carey M, Wu L. Molecular engineering of a two-step transcription amplification (TSTA) system for transgene delivery in prostate cancer. *Mol Ther* 2002; **5**: 223–232.
8. Phillips MI, Tang Y, Schmidt-Ott K, Qian K, Kagiyama S. Vigilant vector: Heart-specific promoter in an adeno-associated virus vector for cardioprotection. *Hypertension* 2002; **39**: 651–655.
9. Tang Y, Schmitt-Ott K, Qian K, Kagiyama S, Phillips MI. Vigilant vectors: Adeno-associated virus with a biosensor to switch on amplified therapeutic genes in specific tissues in life-threatening diseases. *Methods* 2002; **28**: 259–266.
10. Tang Y, Jackson M, Qian K, Phillips MI. Hypoxia inducible double plasmid system for myocardial ischemia gene therapy. *Hypertension* 2002; **39**: 695–698.
11. Tang YL, Tang Y, Zhang YC, Qian K, Shen L, Phillips MI. Protection from ischemic heart injury by a vigilant heme oxygenase-1 plasmid system. *Hypertension* 2004; **43**: 746–751.
12. Tang YL, Qian K, Zhang YC, Shen L, Phillips MI. A vigilant, hypoxia-regulated heme oxygenase-1 gene vector in the heart limits cardiac injury after ischemia-reperfusion in vivo. *J Cardiovasc Pharmacol Ther* 2005; **10**: 251–263.
13. Boussif O, Lezoualc'h F, Zanta MA, Mergny MD, Scherman D, Demeneix B, Behr JP. A versatile vector for gene and oligonucleotide transfer into cells in culture and in vivo: Polyethylenimine. *Proc Natl Acad Sci USA* 1995; **92**: 7297–7301.
14. Iyer M, Salazar FB, Lewis X, Zhang L, Carey M, Wu L, Gambhir SS. Noninvasive imaging of enhanced prostate-specific gene expression using a two-step transcriptional amplification-based lentivirus vector. *Mol Ther* 2004; **10**: 545–552.
15. Lee M, Oh S, Ahn CH, Kim SW, Rhee BD, Ko KS. An efficient GLP-1 expression system using two-step transcription amplification. *J Control Release* 2006; **115**: 316–321.
16. Koshikawa N, Takenaga K. Hypoxia-regulated expression of attenuated diphtheria toxin A fused with hypoxia-inducible factor-1alpha oxygen-dependent degradation domain preferentially induces apoptosis of hypoxic cells in solid tumor. *Cancer Res* 2005; **65**: 11622–11630.
17. Harada H, Hiraoka M, Kizaka-Kondoh S. Antitumor effect of TAT-oxygen-dependent degradation-caspase-3 fusion protein specifically stabilized and activated in hypoxic tumor cells. *Cancer Res* 2002; **62**: 2013–2018.
18. Harada H, Kizaka-Kondoh S, Itasaka S, Shibuya K, Morinibu A, Shinomiya K, Hiraoka M. The combination of hypoxia-response enhancers and an oxygen-dependent proteolytic motif enables real-time imaging of absolute HIF-1 activity in tumor xenografts. *Biochem Biophys Res Commun* 2007; **360**: 791–796.
19. Springer ML, Chen AS, Kraft PE, Bednarski M, Blau HM. VEGF gene delivery to muscle: Potential role for vasculogenesis in adults. *Mol Cell* 1998; **2**: 549–558.
20. Lee RJ, Springer ML, Blanco-Bose WE, Shaw R, Ursell PC, Blau HM. VEGF gene delivery to myocardium: Deleterious effects of unregulated expression. *Circulation* 2000; **102**: 898–901.

21. Nakagawa S, Massie B, Hawley RG. Tetracycline-regulatable adenovirus vectors: Pharmacologic properties and clinical potential. *Eur J Pharm Sci* 2001; **13**: 53–60.
22. Huang Q, Hu JK, Lohr F, Zhang L, Braun R, Lanzen J, Little JB, Dewhirst MW, Li CY. Heat-induced gene expression as a novel targeted cancer gene therapy strategy. *Cancer Res* 2000; **60**: 3435–3439.
23. Yoon JW, Jun HS. Recent advances in insulin gene therapy for type 1 diabetes. *Trends Mol Med* 2002; **8**: 62–68.
24. Dachs GU, Patterson AV, Firth JD, Ratcliffe PJ, Townsend KM, Stratford IJ, Harris AL. Targeting gene expression to hypoxic tumor cells. *Nat Med* 1997; **3**: 515–520.
25. Wang GL, Semenza GL. General involvement of hypoxia-inducible factor 1 in transcriptional response to hypoxia. *Proc Natl Acad Sci USA* 1993; **90**: 4304–4308.
26. Semenza GL. HIF-1 and mechanisms of hypoxia sensing. *Curr Opin Cell Biol* 2001; **13**: 167–171.
27. Jiang BH, Rue E, Wang GL, Roe R, Semenza GL. Dimerization, DNA binding, and transactivation properties of hypoxia-inducible factor 1. *J Biol Chem* 1996; **271**: 17771–17778.
28. Wenger RH. Mammalian oxygen sensing, signalling and gene regulation. *J Exp Biol* 2000; **203**: 1253–1263.
29. Gorlach A, Camenisch G, Kvietikova I, Vogt L, Wenger RH, Gassmann M. Efficient translation of mouse hypoxia-inducible factor-1alpha under normoxic and hypoxic conditions. *Biochim Biophys Acta* 2000; **1493**: 125–134.
30. Semenza GL, Agani F, Feldser D, Iyer N, Kotch L, Laughner E, Yu A. Hypoxia, HIF-1, and the pathophysiology of common human diseases. *Adv Exp Med Biol* 2000; **475**: 123–130.
31. Soitamo AJ, Rabergh CM, Gassmann M, Sistonen L, Nikinmaa M. Characterization of a hypoxia-inducible factor (HIF-1alpha) from rainbow trout. Accumulation of protein occurs at normal venous oxygen tension. *J Biol Chem* 2001; **276**: 19699–19705.
32. Wang F, Sekine H, Kikuchi Y, Takasaki C, Miura C, Heiwa O, Shuin T, Fujii-Kuriyama Y, Sogawa K. HIF-1alpha-prolyl hydroxylase: Molecular target of nitric oxide in the hypoxic signal transduction pathway. *Biochem Biophys Res Commun* 2002; **295**: 657–662.
33. Masson N, Ratcliffe PJ. HIF prolyl and asparaginyl hydroxylases in the biological response to intracellular O(2) levels. *J Cell Sci* 2003; **116**: 3041–3049.
34. D'Angelo G, Duplan E, Boyer N, Vigne P, Frelin C. Hypoxia up-regulates prolyl hydroxylase activity: A feedback mechanism that limits HIF-1 responses during reoxygenation. *J Biol Chem* 2003; **278**: 38183–38187.
35. Dachs GU, Dougherty GJ, Stratford IJ, Chaplin DJ. Targeting gene therapy to cancer: A review. *Oncol Res* 1997; **9**: 313–325.
36. Binley K, Iqball S, Kingsman A, Kingsman S, Naylor S. An adenoviral vector regulated by hypoxia for the treatment of ischaemic disease and cancer. *Gene Ther* 1999; **6**: 1721–1727.
37. Boast K, Binley K, Iqball S, Price T, Spearman H, Kingsman S, Kingsman A, Naylor S. Characterization of physiologically regulated vectors for the treatment of ischemic disease. *Hum Gene Ther* 1999; **10**: 2197–2208.
38. Lee M, Rentz J, Bikram M, Han S, Bull DA, Kim SW. Hypoxia-inducible VEGF gene delivery to ischemic myocardium using water-soluble lipopolymer. *Gene Ther* 2003; **10**: 1535–1542.
39. Lu H, Zhang Y, Roberts DD, Osborne CK, Templeton NS. Enhanced gene expression in breast cancer cells in vitro and tumors in vivo. *Mol Ther* 2002; **6**: 783–792.
40. Lee M, Bikram M, Oh S, Bull DA, Kim SW. Sp1-dependent regulation of the RTP801 promoter and its application to hypoxia-inducible VEGF plasmid for ischemic disease. *Pharm Res* 2004; **21**: 736–741.
41. Choi D, Lee M, Bull DA, Reiss R, Chang CW, Christensen L, Kim SW. Hypoxia-inducible VEGF gene therapy using the RTP801 promoter. *Mol Ther* 2004; **9**: S74–S75.
42. Lee M, Lee ES, Kim YS, Choi BH, Park SR, Park HS, Park HC, Kim SW, Ha Y. Ischemic injury-specific gene expression in the rat spinal cord injury model using hypoxia-inducible system. *Spine* 2005; **30**: 2729–2734.
43. Choi UH, Ha Y, Huang X, Park SR, Chung J, Hyun DK, Park H, Park HC, Kim SW, Lee M. Hypoxia-inducible expression of vascular endothelial growth factor for the treatment of spinal cord injury in a rat model. *J Neurosurg Spine* 2007; **7**: 54–60.
44. Lee M, Ryu JK, Piao S, Choi MJ, Kim HA, Zhang LW, Shin HY, Jung HI, Kim IH, Kim SW, Suh JK. Efficient gene expression system using the RTP801 promoter in the corpus cavernosum of high-cholesterol diet-induced erectile dysfunction rats for gene therapy. *J Sex Med* 2008; **5**: 1355–1364.
45. McGary EC, Rondon IJ, Beckman BS. Post-transcriptional regulation of erythropoietin mRNA stability by erythropoietin mRNA-binding protein. *J Biol Chem* 1997; **272**: 8628–8634.

46. Lee M, Choi D, Choi MJ, Jeong JH, Kim WJ, Oh S, Kim YH, Bull DA, Kim SW. Hypoxia-inducible gene expression system using the erythropoietin enhancer and 3′-untranslated region for the VEGF gene therapy. *J Control Release* 2006; **115**: 113–119.
47. Choi BH, Ha Y, Ahn CH, Huang X, Kim JM, Park SR, Park H, Park HC, Kim SW, Lee M. A hypoxia-inducible gene expression system using erythropoietin 3′ untranslated region for the gene therapy of rat spinal cord injury. *Neurosci Lett* 2007; **412**: 118–122.
48. Scandurro AB, Beckman BS. Common proteins bind mRNAs encoding erythropoietin, tyrosine hydroxylase, and vascular endothelial growth factor. *Biochem Biophys Res Commun* 1998; **246**: 436–440.
49. Levy AP, Levy NS, Goldberg MA. Post-transcriptional regulation of vascular endothelial growth factor by hypoxia. *J Biol Chem* 1996; **271**: 2746–2753.
50. Dibbens JA, Miller DL, Damert A, Risau W, Vadas MA, Goodall GJ. Hypoxic regulation of vascular endothelial growth factor mRNA stability requires the cooperation of multiple RNA elements. *Mol Biol Cell* 1999; **10**: 907–919.
51. Schneider BD, Leibold EA. Effects of iron regulatory protein regulation on iron homeostasis during hypoxia. *Blood* 2003; **102**: 3404–3411.
52. Kim HA, Lee BW, Kang D, Kim JH, Ihm SH, Lee M. Delivery of hypoxia inducible VEGF gene to rat islets using polyethylenimine. *J Drug Target* 2009; **17**: 1–9.
53. Salloum RM, Saunders MP, Mauceri HJ, Hanna NN, Gorski DH, Posner MC, Stratford IJ, Weichselbaum RR. Dual induction of the Epo-Egr-TNF-alpha-plasmid in hypoxic human colon adenocarcinoma produces tumor growth delay. *Am Surg* 2003; **69**: 24–27.
54. Chen R, Meseck M, McEvoy RC, Woo SL. Glucose-stimulated and self-limiting insulin production by glucose 6-phosphatase promoter driven insulin expression in hepatoma cells. *Gene Ther* 2000; **7**: 1802–1809.
55. Chen R, Meseck ML, Woo SL. Auto-regulated hepatic insulin gene expression in type 1 diabetic rats. *Mol Ther* 2001; **3**: 584–590.
56. Lan MS, Wang HW, Chong J, Breslin MB. Coupling of glucose response element from L-type pyruvate kinase and G6Pase promoter enhances glucose responsive activity in hepatoma cells. *Mol Cell Biochem* 2007; **300**: 191–196.
57. Little E, Ramakrishnan M, Roy B, Gazit G, Lee AS. The glucose-regulated proteins (GRP78 and GRP94): Functions, gene regulation, and applications. *Crit Rev Eukaryot Gene Expr* 1994; **4**: 1–18.
58. Gazit G, Kane SE, Nichols P, Lee AS. Use of the stress-inducible grp78/BiP promoter in targeting high level gene expression in fibrosarcoma in vivo. *Cancer Res* 1995; **55**: 1660–1663.
59. Gazit G, Hung G, Chen X, Anderson WF, Lee AS. Use of the glucose starvation-inducible glucose-regulated protein 78 promoter in suicide gene therapy of murine fibrosarcoma. *Cancer Res* 1999; **59**: 3100–3106.
60. Song MS, Park YK, Lee JH, Park K. Induction of glucose-regulated protein 78 by chronic hypoxia in human gastric tumor cells through a protein kinase C-epsilon/ERK/AP-1 signaling cascade. *Cancer Res* 2001; **61**: 8322–8330.
61. Lee AS. The glucose-regulated proteins: Stress induction and clinical applications. *Trends Biochem Sci* 2001; **26**: 504–510.
62. Reddy RK, Dubeau L, Kleiner H, Parr T, Nichols P, Ko B, Dong D, Ko H, Mao C, DiGiovanni J, Lee AS. Cancer-inducible transgene expression by the Grp94 promoter: Spontaneous activation in tumors of various origins and cancer-associated macrophages. *Cancer Res* 2002; **62**: 7207–7212.
63. Thule PM, Liu JM. Regulated hepatic insulin gene therapy of STZ-diabetic rats. *Gene Ther* 2000; **7**: 1744–1752.
64. Lee HC, Kim SJ, Kim KS, Shin HC, Yoon JW. Remission in models of type 1 diabetes by gene therapy using a single-chain insulin analogue. *Nature* 2000; **408**: 483–488.
65. Krones A, Jungermann K, Kietzmann T. Cross-talk between the signals hypoxia and glucose at the glucose response element of the L-type pyruvate kinase gene. *Endocrinology* 2001; **142**: 2707–2718.
66. Yoon JW, Yoon CS, Lim HW, Huang QQ, Kang Y, Pyun KH, Hirasawa K, Sherwin RS, Jun HS. Control of autoimmune diabetes in NOD mice by GAD expression or suppression in beta cells. *Science* 1999; **284**: 1183–1187.
67. Lee M, Han SO, Ko KS, Koh JJ, Park JS, Yoon JW, Kim SW. Repression of GAD autoantigen expression in pancreas beta-Cells by delivery of antisense plasmid/PEG-g-PLL complex. *Mol Ther* 2001; **4**: 339–346.
68. Yang YW, Kotin RM. Glucose-responsive gene delivery in pancreatic Islet cells via recombinant adeno-associated viral vectors. *Pharm Res* 2000; **17**: 1056–1061.
69. Lee M, Han S, Ko KS, Kim SW. Cell type specific and glucose responsive expression of interleukin-4 by using insulin promoter and water soluble lipopolymer. *J Control Release* 2001; **75**: 421–429.

70. Massillon D. Regulation of the glucose-6-phosphatase gene by glucose occurs by transcriptional and post-transcriptional mechanisms. Differential effect of glucose and xylitol. *J Biol Chem* 2001; **276**: 4055–4062.

71. Alam T, Sollinger HW. Glucose-regulated insulin production in hepatocytes. *Transplantation* 2002; **74**: 1781–1787.

72. Ferre P. Regulation of gene expression by glucose. *Proc Nutr Soc* 1999; **58**: 621–623.

73. Li Z, Srivastava P. Heat-shock proteins. *Curr Protoc Immunol* 2004; **Appendix 1**: Appendix 1T.

74. Macario AJ. Heat-shock proteins and molecular chaperones: Implications for pathogenesis, diagnostics, and therapeutics. *Int J Clin Lab Res* 1995; **25**: 59–70.

75. Birnbaum G. Stress proteins: Their role in the normal central nervous system and in disease states, especially multiple sclerosis. *Springer Semin Immunopathol* 1995; **17**: 107–118.

76. Hoshida S, Nishida M, Yamashita N, Igarashi J, Aoki K, Hori M, Kuzuya T, Tada M. Heme oxygenase-1 expression and its relation to oxidative stress during primary culture of cardiomyocytes. *J Mol Cell Cardiol* 1996; **28**: 1845–1855.

77. Sun L, Chang J, Kirchhoff SR, Knowlton AA. Activation of HSF and selective increase in heat-shock proteins by acute dexamethasone treatment. *Am J Physiol Heart Circ Physiol* 2000; **278**: H1091–H1097.

78. Kacimi R, Chentoufi J, Honbo N, Long CS, Karliner JS. Hypoxia differentially regulates stress proteins in cultured cardiomyocytes: Role of the p38 stress-activated kinase signaling cascade, and relation to cytoprotection. *Cardiovasc Res* 2000; **46**: 139–150.

79. Lill R, Neupert W. Mechanisms of protein import across the mitochondrial outer membrane. *Trends Cell Biol* 1996; **6**: 56–61.

80. Gray CC, Amrani M, Yacoub MH. Heat stress proteins and myocardial protection: Experimental model or potential clinical tool? *Int J Biochem Cell Biol* 1999; **31**: 559–573.

81. Chung J, Nguyen AK, Henstridge DC, Holmes AG, Chan MH, Mesa JL, Lancaster GI, Southgate RJ, Bruce CR, Duffy SJ, Horvath I, Mestril R, Watt MJ, Hooper PL, Kingwell BA, Vigh L, Hevener A, Febbraio MA. HSP72 protects against obesity-induced insulin resistance. *Proc Natl Acad Sci USA* 2008; **105**: 1739–1744.

82. Wang J, Yao M, Zhang Z, Gu J, Zhang Y, Li B, Sun L, Liu X. Enhanced suicide gene therapy by chimeric tumor-specific promoter based on HSF1 transcriptional regulation. *FEBS Lett* 2003; **546**: 315–320.

83. Plathow C, Lohr F, Divkovic G, Rademaker G, Farhan N, Peschke P, Zuna I, Debus J, Claussen CD, Kauczor HU, Li CY, Jenne J, Huber P. Focal gene induction in the liver of rats by a heat-inducible promoter using focused ultrasound hyperthermia: Preliminary results. *Invest Radiol* 2005; **40**: 729–735.

84. Rome C, Couillaud F, Moonen CT. Spatial and temporal control of expression of therapeutic genes using heat shock protein promoters. *Methods* 2005; **35**: 188–198.

85. Dammeyer P, Jaramillo MC, Pipes BL, Badowski MS, Tsang TC, Harris DT. Heat-inducible amplifier vector for high-level expression of granulocyte-macrophage colony-stimulating factor. *Int J Hyperthermia* 2006; **22**: 407–419.

86. Rohmer S, Mainka A, Knippertz I, Hesse A, Nettelbeck DM. Insulated hsp70B′ promoter: Stringent heat-inducible activity in replication-deficient, but not replication-competent adenoviruses. *J Gene Med* 2008; **10**: 340–354.

87. Lee YJ, Galoforo SS, Battle P, Lee H, Corry PM, Jessup JM. Replicating adenoviral vector-mediated transfer of a heat-inducible double suicide gene for gene therapy. *Cancer Gene Ther* 2001; **8**: 397–404.

88. Siddiqui F, Li CY, Zhang X, Larue SM, Dewhirst MW, Ullrich RL, Avery PR. Characterization of a recombinant adenovirus vector encoding heat-inducible feline interleukin-12 for use in hyperthermia-induced gene-therapy. *Int J Hyperthermia* 2006; **22**: 117–134.

89. Vekris A, Maurange C, Moonen C, Mazurier F, De Verneuil H, Canioni P, Voisin P. Control of transgene expression using local hyperthermia in combination with a heat-sensitive promoter. *J Gene Med* 2000; **2**: 89–96.

90. Mitra S, Goren EM, Frelinger JG, Foster TH. Activation of heat shock protein 70 promoter with meso-tetrahydroxyphenyl chlorin photodynamic therapy reported by green fluorescent protein in vitro and in vivo. *Photochem Photobiol* 2003; **78**: 615–622.

91. Suda T, Katoh M, Hiratsuka M, Takiguchi M, Kazuki Y, Inoue T, Oshimura M. Heat-regulated production and secretion of insulin from a human artificial chromosome vector. *Biochem Biophys Res Commun* 2006; **340**: 1053–1061.

92. Vilaboa N, Fenna M, Munson J, Roberts SM, Voellmy R. Novel gene switches for targeted and timed expression of proteins of interest. *Mol Ther* 2005; **12**: 290–298.

93. Luna MC, Ferrario A, Wong S, Fisher AM, Gomer CJ. Photodynamic therapy-mediated oxidative stress as a molecular switch for the temporal expression of genes ligated to the human heat shock promoter. *Cancer Res* 2000; **60**: 1637–1644.

94. Walther W, Stein U, Schlag PM. Use of the human MDR1 promoter for heat-inducible expression of therapeutic genes. *Int J Cancer* 2002; **98**: 291–296.

95. Grimm D, Kay MA. Therapeutic short hairpin RNA expression in the liver: Viral targets and vectors. *Gene Ther* 2006; **13**: 563–575.

96. Giering JC, Grimm D, Storm TA, Kay MA. Expression of shRNA from a tissue-specific pol II promoter is an effective and safe RNAi therapeutic. *Mol Ther* 2008; **16**: 1630–1636.

97. Parsons GB, Souza DW, Wu H, Yu D, Wadsworth SG, Gregory RJ, Armentano D. Ectopic expression of glucagon-like peptide 1 for gene therapy of type II diabetes. *Gene Ther* 2007; **14**: 38–48.

98. Carriere V, Le Gall M, Gouyon-Saumande F, Schmoll D, Brot-Laroche E, Chauffeton V, Chambaz J, Rousset M. Intestinal glucose-dependent expression of glucose-6-phosphatase: Involvement of the aryl receptor nuclear translocator transcription factor. *J Biol Chem* 2005; **280**: 20094–20101.

99. Greco O, Marples B, Dachs GU, Williams KJ, Patterson AV, Scott SD. Novel chimeric gene promoters responsive to hypoxia and ionizing radiation. *Gene Ther* 2002; **9**: 1403–1411.

100. Ingram N, Porter CD. Transcriptional targeting of acute hypoxia in the tumour stroma is a novel and viable strategy for cancer gene therapy. *Gene Ther* 2005; **12**: 1058–1069.

101. Kress S, Stein A, Maurer P, Weber B, Reichert J, Buchmann A, Huppert P, Schwarz M. Expression of hypoxia-inducible genes in tumor cells. *J Cancer Res Clin Oncol* 1998; **124**: 315–320.

102. Modlich U, Pugh CW, Bicknell R. Increasing endothelial cell specific expression by the use of heterologous hypoxic and cytokine-inducible enhancers. *Gene Ther* 2000; **7**: 896–902.

103. Matzow T, Cowen RL, Williams KJ, Telfer BA, Flint PJ, Southgate TD, Saunders MP. Hypoxia-targeted over-expression of carboxylesterase as a means of increasing tumour sensitivity to irinotecan (CPT-11). *J Gene Med* 2007; **9**: 244–252.

104. Koshikawa N, Takenaga K, Tagawa M, Sakiyama S. Therapeutic efficacy of the suicide gene driven by the promoter of vascular endothelial growth factor gene against hypoxic tumor cells. *Cancer Res* 2000; **60**: 2936–2941.

105. Inoue M, Mukai M, Hamanaka Y, Tatsuta M, Hiraoka M, Kizaka-Kondoh S. Targeting hypoxic cancer cells with a protein prodrug is effective in experimental malignant ascites. *Int J Oncol* 2004; **25**: 713–720.

106. Isomoto H, Ohtsuru A, Braiden V, Iwamatsu M, Miki F, Kawashita Y, Mizuta Y, Kaneda Y, Kohno S, Yamashita S. Heat-directed suicide gene therapy mediated by heat shock protein promoter for gastric cancer. *Oncol Rep* 2006; **15**: 629–635.

107. Lipinski KS, Djeha AH, Krausz E, Lane DP, Searle PF, Mountain A, Wrighton CJ. Tumour-specific therapeutic adenovirus vectors: Repression of transgene expression in healthy cells by endogenous p53. *Gene Ther* 2001; **8**: 274–281.

108. Braiden V, Ohtsuru A, Kawashita Y, Miki F, Sawada T, Ito M, Cao Y, Kaneda Y, Koji T, Yamashita S. Eradication of breast cancer xenografts by hyperthermic suicide gene therapy under the control of the heat shock protein promoter. *Hum Gene Ther* 2000; **11**: 2453–2463.

Index